Mosby's
COMPREHENSIVE
REVIEW of
NURSING for
NCLEX-RN

17th EDITION

Mosby's COMPREHENSIVE REVIEW of NURSING for NCLEX-RN

Editor

Dolores F. Saxton
RN, BSEd, MA, MPS, EdD

Associate Editors

Patricia M. Nugent
RN, AAS, BS, MS, EdM, EdD

Phyllis K. Pelikan
RN, AAS, BS, MA

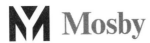 Mosby

An Affiliate of Elsevier Science
St. Louis   London   Philadelphia   Sydney   Toronto

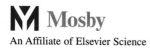

An Affiliate of Elsevier Science

11830 Westline Industrial Drive
St. Louis, Missouri 63146

NOTICE

Pharmacology is an ever-changing field. Standard safety precautions must be followed, but as new research
and clinical experience broaden our knowledge, changes in treatment and drug therapy may become
necessary or appropriate. Readers are advised to check the most current product information provided by the
manufacturer of each drug to be administered to verify the recommended dose, the method and duration of
administration, and contraindications. It is the responsibility of the licensed prescriber, relying on experience
and knowledge of the patient, to determine dosages and the best treatment for each individual patient. Neither
the publisher nor the editor assumes any liability for any injury and/or damage to persons or property arising
from this publication.

Previous editions copyrighted 1999, 1996, 1993, 1990, 1987, 1984, 1981, 1977, 1973, 1969, 1965, 1961, 1958,
1955, 1951, 1949.

NCLEX-RN is a registered trademark of the National Council of State Boards of Nursing, Inc.

Library of Congress Cataloging-in-Publication Data

Mosby's comprehensive review of nursing for NCLEX-RN/editor, Dolores F. Saxton;
associate editors, Patricia M. Nugent, Phyllis K. Pelikan.—17th ed.
     p. cm.
     Includes bibliographical references and index.
     ISBN 0-323-01642-1
     1. Nursing—Examinations, questions, etc. 2, Nursing—Outlines, syllabi, etc.
     I. Title: Comprehensive review of nursing for NCLEX-RN. II. Saxton,
Dolores F. III. Nugent, Patricia Mary, 1994-IV. Pelikan, Phillis K.
     [DNLM: 1. Nursing—Examination Questions. 2. Nursing—Outlines.
     WY 18.2 M8937 2003]
     RT55.M64 2003
     610.73'076—dc21

                              2002028829

Acquisitions Editor: Loren Wilson
Developmental Editor: Nancy L. O'Brien
Publishing Services Manager: Deborah L. Vogel
Project Manager: Claire Kramer
Design Manager: Bill Drone

RT/QWV

Printed in the United States of America.

Last digit is the print number: 9 8 7 6 5 4 3 2 1

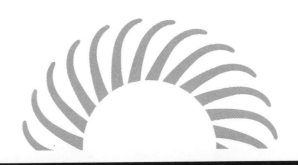

CONTRIBUTING AUTHORS

Jo Ann Schmidt Festa, RNC, AAS, BS, MS, PhD
Professor, Department of Nursing
Nassau Community College
Garden City, New York
President, Hygenia Registered Nursing
     Enterprises, P.C.
Dix Hills, New York

Colleen Glavenspiehs, RN, BS, MSN, DNSc, FNP
Professor, Department of Nursing
Burlington County College
Pemberton, New Jersey

Christina Algiere Kasprisin, RN, MS
Lecturer in Nursing
University of Vermont School of Nursing
Burlington, Vermont

Mary Ann Hellmer Saul, RNCS, AAS, BS, MS, PhD
Professor, Department of Nursing
Nassau Community College
Garden City, New York

Anita Throwe, RN, BSN, MS
Director
Durant Children's Center
Florence, South Carolina

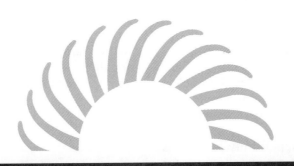

PREFACE

The information in *Mosby's Comprehensive Review of Nursing for NCLEX-RN* has been revised and updated for this seventeenth edition. The progression of subject matter in each area reflects the consistent approach that has been used throughout the book. Information presented incorporates the latest knowledge, newest trends, and current practices in the profession of nursing.

Chapter 1 gives directions on how to study and use the review to prepare for the licensure examination.

The clinical chapters include the components of nursing practice, the health-illness continuum, health resources, nursing practice and the law, and the nurse's role. Highlighted in the section on the nurse's role are those topics the student of today needs to know to function as tomorrow's practitioner: communication, the nursing process, the teaching-learning environment, leadership and management, and critical decision making.

The psychiatric/mental health, childbearing and women's health, pediatric, and medical-surgical chapters incorporate information from the basic sciences, nutrition, pharmacology, and rehabilitation. We continue to present the material in the traditional clinical groupings for we still believe that when preparing for a comprehensive examination, the average student will study all of the distinct parts before attempting to put them together.

Although we believe that in practice the nursing process is continually evolving rather than remaining a clearly defined step-by-step process, we present the content under the following headings: Assessment, Analysis/Nursing Diagnoses, Planning/Implementation, and Evaluation/Outcomes. We believe that this grouping avoids needless repetition, recognizes the abilities of our readers, and reflects current practice.

For every question in this edition and on the CD-ROM we have provided rationales that state the reason why the correct answer is correct, as well as why the incorrect answers are incorrect.

To further assist the user in studying/reviewing by a specific content area, the questions following each chapter have been grouped according to their category of concern. Questions related to nutrition have been integrated into the appropriate category of concern in each clinical area (the specific content within the broad clinical area).

The questions following each chapter are analyzed as to the level of difficulty, critical thinking and professional decision making, step in the nursing process, area of client needs, and category of concern. The 265 questions in each comprehensive test have been analyzed as to the level of difficulty, critical thinking and professional decision making, step in the nursing process, clinical area, area of client needs, and category of concern.

The two comprehensive, integrated tests at the end of the text provide an opportunity to apply material from the specific clinical areas to any nursing situation. These examinations approximate the NCLEX-RN test plan. To parallel the NCLEX-RN, the first 75 questions reflect the minimal testing experience for students taking the NCLEX-RN. The total test of 265 questions reflects the maximum number of questions that a student can take on the NCLEX-RN.

Although the NCLEX-RN is computerized, the information tested remains constant. These tests help students prepare for this experience. The movement from specific learning to general application is educationally sound, and the reader should follow this approach when studying.

A CD-ROM is enclosed that contains all the questions from the book as well as 1000 additional test questions that can be used in both a study and test format. These questions have been analyzed by critical thinking, step in the nursing process, clinical area, and area of client need. To reinforce learned information and build confidence, we suggest that students practice answering questions on this disk to simulate the computerized NCLEX-RN.

All of the questions used in this book have been submitted by outstanding educators and practitioners of nursing. Initially the editorial panel reviewed all questions, selecting the most pertinent for inclusion in a mass field-testing project. Students graduating from baccalaureate, associate degree, and diploma nursing

viii   Preface

programs in various locations in the United States provided a diverse testing group. The results were statistically analyzed. This analysis was used to select questions for inclusion in the book and to provide the reader with a general idea of the level of difficulty of each question.

We would like to take this opportunity to express our sincere appreciation to our many colleagues for their contributions and support. To our editor, Loren Wilson, and our developmental editor, Nancy O'Brien, for their help and support; and last, but not least, to our families for their love and encouragement.

Dolores F. Saxton

Patricia M. Nugent

Phyllis K. Pelikan

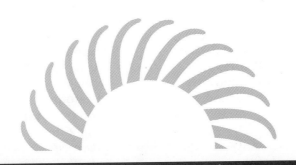

CONTENTS

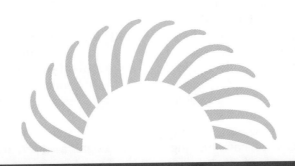

Introduction for Students Preparing for the Licensure Examination

The licensure examination in the United States is integrated and comprehensive. Nursing candidates are required to answer questions that necessitate a recognition and understanding of the physiologic, biologic, and social sciences, as well as the specific nursing skills and abilities involved in a given client situation.

This text contains objective multiple-choice questions. To answer the questions appropriately, a candidate needs to understand and correlate certain aspects of anatomy and physiology, the behavioral sciences, basic nursing, the effects of medications administered, the client's attitude toward illness, and other pertinent factors such as legal responsibilities, leadership and management, and critical thinking. Most questions are based on nursing situations similar to those with which candidates have had experience because they emphasize the nursing care of clients with representative common health problems. Some questions, however, require candidates to apply basic principles and techniques to clinical situations with which they have had little, if any, actual experience.

To prepare adequately for an integrated comprehensive examination, it is necessary to understand the discrete parts that compose the universe under consideration. This is one of the major principles of learning on which *Mosby's Comprehensive Review of Nursing* has been developed.

Using this principle, the text first presents a review of each major clinical area. Each review is followed by questions that test the student's knowledge of principles and theories underlying nursing care in a variety of situations, in a variety of settings, and with a variety of nursing objectives. Rationales for the correct answers and incorrect options follow the questions at the end of each chapter. By reviewing the rationales the student is able to verify information and reinforce knowledge.

Two comprehensive examinations, consisting of 265 questions each, are provided to approximate the NCLEX-RN test plan. To parallel the NCLEX-RN, the first 75 questions in each examination reflect the minimal testing experience for students taking the NCLEX-RN. The total of 265 questions in each test reflects the maximum number of questions that a student will be asked on the NCLEX-RN. Although NCLEX-RN is now computerized, the substance of the test remains constant. The questions require the student to cross clinical disciplines and respond to individual and specific needs associated with given health problems. Rationales are also provided for the correct answers and the incorrect options to these questions.

The following descriptions and the five sample questions on p. 4 are presented to assist in understanding these classifications.

CRITICAL THINKING/PROFESSIONAL DECISION MAKING

The professional nurse's ability to use scientific thinking and to delegate responsibilities to meet desired outcomes is an integral part of all client care situation.

1. **Clinical judgment (CJ).** This includes the organized identification of a problem, collection of data, implementation of a plan of action, and evaluation of the outcomes. Sample questions 1 and 2 reflect this process.
2. **Legal and ethical accountability (LE).** This includes the recognition of the laws and regulations governing the practice of nursing, the state laws, as well as the ethical obligations included in the *American Nurses' Association Code for Nurses.* Sample questions 3 and 5 reflect this process.
3. **Managerial responsibilities (MR).** This includes the delegation of duties, assignment, supervision, and evaluation of licensed and unlicensed assistive personnel, taking into consideration role expectations, level of competence, legal requirements, and institutional policies. It also includes guidance and coordination of all those coming in contact with the client in the health care system extending to the client and the client's significant others. Sample question 4 reflects this process.

PHASES OF THE NURSING PROCESS

This classification reflects the types of behaviors of the nurse.

1. **Assessment (AS).** The assessment phase requires the nurse to obtain objective and subjective data from primary and secondary sources, to identify and group significant data, and to communicate this information to other members of the health team. The information necessary for making nursing decisions is obtained through assessment. Sample question 1 is an assessment question.
2. **Analysis (AN).** This phase requires the nurse to interpret data gathered during the assessment phase. A nursing diagnosis must be made, client and family needs identified, and both short-term and long-term goals/outcomes set related to the identified needs. Sample question 2 is an analysis question.
3. **Planning (PL).** The planning phase requires the nurse to design a regimen with the client, family, and other health team members to achieve goals/outcomes set during the analysis phase. It also requires setting priorities for intervention. Sample question 3 is a planning question.
4. **Implementation (IM).** The implementation phase requires the nurse to provide care designed during the planning phase. The client may be given total care or may be assisted and encouraged to perform activities of daily living or follow the regimen

prescribed by the physician. Implementation also includes activities such as counseling, teaching, and supervising. Sample question 4 is an implementation question.

5. **Evaluation (EV)**. This phase requires the nurse to determine the effectiveness of nursing care. Care is reviewed, the client's response to intervention identified, and a consideration made as to whether the client has achieved the predetermined outcomes and goals. Evaluation also includes appraisal of the client's compliance with the health plan. Sample question 5 is an evaluation question.

CLIENT NEEDS

This classification reflects those health care needs of the client that must be addressed by the nurse.

1. **Support and promotion of physiologic and anatomic equilibrium (PA)**. Meeting this need includes reducing risks that interfere with physiologic or anatomic integrity, promoting comfort and mobility, and providing basic care to assist, modify, or limit physiologic and anatomic adaptations. Sample question 1 reflects this need.

2. **An environment that is safe and conducive to effective therapeutic care (TC)**. The nurse must provide quality, goal-directed care that is coordinated, safe, and effective. Sample questions 4 and 5 reflect this need.

3. **Education and other forms of health promotion to prevent, minimize, or correct actual or potential health problems (ED)**. Fulfilling this need involves supporting optimal growth and development to provide for the achievement of the highest levels of functioning. This includes encouraging use of support systems and self-care directed toward promoting the prevention, recognition, and treatment of disease throughout the life cycle. Sample question 3 reflects this need.

4. **Support and promotion of psychosocial and emotional equilibrium (PS)**. Addressing this need includes supporting individual emotional coping and adapting mechanisms to promote optimal emotional health while limiting or modifying those responses to crises that produce psychopathologic consequences. Sample question 2 reflects this need.

CLINICAL AREA

1. **Medicine/surgery (MS)**. These questions include the care of adult clients who have health problems that may or may not require surgical intervention or invasive techniques. Sample questions 1 and 5 are medical/surgical nursing questions.

2. **Childbearing/women's health (CW)**. These questions include the care of clients preparing for or experiencing childbirth and the common health problems specific to adult women. Sample question 2 is a childbearing and women's health nursing question.

3. **Pediatrics (PE)**. These questions include the care of clients from birth to young adulthood. Sample question 4 is a pediatric nursing question.

4. **Psychiatric/mental health (MH)**. These questions include the care of clients experiencing emotional problems with or without overt psychiatric behavior in all settings. Sample question 3 is a psychiatric/mental health nursing question.

CATEGORY OF CONCERN

This classification reflects specific content within broad clinical areas.

1. **The categories of concern used in medical/surgical and pediatric nursing** include emotional needs related to health problems (EH); respiratory (RE); reproductive and genitourinary (RG); neuromuscular (NM); skeletal (SK); endocrine (EN); integumentary (IT); gastrointestinal (GI); fluid and electrolyte (FE); cardiovascular (CV); blood and immunity (BI); growth and development (GD); and drug-related responses (DR). Sample question 1 reflects information related to cardiovascular content. Sample question 4 reflects information related to growth and development. Sample question 5 reflects information related to blood and immunity content.

2. **The categories of concern used in childbearing and women's health nursing** include emotional needs related to childbearing and women's health (EC); drug-related responses (DR); healthy childbearing (HC); high-risk neonate (HN); high-risk maternal-fetal conditions affecting childbearing (HP); normal neonate (NN); reproductive choices (RC); reproductive problems (RP); and women's health (WH). Sample question 2 reflects information related to healthy childbearing content.

3. **The categories of concern used in psychiatric/mental health nursing** include anxiety, somatoform, and dissociative disorders (AX); crisis situations (CS); dementia, delirium, and other cognitive disorders (DD); disorders first evident before adulthood (BA); disorders of personality (PR); disorders of mood (MO); eating and sleeping disorders (ES); personality development (PD); schizophrenic disorders (SD); substance abuse (SA); emotional disorders related to physical health and childbearing (ED); drug-related responses (DR); and therapeutic relationships (TR). Sample question 3 reflects information related to drug-related responses.

SAMPLE QUESTIONS

1. A client is admitted to the intensive care unit with a diagnosis of Adams-Stokes syndrome. Symptoms most likely include:
   1. Nausea and vertigo
   2. Flushing and slurred speech
   3. Cephalalgia and blurred vision
   4. Syncope and low ventricular rate

2. Two days after the birth of her child a client primarily focuses on her own needs. The nurse recognizes that the client is in the phase of maternal adjustment known as:
   1. Taking-in phase
   2. Letting-go phase
   3. Interdependent phase
   4. Dependent-independent phase

3. When monoamine oxidase (MAO) inhibitors are prescribed, the client should be cautioned against:
   1. Ingesting wines and cheeses
   2. Prolonged exposure to the sun
   3. Engaging in active physical exercise
   4. The use of medications with an elixir base

4. A young boy, age 4, has been hospitalized for fever of undetermined origin (FUO). He screams and becomes uncontrollable as his mother leaves after visiting hours. The best approach is to:
   1. Ignore this outburst
   2. Sit quietly at his bedside
   3. Give him a favorite toy to hold
   4. Hold and pat him even though he struggles

5. After surgery, while receiving a blood transfusion, a client develops chills and headache. The nurse's best action is to:
   1. Lightly cover the client
   2. Notify the physician STAT
   3. Stop the transfusion immediately
   4. Slow the blood flow to keep the vein open

HOW TO USE THIS BOOK IN STUDYING

A. Start in one area. Study the material covered by the section. Refer to other textbooks to find additional details if you are unsure of a specific fact.
B. Answer the questions following the area. As you answer each question, write a few words about why you think that answer was correct; in other words, justify why you selected the answer. If you guess at an answer in this book you should make a special mark to identify it. This will permit you to recognize areas that need further review. It will

also help you to see how correct your "guessing" can be. Remember, on the licensure examination you must answer every question.
C. Record the answer by circling the number you believe is correct.
D. Compare your answers with those provided. If you answered the item correctly, check your reason for selecting the answer with the rationale presented. If you answered the item incorrectly, read the rationale to determine why the one you selected was incorrect. In addition, you should review the correct answer and rationale for each item answered incorrectly. If you still do not understand your mistakes, look up the material pertaining to these questions. You should carefully review all questions and rationales for items you identified as guesses, because you did not have mastery of the material being questioned.
E. Following the rationale for the correct answer you will find a number 1, 2, or 3 in parentheses. These numbers indicate the difficulty of the question and can serve as a guide in your studying. The number 1 signifies that more than 75% of the graduating students in the testing group answered this question correctly; 2 signifies that between 50% and 75% answered it correctly; and 3 that 25% to 50% answered it correctly.
F. In addition to the difficulty level of the question (1, 2, or 3), you will find a grouping of letters that classifies the questions according to the following categories:
   1. *Critical thinking/professional decision making*
      (CJ) Clinical management
      (LE) Legal and ethical accountability
      (MR) Managerial responsibilities
   2. *Nursing process*
      (AS) Assessment
      (AN) Analysis
      (PL) Planning
      (IM) Implementation
      (EV) Evaluation
   3. *Area of client needs*
      (PA) Physiologic and anatomic equilibrium
      (TC) Therapeutic care
      (ED) Education and health promotion
      (PS) Psychosocial and emotional equilibrium
   4. *Category of concern*
      Medical, surgical, and pediatric nursing
      (EH) Emotional needs related to health problems
      (RE) Respiratory
      (RG) Reproductive and genitourinary
      (NM) Neuromuscular
      (SK) Skeletal
      (EN) Endocrine
      (IT) Integumentary

(GI) Gastrointestinal
(FE) Fluid and electrolyte
(CV) Cardiovascular
(BI) Blood and immunity
(GD) Growth and development
(DR) Drug-related responses

Childbearing and women's health nursing

(EC) Emotional needs related to childbearing and women's health
(HC) Healthy childbearing
(HP) High-risk maternal-fetal conditions affecting childbearing
(RC) Reproductive choices
(RP) Reproductive problems
(NN) Normal neonate
(HN) High-risk neonate
(DR) Drug-related responses
(WH) Women's health

Psychiatric/mental health nursing

(BA) Disorders first evident before adulthood
(ES) Eating and sleep disorders
(PR) Disorders of personality
(MO) Disorders of mood
(SD) Schizophrenic disorders
(AX) Anxiety, somatoform, and dissociative disorders
(SA) Substance abuse
(CS) Crisis situations
(DR) Drug-related responses
(TR) Therapeutic relationships
(DD) Dementia, delirium, and other cognitive disorders
(ED) Emotional disorders related to physical health and childbearing
(PD) Personality development

G. For the comprehensive examination, an additional category is added:

Clinical area

(MS) Medicine, surgery
(CW) Childbearing and women's health
(PE) Pediatrics
(MH) Psychiatric/mental health

H. This series of letters will always appear in the same order for each question following the clinical areas and the questions on the comprehensive examination.

I. A few days later, review the area again and retake the questions following it. If you miss the same questions again, you need further study of the material.

J. To study questions for a specific area of content (category of concern), refer to the Table of Contents. Following the clinical review material in each of the clinical areas, there is a list that contains the categories of concern for that clinical area and the pages of the questions that deal with material related to each category. All the questions following the chapter are grouped by the categories of concern.

K. After you have completed the area questions, begin taking the comprehensive test because it will assist you in applying knowledge and principles from the specific clinical area to any nursing situation.
1. Arrange a quiet, uninterrupted time span for each part of the comprehensive test.
2. Avoid spending excessive time on any one question. Most questions can be answered in 1 to 2 minutes.
3. Make educated guesses.
4. Read carefully and answer the question asked; pay attention to specific details in the question.
5. Try putting questions and answers in your own words to test your comprehension.

L. To help analyze your mistakes on the comprehensive examinations and to provide a data base for making future study plans, worksheets follow the Answers and Rationales for Part B of each of the Comprehensive Tests. These worksheets are designed to aid you in identifying and recording errors in the way you process information and to help you identify and record gaps in knowledge.

M. After completing your worksheets, do the following:
1. Identify the frequency with which you made particular errors. As you review material in class notes or this review book, pay special attention to correcting your most common problems.
2. Identify the topics you want to review. It might be helpful to set priorities; review the most difficult topics first so that you will have time to review them more than once.

GENERAL CLUES FOR ANSWERING MULTIPLE-CHOICE QUESTIONS

On a multiple-choice test the question and possible answers are called a test item. The part of the item that asks the question or poses a problem is called the stem. All of the answers presented are called options. One of the options is the correct answer; the remainder are incorrect. The incorrect options are called distractors because their major purpose is to distract the test taker from the correct answer.

A. Read the question carefully before looking at the answers.
1. Attempt to determine what the question is really asking; look for key words.
2. Read each answer thoroughly and see if it completely covers the material asked by the question.
3. Narrow the choices by immediately eliminating answers you know are incorrect.

B. Because few things in life are absolute without exceptions, avoid selecting answers that include words such as always, never, all, every, and none. Answers containing these key words are rarely correct.

C. Attempt to select the answer that is most complete and includes the other answers within it. An example might be as follows:
A child's intelligence is influenced by:
1. A variety of factors
2. Heredity and environment
3. Environment and experience
4. Education and economic factors
The most correct answer is 1 because it includes all the other answers.

D. Make certain that the answer you select is reasonable and obtainable under ordinary circumstances and that the action can be carried out in the given situation.

E. Watch for grammatical inconsistencies. If one or more of the options is not grammatically consistent with the stem, the alert test taker can identify it as a probable incorrect option. When the stem is in the form of an incomplete sentence, each option should complete the sentence in a grammatically correct way.

F. Avoid selecting answers that state hospital rules or regulations as a reason or rationale for action.

G. Look for answers that focus on the client or are directed toward feelings.

H. If the question asks for an immediate action or response, all the answers may be correct, so base your selection on identified priorities for action.

I. Do not select answers that contain exceptions to the general rule, controversial material, or degrading responses.

J. Reread the question if the answers do not seem to make sense, because you may have missed words such as not or except in the statement.

K. Do not worry if you select the same numbered answer repeatedly, because there is usually no pattern to the answers.

L. Mark the number next to the answer you have chosen.

M. Answer every question because on the NCLEX-RN you must answer a question before you move on to the next question.

PREPARING FOR THE LICENSURE EXAMINATION

A few individuals can improve their scores significantly by a highly concentrated period of study immediately before taking an examination. Most, however, profit by spreading their review over a much longer period of time, and the best time to begin studying for the NCLEX-RN is the first class attended.

If you wish to study by using additional practice questions, you may want to purchase *Mosby's Review Questions for NCLEX-RN*. An interactive CD-ROM, *Mosby's NCLEX-RN Review of Nursing,* second edition, is also available for study.

In addition, you may find it beneficial and enlightening to take Mosby's AssessTest by paper and pencil or on computer to evaluate your level of preparation. The AssessTest is a computer-scored, multiple-choice examination designed to test nursing knowledge and evaluate your ability to apply that knowledge in clinical situations. The extensive computer analysis of your performance, which is the most outstanding feature of this test, will help you design effective and efficient plans for further study and review. Identification of your own specific strengths and weaknesses should eliminate much of the anxiety of deciding what material to study by giving you a sense of direction and a means of setting priorities.

If you wish to assess your likelihood of NCLEX success, you may want to take *Mosby's Online Computer Adaptive Test for NCLEX-RN*, which may be obtained by visiting www.mosby.com/NCLEXCAT. This computer adaptive test simulates the NCLEX experience and provides an instant comparison of your individual test performance with that of other RN students in a national norm group.

TAKING THE LICENSURE EXAMINATION

The computerized NCLEX-RN is an individualized testing experience in which the computer chooses your next question based on the ability and competency you have demonstrated on previous questions. The minimum number of questions will be 75 and the maximum 265. You must answer each question before the computer will present the next question, and you cannot go back to any previously answered questions. You have a 1 in 4 (25%) chance of guessing the correct answer; go for it! Remember you do not have to get all the questions correct to pass.

The two most crucial requisites for doing well on the licensure examination are a sound understanding of the subject and the ability to comprehend what is read. Determination to do well and a degree of confidence will further enhance the well-prepared individual's chances of passing. At least three other requirements must be met if an individual's performance is to accurately reflect professional competence:
- First, the candidate must follow explicitly the directions given at the beginning of the test.
- Second, the candidate must read each question carefully before deciding how to answer it.
- Third, the candidate must correctly use the computer to record answers.

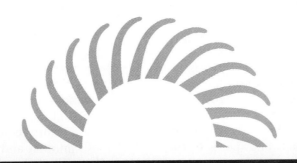

CHAPTER 2

Foundations of Practice

PSYCHOSOCIAL CONCEPTS

CONCEPTS FROM SOCIOLOGY

A. Every human society has institutions for the socialization of its members
   1. Process by which individuals are compelled or induced to conform to the customs of the group
      a. Group establishes rules and codes of conduct governing its members, and these become the norms, values, and mores of the group
      b. Role of members includes specified rights, duties, attitudes, and actions
   2. Controls established through a system of rewards and punishment
      a. Reward leads to acceptance as a member of the group
      b. Punishment for antisocial behavior leads to rejection and separation from the group
B. Development of society requires sanction of group members
   1. Growth takes place in social space
      a. Social boundaries separate one group from another
      b. Barriers to participation are established through mores and customs
   2. Leader's influence is always limited to conditions placed on the leader by the total group
   3. Behavioral roles are established by members of the group
C. A society is a reflection of all the functional relationships that occur among its individual members
   1. Products of group life are a major determinant in an individual's intellect, creativity, memory, thinking, and feeling
      a. Human beings have no memory, thought, or feeling that does not include society
      b. Intellect and creativity can be enhanced or hampered by society
   2. Members of a society have functional and rewarding social contact
      a. Members are accepted and approved and then participate in establishing rules, norms, and values
      b. The nonmembers have, at best, limited social contacts with the members; this causes a segmentation of relationships and provides few rewarding experiences for the nonmembers
D. Society or a group can change because of conflict among members
   1. This conflict is greatest when there is an absence of certain members, an introduction of new members, or a change in leadership
   2. Ensuing reorganization goes through three stages
      a. Tension: caused by conflict
      b. Integration: during which members learn about "the other's" problem
      c. Resolution: during which a reconstruction of the group's norms and values takes place
   3. Resolution of conflict and the restoring of equilibrium
      a. Occurs when people interact with one another and the group is dynamic
      b. Conflicts are not resolved when groups are rigid with fixed ideas

Culture and Health

A. General influences
   1. Culture defines for its people what is important and what is true and real in the world
   2. Ethnocentrism is the belief that one's own culture is generally right or best
   3. The clients' perceptions of health and illness, their help-seeking behavior, and treatment adherence depend on their beliefs, social norms, and cultural values
   4. Age, ethnicity, gender, education, income, and belief system (worldview, religion, or spirituality) make up the sociocultural profile of the client
   5. When clients face increased stressors, suffering, or pain, their belief systems play an even greater role in their lives
   6. Stereotyping, intolerance, stigma, prejudice, discrimination, and racism are common sociocultural stressors experienced by many minority clients
B. Implications for the nurse
   1. Culturally competent nurses are in touch with their own personal and cultural experiences
   2. Nurses must have a holistic perspective to assess the sociocultural context of clients from a different culture
   3. Together, the nurse and the client should agree on the nature of the client's coping responses and set goals and behavioral outcomes within the client's sociocultural context
   4. The degree of compatibility between the client's and the nurse's belief systems often determines a greater satisfaction with treatment, medication compliance, and treatment outcomes
   5. Nurses should expose themselves to cultural diversity and expand their worldviews because this will aid in their ability to provide culturally relevant care

Groups

A. Family is the primary group

1. Helps society to establish and maintain its code of behavior
2. Provides individual family members with:
   a. Strong emotional ties
      (1) Members experience sensory stimuli through close contacts
      (2) Members learn to care about the emotional and physical wellbeing of each other
      (3) Members are responsive to one another's feelings, acts, and opinions
      (4) Members learn empathy by vicariously living the experiences of others
      (5) Members view selves through the eyes of others
   b. A feeling of security by meeting dependent needs
   c. A system of communication: Overt—words; Covert—body language
   d. Role identification and intimacy that helps them to internalize the acceptable behavioral patterns of the group
   e. A spirit of cooperation and competition through sibling interaction
3. Changes that have influenced the family's ability to indoctrinate children with the norms of society
   a. Society has progressed from an agrarian culture through the Industrial Revolution to the Computer Age
      (1) Similarly, families have undergone change from extended to nuclear units, with an increase in numbers of blended and single-parent households
      (2) New social groups were established to replace the extended family
      (3) Electronic influences (computers and television) have weakened the structure of the family
      (4) Increased mobility of individuals reduced contact with extended or separated family members
      (5) Participation in individual activities has grown, thereby reducing time for involvement in family activities
   b. Altered male and female role patterns
      (1) Changing status of women: women are better educated, increased numbers go outside the home to work, and more have an increased role in decision making
      (2) Changing status of men: men are willing to assume homemaking responsibilities, and shared decision making with women has decreased male dominance
      (3) Increased partnership in home and financial management has resulted in less stereotyped sex roles

    (4) Increase in numbers of divorced single parents, both male and female, rearing offspring
    (5) Increase in number of financially independent women conceiving a child or children outside of marriage
  c. Factors resulting in a reduction in the size of families include persons choosing to marry in later adulthood and couples deciding to delay the start of a family until later years, the emphasis on limited population growth, the wide dissemination of birth control information, the legalization of abortions, and an increase in financial cost involved in raising and educating children

B. Peer groups help youth to establish norms of behavior and assist in the rites of passage from the family group to society
   1. Youth learns about society through contact with the peer group
   2. Youth develops further self-concept in contact with other youths
   3. Peer group interaction can produce change in its individual members
   4. Members have a strong loyalty to the peer group because of the reciprocal relationships and other rewards the group offers
   5. Peer group norms may conflict with family or society's norms

C. Crisis intervention groups
   1. Services
      a. Provide assistance for people in crises; clients' previous methods of adaptation are inadequate to meet present needs
      b. The focus of some groups is specific (e.g., poison control, drug-addiction centers, and suicide prevention) or general (e.g., walk-in mental health clinics and hospital emergency services)
      c. Some crisis intervention groups provide service over the phone (e.g., poison control, AIDS hot line, and suicide prevention centers), others help those who are physically present (e.g., hospital emergency services and walk-in mental health clinics)
   2. Success factors
      a. Help requested by the client or family
      b. Addresses the immediate problem
      c. Facilitates exploring feelings
      d. Assists the client in perceiving the event realistically
      e. Maximizes the client's coping mechanisms
      f. Provides assistance in investigating alternative approaches to solve the problem
      g. Identifies support systems

h. Reviews how present situation may help in coping with future crises

i. Provides information about other health resources where the client may receive additional assistance

D. Self-help groups

1. Services

   a. Organized by clients or their families to provide services that are not adequately supplied by previous organizations

   b. Meet the needs of clients and families with chronic problems requiring intervention over an extended period of time

   c. Focus is usually specific (e.g., Gamblers Anonymous); some deal with a range of problems (e.g., Association for Children with Learning Disabilities)

   d. Some are nonprofit (e.g., Alcoholics Anonymous); others are profit making (e.g., Weight Watchers International)

   e. Provide help to people who often are not accepted by society (e.g., addicts, child abusers, mentally ill, obese, or brain injured); many utilize the 12-step program developed by Alcoholics Anonymous

2. Success factors

   a. All members are accepted as equals

   b. All members have experienced similar problems

   c. Members feel a decrease in the sense of isolation that has occurred as a result of their problems

   d. Deal with behavior and changes in behavior rather than with underlying causes of the behavior

   e. Ready supply of human resources available such as: personal resources; help from peers; and finally, extension of self to others as a role model

   f. Each member has identified the problem and wants help in meeting needs—self-motivation

   g. Ritual and language specific to the group and specific to the problems

   h. Leadership remains with the membership

   i. Group interaction

      (1) Identification with peers—sense of belonging

      (2) Group expectations—discipline required of members

      (3) Small steps encouraged and, when attained, reinforced by group

   j. As a member achieves success within the group, he or she often receives reinforcement from outside the group

   k. Participation in 12-step programs is a life-long, continuous process; one is never "recovered" but always "recovering" a day at a time

E. Educational groups

1. Services

   a. Provides health information to change behavior

   b. Meets the needs of clients of families adapting to change

   c. Focus is usually specific (diabetes education group, parenting group)

   d. Majority of educational groups are conducted by health care agencies and are nonprofit

   e. In-service educational groups are also included in this category

2. Success factors

   a. All members have the same educational needs and have experienced similar problems (managing diabetes)

   b. Members experience a decrease in isolation and frustration as knowledge increases

   c. Members have identified the problem and generally are motivated to manage more effectively

   d. Nurse leader is able to educate more people more efficiently using a group format

   e. Members aid each other as they learn together and share information and experiences

   f. Staff attending in-service training become co-teachers of other team members

F. Group membership helps individuals achieve goals that are not attainable through individual effort

1. Types of groups are task oriented, therapy, self-awareness, social

2. Group functional roles include task roles, group building or maintenance roles, individual or self-serving roles

3. Group content refers to the subject matter or task being worked on

4. Group process refers to what is happening among and to group members while working; it deals with morale, feeling tones, influence, competition, conflict

G. Community is a social organization that is considered a secondary group

1. Relationships among members are usually more impersonal

2. Individuals participate in a more limited manner or in a specific capacity

3. The group frequently functions as a means to an end, enables diversified groups to communicate, and helps other groups to identify community problems and possible solutions

4. The secondary group is usually rather large and meets on an intermittent basis; contacts are usually maintained through correspondence

5. Leaders of the community facilitate group interaction because they have a knowledge of the community and its needs and the skill to stimulate others to act
6. Secondary groups help establish laws that are necessary to limit antisocial behavior; they provide diversified groups with a common base of acceptable behavior, but they may favor and protect the vested interests of specific groups within the society

H. Types of roles assumed by members of the group
   1. Harmonizer: brings other group members into accord while reconciling opposing positions
   2. Questioner: asks questions, seeks information, and gives constructive criticism to other group members
   3. Deserter: talks about irrelevant material; is usually disruptive in some manner
   4. Tension reducer: introduces levity when it is needed and appropriate
   5. Encourager: contributes to the ego of others and is a responsive member
   6. Monopolizer: attempts to control group; does not allow others to talk
   7. Clarifier: restates issues for clarification and then summarizes for the group
   8. Opinion giver: uses own experience to back up opinion or belief
   9. Initiator: proposes ideas or topics for discussion and suggests possible solutions for group discussion
   10. Listener: shows interest in the group by expressions on face or by body language while making little or no comment
   11. Negativist: pessimistic, argumentative, and uncooperative
   12. Energizer: pushes the group into action
   13. Aggressor: hostile and aggressive, verbally attacks other group members

Sociology and Health

A. Role of society
   1. Traditionally societies have placed great emphasis on caring for their members when they are ill
   2. Recently society's role in health maintenance and the prevention of disease has been given an increased priority
   3. Society's provision for health maintenance includes:
      a. Establishment of public health agencies for the supervision, prevention, and control of disease and illness, the protection of food, water, and drug supplies, the development of public education programs
      b. Awarding scholarships/grants for health education and research
      c. Development of unemployment insurance programs and workmen's compensation insurance
      d. Establishment of Social Security and Medicare programs; establishment of social welfare services and Medicaid programs
      e. Supervision of medical and hospital insurance programs

B. Health agency as a social institution has:
   1. A bureaucratic structure, a status hierarchy, an increasingly specialized subculture, and an impersonal viewpoint
   2. Policies, rules, and regulations governing behavior of its members

C. Health care agencies as a subculture of society
   1. Employees develop both written and unwritten agencies' policies that:
      a. Set standards of acceptable behavior for both clients and staff
      b. Regulate the hospitalized client's contact with the primary group by limiting visitors
      c. Force both clients and staff to relate to the secondary group
      d. Punish unacceptable behavior by any members of the group, including the client
   2. Folklores and folkways of the health care agencies serve to:
      a. Maintain the mystique of medicine by fostering the use of a unique language and system of symbols
      b. Attach stigmas to various social illnesses, such as AIDS and other sexually transmitted diseases, mental illness, drug addiction, and alcoholism, that are associated with certain patterns of living and acting that are not acceptable to the group
      c. Perpetuate the roles and values of the health team members and maintain the status quo
   3. Health care agencies have several functions
      a. Primary: to help the client regain health and resume a role in society by providing services directed toward:
         (1) Treatment of illness
         (2) Rehabilitation
         (3) Maintenance of health
         (4) Protection of the client's legal rights
      b. Secondary: to help society by providing services directed toward:
         (1) Education of health professionals
         (2) Education of the general public
         (3) Research

D. Delivery of health services: responsibility of the community

1. Members of society become active participants in prevention of illness
2. Community-health centers care for the ill in the home rather than in the hospital
3. Extended care facilities are established with a more communal and homelike atmosphere
4. Nonmedical community leaders take an active role in establishing health policy for society
5. Lay members of the community become involved with health agencies' policies and decisions
6. Health maintenance and treatment are no longer considered a privilege, but the right of all members of society

CONCEPTS FROM PSYCHOLOGY

A. Human beings must be able to perceive and interpret stimuli to interact with the environment
　　1. Perception and cognitive functioning are influenced by:
　　　　a. The nature of the stimuli
　　　　b. Culture, beliefs, attitudes, and age
　　　　c. Past experiences
　　　　d. Present physical and emotional needs
　　2. Individual's personality development is influenced by the ability to perceive and interpret stimuli
　　　　a. Through these processes the external world is internalized
　　　　b. The external world may in turn be distorted by the individual's perceptions
B. Humans must communicate to be able to interact with the environment, and the need to communicate is universal
　　1. Communication is a behavior that is learned through the process of acculturation
　　2. Communication is the avenue used to make needs known and to satisfy needs
　　　　a. Infant uses the cry to bring attention to needs
　　　　b. Hearing is essential to the development of effective speech, because one learns to form words by hearing the words of others
　　　　c. Written word can replace spoken words when face-to-face encounters are impractical, time is essential, and forms are required
　　　　d. Communication cannot be avoided; even with silence, nonverbal communication occurs
　　3. Productive communication depends on the consensual validation of all involved
　　　　a. To understand the intent of the message, each person must be aware of the meaning of the spoken word as well as the inflections in the speaker's voice (verbal and nonverbal communication)
　　　　b. Validation can best be accomplished when participants are empathetic
　　　　c. Language and channels of communication must be adapted to the person and the purpose for which they are intended
　　　　d. Feedback is necessary to evaluate the effectiveness of the words and guide the communication
　　　　e. Written or electronic communication often conveys messages quickly and simultaneously to a greater number of people, in an unemotional manner, and when asked for, one can obtain faster feedback
　　　　f. Satisfaction is enhanced for all involved when lines of communication are kept open
　　4. Barriers to effective communication include:
　　　　a. Variations in culture, language, and education
　　　　b. Problems in hearing, speech, or comprehension: ineffective reception or perception
　　　　c. Refusal to listen to another point of view: inability to evaluate
　　　　d. Use of selective inattention, which may cause an interruption or distortion of the message
　　　　e. Expressive language disorder acquired as a result of a neurologic or medical condition (encephalitis or head trauma)
　　5. Nonverbal behavior communicates the inner feelings of the individual performing the behavior
　　　　a. Facial expression, posture, and body movement may express the anxiety, pain, tension, fear, happiness, joy, or satisfaction the individual is feeling
　　　　b. Nonverbal communication may transmit a different message than the individual's verbal communication (covert versus overt messages)
　　　　c. Confusion arises when there is a difference in the verbal and nonverbal message received
C. Psychologic experiences provide the energy that is transformed into behavior
　　1. Anxiety frequently provides the push that moves people to action because it:
　　　　a. Develops when two goals or needs are in conflict
　　　　b. Is a state of apprehension or tension aroused by impulses from within; tension decreases as anxiety is reduced
　　　　c. Prepares one for action or completely overwhelms and inhibits action
　　2. Anxiety develops in stages that progress from increased alertness to panic
　　3. The sympathetic nervous system prepares the body's physiologic defense for fight or flight by

stimulating the adrenal medulla to secrete epinephrine and norepinephrine

  a. The heartbeat is accelerated to pump more blood to the muscles

  b. The peripheral blood vessels constrict to provide more blood to vital organs

  c. The bronchioles dilate, and breathing becomes rapid and deep to supply more oxygen to the cells

  d. The pupils dilate to provide increased vision

  e. The liver releases glucose for quick energy

  f. The prothrombin time is shortened to protect the body from loss of blood in the event of injury

4. Selye's general adaptation syndrome (GAS) is the body's physiologic adaptation to stress (anxiety); it is a nonspecific response that has three stages: alarm, resistance, and exhaustion

  a. Stress produces wear and tear on the body; it can be internal or external; beneficial or detrimental; and always elicits some response from or change in the individual

  b. The adrenal cortex secretes cortisone during the emergency stage

  c. When stress continues, the increased secretion of cortisone causes the body to go through a resistive stage

  d. If the process continues, the last stage is exhaustion and death

5. Defense mechanisms protect the personality by controlling anxiety and reducing emotional pressures

INFLUENCE OF BASIC NEEDS ON THE PERSONALITY

A. Humanity has certain basic needs that must be satisfied

1. Need to communicate is universal

  a. Through communication, humans maintain contact with reality; validate findings with others to correctly interpret reality; and develop a concept of self in relation to others

  b. Validation is enhanced when communication conveys an understanding of feelings

2. Need for security

  a. An assurance of survival is fundamental: fear emerges when survival is threatened

  b. Initially the infant's security is related to the satisfaction of physical needs and is enhanced when the same individual meets the infant's physical needs in a consistent manner

  c. The infant must also perceive love to feel secure because security is derived from the

perception of self in relation to others; perceived threats to security can result in sibling rivalry

  d. How the individual handles these perceptions influences personality development

3. Need to move from dependence to independence

  a. The infant is dependent on the parents but through learning acquires faculties for independence

  b. There is no real security or deep assurance of survival in being dependent on others because uncertainties always develop

  c. The infant must feel love and security before reaching out to struggle with the environment

  d. When the need for love and security is met, the child is sustained in the failures and hurts associated with learning and independence

  e. Denial of the opportunity or frustration of the drive produces emotional problems

4. Need to develop a self-concept

  a. Self-concept begins to develop early in infancy primarily through parent-child relationship and interactions with significant persons in the environment

  b. Self-concept develops as a result of one's perceptions as to how others see and relate to him/her

  c. Concept of the self is root of security and future developmental needs

  d. Culture and socialization also affect self-concept and personality development

  e. People with positive self-concepts function more effectively; negative self-concept is correlated with personal and social maladjustment

  f. Components of the self include body image, self-ideal, self-esteem, role, and identity

  g. Self-esteem is most threatened during adolescence, which requires difficult task accomplishments

5. Need to find relief from organic discomfort

  a. Through experience one learns to relieve discomfort

  b. Adjustment to illness depends on how the individual adjusts to life

  c. Research reports a relationship between self-reported physical health and self-esteem

  d. Health problems, regardless of type or severity, are associated with significant lower self-esteem than reports of wellness

  e. High self-esteem has been correlated with low levels of anxiety, effective group functioning, and acceptance of others

  f. Low self-esteem is expressed through moderate and severe anxiety levels and reflects negative self-evaluations, feeling of inadequacy, helplessness, and vulnerability

B. Needs of a specific individual at a given time will vary according to internal and external environmental factors

C. The individual attempts to maintain a feeling of safety and comfort in adapting to life's situations by maintaining a feeling of worth and a feeling of being needed by others

RECOGNITION OF FACTORS INFLUENCING CLIENT NEEDS
Type of Condition Affecting the Client

A. Acute illness: caused by a health problem that produces signs and symptoms abruptly and runs a short course; this illness may develop into a long-term illness

B. Chronic illness: caused by a health problem that produces signs and symptoms over time and runs a long course
   1. Exacerbation: period when a chronic illness becomes more active and there is a recurrence of pronounced signs and symptoms of the disease
   2. Remission: period when a chronic illness is controlled and signs and symptoms are reduced or not obvious
   3. Progressive degeneration: continuous deterioration or increased impairment of a person's physical state

C. Terminal illness: death is inevitable in the near future (needs focus on hygiene and physical and emotional comfort)

Client's History

A. Health background
   1. Physiologic: what physical adaptations were manifested in the past
   2. Psychologic: what psychologic methods of adaptation were exhibited in the past

B. Sociocultural background
   1. Religion: particular denomination and/or specific beliefs
   2. Ethnic group
   3. Occupation
   4. Economic status
   5. Family members, significant others, and/or personal resources
   6. Race
   7. Educational background
   8. Environment: urban versus rural; private home versus apartment
   9. Social status
   10. Lifestyle

CLIENT FACTORS INFLUENCING NURSING CARE

A. Hierarchy of needs
   1. Need to survive: physiologic needs for such things as air, food, and water
   2. Need for safety and comfort: physical and psychologic security
   3. Interpersonal needs: social needs for love, acceptance, status, and recognition
   4. Intrapersonal needs: self-esteem and self-actualization

B. Developmental level
   1. Infant: must adapt to a totally new environment; the stress from the transition from intrauterine to extrauterine living is compounded for the infant with a congenital problem
   2. Child: maturation involves physical, functional, and emotional growth; it is an ever-changing process that produces stress; disabilities will provide additional factors that may quantitatively or qualitatively affect maturation
   3. Adolescent: is experiencing a physical, psychologic, and social growth spurt; the individual is asking, "Who am I?" on the way to developing a self-image; limitations provide additional stress during identity formation
   4. Adult: is expected to be independent and productive, to provide for self and family; if one cannot partially or totally accomplish this, additional stress occurs
   5. Aged: our society tends to venerate youth and deplore old age; many elderly persons are experiencing multiple stresses (loss of loved ones, changes in usual lifestyle, loss of physical vigor, and, for many, the thought of approaching death) at a time when their ability to adapt is compromised by the anatomic, physiologic, and psychologic alterations that occur during the aging process

C. Personal resources
   1. Level of self-esteem: attitude that reflects the individual's perception of self-worth; it is a personal subjective judgment of oneself; influenced by loss of independence and changing role
   2. Experiential background: knowledge derived from one's own actions, observations, or perceptions; maturation, culture, and environment influence the individual's experiential foundation
   3. Intelligence: genetic intellectual potential; amount of formal/informal education; level of intellectual development; and the ability to reason, conceptualize, and translate words into actions

4. Level of motivation: internal desire or incentive to accomplish goals
5. Values: factors that are important to the individual
6. Religion: deep personal belief in a higher force than humanity
7. Social interaction: ability to clearly communicate needs and desires to others
8. Stress control: development of varied effective coping skills

COMMUNICATION

A. The reciprocal exchange of information, ideas, beliefs, feelings, and attitudes between two persons or among a group is the definition of communication
B. Recognition of what is communicated is basic for the establishment of a therapeutic nurse-client relationship
C. Clear and accurate communication among members of the health team, including the client, is vital to support the client's welfare
D. A person cannot avoid communicating; all behavior, even silence, has meaning, and nonverbal communication occurs even with silence
E. For communication to occur, there must be a sender, a message, a receiver, feedback, and context or setting in which the interaction takes place

Nursing Responsibilities in Promotion of Productive Communication

A. Effective communication requires skill in both sending and receiving messages
   1. Verbal relates to anything associated with the spoken word; includes speaking, writing, the use of language or symbols, and arrangements of words or phrases
   2. Nonverbal relates to messages sent and received without the use of words and is expressed through appearance, body motions, use of space, and nonverbal sounds
   3. Both levels, verbal and nonverbal, send and receive messages during every interaction
   4. Therapeutic communication techniques are skills that allow the nurse to effectively interact to achieve client outcomes
B. Recognize the high stress-anxiety potential of most health settings created in part by: health problem itself; treatments and procedures; exclusive behavior of personnel; strange environment; change in lifestyle, body image, and self-concept; inability to use normal coping skills such as exercise or talking with friends
C. Recognize the intrinsic worth of each person: listen, consider wishes when possible, and offer explanations; avoid stereotyping, snap judgments, and unjustified comparisons; be nonjudgmental and nonpunitive in response and behavior; spend time with the client to convey acceptance and client's worth
D. Be aware that each individual must be treated as a whole person
E. Recognize that all behavior has meaning and usually results from the attempt to cope with stress or anxiety
   1. Be aware of importance of value systems
   2. Be aware of significance of cultural differences
   3. Be sensitive to personal meaning of experiences to clients
   4. Recognize that giving information may not alter the client's behavior
   5. Recognize the defense mechanisms the individual is using
   6. Recognize own anxiety and cope with it
   7. Search for patterns of adaptation on which to base action
   8. Recognize that client's previous patterns of behavior may become inadequate under stress: health problems may produce a change in family or community constellations; health problems may lead to change in self-perception and role identity
   9. Be aware that behavioral changes are possible only when the individual has other defenses to maintain equilibrium
F. Help the client to accept the health problem and its consequences
G. Identify the individual's needs and determine priority for care
H. Maintain an accepting, open environment: accept the client but set limits on inappropriate behavior; identify and face problems honestly; value the expression of feelings; be nonjudgmental
I. Encourage client participation in decision making when possible
J. Recognize the client is a unique person
   1. Use names rather than labels such as room numbers or diagnoses; maintain the client's dignity; be courteous toward the client, family, and visitors
   2. Protect the client's privacy; permit personal possessions where practical
   3. Explain at the client's level of understanding and tolerance
   4. Encourage expression of feelings
   5. Approach the client as a person with difficulties, not as a "difficult" person
K. Support a social environment that focuses on client needs: use problem-solving techniques that are client centered; be flexible in carrying out routines and policies; be discreet in the use of power and maintain confidentiality; recognize that use of medical jargon can isolate the client

LEADERSHIP

TYPES OF LEADERSHIP

A. Leadership is the process of influencing the actions of an individual or group toward specific goals in a particular situation

B. Type of leadership in a group depends on the needs of the group members as well as the personality of the leader; role is influenced by the leader, the environment, and the cultural climate of the organization

1. Authoritarian or autocratic leader: controlling and uses leadership role for power; leader makes all the decisions, which are then handed down to the membership; little communication and interrelating between leader and group; leader sets the goals, plans, makes the decisions, and evaluates the action taken

2. Democratic leader: fair and logical, uses the leadership role to stimulate others to achieve a collective goal; the leader encourages interrelating among members by relating to all members; weaknesses as well as strengths are accepted; the contributions of all members are fostered and utilized; responsibilities for action taken are shared between the leader and the group

3. Emotional leader: reflects the feeling tones, norms, and values of the group

4. Laissez-faire leader: passive and nondirective; assumes participant-observer role and exerts little control or guidance over group behavior; input and control are minimal, permitting individual members to set independent goals

5. Bureaucratic leader: rigid and assumes a role that is determined by formal criteria or rules that are inherent in the organization and frequently unrelated to the present group; the leader is not emotionally involved and avoids interrelating with the group members

6. Charismatic leader: can assume any of the above behaviors, because the group attributes supernatural power to this person or the office and frequently follows directions without question

7. The effective leader modifies style to fit changing circumstances, problems, and people (e.g., autocratic style is appropriate in an emergency situation; democratic style is appropriate when group acceptance and participation are essential; and laissez-faire leadership is appropriate when group members are knowledgeable and capable of self-direction)

PRINCIPLES OF LEADERSHIP

A. Interpersonal influence depends on a knowledge of human behavior and a sensitivity to others in terms of feelings, values, and problems

1. Explore and understand personal attitudes, feelings, and values

2. Project self into the place of the individuals being led

3. Seek information from members

B. Communication is an essential component of leadership

1. Effective communication depends on the use of the appropriate medium; it may be verbal, written, and/or nonverbal; it may be formal or informal; and it should have two directions: up and down the chain of command and among equals

2. Communication style can affect the person or persons with whom the leader communicates
   a. Meanings or ideas communicated should be received or intended without distraction
   b. People react to communication differently
   c. Written communication should be in language that is understood by the person or persons intended (e.g., ancillary personnel should have a written assignment that does not require them to make judgments)
   d. Verbal communication can be influenced by facial expressions, body movement, and tone of voice

3. Effectiveness of communication can be influenced by inappropriate timing; the information communicated may be correct, but the time may be wrong; ascertain readiness

C. Leader's success is influenced by the ability to respond to group needs and by members' perceptions of effectiveness

1. A role is composed of a number of expectations for the behavior of an individual in a specific position or status classification; the role a person plays may influence the dynamics of the group positively or negatively, depending on whether the role is serving the individual's or the group's needs; some roles are task oriented and help the group directly in doing the assignment; other roles are more process oriented and help the group communicate effectively
   a. Any individual's role consists of a number of expectations and relationships
   b. The nurse leader, by virtue of behavior and status, can influence the perceptions of peers, clients, and colleagues

2. Power is a leader's source of influence

3. Power may be professional or positional
   a. Positional power: acquired through the position the leader has in the hierarchy of the organization
   b. Professional power: acquired through the knowledge or expertise displayed by the leader and/or perceived by the followers

D. Leadership moves from one person to another as changes in the situation occur
   1. The nurse's expertise about a specific client care problem, along with the availability of other resources, can place the nurse in the position of providing leadership for a group
   2. A member of another discipline may assume the role of leadership in specific situations (e.g., the home health nurse coordinates the team's efforts to meet the client's rehabilitation needs)
E. Leadership process requires the use of critical thinking skills associated with problem solving: interpretation, analysis, evaluation, inference, and explanation lead to effective decision making
   1. Decision making requires knowledge about and skill in solving the problem; participative decision making lends itself to the quality of the decision made, improves relationships, and influences the readiness of an individual or group to accept change (e.g., the client or the family should have the opportunity to participate in the development of the client's plan of care; unit staff may decide which primary nurse or team leader should care for a newly admitted client)
   2. Effective delegation of responsibilities is inherent in effective leadership; delegation of work requires matching the task with the appropriate position and providing guidance and coordination to ensure effective completion of duties
F. Need for change should be understood by those effecting the change, as well as those affected by the change
   1. Movement from goal setting to goal achievement involves change
   2. Resistance to change is normal and should be expected and addressed in planning
   3. Process of change includes communication, planning, participation, and evaluation by the individual or group affected
   4. Change is more acceptable when it has been planned, has not been dictated but follows a sequence of impersonal principles, follows a number of successful rather than unsuccessful series of changes, is initiated after other changes have been absorbed rather than during the confusion of a major change, does not threaten security, and the individuals or groups affected have participated in its creation
G. Effective use of leadership is conducive to accomplishing the goals of the group; an evaluation process is necessary if the results of efforts to attain the identified short-term and long-term goals are to be interpreted accurately; the evaluation process should be ongoing and the climate in which the evaluation process occurs influences its success

NURSING PRACTICE AND THE LAW

TORTS AND CRIMES IMPORTANT TO NURSES

A. Torts
   1. Violations of civil law against a person or a person's property
      a. Commission: inappropriate action
      b. Omission: lack of appropriate action
   2. Unintentional torts
      a. Negligence: measurement of negligence is "reasonableness;" involves exposure of person or property of another to unreasonable risk of injury by acts of commission or omission
      b. Malpractice: negligence performed in professional practice; any unreasonable lack of skill in professional duties or illegal or immoral conduct that results in injury to or death of the client
      c. Examples of malpractice/negligence include leaving sponges inside a client; causing burns; medication errors; failure to prevent falls; incompetent assessment leading to subsequent inappropriate actions; improper identification of clients; and carelessness in caring for a client's property
   3. Tort different from crime, but serious tort can be tried as both civil and criminal action
   4. Reasonableness and prudence in actions are usually determining factors in a judgment
   5. Nurse responsible for own acts; employer may also be held responsible under the doctrine of *respondeat superior*; when responsibility is shared, nursing actions must lie within the scope of employment and legislation relating to nursing practice (such as Nurse Practice Acts)
   6. Elements essential to prove negligence:
      a. Legally recognized duty of care to protect others against unreasonable risk
      b. Failure to perform according to the established standard of conduct and care, which becomes breach of duty
      c. Damage to the client, which can be physical, emotional, and/or mental; no physical harm is necessary to establish liability for an intentional tort
      d. Connection between defendant's conduct and the resulting injury referred to as "proximate cause" or "remoteness of damage"
   7. Good Samaritan Laws protect health care professionals who administer first aid in an emergency unless gross negligence or failure to meet a level of care expected of a reasonably prudent professional

8. Intentional torts occur when a person does damage to another person in a willful, intentional way and without just cause and/or excuse
   a. Assault: mental or physical threat includes knowingly threatening or attempting to do violence to another or forcing a medication or treatment on a person who does not want it so long as touching does not occur
   b. Battery: actually touching or wounding a person in an offensive manner with or without the intent to do harm
   c. Fraud: false presentation of facts purposefully to create deception; includes presenting false credentials for licensure or employment
   d. Invasion of privacy: concerns privileged communication and privacy
      (1) Encroachment or trespass on another's body includes any unnecessary exposure or discussion of the client's case unless authorized, unwarranted operations, and unauthorized touching
      (2) False imprisonment, even without force or malicious intent, includes the intentional confinement without authorization; the threat of force, or confining structures and/or clothing; the charge is not false imprisonment if it is necessary to protect an emotionally disturbed person from harming self or others
      (3) Defamation concerns communications, even if true, that cause a lowering of opinion of the person; includes slander (oral) and libel (written, pictured, telecast), both of which are dependent on communication to a third party
B. Crimes
   1. Crime: an intentional wrong that violates societal law punishable by the state; the state is the complainant
      a. Felony: serious crime such as murder punishable by a prison term
      b. Misdemeanor: less serious crime that is punishable by a fine and/or a short-term imprisonment
   2. Commission of a crime requires committing a deed contrary to criminal law or failing to act when there is a legal obligation to act
   3. Criminal conspiracy occurs when two or more persons agree to commit a crime
   4. Giving aid to another in the commission of a crime makes the person equally guilty if awareness is present that a crime is being committed
   5. Ignorance of the law is usually not an adequate defense
   6. Search warrants are required before property can be searched
   7. Administration of narcotics by a nurse is legal only when prescribed by a physician; possession or sale of a controlled substance by a nurse is illegal
   8. If a nurse knowingly administers a drug that causes a major disability or death, a crime may be charged

CLIENT'S RIGHTS

A. Clients have the right to choose their own doctor, hospital, or medical insurance based on availability and ability to meet costs free of discrimination, to be given treatment in an emergency, to receive a proper standard of care, to execute informed consent, to decide whether to be used for research or teaching, to be treated in confidentiality, and to have their personal property protected; in addition, mentally competent clients have the legal right to refuse treatment and the right to make a choice even if it is choosing to die rather than receive identified treatments
B. Statutory restrictions may be imposed on the client's rights (e.g., rights of clients to use specific health resources)
C. The United States government has set stringent rules about the use of human subjects in research

Informed Consent

A. Consent is essential for any treatment, except in an emergency where failure to institute treatment may constitute negligence; routine procedures are covered by a consent signed at admission
B. In an emergency situation, two physicians may sign consent for the client when failure to intervene may cause death; when the common law permits administration of health care to unconscious or mentally incompetent persons in an emergency situation; when family members voice opposition a court order may be required
C. Informed consent makes a competent decision possible for a client, who has the final decision, to enter into a shared contract with a health care provider or institution
D. Essential elements of legally effective consents are that the consent is voluntary; authorizes the specific treatment or care and the person giving the treatment or care; is given by a person with the legal and mental capacity to consent based on an informed decision; clients 18 years or older and emancipated minors are legally able to give consent
E. The informed consent must include an explanation of the treatment to be done with a presentation of the advantages and disadvantages and a description of possible alternatives; there must be time for decision making with an absence of undue pressure; the explanation and decision making must occur before sedation is given

Death with Dignity: Legal, Ethical, and Emotional Issues

A. Legal and ethical guidelines for making professional decisions in situations for which intensive treatment and resuscitative measures may not be appropriate are being developed
1. Underlying problems include the public concern that terminal illness is not managed appropriately by the health care team; newer treatment protocols and technologic support are used unnecessarily to prolong the dying process; and whether clients are provided with the opportunity to express desires about death with dignity while they are competent
2. Death with dignity in health care settings includes two fundamental questions, namely, who has control over one's life and the demonstration of respect for the worth of the individual as a unique being
3. Laws must empower clients to have as much control as possible over their care and activities, recognizing that pain, increasing helplessness, and hopelessness lead to despair
4. The use of living wills, "do not resuscitate" orders, and life-sustaining treatment protocols constitutes some of the most highly debated legal/ethical issues in health care
5. The ethical/medical problems that exist require the education of an interested public about living wills through literature distribution and discussions, the use of quality management to include assessment of the appropriate care of terminally ill clients, and an increased availability and accessibility of palliative care services
B. Criteria of death: individual states have increasingly been forced to define death (many using signs of brain death as the indicator) and define when death occurs
C. Do not resuscitate (DNR) status
1. All health care institutions are required to have DNR procedures to meet accreditation standards; standards for home care from the Joint Commission on Accreditation of Health Care Organizations include "a statement regarding the need to document discussions with patients and significant others about life-sustaining measures"
2. Documentation of DNR status includes progress notes of all DNR discussions and decisions and DNR orders in the client's cumulative medical record if the client wishes not to be resuscitated
3. Most important factors considered are the client's wishes, the prognosis, the client's ability to cope, and whether cardiopulmonary resuscitation (CPR) will provide benefits sufficient to make it worthwhile

4. In many states, the right to request a DNR status is mandated within the Patient's Bill of Rights, and hospitals must also provide education on the issue of DNR to clients and families
5. A DNR order must be a team decision and the client and the family must be included in the decision-making process when possible
D. Advanced directives
1. Concepts
   a. Living wills allow clients to state their wish to die in certain situations and not prolong life by using medications, artificial means, or heroic measures; the living will sets forth the client's wishes regarding health care decisions; it includes which medical procedures are authorized or declined
   b. A health care proxy designates an agent to make health decisions according to the client's plans or wishes; it includes the power of not giving or stopping treatment necessary for life when the client is unable to do so
2. Advantages associated with living wills and health care proxies are that they permit expression of the person's preferences; promote communication between the person and caregivers; foster respect for the client as a person; and support the belief that clients have the right to self-determination
3. The Patient's Self-Determination Act of 1991 mandates that health care agencies receiving Medicare and Medicaid reimbursement advise clients of their right to advanced directives

THE NURSE'S RIGHTS AND RESPONSIBILITIES

A. Nurses must practice in accordance with standards of the profession
B. Nurses must intervene to protect clients from incorrect, unethical, and/or illegal actions by any person delivering health care
C. Nurses must participate in and promote the growth of the profession
D. Nurses must attempt to increase knowledge and experience
E. Nurses must maintain competence through professional continuing education
F. Nurses must report any suspected child abuse to the appropriate authority; this reporting is mandatory and does not incur legal jeopardy
G. Ethical principles
1. Are broader and more universal than laws
2. Ethical values address what is right or wrong or what the nurse's duties and obligations are
3. Ethical issues become legal issues through court case decisions or by legislative enactment

4. Ethical principles cannot override laws
H. American Nurses Association (ANA) *Code for Nurses*
   1. Provides general guidelines for nurses dealing with ethical issues
   2. Laws override ethical principles

REHABILITATION

A. Focuses on interventions that improve the quality of life rather than saving life; health care resources often are allocated more for critical care than rehabilitation
B. Concerns establishing function that is lost while expanding, maintaining, and supporting the limited remaining function
C. Assists people in attaining their maximum level of wellness on the continuum after a negative change in health
D. Immediate or potential rehabilitation needs exhibited in all health problems
E. Concerns all levels of prevention: primary, secondary, and tertiary
F. Not an isolated process; it involves the client, family, health team, community, and society
G. The client is the primary rehabilitator; professional health team members assist the client and family with the process of self-rehabilitation
H. Health problems that cause disabilities are socially significant because of the number of people affected, economic cost and loss, distress of personal suffering, and conditions in society that increase their incidence
I. More individuals are candidates for rehabilitation than ever before because of:
   1. Advances in technology
   2. Increased survival rates from birth defects, traumatic injuries, and infection
   3. Aging of society and more chronic illness

THE NURSING PROCESS

A. Assessment
   1. Collection of personal, social, medical, and general data
   2. Determination of current health status from the physical assessment
B. Analysis/nursing diagnoses
   1. Classification of data: screening, organizing, and grouping significant related information
   2. Definition of client's problem: determining an appropriate nursing diagnosis (definitive statements of the client's actual or potential difficulties), concerns, or deficits that can be altered by nursing interventions

C. Planning
   1. Establish client outcomes
      a. Outcomes are stated as expected changes in the client's behavior, activity, or physical state
      b. Outcomes must be objective, realistic, measurable, and include a realistic period for accomplishment to determine if the outcome has been achieved
   2. Client, family/significant others, and nurse collaborate with appropriate health team members to formulate the plan to reach the identified outcome
D. Implementation: the actual administration of the planned care
E. Evaluation/outcome and revision of care
   1. If outcome is not reached in specified time, the client is reassessed to discover the reason
   2. Reordering of priorities as necessary because process of evaluation is ongoing

TEACHING-LEARNING PROCESS

A. Learning: involves a change in or acquisition of new behavior and takes place within the individual
   1. Cognitive: knowledge
   2. Psychomotor: skill performance
   3. Affective: attitudes, emotions
B. Motivation; desire for change in response to an identified need
   1. Intrinsic motivation: motivation that comes from within; preferred to extrinsic motivation
   2. Extrinsic motivation: motivation that comes from outside the learner
   3. Readiness to learn (physical, emotional, and cognitive)
      a. Awareness of health problem and implications
      b. Willingness to ask questions
      c. Demonstration of indirect health-seeking behaviors
      d. Absence of acute distress reactions (e.g., severe anxiety and pain inhibit learning)
   4. Culture (e.g., language, values, beliefs)
   5. Physical abilities (e.g., vision, hearing)
   6. Cognitive ability (e.g., intelligence, developmental level, education)
   7. Support systems
C. Teaching: activities that result in learning
   1. Involve client and family to individualize teaching plan
   2. Exhibit nonjudgmental attitude
   3. Build on client's prior knowledge
   4. Incorporate multiple strategies that involve multiple senses (e.g., discussion, demonstration, practice, role playing, discovery, audiovisual aids, computer-assisted instruction)

5. Establish short-term achievable learning objectives to maintain motivation
6. Use positive reinforcement; learning by success or positive rewards is preferable to learning by failure or negative rewards
7. Establish an environment conducive for learning (e.g., safe, limited noise, reduced distractions)
8. Evaluate client learning
   a. Observation of behavior
   b. Written tests
   c. Self reports

MEDICATION ADMINISTRATION

DRUG EFFECTS

A. Desired effect (therapeutic effect): the action for which the drug is given
B. Adverse effect: a harmful unintended reaction to a drug
C. Toxic effect: a serious adverse effect that occurs when the plasma concentration of the drug reaches a dangerous, life-threatening level
D. Side effect: a response that is unrelated to the primary action of the drug
E. Cumulative action: the increased activity demonstrated by a drug when repeated doses accumulate in the body and exert a greater biologic effect than the initial dose
F. Drug dependence: the physical or psychological reliance on a chemical agent resulting from continued use, abuse, or addiction
G. Hypersensitivity reaction: an abnormal, excessive response to a drug
H. Idiosyncratic response: an individual's unique sensitivity to a drug that is an unpredictable, highly individualized response
I. Paradoxical reaction: a response to a drug that contrasts sharply with the usual, expected response
J. Tolerance: the ability to endure ordinarily injurious amounts of a drug or the lowering of the effect obtained from an established dose that requires raising the dose to a possibly toxic level to maintain the same effect
K. Drug allergy: a hypersensitive response to an allergen to which the individual has been exposed and has developed antibodies; usually occurs when drugs contain protein sources or combine with body protein to induce an allergen-antibody reaction
   1. Anaphylaxis: life-threatening episode of bronchial constriction and edema that obstructs the airway and causes generalized vasodilation that depletes circulating blood volume; occurs when an allergen is administered to an individual having antibodies produced by prior use of the drug
   2. Urticaria: generalized pruritic skin eruptions or giant hives
   3. Angioedema: fluid accumulation in periorbital, oral, and respiratory tissues
   4. Delayed-reaction allergies: rash and fever occurring during drug therapy

FACTORS INFLUENCING DOSAGE AND RESPONSE

A. Individual factors: age, weight, sex, height, physiologic status, and genetic and environmental factors affect dosage and response
B. The therapeutic index (TI) is used as a guide to the safe dosage range (a low TI provides a narrow margin of safety) but the individual factors must be considered
C. Concentration and duration of drug action are affected by:
   1. Characteristics of the drug and the rate of absorption, distribution, biotransformation, and excretion
   2. Drug affinity for particular tissues, immaturity of enzymes required for metabolism of the drug, or depressed function of tissues naturally metabolizing or excreting the drug
D. Membrane barriers (e.g., placental or blood-brain) may block or selectively pass the drug from the circulating fluids to protected areas

DRUG INTERACTIONS

A. Drugs and foods may interact to affect the therapeutic plan adversely
B. Drug antagonism: opposing effects of two drugs at receptor sites in body tissues
   1. Chemical antagonism: combining or binding of two drugs causing inactivation
   2. Pharmacologic antagonism: competition of two drugs for a receptor that may allow the weaker drug to block access by the more potent drug
   3. Physiologic antagonism: opposing action on physiologic systems that allows cancellation of action by either drug
C. Combined or concurrent action of two drugs can increase the therapeutic or adverse effects of either drug
   1. Synergism: interaction of drugs at common receptor sites that alters metabolism or excretion and enhances the effect of drugs
   2. Potentiation: intensified action occurring when two drugs are administered concurrently that is greater than when either drug is administered alone

NURSING RESPONSIBILITIES

A. Recognize that the administration of medications is a dependent function requiring a legally written order and knowledge of the medication's cause and effect

B. Know the common symbols, equivalents, abbreviations, and route of administration of medications

C. Monitor serum-drug levels for attainment of therapeutic level, toxic level, and peak and trough levels

D. Use independent judgment before administering a medication by assessing:
   1. The client's needs
   2. Untoward or toxic manifestations of earlier doses
   3. Compatibility of medications with other medications and substances in the diet

E. Ensure that the right medication is given to the right client at the right time, in the right dose, and by the right route

F. Recognize that the client has the right to refuse medication

G. For assistance with calculation of solutions and dosages, refer to a math for medication text

H. Common routes
   1. Oral
      a. Most common, convenient, and least expensive
      b. Absorption is slow and may be unpredictable; may cause gastrointestinal irritation
      c. Preparations include tablets, capsules, pills, powders, or liquids
         (1) Sustained-release or enteric-coated preparations should not be crushed or broken
         (2) Suspensions should be shaken well before pouring
   2. Sublingual: placed under tongue; absorbed rapidly directly into bloodstream
   3. Parenteral: requires use of sterile technique
      a. Intradermal: small volume (usually 0.1 ml) under epidermis; most commonly used for allergy and tuberculin testing
      b. Subcutaneous: 0.5 to 2 ml into tissues just below skin
      c. Intramuscular: up to 3 ml into muscle; sites include ventrogluteal, dorsogluteal, vastus lateralis, rectus femoris, and deltoid
      d. Intravenous: given directly into a vein by continuous infusion, bolus (push), or intravenous piggyback
   4. Transdermal preparations

I. Clearly and accurately record and report the administration of medications and client's response

FOUNDATIONS OF PRACTICE
REVIEW QUESTIONS

1. The best definition of a tort is:
   1. The application of force to the person of another by a reasonable individual
   2. An illegality committed by one person against the property or person of another
   3. Doing something that a reasonable person under ordinary circumstances would not do
   4. An illegality committed against the public and punishable by the law through the courts

2. A client is placed on a stretcher and restrained with straps while being transported to the x-ray department. A strap breaks, and the client falls to the floor, sustaining a fractured arm. Later the client states, "The strap was worn just at the very spot where the strap snapped." The nurse is:
   1. Exempt from any lawsuit because of the doctrine of *respondeat superior*
   2. Totally and singly responsible for the obvious negligence because of failure to report defective equipment
   3. Liable, along with the employer, for misapplication of equipment or use of defective equipment that harms the client
   4. Completely exonerated, because only the hospital, as principal employer, is primarily responsible for the quality and maintenance of equipment

3. A 2-year-old child is admitted to the hospital with a diagnosis of pneumonia and is given antibiotics, fluids, and oxygen. The child's temperature continues to rise until it reaches 103° F (39.4° C). The nurse calls the physician at the mother's request, but the physician sees no cause for alarm or change in treatment, even though the child has a history of convulsions during previous periods of high fever. Although concerned, the nurse takes no further action. Later the child has a convulsion that results in neurologic impairment of the left arm and leg. Legally:
   1. The physician's decision takes precedence over the nurse's concern
   2. The nurse's failure to further question the physician placed the child at risk
   3. The physician is totally responsible for the client's health history and treatment regimen

4. High temperatures are common in children, and this situation presented little cause for undue concern

4. The primary purpose for regulating nursing practice is to protect:
   1. The public
   2. Practicing nurses
   3. The employing agency
   4. Professional standards

5. A client with coronary artery disease has a sudden episode of cyanosis and a change in respirations. The nurse starts oxygen administration immediately. In this situation:
   1. Oxygen had not been ordered and therefore should not be administered
   2. The nurse's observations were sufficient to begin administration of oxygen
   3. The symptoms were too vague for the nurse to diagnose a need for oxygen
   4. The physician should have been called for an order before oxygen was begun

6. A 15-year-old is taken to the emergency room of the local hospital after stepping on a nail. The puncture wound is cleansed and a sterile dressing applied. The nurse asks if the adolescent has been immunized against tetanus. The reply is affirmative. Penicillin is administered, and the adolescent is sent home with instructions to return if there is any change in the wound area. A few days later, the adolescent is admitted to the hospital with a diagnosis of tetanus. Legally:
   1. Hospital protocol should govern treatment in emergency care
   2. The nurse's judgment was adequate in view of the client's symptoms
   3. Assessment by the nurse was incomplete and the treatment was inadequate
   4. The possibility of tetanus could not have been foreseen, because the adolescent had been immunized

7. An example of an intentional tort would be:
   1. Malpractice
   2. Negligence
   3. Breach of duty
   4. False imprisonment

8. A 3-year-old with eczema of the face and arms has not heeded the nurse's warnings to "stop scratching—or else!" The nurse finds the toddler scratching so intensely that the arms are bleeding. With great flurry, the nurse ties the toddler's arms to the crib sides, saying, "I'm going to teach you one way or another." In this situation, the nurse:
   1. Has merely done the job with considerable accountability
   2. Has used actions that can be interpreted as assault and battery
   3. Had to protect the toddler's skin and acted as any reasonably prudent nurse would do
   4. Tried to explain to the toddler and rightly expected the toddler to understand and cooperate

9. When teaching about child abuse, the nurse tells a parent group that the best legal definition of assault is:
   1. Threats to do bodily harm to the person of another person
   2. The application of force to another person without lawful justification
   3. A legal wrong committed by one person against the property of another
   4. A legal wrong committed against the public and punishable by law through the state and courts

10. When teaching staff about the legal terminology used in child abuse, the nurse emphasizes that the term battery means:
    1. A legal wrong committed by one person against the property of another
    2. Maligning the character of an individual while threatening to do bodily harm
    3. The application of force to the person of another person without lawful justification
    4. Doing something that a reasonable person with the same education or preparation would not do

11. A toddler screams and cries noisily after parental visits, disturbing all the other children. When the crying is particularly loud and prolonged, the nurse puts the crib in the storeroom and closes the door. The toddler is left there until the crying ceases, a matter of 30 or 45 minutes. Legally:
    1. The child needed to have limits set to control the crying
    2. The child had a right to remain in the room with the other children
    3. Keeping the child segregated alone for more than 30 minutes was too long
    4. The other children had to be considered, so the child needed to be removed

12. A client is admitted with the diagnosis of possible placenta previa. The nurse begins IV fluids, administers oxygen, and draws blood for laboratory tests as ordered. The client's apprehension is increasing, and she asks the nurse what is happening. The nurse tells her not to worry, that she is going to be all right, and everything is under control. The nurse's statements are:
    1. Adequate, because all preparations are routine and need no explanation
    2. Proper, because the client's anxieties would be increased if she knew the dangers
    3. Correct, because only the physician should explain why treatments are being done
    4. Questionable, because the client has the right to know what treatment is being given and why

13. When obtaining consent for surgery, initially the nurse should:
    1. Explain the risks involved in the surgery
    2. Explain that obtaining the signature is routine for any surgery
    3. Evaluate if the client's knowledge level is sufficient to give consent
    4. Witness the signature because this is what the nurse's signature documents

14. A client who has been told she needs a hysterectomy for cervical cancer is upset about being unable to have more children. The nurse should:
    1. Evaluate her willingness to pursue adoption
    2. Encourage her to focus on her own recovery
    3. Emphasize that she does have two children already
    4. Ensure that all treatment options have been explored

15. The family of an elderly, aphasic client complains that the nurse failed to obtain a signed consent before inserting an indwelling catheter to measure hourly output. This is an example of:
    1. A catheter inserted for the client's benefit
    2. A treatment that does not need a separate consent form
    3. Treatment without consent of the client, which is an invasion of rights
    4. Inability to obtain consent for treatment because the client was aphasic

16. The spouse of a comatose client who has severe internal bleeding refuses to allow transfusions of whole blood because they are Jehovah's Witnesses. The nurse involved in this situation should:
    1. Phone the physician for a special administrative order to give the blood under these circumstances
    2. Have the spouse sign a treatment refusal form and notify the physician so that a court order can be obtained
    3. Gently explain to the spouse why the transfusion is necessary, emphasizing the implications of not having the transfusion
    4. Institute the blood transfusion anyway, because the physician ordered it and the client's survival depends on volume replacement

17. A client is voluntarily admitted to the psychiatric unit. Later the client develops severe pain in the right lower quadrant and is diagnosed as having acute appendicitis. When preparing the client for an appendectomy the nurse should:
    1. Have two nurses witness the operative consent as the client signs it
    2. Have the surgeon and the psychiatrist sign for the surgery, because it is an emergency procedure
    3. Phone the client's next of kin to come in to sign the consent form because the client is on the psychiatric unit
    4. Ask the client to sign the preoperative consent form after being informed of the procedure and required care

18. In relation to obtaining an informed consent from a 17-year-old adolescent, the nurse should remember that the adolescent:
    1. Does not have the legal capacity to give consent
    2. Is not able to make an acceptable or intelligent choice
    3. Is able to give voluntary consent when parents are not available
    4. Will most likely be unable to choose between alternatives when asked to consent

19. A client with rheumatoid arthritis does not want cortisone even if it is prescribed and informs the nurse of this. Later the nurse attempts to administer cortisone that has been ordered by the physician. When the client asks what the medication is, the nurse gives an evasive answer. The client takes the medication and later finds that it was cortisone. The client states an intent to sue. The decision in this suit would take into consideration the fact that:
    1. The nurse should have notified the physician
    2. The nurse is required to answer the client truthfully
    3. The client has insufficient knowledge to make such a decision
    4. The physician's order takes precedence over a client's preference

20. When assessing a client with an acute anxiety reaction, the most significant legal factor for the nurse to explore is the client's:
    1. Physical status
    2. Available support systems
    3. Past behavior under stress
    4. Perception of the current situation

21. The physician prescribes "NPO after midnight" for a hospitalized client who is scheduled for a diagnostic test. The morning of the test the client eats breakfast. The test is canceled and the client must stay an extra day. The client is very disturbed and insists on not paying for the additional day because of the error. In situations such as this:
    1. The client is responsible for the hospital bill and must pay
    2. A full explanation of tests or treatments is the right of the client
    3. The order should have been written more clearly by the physician
    4. Things go wrong, and hospital personnel are not responsible unless there is gross negligence

22. Twenty-four hours after a cesarean delivery a client elects to sign herself and her baby out of the hospital because of difficulty at home with her 2-year-old son. Staff members have been unable to contact her physician. The client arrives at the nursery dressed and ready to leave and asks that her infant be given to her to dress and take home. Appropriate nursing action would be:
    1. Explain to the client that her infant must remain in the hospital until signed out by the physician and that she must leave the baby in the nursery
    2. Allow the client time with the baby to cuddle him before she leaves, but emphasize that the baby is a minor and legally must remain until orders are received
    3. Tell the client that under the circumstances hospital policy prevents the staff from releasing the infant into her care, but she will be informed when the infant is discharged
    4. Give the baby to the client to take home, making sure that she receives information regarding care and feeding of a 2-day-old infant and any potential problems which may develop

23. A female client is hospitalized because of a severe depression. While at home she refused to eat, stayed in bed most of the time, and did not talk with family members. Finally, unable to cope with the problem, her husband took her to the hospital. Here the symptoms persist, and she will not leave her room. The nurse caring for her attempts to talk to her, asking questions but receiving no answers. Finally, in exasperation, the nurse tells the client that if she does not respond she will be left alone. The nurse:
    1. Recognizes that the client has the right to make the decision
    2. Attempts to use reward and punishment to motivate the client
    3. Is really assaulting the client and should have refrained from this
    4. Should get her involved in group therapy rather than attempting one-to-one therapy

24. A newborn is admitted to the nursery. During the newborn assessment the nurse notes that the temperature, pulse, and respirations are within normal range. Other physical characteristics are also normal. The nurse records all observations on the baby's chart. The nurse's actions were:
    1. Correct, because the nurse met the requirements set forth in the Nurse Practice Act
    2. Incorrect, because making this type of medical diagnosis is not within the purview of the nurse
    3. Correct, because the assessment by the nurse is not equivalent to the physician's assessment
    4. Incorrect, because the initial assessment of the infant's physical status is the responsibility of the physician

25. Nurses are protected from all legal action when they:
    1. Offer health teaching regarding family planning
    2. Offer first aid at the scene of an automobile-bus accident
    3. Administer CPR measures on an unconscious child pulled from a swimming pool
    4. Report incidents of suspected child abuse to the appropriate authorities identified in legislation and policies

26. A client with a history of emphysema is now terminally ill with cancer of the esophagus. The client is weak, dyspneic, emaciated, and apathetic. The plan of care includes a soft diet, modified postural drainage, and nebulizer treatments. The nursing care plan for this client should give priority to:
    1. Intake and output
    2. Diet and nutrition
    3. Hygiene and comfort
    4. Body mechanics and posture

27. A terminally ill client is visited frequently by the spouse, a 16-year-old daughter, and a 20-year-old son. In view of the client's extreme weakness and dyspnea, nursing care plans should include:
    1. Allowing self-activity whenever possible
    2. Encouraging family members to feed and assist the client
    3. Limiting family visiting hours to the evening before the client sleeps
    4. Planning all necessary care at one time with long rest periods in between

28. When preparing a client for ambulation with crutches, the nurse should recognize the need for further teaching when the client states, "I must practice:
    1. Sitting down and standing up."
    2. Ambulating several hours a day."
    3. Standing and maintaining balance."
    4. Doing active exercises for muscle strengthening."

29. Rehabilitation plans for a client who has paraplegia as a result of spinal cord severance:
    1. Should be left up to the client and the client's family
    2. Should be considered and planned for early in the client's care
    3. Are not necessary, because the client will return to former activities
    4. Are not necessary, because the client will probably not be able to work again

30. A client is transferred to a rehabilitation unit following a CVA. A basic concept about rehabilitation is:
    1. Rehabilitation needs are best met by the client's family and community resources
    2. Rehabilitation is a specialty area with unique methods for meeting the client's needs
    3. Rehabilitation needs, immediate or potential, are exhibited by all clients with a health problem
    4. Rehabilitation is unnecessary for clients returning to their usual activities following hospitalization

31. The nursing process can be defined as the:
    1. Implementation of nursing care by the nurse
    2. Steps the nurse employs to provide nursing care
    3. Process the nurse uses to determine nursing goals
    4. Activities a nurse employs to identify a client's problem

32. To utilize the nursing process, the nurse must first:
1. Identify goals for nursing care
2. State the client's nursing needs
3. Obtain information about the client
4. Evaluate the effectiveness of nursing actions

33. A nursing diagnosis represents the:
1. Proposed plan of care
2. Client's health problems
3. Assessment of client data
4. Actual nursing intervention

34. The nurse who collaborates directly with the client to establish and implement a plan of care is the:
1. Primary nurse
2. Nurse clinician
3. Clinical specialist
4. Nurse coordinator

35. The determining factor in the revision of a nursing care plan is the:
1. Time available for care
2. Validity of the diagnoses
3. Method for providing care
4. Effectiveness of the interventions

36. A need for cognitive learning becomes apparent when an adolescent, newly diagnosed as having diabetes mellitus, asks:
1. "What is diabetes?"
2. "Can I still be a cheerleader?"
3. "How do I give myself an injection?"
4. "When do I test my blood for glucose?"

37. Developing independence is a primary goal for a client with hemiplegia. The nurse can motivate the client by:
1. Establishing long-range goals for the client
2. Reinforcing success in tasks accomplished
3. Pointing out errors and helping to correct them
4. Demonstrating ways the client can regain independence

38. A client is receiving an antihypertensive drug intravenously for control of severe hypertension. The client's blood pressure is unstable and is at 160/94 before the infusion. Fifteen minutes after the infusion is started the blood pressure rises to 180/100. The response to the drug would be described as a(n):
1. Allergic response
2. Synergistic response
3. Paradoxical response
4. Individual hypersusceptibility

39. Occurrence of an anaphylactic reaction after receiving penicillin indicates that the client has:
1. An acquired atopic sensitization
2. Passive immunity to the penicillin allergen
3. Antibodies to penicillin developed after earlier use of the drug
4. Developed potent bivalent antibodies when the IV administration was started

40. A 35-year-old professional golfer is brought to the emergency room for a bee sting. The client has a history of allergies to bees and is having trouble breathing. The nurse is aware that this client can expire from:
1. Ischemia
2. Asphyxia
3. Lactic acidosis
4. Antihistamenia

41. A client has an anaphylactic reaction within the first half hour after an IV infusion containing ampicillin is started. The nurse understands that the symptoms occurring during an anaphylactic reaction are the result of:
1. Respiratory depression and cardiac standstill
2. Constriction of capillaries and decreased cardiac output
3. Bronchial constriction and decreased peripheral resistance
4. Decreased cardiac output and dilation of major blood vessels

42. At the conclusion of visiting hours, the mother of a 14-year-old female scheduled for orthopedic surgery the following day hands the nurse a bottle of capsules and says, "These are for my daughter's allergy. Will you be sure she takes one about 9 tonight?" The nurse's best response would be:
1. "One capsule at 9 PM? Of course, I will give it to her."
2. "Did you ask the doctor if she should have this tonight?"
3. "I am certain the doctor knows about your daughter's allergy."
4. "I will ask your daughter's doctor to write an order so I can give this medication to her."

43. The physician orders filgrastim (Neupogen) 5 mcg/kg per day by injection for a client who weighs 132 pounds. The vial label reads Neupogen 300 mcg/ml. The nurse should administer:
1. 0.5 ml
2. 0.75 ml
3. 1.0 ml
4. 1.25 ml

44. An infant is to receive thyroxine sodium, 0.35 mg qd po. The medication is available in elixir form, 0.25 mg/ml. The nurse should administer:
1. 0.6 ml
2. 1.0 ml
3. 1.4 ml
4. 1.6 ml

45. The physician orders atropine, gr 1/300 IM pre-operatively for a 7-year-old with excessive respiratory secretions who is scheduled to have an exploratory laparotomy. The vial reads "atropine 0.4 mg/ml." The nurse should administer:
1. 0.25 ml
2. 0.5 ml
3. 0.75 ml
4. 1.0 ml

46. A 9-year-old is about to have surgery. The physician orders meperidine (Demerol), 20 mg, IV preoperatively. The container reads "50 mg/ml." The nurse should administer:
1. 0.4 ml
2. 0.6 ml
3. 0.8 ml
4. 1.0 ml

47. The physician orders 375 mg ampillin IV q6h for a 5-month-old with recurring respiratory infections. The drug is supplied as 500 mg of powder in a vial. The directions are to mix the powder with 1.8-ml diluent, which yields 250 mg/ml. The nurse should administer:
1. 0.75 ml
2. 1.25 ml
3. 1.50 ml
4. 1.75 ml

48. A client is scheduled to receive phenytoin (Dilantin) 100 mg, orally at 6 PM but is having difficulty swallowing capsules. The nurse should:
1. Insert a rectal suppository containing 100 mg phenytoin
2. Open the capsule and sprinkle the powder in a cup of water
3. Administer 4 ml of phenytoin suspension containing 125 mg/5 ml
4. Obtain a change in the prescribed administration route to allow IM administration

49. A pregnant client is now in the third trimester. The client tells the nurse she wants to have general anesthesia for delivery. The nurse's best response would be:
1. "You are worried about too much pain?"
2. "You want general anesthesia for delivery?"
3. "I will tell your doctor about this request."
4. "I can understand that; labor is uncomfortable."

50. When promoting affective learning (developing attitudes) in a client with a newly diagnosed disease, the nurse must first consider the influence of the:
1. Client's past experiences
2. Total stress of the situation
3. Client's personal resources
4. Type of onset of the disease

51. When evaluating the appropriateness of a response by a family member in the developing awareness stage of grief, the nurse must be aware of the family's:
1. Personality traits
2. Educational levels
3. Cultural background
4. Past experience with death

52. Groups are important in the emotional development of the individual because they:
1. Always protect their members
2. Are easily identified by their members
3. Go through the same developmental phases
4. Identify acceptable behavior for their members

53. For an emotional balance the individual always needs:
1. Family, work, and play
2. Security and social recognition
3. Biologic satisfaction and social acceptance
4. Individual recognition and group acceptance

54. To help parents cope with the behavior of young school-aged children, the nurse suggests that it would help if they:
1. Avoid asking specific questions
2. Give the child a detailed list of expectations
3. Be consistent and firm about established rules
4. Allow the child to set up his or her own routines

55. The family is most important in the emotional development of the individual because it:
1. Provides support for the young
2. Gives rewards and punishment
3. Helps one to learn identity and roles
4. Reflects the mores of a larger society

56. The nurse is aware that clients attending Alcoholics Anonymous meetings will be required to:
1. Attend weekly meetings and speak aloud
2. Maintain controlled drinking after six months
3. Promise to attend at least 12 meetings yearly
4. Acknowledge their alcoholism and their inability to control it

57. Self-help groups such as Alcoholics Anonymous are successful because they meet the client's need to:
1. Grow
2. Belong
3. Be trusted
4. Be independent

58. When providing group therapy, the nurse must focus on:
1. Jointly experienced stress
2. Behavior of individual members
3. Confrontation between members
4. Personal feelings affecting behavior

59. Communication ties people to their:
1. Social surroundings
2. Physical surroundings
3. Materialistic surroundings
4. Environmental surroundings

60. The effectiveness of nurse-client communication is best validated by:
1. Client feedback
2. Medical assessments
3. Health team conferences
4. Client's physiologic adaptations

61. A client becomes openly hostile when learning that amputation of a gangrenous toe is being considered. The best indication that the nurse's interaction has been therapeutic would be:
1. An increase in physical activity
2. A relaxation of tensed muscles
3. An absence of further outbursts
4. A denial that further discussion is necessary

62. During a group therapy session, a female client interrupts a male client. When the female client finishes talking, the male client is sitting rigidly, looks angry, and says, "I'm so glad that you feel like talking today." It would be most therapeutic for the nurse to:
1. State that it appears that the two clients are not getting along
2. Agree with the male client that it is good to have the female client talk
3. Comment on the male client's angry behavior and his use of pleasant words
4. Ignore the male client's comments and speak with him privately about his hostility

63. Mentally healthy individuals can be defined as those who:
1. Have insight into their own problems
2. Do not exhibit pathological symptoms
3. Are able to meet their own basic needs
4. Are free from both physical and emotional problems

64. Since people need some gratifying communication to learn, to grow, and to function in a group, all events that significantly curtail communication will eventually produce:
1. Withdrawal
2. Severe disturbances
3. Some degree of mental deficiency
4. Further attempts to increase communication

65. The stage of sleep associated with psychologic rest is:
1. Stage 1
2. Stage 4
3. REM sleep
4. NREM sleep

66. While talking with the nurse about the problem of not being able to make friends, a teenager begins to cry. At this time it would be most therapeutic for the nurse to:
1. Sit quietly with the client
2. Point out how the client can change this
3. Tell the client that crying isn't helping
4. Suggest that they play a game of Scrabble

67. A client with a history of hypertension is hospitalized with a transient ischemic attack (TIA). The client has been told to stop smoking. The nurse discovers a pack of cigarettes in the client's bathrobe. The best course of action to take at this time is to:
1. Let the client know they were found
2. Discard them without making comments
3. Report the situation to the head nurse
4. Call the physician and request directions

68. When planning care for the parents of a newborn with abnormalities, the nurse should be aware that the parents are better able to cope with this problem if informed:
1. When bringing the baby to the mother for the first time
2. When the parents ask if something is wrong with their baby
3. Right after delivery while the mother is still in the delivery room
4. After the first 24 hours, when the mother's strength has returned

69. A condyloma has been identified during a yearly gynecological examination. While awaiting the biopsy report prior to its removal, the client indicates to the nurse that she is fearful of cervical cancer. The best response by the nurse would be:
    1. "Worrying today is not going to help the situation."
    2. "It is very upsetting to have to wait for a biopsy report."
    3. "Of course you don't have cancer; a condyloma is always benign."
    4. "No operation is done without specimens being sent to the laboratory first."

70. A female client is admitted for surgery. Although not physically distressed, the client appears apprehensive and alienated. A nursing action that may help the client to feel more at ease includes:
    1. Telling her that everything is all right
    2. Giving her a copy of hospital regulations
    3. Orienting her to the environment and unit personnel
    4. Reassuring her that staff will be available if she becomes upset

71. An obstetric client with a history of three spontaneous abortions is now 16 weeks pregnant and attending the high-risk clinic. The client expresses concerns about remaining at home during this pregnancy. The nurse should question the client to determine her knowledge of:
    1. Causes of spontaneous abortion
    2. Signs and symptoms of spontaneous abortion
    3. Interrelationship among rest, normal delivery, and diet
    4. Current status of pregnancy and availability of support system

72. A client with preeclampsia with two preschool children is prescribed bed rest at home. To help stimulate compliance, plans for the client's care should include:
    1. A suggestion to find a housekeeper
    2. An explanation as to why bed rest is necessary
    3. A warning of the risks involved in noncompliance
    4. A contract that 4 hours of nap time will meet the requirement

73. A nurse is assigned to introduce a client who has a PhD to the other clients. The client tells the nurse, "I wish to be called Doctor." The nurse could best respond:
    1. "Why do you insist on being called Doctor?"
    2. "That's fine; that is how I will introduce you then."
    3. "All the clients here call one another by their first names."
    4. "I can't do that. It's better if the other clients do not know you are a doctor."

74. "But you don't understand" is a common statement associated with adolescents. The best response by the nurse when communicating with an adolescent would be to say:
    1. "I don't understand..."
    2. "I would like to understand; let's talk."
    3. "I guess you're right; tell me what's going on from your perspective."
    4. "I'm not sure I have to. I believe it's you who has to understand and comply."

75. The emotional responses of a client with a left CVA would be most influenced by the:
    1. Cause of the CVA
    2. Care the client is receiving
    3. Client's premorbid personality
    4. Ability of the client to understand the illness

FOUNDATIONS OF PRACTICE

ANSWERS AND RATIONALES

1. 2 An individual is held legally responsible for actions committed against another individual or an individual's property. (3; LE; AN; TC; EH)
1 This is related to battery, which involves physical harm.
3 This is the definition of negligence.
4 This is the definition of a crime.

2. 3 The nurse was negligent in using a stretcher with worn straps. Such an oversight did not reflect the actions of a reasonably prudent nurse. (2; LE; EV; TC; EH)
1 The nurse is responsible for own actions and must ascertain the adequate functioning of equipment.
2 The hospital shares responsibility for safe, functioning equipment.
4 The nurse is responsible for determining the safety of hospital equipment.

3. 2 Since part of a nurse's responsibility is to foresee potential harm and prevent risks, it is imperative that the nurse not only take a health history and perform a physical assessment on each client, but act to ensure the safety of the client. (3; LE; EV; TC; NM)
1 This is not true and cannot be accepted as a rationale for inaction.
3 The nurse and physician share interdependent roles in the assessment and care of clients.
4 High temperatures are common in children but are nonetheless a valid cause for concern.

4. 1 Each state or province is charged with the responsibility of protecting the health and welfare of its populace, which it does by regulating nursing practice. (2; LE; AN; TC; EH)
2 Although the members of the profession can also benefit from a clear description of their role, this is not the primary purpose of the law.
3 The employing agency does assume responsibility for its employees and therefore benefits from maintenance of standards, but this is not the purpose of the law.
4 Professional standards are established by the profession to ensure quality care for the public.

5. 2 The Nurse Practice Act states that nurses diagnose and treat human responses to actual or potential health problems. Administration of oxygen in an emergency situation is within the scope of nursing practice. (2; LE, EV; PA; CV)
1 Because the client's symptoms reflected an immediate need for oxygen, postponement of treatment could result in further deterioration of the client's condition.
3 Same as answer 1.
4 Same as answer 1.

6. 3 The nurse's data collection was not adequate because no questions were asked concerning the recency of the previous tetanus inoculation. The nurse failed to support the life and well-being of a client. (3; LE; EV; TC; NM)
1 This is usually a clinical decision.
2 The nurse's assessment was not thorough in regard to determining the recency of immunization.
4 It was essential to determine the recency of the immunization; for a "tetanus-prone" wound, like a puncture from a rusty nail, some form of tetanus immunization is usually given.

7. 4 False imprisonment is a wrong committed by one person against another in a willful intentional way without just cause and/or excuse. (3; LE; AN; TC; EH)
1 Malpractice, which is professional negligence, is classified as an unintentional tort.
2 Negligence is an unintentional tort.
3 Breach of duty is an unintentional tort.

8. 2 Assault is a threat or an attempt to do violence to another, and battery means touching an individual in an offensive manner or the actual injuring of another person. (1; LE; EV; PS; EH)
1 The nurse's behavior demonstrates anger and has not taken into account the growth and development needs of this age.
3 Although the behavior (scratching) needs to be decreased, this can be done through mittens so as not to immobilize a child of this age.
4 A 3-year-old does not have the capacity to understand cause (scratching) and effect (bleeding).

9. **1** Assault is a threat or an attempt to do violence to another. (3; LE; IM; ED; EH)
   2 This is not the appropriate legal definition of assault.
   3 Assault implies harm to persons rather than property.
   4 This definition is too broad to describe assault.

10. **3** Battery means touching in an offensive manner or the actual injuring of another person. (2; LE; IM; ED; EH)
   1 Battery refers to harm against persons instead of property.
   2 Battery refers to actual bodily harm rather than threats of physical or psychologic harm.
   4 This definition is too broad to describe battery.

11. **2** A client cannot legally be locked in a room (isolated) unless there is a threat of danger involved either to the client or to other clients. (2; LE; EV; ED; EH)
   1 This is a reaction to separation from the mother, which is common at this age.
   3 The action is illegal, not permitted for any length of time.
   4 Crying, although irritating, will not harm the other children.

12. **4** The client's rights were violated. All clients have the right to a complete and accurate explanation of treatment. (1; LE; AN; PS; HP)
   1 All preparations or procedures should be explained because they are not routine to the client.
   2 The Patient's Bill of Rights states that the client should be informed.
   3 When administering treatment, the nurse is responsible for explaining to the client what the treatment is and why it is being done.

13. **3** Informed consent means the client must comprehend the surgery, the alternatives, and the consequences. (1; LE; EV; ED; EH)
   1 This explanation is not within nursing's domain.
   2 Although this is true, it does not determine the client's ability to give informed consent.
   4 Although this is true, initially the nurse should assess the client's knowledge in relation to the surgery.

14. **4** Although a hysterectomy may be performed, conservative management may include cervical conization and laser treatment that would not preclude future pregnancies; clients have a right to be informed by their physician of all treatment options. (2; LE; IM; PS; EH)

   1 This currently is not the issue for this client.
   2 This denies the validity of the client's feelings.
   3 Same as answer 2.

15. **2** This is considered a routine procedure to meet basic physiologic needs and is covered by a consent signed at the time of admission. (3; LE; EV; TC; RG)
   1 Although the catheter provides assessment information, it is not directly beneficial to the client at this time.
   3 This treatment does not require special consent.
   4 Same as answer 3.

16. **2** The client is unconscious. Although the spouse can consent, there is no legal power to refuse a treatment for the client unless previously authorized to do so by a power of attorney or a health care proxy; the court can make a decision for the client. (2; LE; IM; TC; BI)
   1 This alternative is without legal basis, and the nurse could be held liable.
   3 Explanations would not be effective at this time and will not meet the client's needs.
   4 Same as answer 1.

17. **4** There is no evidence of incompetence. Because the client has not been certified as incompetent, the right of informed consent is retained. (3; LE; IM; TC; EH)
   1 The client can sign the consent, and the client's signature requires only one witness.
   2 Because there is no evidence of incompetence, the client should sign the consent.
   3 Same as answer 2.

18. **1** An individual is legally unable to sign a consent until the age of 18 years. The only exception is the emancipated minor, a minor who is self-sufficient or married. (1; LE; AN; ED; EH)
   2 Although the adolescent is capable of intelligent choices, it is the legality, not the acceptability or intelligence of the choice, that is at issue.
   3 Parents or guardians are legally responsible under all circumstances unless the adolescent is an emancipated minor.
   4 Adolescents have the capacity to choose between alternatives, but not the legal right in this situation.

19. **2** The client has a right to know what medication is being administered (informed consent). This also constitutes an invasion of the client's rights. (2; LE; AN; TC; EH)
  1 The physician should have been notified only after the nurse had interviewed the client to determine the reasons for the decision; this would have been the time to impart the appropriate information.
  3 This cannot be determined from the situation described; the client should have been questioned about the reasons for refusing the drug to determine the level of understanding.
  4 The client has a right to refuse treatment and a right for an explanation of treatment before its administration; that client's right takes precedence over the physician's order.

20. **4** The way the client perceives the situation is most significant to the experience. (2; LE; AS; TC; AX)
  1 This may or may not have an effect on the situation.
  2 This is important, but not as significant as the client's perception of the situation.
  3 This may or may not have an effect on the situation.

21. **2** This is negligence. The client should have been informed. (2; LE; EV; TC; EH)
  1 The hospital should assume the added expense incurred as a result of the negligent actions of its employees.
  3 The physician wrote an appropriate, clear order. The nurse was negligent in carrying it out.
  4 The staff is liable for negligent actions.

22. **4** When the client signs herself and the baby out of the hospital, she is legally responsible for her infant and must be given the baby. (3; LE; IM; ED; EC)
  1 The baby belongs to the mother and can leave with the mother when she signs them out.
  2 The mother is the baby's guardian and may take the baby with her when she leaves.
  3 The baby is under the guardianship of the mother and may leave with the mother.

23. **3** The nurse's response really was a threat by attempting to put pressure on the client to speak or be left alone. (2; LE; IM; TC; MO)
  1 The statement reflects an insensitivity to, rather than a recognition of, the client's rights.
  2 This is not reward and punishment, which is used in behavior modification therapy.
  4 The client is not ready at this stage for group involvement; the nurse must start with a one-to-one relationship.

24. **1** The Nurse Practice Act requires nurses to diagnose human responses. (2; LE; EV; TC; NN)
  2 This is physical assessment, not medical diagnosis, and is within the nurse's role.
  3 Assessment should not differ if done by the nurse.
  4 Fortunately not true, because the physician may not be present; the nurse is capable of making a physical assessment.

25. **4** The reporting of possible child abuse is required by law, and the nurse's identity can remain confidential. (2; LE; AN; TC; EH)
  1 The nurse is functioning in a professional capacity and therefore can be held accountable.
  2 Although the Good Samaritan Act protects health professionals, the nurse would still be responsible for acting as any reasonably prudent nurse would in a similar situation.
  3 Same as answer 2.

26. **3** Because the client's condition is described as terminal, the nursing priority should be directed toward providing comfort. (1; CJ; PL; TC; RE)
  1 Although these are important aspects of nursing care, provision of comfort retains priority in the care of a dying client.
  2 Same as answer 1.
  4 Same as answer 1.

27. **2** Because family members are old enough to understand the client's needs, they should be encouraged to participate in the care. (3; CJ; PL; TC; RE)
  1 Self-care increases oxygen utilization, increasing fatigue and dyspnea.
  3 This deprives the client of a support system.
  4 Overworking the client causes undue fatigue and dyspnea; frequent rest periods should be incorporated into the plan.

28. **2** Practicing ambulation without proper preparation (e.g., ambulation techniques and strengthening the involved muscle groups) would not be helpful in the rehabilitation process and could exhaust the client (1; CJ; EV; ED; SK)
  1 Because different muscle groups are utilized, the client must be instructed even about what seem to be simple maneuvers; transfer from a sitting to a standing position must be accomplished before ambulation.
  3 Before ambulation the individual must be able to maintain balance.
  4 The muscles used for crutch walking are different from those used in normal ambulation; therefore they must be strengthened by active exercises before ambulation.

29. **2** To promote optimism and facilitate smooth functioning, all rehabilitation should begin on admission to the hospital. (1; MR; PL; TC; NM)
   1 Although the client and family should be included in planning, they are often unaware of the options available in the health care system; the nurse should be available to provide the necessary information and support.
   3 Because paralysis is permanent, alterations in normal lifestyle are required.
   4 Because the paralysis is permanent, rehabilitation plans should be made.

30. **3** All nursing intervention aims to assist an individual in maximizing capabilities and coping with modifications in lifestyle. (2; MR; AN; PA; NM)
   1 All resources, including the private physician and acute care facilities, that can be beneficial to client rehabilitation should be utilized.
   2 Rehabilitation is a commonality in all areas of nursing practice.
   4 Rehabilitation is necessary to help clients return to a previous level of functioning after both illness and surgery.

31. **2** The nursing process is a step-by-step process that scientifically provides for a client's nursing needs. (2; CJ; AN; TC; EH)
   1 This is incomplete; implementation of care is one aspect of the nursing process.
   3 This is incomplete; goal establishment is one aspect of the nursing process.
   4 This is incomplete; the nursing process goes beyond identification of a problem.

32. **3** The initial step in any process using problem solving is the collection of data. (1; CJ; AS; TC; EH)
   1 Goals are set after nursing needs are established.
   2 Nursing needs can be determined only after assessment.
   4 Evaluation is the last phase of the nursing process.

33. **2** Nursing diagnosis defines an actual or potential health problem faced by the client. (1; CJ; AN; TC; EH)
   1 This is the plan of care made before implementation; it follows the nursing diagnosis but is not part of it; it is a step in the nursing process.
   3 This is part of data collection before making the nursing diagnosis; it is the first step of the nursing process.
   4 Intervention follows the nursing diagnosis; it is part of the nursing process but not part of the nursing diagnosis.

34. **1** The primary nurse provides or oversees all aspects of care, including assessment, implementation, and evaluation of that care. (2; MR; AN; TC; EH)
   2 A clinician is an expert teacher or practitioner in the clinical area.
   3 The title given to a specially prepared nurse for one very specific clinical role.
   4 The nurse coordinator oversees all the staff and clients on a unit and coordinates care.

35. **4** When a plan does not effectively produce the desired outcome, the plan should be changed. (2; CJ; AN; TC; EH)
   1 Time is not relevant in the revision of a care plan.
   2 Client response is the determinant, not the nursing diagnosis.
   3 Various methods may have the same outcome; effectiveness is most important.

36. **1** The acquiring of knowledge or understanding aids in developing concepts rather than skills or attitudes and is a basic learning task in the cognitive domain. (2; CJ; AN; ED; EN)
   2 The acquiring of values and self-realization is in the affective domain.
   3 The acquiring of skills and tasks is psychomotor learning.
   4 Same as answer 3.

37. **2** Success is a basic motivation for learning. People receive satisfaction when a goal is reached. The more frequent the success, the greater is their satisfaction, which in turn motivates them to continue striving toward realistic goals. (2; CJ; PL; TC; NM)
   1 Progress toward long-range goals is often not readily apparent and may tend to discourage a client.
   3 Constructive criticism is an important aspect in client teaching; but if not tempered with praise, it is discouraging.
   4 An important part of teaching, but this will not necessarily motivate the client to attempt them.

38. **3** A paradoxical response to a drug is directly opposite the desired therapeutic response (3; CJ; EV; PA; DR)
   1 An allergic response induces an allergen-antibody reaction.
   2 This response involves drug combinations that enhance each other.
   4 This is a response to a drug that is more pronounced than the response observed in most of the population.

39. 3 Hypersensitivity results from the production of antibodies in response to exposure to certain foreign substances (allergens). Earlier exposure is necessary for the development of these antibodies. (3; CJ; AN; PA; BI)

1 This is not a sensitivity reaction to penicillin; hay fever and asthma are atopic conditions caused by atopens.
2 It would be an active immunity.
4 Antibodies have been developed in a prior exposure to the allergen, in this case penicillin.

40. 2 Hypersensitivity can result in anaphylaxis; edema of the respiratory system can result in respiratory obstruction and respiratory arrest. (2; CJ; AN; TC; BI)

1 This is unrelated to anaphylaxis.
3 This is associated with excessive exercise not anaphylaxis.
4 There is no condition called antihistamenia.

41. 3 Hypersensitivity to a foreign substance can cause an anaphylactic reaction. Histamine is released, causing bronchial constriction, increased capillary permeability, and dilation of arterioles. This decreased peripheral resistance is associated with hypotension and inadequate circulation to major organs. (3; CJ; AN; PA; BI)

1 These are the problems that result from bronchial constriction and vascular collapse.
2 Arterioles dilate, capillary permeability increases, and eventually vascular collapse occurs.
4 Dilation of arterioles occurs.

42. 4 By law, a nurse cannot administer medications without a prescription from a legally licensed individual. This is a dependent function of the nurse. (1; LE; IM; TC; DR)

1 The nurse cannot distribute medication without a legal order.
2 The nurse must get an order for the medication and cannot accept the parent's information alone.
3 The nurse should not assume that the physician is aware of the problem.

43. 3 When 132 pounds is converted it equals 60 kg; the physician has ordered 5 mcg/kg or 5 × 60 = 300 mcg; this amount would be contained in 1 ml from the vial. (2; LE; AN; TC; DR)

1 This would provide less than the ordered dose.
2 Same as answer 1.
4 This would provide more than the ordered dose.

44. 3 $\frac{0.35 \text{ mg}}{0.25 \text{ mg}} \times \frac{X \text{ ml}}{1 \text{ ml}} = 1.4 \text{ m}$ (2; LE; AN; TC; DR)

1 This is too low.
2 Same as answer 1.
4 This is too high.

45. 2 Convert grains to milligrams (gr 1/300 = 0.2 mg); then use the formula:
$$\frac{0.2 \text{ mg}}{0.4 \text{ mg}} \times \frac{X \text{ ml}}{1 \text{ ml}}$$
0.4 X = 0.2
X = 0.5 ml (This will contain the desired 0.2 mg atropine.) (3; LE; AN; TC; DR)

1 This amount is too little according to calculations.
3 This amount is too much according to calculations.
4 Same as answer 3.

46. 1 $\frac{20 \text{ mg}}{50 \text{ mg}} \times \frac{X}{1 \text{ ml}}$
50 X = 20
X = 0.4 ml (1; LE; AN; TC; DR)

2 This calculation is too high.
3 Same as answer 2.
4 Same as answer 2.

47. 3 $\frac{250 \text{ mg}}{1 \text{ ml}} \times \frac{375 \text{ mg}}{X \text{ ml}}$
250 X = 375
X = 1.5 ml (2; LE; AN; TC; DR)

1 This is too little.
2 Same as answer 1.
4 This is too much.

48. 3 When an oral medication is available in a suspension form, the nurse should use it for clients who cannot swallow capsules. (3; LE; IM; TC; DR)

1 The route of administration cannot be altered without physician approval.
2 Because a palatable suspension is available, it is a better alternative than opening the capsule.
4 Intramuscular injections should be avoided because of related risks of tissue injury and infection.

49. 2 Paraphrasing encourages the client to express the rationale for this request. (2; CJ; IM; PS; EC)

1 This is making an assumption without enough information; the nurse should respond with an open-ended question.
3 Although this request would be forwarded to the physician, the reason for the choice of general anesthesia should be explored.
4 This statement can further raise the client's anxiety.

50. **1** Past experiences have the most meaningful influence on present learning. (2; CJ; PL; PS; ED)
    2 Although this consideration affects learning, its influence is not as great as that of all past experiences.
    3 Same as answer 2.
    4 Same as answer 2.

51. **3** In this stage the degree of anguish experienced or expressed is set or imposed by the cultural background of the individual. (2; CJ; EV; PS; CS)
    1 Although this factor does enter into the grief process, it is not as important in the developing awareness stage as cultural background.
    2 Educational level has no relationship to the grieving process.
    4 Past experience with death has no relationship to the appropriateness of an individual's present response.

52. **4** Learning from others occurs in a group setting and is reinforced by group acceptance of the norms. Group pressure is peer pressure, which is more easily accepted if the individual wants to stay in the group. (1; CJ; AN; ED; PD)
    1 One member of a group can be the target of hostility.
    2 This is not necessarily so; the group may not be easily identified by its members.
    3 Groups do not go through the same developmental phases as individuals.

53. **4** A sense of one's self and a feeling of belonging form the basis for mental health, because they provide comfort with self and group. (3; CJ; AN; PS; PD)
    1 A person could have emotional balance without all three.
    2 A person needs security but can do without social recognition.
    3 A person needs to have biologic needs met; one does not need social acceptance; the group providing acceptance may not be acceptable to society or to the individual.

54. **3** Because of a short attention span and distractibility, a specific limit setting consistently employed is crucial toward providing an environment that promotes concentration, prevents confusion, and minimizes conflicts for the child. (1; MR; IM; PS; EH)
    1 Questions are appropriate as long as judgments are not made about the answers.
    2 Some children have difficulty reading.

4 Parents need to assist child with routine tasks; this age child may not be concerned with time frames.

55. **3** Socialization, values, and role definition are learned within the family and help develop a sense of self. Once established in the family, the child can more easily move into society. (1; CJ; AN; ED; PD)
    1 This is true, but not as important as identity and roles in relation to emotional development.
    2 This is only a very small aspect of the family's influence.
    4 Same as answer 2.

56. **4** A major premise of AA is that in order to be successful in achieving sobriety, clients with alcohol abuse problems must acknowledge their inability to control the use of alcohol. (2; CJ; AN; PS; SA)
    1 There are no rules of attendance or speaking at meetings, although both actions are strongly encouraged.
    2 This is not part of AA; this group strongly supports total abstinence for life.
    3 There are no rules of attendance at meetings; the member is strongly encouraged to attend as often as possible.

57. **2** Self-help groups are successful because they support a basic human need for acceptance. A feeling of comfort and safety and a sense of belonging may be achieved in a nonjudgmental, supportive, sharing experience with others. (2; MR; AN; TC; TR)
    1 If the client had a need to grow, AA would probably not be able to meet this need.
    3 AA would not meet the client's need to be trusted.
    4 On the contrary, AA meets dependency needs rather than focusing on independence.

58. **4** Group therapy should focus on the present and how current problems and feelings are affecting current behavior. In the group setting the individual members have the opportunity to receive feedback on their behavior. (2; CJ; PL; PS; TR)
    1 The nurse focuses not on the stress itself, but on how to deal with the stress.
    2 The focus is the feelings behind the behavior with which others can identify.
    3 The nurse must protect individual group members from confrontation until certain that they are strong enough to deal with it.

59. 1 Socialization occurs through communication with others. Without some form of communication there can be no socialization. (1; CJ; AN; PS; PD)
  2 People interact with other social beings, not with inanimate objects.
  3 Same as answer 2.
  4 Same as answer 2.

60. 1 Feedback permits the client to ask questions and express feelings and allows the nurse to verify client understanding. (2; CJ; EV; PS; EH)
  2 Medical assessments do not necessarily include nurse-client relationships.
  3 Team conferences are subject to all members' evaluations of a client's status.
  4 Nurse-client communication should be evaluated by the client's verbal and behavioral responses.

61. 2 Relaxation of muscles and facial expression are examples of nonverbal behavior; nonverbal behavior is a better index of feelings because it is less likely to be consciously controlled. (2; CJ; EV; PS; EH)
  1 Increased activity may be an expression of anger or hostility.
  3 Clients may suppress verbal outbursts despite feelings and become withdrawn.
  4 Refusing to talk may be a sign that the client is just not ready to discuss feelings.

62. 3 Commenting on the incongruent verbal and nonverbal behavior may lead to a growth experience for the client and the group. (2; MR; IM; PS; TR)
  1 It is better to focus on behaviors and feelings than personalities and relationships.
  2 Agreement with the statement ignores the covert message, which should be explored to help the client and the group.
  4 For the group to be a growth process for this client, feelings and behaviors must be explored within the group.

63. 3 It is the inability to meet these needs that will cause a person to become mentally ill. (2; CJ; AS; PS; TR)
  1 This is not necessary to be mentally healthy.
  2 To be considered mentally healthy a person must be more than just free from illness.
  4 This would rule out most of the population.

64. 2 The individual who cannot communicate cannot test reality. Without this connection to others or reality, severe emotional problems will develop. (2; MR; AN; PS; TR)

  1 Lack of communication can lead to isolation and withdrawal, but this response is too narrow because a variety of problems usually develop.
  3 Without the stimulation of communication, mental dullness or slowness will occur, not mental deficiency.
  4 There is a frustration and inability to foster communication.

65. 3 REM (rapid eye movement) sleep is necessary for psychologic coping. The nurse should be aware that some medications affect this sleep stage and thereby alter emotional health. (2; CJ; AN; PA; NM)
  1 The individual is just drifting off to sleep.
  2 The individual is in a deep sleep and is difficult to arouse.
  4 NREM sleep consists of stages 1 through 4 and supports the recuperative functions assigned to sleep.

66. 1 Sitting quietly with the client gives the message that the nurse cares and accepts the client's feelings. (1; CJ; IM; PS; BA)
  2 Helping the client explore reasons is more therapeutic than giving advice.
  3 This is negating feelings and the client's right to cry when upset.
  4 This in effect closes the door on any further communication of feelings.

67. 1 An honest nurse-client relationship should be maintained so that trust can develop. (1; CJ; IM; TC; EH)
  2 This does nothing to establish communication about feelings or motivation behind behavior.
  3 Although other health team members may need to be informed eventually, the initial action should concern only the nurse-client relationship.
  4 Same as answer 3.

68. 3 The parents should be informed of the birth of a child with an abnormality as early as possible, preferably in the delivery room when staff is present to support and assist them in mobilizing resources; this approach prevents fantasizing about the problem. (2; CJ; PL; PS; EC)
  1 This may be too much of a shock if the mother is not aware of the defect.
  2 The parents may not ask and providing the information should not be delayed.
  4 Crisis intervention should not be delayed; immediately informing the parents improves coping abilities.

69. 2 This recognizes the client's feelings of anxiety are valid. (2; CJ; IM; PS; RG)

1 This does not recognize the client's concerns and may inhibit the expression of feelings.

3 This is false reassurance. Although a condyloma is a benign wart, the papilloma virus that causes it can bring about neoplastic changes in the cervical tissue, which if not interrupted lead to cervical carcinoma.

4 This is not true and does not recognize the client's concerns.

70. 3 Orienting the client to the hospital provides knowledge that may reduce the strangeness of the environment, and introducing staff members lets the client know who will be providing care. (2; MR; IM; PS; TR)

1 This may be false reassurance, because no one can guarantee that everything will be all right.

2 This would be part of orienting the client to the unit.

4 This implies that staff members are available only if the client becomes upset.

71. 4 This would assist the client to focus on reality and help reduce anxiety. (2; MR; AS; PS; EC)

1 The actual causes of spontaneous abortion are not known.

2 This would add to the client's anxiety; after three abortions the client knows the symptoms.

3 This is too broad; these are unrelated to the concerns about abortion.

72. 2 Clients who understand the "why" of treatment are more likely to comply. (2; CJ; PL; TC; EC)

1 This may be an unrealistic suggestion; more data should be obtained to see if this is feasible.

3 This is a negative approach; the nurse should reinforce benefits of compliance rather than risks of noncompliance.

4 This would not meet the requirement for bed rest.

73. 2 The client has the right to make this decision and the staff should accept the client's wishes. (2; CJ; IM; PS; TR)

1 The client is a doctor, and the nurse's statement attacks the client's self-concept.

3 It helps support clients' dignity by addressing them as they wish.

4 For whom is it better—the staff, the other clients, or the client?

74. 2 This response attempts to open the communication process. (2; CJ; IM; PS; BA)

1 Restating only serves to entrench each communicant's position and does little to open the flow of communication.

3 This serves to reinforce a negative statement and provides for listening but not for clarification of the issue.

4 This is authoritative and closes down the flow of communication.

75. 3 Although the client who has suffered a CVA may be emotionally labile, the major factors determining the reaction to illness are past experiences and coping mechanisms. (1; CJ; AS; PS; EH)

1 The cause of the CVA has no effect on the client's emotional response to the disease.

2 Although care is important, basic coping mechanisms and personality are already established.

4 Emotional response does not depend on one's ability to understand the underlying physiologic causes of disease.

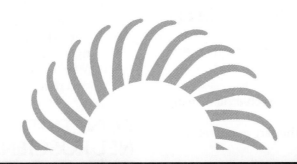

CHAPTER 3

Psychiatric/Mental Health Nursing

LEGAL CONCEPTS RELATED TO PSYCHIATRIC/MENTAL HEALTH NURSING

MENTAL HEALTH LAWS

A. A fundamental component of psychiatric nursing is understanding the legal framework, in any given state, that is used to regulate the care and treatment of clients with mental illness
B. Adherence to the *Patient's Bill of Rights* is essential
C. Laws are specific in addressing what is wrong in a particular society
D. Types of hospital admissions
   1. Voluntary admission—client of lawful age may apply in writing (standard admission form) for admission to a public or private psychiatric hospital
      a. Voluntary admission is similar to a medical hospitalization
      b. All civil rights are retained
   2. Involuntary admission (commitment)—client has not requested
      a. Most state laws permit commitment of the mentally ill based on the following:
         (1) Dangerous to self or others
         (2) Mentally ill and in need of treatment
         (3) Unable to provide for own basic needs
   3. Emergency hospitalization—is used to control an immediate threat by an acutely ill person to self or others
      a. There is a time limit governing the length of commitment (48 to 72 hours)
      b. The purpose is to detain only until proper legal action is initiated, which provides for additional hospitalization
   4. Observational hospitalization—this type of commitment allows for short-term diagnosis and therapy. No emergency situation need occur
      a. Length of time varies according to states' laws
      b. If the length of time runs out before the client is ready for discharge, a petition can be filed for long-term commitment
   5. Formal commitment—a long-term commitment allows for an indefinite time or until the client is ready for discharge
      a. Client retains right to a lawyer and right to request a court hearing
      b. Periodic reviews for long-term hospitalization may be made every 3, 6, or 12 months
E. Nursing responsibilities
   1. Implement care that meets the *Scope and Standard of Psychiatric-Mental Health Clinical Nursing Practice* as described by the ANA
   2. Stay current with skills and knowledge base
   3. Keep accurate and concise nursing notes
   4. Maintain client/family confidentiality
   5. Know the laws governing practice within the state, the rights and duties of the nurse, and the rights of the client
   6. Maintain current malpractice liability insurance coverage

CONCEPTS FROM NEUROSCIENCE

NEUROPHYSIOLOGIC THEORY OF BEHAVIOR

A. Research with an emphasis on neurobiologic information has focused on the structure and function of the brain and nervous system and their relationship to health and illness
B. Considerable knowledge gaps still exist as to the specific mechanisms of causation for many psychiatric disorders
C. There is general acceptance that there is no real division between the mind and body, the mental and the physical, and the brain and thought
D. The brain, like other body organs, is vulnerable to disease
E. Neuroscience encompasses anatomy, physiology, biochemistry, genetics, neuroimaging, physics, pharmacology, neurology, neurosurgery, immunology, psychiatry, psychology, electronics, and computer science
F. Structure and function of the brain
   1. The reader is encouraged to review texts on basic anatomy and physiology or neurophysiology for a more detailed review
      a. The brain weighs about 3 pounds and is composed of trillions of groups of cells that have formed structures
      b. About 100 billion brain cells form groups of neurons that are arranged in networks
      c. Neurons communicate with each other via neurotransmission, which affects body functions, consciousness, intelligence, creativity, memory, and emotion
      d. Neurotransmission plays a key role in understanding various brain functions and how biochemical interventions (medications) affect brain activity and behavior
      e. Neurotransmitters are chemical messengers of the nervous system manufactured in one neuron, released from the axon into the synapse, and received by the dendrite of the next neuron
      f. Communication between brain cells occurs via this neurotransmission process

g. Signals given by the neurotransmitter either excite or inhibit cell firing

h. After release into the synapse and communication with receptor cells, the neurotransmitter chemicals are transported back from the synapse into the axon, where they are stored or metabolized and inactivated by enzymes

i. This process of neurotransmitters returning to the presynaptic cell is known as reuptake

j. Glial cells are support cells from myelin sheaths, thought to remove excessive transmitters and ions from extracellular spaces in the brain, provide glucose to some nerve cells, and direct the flow of blood and oxygen to various parts of the brain

k. Cerebral spinal fluid (CSF) is found in several chambers within the brain; its purpose is to bathe the brain with nutrients and cushion the brain within the skull; it exits through the blood

2. Neurotransmitters perform vital brain functions, and their absence or excess can play a major role in brain disease and behavioral disorders

a. Generally, neurotransmitters fall into one of two categories: small amine molecules and peptides

b. Amines are neurotransmitters that are synthesized from amino molecules such as tyrosine, tryptophan, and histidine that are found in various brain regions

c. Amines affect learning, emotions, and motor control

d. Peptides are chains of amino acids found throughout the body; their role as neurotransmitters is not well defined

e. Low concentrations of peptides appear in the CNS, but they are very potent

f. They appear to play a secondary role in neurotransmission, that of modulating the messages of the amines

G. Genetics of mental illness

1. The search for a genetic cause of mental illness has been inconclusive

2. The only gene that has been linked to mental illness affects people before age 65 with a rare form of Alzheimer's disease (AD); it affects only 10% of the people with AD

3. Genetic studies continue; however, clinical implications are not defined and limits the information that can be provided to clients and their families

H. Psychoimmunology

1. This relatively new field explores the psychologic influences on the nervous system's control of immune responsiveness

2. Efforts to match specific stressors to specific diseases have not generally been successful; stress is recognized as a basis for understanding the development and course of many illnesses

3. Evidence shows that psychosocial stressors temporarily impair the immune responses and thus contribute to the development of a variety of illnesses

4. Research has demonstrated that suppression of WBC reproduction occurs following sleep deprivation, marathon running, space flight, death of a loved one, and during depression

5. The body's natural killer cells are thought to play a role in tumor surveillance and control of viral infections; when compromised, they are less effective

I. Biologic components of mental illness

1. The knowledge base continues to expand through neurobiologic research

2. Clinical implications of neuroscientific research:

a. Schizophrenia—cause is unknown, but it is believed that at least one biologic cause exists

(1) Genetics—there is a 1% lifetime risk in the general population

(2) No specific gene for schizophrenia has been identified

(3) Several distinct brain regions are involved that affect thought, perceptions, emotions, movement, and behavior

(4) Biochemistry has been implicated and includes

(a) An excess of the neurotransmitter dopamine

(b) An imbalance between dopamine and other neurotransmitters, especially serotonin

(c) Problems in the dopamine receptor systems

(5) Brain imaging focuses on two areas of the brain

(a) The frontal cortex (involved with negative symptoms)

(b) The limbic system within the temporal lobes (involved with positive symptoms)

(c) Imaging studies are continuing to provide data that link abnormal brain structure and function with etiology and symptomatology

b. Mood disorders—neuroscientific research has identified biologic markers for mood disorders and psychopharmacologic interventions have provided for greater specificity, fewer side effects, and better outcomes

(1) Genetics—mood disorders tend to be familial and inherited

(2) The lifetime risk for a mood disorder in the general population is 6%

(3) The lifetime risk for relatives of people with depression is 20%

(4) The lifetime risk for relatives of people with mania is 24%

(5) No clear genetic mapping is available

(6) Research into mood disorders reveals a complex picture of genetic and environmental interaction, not a single-gene theory

(7) The amounts of balance of norepinephrine and serotonin remain unquestioned as to the pathophysiology of mood disorders

(8) The effects of antidepressants regulate the norepinephrine and/or serotonin systems suggesting that psychopharmacology can restore more efficient regulation of these two systems

(9) Brain imaging, although inconclusive, found larger ventricles in clients with affective disorders when compared with control study groups

c. Panic disorder—neurologic studies of anxiety have helped in understanding and treating anxiety disorders

(1) Genetics—there appears to be a genetic component, although research also indicates that traumatic events and stress are important components in anxiety disorders

(2) Family studies have shown 8% to 20% among first-degree relatives of people with this disorder as compared with the control study group with a risk of 2% to 4%

(3) Studies have been able to distinguish between pain disorder and other types of anxiety disorders; this suggests a separate mechanism for inheritance of each type of anxiety disorder

(4) Biochemical—studies indicate a dysfunction in multiple systems as opposed to isolation of one neurotransmitter

(a) Systems involved in panic and anxiety disorders related to gamma-aminobutyric acid, serotonin, cholecystokinin, and the hypothalamic pituitary-adrenal axis

(b) Specific antianxiety drugs are used to control anxiety behaviors and are effective

(c) Clinically, people with panic disorders have noted the panic effect of caffeine and chocolate; caffeine affects a variety of neurotransmitters and blocks the receptors for the inhibitory neurotransmitter adenosine

(5) Biological—it is accepted that an individual's general health status affects the predisposition to anxiety

(a) Anxiety accompanies many physical disorders

(b) Coping abilities are thought to be impaired by toxic influences, nutritional deficiencies, reduced blood supply, hormonal shifts, and some physical disorders

(c) Fatigue increases irritability and seems to contribute to anxiety

(6) Brain imaging remains inconclusive; data provided through CT and MRI scans have shown brain underdevelopment or atrophy, particularly in the frontal and temporal lobes of people with panic disorders

(a) Significance of these data is unknown

(b) Laboratory challenge test findings support a biologic component to panic disorders

(c) Further research is essential to clarify the mechanisms that cause anxiety disorders

d. Alzheimer's disease—causes are unknown; research continues because this disease is the most disabling psychiatric disorder of adulthood

(1) It is thought that genetics is involved in perhaps 10% of all early age onset of AD

(2) Before age 65, DNA mutations occur with chromosomes 1, 14, and 21

(3) Between 40 and 50 years of age people with Down syndrome are affected; they have 3 rather than 2 copies of chromosome 21

(4) Research to explore the link between a cholesterol-transporting protein, Apo-E, and AD; developing AD may hinge on which combination of Apo-E is inherited

(5) Biochemical—almost every neurotransmitter has been somehow implicated in AD; so research of the cholinergic hypothesis continues

(a) Acetylcholine is consistently reduced in AD

(b) Research that focuses on understanding the molecular mechanism underlying AD continues so that drugs can be designed to block these processes

(c) Cholinergic inhibitors tacrine (Cognex) and donepezil (Aricept) slow the breakdown of acetylcholine

(6) To date, brain imaging is not conclusive for diagnosing AD; it is helpful in ruling out space-occupying lesions, infarcts, or infections as causes of dementia

   (a) It is useful to detect changes in cortical atrophy, ventricular enlargement, loss of temporal lobe volume, and brain weight loss, all indications of early-onset AD

   (b) Only age-related changes can be detected in persons developing late-onset AD (over age 75)

DEVELOPMENT OF THE PERSONALITY

DEFINITION

A. Sum of all traits that differentiate one individual from another
B. Total behavior pattern of an individual through which the inner interests are expressed
C. The individual's unique and distinctive way of behaving and interacting with others
D. Constellation of defense mechanisms for dealing with inner and outer pressures
E. A functional role within a family system
F. Emergence of personality occurs around 2 years of age

FACTORS INVOLVED IN PERSONALITY DEVELOPMENT

A. Behavior is a learned response that develops as a result of past experiences and genetic and psychologic factors
B. To protect the individual's emotional well-being, these experiences are organized in the psyche on three different levels
   1. Conscious: composed of past experiences, easily recalled, that create little if any emotional discomfort and tend to be somewhat pleasant
   2. Subconscious: composed of material that has been deliberately pushed out of the conscious but can be recalled with some effort
   3. Unconscious: contains the largest body of material; greatly influences behavior
      a. This material cannot be deliberately brought back into awareness because it is usually unacceptable and painful to the individual
      b. If recalled, it is usually disguised or distorted, as in dreams or slips of the tongue; however,

it is still capable of producing high levels of anxiety

c. According to Freud the personality consists of three parts: the id, ego, and superego
   (1) Id is the unconscious instincts, impulses, and urges; it is totally self-centered
   (2) Ego is the conscious self, the "I" that deals with reality; the part of the personality that is shown to the environment
   (3) Superego controls, inhibits, and regulates impulses and instincts whose uncontrolled expression would endanger the emotional well-being of the individual and the stability of the society; incorporates parental, religious, and societal values

FORMATION OF PERSONALITY

A. Personality of an individual develops in overlapping stages that shade and merge together
   1. Certain goals must be accomplished during each stage in the development from infancy to maturity if needs are to be met and mental health maintained
   2. If these goals are not accomplished at specific periods, the basic structure of the personality will be weakened
   3. Factors in each stage persist as a permanent part of the personality
   4. Each stage has particular frustrations and major traumas that must be overcome
   5. Successful resolution of the conflicts associated with each stage is essential to development
   6. Childhood identifications are integrated with basic drives, native endowments, and opportunities offered in social roles
   7. Unresolved conflicts remain in the unconscious and may, at times, result in maladaptive behavior
   8. Personality is capable of change throughout life
B. Psychodynamic theory (Freud)
   1. Psychodynamic theories propose that human behavior is largely governed by motives and drives that are internal and often unconscious
   2. Freud believed that development proceeds best when children's psychosexual needs at each stage are met, but not exceeded; the stages are:
      a. Oral (birth–1 year)—psychosexual needs gratified orally; unable to delay gratification; begins to develop self-concept from the responses of others
      b. Anal (1-3 years)—bladder and bowel training occurs; this interferes with instinctual impulses; struggle of giving of self and breaking the symbiotic ties to mother; as the ties

are broken, the child learns independence; struggle with toilet training creates conflict between child's needs and parents' desires

 c. Phallic (3-5 years)—psychosexual energy directed to genitals (oedipal); values and rules learned from parents; guilt and self-esteem develop; incestuous desire for opposite sex parent develops and creates fear and guilt feelings; desires are repressed, and introjection and role identification with parent of the same sex occurs

 d. Latency (6-12 years)—Mastery of learning; relationships with same sex peers develop; sex instincts are relatively quiet

 e. Genital (12 years and beyond)—Period of sexual maturity in which psychosexual needs are directed toward heterosexual relationships; sexual activity increases; sexual identity is strengthened or attacked

C. Psychosocial theory (Erikson)

 1. Psychosocial theory attributes development to social interactions and relationships that occur throughout the lifespan

 2. Erikson believed that development results from social aims or conflicts arising from feelings, parent-child interactions, and social relationships

 3. Eight major crises or conflicts need to be faced during a lifetime; each stage is marked by a struggle between two opposing tendencies, both of which are experienced by the individual. Stages are:

 a. Trust vs. mistrust (birth to 1 year)—Infant develops a sense of whether the world can be trusted; child learns to depend on satisfaction that is derived from this care, and, when the need is met, trust develops. Psychosocial strength: Hope

 b. Autonomy vs. shame and doubt (1-3 years)—Child develops first sense of self as independent or as shameful and doubtful; the struggle of holding on to or letting go; an internal struggle for self-identity; love versus hate. Psychosocial strength: Will

 c. Initiative vs. guilt (3-6 years)—Child learns ability to try new things and learns how to handle failure; period of intensive activity, play, and consuming fantasies where child interjects parents' social consciousness. Psychosocial strength: Purpose

 d. Industry versus inferiority (6-12 years)—Child learns how to make things with others and strives to achieve success. Psychosocial strength: Self-worth

 e. Identity vs. confusion (puberty to young adulthood)—Adolescent determines own sense of self. Psychosocial strength: Fidelity

 f. Intimacy vs. isolation (young adulthood)—Person makes commitment to another; moves from the relative security of self-identity to the relative insecurity involved in establishing intimacy with another; isolation and self-absorption occur if unsuccessful. Psychosocial strength: Love

 g. Generativity vs. stagnation (middle adulthood)—Person seeks to guide the next generation or risks feelings of personal incompleteness. Psychosocial strength: Care

 h. Integrity vs. despair (late life)—Older adult seeks a sense of personal accomplishment, adapts to triumphs and disappointments with a certain ego integrity and accepts death, or falls into despair. Psychosocial strength: Wisdom

D. Interpersonal theory (Sullivan)

 1. Development results from interpersonal relationships with others in maximizing satisfaction of needs while minimizing insecurity

 2. Believed that development results from interpersonal relationships in the infancy, childhood, juvenile, preadolescent, adolescent, and late adolescent eras

 a. Infancy era (0-2 years): Learns to differentiate self from others; through trial and error, learns from parental interactions to rely on others to gratify needs and satisfy wishes; develops a sense of basic trust, security, and self-worth when this occurs; ends with language development

 b. Childhood era (2-6 years): Language development allows for education; development of body image and self-perception; self-esteem develops with sublimation; child learns to communicate needs through the use of words and the acceptance of delayed gratification and interference with wish fulfillment (expression of impulses in socially acceptable ways or develops a feeling of living among enemies)

 c. Juvenile era (6-10 years): Relations with peers allow child to see self objectively; develops conscience; behavior is connected to others' opinions; organizes and uses experiences in terms of approval and disapproval received; begins using selective inattention and disassociates those experiences that cause physical or emotional discomfort and pain

 d. Preadolescent era (10-13 years): Develops same-sex friends; moves from egocentrism to love; able to form satisfying relationships and work with peers; uses competition, compromise, and cooperation

e. Adolescent era (13-17 years): Interest in sexual activity; learns how to establish satisfactory relationships with members of the opposite sex; if attractions are severely discouraged or thwarted by adults, the adolescent will feel insecure and lonely

f. Late adolescent era (17-19 years): Personality integration; able to integrate the needs of society without becoming overwhelmed with anxiety; inability to achieve personality integration results in regression and egocentrism for life

g. Young adulthood: becomes economically, intellectually, and emotionally self-sufficient

h. Older adulthood: learns to be interdependent and assumes responsibility for others

i. Senescence: develops an acceptance of responsibility for what life is and was and of its place in the flow of history

E. Cognitive development (Piaget)
1. Sensorimotor stage (infancy-toddler): infant develops physically with a gradual increase in the ability to think and use language; progresses from simple reflex responses through repetitive behaviors to deliberate and imaginative activity
2. Preoperational thought stage (preschool): child learns to imitate and play; begins to use symbols and language although interpretation is literal
3. Preoperational thought stage continues (school age): child begins to understand relationships and develops basic conceptual thought and intuitive reasoning
4. Concrete operational thought stage (pre-adolescent): thinking is more socialized and logical with increased intellectual and conceptual development; begins problem solving by use of inductive reasoning and logical thought
5. Formal operational stage (adolescent): develops true abstract thought by application of logical tests; achieves conceptual independence and problem-solving ability

ANXIETY AND BEHAVIOR

A. Anxiety
1. Is a diffuse feeling of uneasiness, uncertainty, and helplessness that occurs as a result of a threat to an individual's self-concept, esteem, or identity
2. Is a normal response to a threat or stressors
3. Is different from fear, which has a specific source or object that can be identified and described
4. Is an emotion, is subjective in nature, and is without a specific object
5. Is related to one's culture, because culture influences one's values
6. Causes are uncertain, but research indicates a combination of physical, psychosocial, and environmental factors

B. Levels of anxiety
1. Mild—alertness level: automatic response of the central nervous system that prepares the body for danger by regulating internal processes and concentrating all energies for internal activity; perceptual field is increased
2. Moderate—apprehension level: response to anticipation of short-term threat that prepares the individual for efficient performance; perceptual field is narrowed as focus is on the immediate concern
3. Severe—high anxiety level: focus is on a specific detail and behavior is aimed at relieving anxiety; needs much direction by others to focus on another detail or area; marked reduction in the perceptual field limits cognitive abilities
4. Panic—extreme level: involves the disorganization of the personality and is associated with dread and terror; communication abilities and problem solving are nonexistent; even with direction the person has great difficulty following commands; perceptual field is distorted; prolonged period of panic results in exhaustion and death; therefore intervention is essential

C. Behavioral defenses against anxiety
1. Consciously directed, task-oriented behaviors that are deliberate attempts to problem solve, resolve conflicts, and gratify; they tend to comprise the individual's deliberate effort to maintain control, reduce tension, and limit anxiety; they include attack, withdrawal, and compromise behaviors:
   a. Attack behavior—an attempt to overcome obstacles to satisfy a need
      (1) Constructive behaviors reflect use of problem-solving behaviors
      (2) Destructive behaviors are usually accompanied by feelings of anger and hostility and may violate rights, property, and well-being of others
   b. Withdrawal behavior can be expressed physically or psychologically
      (1) Physical withdrawal involves removing oneself from the source of threat
      (2) Psychologic withdrawal occurs when one admits defeat, becomes apathetic, or lowers aspirations; when this behavior isolates the person or interferes with work production, it causes additional problems

c. Compromise is essential in situations that cannot be resolved through attack or withdrawal; it occurs by changing usual methods of operating, altering goals, or adjusting personal needs
   (1) Compromise behaviors are usually constructive and are noted in approach-approach and avoidance-avoidance situations
   (2) Compromise solutions can later offer opportunities for renegotiation or adapting different coping mechanisms
2. Task-oriented reactions and effective problem solving is influenced by the expectation of some degree of success and upon drawing on one's past successes to deal with current stressful situations
3. Problem solving perseverance and the belief that one can endure the discomfort helps one find the courage to deal with anxiety
4. Task-oriented reactions are not always successful in coping with stressful situations, therefore ego-oriented reactions (defense mechanisms) are often used to protect the self

PERSONALITY DEFENSES

Defense Mechanisms

A. Defense mechanisms provide initial protection for the personality; they operate on unconscious levels
B. Defense mechanisms are most helpful in dealing with mild and moderate levels of anxiety because they offer protection from feelings of inadequacy and worthlessness; when used to extreme they can distort reality, impede interpersonal relationships, and limit productivity
C. Identifiable patterns of response begin to form when individuals respond to most situations they encounter with the same type of behavior
D. Commonly used normal defense mechanisms that help an individual to deal with reality are:
   1. Compensation: the individual makes up for a perceived lack in one area by emphasizing capabilities in another
   2. Compromise: reciprocal give-and-take necessary in many relationships to salvage some part of the situation or the goal
   3. Identification: the individual internalizes characteristics of an idealized person
   4. Rationalization: the individual makes acceptable excuses for behavior and feelings; attempts to explain behavior by logical reasoning
   5. Sublimation: a socially acceptable behavior is substituted for an unacceptable instinct; this mechanism is used when the expression of these instincts would prove a threat to the self

6. Substitution: the individual replaces one goal for another
E. In addition to the normal defenses, all individuals may use compensatory-type defenses in times of stress; these, when used in moderation, are adaptive; if used to excess, they frequently create greater emotional problems
   1. As the use of these compensatory defenses increases and encompasses more of the individual's life, contact with reality is interrupted and distortions begin
   2. These patterns of behavior are considered deviations and are usually looked on as symptoms of emotional problems
      a. Conversion: emotional conflict is unconsciously changed into a physical symptom that can be expressed openly and without anxiety
      b. Denial: emotional conflict is blocked from the conscious mind and the individual refuses to recognize its existence
      c. Displacement: emotions related to an emotionally charged situation or object are shifted to a relatively safe substitute situation or object
      d. Fantasy: conscious distortion of unconscious wishes and needs to obtain gratification and satisfaction
      e. Intellectualization: use of thinking, ideas, or intellect to avoid emotions
      f. Introjection: complete acceptance of another's opinions and values as one's own
      g. Projection: unconscious denial of unacceptable feelings and emotions in oneself while attributing them to others
      h. Reaction formation: the individual unconsciously reverses unacceptable feelings and behaves in the exact opposite manner
      i. Regression: return to an earlier stage of behavior when stress creates problems at the present stage
      j. Repression: involuntary exclusion from consciousness of those ideas, feelings, and situations that are creating conflict and causing discomfort
      k. Suppression: voluntary exclusion from consciousness of those ideas, feelings, and situations that are creating conflict and causing discomfort
      l. Dissociation: separation of any group of mental or behavioral processes from the rest of the individual's consciousness or identity
      m. Undoing: act or communication that partially negates a previous one
      n. Splitting: viewing others or situations as either all good or all bad; failure to integrate the positive and negative qualities in oneself

MOTIVATION AND BEHAVIOR

A. All behavior is motivated
   1. Motive always implies some purpose
   2. Social motives are often changed through learning
   3. Symbolic rewards are the major factors in learning
   4. Social approval is an important form of symbolic reward
B. Behavior and emotions
   1. Emotions act as motives for behavior, because they often involve a reaction to some external situation
   2. Behavior is always accompanied and often controlled by the emotions
   3. Emotions may facilitate or hinder the learning process
   4. Emotions exert a strong influence on the thinking process
C. Automatic behavior
   1. Is the predetermined or repetitive type behavior that has been used successfully in prior situations
   2. Requires little effort or thought
   3. Is adapted to definite situations and can be difficult to alter if the situation changes
   4. Is integrated with cognition in the functioning of a mature and independent adult
D. Life is a continually changing process, and when these changes occur in areas of significance they often produce rather distinct emotional responses; these changes include:
   1. Resistance to change: the individual hesitates to accept or adapt to the change and may attempt to deny its occurrence or reject its outcome
   2. Regression: the individual returns to an earlier type of behavior that, at the time, provided some satisfaction and gratification and now provides an escape from the unacceptable or anxiety-producing situation
   3. Acceptance and progression: the individual adapts to the change and expends energy on outside objects rather than self-centered aims
E. Maslow's humanistic theory, a nondevelopmental theory, postulates that people are guided by a variety of needs, from basic physiologic ones to self-actualization, the need to achieve one's full potential
   1. The existence of unmet needs and the desire to achieve optimum self-potential are fundamental sources of human motivation. Needs are:
      a. Physiologic—satisfying needs for oxygen, water, food, shelter, sleep, and relief of sexual tension
      b. Safety—avoiding harm and achieving security and safety
      c. Love and belonging—giving and receiving affection, developing companionship, group acceptance
      d. Esteem and recognition—achieving recognition from others leads to self-esteem and prestige; work success
      e. Self-actualization—achieving one's own unique potential
   2. With the gratification of basic needs, other higher needs emerge, driving one toward self-potential

DYSFUNCTIONAL PATTERNS OF BEHAVIOR

Withdrawn Behaviors

A. Definition: pathologic retreat from or an avoidance of people and the world of reality
   1. Schizophrenia, the most common psychosis, is characterized by distorted thinking, perceptions, and behaviors
   2. Other psychotic disorders include brief psychotic disorder, delusional disorder, and psychoses related to medical conditions and drug use
   3. All these disorders involve a change in the individual's perception of reality
B. Psychoanalytic model and developmental factors
   1. Thought to be caused by a basic character flaw in combination with poor family relationships
   2. Failure to accomplish developmental tasks such as trust or intimacy
   3. Faulty reality interpretation and cognitive processing
   4. Interpersonal relationships create a source of anxiety
   5. Prolonged high anxiety results in loss of interest in interpersonal relationships and reality testing
   6. Extreme sensitivity, narcissism, and introversion develop
C. Neurobiologic factors: see Neurobiologic perspective—etiology under Schizophrenic Disorders. Neurobiologic cause of psychoses is becoming more and more convincing
D. Stress/disease/trauma model
   1. Studies note the effects of stress during the gestational period of development
   2. Immune reactions affected by viral infections and malnutrition during pregnancy are thought to contribute to childhood schizophrenia
   3. Use of cocaine and other drugs during pregnancy has been linked to schizotypal behaviors in children of users
   4. Communication patterns are more destructive, critical, and hostile than supportive and protective

E. Cultural and environmental theories
1. All socioeconomic groups and cultures affected
2. Limited or absent social support of family
3. Changes in social roles
F. Learning theories and behavioral models
1. Irrational problem-solving methods, distorted thinking, deficient communication patterns learned from parents
2. Generalized social interactions learned from significant others
G. Compensatory mechanisms used to reduce and avoid stress include fixation; projection; reaction formation; regression; rigidity, compulsiveness; and withdrawal
H. Effect of compensatory mechanisms on behavior: isolation and failure to test reality result in greater distortions of reality

Projective Behaviors

A. Definition: a continual denial of one's own feelings, faults, failures, and emotions while continually attributing them to others
B. Psychoanalytic model and developmental factors
1. Parents set extremely high demands and continually raise expected standards of performance
2. Expectations of failure are fostered, creating feelings of inadequacy and feelings of inferiority
3. Childhood experiences continue to reinforce these feelings and chronic insecurity, suspiciousness, and extreme sensitivity develop
4. Feelings of hostility develop and cannot be expressed
5. Inability to establish relationships with others interferes with reality testing
6. The individual develops a rigid, structured, narcissistic personality
7. Competitive society fosters and supports projective patterns of behavior
C. Neurobiologic factors: See Neurobiologic perspective—etiology under Delusional (Paranoid) Disorders
D. Compensatory mechanisms used to reduce and avoid stress include delusions; denial; displacement; ideas of reference; projection; rationalization; and rigidity
E. Effects of compensatory mechanisms on behavior
1. The individual is unable to tolerate suspense, prolonged anxiety, or tension
2. Unacceptable impulses and wishes are denied and faults and failures are disclaimed for self and attributed to others
3. Delusional ideas develop and begin to dominate behavior
4. Ideas of reference result in continual misinterpretation of events
5. Delusions become more systematized and spread out

6. Social, marital, or work problems can result from delusional beliefs

Aggressive Behaviors

A. Definition: physical, symbolic, or verbal behavior that is forceful or hostile and enacted to intimidate others; aggression occurs on a continuum ranging from verbal angry affect to physical aggression directed at a person and/or the environment
B. Psychoanalytic model and developmental factors
1. Aggressive behavior is the result of instinctual drives; Freud proposed that two primary drives influence behavior: the life force expressed through sexuality, and the death force expressed through aggression; the more powerful life force usually prevails
2. Research has not supported this theory
3. Inherent in this theory is that humans are innately aggressive and it negates choice and discourages individual responsibility
4. Aggression is viewed as a learned behavior; if the positive results outweigh the negative consequences, then there is little reason to stop using the behavior
5. Socialization for gratification or considering the rights of others along with one's own has not occurred
6. Research studies indicate a history of family violence is a major correlate of aggression; the behavior may have been modeled in family life of a child
7. Severe emotional deprivation or overt rejection in childhood contributes to defects in trust and self-esteem
8. Organic brain damage, mental retardation, or learning disabilities may impair capacity to deal with frustration
C. Neurobiologic factors
1. Research has focused on three areas of the brain believed to be involved in aggression: the limbic system, the frontal lobe, and the hypothalamus
2. Damage to the limbic system may result in an increase or decrease in the potential for aggressive behavior; the amygdala mediates the expression of rage or fear
3. Damage to the frontal lobe can result in impaired judgment, personality changes, difficulty with decision making, inappropriate conduct, and aggressive outbursts
4. The hypothalamus, at the base of the brain, serves as the alarm system; when there is impairment of the hypothalamus-pituitary-adrenal axis feedback system the entire system responds more vigorously to all provocations
5. Neurotransmitters most often associated with aggressive behavior are norepinephrine, sero-

tonin, dopamine, acetylcholine and the amino acid gamma-aminobutyric acid (GABA)

D. Sociocultural factors
1. Cultural theories state that aggressive acts are a product of cultural values, beliefs, norms, and rituals
2. Social and cultural factors influence aggressive behaviors
3. Physical crowding and extremes of heat appear to be related to increased violence
4. Behaviors associated with aggression are often used to achieve fame, fortune, and power
5. Gender violence (domestic violence) is seen in many cultural and social settings

E. Compensatory mechanisms used to reduce and avoid stress include denial; displacement; hostility that can be directed on self or the environment; rigidity; projection; and repression

F. Effects of compensatory mechanisms on behavior
1. Need for approval results in compliance to demands
2. Necessary compliance creates resentment
3. Hostility develops and fosters feeling of guilt
4. Self-doubt increases anxiety and tension
5. Increased anxiety and tension reduce interpersonal relationships and reality testing
6. Overwhelming anxiety may precipitate an episode of delusions and/or hallucinations

Anxiety-Based Behaviors

A. Definition: a vague, subjective nonspecific feeling of uneasiness, tension, apprehension, occasional dread or pending doom; occurs as a result of a threat to one's being, self-esteem, or identity; includes panic attack and disorders of panic, phobias, post-traumatic stress, acute distress, generalized anxiety, obsessive-compulsive and somatoform disorders
1. Characterized by many fears, anxieties, and/or physical symptoms with or without physical cause
2. It is a universal experience, an integral part of human existence, and occurs on a continuum
3. Behaviors related to anxiety include physiologic, behavioral, cognitive, and affective responses

B. Psychoanalytic model and developmental factors
1. Freud initiated the study of anxiety, and viewed anxiety as a warning to the ego of danger from internal or external threats; anxiety was later viewed as primary (a state of tension or a drive produced by external causes) and secondary (the emotional conflict that occurs between the id and the superego)
2. Epidemiological and family studies show an increase in anxiety disorders among relatives; some disorders are similar and others differ

3. Interpersonal theory explains anxiety in terms of interactions with others who give or withhold approval
a. Anxiety is first conveyed by the mother to the infant
b. During childhood, the child realizes discomfort is a result of one's own actions
c. Developmental traumas such as separations and losses can lead to vulnerabilities
d. Later, chronic insecurity, anxiety, and apprehension are perceived when threatened by loss
e. Relationship exists between low self-esteem and susceptibility to anxiety
f. Constant struggle to gain reassurance and security
4. Behavioral model involves cognition and explains anxiety as physiologic and cognitive responses to external stimuli
a. Based on learning theory, the etiology of anxiety is a generalization from an earlier traumatic experience to a benign setting or object
b. Anxiety then occurs when a conditioned individual encounters a signal that "predicts" a painful or feared event
c. Satisfaction is gained from a behavior and substituted for the satisfaction desired but not obtained through interpersonal relations

C. Neurobiologic factors involve dysfunction in multiple systems as opposed to the isolation of one particular neurotransmitter abnormality; these systems entail the GABA, norepinephrine, serotonin, and cholecystokinin; the biochemical theory provides a framework for symptom development and pharmocotherapeutic intervention

D. Compensatory mechanisms used to reduce anxiety and avoid stress include:
1. Task-oriented reactions are deliberate attempts to solve problems, resolve conflict, and gratify needs; reactions include attack, withdrawal, and compromise behaviors
2. Ego defenses are utilized when task-oriented behaviors are unsuccessful: conversion; compensation; denial; displacement; intellectualization; malingering; rationalization; regression; rigidity; and compulsiveness
3. When ego defenses are overused or used unsuccessfully, physiologic and psychologic symptoms commonly associated with emotional illness occur

Socially Aggressive Behaviors

A. Definition: maladjustive response resulting from a defect in the development of the personality that is characterized by peculiar actions or misbehavior

B. Developmental factors
1. Approval and disapproval do not appear sufficiently strong in childhood to influence the behavior along accepted patterns
2. Long history of maladjustment that creates more problems as child matures and standards for acceptable behavior are increased
3. The individual may show a history of severe emotional trauma in early life that interferes with emotional development
4. Parents frequently provide a cold, emotionally sterile environment

C. Psychoanalytic model and developmental factors
1. Freudian theory postulates if individuals have difficulty during the genital stage, their sense of self and ability to relate to others will be compromised; attainment of goals or values is thwarted
2. The capacity for relatedness results from a developmental process
   a. Interference with this process decreases the ability to develop healthy interpersonal relationships
   b. Basic trust in the parent(s) leads to establishing trust with others; failure to develop trust can lead to suspicious attitudes toward others
   c. A child who is treated as an object may become an adult who treats others as objects
   d. Security may be found in material possessions rather than through caring relationships

D. Neurobiologic factors: See Neurobiologic perspective—etiology under Personality Disorders

E. Compensatory mechanisms used to reduce anxiety and avoid stress include denial; displacement; hostility; regression; rejection; projection; rationalization; splitting; and repression

F. Effects of compensatory mechanisms on behavior; the individual
1. Appears competent but is usually unreliable; lacks a sense of responsibility
2. Has the potential to succeed but shows a history of repeated failure
3. Lacks perseverance, honesty, and sincerity
4. Is egocentric and unable to sustain emotional relationships
5. Experiences no remorse or shame
6. Is explosive under pressure
7. Is unable to tolerate criticism
8. Fails to profit from past experiences and cares little about the consequences of present acts
9. Has impaired judgment, which usually creates problems and brings the individual into conflict with society; usually classified as personality disturbances

Addictive Behaviors

A. Definition: repeated or chronic use of alcohol or drugs with a resulting dependency on these substances; described by DSM-IV-TR, refers to continued use of these substances despite the occurrence of related problems

B. Psychoanalytic model and developmental factors
1. Early psychoanalytic perspective viewed the substance abuser as regressed and fixated at the pregenital, oral levels of psychosexual development
2. Need gratification is satisfied through oral behaviors (smoking, ingestion of food or substances)
3. Interpersonal theories focused on the dependent personality type with an inability to delay satisfaction and an infantile need for immediate gratification
   a. Feelings of loneliness and isolation develop
   b. Chronic anxiety, fears, and low tension tolerance develop as a result of early relationships and feelings of inadequacy in interpersonal relationships
   c. Struggle for independence yet unconsciously desire to be dependent
   d. Impulsiveness and resentment of responsibility
4. Some substance abusers have psychologic problems related to childhood/family experiences
5. Generally, psychologic theories are becoming less well accepted and are considered insufficient to explain the need for excessive substance use

C. Neurobiologic factors: See Neurobiologic perspective—etiology under Substance Related Disorders

D. Compensatory mechanisms used to reduce anxiety and avoid stress include addiction; denial and minimization of amount of drugs or alcohol used; projection; rationalization; and repression

E. Effects of compensatory mechanisms on behavior
1. Ego defenses reduce anxiety
2. Literature indicates individuals with personality disorders have a higher incidence of dual diagnoses (e.g., borderline personality and substance abuse)
3. Substance abuse reduces inhibitory self-control
4. Drugs or alcohol use allows for expression of inner feelings but increases guilt and requires more substance to relieve the guilt
5. The individual becomes increasingly less efficient and devotes less energy to goals and ambitions
6. Dependency and tolerance develop and the substances are needed in increasing amounts to achieve the same dulling of reality
7. Once dependent, the disease continues to progress and can be fatal

Self-Destructive Behaviors

A. Definition: chronically indulging in self-destructive behavior by noncompliance with medical regimens; habitually abusing food, drugs, alcohol, or nicotine; or engaging in high-risk activities

B. Neurobiologic factors: See Neurobiologic perspective—etiology under Mood Disorders

C. Psychoanalytic model and developmental factors

    1. At the turn of the century, Freud viewed self-destruction as hostility directed inward toward the internalized love object; later expanded to include guilt

    2. Menninger described several sources of suicidal impulses as the wish to kill, the wish to be killed, and the wish to die

    3. Jung wrote that the suicidal person had an unconscious wish for spiritual rebirth after feeling that life had lost meaning

    4. Developmental factors:

        a. Failure to develop security and self-worth and little hope for the future

        b. Sense of isolation; inconsistent, superficial interpersonal relationships and difficulty with goal attainment

        c. Inconsistent relationship with parents with a lack of firm standards for reward or punishment and variations between verbal and nonverbal communications

    5. Family history of suicide is a significant risk factor for self-destructive behavior; explanations include identification, family stress, and possible genetic factors

D. Interpersonal theory: suicide is viewed as a failure to work with or resolve interpersonal conflict

    1. Self-injury may result from pattern interactions that leave one feeling guilty and worthless

    2. Negative feelings are internalized and later with a lack of secure attachments self-destructive behavior can result

E. Compensatory mechanisms used to reduce anxiety and avoid stress include denial; identification; magical thinking; rationalization; regression; rigidity

F. Effects of compensatory mechanisms on behavior

    1. Greater risk of self-destructive behavior

    2. Greater risk of suicide

        a. Talking, threatening, or planning suicide in either very vague or specific terms throughout planning

        b. Making a suicide attempt in an acute crisis state by seriously and deliberately executing a plan

        c. The suicide is completed, but there is difficulty in determining whether the act was accidental or deliberate (e.g., autoeroticism practiced by adolescents; reckless driving)

        d. Cluster suicide: suicidal acts carried out by adolescents knowing or reading about similar acts

    3. Completed suicide represents the total failure of adaptive coping mechanisms

PSYCHOLOGIC FACTORS AND PHYSICAL HEALTH

A. Category of psychophysiologic disruptions in which organic impairment is evident

B. Anxiety stimulates the autonomic nervous system, and the nervous and endocrine impulses appear to center on one particular organ, creating actual physical illness and changes in the tissue structure

C. Selye's stress theory has helped to identify mental-physical interactions

D. Predisposing factors are described from biologic, psychologic, and sociocultural perspectives; precipitating stressors include any experience the individual interprets as stressful

E. The stress is often unrecognized consciously; if recognized, individuals are unable to relate this to the physical symptoms of the psychophysiologic disorder

F. Each person has a "shock organ" that is genetically vulnerable to stress (some are prone to cardiac illness; others may react with gastrointestinal distress or skin rashes; or other problems)

G. Physical conditions affected by psychologic factors

    1. Cardiovascular

        a. Migraine headaches

            (1) Psychosocial factors can influence headaches; most often they occur in persons who have "perfectionist" tendencies

            (2) Dietary triggers are also associated; they include chocolate, cheese, citrus fruits, coffee, pork, and dairy products

            (3) Skipping meals may lower blood sugar, which may also lead to headaches

        b. Primary hypertension

            (1) Anxiety and other environmental stressors are believed to contribute to the etiology

            (2) Genetics, obesity, and arteriosclerosis also contribute

        c. Angina

            (1) Exertion, stressors, and cold exposure are known to precipate angina

            (2) Angina may occur following periods of fatigue, anxiety, or after eating a large meal

    2. Musculoskeletal

        a. Rheumatoid arthritis

(1) The etiology of RA is unknown and may be caused by a combination of factors

(2) Onset often coincides with stress (anxiety), exposure to temperature extremes, fatigue and acute infections; all deplete the physical and emotional reserves

b. Idiopathic low back pain

(1) Anxiety and fear often create a tightening of muscles

(2) This aggravating factor is noted in musculoskeletal disorders in which tension and spasm are involved (arthritis, backache, tension headache)

3. Respiratory

a. Hyperventilation syndrome

(1) Panting occurs with tension and excitement and this forced respiration can produce a decrease CO_2 resulting in giddiness, dizziness, syncope, convulsions, or coma

(2) Other factors that may overstimulate the respiratory center include CNS lesions, trauma, fever, exercise, extreme emotional stress, and severe pain

b. Asthma

(1) Stress and tension appear to create increased secretions and airway spasms

(2) Other precipitating factors are changes in environmental temperature, strong odors, stress, emotion, exercise, and exposure to allergens

(3) It is believed that individuals with asthma tend to exhibit a strong desire for protection and dependency yet fear rejection or engulfment

4. Gastrointestinal

a. Eating disorders

(1) Maladaptive eating disorders include anorexia nervosa, bulimia, and binge eating disorders

(2) Biologic, psychologic, and sociocultural factors are all involved in the regulation and control of food intake

b. Peptic ulcer

(1) Previously thought to be related to stresses in life, particularly those concerned with conflicts between passivity and aggression

(2) Found to be associated with *H. pylori* infections

c. Ulcerative colitis

(1) Parasympathetic stimulation of the lower bowel produces an enzyme that interferes with the protective coating of the mucosa and submucosa

(2) May occur as a reaction to a variety of stresses but most often in situations that demand accomplishment and arouse fear of not succeeding

5. Skin—neurodermatitis, psychic factors appear to dominate dermatitis factitia, pruritus, and psoriasis

a. Excitability and arousal of the CNS due to an emotional upset can intensify the vasomotor and sweat responses in the skin

b. This intensification leads to the itch-scratch cycle

6. Genitourinary—impotence, frigidity, and premenstrual syndrome may occur under stress; any experience that an individual interprets as stressful may lead to a psychophysiologic response

a. The etiology of the problem must be determined

b. Assess for environmental and occupational agents and pharmacologic agents

H. Therapy: must be directed toward both the physical and emotional problems

General Nursing Care of Clients with Physical Conditions Related to Psychogenic Factors

A. Reduce emotional stressors when possible

B. Explain all procedures carefully and allow client time for questions

C. Provide the client with talking time

D. Avoid conversational topics that appear to stimulate conflict for the client

E. Anticipate a variety of coping mechanisms such as repression, denial, regression, and compensation

F. Interventions include psychologic approaches, client education, and physiologic support

G. The expected outcome of nursing care is that the individual will express feelings verbally rather than through the development of physical symptoms

NURSING IN PSYCHIATRY

BASIC PRINCIPLES OF PSYCHIATRIC NURSING

A. These principles:

1. Are by necessity general in nature

2. Form the guidelines for the emotional care of all clients and the prevention of emotional disequilibrium

B. When caring for clients, the nurse should attempt to:

1. Accept and respect people as individuals and strive to separate the person from the abhorrent behavior

2. Limit or reject inappropriate behavior without rejecting the individual
3. Recognize that all behavior has meaning and is meeting the needs of the performer regardless of how distorted or meaningless it appears to others
4. Accept the dependency needs of individuals while supporting and encouraging moves toward independence; build on ego strengths
5. Help individuals set appropriate limits for themselves or set limits for them when they are unable to do so
6. Encourage individuals to express their feelings in an atmosphere free of reprisal or judgment
7. Recognize that individuals need to use their defenses until other defenses can be substituted
8. Recognize how feelings affect behavior and influence relationships
9. Recognize that individuals frequently respond to the behavioral expectations of others: family, peers, authority (staff)
10. Recognize that all individuals have a potential for movement toward higher levels of emotional health

THERAPEUTIC NURSE-CLIENT RELATIONSHIPS

A. Phases
1. Preinteraction: this phase begins before the nurse's initial contact with client
   a. Self-exploration regarding misconceptions and prejudices of the general public and acknowledging one's own feelings, fears, personal values, and attitudes should occur before contact; self-awareness is a necessary task before one can establish mutuality with others.
   b. Additional tasks of this phase include gathering data about the client, and planning for the first interaction with the client
2. Orientation or introductory: the nurse, who initially is in the role of stranger, establishes a trust relationship that the client tests by discussing only what he or she wishes to discuss; clients are never pushed to discuss areas of concern that are upsetting to them
   a. Introduction of nurse, educational background, and purpose of meeting need to be clarified
   b. Contract outlining mutually agreed on goals should be set
   c. Confidentiality issues must be discussed and patient rights must be upheld
   d. Termination begins during the orientation phase

3. Working: the nurse and the client discuss areas of concern and the client is helped to plan, implement, and evaluate a course of action
   a. Transference and countertransference may become an issue
   b. Anxiety levels may rise, acting out behaviors can and does occur, and denying is expected
   c. Problems should be discussed and resolved
   d. New adaptive behaviors can be learned
4. Termination: the end of the therapeutic relationship between the nurse and the client; the time parameters should be set within the first or second session; meetings spaced farther and farther apart near the end will facilitate termination
   a. Goals and objectives achieved should be summarized
   b. Adaptive behaviors should be reinforced
   c. Feelings and experiences for both client and nurse should be shared
   d. Rejection, anger, regression, or other negative behaviors may be expressed as a means of handling the loss (relationship termination)
   e. Plans for help in future and a list of agency resources should be provided
B. Themes of communication: recurring thoughts and ideas that give insight into what an individual is feeling and tie the communication together
   1. Content: conversation may appear superficial but careful attention to the underlying theme helps the nurse identify problem areas while providing insight into the client's self-concept
   2. Mood: emotion or affect that the client communicates to the nurse; includes personal appearance, facial expressions, and gestures that reflect the client's mood and feelings
   3. Interaction: how the client reacts or interacts with the nurse; includes how the client relates and what role he or she assumes when communicating with the nurse and others
C. Fundamental requirements of a therapeutic relationship
   1. Ability to communicate therapeutically requires a basic understanding and use of interviewing techniques in developing a trusting relationship through:
      a. Open-ended rather than probing questions
      b. Reflection of words and feelings and paraphrasing
      c. Acceptance of the client's behavior
      d. Nonjudgmental, objective attitude
      e. Focusing on the emotional needs of the client
      f. Having a therapeutic goal for the interview
   2. Recognition that an individual has potential for growth

a. Individuals need to learn about their own behavior in relation to others

b. Exchanging experiences with others provides a new learning environment and the reassurance that reactions are valid and feelings shared

c. Participating with groups increases knowledge of interpersonal relationships and helps individuals to identify strengths and resources

d. The identification of the individual's strengths and resources helps to convey the expectation of growth

3. Recognition that an individual needs to be accepted

a. Acceptance is an active process designed to convey respect for another through empathetic understanding

b. Acceptance of others implies and requires acceptance of self

c. To be nonjudgmental, one must become aware of one's own attitudes and feelings and their effect on perception

d. Acceptance requires that individuals be permitted and even encouraged to express their feelings and attitudes even though they may be divergent from the general viewpoint
   (1) Individuals should be encouraged to express both positive and negative feelings
   (2) This encouragement must occur on both the verbal and nonverbal level

e. Acceptance means showing interest in another person; interest requires:
   (1) Face-to-face contact and careful listening to what the person has to say
   (2) Developing an awareness of the other person's likes and dislikes
   (3) Attempting to understand another's point of view
   (4) Using nonverbal as well as verbal expressions of acceptance

f. Acceptance requires the development of interpersonal techniques that encourage others to express problems; the listener's:
   (1) Reflection of feelings, attitudes, and words help the speaker to identify feelings
   (2) Open-ended questions permit the speaker to focus on problems
   (3) Paraphrasing assists the speaker in clarifying statements
   (4) Use of silence provides both the listener and the speaker with the necessary time for thinking over what is being discussed

g. Acceptance requires the recognition of factors that block communication, such as:

   (1) Any overt/covert response that conveys a judgmental or superior attitude
   (2) Direct questions that convey an invasive or probing attitude
   (3) Ridicule that conveys a hostile attitude
   (4) Talking about one's own problems and not listening, which conveys a self-serving attitude and loss of interest in the speaker

D. Recognition of behavioral changes that result from physical illness

1. Anxiety, fear, and depression occur whenever there is a major health problem

a. Body image and feelings of being in control of one's body have their basis in early development; struggle to maintain independence continues

b. Anxiety develops whenever a real or imagined threat to the body image occurs

2. Signs of the anxiety, fear, and depression associated with illness are variable and include:

a. Indifference to symptoms: usually related to failure to accept the occurrence of a health problem

b. Denial of reality: usually related to attempts to maintain stability and integrity of the personality

c. Reaction formation: usually related to attempts to block the reality from consciousness and acting as if nothing is wrong

d. Failure to keep appointments and noncompliant with treatment plan: usually related to fear of finding additional problems or admitting there is something wrong

e. Overconcern with body functions and symptoms: usually related to fear of death

f. Asking many questions and offering many complaints: usually related to attempts to keep a staff member by the bedside because of fears associated with illness; fear of abandonment

g. Constantly ventilating feelings

3. Emotional needs of the ill person include:

a. Security of continuous relationships with friends and family members

b. Some control to achieve feelings of self-worth and self-esteem

c. Assistance in accepting the dependent role

d. Self-protection, disbelief, denial, avoidance and/or intellectualization; with developing awareness of the implications of illness the individual defends the self further by use of anger, depression, and/or joking

e. Assistance in resolving conflicts while maintaining security

f. Assistance in refocusing inner resources

g. Contact with the reality of the external world
4. To help the individual maintain the self-concept during illness, the nurse must understand the normal emotional stages of illness
   a. Denial: individuals cannot believe it is happening and seek other opinions to collaborate their feelings
   b. Anger: something has happened that one cannot control
   c. Bargaining: promising to be a better person or behave differently if given another chance
   d. Depression: one grieves for loss or expected loss
   e. Realization: with developing realization of implications of illness, the individual reorganizes self-feelings and restructures relationships with family and society
   f. Resolution: the individual begins to accept the consequences of the illness and acknowledges feelings about self and further changes that must be made
   g. Acceptance and adaptation to the illness: this stage can only be reached when the individual has resolved the conflicts that developed during the earlier stages
5. Common reactions occur to the change in body image associated with many health problems
   a. Attitudes toward one's body and self-concept greatly influence response
   b. Fear is a universal response; individual may focus on fear of: death; pain; incapacitation; disfigurement; altered self-concept; rejection of loved ones
   c. Questioning is a universal response; the individual may focus on: "This cannot be happening to me"; "Is this really happening to me?"; "What did I do to deserve this?"; "Why am I being punished?"
   d. Grief and mourning are universal responses; the individual may focus on: what was in the past; what could have been in the future; missed opportunities; a magnified view of the loss; avoiding interpersonal contacts
6. Extent of actual or perceived change in body image
   a. Obvious reminder of disability to self and others; loss of body part or altered function; need for a prosthesis (e.g., breast, leg, or eye); need for hardware (e.g., pacemaker, hearing aid, or wheelchair); extent of disability or limitation; need for medication
   b. Value placed on loss by self or society
   c. Image as "no longer whole" or "different"
   d. Type of loss: perception of body part, function, or disease as being good, pleasing, clean, or repulsive or dirty
      (1) Symbols of sexuality; breast, uterus, prostate, heart
      (2) May lack social acceptability; colostomy or mental illness, incontinence, cancer, tuberculosis, AIDS, or drug abuse
      (3) Impairment of senses and/or ability to communicate; laryngectomy, aphasia, deafness, or blindness
      (4) Altered body image resulting from anatomic changes; amputation of body parts
7. Caring for a dying client involves caring for the body, mind, and spirit; acceptance of death by the client may result in gradual detachment from the environment
   a. First an understanding and acceptance of the nurse's own feelings, beliefs, and fear about death are essential; as well as recognition of the client's behavior associated with the stages of death and dying (denial and shock, anger, bargaining, depression, and acceptance)
   b. The nurse must help the family understand the client's feelings as well as assisting him or her to recognize the client's behavior associated with the stages
   c. The last stages of life should be viewed as a positive rather than negative achievement; the nurse can provide acceptance by being available to the client and family

 # RELATED PHARMACOLOGY

PSYCHOTROPIC MEDICATIONS

A. Chemicals that produce profound effects on the mind, emotions, and body
B. Within one decade (1950s) three major classes of psychotropic drugs—antimanic, antipsychotic, and antidepressant—were developed
C. These compounds significantly advanced the treatment of bipolar illness, psychosis, and depression
D. The decrease in state hospital census has been attributed to the introduction of psychotropic drugs
E. Include antianxiety or anxiolytic agents; antipsychotic or neuroleptic agents; antidepressants, antimanic, and mood-stabilizing agents; and sedative and hypnotic agents
F. The safety of psychotropic drugs during pregnancy is of concern; consult with psychiatrist and pharmacist before administration

Antianxiety or Anxiolytic Medications
Description
A. Used for the treatment of anxiety and also useful in the induction of sleep

B. Exert a general depressing effect on the CNS, many also exert skeletal muscle-relaxant and anticonvulsant effects
C. Anxiolytics are available in oral and parenteral (IM, IV) preparations
D. Used when the individual has difficulty in coping with environmental stresses and accomplishing daily activities
E. Benzodiazepines enhance the GABA activity (the primary inhibitory neurotransmitter in the brain) resulting in further opening of the chloride ion channel and a further inhibition of neuronal activity; (a decrease in the firing rate of neutrons results in lowering of anxiety)

Types
A. Benzodiazepines
  1. Alprazolam (Xanax)
  2. Clonazepam (Klonopin)
  3. Chlordiazepoxide (Librium)
  4. Clorazepate (Tranxene)
  5. Diazepam (Valium)
  6. Flurazepam (Dalmane)
  7. Halazepam (Paxipam)
  8. Lorazepam (Ativan)
  9. Oxazepam (Serax)
  10. Quazepam (Doral)
  11. Temazepam (Restoril)
  12. Triazolam (Halcion)
  13. Prazepam (Centrax)
B. Nonbarbituate, nonbenzodiazepine
  1. Chloral hydrate (Noctec)
  2. Ethchlorvynol (Placydyl)
  3. Diphenhydramine (Benadryl)
  4. Doxylamine (Unisom)
  5. Hydroxyzine (Atarax, Vistaril)
  6. Zolpidem (Ambien)
  7. Buspirone (Buspar)
C. Antidepressants indicated for anxiety
  1. Clomipramine (Anafranil)
  2. Fluvoxamine (Luvox)
  3. Paroxetine (Paxil)
  4. Sertraline (Zoloft)
  5. Venlafaxine (Effexor XR)
  6. Fluoxetine (Prozac)

Precautions
A. Drug interactions: drugs potentiate depressant effects of alcohol or sedatives
B. Tolerance to the sedative and hypnotic effects develops eventually with all these drugs, although it develops more slowly with the benzodiazepines than other drugs
C. All of these drugs, if taken in large enough doses or for extended time periods, can lead to physical and emotional dependence
D. Tolerance can contribute to self-medication and dosage escalation

E. Adverse side effects are related to diminished mental alertness; caution about driving or operating hazardous machinery until tolerance develops
F. A drop in BP of 20 mm Hg (systolic) on standing warrants withholding the drug and notifying the physician
G. Benzodiazepine use should not be abruptly discontinued to avoid a withdrawal syndrome
H. Physical withdrawal symptoms can occur any time these drugs are taken continuously for more than 2 weeks; signs and symptoms closely resemble the original sleep or anxiety complaints
I. Clients treated with Buspar need education regarding the antianxiety effects not apparent for 3 to 6 weeks; this is a longer lag time than other drugs in this category; caffeine can worsen symptoms of anxiety; it is thought to interfere with medications used to treat these disorders

Nursing Care of Clients Receiving Antianxiety or Anxiolytic Medications

A. Assess the client's medication history, knowledge level and use of current medications (prescribed, over-the-counter, and illicit drugs), medication allergies, and pattern of alcohol, tobacco, and herbal use because all may interfere with anxiolytics
B. Explore the client's perceptions and feelings about medications; clarify misinformation, fears, etc.
C. Review psychotropic drug references for current information
D. Plan for client education regarding benzodiazepines should include:
  1. Over-the-counter drugs may increase potency
  2. Until tolerance develops driving or working with machinery should be avoided
  3. CNS depressants and alcohol potentiate effects
  4. Drug should not be discontinued abruptly
  5. If prior assessment reveals use of herbal or related products (St. John's wort, kava, ginseng, etc.) consult with psychiatrist and pharmacist
E. Monitor the effects of medication (effects on target symptoms, side effects, and adverse reactions)
F. Administer medications as prescribed
G. Teach the client about the medication; desired effect; side effects, food, herbal, and activity restrictions; and lag period between onset of treatment and symptom remission
H. Supplement verbal teaching with appropriate written or audiovisual materials
I. Administer controlled substances according to schedule restrictions
J. Evaluate client's response to medications and understanding of teaching

Neuroleptics (Antipsychotic Agents)
Description
A. Used to treat psychotic symptoms; that is, symptoms of being out of touch with reality; makes client more amenable to therapy
B. Act by blocking dopamine receptors in the CNS; they can also block the muscarinic receptors for acetylcholine and the alpha receptors for norepinephrine
   1. Positive symptoms of schizophrenia respond to traditional antipsychotic drugs
   2. Negative symptoms of schizophrenia are more responsive to the newer atypical antipsychotic drugs
C. Available in oral and parenteral (IM, IV) preparations
D. Effective in treating symptoms of psychosis noted in schizophrenia, schizophreniform disorder, schizoaffective disorder and delusional disorder
E. Action of drug is to diminish psychotic symptoms (hallucinations, delusions, and grossly disorganized speech and behavior)
F. May be prescribed in conjunction with benzodiazepines, which is thought to minimize the dose of neuroleptics and diminish the potential for tardive dyskinesia
G. Antipsychotic effects usually occur within 1 to 2 weeks after initiating treatment

Types
A. Traditional drugs—Phenothiazines
   1. Aliphatics: Chlorpromazine (Thorazine)
   2. Piperidines: mesoridazine (Serentil); thioridazine (Mellaril)
   3. Piperazines
      a. Fluphenazine (Prolixin, Permitil)
      b. Perphenazine (Trilafon)
      c. Prochlorperazine (Compazine)
      d. Trifluoperazine (Stelazine)
B. Butyrophenones: droperidol (Inapsine); haloperidol (Haldol)
C. Thioxanthenes: chlorprothixene (Taractan); thiothixene (Navane)
D. Dibenzoxapine: loxapine (Loxitane)
E. Dihydroindolone: molindone (Moban)
F. Diphenylbutylpiperidine: pimozide (Orap)
G. Atypical drugs
   1. Dibenzodiazepine: clozapine (Clozaril); quetiapine (Seroquel)
   2. Benzisoxazole: risperidone (Risperdal); ziprasidone (Zeldox)
   3. Thienobenzodiazepine: olanzapine (Zyprexa)

Precautions
A. Drug interactions: potentiate the action of alcohol, barbiturates, antihypertensives, and anticholinergics; concomitant use should be avoided if possible; antipsychotic medications should be temporarily discontinued when spinal or epidural anesthesia is necessary
B. Adverse effects: agranulocytosis (manifested by cold or sore throat), jaundice (hepatotoxicity), signs of extrapyramidal tract irritation, drowsiness (highest incidence in initial days of therapy because of CNS depression), orthostatic hypotension (CNS depression), constipation and urinary retention (anticholinergic effects), anorexia (depressed appetite center), hypersensitivity reactions (tissue fluid accumulation, photoallergic reaction, impotence, cessation of menses or ovulation), cardiac toxicity (direct toxic effect); notify physician and withhold the medication if any adverse effects are noted
   1. Extrapyramidal side effects (EPS)
      a. Dystonia: occurs early in treatment, possibly after initial dosage; involves grimacing, torticollis, intermittent muscle spasms
      b. Pseudoparkinsonism: resembles true Parkinsonism (tremor, masklike facies, drooling, restlessness, festinating gait, rigidity)
      c. Akathisia: motor agitation (restless legs, "jitters," nervous energy); most common of all EPS
      d. Akinesia: fatigue, weakness (hypotonia), painful muscles, anergy (lack of energy)
      e. Tardive dyskinesia: late appearing after prolonged use of antipsychotic drugs; not related to dopamine-acetylcholine imbalance; most severe effect characterized by involuntary movements of face, jaw, and tongue; lipsmacking, grinding of teeth, rolling or protrusion of tongue, tics, diaphragmatic movements that may impair breathing; condition disappears during sleep; antiparkinsonian drugs ineffective and condition is usually irreversible; all antipsychotics stopped to see if symptoms subside
      f. Neuroleptic malignant syndrome: infrequent yet extreme condition occurring in severely ill clients and is believed to be the result of dopamine blockage in the hypothalamus; associated with high-potency antipsychotic drugs, especially when given in a large loading dose; symptoms are hyperthermia (cardinal symptom), muscular rigidity, tremors, impaired ventilation, muteness, altered consciousness, unstable blood pressure, and autonomic hyperactivity
   2. Antiparkinsonian drugs: block the extrapyramidal symptoms
      a. Anticholinergics: benztropine (Cogentin); trihexyphenidyl (Artane); procyclidine (Kemadrin); biperiden (Akineton)
      b. Antihistamine; diphenhydramine (Benadryl)

c. Others
   (1) Amantadine (Symmetrel)
   (2) Benzodiazepines (Lorazepam, Diazepam, Clonazepam), useful for akinesia and akathisia
   (3) Propranolol (Inderal), useful for treatment of EPS
   (4) Clonidine (Catapres), useful for treatment of EPS
   (5) Nifedipine (Procardia), useful for treatment of tardive dyskinesia
   (6) Verapamil (Calan), useful for treatment of tardive dyskinesia
   (7) Bromocriptine (Parlodel), useful for treatment of neuroleptic malignant syndrome
   (8) Amantadine (Symmetrel), useful for treatment of neuroleptic malignant syndrome
   (9) Ethopropazine, useful for the treatment of acute dystonic reactions

Nursing Care of Clients Receiving Antipsychotic Agents

A. Monitor for signs of hepatic toxicity (e.g., jaundice)
B. Monitor for signs of infection (e.g., sore throat)
C. Monitor blood pressure in standing and supine positions
   1. Assist client to get out of bed slowly (dangle feet before ambulating)
   2. Assess for hypotension and tachycardia (which is usually a reflex response to hypotension)
   3. If hypotension occurs, monitor by measuring BP before each dose is given
   4. Consult physician as to safe BP systolic/diastolic parameters for each client
D. Offer sugar-free chewing gum or hard candy to increase salivation and relieve dry mouth
E. Assist with ambulation as necessary; keep siderails up when nonambulatory
F. Assess for extrapyramidal symptoms (antiparkinsonism agent may be prescribed to decrease symptoms)
G. Monitor blood work during long-term therapy (periodic CBC, chemistry analysis; weekly WBC if administering Clozapine)
H. Monitor dietary intake to avoid weight loss resulting from caloric expenditure caused by extrapyramidal symptoms
I. Instruct client to:
   1. Avoid administration with other CNS depressants, including concurrent use of alcohol
   2. Avoid engaging in potentially hazardous activities
   3. Avoid exposure to direct sunlight; wear protective clothing and sunglasses outdoors
   4. Recognize extrapyramidal symptoms and report their occurrence to the physician immediately
   5. Avoid changing positions rapidly
   6. Notify physician if sore throat, fever, or weakness occurs; avoid crowded, potentially infectious places
   7. Increase water intake and eat high-fiber diet to avoid constipation
   8. Expect weight gain (diet pills should not be taken); control weight with appropriate diet
   9. Avoid mixing neuroleptics with certain juices or liquids (coffee, tea, or cola beverages may decrease effectiveness of drug)
   10. Avoid antacids or take 1 to 2 hours after antipsychotic drug is taken (antacids decrease absorption of antipsychotics)
   11. Avoid smoking because it decreases serum levels of antipsychotics
J. Use precautions to avoid drug contact with skin; can cause contact dermatitis
K. Recognize that drug noncompliance is common; consult physician about use of longer-acting drugs such as Prolixin
L. Evaluate client's response to medication and understanding of teaching

Antidepressants
Description
A. The primary clinical indication for use of antidepressant drugs is major depressive illness; also used in the treatment of panic disorder, narcolepsy, and in attention deficit disorders and enuresis in children
B. Selective serotonin reuptake inhibitors, with their low side effect profile, are being used to treat eating disorders and obsessive-compulsive disorder
C. Antidepressant drugs affect the neurotransmitters norepinephrine (NE) and/or serotonin (SR) by partially blocking their reuptake; roles for other neurotransmitters are unclear and under study
D. Available in oral and parenteral (IM) preparations
E. Psychopharmacologic treatment is based on the restoration of normal levels of neurotransmitter systems by blocking the uptake in the presynaptic nerve ending, inhibiting breakdown, stimulating the release, and reducing stimulation at the site of the postsynaptic beta receptors (i.e., downregulation)
F. All antidepressant drugs must be taken for 3 to 4 weeks before therapeutic response occurs
G. Monoamine oxidase inhibitors (MAOIs) elevate norepinephrine levels in brain tissues by interfering with the enzyme MAO; act as psychic energizers

Types
A. Tricyclic drugs (TCAs) or nonselective cyclic
   1. Amitriptyline (Elavil, Endep)

2. Clomipramine (Anafranil)
3. Desipramine (Norpramin)
4. Doxepin (Sinequan, Triadapin)
5. Imipramine (Tofranil)
6. Maprotiline (Ludiomil)
7. Nortriptyline (Aventyl, Pamelor)
8. Protriptyline (Vivactil, Triptal)
9. Trimipramine (Surmontil)
B. Monoamine oxidase inhibitors (MAOIs): isocarbox-azid (Marplan); phenelzine sulfate (Nardil); tranyl-cypromine sulfate (Parnate); selegiline (Eldepryl)
C. Selective serotonin reuptake inhibitors (SSRIs): fluoxetine (Prozac daily or weekly); fluvoxamine (Luvox); paroxetine (Paxil); sertraline (Zoloft); citalopram (Celexa)
D. Atypical new generation drugs
  1. Bupropion (Wellbutrin)
  2. Bupropion SR (Wellbutrin SR, Zyban)
  3. Venlafaxine (Effexor)
  4. Venlafaxine XR (Effexor XR)
  5. Nefazodone (Serzone)
  6. Trazodone (Desyrel)
  7. Mirtazapine (Remeron)

Precautions
A. Tricyclic antidepressants (TCAs)
  1. Drug interactions: potentiate effects of anti-cholinergic drugs and CNS depressants (e.g., alcohol and sedatives)
  2. Adverse effects: orthostatic hypotension, skin rash, drowsiness, dry mouth, blurred vision, constipation, urine retention, tachycardia, CNS stimulation in elderly clients (excitement, restlessness, incoordination, fine tremor, nightmares, delusions, disorientation, insomnia)
  3. TCAs should not be given to clients with narrow-angle glaucoma
  4. TCAs are contraindicated during recovery phase of myocardial infarction or when client's history indicates cardiac dysrhythmias and cardiac conduction defects
  5. There should be a minimum of 14 days between switching the TCA-resistant client to MAOIs to avoid hypertensive crisis
  6. Abrupt discontinuation of TCAs can cause nausea, headache, and malaise
B. Monoamine oxidase inhibitors (MAOIs)
  1. Drug interactions: MAOIs potentiate the effects of alcohol, barbiturates, anesthetic agents (cocaine), antihistamines, narcotics, corticoids, anticholinergics, and sympathomimetic drugs
  2. Drug-food interactions: hypertensive crisis with vascular rupture, occipital headache, palpitations, stiffness of neck muscles, emesis, sweating, photophobia, and cardiac dysrhythmias may occur when neurohormonal levels are elevated by ingestion of foods with high tyramine content (pickled herring, beer, wine, chicken livers, aged or natural cheese, chocolate, caffeine, cola, licorice, avocados, bananas, and bologna)
  3. Adverse effects: orthostatic hypotension (CNS effect); skin rash (hypersensitivity); drowsiness (CNS depression); dry mouth, blurred vision, urinary retention, tachycardia (anticholinergic effect); sexual dysfunction (autonomic effect); nightmares, delusions, disorientation, insomnia (CNS stimulation)
C. Selective serotonin reuptake inhibitors (SSRIs)
  1. Usually these drugs are administered before noon to avoid insomnia or sleep disturbances
  2. Drug interactions: may interact with tryptophan; question concomitant use of diazepam, warfarin, and digoxin; should be discontinued 4 to 6 weeks before switching to MAOIs
  3. Adverse effects: insomnia, headache, dry mouth, sexual dysfunction, anxiety, diarrhea and other gastrointestinal complaints
D. Atypical new generation drugs
  1. Mild anticholinergic side effects noted
  2. Adverse effects: increased appetite, weight gain, and sleep disturbances
  3. Bupropion (Wellbutrin) is thought to affect dopamine reuptake and agitation is sometimes produced

Nursing Care of Clients Receiving Antidepressants

A. Assess for effectiveness of drug action
B. Maintain suicide precautions, especially as depression begins to lift; carefully monitor serum glucose in diabetics
C. Instruct client to:
  1. Change positions slowly
  2. Avoid engaging in hazardous activities
  3. Utilize sugar-free chewing gum or hard candy to stimulate salivation
  4. Check with physician before taking all OTC preparations, alcohol, and cough or herbal medicines (St. John's wort)
  5. Expect therapeutic effect to be delayed; may take less than 3 weeks with MAOIs and 3 to 4 weeks with other antidepressants
D. MAOIs
  1. Maintain dietary restrictions; avoid foods containing tyramine; provide for nutritional education
  2. Monitor client for occurrence of hypertensive crisis (occipital headache, palpitations, and stiff neck)
E. Avoid concurrent administration of adrenergic drugs; limit or eliminate caffeine use to prevent exacerbation of depression

F. Monitor for self-destructive behavior, particularly during the second week of drug therapy when suicidal ideation remains and energy increases
G. Evaluate client's response to medication and understanding of teaching
H. Recommend Prozac weekly capsule (90 mg) to treat noncompliant clients

Antimanic and Mood-Stabilizing Agents

Description
A. Used to control the manic episode of mood disorders and for maintenance in clients with a history of mania
B. Lithium affects the neurotransmitters of multiple systems including dopamine, norepinephrine, serotonin, acetylcholine, and GABA
C. Antimanic agents are available in oral capsules and tablets, both regular and sustained-release forms, and in concentrates
D. Improves productivity by decreasing psychomotor activity or response to environmental stimuli

Types
A. Antimanic agents and mood stabilizers
  1. Lithium carbonate (Eskalith, Lithotabs, Lithane, Lithonate)
  2. Lithium carbonate sustained release (Eskalith C-R, Lithobid)
  3. Lithium citrate concentrate (Cibalith-S)
B. Alternative antimanic agents and mood stabilizers
  1. Carbamazepine (Tegretol)
  2. Valproate (Depakene, Depakote)

Precautions
A. Drug interactions: diuretics increase the reabsorption of lithium resulting in possible toxic effects; haloperidol and thioridazine when given with these drugs can result in encephalopathic syndrome; sodium bicarbonate or sodium chloride increase the excretion of lithium
B. Drug-food interaction: restriction of sodium intake increases drug substitution for sodium ions, which causes signs of hyponatremia (nausea, vomiting, diarrhea, muscle fasciculations, stupor, seizures); therefore salt intake must be maintained; daily intake of over 250 mg of caffeine, as well as lithium, decreases effect of antianxiety drugs
C. Adverse effects: excess voiding and extreme thirst caused by drug suppression of antidiuretic hormone (ADH) function, which causes dehydration; slurred speech, disorientation, confusion, cogwheel rigidity, ataxia, renal failure, respiratory depression, and coma are toxic side effects; toxic effects can easily occur because the difference between the therapeutic level and toxic level is slight
D. One to two weeks of treatment will be necessary to achieve a clinical response; antipsychotic agents or benzodiazepines may be used in combination with lithium to control manic symptoms

Nursing Care of Clients Receiving Antimanic and Mood-Stabilizing Agents
A. Recognize that therapeutic effects will be delayed for several weeks
B. Recognize that dehydration and hyponatremia predispose to lithium toxicity
C. Assess therapeutic blood levels (0.6 to 1.2 mEq/L) during course of therapy; levels above 2.0 mEq/L show significant toxicity
D. Recognize that lithium is the drug of choice, but other agents such as carbamazepine or valproate may be used to treat acute mania
E. Avoid concurrent administration of adrenergic drugs
F. Maintain normal sodium intake during course of therapy
G. Encourage increased fluid intake; limit amount of caffeine
H. Supervise ambulation if necessary
I. Administer with meals to reduce GI irritation
J. Teach the client that the nausea, polyuria, and thirst that occur initially will subside after several days
K. Teach client and family to observe for signs of toxicity (diarrhea, vomiting, drowsiness, muscular weakness, ataxia, confusion, and tonic-clonic seizures)
L. Evaluate client's response to medication and understanding of teaching
M. Maintenance lithium regimen
  1. Monitor serum blood levels weekly for first month; then at 3- to 6-month intervals; reassess renal status and lithium level q6 months
  2. Yearly, reassess thyroid function and ECG; more often if symptoms are noted
N. Monitor dietary intake (provide finger foods, snacks, and liquid supplements)
O. Refer pregnant woman to health care provider; cessation of lithium during pregnancy is recommended to avoid teratogenic effects during first trimester
P. Evaluate client's response to medication and understanding of teaching

Sedative and Hypnotic Agents

Description
A. Benzodiazepines have almost entirely replaced the barbiturates in the treatment of anxiety and sleep disorders; sedative and hypnotic agents are primarily used in general medicine rather than psychiatry
B. Insomnia and hypersomnia, narcolepsy, and parasomnias, periodic leg movements (nocturnal myoclonus), and sleep apnea are among the disorders that are responsive to these agents
C. Specific psychiatric conditions do predispose clients to insomnia (mood disorders, anxiety, and dementias)

D. Central nervous system depressants have anti-anxiety effects in low dosages, produce sleep in high dosages, and general anesthetic-like states in very high dosages

E. All hypnotic drugs probably alter either the character or the duration of REM sleep

F. Sedatives reduce nervousness, excitability, and irritability without causing sleep, but a sedative can become a hypnotic in large doses

G. Hypnotics cause sleep and have a more potent effect on the CNS than sedatives

H. Sedative-hypnotics are classified chemically into three groups: barbiturates, benzodiazepines, and nonbenzodiazepines

Types
A. Benzodiazepines: see antianxiety agents
B. Barbiturates: amobarbital (Amytal); butabarbital (Butisol); pentobarbital (Nembutal); phenobarbital (Luminal); secobarbital (Seconal)
C. Antidepressant: trazodone (Desyrel)
D. Acetylenic alcohols: ethchlorvynol (Placidyl)
E. Piperidinediones: glutethimide (Doriden); methyprylon (Noludar)
F. Chloral derivative: chloral hydrate (Noctec)
G. Antihistamines: diphenhydramine (Benadryl); hydroxyzine (Atarax)
H. Beta-adrenergic blocker: propranolol (Inderal)
I. Anxiolytic: buspirone (Buspar)
J. Nonbenzodiazepine hypnotics: zolpidem (Ambien); zaleplon (Sonata)

Precautions
A. Sedative-hypnotic preparations are generally intended for either occasional or short-term use
B. Hypnotic drugs have undesirable effects (physiologic addiction, fatal overdose potential, and dangerous interactions with other drugs)
C. Barbiturate sedatives also speed up the metabolism of anticoagulants because they induce liver enzyme synthesis
D. Buspirone appears to be a potent antianxiety agent with no addictive potential; it is not effective in the management of drug or alcohol abuse
E. Chloral hydrate and paraldehyde are not used for treatment of alcohol withdrawal because of toxic effects; paraldehyde is sometimes used for treating status epilepticus when other drugs have failed
F. The sedative-hypnotics are CNS depressants
G. Tolerance develops to sedative and hypnotic agents; therefore, the client in the outpatient setting may resort to increasing doses to produce the desired effect
H. If taken in large dosages or for a long time period, physical and emotional dependence occurs
I. Once physical dependence has developed, abrupt discontinuation of sedative-hypnotics leads to withdrawal

1. Withdrawal characteristics: insomnia, weakness, muscle tremors, anxiety, irritability, sweating, anorexia, fever, nausea and vomiting, headache, incoordination, and restlessness
2. After a few more days, severe symptoms of withdrawal may develop: postural hypotension, tinnitus, incoherence, delirium, psychosis, seizures, status epilepticus, cardiovascular collapse, loss of temperature regulation, and/or death

J. To avoid withdrawal, it is important to slowly and gradually taper the dose with the same drug or one that is cross-tolerant
K. Excess ingestion
1. Any of the sedative-hypnotics may cause unconsciousness, coma, and death
2. Addiction to these drugs alone or in combination has increased
3. Removal of the drug from the stomach by aspiration, resuscitative measures (assisted ventilation, cardiac massage), hemodialysis of diffusible drug, vasopressor administration to counteract vascular collapse, and correction of acidosis
4. Follow-up drug supervision to avoid repetition of the problem
5. Initiate psychotherapy for depressed clients
L. Refer to antianxiety agent precautions for additional information

Nursing Care of Clients Receiving Sedative-Hypnotics
A. Assess for history of drug or alcohol abuse or suicide attempts by overdose because of the increased risk of abuse
B. Assess for pregnancy and breastfeeding, as safe use has not been established
C. Explore the client's perceptions and feelings about medications; clarify any misinformation, fears, etc.
D. Review drug reference for current information about specific sedative-hypnotic
E. Plan for client teaching about specific sedative-hypnotic agent; institute safety precautions
F. Administer medication and monitor the response
G. Assess for undesired effects (respiratory depression, increased sedation, and hypotension)
H. Teach the client about the agent and its correct use
I. Supplement verbal teaching with appropriate written or audiovisual materials
J. Administer controlled substances according to schedule restrictions
K. Evaluate client's response to medication and understanding of teaching
L. Refer to nursing care of clients receiving antianxiety agents

CLASSIFICATION OF MENTAL DISORDERS*

A. Disorders usually first diagnosed in infancy, childhood, or adolescence
   1. Mental retardation
   2. Learning disorders
   3. Motor skills disorders
   4. Communication disorders
   5. Pervasive developmental disorders
   6. Attention-deficit and disruptive behavior disorders
   7. Feeding and eating disorders (infancy or early childhood)
   8. Tic disorders
   9. Elimination disorders
   10. Others disorders
B. Delirium, dementia, and amnestic and other cognitive disorders
   1. Delirium
   2. Dementia
   3. Amnestic disorders
C. Mental disorders resulting from a general medical condition
D. Substance-related disorders
   Types: alcohol, amphetamine, caffeine, cannabis, cocaine, hallucinogen, inhalant, nicotine, opioid, phencyclidine, sedative, hypnotic, or anxiolytics and polysubstances
      a. Substance-use disorders are concerned with substance dependence and abuse
      b. Substance-induced disorders are concerned with mental disorders resulting in intoxications; withdrawal; delirium; hallucinations; and delusional, sleep, and sexual disorders
E. Schizophrenia and other psychotic disorders
F. Mood disorders
   1. Depressive disorders
   2. Bipolar disorders
G. Anxiety disorders
H. Somatoform disorders
I. Factitious disorders
J. Dissociative disorders
K. Sexual and gender identity disorders
L. Eating disorders
   1. Anorexia nervosa
   2. Bulimia nervosa
M. Adjustment disorders
N. Personaltiy disorders
O. Sleep disorders

Adapted from *Diagnostic and statistical manual of mental disorders* (test revision), ed 4, Washington, DC, 2000, American Psychiatric Association.

DISORDERS USUALLY FIRST EVIDENT IN INFANCY, CHILDHOOD, OR ADOLESCENCE

FUNDAMENTAL PRINCIPLES WHEN CARING FOR CLIENTS WITH DISORDERS USUALLY FIRST EVIDENT IN INFANCY, CHILDHOOD, OR ADOLESCENCE

A. Recognize that all children, especially these children, require:
   1. Protection from danger
   2. Love and acceptance
   3. Basic physiologic needs to be met
   4. Meaningful relationships
   5. An opportunity to explore the environment
B. Direct care toward helping the child grow up emotionally by:
   1. Establishing a favorable environment in which the child can gain or regain a favorable equilibrium
   2. Establishing a constructive relationship
   3. Helping the child to see self as a worthwhile person
   4. Recognizing that the behavior has meaning for the child
   5. Being as realistic and as truthful as possible when dealing with the child
   6. Attempting to establish trust
   7. Setting limits that are as realistic as possible but as firm as necessary
   8. Pointing out reality, but accepting the child's views of it while pointing it out
   9. Being consistent both in approach and in rules and regulations
   10. Making all explanations as clear as possible and at the appropriate cognitive developmental level
   11. Supporting and encouraging the child's moves toward independence but allowing dependency when necessary

▼ MENTAL RETARDATION

See Mental Retardation in Pediatric Nursing

▼ LEARNING DISORDERS

Data Base

A. Etiologic factors
   1. Theories as to the cause are being studied; however, no one definitive cause has been established

2. Learning disorders (LD) are frequently found in association with a variety of medical conditions (lead poisoning, fetal alcohol syndrome, fragile X syndrome)
3. Although genetic predisposition, perinatal injury, neurologic and general medical conditions may be associated, the presence of such conditions does not invariably predict the learning disorder

B. Behavioral/clinical findings
   1. Achievement on individually administered, standardized tests in reading, mathematics, or written expression is substantially below (defined as 2 or more standard deviations between achievement and IQ) that expected for age, schooling, and level of intelligence
   2. Disorders of written expression and mathematics commonly occur in combination with a reading disorder
   3. Demoralization, lower self-esteem, and deficits in social skills may be associated
   4. Approximately 5% of students in public schools are identified as having a learning disorder
   5. Employment difficulties and social adjustment are noted in adolescence and adulthood
   6. LD must be differentiated from normal variations in academic attainment and from scholastic difficulties resulting from lack of opportunity, poor teaching, or cultural factors
   7. Impaired vision or hearing should be investigated through visual screening and audiometric testing
   8. Disorders may persist into adulthood

C. Therapeutic interventions
   1. Accept child and focus on strengths to raise self-esteem
   2. Identify learning deficits early
   3. Minimize long-term consequences
      a. Treatment of associated problems
      b. Infant, child stimulation
      c. Parent education

Nursing Care of Clients with Learning Disorders

A. ASSESSMENT
   1. Determine attainment or delay of developmental milestones (motor, language, social, etc.)
   2. Observe parent behavior and attitude
      a. Expectations
      b. Acceptance or rejection
      c. Encouragement or pressure
   3. Social history
      a. Social activities
      b. Peer and sibling relationships
      c. Developmental history of personal and social relationships

   d. Ascertain specific and outstanding accomplishments
   4. Medical history
      a. Vision
      b. Hearing
      c. General health
      d. Pregnancy, neonatal, and birth data
      e. Past illness
      f. Family history

B. ANALYSIS/NURSING DIAGNOSES
   1. Anxiety related to a frequent lack of success, the inability to meet expectations of others, and the failure to develop meaningful relationships
   2. Impaired verbal communication related to cerebral deficits and psychologic barriers
   3. Interrupted family processes related to disturbed family interactions and the disturbed behavior of infant, child, or adolescent
   4. Risk for injury related to sensory deficits, altered judgment, and sensorimotor deficits
   5. Disturbed thought processes related to an inability to evaluate reality, a disturbed interpretation of environment, disturbed mental activities, an altered sensory perception, reception, and transmission, and inattention and impulsivity

C. PLANNING/IMPLEMENTATION
   1. Refer to Fundamental Principles When Caring for Clients with Disorders Usually First Evident in Infancy, Childhood, or Adolescence
   2. Provide activities consistent with disorder
   3. Refer for diagnostic evaluation of specific learning disorder based upon assessments
   4. Provide guidance, supervision, and habilitation
   5. Maintain routines based on the child's usual schedule
   6. Set consistent and firm limits for behavior
   7. Refer for remediation
   8. Develop a trusting relationship with the child and family
   9. Assist the parents to gain an accurate understanding of their child's strengths and weaknesses

D. EVALUATION/OUTCOMES
   1. Participates in school and home activities
   2. Follows directions
   3. Carries tasks to completion
   4. Benefits from remediation

▼ MOTOR SKILLS DISORDERS

Data Base
A. Etiologic factors
   1. No definitive cause for motor impairment has been established for developmental coordination disorder

2. No specific neurologic disorders are present
3. Lack of coordination can continue through adolescence and adulthood

B. Behavioral/clinical findings
1. A marked impairment in the development of motor coordination that interferes with academic achievement or activities of daily living
2. Coordination difficulties are not related to child's medical condition
3. If mental retardation is present, the motor difficulties are in excess of those usually observed
4. First noted when child attempts motor tasks such as running, holding a knife and fork, buttoning clothes, or playing ball games
5. Performance in daily activities requiring motor coordination is substantially below that expected for chronologic age and measured IQ

C. Therapeutic interventions
1. Direct activities toward the developmental level of the child
2. Identify motor skills deficits early
3. Accept child; develop trusting relationship
4. Assist with academic achievement or activities of daily living only as required
5. Reward achievement of motor milestones (walking, crawling, sitting, improved handwriting, etc.)

Nursing Care of Clients with Motor Skills Disorders

A. ASSESSMENT
1. Developmental screening for delayed milestones
2. Associated illness/risk factors
3. Visual acuity
4. Play activities
5. Child's response to lack of coordination

B. ANALYSIS/NURSING DIAGNOSES
1. Anxiety related to a frequent lack of success, the inability to meet expectations of others, and the failure to develop meaningful relationships
2. Ineffective coping related to an inadequate support system, a personal vulnerability, an inability to meet basic needs and role expectations, and a poorly developed or inappropriate use of defense mechanisms
3. Risk for injury related to sensory deficits, altered judgment, and sensorimotor deficits
4. Risk for falls related to impairment in motor coordination (gross motor skills) and sensorimotor deficits

C. PLANNING/IMPLEMENTATION
1. Teach need for prevention of injury from falls
2. Encourage exercises such as swimming
3. Foster independence by emphasizing abilities and achievements rather than limitations

4. Help parents to cope with child's lack of coordination

D. EVALUATION/OUTCOMES
1. Maintains or increases mobility
2. Participates in desired activities
3. Verbalizes positive self-image
4. Engages in activities suitable to interests, capabilities, and developmental level

▼ COMMUNICATION DISORDERS

Data Base

A. Etiologic factors
1. Diagnosis should be based on standardized measures or thorough functional assessment of language ability; assessment must be culturally relevant for the individual
2. Developmental type: inability to begin or interruption in normal patterns of speech in the absence of physiologic causes
3. Acquired type: impairment in expressive language from a physiologic cause (brain tumor, stroke, head trauma), which may occur at any age, with sudden onset
4. Two common types
   a. Cluttering: abnormally rapid, erratic, dysrhythmic speech patterns that make communication very difficult to follow
   b. Stuttering: frequent repetition of sounds or syllables impairing speech fluency although child has normal laryngeal skills; usually occurring at the beginning of a word or phrase

B. Behavioral/clinical findings
1. Presence of faulty speech patterns that are persistent and increased by stress
2. Anxiety
3. Avoidance of social situations
4. Loss of self-esteem

C. Therapeutic interventions
1. Speech therapy
2. Counseling to reduce anxiety
3. Provision of positive environment during diagnostics and treatments

Nursing Care of Clients with Communication Disorders

A. ASSESSMENT
1. Characteristics, pattern, and onset of speech disorder
2. Factors or situations that precipitate disturbed speech patterns
3. Level of self-esteem
4. Levels of anxiety and frustration
5. Family history of speech disorders

B. **ANALYSIS/NURSING DIAGNOSES**
1. Anxiety related to a frequent lack of success, an inability to meet expectations of others, and a failure to develop meaningful relationships
2. Risk for situational low self-esteem related to difficulty with receptive or expressive language skills or the articulation of speech
3. Ineffective coping related to an inability to meet role expectations and a poorly developed or inappropriate use of defense mechanisms
4. Chronic low self-esteem related to perceptual or cognitive impairment, emotional dysfunction, disturbed relationships, and a frequent lack of success
5. Disturbed thought processes related to altered sensory perception, reception, and transmission, and inattention and impulsivity

C. **PLANNING/IMPLEMENTATION**
1. Refer to Fundamental Principles When Caring for Clients with Disorders Usually First Evident in Infancy, Childhood, or Adolescence
2. Encourage client to adhere to speech therapy routine
3. Allow individual time to verbalize; do not complete word or sentence
4. Avoid nonverbal behavior that implies impatience to the client

D. **EVALUATION/OUTCOMES**
1. Demonstrates a decrease in speech-pattern disturbances
2. Demonstrates increased participation in social and public situations
3. Exhibits an increase in self-esteem
4. Continues with prescribed therapy

▼ PERVASIVE DEVELOPMENTAL DISORDERS (AUTISTIC DISORDERS)

Data Base

A. Etiologic factors
1. Many theories regarding cause are being studied; however, no definitive cause has been established
2. Viewed as a behavioral disorder resulting from abnormal brain function
3. Severe and pervasive impairment in reciprocal social interaction and communication skills, usually accompanied by stereotypical behavior, interests, and activities

B. Behavioral/clinical findings
1. An alienation or withdrawal from reality, usually evident before age 3
2. Autism is more common among siblings than in the general population
3. Autistic infant or child appears indifferent to, or has an aversion to, affection and physical contact

4. A small percentage of autistic children develop seizure disorders and/or schizophrenia
5. Impairments are noted in both verbal and nonverbal communication
6. Puberty can be a crucial stage for showing improvement or further deterioration
7. Adheres to routines and rituals with aversion to minor changes
8. A defect in the adaptive, inhibitory, and steering mechanisms of the personality
9. Interference with intellect may be so profound, child appears mentally retarded
10. Lack of meaningful relationships with outside world
11. Adheres to patterns of stereotypical and repetitive motor mannerisms
12. Turning to inanimate objects and self-centered activity for security
13. Symptoms associated with severe autism include:
    a. Profound apathy
    b. Looseness of association
    c. Autistic thinking
    d. Ambivalence
    e. Absence of communication skills
    f. Poor grasp of reality
    g. Bizarre, unpredictable, uncontrolled behavior
    h. Inability to relate to others
    i. Total interference with intellectual functioning
    j. Stereotypic body movements (rocking, spinning) and same routines
    k. Increased withdrawal is often signaled by a refusal of food

C. Therapeutic interventions
1. Psychotherapy directed toward the developmental level of the child: play, group, or individual therapy
2. Medications: neuroleptics, stimulants, and lithium provide some reduction of symptoms
3. Removal from the home situation may be necessary, although day school situations frequently provide enough relief so that hospitalization can be avoided

Nursing Care of Clients with Autistic Disorders

A. **ASSESSMENT**
1. Behavior associated with autism
2. Rejection of physical contact with others
3. Preference for inanimate, spinning, shiny objects
4. Behavior directing emotional energy inward rather than toward the external environment

B. **ANALYSIS/NURSING DIAGNOSES**
1. Anxiety related to failure to develop meaningful relationships and separation from parents

2. Impaired verbal communication related to delay or absence, or repetitive use of language
3. Ineffective coping related to an inability to meet role expectations and a poorly developed or inappropriate use of defense mechanisms
4. Interrupted family processes related to the failure of infant, child, or adolescent to meet role expectations
5. Impaired social interaction related to lack of responsiveness or interest in others
6. Risk for self-mutilation related to an inability to discharge emotions verbally, and the misinterpretation of stimuli

C. PLANNING/IMPLEMENTATION
1. Refer to Fundamental Principles When Caring for Clients with Disorders Usually First Evident in Infancy, Childhood, or Adolescence
2. Accept child's need to push away but continue to make physical contact on a regular basis
3. Provide a consistent routine for activities of daily living
4. Maintain a consistent familiar environment
5. Use picture and letter boards to assist in communication; participate in child's activities
6. Set consistent and firm limits for behavior
7. Prevent acts of self-destructive behavior
8. Support family's decision for homecare or institutionalization
9. Encourage verbalization of feelings
10. Help child establish self-boundaries by using child's name and personal pronouns and identifying belongings
11. Provide parents with a list of available community resources

D. EVALUATION/OUTCOMES
1. Sits in a group
2. Decreases self-destructive behaviors
3. Limits inappropriate behavior
4. Increases use of first-person speech
5. Uses less stereotyped and repetitive motor behaviors
6. Depending on age, attends a therapeutic nursery program, a day treatment program, or special education classes in public schools in compliance with the American Disabilities Act

▼ ATTENTION-DEFICIT HYPERACTIVITY DISORDERS

Data Base
A. Etiologic factors
1. Diagnosis difficult, because the pathology must be separated from normal disturbances that occur during this period of life
2. Evident before 7 years of age; lasting at least 6 months
3. Thought to have a neurobiologic basis, sometimes complicated by family dynamics and progressive consequences of related learning problems
B. Behavioral/clinical findings
1. Inappropriately inattentive
2. Excessive impulsiveness
3. Short attention span; easy distractibility
4. Squirming and fidgeting
5. Hyperactivity may or may not be present
6. Difficulty organizing tasks and activities
7. Symptoms persist although adolescents usually become more goal directed and less impulsive
C. Therapeutic interventions
1. Psychologic counseling
2. Psychotropic medications; methylphenidate hydrochloride (Ritalin) is frequently used
3. Teach and model more adaptive coping behaviors

Nursing Care of Clients with Attention-Deficit Hyperactivity Disorder
A. ASSESSMENT
1. History of child's behavior from parents, teachers, and guidance counselor to include results of psychometric testing
2. Behavior reflecting impulsiveness and pattern of inattention
3. Difficulty in following instructions
4. Inability to sit without fidgeting or moving about
5. Easy distractibility by extraneous stimuli
B. ANALYSIS/NURSING DIAGNOSES
1. Anxiety related to an inability to meet expectations of others
2. Impaired verbal communication related to psychologic barriers
3. Interrupted family processes related to the disturbed behavior of infant, child, or adolescent
4. Disturbed sleep pattern related to emotional dysfunction
5. Disturbed thought processes related to inattention and impulsivity
6. Ineffective role performance related to short attention span, and difficulty organizing and completing work tasks
C. PLANNING/IMPLEMENTATION
1. Refer to Fundamental Principles When Caring for Clients with Disorders Usually First Evident in Infancy, Childhood, or Adolescence
2. Plan activities to provide a balance between energy expenditure and quiet time
3. Set realistic, attainable goals

4. Structure situations to provide less stimulation (play with only one other child rather than a group)
5. Provide firm and consistent discipline; ignore temper tantrums
6. Provide exercises in perceptual-motor coordination and balance
7. Structure learning experience to utilize the child's ability
8. Provide opportunities so the child can experience success and satisfaction
9. Administer drugs such as methylphenidate (Ritalin) or dextroamphetamine sulfate (Dexedrine)

D. EVALUATION/OUTCOMES
1. Participates in school and home activities
2. Carries tasks to completion
3. Follows directions

▼ UNSPECIFIED CONDUCT DISORDERS

Data Base
A. Etiologic factors
   1. The child may be socialized or undersocialized
   2. The child may be aggressive or nonaggressive
   3. Relabeled antisocial personality disorder after age 18
   4. Theories subscribe to both genetic and environmental components
B. Behavioral/clinical findings
   1. Behavior is destructive to the child's own general aims and falls into four main groupings
      a. Aggression toward people and animals
      b. Destruction of property
      c. Deceitfulness or theft
      d. Serious violations of rules
   2. Behavior is repeated despite rational arguments to the contrary and punishment
   3. Behavior leads to getting caught and punished
   4. Behavioral disturbance causes significant impairment in social, academic, or work performance
   5. Onset may occur as early as age 5 or 6, but is usually in late childhood or early adolescence
C. Therapeutic interventions
   1. Psychologic counseling
   2. Milieu therapy

Nursing Care of Clients with Conduct Disorders
A. ASSESSMENT
1. History of behavior and onset from family's and teachers' perspectives
2. Repetitive and persistent pattern of aggressive conduct toward others
3. Aggressive conduct toward animals

4. Nonaggressive conduct that causes property loss or damage
5. Deceitfulness or theft
6. Serious violations of rules
7. Inability to attain and maintain friendships
8. Parents' expectations of child and family functioning

B. ANALYSIS/NURSING DIAGNOSES
1. Anxiety related to a frequent lack of success, the inability to meet expectations of others, and the failure to develop meaningful relationships
2. Impaired parenting related to frustration in not being effective in dealing with child's disruptive and aggressive behaviors
3. Impaired verbal communication related to psychologic barriers
4. Disabled family coping related to the child's abusive or destructive behavior
5. Ineffective coping related to an inability to meet role expectations, and a poorly developed or inappropriate use of defense mechanisms
6. Risk for violence: self-directed or directed at others related to the inability to discharge emotions verbally and the inability to control aggression

C. PLANNING/IMPLEMENTATION
1. Refer to Fundamental Principles When Caring for Clients with Disorders Usually First Evident in Infancy, Childhood, or Adolescence
2. Utilize a firm system of rewards and punishments within set limits
3. Provide for consistency and avoid manipulation
4. Create opportunities for success in sports or recreation activities
5. Involve family in parenting management training
6. Use life lessons and games to teach delayed gratification
7. Use positive reinforcement for child's strengths and abilities

D. EVALUATION/OUTCOMES
1. Decreases destructive acts directed at self or others
2. Demonstrates appropriate behavior
3. Parents express realistic expectations of child
4. Is able to delay gratification
5. Gains a realistic self-appraisal of strength and weaknesses

▼ FEEDING AND EATING DISORDERS OF INFANCY OR EARLY CHILDHOOD

Data Base
A. Etiologic factors

1. Persistent feeding and eating disturbances (include pica and rumination disorders) result in failure to gain weight or significant loss of weight over 1 month
2. Refer to Failure to Thrive (FTT) in Pediatric Nursing
3. Disturbance is not due to organic medical conditions
4. Mental retardation has been associated with pica and rumination disorders

B. Behavioral/clinical findings
   1. Refer to Failure to Thrive in Pediatric Nursing
   2. Onset in the first year, but can also develop in children ages 2 to 3 years
   3. Irritability and difficulty in consoling, especially during feeding
   4. Developmental delays are common
   5. Inadequate caloric intake may exacerbate irritability, developmental lags, and malnutrition
   6. Parental psychopathology and child abuse or neglect

C. Therapeutic interventions
   1. Provide sufficient nutrients to achieve a rate of growth greater than expected
   2. Attempt to limit behavioral outbursts during feedings
   3. Help parents to care for child to promote bonding

Nursing Care of Clients with Feeding and Eating Disorders of Infancy or Early Childhood

A. **ASSESSMENT**
   1. Accurate height and weight
   2. Feeding behavior
   3. Developmental level
   4. Parent-child behavior
   5. Screening for anemia, low serum albumin, and total protein levels

B. **ANALYSIS/NURSING DIAGNOSES**
   1. Interrupted family process related to disturbed infant or child behavior
   2. Imbalanced nutrition: less or more than body requirements related to a dysfunctional emotional conditioning in relationship to food
   3. Imbalanced nutrition: less than body requirements related to the feeding or eating disorder
   4. Delayed growth and development related to physical or social neglect
   5. Disorganized infant behavior related to feeding difficulties, "fussy baby," and irritability associated with feeding times
   6. Deficient knowledge related to lack of information regarding age-appropriate diet and consoling strategies

C. **PLANNING/IMPLEMENTATION**
   1. Refer to Failure to Thrive in Pediatric Nursing

2. Record daily weights and accurate caloric intake
3. Review lab values to rule out anemia and other low values
4. Observe parent-infant/child feeding process
5. Model appropriate feeding and consoling behaviors
6. Observe child for pica or rumination (regurgitation and swallowing) behaviors

D. **EVALUATION/OUTCOMES**
   1. Achieves expected growth curve and development milestones
   2. Decreases problematic behaviors during feeding times
   3. Parents demonstrate ability to care for child

▼ TIC DISORDERS

Data Base

A. Etiologic factors
   1. Classified as a rapid, recurrent, nonrhythmic, stereotyped motor movement or vocalization involving a few or many muscle movements and vocal tics
   2. Familial or autosomal-dominant patterns exist in high percentage of tic disorders
   3. Types
      a. Tourette's disorder
      b. Chronic motor or vocal
      c. Transient
      d. Unspecified
   4. Duration, variety of tics, and age of onset differentiate types
      a. Tourette's disorder: duration of more than 12 months, onset before age 18, and evidence of multiple motor and at least one vocal tic
      b. Chronic motor or vocal disorder: each has a duration of more than 12 months; evidence of single or multiple motor or vocal tics, but NOT both; onset before age 18
      c. Transient disorder: evidence of motor and/or vocal tics lasting for at least 1 month, but no more than 12 consecutive months; onset before age 18
      d. Unspecified disorder: does not meet criteria for other types; may last longer than 1 month or have an onset after 18 years of age

B. Behavioral/clinical findings
   1. Involuntary, uncontrolled, multiple, rapid movements of muscles such as eye blinking, twitching, and head shaking that occur in bouts throughout the day
   2. Involuntary production of sounds such as throat clearing, grunting, barking, or the utterance of socially unacceptable words is usually associated with Tourette's disorder

3. Can be controlled for short duration; not usually present during sleep; increased during times of stress
4. More common in males than females
5. Tics are not due to physiologic effects of substances (stimulants) or a general medical condition

C. Therapeutic interventions
1. Treat any precipitating factor such as head injury, psychoactive substance intoxication, or infection
2. Supportive individual or group counseling
3. Medications such as sedatives or anticonvulsants may be prescribed, usually have minimal effect; CNS stimulants should be avoided because they increase symptoms in most individuals

Nursing Care of Clients with Tic Disorders

A. ASSESSMENT
1. History, onset, and presence of behavior associated with tic disorders
2. Exacerbation of tics by stress
3. Decreased tic activity during sleep
4. History of psychoactive substance use to determine if tic disorder is related to intoxication
5. History of central nervous system trauma, infection, or degeneration
6. Family history of tic disorder
7. History of neuroleptic agents to determine if tics are direct physiologic consequence of medications (medication-induced movement disorder would be the appropriate label)

B. ANALYSIS/NURSING DIAGNOSES
1. Anxiety related to the inability to meet expectations of others
2. Disturbed body image related to uncontrollable body movements and production of sounds
3. Impaired adjustment related to pattern of motor movements and socially stigmatizing vocal tics
4. Risk for injury related to sensorimotor deficits

C. PLANNING/IMPLEMENTATION
1. Refer to Fundamental Principles When Caring for Clients with Disorders Usually First Evident in Infancy, Childhood, or Adolescence
2. Accept behavior, recognizing it is often uncontrollable
3. Help client to identify precipitating factors
4. Support client's attempts to control tic

D. EVALUATION/OUTCOMES
1. Demonstrates a decrease in tic behavior
2. Accepts presence of tic
3. Functions socially despite presence of tic
4. Family members with Tourette's disorder respond positively to advice regarding genetic counseling

▼ ELIMINATION DISORDERS

Data Base
A. Etiologic factors
1. Functional encopresis: involuntary or intentional defecation in inappropriate places, including clothing
2. Functional enuresis: involuntary or intentional micturition in inappropriate places, including clothing

B. Behavioral/clinical findings
1. These disorders are more common in males than females
2. No identifiable physical problems are present
3. Chronologic age is at least 4 years or equivalent developmental level
4. Can occur before bladder training has been accomplished (primary) or after a period of controlled continence (secondary)
5. Nocturnal bedwetting is most frequent; child may or may not be aware of voiding or recall a dream about the act of urinating
6. Loss of self-esteem; anxiety and rejection by peers may cause child to avoid situations (camp, school)

C. Therapeutic interventions
1. Psychotherapy
2. Medications such as tricyclic antidepressants for children over the age of 5 to treat enuresis
3. Bowel retraining program

Nursing Care of Clients with Elimination Disorders

A. ASSESSMENT
1. History of toileting behaviors
2. History of school or family difficulties
3. Level of self-esteem
4. Secondary gains achieved by behavior

B. ANALYSIS/NURSING DIAGNOSES
1. Anxiety related to a frequent lack of success and an inability to meet others' expectations
2. Risk for impaired parenting related to child's pattern of disturbed behavior (encopresis or enuresis) not responding to discipline or other control measures
3. Feeding, bathing/hygiene, dressing/grooming, toileting self-care deficit related to emotional dysfunction
4. Chronic low self-esteem related to emotional dysfunction, disturbed relationships, and a frequent lack of success
5. Disturbed sleep pattern related to emotional dysfunction

C. PLANNING/IMPLEMENTATION
1. Refer to Fundamental Principles When Caring for Clients with Disorders Usually First Evident in Infancy, Childhood, or Adolescence

2. Change linen and clothing in a nonjudgmental manner to avoid further embarrassment for the client
3. Recognize and accept the fact that the act is usually not motivated by hostility
4. Help parents deal with feelings such as guilt, failure, or anger

D. EVALUATION/OUTCOMES
1. Demonstrates a decrease in encopresis or enuresis
2. Exhibits an increase in self-esteem
3. Verbalizes understanding that behavior is neither good nor bad but solution requires outside assistance
4. Parents verbalize understanding that behavior is related to an emotional problem, not hostility

▼ ANXIETY DISORDERS OF INFANCY, CHILDHOOD, AND ADOLESCENCE

Data Base
A. Etiologic factors
   1. Separation anxiety disorder
      a. Excessive anxiety centered on harm befalling self, family, or those to whom child has attachment
      b. Equally common in males and females
      c. Begins in infancy (oral phase of development)
   2. School phobia
      a. Severe anxiety about attending school
      b. Often accompanied by psychophysiologic symptoms
      c. Onset any time during early school years
      d. Interferes with educational, social, and occupational achievement
   3. Selective mutism
      a. Persistent failure to speak in specific social situations
      b. Interferes with educational, social, and occupational achievement
      c. Onset usually before age 5
   4. Reactive attachment disorder
      a. Disturbed or developmentally inappropriate behavior
      b. Onset before age 5
B. Behavioral/clinical findings
   1. Separation anxiety disorder
      a. Problems with sleeping unless near the person to whom child has attachment
      b. Refusal to attend school in order to remain near the person to whom child has attachment
      c. Physical complaints of headaches and stomachaches when separation is anticipated
   2. School phobia
      a. Overwhelming shyness and insecurity causes severe anxiety about attending school
      b. Physical complaints or vague symptoms often used to justify nonattendance
      c. Anxiety often severe in response to attempts to force attendance
   3. Selective mutism
      a. Avoidance of speaking in social environments outside the home
      b. Social involvement limited to family members or people who are familiar to the child
      c. Excessive shyness and timidity when confronted with strangers
   4. Reactive attachment disorder
      a. Psychosocial deprivation resulting in child's failure to initiate or respond to most social interactions
      b. Difficulty in choice of attachment figures
      c. Onset in the first several years of life; begins before age 5
C. Therapeutic interventions
   1. Psychotherapy: in children, usually in the form of play therapy
   2. Psychopharmacology may be helpful (stimulants and antianxiety agents)

Nursing Care of Clients with Anxiety Disorders of Infancy, Childhood, and Adolescence
A. ASSESSMENT
1. History of child's behavior from parents and teachers
2. Presence of sleep disturbances
3. Interpersonal functioning with others
4. Physical complaints
5. History of attendance at school
6. Child's appearance and behavior

B. ANALYSIS/NURSING DIAGNOSES
1. Anxiety related to the inability to meet expectations of others and a failure to develop meaningful relationships
2. Ineffective coping related to the poorly developed or inappropriate use of defense mechanisms
3. Parental role conflict related to protective behaviors vs. societal demands (child's attachment need vs. school attendance anxiety)
4. Feeding, bathing/hygiene, dressing/grooming, toileting self-care deficit related to emotional dysfunction
5. Chronic low self-esteem related to emotional dysfunction and disturbed relationships
6. Disturbed sleep pattern related to emotional dysfunction

C. PLANNING/IMPLEMENTATION
1. Refer to Fundamental Principles When Caring

for Clients with Disorders Usually First Evident in Infancy, Childhood, or Adolescence

2. Provide consistent caregivers
3. Introduce child to new situations gradually; permit child to bring a familiar, comforting toy
4. Allow parent to stay with child as long as possible
5. Return child to school as soon as possible
6. Involve family in multifamily therapy to work through problems of daily life and to gain new information, and more adaptive coping skills

D. EVALUATION/OUTCOMES
1. Demonstrates a decrease in sleep disturbances
2. Attends school on a consistent basis
3. Verbalizes fewer physical complaints
4. Develops relationships outside of family members and the home environment
5. States a decrease in episodes of anxiety and worry
6. Behaviors of family members show a decline in overprotection of child

DELIRIUM, DEMENTIA, AMNESTIC, AND OTHER COGNITIVE DISORDERS

Disorders associated with actual temporary or permanent changes in brain tissue

FUNDAMENTAL PRINCIPLES WHEN CARING FOR CLIENTS WITH DELIRIUM, DEMENTIA, AMNESTIC, AND OTHER COGNITIVE DISORDERS

A. Provide a safe, familiar environment; provide direct supervision as necessary; provide a consistent caregiver to foster trust
B. Continually orient the client to time, date, and place
C. Keep client involved in reality and in the home situation as long as possible
D. Allow client to assume as much responsibility for self-care as possible
E. Provide a quiet environment; reduce stimuli; help client maintain relationships
F. Plan care so the staff approaches these clients when they appear receptive
G. Attempt to follow familiar routines; keep the schedule of activities flexible to make use of the client's lability of mood and easy distractibility
H. Encourage adequate nutritional intake; monitor intake and output
I. Provide diversional activities including exercises that the client enjoys and can handle
J. Observe for changing physiologic and neurologic symptoms

K. Prevent physical harm related to confusion, aggression, or fluid and electrolyte imbalance
L. Support family caregivers; maintain nonjudgmental attitude
M. Help provide some relief from responsibility of total care; refer to community agencies that provide homecare helpers or respite care if appropriate
N. Support the family's decision to place client in a nursing home

▼ DELIRIUM

Data Base
A. Etiologic factors
1. Syndromes from which the client usually recovers, because the changes may be reversible and temporary
2. Delirium is always secondary to some physical disorder or drug toxicity
3. Clinical manifestations develop over a short period (hours or days) and cognitive impairment fluctuates during a 24-hour period
4. Delirium that becomes more pronounced in the evening is referred to as sundowning
5. Stressors
   a. Infection
      (1) Intracranial or nervous system (e.g., meningitis or encephalitis)
      (2) Systemic or toxic (e.g., AIDS, acute or chronic respiratory disorders)
   b. Trauma to the head
   c. Circulatory disturbances resulting in impairment of blood flow to the brain
   d. Metabolic disorders: electrolyte imbalance (e.g., dehydration, diarrhea, vomiting), fever
   e. Ingestion of psychoactive substances or the accumulative CNS effect of prescribed medications
   f. Multiple etiologies (e.g., combination of medical condition and substance interaction)
B. Behavioral/clinical findings
1. Delirium and its accompanying confusion, hallucinations, and delusions
2. Disorientation and confusion as to time, place, identity
3. Memory defects for both recent and remote events and facts
4. Slurring or rapid speech may occur along with an indistinct pronunciation or use of words
5. Tremors, incoordination, imbalance, and incontinence may develop
6. Physical symptoms such as depressed respiration, cardiac irregularities, and gastrointestinal changes may occur
C. Therapeutic interventions

1. Reduction of causative agent such as fever or toxins
2. Prevention of further damage
3. Provision of diet high in calories, protein, and vitamins
4. Prescription of mild sedatives if necessary
5. Provision of a safe environment

Nursing Care of Clients with Delirium
A. ASSESSMENT
1. History of onset and progression of symptoms from family members
2. Orientation to time, place, and person
3. Occurrence of memory defects
4. Mood swings or behavior associated with delirium
5. State of consciousness
B. ANALYSIS/NURSING DIAGNOSES
1. Risk for injury related to confusion as evidenced by sensory or perceptual deficits
2. Impaired verbal communication related to progressive cerebral impairment and progressive neurologic losses
3. Acute confusion related to global changes and disturbances in attention, cognition, and psychomotor level of consciousness
4. Chronic confusion related to changes in brain tissue resulting in impairment of intellect and personality
5. Disturbed sleep pattern awake or disoriented during the night
6. Impaired environmental interpretation syndrome related to difficulty recognizing familiar people or places and experiencing illusions and delusions
7. Impaired memory related to neurologic disturbances and dysfunctions
8. Feeding, bathing/hygiene, dressing/grooming, toileting self-care deficit related to cognitive or sensory impairment and the increasing inability to carry out activities of daily living
9. Risk for violence; self-directed or directed at others, related to sensory perceptual alterations and toxic reactions in or progressive deterioration of cerebral tissue
C. PLANNING/IMPLEMENTATION
1. Refer to Fundamental Principles When Caring for Clients with Delirium, Dementia, and Amnestic and Other Cognitive Disorders
2. Implement measures as ordered to reduce causative factors
3. Reassure family members that symptoms associated with the delirium may subside
4. Provide one-to-one caregiver assignment during restless or agitated periods

D. EVALUATION/OUTCOMES
1. Remains free from injury
2. Remains oriented to time, place, and person
3. Assumes increased responsibility for self-care
4. Maintains a diet high in calories, protein, and vitamins
5. Avoids intake of pharmacologic substance associated with delirium
6. Continues to visit health care provider for treatment and amelioration of underlying cause

▼ DEMENTIA

Data Base
A. Etiologic factors
1. Dementia may be progressive, static, or remitting
2. Alzheimer's disease and vascular disease are two most common causes
3. Stressors
   a. Prenatal injury or malformation (e.g., hydrocephalus, microcephalus, neurosyphilis)
   b. Infections such as tertiary syphilis
   c. Trauma in which a head injury results in permanent brain damage
   d. Circulatory disturbances causing anoxia and permanent brain damage (e.g., cerebral arteriosclerosis, CVA)
   e. Nutritional deprivation of brain cells (e.g., pellagra)
   f. Damage may result from generalized diseases (e.g., multiple sclerosis, hepatolenticular disease, Huntington's chorea, Parkinson's disease, AIDS)
   g. Damage resulting from pressure of brain tumors
   h. Toxins
B. Behavioral/clinical findings
1. Memory impairment (recall or learning)
2. One or more of the following
   a. Aphasia (language disturbance)
   b. Apraxia (impaired motor activities)
   c. Agnosia (inability to recognize familiar objects)
   d. Disturbance in planning, organizing, sequencing, and abstracting
C. Therapeutic interventions
   The same as those for delirium with greater emphasis on preventing further damage

Nursing Care of Clients with Dementia
A. ASSESSMENT
1. History of onset and progression of symptoms from family

2. Physical and emotional status in relation to needs associated with nutrition, fluid and electrolyte status, and safety
3. History of premorbid personality from family
4. History of impaired memory
5. History of hallucinations (visual) and delusions (persecution)

B. ANALYSIS/NURSING DIAGNOSES

1. Anxiety related to recognized early memory loss, threat to self-concept, and motor and sensory loss
2. Acute confusion related to: abrupt onset or global changes and disturbances in attention, cognition, and psychomotor level of consciousness and changes in the wake/sleep cycle resulting from dementia
3. Chronic confusion related to: changes in brain tissue resulting in impairment of intellect and personality, and decreased intellectual capacity resulting in disturbances in memory, orientation, and behavior
4. Caregiver role strain related to progressive increase in care for family member with dementia that eventually becomes overwhelming
5. Impaired home maintenance management related to impaired mental status and the progressive inability to carry out activities of daily living
6. Risk for injury related to cognitive deficits and psychomotor deficits
7. Impaired memory related to neurologic disturbances and dysfunctions
8. Feeding, bathing/hygiene, dressing/grooming, toileting self-care deficit related to cognitive or sensory impairment and an increasing inability to carry out activities of daily living
9. Disturbed thought processes related to an inability to transmit messages and the destruction of cerebral tissue

C. PLANNING/IMPLEMENTATION

1. Refer to Fundamental Principles When Caring for Clients with Delirium, Dementia, and Amnestic and Other Cognitive Disorders
2. Toilet client frequently
3. Feed the client who is not able to feed self
4. Protect client from self and environment
5. Support client's attempts at independence
6. Support family's decisions regarding present and future care of client

D. EVALUATION/OUTCOMES

1. Remains free from injury
2. Maintains maximal potential for as long as possible
3. Family utilizes community resources as necessary

▼ DEMENTIA OF THE ALZHEIMER'S TYPE

Data Base

A. Etiologic factors
1. Primary degenerative dementia with late onset: occurs after age 65
2. Primary degenerative dementia with early onset: occurs before age 65
3. About 10% of Alzheimer's disease is related to genetic mutations.
4. Decreased levels of acetylcholine; cell loss and subsequent disruption in the cholinergic system is extensive; glutamate and peptide transmitters are affected in specific brain regions
5. Characteristics
   a. Atrophy of brain accompanied by widened cortical sulci and enlarged cerebral ventricles
   b. Microscopic brain changes include senile plaques and a granulovascular degeneration of neurons
   c. Believed to be related to the brain's inability to produce sufficient neurotransmitters that transmit messages through the brain
6. Stressors
   a. Aluminum deposits found in the brains of clients with Alzheimer's disease was thought to be a factor; research has not supported this theory
   b. Immunologic defect suspected because of higher titers of antibodies in clients with Alzheimer's disease
   c. Chromosomal defect linked to Down syndrome
   d. Previous severe head injury with unconsciousness
B. Behavioral/clinical findings
1. Memory impairment (recall or learning)
2. One or more of the following:
   a. Aphasia (language disturbance)
   b. Apraxia (impaired motor activities)
   c. Agnosia (inability to recognize familiar objects)
   d. Disturbance in planning, organizing, sequencing, and abstracting
3. More common in females than males; appears to have a familial or genetic predisposition
4. Differs from normal changes associated with aging
5. Dementia has an insidious onset with symptoms following a progressively downhill course; changes are unrelated to any other specific cause
6. Progression moves from mild forgetfulness for recent events to mutism, inability to carry out any activities of daily living, and incontinence; degeneration usually ends in a vegetative state and coma; disease is 100% fatal and death

usually occurs within 8 to 10 years after onset of symptoms; currently the fourth leading cause of death in the United States

C. Therapeutic interventions
   1. Ruling out causes such as fluid and electrolyte or vitamin deficiencies, excessive medication, exogenous poisons, or metabolic disorders
   2. Provision of supportive care including adequate nutrition with supplemental vitamins
   3. Assess effectiveness of prescribed chemical agents used to increase acetylcholine
     a. Tacrine (Cognex)
     b. Donepezil (Aricept)
     c. Rivastigmine (Exelon)
   4. Admission to a total care institution when necessary

Nursing Care of Clients with Dementia of the Alzheimer's Type

A. ASSESSMENT
   1. History of progressive memory loss and regressive behaviors
   2. History of progressive degeneration of mental, emotional, social, and physical abilities
   3. Physical and emotional status in relation to needs associated with nutrition, fluid and electrolyte status, and safety
   4. History of previous head injury with loss of consciousness
   5. History of medications used by client

B. ANALYSIS/NURSING DIAGNOSES
   1. Anxiety related to recognized early memory loss, threat to self-concept, and motor and sensory loss
   2. Caregiver role strain related to dealing with progressive degeneration
   3. Impaired verbal communication related to progressive cerebral impairment
   4. Acute confusion related to abrupt onset or global changes and disturbances in attention, cognition, and psychomotor level of consciousness and changes in the wake/sleep cycle resulting from dementia
   5. Chronic confusion related to changes in brain tissue resulting in impairment of intellect and personality, and decreased intellectual capacity resulting in disturbances in memory, orientation, and behavior
   6. Compromised family coping related to role changes secondary to family member's inability to function independently and progressive degeneration
   7. Impaired home maintenance management related to impaired mental status and the progressive inability to carry out activities of daily living
   8. Risk for injury related to cognitive deficits and psychomotor deficits

   9. Impaired memory related to neurologic disturbances and dysfunctions
  10. Feeding, bathing/hygiene, dressing/grooming, toileting self-care deficit related to cognitive or sensory impairment and an increasing inability to carry out activities of daily living
  11. Disturbed thought processes related to an inability to transmit messages and the destruction of cerebral tissue
  12. Wandering related to moderate or severe stage of Alzheimer's disease

C. PLANNING/IMPLEMENTATION
   1. Refer to Fundamental Principles When Caring for Clients with Delirium, Dementia, and Amnestic and Other Cognitive Disorders
   2. Refer to Planning/Implementation under Nursing Care of Clients with Dementia

D. EVALUATION/OUTCOMES
Refer to Evaluation/Outcomes under Nursing Care of Clients with Dementia

▼ AMNESTIC DISORDERS

Data Base
A. Etiologic factors
   1. Disturbance in memory related to medical condition (head trauma, stroke)
   2. Disturbance in memory related to persistent effects of substance (drug abuse, medication, or toxin exposure)
B. Behavioral/clinical findings
   1. Impaired ability to learn new information
   2. Difficulty recalling previously learned information or past events
   3. No evidence of anxiety related to a traumatic event
   4. Impaired social and occupational functions
C. Therapeutic interventions: same as those for dementia with emphasis on determining causative agent

Nursing Care of Clients with Amnestic Disorders
A. ASSESSMENT
   1. History of onset and progression of symptoms from family
   2. Physical and emotional status
   3. History of previous functioning level

B. ANALYSIS/NURSING DIAGNOSES
Refer to Analysis/Nursing Diagnoses under Nursing Care of Clients with Dementia of the Alzheimer's Type

C. PLANNING/IMPLEMENTATION
   1. Refer to Fundamental Principles When Caring for Clients with Delirium and Dementia, and Amnestic and Other Cognitive Disorders
   2. Maintain the client in a safe environment
   3. Support the client's attempts at independence

4. Assist with health care team's efforts to identify causative agent
5. Support client and family regarding present and future care decisions

D. EVALUATION/OUTCOMES
1. Demonstrates remission of amnesia
2. Returns to previous level of functioning
3. Family utilizes community resources

▼ SUBSTANCE-INDUCED PERSISTING AMNESTIC DISORDERS

Data Base

A. Etiologic factors
1. Nervous system, particularly the CNS, directly affected by substances taken nonmedically (alcohol, opiates, barbiturates, cocaine, etc.); by toxin exposure (lead, mercury, carbon monoxide, industrial solvents, and insecticides); and by heavy use of medications (sedatives, hypnotics, or anxiolytic drugs)
2. Occurs in individuals with substance-abuse disorders
3. Behavioral changes may be related to a vitamin deficiency such as thiamine, especially in long-term alcohol abuse such as Korsakoff's syndrome
4. Memory disturbance persists long after drug or toxin exposure has ended

B. Behavioral/clinical findings
1. Specific neurologic and psychologic signs and maladaptive behavior such as euphoria; dysphoria; apathy; confabulation; psychomotor agitation, excitement, or depression; hypervigilance; and fighting or violent behavior
2. Symptoms of dementia or delirium may be present depending on the substance used
3. Physical symptoms such as depressed respiration, cardiac irregularities, and gastrointestinal changes may occur
4. Memory disturbance causes significant impairment in social and work activities and represents a decline in previous level of function
5. Impairment in ability to learn new information or to recall previously learned information

C. Therapeutic interventions: refer to Delirium

Nursing Care of Clients with Substance-Induced Persisting Amnestic Disorders

A. ASSESSMENT
1. History, physical examination, or laboratory findings related to drug abuse or toxin exposure
2. History of symptom onset (rapid/slow)
3. Orientation to time, place, and person
4. Ability to have short-term and long-term recall
5. Level of consciousness and stimulation necessary to evoke a response
6. Physiologic status

B. ANALYSIS/NURSING DIAGNOSES
1. Caregiver role strain related to dealing with progressive degeneration
2. Impaired verbal communication related to progressive cerebral impairment, progressive neurologic losses, and/or withdrawal from others
3. Acute confusion related to global changes and disturbances in attention, cognition, and psychomotor level of consciousness
4. Chronic confusion related to changes in brain tissue resulting in impairment of intellect and personality and a long-standing decreased intellectual capacity resulting in disturbances in memory, orientation, and behavior
5. Impaired home maintenance management related to impaired mental status and a progressive inability to carry out activities of daily living
6. Risk for injury related to cognitive deficits and psychomotor deficits
7. Impaired memory related to neurologic disturbances and dysfunctions
8. Imbalanced nutrition: less than body requirements related to confusion, depression, and/or anorexia
9. Disturbed sensory perception (visual, auditory, kinesthetic, gustatory, tactile, olfactory) related to progressive cerebral impairment and progressive neurologic losses
10. Disturbed thought processes related to destruction of cerebral tissue
11. Risk for violence: self-directed or directed at others related to sensory perceptual alterations and toxic reactions in or progressive deterioration of cerebral tissue

C. PLANNING/IMPLEMENTATION
1. Refer to Fundamental Principles When Caring for Clients with Delirium, Dementia, and Amnestic and Other Cognitive Disorders
2. Refer to Planning/Implementation under Nursing Care of Clients with Dementia and Nursing Care of Clients with Delirium

D. EVALUATION/OUTCOMES
1. Abstains from injurious substances
2. Reduces maladaptive behavior
3. Remains free from injury
4. Remains cognitively stable or slightly improves

▼ MENTAL DISORDERS DUE TO A GENERAL MEDICAL CONDITION

Refer to specific conditions in Medical-Surgical Nursing as well as Delirium, Dementia, and Amnestic and Other Cognitive Disorders

SUBSTANCE RELATED DISORDERS

Definitions*

A. Substance refers to a drug of abuse, a medication, or a toxin

B. Substance abuse: maladaptive pattern of drug use leading to impairment or distress, as manifested by one or more of the following occurring within a 12-month period
 1. Failure to fulfill major roles
 2. Use in hazardous situations
 3. Recurring related legal problems
 4. Continued use despite social or interpersonal problems

C. Substance intoxication: a reversible substance-specific syndrome caused by recent ingestion of, or exposure to, a substance resulting in maladaptive behavior or psychologic changes from effect on the CNS

D. Substance withdrawal: development of a substance-specific syndrome resulting from cessation or reduction in substance use that has been heavy or prolonged
 1. Impairment in role functioning (social, school, or occupational)
 2. Symptoms are not from another mental disorder

E. Substance tolerance: the need for greatly increased amounts of the substance to achieve the desired effects, or a markedly diminished effect with the continued use of the same amount of substance

F. Polysubstance abuse: abuse of two or more drugs or of alcohol and drugs

G. Potentiation: two or more substances interact in the body to produce an effect greater than the sum of the effects of each substance taken alone

H. Substance dependence: the continued use of a substance despite significant related problems in cognitive, physiologic, and behavioral components; spending more time in getting, taking, and recovering from the substance; continuous abuse despite knowledge of physical or psychological problems or awareness of complications resulting from continued use

▼ ALCOHOL ABUSE

Data Base

A. Etiologic factors
 1. Depressant of major brain functions (mood cognition, attention, concentration, insight, judg-

*Adapted from *Diagnostic and statistical manual of mental disorders* (text revision), ed 4, Washington, DC, 2000, American Psychiatric Association.

ment memory, affect) resulting in diminished emotional rapport with others
 2. Alcohol is a CNS depressant that is dose dependent and ranges from lethargy, unconsciousness, coma, respiratory distress, to death
 3. Causation theories range form genetic, stress, environmental to interpersonal factors; none fully explains causation
 4. Neurobiologic perspective
  a. The biologic or genetic theory continues to be researched
  b. Some research has identified subtypes of alcoholism; one type is associated with early onset, inability to abstain, and an antisocial personality; another is a later onset, after age 25, inability to stop drinking once started, and a passive-dependent personality; this latter type seems more to be influenced by the environment
  c. Some researchers subscribe to the single genetic transmission; others believe that complex genetic factors are involved in alcoholism
  d. Biologic differences in the response to alcohol may influence susceptibility
  e. Further research is necessary before conclusive results are known

B. Behavioral/clinical findings
 1. Intoxication: state in which coordination or speech is impaired and behavior is altered
 2. Episodic excessive drinking: becoming intoxicated as infrequently as four times a year; episodes may vary in length from hours to days or weeks
 3. Habitual excessive drinking: becoming intoxicated more than 12 times a year or being recognizably under the influence of alcohol more than once a week even though not considered intoxicated
 4. Alcohol addiction: direct or strong presumptive evidence of dependence on alcohol; demonstrated by withdrawal symptoms (nausea, hypertension, anorexia) or by the inability to go for a day without drinking; when there is a history of heavy drinking for 3 or more months, the individual is considered addicted to alcohol
 5. Early symptoms of alcoholism: frequent drinking sprees, increased intake, drinking alone or in the early morning, occurrence of blackouts

C. Therapeutic interventions
 1. Should be multifaceted social and medical; involves psychotherapy (group, family, and individual counseling)
 2. Self-help groups such as Alcoholics Anonymous

3. Negative conditioning with disulfiram (Antabuse) appears to help but never given without the client's full knowledge, understanding, and consent
4. Naltrexone hydrochloride (Trexan, ReVia) to help overcome the craving for alcohol
5. Clients can be assisted only when they admit they need help
6. Relaxation therapy
7. Physical needs must be met because dietary needs have often been ignored for long periods

Nursing Care of Clients with Alcohol Abuse

A. ASSESSMENT

1. History of alcohol use/abuse from client and family if available; screen using the CAGE questionnaire
2. Blood alcohol level (BAL)
3. Data collection pertaining to substance dependence and psychiatric impairment
4. Client's perception of the problem
5. Sleep patterns and withdrawal symptoms
6. Physical and emotional status in relation to needs associated with nutrition, fluid and electrolyte status, and safety
7. Why client is seeking treatment at this time

B. ANALYSIS/NURSING DIAGNOSES

1. Anxiety related to threat to self-concept, inability to deal with responsibility, feelings of inadequacy
2. Impaired verbal communication related to mental confusion or CNS depression because of substance use
3. Acute confusion related to global changes and disturbances in attention, cognition, and psychomotor level of consciousness and changes in the wake/sleep cycle resulting from substance use
4. Chronic confusion related to changes in brain tissue resulting in impairment of intellect and personality, long-standing decreased intellectual capacity resulting in disturbances in memory, orientation, and behavior
5. Defensive coping related to denial of obvious problem, projection of blame/responsibility, rationalization of failures, and lack of participation in treatment or therapy
6. Dysfunctional family processes related to alcoholism and others enabling behaviors
7. Ineffective health maintenance related to lack of self-care (hygiene, grooming, nutrition)
8. Defensive coping related to denial of alcoholism and its impact on pattern on life
9. Risk for injury related to altered cerebral or perceptual function, judgment, and mobility

10. Risk for loneliness related to social isolation from family and friends resulting from total involvement with addicting substance
11. Impaired memory related to neurologic disturbances and dysfunctions
12. Noncompliance with abstinence and supportive therapy related to inability to stop using substance because of dependence and refusal to alter lifestyle
13. Imbalanced nutrition: less than body requirements, related to a lack of interest in food, satiety of hunger by use of "empty calories" in alcohol, chemical dependence
14. Chronic low self-esteem related to inability to meet role expectations, feelings of inadequacy and expectation of failure, and negative feelings about self
15. Risk for self-mutilation related to intake of mind-altering substances
16. Disturbed sensory perceptions (visual, kinesthetic, tactile) related to intake of mind-altering substances
17. Risk for violence: self-directed or directed at others, related to intake of mind-altering substances, misinterpretation of stimuli, and feelings of suspicion or distrust

C. PLANNING/IMPLEMENTATION

1. Provide a well-controlled, alcohol-free environment; explain unit routines
2. Plan a full program of activities but provide for adequate rest; environment should be well lit and quiet
3. Support the client without criticism or judgment
4. Expect and accept lapses as client is changing a long-term habit; assist with ADL as necessary
5. Avoid attempting to talk client out of problem or making client feel guilty
6. Accept the smooth facade that the client may present while approaching the lonely and fearful individual behind it
7. Monitor visitors because they may supply the client with alcohol
8. Accept failures without judgment or punishment
9. Recognize that the development of DTs and hallucinations are frightening; stay with and support client
10. Accept hostility without criticism or retaliation
11. Recognize ambivalence and limit the need for decision making
12. Maintain the client's interest in a therapy program
13. Refer to an appropriate 12-step group such as AA, NA, or CODA

D. EVALUATION/OUTCOMES
1. Recognizes, accepts, and seeks treatment for problem
2. Accepts responsibility for problem without blaming others
3. Achieves optimal physiologic and nutritional status
4. Learns new, more self-preserving coping mechanisms
5. Verbalizes feelings and situations that pose increased risk of alcohol use
6. Enters into and continues with community-based self-help program
7. Maintains abstinence from alcohol and chemical substances
8. Demonstrates responsibility in meeting own health care needs

▼ DRUG ABUSE

Data Base
A. Etiologic factors
1. Misuse of drugs, usually by self-administration, in such a way as to bring about physical, emotional, or behavioral changes and a blurring of reality
2. Stressors: premorbid personality, utilizing compensatory mechanisms of the addictive pattern of behavior
B. Behavioral/clinical findings
1. Needle marks on limbs, or between toes, can lead to infections (e.g., endocarditis, hepatitis, or HIV)
2. Addicted individuals may tend to wear long-sleeved shirts, even in warm weather
3. Yawning, lacrimation, rhinorrhea, and perspiration appear 10 to 15 hours after the last opiate injection; unrealistic high; pronounced depression
4. Severe abdominal cramps if too much time has elapsed between opiate injections or inhalation
5. Physical examination may reveal an underweight, malnourished individual with multiple dental caries and depressed CNS functioning
6. Job or academic failure; marital conflicts; poor reality testing; personality change
7. History of violent acting out with total disregard for human life or suffering
8. History of stealing to support habit
9. Cocaine snorting leads to nasal septum destruction, hoarseness, and throat infections
10. Inability to maintain activities of daily living or fulfill role obligations
11. Marked tolerance with a progressive need for higher doses to achieve desired effects
12. Marked letdown with progression to severe depression after cocaine use
13. Hallucinations, hypervigilance, increased sexual activity, and paranoid ideation with cocaine use
14. Techno drugs: ecstasy (MDMA, methylenedioxymethamphetamine) and ketamine resemble amphetamine effects; they are also known as recreational drugs
    a. Adverse effects of psychostimulants can cause hyperthermia, acute renal failure, depression, panic, psychosis, and cardiovascular collapse
    b. Sleep disorders, depression, high anxiety levels, hostility, and impulsiveness are all associated with recreational drug use
    c. Sexual assault-rape drug, flunitrazepam (Rohypnol) produces disinhibition and voluntary muscle relaxation along with anterograde amnesia; alcohol potentiates the effects
C. Therapeutic interventions
1. Treatment for drug overdose
   a. Narcotic antagonists
      (1) Nalorphine (Nalline), a partial antagonist, or naloxone (Narcan), a pure antagonist, will improve respiratory rate, although they may not affect level of consciousness
      (2) Nalline will increase respiratory depression if barbiturates have also been used, so Narcan is the drug of choice when in doubt about the substance used
      (3) These antagonists completely or partially reverse narcotic depression and may produce an acute abstinence (withdrawal) syndrome by blocking the euphoric and physiologic effects of the narcotic
      (4) Symptoms of respiratory depression can recur when naloxone (Narcan) is metabolized
   b. Gastric lavage may be done if substance had been taken orally within the past several hours
2. Treatment for withdrawal symptoms
   a. Antidepressants seem to block the "high" from stimulant abuse and diminish the craving for the substance
   b. Clonidine (Catapres) suppresses narcotic withdrawal symptoms and decreases adrenergic excess while opiate receptors return to normal levels
      (1) Heroin addicts who are first stabilized on methadone before detoxification do better than those who go directly from heroin to Catapres
      (2) Catapres should not be used in those individuals who also abuse alcohol or

those who have unstable psychiatric or cardiovascular conditions

3. Methadone maintenance for opiate addiction: programs do not treat addiction, but change the addiction from an illegal drug to a legal drug, which is administered under supervision; has proved successful only in individuals with long-standing addictions
   a. Reduction in dosage can cause withdrawal symptoms
   b. Withdrawal symptoms begin to develop in 8 hours, reaching a peak in 3 days
   c. Methadone is approved for treatment of pregnant opioid addicts
   d. L-ALPHA acetylmethadol (LAAM) is an alternative to methadone; its 3-day effectiveness increases independence; it is an addictive narcotic with effects similar to morphine
4. High-calorie, high-protein, high-vitamin diet because of poor eating habits
5. Treatment in groups run by ex-addicts
6. Therapeutic community setting
7. Psychotherapy and family therapy on an outpatient basis
8. Vocational counseling

Nursing Care of Clients with Drug Abuse

A. ASSESSMENT
1. History of drugs being used
2. Urine toxicology screen and HIV test
3. Drug abuse screening test (DAST)
4. History of length and pattern of drug dependence
5. Time since last dose was taken
6. Physical status of the client for signs and symptoms of drug dependence; nutritional status
7. Symptoms of drug overdose or withdrawal
8. Degree of difficulty sustained by client in relation to family members, job, school, etc.
9. Why client is seeking treatment at this time
10. Pending criminal charges
11. Presence of hallucinations, paranoid ideation, and depression (often associated with cocaine use)
12. Potential for violence toward others or self
13. Relationship between substance use and psychiatric disorders (known as dual diagnosis)

B. ANALYSIS/NURSING DIAGNOSES
1. Anxiety related to threat to self-concept, inability to deal with responsibility, feelings of inadequacy
2. Impaired verbal communication related to mental confusion or CNS depression because of substance use
3. Acute confusion related to global changes and disturbances in attention, cognition, and psychomotor level of consciousness and changes in the wake/sleep cycle resulting from substance use
4. Chronic confusion related to changes in brain tissue resulting in impairment of intellect and personality, long-standing decreased intellectual capacity resulting in disturbances in memory, orientation, and behavior
5. Defensive coping related to denial of obvious problem, projection of blame/responsibility, rationalization of failures, and lack of participation in treatment or therapy
6. Dysfunctional family processes related to anger and frustration associated with client's negative response to attempts at assistance or support
7. Ineffective denial related to inability to admit impact of problem on pattern of life
8. Risk for injury related to altered cerebral or perceptual function, judgment, and mobility
9. Risk for loneliness related to social isolation from family and friends resulting from total involvement with addicting substance
10. Impaired memory related to neurologic disturbances and dysfunctions
11. Noncompliance with abstinence and supportive therapy related to inability to stop using substance because of dependence and refusal to alter lifestyle
12. Imbalanced nutrition: less than body requirements related to a lack of interest in food and chemical dependence
13. Self-esteem disturbance related to inability to meet role expectations, feelings of inadequacy and expectation of failure, and negative feelings about self
14. Risk for self-mutilation related to intake of mind-altering substances
15. Disturbed sensory perception (visual, kinesthetic, tactile) related to intake of mind-altering substances
16. Risk for violence: self-directed or directed at others, related to intake of mind-altering substances, misinterpretation of stimuli, and feelings of suspicion or distrust of others

C. PLANNING/IMPLEMENTATION
1. Set firm controls and keep area drug free when the client is hospitalized
2. Keep atmosphere pleasant and cheerful but not overly stimulating
3. Contribute to the client's self-confidence, self-respect, and security in a realistic manner
4. Walk the fine line between a relatively permissive and a firm attitude
5. Expect and accept evasion, manipulative behavior, and negativism, but require the client to shoulder certain standards of responsibility

6. Accept the client without approving the behavior
7. Do not permit the client to become isolated
8. Introduce the client to group activities as soon as possible; evaluate client's response to group interaction
9. Protect clients from themselves and others
10. Refer to appropriate 12-step group such as NA, AA, or CODA

D. EVALUATION/OUTCOMES
1. Recognizes, accepts, and seeks treatment for problem
2. Accepts responsibility for problem without blaming others
3. Achieves optimal physiologic and nutritional status
4. Learns new, more self-preserving coping mechanisms
5. Verbalizes feelings and emotions
6. Enters into and continues with community-based self-help program
7. Abstains from all mood-altering chemicals

SCHIZOPHRENIA AND OTHER PSYCHOTIC DISORDERS

Group of disorders characterized by psychosis, that may be acute and short-term or chronic and debilitating; includes schizophrenia, delusional paranoid and schizoaffective disorders; brief psychotic and shared psychotic disorders; psychotic disorders caused by medical conditions; and substance-induced psychotic disorders

▼ SCHIZOPHRENIC DISORDERS

Data Base
A. Etiologic factors
1. Foremost etiology today is the biologic perspective (neuroanatomy, genetics, endocrinology, and immunology all produce symptoms; trauma and disease as causation continue to be researched)
2. Biologic components
   a. Heredity and genetics
   b. Neuroanatomic differences and neurochemicals; e.g., dopamine hyperactivity
      (1) Structure and function of nervous system
      (2) Teratogenic drug exposure
      (3) Neuroanatomic differences in brain
   c. Neurotransmitter function: abnormal neurotransmitter–endocrine interactions
   d. Immunologic factors: viral exposure during pregnancy

   e. High arousal levels from stress, disease, drugs, and trauma
      (1) Stress such as bombardment of stimuli from life events may contribute to relapse and return of symptoms
      (2) Diseases such as prenatal virus exposure; encephalitis
      (3) Trauma from birth complications, head trauma, childhood accidents
      (4) Drugs such as cannabis and cocaine
3. Psychosocial considerations are significant; causative models postulate that vulnerability interacts with stressful environmental influences to produce the symptoms of schizophrenia
4. Onset in men is usually between ages 18 and 25 years; onset for women is later, between 25 and 35 years; approximately 3% to 10% of women have age onset after 40; incidence of schizophrenia slightly higher in men
5. Chronic insecurity and an almost total failure in interpersonal relationships develops
6. Etiology still unknown; however, a consistent finding through MRI studies shows an enlargement of the ventricles
7. Regardless of the ultimate etiology, a disturbed relationship with the environment and the family is an almost universal characteristic
8. Course of the disease: either acute or chronic; although it can stop or retrogress at any point, the disorder does not appear to permit a full restoration of integrity of the personality

B. Behavioral/clinical findings
1. Primary symptoms are often referred to as "the 4 A's"
   a. Disturbances in association, affect (flattened affect), ambivalence, and autistic thinking
   b. Additional "A's" include attention defects and activity disturbances
2. Characteristic symptoms generally fall into two broad categories: positive (additional behaviors) and negative (deficits of behaviors)
   a. Positive symptoms include delusions, hallucinations, thought disorders, disorganized speech, bizarre behavior, and inappropriate affect
   b. Negative symptoms include the A's: affect flattening, apathy/avolition, anhedonia, and attention deficit
3. Problems in cognitive functioning involve attention deficits, memory disturbance, abstract concept formation, decision making, and problem solving
4. Alterations in mood symptoms are dysphoria, suicidality, and hopelessness
5. Social and occupational role dysfunction
6. Duration of at least 6 months

C. Types
1. Although historically much time and effort were directed toward identifying types of schizophrenia, it should be recognized that the classification is not static; there is a great deal of overlapping symptomatology; individuals diagnosed as being in one classification frequently are diagnosed at a later time in another classification
2. Paranoid type: uses delusions of persecutory or grandiosity, or both, less often noted are delusional themes of jealousy, religiosity, or somatization
3. Disorganized type: uses disorganized speech and behavior and exhibits flat or inappropriate behavior; does not exhibit catatonic behaviors (psychomotor or language mimic)
4. Catatonic type: features marked psychomotor disturbance that may involve motor immobility (waxy flexibility), excessive motor activity, extreme negativism, mutism, posturing, echolalia, or echopraxia
5. Undifferentiated type: demonstrates delusions, hallucinations, disorganized speech, disorganized behavior, and does not demonstrate behaviors usually observed in paranoid, disorganized, or catatonic types
6. Residual type: criteria for schizophrenia and subtypes listed above are not met; there is continuing evidence of negative symptoms and two or more of these characteristic symptoms (delusions, hallucinations, disorganized speech, and gross disorganization)

D. Therapeutic interventions
1. Psychotherapy (individual, family, and group counseling)
2. Motivational therapy
3. Occupational and vocational therapy
4. Day-care treatment programs in community settings that foster interpersonal relationships
5. Paranoid schizophrenia appears to be the most responsive to treatment when compared to courses of other subtypes
6. Pharmacologic therapy: positive symptoms respond to traditional antipsychotic drugs; negative symptoms respond more effectively to atypical drugs (see Related Pharmacology)

Nursing Care of Clients with Schizophrenic Disorders

A. ASSESSMENT
1. History of start of disorder from client and family if available
2. Presence of delusional ideation (fixed false belief) and/or hallucinations (perceived stimuli without external stimuli)
3. Presence of suspiciousness and/or feelings of paranoia; may fear other clients and staff
4. History of work and social functioning
5. Presence of precipitating or current stress factors
6. Unclear or incomplete client and family communication patterns
7. Physiologic status

B. ANALYSIS/NURSING DIAGNOSES
1. Anxiety related to disturbed thought processes, pervasive ambivalence, mistrust of others, and difficulty in dealing with reality
2. Impaired verbal communication related to inappropriate use of words and unique patterns of speech, anxiety, and disturbed and disruptive thought processes
3. Risk for caregiver role strain related to disturbed behavior
4. Acute confusion related to abrupt onset or global changes and disturbances in attention, cognition and psychomotor level of consciousness, and changes in the wake/sleep cycle resulting from disturbed thinking patterns
5. Chronic confusion related to changes in functioning resulting in impairment of intellect and personality and long-standing decreased intellectual functioning resulting in disturbances in memory, orientation, and behavior
6. Compromised family coping: compromised or disabling, related to ambivalent family relationships and abusive or destructive behavior
7. Ineffective coping related to inability to meet basic needs, poorly developed or inappropriate use of defense mechanisms, and an inability to meet role expectations
8. Disturbed personal identity related to altered thought processes, detachment from reality, and the lack of boundaries between self and environment
9. Risk for injury related to sensory or perceptual deficits, cognitive or psychomotor deficits, and altered judgment
10. Feeding, bathing/hygiene, dressing/grooming, toileting self-care deficit related to perceptual or cognitive impairment, emotional dysfunction, and an increasing inability to carry out activities of daily living
11. Disturbed sensory perception (visual, auditory, kinesthetic, gustatory, tactile, olfactory) related to emotional misinterpretation of stimuli and inability to test reality
12. Impaired social interaction related to withdrawal, delusions and hallucinations, and distrust of others
13. Disturbed sleep pattern related to emotional dysfunction and the side effects of psychotropic drugs

14. Disturbed thought processes related to an inability to evaluate reality, a disturbed interpretation of environment, disturbed mental activities, and altered sensory perception, reception, and transmission
15. Risk for violence: self-directed or directed at others, related to feelings of suspicion or distrust of others, an inability to discharge emotions verbally, misinterpretation of stimuli, and disturbed thought processes

C. PLANNING/IMPLEMENTATION
1. Observe for adverse drug reactions whenever large doses of antipsychotic medications are being administered
2. Teach client to recognize and report extrapyramidal side effects to avoid physical discomforts
3. Administer antiparkinsonian agents to minimize EPS
4. Encourage the client to follow a plan of organized activity and the prescribed drug regimen
5. Encourage the client to continue medications even after symptoms abate
6. Respect the client as a human being with both dignity and worth
7. Accept the client at his or her present level of functioning; set limits on unacceptable behavior
8. Avoid trying to argue the client out of delusions or hallucinations
9. Accept that the client's hallucinations and delusions are real and possibly frightening; stay with and support client
10. Attempt to direct client's need to expiate guilt into safe expression
11. Encourage the development of interpersonal relationships between the client and others; help client learn to trust
12. Point out reality to the client but do not impose staff's concept of reality
13. Recognize that the client's ability to test reality is distorted by pathologic use of defenses
14. Recognize safety of the client, especially during acute phase; safety remains the highest priority because of poor judgment

D. EVALUATION/OUTCOMES
1. Remains free from adverse side effects of psychotropic drug regimen
2. Continues taking prescribed medications
3. Exhibits a decrease in hallucinations
4. Differentiates between hallucinations and reality
5. Remains free from injury to self and others
6. Demonstrates a reduction in anxiety through verbalizations or body language
7. Continues therapy after discharge

▼ DELUSIONAL (PARANOID) DISORDERS

Data Base
A. Etiologic factors
1. Individuals who demonstrate the suspiciousness and delusions common to paranoid conditions but do not exhibit the thinking and behavioral disorganization or the personality disintegration found in the other psychoses
2. Premorbid personality: uses the compensatory mechanisms of the projective pattern of behavior
3. Paranoid defenses considered by some to be a protective mechanism against unconscious homosexuality or overt hostility
4. Neurobiologic perspective
   a. The exact nature of the physiologic disruption is not well defined; it is thought that psychotic disorders involve an abnormality in the transmission of neural impulses, and that the difficulty occurs at the synaptic level and involves neurochemicals such as dopamine, serotonin, and norephinedrine
   b. Neurologic and cognitive impairments are less and prognosis seems better
   c. See Biologic Components under Schizophrenic Disorders
5. Cultural and religious background must be taken into account because variations exist in cultures and subcultures
B. Behavioral/clinical findings
1. Exhibits a rather elaborate, highly organized paranoid delusional system while preserving other functions of the personality
2. Apart from the impact of the delusions, thinking and functioning is not interfered with, nor is it bizarre
3. Personality function continues
4. Delusions are drawn from real-life situations and have a coherent theme
5. Hallucinations are not prominent; if present they are usually auditory and are related to the delusional theme
6. Predominant theme of delusions determines type of paranoia (e.g., grandiose, jealous, persecutory)
7. Intellectual and occupational functioning less impaired than social or marital relationships
C. Types
1. Erotomanic: delusion that another person is in love with the client; idealized, romantic love or spiritual union rather than sexual attraction is basic to this type
2. Grandiose: theme centers around client having some great (but unrecognized) talent or insight

or having made an important discovery; less commonly, the individual claims a special relationship with a prominent person or claims to be a prominent person

3. Jealous: unfaithfulness in one's spouse or lover based upon incorrect inferences is the central theme of this type

4. Persecutory: delusion that one is being conspired against, spied upon, cheated, followed, poisoned or drugged, maligned, harassed, or obstructed in the pursuit of long-term goals

5. Somatic: delusions involving bodily functions or sensations

D. Therapeutic interventions

1. Pharmacotherapy with neuroleptics considered most helpful (see Related Pharmacology)

2. Individual psychotherapy may provide some relief of symptoms

3. The course of paranoid disorders varies but is more hopeful than other psychotic disorders, because they are most responsive to treatment

Nursing Care of Clients with Delusional (Paranoid) Disorders

A. ASSESSMENT

1. History of start of disorder from client and family if available

2. Presence of hallucinations and delusional ideation; may constitute a danger to self or others

3. Presence of suspiciousness; paranoid feelings are usually limited to specific areas in the client's life

4. Absence of odd or bizarre behavior and other criteria related to schizophrenia

5. Social and marital functioning

B. ANALYSIS/NURSING DIAGNOSES

1. Anxiety related to disturbed thought processes about specific areas, mistrust of others, difficulty in dealing with certain aspects of reality, and threats to security

2. Ineffective coping related to poorly developed or inappropriate use of defense mechanisms

3. Risk for loneliness related to mistrust of others and threats to security

4. Self-esteem disturbance related to perceptual or cognitive impairment, feelings of grandiosity, and/or feelings of persecution

5. Disturbed thought processes related to misinterpretations of events

6. Risk for violence: directed at others, related to feelings of suspicion or distrust of others and misinterpretation of stimuli

C. PLANNING/IMPLEMENTATION

1. Provide an environment with some intellectual challenges that do not threaten security

2. Avoid counteraggression and retaliation against the client

3. Accept and recognize the client's need for a superior attitude

4. Meet sarcasm and ridicule in a matter-of-fact manner

5. Guard the client's self-esteem from attack by other clients

6. Accept the client's misinterpretations of events

7. Point out reality but do not directly challenge the client's delusions

D. EVALUATION/OUTCOMES

1. Continues to function in society

2. Avoids factors that stimulate delusional thinking

▼ SCHIZOAFFECTIVE DISORDER

Data Base

A. Etiologic factors

1. This disturbance is unrelated to the direct physiologic effects of a substance or medication or a general medical condition

2. An interrupted period of illness including a major depressive episode or manic episode concurrent with symptoms of schizophrenia (delusions or hallucinations, disorganized speech or behavior, and negative symptoms)

3. Occurs in early adulthood

B. Behavioral/clinical findings

1. Demonstrates a mixture of symptoms from both schizophrenia and mood disorders

2. The thought processes and bizarre behavior appear schizophrenic, but there is usually marked elation or depression; often proves to be basically schizophrenic in nature

C. Therapeutic interventions

1. Antipsychotic or antidepressant agents may be used to treat symptoms

2. Therapy depends on the type and severity of the symptoms exhibited

Nursing Care of Clients with a Schizoaffective Disorder

See Nursing Care of Clients with Schizophrenic Disorders and Bipolar Disorders (Depressive/Manic Episode)

MOOD DISORDERS

Characterized by a disturbance of mood, encompassing two emotional extremes; individual demonstrates the vehement energy of mania, the despair and lethargy of depression, or both

FUNDAMENTAL PRINCIPLES WHEN CARING FOR CLIENTS WITH MOOD DISORDERS

A. Monitor nutritional intake and elimination
B. Keep the environment nonchallenging and nonstimulating
C. Observe children or adolescents for irritable mood and observe adults for depressive episodes
D. Protect the client against suicide during the entire episode; keep under constant observation if necessary
E. Keep activities simple, uncomplicated, and repetitive in nature; they should be of short duration and should require little concentration
F. Observe for adverse effects of drugs; monitor lithium blood levels weekly and white cell count less often
G. Encourage the client to continue medications even after symptoms abate
H. Caution and teach the client regarding special dietary precautions with lithium and the MAO inhibitors
I. Plan for follow-up support and supervision

▼ BIPOLAR DISORDERS

Data Base

A. Presence of one or more manic or hypomanic episodes in a client with a history of depressive episodes
  1. Hypomanic episode: a distinct period of elevated or irritable mood that is clearly different from the nondepressive mood; duration at least 4 days; hypomania is mood elation with higher than usual activity and social interaction, but not as expansive as full mania
  2. The predominant mood is elevated or irritable, accompanied by one or more of these symptoms: hyperactivity, lack of judgment with no regard for consequences, pressured speech, flight of ideas, distractibility, inflated self-esteem, and hypersexuality
  3. Although the functioning level is altered, there is no marked impairment
  4. Mania is an elevated, expansive, or irritable mood accompanied by hyperactivity, grandiosity, and loss of reality
B. Neurobiologic perspective
  1. Neurotransmitters, or certain chemicals in the brain that regulate mood, have been identified (serotonin, dopamine, norepinephrine, and gamma amino butric acid)
  2. Research suggests this disorder results from complex interactions among chemicals, including neurotransmitters and hormones

  3. Family and twin studies suggest a genetic component, but the modes of transmission have not been identified
  4. Biologic rhythms and physiology related to depression show abnormal sleep EEGs, sensitivity to absence of sunlight, and circadian rhythm disturbance.
  5. Physiologic theory postulates that mood may also respond to drugs or a variety of physical illnesses
    a. Drugs associated with depressive status: alcohol, sedative-hypnotics, amphetamine withdrawal, glucocorticoids, propranolol, resperine, and steroidal contraceptives
    b. Drugs associated with manic status: cocaine, MAOIs, tricyclic antidepressants, steroids, and levodopa
    c. Physical illness, such as stroke, Cushing's disease, and some endocrine disorders can lead to depressive episodes
C. Generally occurs between 20 and 40 years of age, although it has been reported in clients older than 50 years
D. Usually a response to a loss, change in life events, or role change
E. Increased levels of norepinephine, dopamine, and serotonin in acute mania
F. Decreased levels of norepinephine, dopamine, and serotonin in depression
G. Cyclic, periodic episodes of acute self-limiting mood swings; can be all manic, all depressed, or mixed manic and depressed
H. Resumption of customary activities between episodes
I. Obesity a frequent precursor of an attack; onset can be slowed or modified by dieting

▼ DEPRESSIVE EPISODE OF A BIPOLAR DISORDER

Data Base

A. Etiologic factors
  See Data Base under Bipolar Disorder
B. Behavioral/clinical findings
  1. Prime symptoms are either a depressed mood or loss of interest or pleasure, occurring during a 2-week period, with a change in level of functioning, plus five or more of the following: change in weight, insomnia, psychomotor agitation or retardation, fatigue, worthless feelings or inappropriate guilt, concentration difficulties, death thoughts, suicidal ideation, or suicidal attempt
  2. Orientation and logic unaffected
  3. Sex drive decreased

4. Constipation and urinary retention may occur
5. Depression and suicidal gestures may increase as anniversary of loss of loved object nears
C. Therapeutic interventions
1. Dexamethasone suppression test (DST): used to identify depressed clients who may be responsive to antidepressant drug therapy or electroconvulsant therapy (ECT)
2. Electroconvulsive therapy to reduce depression; drugs such as succinylcholine chloride (Anectine), a depolarizing muscle relaxant causing paralysis, are used to reduce the intensity of muscle contractions during the convulsive stage; used most often for clients with recurrent depressions, delusions, suicidal ideation, and those who are resistant to drug therapy; may cause temporary memory loss
3. High-protein, high-carbohydrate diet is provided for energy; dietary supplements may be necessary
4. Psychotherapy
5. Pharmacologic approach in depressive phase: antidepressant drugs that increase the level of norepinephrine at subcortical neuroeffector sites (see Related Pharmacology)

Nursing Care of Clients During a Depressive Episode of a Bipolar Disorder

A. ASSESSMENT
1. Presence of feelings of worthlessness, guilt, and suicidal ideation or acting out; presence of a plan increases the danger of suicide
2. Presence of depressed mood, loss of interest or pleasure, and slowing of psychomotor activity
3. Weight for recent changes and to establish a baseline
4. Changes in sleep patterns
5. Changes in the ability to concentrate

B. ANALYSIS/NURSING DIAGNOSES
1. Anxiety related to disturbed thought processes, difficulty in dealing with reality and feelings of failure and unworthiness
2. Impaired verbal communication related to lethargy, psychomotor depression, and an inability to verbalize feelings and thoughts
3. Dysfunctional grieving related to actual or perceived object loss
4. Risk for injury related to impaired judgment
5. Risk for loneliness related to feelings of depression that can become contagious, keeping others at a distance
6. Imbalanced nutrition: less than body requirements, related to a lack of interest in food and feelings of unworthiness
7. Ineffective role performance related to emotional dysfunction and feelings of inadequacy

8. Feeding, bathing/hygiene, dressing/grooming self-care deficit related to disinterest in activities of daily living
9. Self-esteem disturbance related to disturbed sensory perceptions resulting in somatic delusions and feelings of inadequacy
10. Disturbed sleep pattern related to emotional dysfunction and side effects of psychotropic drugs
11. Social isolation related to object loss and alterations in mental function
12. Disturbed thought processes related to impaired judgment, an impaired ability to make decisions, an altered attention span, and an overinvolvement with or withdrawal from environment
13. Risk for violence: self-directed or directed toward others, related to the inability to discharge emotions verbally, disturbed thought processes, and feelings of unworthiness

C. PLANNING/IMPLEMENTATION
1. See Fundamental Principles When Caring for Clients with Mood Disorders
2. Accept client's inability to carry out daily routines; assist with ADLs
3. Set expectations that can be achieved by the client
4. Help client express hostility and accept client's responses without rejection
5. Provide realistic praise whenever possible
6. Involve client in simple repetitious tasks and activities
7. Accept client's feelings of worthlessness as real; client's feelings should not be denied, condoned, or approved
8. Protect client against suicidal acting out, especially when the depression begins to lift; suicide is a real and ever-present danger throughout the entire illness
9. Spend time with client to demonstrate staff's recognition of client's worth
10. Recognize that client has ambivalence about suicide and is fearful of feelings
11. Teach client about ECT treatments; stay with client following treatment; orient as necessary

D. EVALUATION/OUTCOMES
1. Avoids acting out suicidal ideation
2. Verbalizes feelings
3. Verbalizes increased feelings of self-worth
4. Continues prescribed treatment regimen
5. Returns to preillness level of function

▼ MANIC EPISODE OF A BIPOLAR DISORDER

Data Base
A. Etiologic factors
See Data Base under Bipolar Disorder

B. Behavioral/clinical findings
   1. Abnormally and persistently elevated, expansive, or irritable mood for a duration of 1 week
   2. Three or more of the following symptoms are noted: grandiosity, insomnia, verbosity, flight of ideas, distractibility, increase in goal-directed behavior or psychomotor agitation, excessive involvement in pleasurable activities without regard for consequences
   3. Marked impairment in occupational and social activities and in relationships
   4. Extreme overactivity requires hospitalization to prevent harm to self or others
   5. Marked impairment in functioning
   6. Symptoms are unrelated to a general medical condition or physiologic effects of a substance
C. Therapeutic interventions
   1. High-protein, high-carbohydrate diet is provided for energy; handheld foods should be available
   2. Psychotherapy
   3. Pharmacologic approach: improves productivity by decreasing psychomotor activity or response to environmental stimuli (see Related Pharmacology)

Nursing Care of Clients During the Manic Episode of a Bipolar Disorder

A. ASSESSMENT
   1. Rapid increase in manic behavior
   2. Presence of elevated mood
   3. Increased psychomotor agitation
   4. Impairment in functioning
   5. Feelings of grandiosity and euphoria
   6. Nutrition, hygiene, and rest patterns
   7. Danger to self or others
   8. Physiologic status

B. ANALYSIS/NURSING DIAGNOSES
   1. Anxiety related to disturbed thought processes and difficulty in dealing with reality and feelings of failure and unworthiness
   2. Impaired verbal communication related to pressured speech and psychomotor activity
   3. Risk for injury related to impaired judgment
   4. Risk for loneliness related to disturbing behavior that keeps people at a distance
   5. Imbalanced nutrition: less than body requirements, related to hyperactivity and excessive expenditure of calories, an inability to sit down long enough to eat, and a lack of interest in food
   6. Ineffective coping related to intrusive and taunting behaviors
   7. Self-esteem disturbance related to emotional dysfunction and feelings of grandiosity
   8. Disturbed sleep pattern related to emotional dysfunction and side effects of psychotropic drugs
   9. Social isolation related to alterations in mental function
   10. Disturbed thought processes related to impaired judgment, impaired ability to make decisions, altered attention span, and an overinvolvement with or withdrawal from environment
   11. Risk for violence: self-directed or directed toward others, related to the inability to discharge emotions verbally, disturbed thought processes, and feelings of unworthiness

C. PLANNING/IMPLEMENTATION
   1. See Fundamental Principles When Caring for Clients with Mood Disorders
   2. Accept client while rejecting objectionable behavior
   3. Permit expression of hostility and ambivalence without reinforcement of guilt feelings; usually precipitated by anxiety
   4. Approach in a calm, collected manner and maintain self-control
   5. Set limits for behavior
   6. Communicate in a nonargumentative manner
   7. Use client's easy distractibility to interrupt hyperactive behavior to avoid injury and exhaustion
   8. Advise all caregivers to approach client in a consistent manner
   9. Prevent physical exhaustion and maintain physical health; provide foods that can be eaten on the run
   10. Maintain environmental safety for client, other clients, and staff
   11. Direct and channel client's energy into safe, controlled activities
   12. Maintain client's contact with reality by helping with grooming and dressing
   13. Monitor medications and side effects
   14. Educate family as to early symptoms of hypomanic episode

D. EVALUATION/OUTCOMES
   1. Exhibits a decrease in manic behavior
   2. Verbalizes feelings of increased self-worth
   3. Displays improvement in judgment
   4. Decreases use of caustic humor
   5. Relaxes more readily
   6. Maintains adequate nutrition
   7. Adheres to medication regimen
   8. Demonstrates an absence of destructive behaviors

▼ MAJOR DEPRESSION

Data Base
A. Etiologic factors
   1. See Data Bases under Bipolar Disorder and Depressive Episode of a Bipolar Disorder

2. Neurotransmitter dysregulation includes serotonin, norepinephrine, dopamine, acetylcholine, and GAMBA systems; neuropeptides are also altered, including corticotrophin-releasing hormones
3. Individuals with chronic or severe general medical conditions are at increased risk
4. Psychosocial stressors associated with a major loss play a significant role in first or second depressive onset
5. Familial history among close biologic relatives increases risk for this disorder
6. Onset usually occurs in late 20s, but may occur across the life span

B. Behavioral/clinical findings
1. Diminished interest or pleasure in all activities
2. Decreased appetite with weight loss, or overeating with weight gain
3. Psychomotor retardation
4. Anxiety, tearfulness, fearfulness, and hopelessness
5. Insomnia or hypersomnia
6. Feelings of worthlessness
7. Inappropriate guilt
8. Interruption in thinking and concentration that may interfere with occupational and social functioning
9. Recurrent thoughts of death; suicidal ideation with or without a specific plan to carry it out
10. Associated with high mortality rates, especially in individuals older than 55 years

C. Therapeutic interventions
See Fundamental Principles When Caring for Clients with Mood Disorders

Nursing Care of Clients with Major Depression

A. See Fundamental Principles When Caring for Clients with Mood Disorders
B. See Nursing Care of Clients During the Depressive Episode of a Bipolar Disorder

▼ MAJOR DEPRESSION—MELANCHOLIC TYPE

Data Base

A. Etiologic factors
1. Frequently there is a history of a previous major depressive episode
2. Depression can be expressed through psychomotor retardation or agitation; usually rigid, inflexible, overassertive, overconscientious, overly meticulous, and worrisome with few outside interests
3. Depression occurs after 40 years of age and before 60 years of age

4. Precipitating factors such as the marriage of children, loss of a job, breakup of a marriage, or death of a partner frequently are identified
5. Depression often closely related to the menopause or climacteric; hormonal and endocrine changes are considered by many to play an important role, although current thinking does not make a distinction between this depression and depressions occurring at other periods of life
6. See Data Base for Major Depression

B. Behavioral/clinical findings
Loss of interest or lack of reactivity to usually pleasurable stimuli, plus three or more of the following: distinct quality of the depressed mood, morning depression that is worse than other times, early morning awakening, psychomotor agitation or retardation, significant anorexia or weight loss, excessive or inappropriate guilt

C. Therapeutic interventions
1. Treatment with antidepressant medications and psychotherapy; with recurring episodes anticipate treatment with ECT and maintenance medications
2. See Depressive Episode of Bipolar Disorder

Nursing Care of Clients with a Major Depression—Melancholic Type

A. See Fundamental Principles When Caring for Clients with Mood Disorders
B. See Nursing Care of Clients During the Depressive Episode of a Bipolar Disorder

▼ CYCLOTHYMIC DISORDER

Data Base

A. Etiologic factors
1. There are numerous hypomanic episodes dispersed with periods of depressed mood and lack of interest in pleasurable activities
2. No evidence of true manic or major depressive episodes
3. Symptom-free intervals are generally shorter than 2 months' duration
4. The mood disturbance is not due to physiologic effects of substances or to a medical condition
5. Duration: at least 2 years in adults; in children/adolescents, mood can be irritable for at least 1 year

B. Behavioral/clinical findings
1. Alternating mood swings between elation and sadness; apparently unrelated to external environment
2. Individual is regarded as temperamental, moody, unpredictable, inconsistent, or unreliable
3. Mood swings do not demonstrate great emotional intensity

4. Refer to Data Base under Bipolar Disorder for hypomanic symptoms
C. Therapeutic interventions
   1. Often unnecessary; if required, same as for Depressive or Manic Episode of Bipolar Disorder
   2. Medication often unnecessary; if required, same as for Depressive or Manic Episode of Bipolar Disorder

Nursing Care of Clients with a Cyclothymic Disorder

A. See Fundamental Principles When Caring for Clients with Mood Disorders
B. See Nursing Care of Clients During the Depressive Episode of a Bipolar Disorder
C. See Nursing Care of Clients During the Manic Episode of a Bipolar Disorder

▼ DYSTHYMIC DISORDER

Data Base

A. Etiologic factors
   1. Biochemical theories continue to be researched
   2. Genetic transmission theories of mood disorders are derived from family studies
   3. Depression is real and suicide can occur
   4. Feelings of guilt or brooding about the past
B. Behavioral/clinical findings
   1. Depressed mood for most of day
   2. Duration: at least 2 years in adults; in children and adolescents, mood can be irritable for at least 1 year
   3. Two or more of the following: poor appetite or overeating, insomnia, low energy or fatigue, low self-esteem, concentration/problem-solving difficulties, feelings of hopelessness
   4. Impairment in social, occupational, and other roles
   5. No evidence of manic or hypomanic episodes in present or past history
   6. In children/adolescents the symptoms noted are irritability and depression; low self-esteem, poor social skills, and pessimism; school performance and social interactions are impaired
C. Therapeutic interventions
   1. Often unnecessary; if required, same as for Depressive Episode of Bipolar Disorder
   2. Medication often unnecessary; if required, same as for Depressive Episode of Bipolar Disorder

Nursing Care of Clients with a Dysthymic Disorder

A. See Fundamental Principles when Caring for Clients with Mood Disorders

B. See Nursing Care of Clients During the Depressive Episode of a Bipolar Disorder

ANXIETY DISORDERS

Most common of all psychiatric disorders resulting in considerable distress and functional impairment; rarely treated in inpatient psychiatric settings. Rigid, repetitive, and ineffective behaviors are used to try to control anxiety; there is no great deficit in reality testing or severe antisocial behavior

FUNDAMENTAL PRINCIPLES WHEN CARING FOR CLIENTS WITH ANXIETY DISORDERS

A. Establish a trusting relationship
B. Accept symptoms as real to the individual
C. Attempt to limit the use of defenses, but do not stop them until the individual is ready to give them up
D. Encourage the individual to develop a balance between work and play so anxiety is lessened
E. Help the individual develop better ways of handling anxiety-producing situations through problem solving
F. Accept physical symptoms but do not emphasize or call attention to them
G. Reduce demands on the individual as much as possible
H. Recognize when anxiety is interrupting ability to think clearly
I. Intervene to protect client from acting out on impulses that may harm self or others; recognize client is acting out because of fear, not antisocial behavior
J. Determine comorbidity of anxiety disorders and depression because they frequently occur simultaneously

▼ PANIC DISORDERS

Data Base

A. Etiologic factors
   1. Biochemical and genetic theories are most often cited as the underlying cause of anxiety disorders; no one gene or biochemical dysfunction has been singled out
   2. Recurrent attacks of severe anxiety may not be associated with a stimulus but can occur spontaneously
   3. Development of symptoms usually permits some measure of social adjustment
   4. Onset varies, most often noted between late adolescence and mid 30s; a small number of cases begin in childhood, or after age 45

5. Early life rigid and orderly
6. Pressures of decision making regarding lifestyle that occur in the early adult years seem to act as precipitating factors
7. Discrete periods of intense discomfort or fear for more than 1 month in duration

B. Behavioral/clinical findings

Period of intense fear or discomfort resulting in four or more of the following symptoms: palpitations or accelerated heart rate, sweating, trembling or shaking, shortness of breath, feelings of choking, chest pain or discomfort, nausea or abdominal distress, depersonalization, fear of losing control, fear of dying, paresthesias, and chills or hot flashes

C. Therapeutic interventions
1. Complete medical workup to reassure the individual and rule out illness
2. Psychotherapy, family therapy, group therapy
3. Sedatives and antianxiety agents useful when client is unable to cope or accomplish daily activities

Nursing Care of Clients with Panic Disorders

A. ASSESSMENT
1. Increase in somatic symptoms and complaints
2. Interference in activities of daily living and social and occupational functioning
3. Situational triggers may or may not precipitate the onset of an attack
4. Determine if panic symptoms relate to an agoraphobic situation

B. ANALYSIS/NURSING DIAGNOSES
1. Anxiety related to a threat to security or self-concept, or a recall of traumatic experiences
2. Ineffective coping related to an inability to meet role expectations or a pervasive anxiety and fear
3. Decisional conflict related to pervasive anxiety
4. Fear related to feelings of panic, altered judgment, and pervasive anxiety
5. Risk for injury related to flight from the stress-producing object or situation, feelings of panic, and altered judgment
6. Powerlessness related to overwhelming, pervasive anxiety
7. Impaired adjustment related to pervasive anxiety and an inability to meet role expectations
8. Impaired social interaction related to pervasive anxiety and irrational fear
9. Risk for violence: self-directed or directed toward others, related to altered judgment and pervasive anxiety and fear

C. PLANNING/IMPLEMENTATION
1. See Fundamental Principles When Caring for Clients with Anxiety Disorders

2. Remain with client during an attack
3. Do not get caught up in client's panic; remain calm and in control of the situation
4. Recognize that clients usually have less anxiety in private rooms with decreased environmental stimulation

D. EVALUATION/OUTCOMES
1. Identifies situations that increase anxiety
2. Demonstrates increased use of anxiety-reducing behaviors
3. Follows prescribed treatment regimen
4. Reports a decreased number of panic attacks

▼ PHOBIC DISORDERS

Data Base

A. Etiologic factors
1. Multiple theories as to the cause (genetic, psychologic, developmental, and environmental) are being studied; etiology remains unverified
2. Development of the phobia usually permits some measure of social adjustment
3. Onset begins in childhood; traumatic phobias can occur throughout the life span
4. Early life rigid and orderly
5. Pressures of decision making regarding lifestyle that occur in the early adult years seem to act as precipitating factors
6. Anxiety unconsciously transferred to an inanimate object or situation, which then symbolically represents the conflict and can be avoided
7. Anxiety is severe if the object, situation, or activity cannot be avoided

B. Behavioral/clinical findings
1. Anxiety appears when clients find themselves in places that threaten their sense of security
2. Attempts are made to avoid these distressing situations
3. Depending on the phobic object, the individual's lifestyle is often greatly limited
4. Fear of being trapped, embarrassed, or humiliated in social situations
5. Adults recognize that the fear is excessive or unreasonable

C. Types
1. Agoraphobia: fear of being alone or in public places where help would not be immediately available if necessary; includes tunnels, bridges, crowds, buses, and trains
2. Social phobia: fear of public speaking or situations in which public scrutiny may occur
3. Specific phobia: fear of a specific object, animal, or situation

D. Therapeutic interventions

1. Same as Panic Disorders
2. Behavior modification: a counter-conditioning technique to overcome fears by gradually increasing exposure to the feared object, situation, or animal (desensitization)
3. Pharmacologic and cognitive therapies

Nursing Care of Clients with Phobic Disorders

A. ASSESSMENT
1. Behaviors associated with anxiety disorders
2. Presence, type, and duration of phobia (at least 6 months)
3. Interference in activities of daily living and social and occupational functioning
4. Behaviors used to avoid phobic object or stress-producing situations

B. ANALYSIS/NURSING DIAGNOSES
1. Anxiety related to a threat to security and self-concept and feelings of inadequacy
2. Ineffective coping related to inability to meet role expectations, difficulty in meeting basic needs, and a pervasive anxiety and fear
3. Fear related to pervasive anxiety
4. Risk for injury related to flight from the stress-producing object or situation
5. Powerlessness related to overwhelming, pervasive anxiety
6. Impaired social interaction related to pervasive anxiety and irrational fear
7. Risk for violence: self-directed or directed toward others, related to altered judgment and pervasive anxiety and fear

C. PLANNING/IMPLEMENTATION
1. See Fundamental Principles When Caring for Clients with Anxiety Disorders
2. Recognize client's feelings about phobic object or situation
3. Provide constant support if exposure to phobic object or situation cannot be avoided
4. Assist with relaxation techniques to control or diminish anxiety levels

D. EVALUATION/OUTCOMES
1. Tolerates desensitization process
2. Deals with anxiety-producing object or situation effectively
3. Follows prescribed treatment regimen
4. Utilizes relaxation techniques to diminish anxiety

▼ OBSESSIVE-COMPULSIVE DISORDERS (OCD)

Data Base
A. Etiologic factors
1. Decreased levels of serotonin

2. OCD is a chronic anxiety disorder that responds to different treatment strategies
3. With stress, symptoms of thoughts, impulses, and images worsen
4. Pressures of decision making regarding life-style that occur in the early adult years seem to act as precipitating factors
5. Unconscious control of anxiety by the use of rituals and thoughts
6. Either obsessions or compulsions are recognized as excessive and interfere with daily activities
7. Some evidence that early life patterns were rigid and orderly

B. Behavioral/clinical findings
1. Major defensive mechanisms utilized are isolation, undoing, and reaction formation
2. Thoughts persist and become repetitive and obsessive
3. Some research notes that compulsive behavior precedes obsessive thinking
4. Client is indecisive and demonstrates a striving for perfection and superiority
5. Intellectual and verbal defenses are used
6. Anxiety and depression may be present in various degrees, particularly if rituals are prevented
7. Adults experiencing this disorder usually recognize that obsessions or compulsions are excessive or unreasonable; children do not have this insight
8. Obsessions or compulsions interfere with activities of daily living, occupation, social activities, or relationships and consume more than 1 hour per day
9. OCD symptoms are similar in adults and children

C. Therapeutic interventions
1. Refer to Panic Disorders for similarities
2. Behavior modification to attempt to limit the length and/or frequency of ritual
3. Cognitive therapy
4. Pharmacologic treatment: clomipramine (Anafranil) and fluvoxamine (Luvox) to control symptoms
5. Electroconvulsive therapy (ECT) when depressive suicidal ideation has not abated with psychotropic medications

Nursing Care of Clients with Obsessive-Compulsive Disorders

A. ASSESSMENT
1. Behavior associated with anxiety disorders
2. Type and use of ritual or obsession
3. Level of interference in life style
4. Degree of anxiety experienced by the client
5. Extent of danger inherent in the ritual or obsession

B. ANALYSIS/NURSING DIAGNOSES

1. Anxiety related to a threat to security and self-concept
2. Ineffective coping related to an inability to meet role expectations, difficulty in meeting basic needs, and pervasive anxiety and fear
3. Decisional conflict related to pervasive anxiety and altered judgment
4. Risk for injury related to altered judgment
5. Powerlessness related to overwhelming, pervasive anxiety
6. Ineffective role performance related to pervasive anxiety and an inability to meet role expectations
7. Impaired social interaction related to pervasive anxiety and irrational fear
8. Risk for violence: self-directed or directed toward others, related to pervasive anxiety and fear

C. PLANNING/IMPLEMENTATION

1. See Fundamental Principles When Caring for Clients with Anxiety Disorders
2. Recognize that the client understands that the ritual has no rational basis but cannot control it
3. Allow the client to continue the ritual but attempt to limit the length and frequency of the ritual
4. Support clients in their attempt to reduce dependency on the ritual
5. Role model appropriate behavior and discuss adaptive responses with client

D. EVALUATION/OUTCOMES

1. Demonstrates decrease in need to perform ritual or continue obsession
2. Controls anxiety without ritual or obsession
3. Follows prescribed treatment regimen
4. Learns new adaptive coping responses
5. Decreases use of anxiety-binding activities and increases time in completing tasks of daily living, social/recreational activities

▼ POSTTRAUMATIC STRESS DISORDERS

Data Base

A. Etiologic factors

1. Follows a devastating event that is outside the range of usual human experience (e.g., rape, assault, military combat, hostage situations)
2. Individual's response must involve intense fear, helplessness, or horror; in children the response must involve disorganized or agitated behaviors
3. The traumatic event is persistently reexperienced as flashbacks, distressing dreams, sense of reliving the experience, or exposure to situations that foster recall of the event (including anniversaries)

B. Behavioral/clinical findings

1. Exposure to a traumatic event resulting in actual death, threatened death, or serious injury to others or self and/or responding to the event with intense fear, helplessness, or horror; onset at any age
2. Feeling of isolation and detachment
3. Difficulty sleeping
4. Violent outbursts of anger
5. Depression
6. Interrupted concentration
7. Hypervigilance
8. Avoidance of associated stimuli
9. Duration of disturbance more than 1 month
10. Neurobiology of PTSD does not follow stress response, study indicates a hyperresponsiveness to a variety of stimuli

C. Therapeutic interventions

1. Same as Panic Disorders
2. Behavior modification to provide controlled exposure to recall of the event
3. Supportive therapy
4. Use of Eye Movement, Desensitization, Reprocessing techniques (EMDR)
5. Imagery, relaxation, and meditation may also be useful

Nursing Care of Clients with Posttraumatic Stress Disorders

A. ASSESSMENT

1. Behavior associated with anxiety disorders
2. History of traumatic experience
3. Sleep-pattern disturbances
4. Screening for symptoms of major depression, phobias, and substance abuse
5. Presence of depression, outbursts of anger, and/or decreased concentration

B. ANALYSIS/NURSING DIAGNOSES

1. Anxiety related to threat to security and self-concept and recall of traumatic experiences
2. Ineffective coping related to an inability to meet role expectations, and pervasive anxiety and fear
3. Fear related to feelings of panic, altered judgment, and pervasive anxiety
4. Risk for injury related to flight from the stress-producing object or situation, feelings of panic, and altered judgment
5. Powerlessness related to overwhelming, pervasive anxiety
6. Compromised family coping related to disturbed relationships, pervasive anxiety, and an inability to meet role expectations

7. Impaired social interaction related to pervasive anxiety
8. Post-trauma response related to unusual life experience causing avoidance of traumatic-associated stimuli and a numbing of general responsiveness
9. Risk for violence: self-directed or directed toward others, related to pervasive anxiety and fear

C. PLANNING/IMPLEMENTATION
1. See Fundamental Principles When Caring for Clients with Anxiety Disorders
2. Stay with client when memory of the event returns to the conscious level
3. Protect client from acting out violently with disregard for safety of self or others

D. EVALUATION/OUTCOMES
1. Uses coping mechanisms to more realistically deal with the traumatic event
2. Verbalizes decrease in dreams or flashbacks regarding the traumatic event
3. Follows prescribed treatment regimen
4. Demonstrates new adaptive ways of coping with anxiety

▼ GENERALIZED ANXIETY DISORDERS

Data Base
A. Etiologic factors
1. Psychologic, behavioral, and psychobiologic theories are all offered; the latter theory is most promising
2. Development of the anxiety usually permits some measure of social adjustment
3. Commonly begins in early 20s as a result of environmental factors in childhood
4. Early life rigid and orderly
5. Pressures of decision making regarding lifestyle that occur in the early adult years seem to act as precipitating factors
6. Excessive anxiety and worry about at least two life situations
B. Behavioral/clinical findings
1. Excessive anxiety and worry about a number of events or activities for a 6-month duration
2. Unable to control the worry
3. Anxiety and worry associated with three or more of the following symptoms: restlessness or feeling on edge, easily fatigued, difficulty concentrating, irritability, muscle tension, and sleep disturbance
4. Impairment in social or occupational relationships caused by anxiety, worry, and physical symptoms
5. Anxiety is not due to direct physiologic effects of substances or a medical condition

6. Symptoms of autonomic hyperarousal (tachycardia, shortness of breath, and dizziness) are less prominent than in other anxiety disorders
C. Therapeutic interventions
Same as Panic Disorder

Nursing Care of Clients with Generalized Anxiety Disorders
A. See Fundamental Principles When Caring for Clients with Anxiety Disorders
B. See Nursing Care of Clients with a Panic Disorder

SOMATOFORM DISORDERS

FUNDAMENTAL PRINCIPLES WHEN CARING FOR CLIENTS WITH SOMATOFORM DISORDERS
A. Establish a trusting relationship
B. Recognize a pattern of multiple recurring clinically significant somatic complaints; symptoms are real to client
C. Attempt to limit the use of defenses, but do not stop them until the individual is ready to give them up
D. Encourage the individual to develop a balance between work and play so anxiety is lessened
E. Help the individual develop better ways of handling anxiety-producing situations through problem solving
F. Accept physical symptoms but do not emphasize or call attention to them
G. Minimize sick-role behavior
H. Help client identify and label needs met by symptoms

▼ CONVERSION DISORDERS

Data Base
A. Etiologic factors
1. Anxiety unconsciously converted to physical symptoms that are not under voluntary control; these symptoms permit the individual to avoid some unacceptable activity
2. Development of symptoms usually permits some measure of social adjustment
3. Generally begins before 30 years of age
4. Early life often rigid and orderly; physical illness frequently used by the family as an excuse for problems
5. Pressures of decision making regarding lifestyle in the early adult years seem to be precipitating factors
B. Behavioral/clinical findings

1. Presence of symptoms or deficits affecting voluntary motor or sensory function
2. Conflicts or stressors, usually dependence vs independence, precede the initiation or exacerbation of symptoms or deficits (paralysis, blindness, deafness)
3. Noticeable lack of concern about the problem; this lack of concern has been labeled "la belle indifférence"
4. Impairment may vary over different episodes and does not follow anatomic structure; paralysis or numbness may circle the foot or arm instead of beginning at the joint and is known as stocking-and-glove anesthesia
5. The individual appears relieved by symptoms and demonstrates little anxiety when observed
6. The symptom or deficit is not related to an underlying medical condition, to substances, or to a cultural norm

C. Therapeutic interventions
1. Complete medical workup to rule out medical problems
2. Psychotherapy, family therapy, group therapy as necessary to resolve severe emotional problems
3. Pharmacologic approach: antianxiety agents rarely helpful; antidepressants (SSRIs) appear to more effective

Nursing Care of Clients with Conversion Disorders

A. ASSESSMENT
1. Presence of physical symptoms with no physiologic basis
2. Level of concern regarding physical symptoms
3. Degree of impairment
4. Level of anxiety

B. ANALYSIS/NURSING DIAGNOSES
1. Anxiety related to a threat to security, self-concept, and an inability to meet role expectations
2. Ineffective coping related to development of physical problems to escape stressful situations and control anxiety and an inability to accept that symptoms lack a physiologic basis
3. Disturbed body image related to passive acceptance of disabling symptoms that would alter body image and an inability to meet idealized role expectations and performance
4. Risk for injury related to feeling that the physiologic problem is real and an inability to overcome perceived physiologic problem
5. Impaired adjustment related to fear of assuming adult responsibilities, evidence by pattern of somatic complaints

C. PLANNING/IMPLEMENTATION
See Fundamental Principles When Caring for Clients with Somatoform Disorders

D. EVALUATION/OUTCOMES
1. Reduces need to develop physical symptoms to decrease anxiety
2. Develops a balance between work and play
3. Uses problem solving rather than physical symptoms to handle anxiety-producing situations

▼ BODY DYSMORPHIC DISORDERS

Data Base
A. Etiologic factors
1. Preoccupied with a defect in appearance, either imagined or exaggerated if a slight defect is present (not of delusional intensity)
2. Onset usually during adolescence, but can begin in childhood; lasts for several years
3. No predisposing factor in early life or family patterns has been identified

B. Behavioral/clinical findings
1. History of multiple visits to plastic surgeons to correct imagined defects
2. Preoccupation with imagined deficit causes avoidance or impairment in social and occupational relationships
3. Often exhibits symptoms of depression or obsessive-compulsive personality traits

C. Therapeutic interventions
Same as Conversion Disorder

Nursing Care of Clients with Body Dysmorphic Disorders

A. ASSESSMENT
1. Preoccupation with imagined physical defects
2. History of medical and surgical therapies to correct imagined defects
3. Ability to handle stressful situations
4. Level of anxiety

B. ANALYSIS/NURSING DIAGNOSES
1. Anxiety related to a threat to security, self-concept, and an inability to meet role expectations
2. Ineffective coping related to development of physical problems to escape stressful situations and control anxiety and an inability to verbalize feelings
3. Disturbed body image related to an inability to meet idealized role expectations and performance
4. Risk for injury related to feeling that the physiologic problem is real and an inability to overcome perceived physiologic problem

5. Chronic low self-esteem related to exaggerated focus on negative physical appearance that limits the attainment of one's ideal image

C. PLANNING/IMPLEMENTATION
See Fundamental Principles When Caring for Clients with Somatoform Disorders

D. EVALUATION/OUTCOMES
1. Recognizes that emphasis on physical defect is exaggerated
2. Uses problem solving rather than physical defect to handle anxiety-producing situations
3. Accepts and is comfortable with self

▼ HYPOCHONDRIASIS

Data Base
A. Etiologic factors
1. Preoccupation with the belief that one has a serious illness because of how physical symptoms are interpreted
2. A positive medical evaluation does not allay fears
3. Knowledge of symptoms associated with a given disease aids in the client's developing a similar set of symptoms, leading them to conclude that they have the disease
4. Psychosocial stresses are believed to lead to development of this disorder
5. Usually begins between 20 and 30 years of age; can occur across the life span
B. Behavioral/clinical findings
1. Misinterpretation and exaggeration of physical symptoms
2. Inability to accept reassurance even after exhaustive testing and therapy; leads to "doctor-shopping"
3. History of repeated absences from work
4. Duration of disturbance is at least 6 months
5. Adoption of sick role and invalid lifestyle
C. Therapeutic interventions
Same as Conversion Disorder

Nursing Care of Clients with Hypochondriasis
A. ASSESSMENT
1. Level of preoccupation with symptoms
2. Past and present degree of interference with functioning related to symptoms
3. Duration and degree of disability associated with symptoms
4. History of precipitant stressors associated with death of a significant person

B. ANALYSIS/NURSING DIAGNOSES
1. Anxiety related to a threat to security, self-concept, and an inability to meet role expectations

2. Ineffective coping related to development of physical problems to escape stressful situations and control anxiety and an inability to accept that the symptoms lack a physiologic basis
3. Disturbed body image related to an inability to meet idealized role expectations and performance
4. Impaired adjustment related to passive acceptance of disabling symptoms that would alter body image, an inability to meet idealized role expectations and performance, and a preoccupation with physical symptoms

C. PLANNING/IMPLEMENTATION
See Fundamental Principles When Caring for Clients with Somatoform Disorders

D. EVALUATION/OUTCOMES
1. Accepts that there is no physical basis for the symptoms
2. Uses more effective coping mechanisms to deal with anxiety
3. Accepts need to continue therapy even after condition has improved

FACTITIOUS DISORDERS

These disorders are characterized by physical or psychologic symptoms that are intentionally produced or feigned to enable one to assume the sick role. Therefore the client with a factitious disorder will "doctor shop," present for treatment in multiple emergency departments, and generally not be admitted to a psychiatric facility.

A factitious disorder must be distinguished from a true medical condition through a medical workup; the nurse's role is to assist with this process. Medical/Surgical Nursing and the Somatoform Disorders discussed in this chapter may be useful to help distinguish physiologic from intentional conditions.

The DSM-IV-TR does not classify specific factitious disorders, but malingering, Munchausen syndrome, and Munchausen syndrome by proxy clearly fall within this category.

Malingering is defined as making a conscious attempt to deceive others by pretending to have a false or exaggerated symptoms(s). Back pain and recurrent headaches are two chief complaints expressed by many clients who seek medical attention. Commonly, little or no improvement is made in comfort or symptom management. Many medical providers believe these clients are "acting ill" for secondary gains.

The term Munchausen syndrome is used to describe clients who intentionally cause their own illness. The deceptions may involve self-mutilation, fever, hemorrhage, hypoglycemia, seizures, nonhealing wounds, and abdominal or back pain. One commonality in clients who intentionally cause their own illness is their close ties (usually employment at some time) in some aspect of the health care industry. Nursing staff may feel anger toward the client for having been tricked by the feigning of illness. The client is in need of psychiatric treatment. When this isn't forthcoming, a later pattern of Munchausen syndrome by proxy can and does occur.

Munchausen syndrome by proxy is the term used when a parent (usually the mother) creates an illness in the child. The mother falsifies illness in the child through simulation or production of illness, then takes the child for medical care and claims no knowledge of the etiology. The most common reasons these parents seek medical attention are for bleeding, seizures, apnea, diarrhea, vomiting, fever, and rash. Often, when under supervision of other caretakers, the child exhibits no symptoms. The goal of the offending parent is to seek recognition from the medical providers. Many times there is indifference in the parent toward the child's pain and anguish. Sometimes the parent may actually encourage the medical provider to perform invasive tests and procedures that may be unnecessary. The mother is very involved in the child's care while hospitalized, and the father rarely visits or take an active interest. Munchausen syndrome by proxy is a form of physical abuse, and the child must be protected.

Psychiatric care is necessary for all clients whose behavior patterns fall within the category of a factitious disorder.

DISSOCIATIVE DISORDERS

These disorders are characterized by either a sudden or gradual disruption in the usual integrated functions of consciousness, memory, identity, or perception of the environment

FUNDAMENTAL PRINCIPLES WHEN CARING FOR CLIENTS WITH DISSOCIATIVE DISORDERS

Refer to Fundamental Principles When Caring for Clients with Anxiety Disorders

Data Base
A. Etiologic factors
1. Inability to recall important personal information usually of a traumatic or stressful nature
2. Gaps are reported in recalling aspects of an individual's life history
3. Gaps are usually related to traumatic episodes
B. Behavioral/clinical findings
1. The disruption may be transient or may become a well-established pattern
2. Development of these disorders is often associated with exposure to a traumatic event
3. Sexual abuse during childhood is a frequent contributing factor
4. Types
   a. Dissociative amnesia: characterized by an inability to recall important personal information, usually of a traumatic or stressful nature as distinguished from ordinary forgetfulness
   b. Dissociative fugue: characterized by sudden, unexpected travel accompanied by an inability to recall one's past and identity confusion or the assumption of a new identity
   c. Dissociative identity disorder: characterized by coexistence of two or more distinct personalities within an individual
   d. Depersonalization disorder: characterized by a persistent or recurrent feeling of being detached from one's mental processes or body that is accompanied by intact reality testing
C. Therapeutic interventions
1. Complete medical workup to rule out possibility of organic causes (e.g., brain tumor versus dissociative disorder)
2. Psychotherapy, individual and family
3. Development of more effective and satisfying ways to handle anxiety

Nursing Care of Clients with Dissociative Disorders
A. **ASSESSMENT**
1. Identity
2. Memory
3. Consciousness
4. Physical condition
5. Psychosocial component to discover fundamental anxiety source
6. History of emotional trauma in childhood from client (if possible) and family
7. Suicidal risk
8. Recent use of alcohol or drugs
B. **ANALYSIS/NURSING DIAGNOSES**
1. Anxiety related to a threat to security and self-concept
2. Ineffective coping related to an inability to meet role expectations and pervasive anxiety and fear
3. Risk for injury related to altered judgment
4. Ineffective role performance related to feelings of inadequacy and hostility, disturbed relationships, and an inability to meet role expectations
5. Chronic or situational low self-esteem related to feelings of inadequacy and hostility, disturbed relationships, pervasive anxiety, and an inability to meet role expectations

6. Post-trauma response related to experiencing an event that is outside of usual human experience
7. Disturbed sensory perception related to sudden memory loss, disorientation, loss of personal identity, and an alteration in state of consciousness
8. Disturbed personal identity related to sudden memory loss, disorientation, loss of personal identity, and an alteration in state of consciousness

C. PLANNING/IMPLEMENTATION
1. See Fundamental Principles When Caring for Clients with Anxiety Disorders
2. Assist with treatment plan to alleviate the troublesome symptoms
3. Reinforce usual coping styles
4. Provide for family therapy
5. Assist with problem solving
6. Encourage involvement in long-term therapy

D. EVALUATION/OUTCOMES
1. Recalls and identifies past experiences correctly
2. Verbalizes increased satisfaction with family and work relationships
3. Ceases incidents of being absent without explanation
4. Develops more effective coping mechanisms to deal with anxiety

SEXUAL AND GENDER IDENTITY DISORDERS

Changing social and cultural mores have caused many of the sexual behaviors that were once considered deviations to be removed from the list of "abnormal practices." Today sexual activities are considered abnormal only if they are directed toward anything other than consenting adults or are performed under unusual circumstances.

FUNDAMENTAL PRINCIPLES WHEN CARING FOR CLIENTS WITH SEXUAL AND GENDER IDENTITY DISORDERS

A. Accept the individual as a person in emotional pain
B. Avoid punitive remarks or responses
C. Protect the individual from others
D. Set limits on the individual's sexual acting out
E. Provide diversional activities

▼ PARAPHILIAS

Data Base
A. Etiologic factors

1. Sexual urges or fantasies that are directed toward nonhuman objects, infliction of pain to self, partner, children, or other nonconsenting individuals for at least 6 months' duration
2. Diagnosis is made when the individual has acted on urges or is extremely distressed by the urges
3. Sexual arousal accompanies paraphiliac fantasies or stimuli
4. Person may or may not be able to function sexually without the paraphiliac fantasy or stimuli
5. May be symptomatic of other personality or psychiatric disorders
6. May occur as a behavior aberration or a disordered personality
7. Onset of fantasies and related behaviors may begin in childhood or early adolescence and becomes more defined in adulthood

B. Types and behavioral/clinical findings
1. Fetishism: substitution of an inanimate object for the genitals
2. Transvestic fetishisms: wearing clothes of the opposite sex to achieve sexual pleasure
3. Exhibitionism: sexual pleasure obtained by exposing the genitals
4. Pedophilia: attraction to children as sex objects
5. Voyeurism: sexual gratification obtained by watching the sexual play of others
6. Sadism: sexual gratification obtained from cruelty to others; used as a substitute for or an accompaniment to the sex act
7. Masochism: sexual gratification obtained from self-suffering; used as a substitute for or an accompaniment to the sex act
8. Frotteurism: sexual pleasure obtained by touching or rubbing against a nonconsenting person; usually occurs in crowds or on public transportation
9. Necrophilia: sexual gratification obtained from sexual relations with a corpse
10. Telephone scatologia: sexual gratification from or during lewdness on the telephone

C. Therapeutic interventions
1. Rather unsuccessful with these individuals unless they really want to change
2. If change is desired, psychotherapy may be effective treatment models
   a. Cognitive therapy
   b. Behavioral therapy

Nursing Care of Clients with Paraphilias
A. ASSESSMENT
1. History of sexual behavior
2. Presence of other psychosocial difficulties
3. Level of anxiety regarding sexual behavior

4. Pending criminal charges
5. Why client is seeking treatment at this time
6. Potential for violence toward others or self

B. ANALYSIS/NURSING DIAGNOSES

1. Anxiety related to threat to security, fear of discovery, and conflict between sexual desires and societal norms
2. Disturbed body image related to feelings about size and functioning of genitalia and ineffective past sexual functioning
3. Ineffective coping related to inability to meet basic sexual needs and sexual role expectations and poor self-esteem
4. Risk for infection related to frequent changes in sexual partners and sadistic or masochistic acts
5. Risk for injury related to retaliation for sexual behavior or sadistic or masochistic acts
6. Ineffective sexuality patterns related to an inability to achieve sexual satisfaction without the use of paraphiliac behaviors
7. Risk for violence: directed toward others or self, related to choice of sex objects or obtaining sexual gratification by inflicting or receiving physical abuse

C. PLANNING/IMPLEMENTATION

See Fundamental Principles When Caring for Clients with Sexual and Gender Identity Disorders

D. EVALUATION/OUTCOMES

1. Ceases socially unacceptable behavior
2. Seeks and continues long-term therapy
3. Limits paraphiliac behavior to consenting adults
4. Utilizes safer sex techniques

▼ SEXUAL DYSFUNCTION

Data Base

A. Etiologic factors
   1. Inhibition or interference with the desire, excitement, orgasm, or resolution phases of the sexual response cycle
   2. Dysfunction is psychogenic, but it may begin with a physiologic basis
   3. Dysfunction can be lifelong or acquired
   4. Dysfunction can be generalized or situational
B. Types and behavioral/clinical findings
   1. Sexual desire disorders: deficient, absent, or extreme aversion to and avoidance of sexual activity
   2. Sexual arousal disorders: partial or complete failure to achieve a physiologic or psychologic (subjective) response to sexual activity
   3. Orgasm disorders: delay in or absence of orgasm or premature ejaculation

4. Sexual pain disorders: recurrent or persistent genital pain before, during, or after sexual activity

C. Therapeutic interventions
   1. Treatment of underlying physiologic cause if present
   2. Sexual counseling for client and partner

Nursing Care of Clients with a Sexual Dysfunction

A. ASSESSMENT

1. Feelings about inability to function sexually
2. Expectations regarding sexual ability
3. Effect of sexual dysfunction on relationship with significant other

B. ANALYSIS/NURSING DIAGNOSES

1. Anxiety related to threat to security and fear of discovery
2. Disturbed body image related to feelings about size and functioning of genitalia and ineffective past sexual functioning
3. Ineffective coping related to inability to meet basic sexual needs and sexual role expectations and poor self-esteem
4. Sexual dysfunction related to lack of sex education, lack of communication with partner regarding individual responses, ineffective sexual techniques, physical (illness, injury, surgery, medication), or substance abuse (addiction) contributing to sexual dysfunction, feelings of vulnerability, value conflict, and actual or perceived sexual limitations

C. PLANNING/IMPLEMENTATION

1. See Fundamental Principles When Caring for Clients with Sexual and Gender Identity Disorders
2. Recognize that the problem is real to the client regardless of age
3. Recognize that the desire to function sexually does not diminish with age

D. EVALUATION/OUTCOMES

1. Reports an increased satisfaction in sexual functioning
2. Reports sexual ability approaches sexual expectations

▼ GENDER IDENTITY DISORDERS

Data Base

A. Etiologic factors
   1. Origins of GID unknown
   2. Persistent discomfort with one's assigned gender and a feeling that it is inappropriate or inaccurate
   3. Persistent repudiation of current gender anatomy

4. Preoccupation with activities and clothing of opposite gender
5. Intense desire to be the opposite sex

B. Behavioral/clinical findings
   1. Child gender identity disorders
      a. Most children are firmly committed to gender role expectations as early as 18 months
      b. Manifested by four or more of these behaviors:
         (1) Intense discomfort with own gender and desires to be the opposite sex or believes that he or she is the opposite sex
         (2) Preference for cross-dressing
         (3) Participates in activities associated with the opposite sex
         (4) Demonstrates strong and persistent preference for cross-sex roles in make-believe play or fantasies
         (5) Prefers playmates of opposite sex
   2. Adolescent/adult gender identity disorders
      a. Educational problems
      b. Manifested by these behaviors:
         (1) Stated desire to be the other sex
         (2) Frequently cross-dresses
         (3) Desires to live or be treated as the other sex
         (4) Belief that one has the typical feelings and reaction of the other sex
         (5) Persistent discomfort with gender
         (6) Preoccupation with getting rid of primary and secondary sex characteristics
         (7) Disturbance causes impairment in social and occupational relationships

C. Therapeutic interventions
   1. Individual or group psychotherapy
   2. Antianxiety medication if necessary
   3. Monitoring of children/adolescents over an extended period of time to aid in diagnosing

Nursing Care of Clients with Gender Identity Disorders

A. ASSESSMENT
1. Distress about assigned sex role
2. Behaviors, social habits, and cross-dressing inappropriate for sexual gender
3. Preoccupation with becoming, being, or behaving as the opposite sex
4. History of sexual orientation (asexual, homosexual, bisexual, heterosexual)
5. Presence of depressive behaviors and suicidal ideation

B. ANALYSIS/NURSING DIAGNOSES
1. Anxiety related to threat to security, fear of discovery, and conflict between sexual desires and societal norms
2. Disturbed body image related to a strong and persistent cross-gender identification and discomfort with one's assigned sex
3. Ineffective coping related to inability to meet basic sexual needs and sexual role expectations and poor self-esteem
4. Risk for infection related to frequent changes in sexual partners
5. Risk for injury related to retaliation for sexual behavior
6. Sexual dysfunction related to value conflict
7. Social isolation related to others' reaction to cross-dressing, leading to low self-esteem and school or work difficulties

C. PLANNING/IMPLEMENTATION
1. See Fundamental Principles When Caring for Clients with Sexual and Gender Identity Disorders
2. Accept and understand client's discomfort with gender
3. Accept own feelings about client's cross-dressing
4. Encourage client to become involved with support groups
5. Be aware that if discomfort or depression is severe, self-mutilation and suicide are possibilities
6. Assist client to sort out solution (acceptance, suppression, information regarding surgical sex reassignment)

D. EVALUATION/OUTCOMES
1. Verbalizes increased comfort with self
2. Ultimately accepts gender or explores surgical options
3. Participates in support groups

EATING DISORDERS

Eating behaviors and perceptions of body shape and weight are severely disturbed in these disorders; anorexia and bulimia nervosa may be present in the same client or exist separately

FUNDAMENTAL PRINCIPLES WHEN CARING FOR CLIENTS WITH EATING DISORDERS

A. Recognize that adolescent or adult requires:
   1. Basic physiologic and safety needs to be met
   2. Acceptance
   3. Meaningful relationships
   4. Limit setting on manipulative behavior
   5. Monitoring during and after meal time
   6. An awareness of type, amount, and patterns of food eaten (food diary)

7. Consult with nutritionist to determine adequate dietary regimen
B. Direct care toward helping the individual to mature by:
   1. Establishing a constructive relationship
   2. Promoting self-worth
   3. Setting limits that are realistic
   4. Being consistent in approach and in rules and regulations
   5. Supporting and encouraging independence
   6. Learning more effective ways of coping
   7. Participating in individual and family therapy

▼ ANOREXIA NERVOSA

Data Base
A. Etiologic factors
   1. Decreased levels of norepinephrine, serotonin, and dopamine
   2. Combination of genetic, neurochemical, developmental, characteriological, social, cultural, and familiar factors cited
   3. More common in females
   4. Avoidance of food may result from excessive concern with obesity
   5. Apparent failure to separate from mother and become autonomous; unconscious fear of growing up
   6. Onset usually during adolescence through young adulthood; less common in elderly
B. Behavioral/clinical findings
   1. Weigh less than 85% of expected weight
   2. Distorted self-image; appear fat to themselves even when emaciated
   3. Intense fear of becoming fat, even though underweight
   4. May have history of compulsive traits such as rigidity, ritualistic behavior, and meticulousness
   5. Usually very manipulative
   6. Usually high achievers academically
   7. Frequent discord in family relationships, especially with mother
   8. Often interested in food and cooking in general; serves as a control strategy
   9. Cessation of menses in females
   10. Inability to sustain self-starvation may result in bulimic episodes (binging of food followed by self-induced vomiting)
   11. Fatigue or hyperactivity
   12. Feeling of fullness after small intake
   13. Nausea
   14. Constipation
   15. Emaciation
   16. Hypotension
   17. Low blood glucose
   18. Anemia
   19. Low BMR
   20. Subtypes:
      a. Restricting type: weight loss is accomplished through dieting, fasting, or excessive exercise
      b. Binge eating/purging type: weight loss is accomplished through binge eating or purging (or both); use of self-induced vomiting and misuse of laxatives, diuretics, or enemas on weekly basis
C. Therapeutic interventions
   1. Unified team approach
   2. Behavior modification techniques that focus on client's responsibility for weight gain
   3. Time limit on meals
   4. Use of nasogastric tube if weight loss is so great or fluid and electrolyte imbalance is so severe that it causes a threat to life
   5. Psychotherapy focusing on self-image
   6. Group and cognitive therapy
   7. Family therapy with all members of family involved
   8. Gradual increase in calories and protein under guidance of nutritionist
   9. Antidepressants have been helpful especially with comorbid depression

Nursing Care of Clients with Anorexia Nervosa
A. ASSESSMENT
   1. Complete physical and dental examination to rule out associated medical complications of eating disorder
      a. Involved systems are CNS, renal, hematologic, gastrointestinal, metabolic, endocrine, and cardiovascular
      b. Skin, hair, and nutritional status
   2. Weight and height
   3. Signs of fluid and electrolyte imbalance
   4. History of amenorrhea
   5. Indulgence in excessive exercise
   6. Behavior reflecting obsessiveness with food
   7. History of stringent control of intake of food
   8. Depressive mood
   9. Motivation to change maladaptive eating patterns
B. ANALYSIS/NURSING DIAGNOSES
   1. Anxiety related to low self-concept, feelings of inferiority, and unmet dependency needs
   2. Disturbed body image related to unrealistic appraisal of body size, underestimating food requirements and a desire for slimness
   3. Ineffective family coping: compromised, related to overprotection and unwillingness to allow client to separate (meet developmental tasks), unrealistic expectations, and an inability to cope with client's eating disorder

4. Risk for fluid volume deficit related to inadequate intake and purging
5. Ineffective coping related to deficits in self-care activities, altered role performance, quest for thinness, and delay in mastery of developmental tasks
6. Ineffective health maintenance related to inadequate health practices, health beliefs, alterations in self-image, preoccupation with food, and a denial of one's own hunger
7. Imbalanced nutrition: less than body requirements, related to a disturbed body image and a dysfunctional emotional conditioning in relationship to food

C. PLANNING/IMPLEMENTATION

1. Refer to Fundamental Principles When Caring for Clients with Eating Disorders
2. Develop a therapeutic environment
3. Establish a behavior modification program
4. Help client identify feelings
5. Briefly discuss dietary modification with the client in a nonthreatening manner
6. Encourage diet high in nutrient-dense foods
7. Do not focus on eating or weight loss

D. EVALUATION/OUTCOMES

1. Maintains dietary intake adequate to meet daily caloric requirements
2. Reaches and maintains appropriate body weight
3. Develops realistic body image
4. Identifies and verbalizes feelings
5. Accepts role of young adult
6. Resolves separation and individuation issues

▼ BULIMIA NERVOSA

Data Base

A. Etiologic factors
  1. Most common in adolescent through 30-year-old population
  2. More common in females
  3. Obesity is frequently found in parents or siblings
  4. Predisposition to depression
  5. Discord in family relationships
  6. Obsession with food results from a morbid fear of obesity and the pathologic need to binge

B. Behavioral/clinical findings
  1. Compulsive eating binges characterized by rapid consumption of excessive amounts of high-caloric foods in brief periods followed by induced purging (vomiting, enemas, laxatives, or diuretics)
  2. Periods of severe dieting or fasting between binges
  3. Sporadic vigorous exercising between binges
  4. Weight may be within normal range with frequent fluctuations above or below normal range because of alternating binges and fasts
  5. Lack of control over eating during episode
  6. Depression and self-deprecating thoughts follow binges
  7. Bingeing and purging pattern occurring at least biweekly, for past 3 months
  8. Extroverted
  9. Possible intermittent substance abuse
  10. Very concerned with body image and appearance
  11. Repeated attempts to control or lose weight
  12. Subtypes
    a. Purging type: engages in purging behaviors
    b. Nonpurging type: uses fasting or excessive exercise, not purging

C. Therapeutic interventions
  1. See Therapeutic Interventions under Anorexia Nervosa, except for 4
  2. Treat the depression that is the most frequently observed psychologic concomitant condition associated with bulimia

Nursing Care of Clients with Bulimia Nervosa

A. ASSESSMENT

1. Behavior indicative of purging such as self-induced vomiting and use of enemas, laxatives, and diuretics
2. Obsession with excessive exercise
3. Pattern and duration of binging
4. Overconcern with body weight and shape
5. Physiologic changes such as dental caries, chipped teeth, enlarged paratoid glands, calluses, or scars on knuckles from induced vomiting
6. Signs of fluid and electrolyte imbalances
7. Weight and height
8. History of consuming tremendous amounts of calories in a short period of time
9. Symptoms of depression or obsessive-compulsive behaviors
10. Substance abuse, pattern, drug(s) duration

B. ANALYSIS/NURSING DIAGNOSES

1. Anxiety related to low self-concept and feelings of inferiority
2. Disturbed body image related to unrealistic appraisal of body size and a desire for slimness
3. Ineffective family coping: compromised, related to unrealistic expectations and an inability to cope with client's eating disorder
4. Risk for fluid volume deficit related to purging
5. Ineffective coping related to deficits in self-care activities, altered role performance, quest for thinness, and shame and guilt over secret binges

6. Ineffective health maintenance related to inadequate health practices and alterations in self-image
7. Imbalanced nutrition: less than body requirements related to self-induced vomiting and purging
8. Imbalanced nutrition: more than body requirements, related to an abnormality in amount of food consumed and a dysfunctional emotional conditioning in relationship to food
9. Self-esteem disturbance related to low self-confidence, feelings of inferiority, and unrealistic expectations of self and others

C. **PLANNING/IMPLEMENTATION**
1. See Fundamental Principles When Caring for Clients with Eating Disorders
2. Provide a nonjudgmental, accepting environment
3. Set realistic limits; keep client under close observation to prevent purging
4. Encourage verbalization of feelings
5. Help client to identify feelings associated with binging and purging episodes
6. Shift focus from food, eating, and exercise to emotional issues

D. **EVALUATION/OUTCOMES**
1. Limits dietary intake to caloric requirements
2. Reduces episodes of binging
3. Reduces episodes of purging
4. Identifies feelings
5. Verbalizes emotions and needs
6. Exhibits no depressive symptoms

SLEEP DISORDERS

A common problem in adults, rarely treated in an inpatient psychiatric setting, can present as a symptom of depressive, manic, or anxiety disorders. Sleep consists of two distinct states: REM (rapid eye movement), also called dream sleep, and NREM (non-REM) sleep, which is divided into four stages. Sleep is a cyclic phenomenon with restorative qualities. The dreaming that occurs during sleep is also helpful to gain insights, solve problems, work through emotional reactions, and prepare for the future. Sleep disorder is a condition or problem that repeatedly disrupts pattern of sleep leading to diminished performance.

Data Base

A. Etiologic factors
1. Normal sleep cycle evolves throughout the life cycle and becomes decreased with age
2. Disorder from which the client usually recovers, because the changes may be reversible and temporary if treated
3. Neuroendocrine arousal system thought to release corticosteroids by the hypothalamic-pituitary-adrenal axis, as well as stimulation of the neurotransmitter system producing norepinephrine and serotonin
4. Genetic factors show a biologic tendency may be inherited (e.g., light sleepers in a family); no single gene has been identified
5. Environmental factors thought to contribute to sleep disturbances, such as jet lag, shift work, and fast pace of life
6. Biologic factors such as cardiovascular, endocrine, psychiatric, infections, cough related to pulmonary disease, pain, use of stimulants, and side effects of many medications and drug interaction all contribute to sleep-related problems
7. Impaired function results from sleep deprivation

B. Behavioral/clinical findings
1. Onset usually begins in young adulthood; more prevalent with increasing age
2. Difficulty initiating or maintaining sleep, or nonrestorative sleep, for at least 1 month
3. Depression is usually associated with fragmented sleep patterns
4. Sleeplessness is a cardinal feature noted in manic disorders; it is an early sign of impending mania in bipolar disorders
5. Abuse of alcohol, stimulants, heavy smoking, and use of (OTC) cold remedies cause decreased total sleep time
6. Anxiety can precipitate insomnia

C. Types (primary and secondary sleep disorders)
1. Primary
   a. Insomnia—disorder of initiating or maintaining sleep; anxiety and depression are major causes
   b. Parasomnias—disorders associated with sleep stages (sleepwalking, night terrors, nightmares, restless leg syndrome, and enuresis); most common in children
2. Secondary
   a. Sleep disorders related to mental disorders—noted in this category are anxiety-related disorders, depressive disorders, and manic episodes
   b. Substance-induced sleep disorders—included in this subclass are conditions related to intoxication, periods of withdrawal, use of stimulants, and side effects of many medications
   c. Sleep disorders related to general medical conditions—etiology must be established through history, physical examination, or laboratory findings in this subclass; medical conditions noted are degenerative neurologic

disease, cardiovascular, endocrine, infections, and pain from musculoskeletal diseases

D. Therapeutic interventions
1. Promote comfort
2. Teach sleep hygiene practices
3. See Hypnotic/Sedative agents
4. Sedatives/hypnotics should be avoided, especially in the elderly
5. See Benzodiazepines and Nonbenzodiazepine drug categories
6. Anticipate short-term use of benzodiazepines/nonbenzodiazepines

Nursing Care of Clients with Sleep Disorders

A. **ASSESSMENT**
1. History of onset, duration, and sleep patterns
2. Daily routines, night rituals
3. Diet and physical activity
4. Stressors
5. Level of daytime alertness, nap patterns
6. Restless leg movement, snoring
7. Drug, alcohol, caffeine, nicotine use
8. Pharmacologic or herbal remedies

B. **ANALYSIS/NURSING DIAGNOSES**
1. Sleep deprivation related to difficulty initiating or maintaining sleep, or nonrestorative sleep
2. Disturbed sleep pattern related to personal stressors, or high anxiety levels, evidenced by difficulty falling asleep and frequent awakening during the nights
3. Ineffective coping related to excessive sleepiness or insomnia that affects one's abilities to meet social, work, or family expectations
4. Fatigue related to sleep cycle changes that cause low energy levels and interference with desired lifestyle activities
5. Risk for activity intolerance related to chronic insomnia resulting in diminished creativity and a lessening of response to stimuli

C. **PLANNING/IMPLEMENTATION**
1. Provide a quiet, restful environment; demonstrate relaxation techniques
2. Plan care when client is receptive
3. Encourage adequate nutrition
4. Obtain a diet recall to assess food/liquid intake and caffeine consumption
5. Instruct client to avoid stimulants (coffee, tea, chocolate, nicotine, and OTC cold remedies) at bedtime
6. Establish a daily exercise regimen during the day hours to reduce stress
7. Provide diversional activities during the day to avoid napping
8. Instruct client to eat a larger meal at noon rather than at dinner
9. Establish set sleep patterns and promote effec-

tive sleep hygiene practices
10. Promote comfort and control physical disturbances at night
11. Assist with ruling out medical conditions that contribute to sleep-related problems

D. **EVALUATION/OUTCOMES**
1. Deals with anxiety-producing situations effectively
2. Develops coping skills
3. Uses relaxation techniques
4. Limits use of stimulants
5. Reports restorative sleep
6. Reports improved sense of well-being

ADJUSTMENT DISORDERS

These disorders are characterized by a short-term disturbance in mood or behavior with nonpsychotic manifestations resulting from identifiable stressors; the severity of the reaction is not predictable by the severity of the stressors

Data Base

A. Etiologic factors
1. Problematic response to life events, either developmental or situational stressors
2. Interaction of personality, crisis, developmental factors, and cultural influences should be considered
3. No apparent underlying mental disorder in these individuals, although present behavior may be extremely disturbed
4. The individual seems to have the capacity to adapt to the overwhelming stress when given the time to do so
5. Problems with distortions or interruptions in thinking processes and decision making tend to resolve themselves

B. Behavioral/clinical findings
1. Infancy: extremely upset; demonstrating grief when separated from mother
2. Childhood: regression to an earlier level of development when a new sibling arrives; intense anxiety on entering school
3. Adolescence: struggle for independence; leads to hypersensitivity and frequent episodes of heightened anxiety
4. Adult life: heightened anxiety in response to the stressors associated with marriage, pregnancy, divorce, change of employment, purchase of a house, etc.
5. Later life: menopause and climacteric, plan for retirement, "loss" of children to marriage, and death of a mate all serve to produce extreme stress situations

6. Onset begins within 3 months of stressors
7. Causes significant impairment in social and occupational functioning
8. Duration of disorder lasts no longer than 6 months after stress has ceased
9. Onset may occur at any age; commonly noted in children and adolescents

C. Therapeutic interventions
   Determine the underlying cause of the conflict and work toward resolution

Nursing Care of Clients with Adjustment Disorders

A. **ASSESSMENT**
   1. Individual's perception of problem
   2. Factors impinging upon current situation
   3. Individual's personal strengths and support system
   4. Level of anxiety
   5. Identification of type(s) of stressors and onset

B. **ANALYSIS/NURSING DIAGNOSES**
   1. Anxiety related to inability to handle overwhelming stress effectively and a threat to self-concept and security
   2. Ineffective coping related to overwhelming environmental stress, which is usually resolved over time, failure of support system, and the developmental level
   3. Chronic low self-esteem related to overwhelming stress and an inability to cope
   4. Ineffective role performance related to overwhelming stress, an inability to cope, and social withdrawal

C. **PLANNING/IMPLEMENTATION**
   1. Help the client and/or parents recognize and accept that a problem exists
   2. Support and avoid humiliation of the individual
   3. Maintain client safety
   4. Encourage the identification and use of support systems
   5. Attempt to minimize environmental pressures
   6. Allow the client time to recover personal resources

D. **EVALUATION/OUTCOMES**
   1. Reorganizes defenses
   2. Utilizes support system
   3. Verbalizes a decrease in anxiety
   4. Develops more effective coping

PERSONALITY DISORDERS

These disorders are extreme exaggerations of personality traits or styles that often define the uniqueness of the individual; under stress they manifest patterns of inflexibility, maladaptive emotional responses, and

functioning impairments. A personality disorder, according to the DSM IV-TR is an "enduring pattern of inner experiences and behavior that deviates markedly from the expectations of the individual's culture, is pervasive and inflexible, has an onset in adolescence or early adulthood, is stable over time, and leads to distress or impairment."

Data Base

A. Etiologic factors
   1. Psychodynamic theory postulates that individuals with personality disorders have deficits in psychosexual development or failure to achieve object constancy
   2. Neurobiologic perspective
      a. Research evidence suggests that the development of the major personality disorders is determined by environmental factors that interact with biologic factors such as inability to tolerate anxiety, aggressiveness, and genetic vulnerability to certain affects
      b. Family and twin studies are demonstrating a strong genetic influence; this suggests some connection between biologic factors and personality organization
      c. Study findings suggest a structural brain deficit in antisocial personality disorder that may cause low arousal, low fear, lack of conscience, and deficits in decision making
      d. Further research is needed to clarify the role of inheritance and brain structure and function in the development of personality disorders
   3. Sociocultural factors (isolation and family instability) can also influence the ability to establish and maintain relatedness
   4. Relationship problems develop early in life, and often move through predictable stages ranging from idealization and over-evaluation and ending with rationalization, devaluation and rejection of the other person
   5. Premorbid personality of individuals demonstrating any of the 10 classified and 2 not otherwise specified personality disturbances* resembles the compensatory mechanisms associated with the pathologic counterpart

B. Types and behavioral/clinical findings
   1. Antisocial personality disorder
      a. Chronic lifelong disturbances that conflict with society's laws and customs
      b. Unable to postpone gratification

*Adapted from *Diagnostic and statistical manual of mental disorders* (text revision), ed 4, Washington, DC, 2000, American Psychiatric Association.

   c. Randomly act out their aggressive egocentric impulses on society
   d. Do not profit from past experience or punishment; live only for the moment
   e. Have the ability to ingratiate themselves but "do not wear well"
   f. Are in contact with reality but do not seem to care about it or people
2. Avoidant personality disorder
   a. Social discomfort and timidity
   b. Loner; unwilling to get involved with others
   c. Fear of negative evaluation from others
3. Borderline personality disorder
   a. Unstable and intense interpersonal relationships
   b. Impulsive, unpredictable behavior that is potentially self-destructive
   c. Marked mood shifts
   d. Identity disturbance
   e. Chronic feeling of emptiness
   f. History of parental abuse or neglect in early childhood; sexual abuse by nonparents
4. Dependent personality disorder
   a. Unable to make decisions
   b. Lack of self-confidence
   c. Dependent and submissive
   d. Induces others to assume responsibility
5. Histrionic personality disorder
   a. Emotional instability and hyperexcitability
   b. Extroverted and directed toward gaining attention
   c. Vain and deliberately manipulative
6. Narcissistic personality disorder
   a. Overblown sense of importance
   b. Strong need for attention and admiration
   c. Relationships marked by ambivalence
   d. Preoccupation with appearance
7. Obsessive-compulsive personality disorder
   a. Rigidity, overconscientiousness, inordinate capacity for work
   b. Driven by obsessive concerns
   c. Behavior contains many rituals that the client cannot control
8. Paranoid personality disorder
   a. Frequent use of projective mechanisms
   b. Suspiciousness, fear, irritability, and stubbornness
   c. Reality testing not greatly impaired
9. Schizoid personality disorder
   a. Avoidance of meaningful interpersonal relationships; prefers solitary activities
   b. Use of autistic thinking, emotional detachment, and daydreaming
   c. Introverted since childhood but maintaining fair contact with reality
   d. Asexual
10. Schizotypal personality disorder

   a. Unattached, withdrawn
   b. Affectively and intellectually diminished
   c. Frequently part of the vagabond or transient groups of society
   d. Behavior or appearance that is odd, eccentric, or peculiar
11. Personality disorder not otherwise specified (components of mixed disorders, passive-aggressive, or depressive personality disorder)
   a. Does not meet criteria for a specific personality disorder
   b. Generally has features of more than one specific type (mixed disorders)
   c. Causes clinically significant distress of functional impairment beginning in early adulthood
   d. Also included are depressive and passive-aggressive personality disorders
      (1) Depressive personality disorder characteristics include five or more of the following:
         (a) Usual mood dominated by dejection, gloom, unhappiness
         (b) Low self-esteem
         (c) Critical and negativistic toward others
         (d) Pessimistic
         (e) Prone to feelings of guilt and remorse
      (2) Passive-aggressive personality disorder characteristics include four or more of the following:
         (a) Passively resists fulfilling social and occupational tasks
         (b) Complains of not being understood or appreciated
         (c) Sullen and argumentative
         (d) Envious of and resentment toward others more fortunate
         (e) Exaggerates and complains of personal misfortune
         (f) Alternates between hostile defiance and contrition
      (3) Both of these disorders deleted from DSM-IV-TR for further study; included here as a reminder of a negativistic traits
C. Therapeutic interventions
   1. Individual, group, and family psychotherapy
   2. Crisis intervention when necessary
   3. Vocational and occupational therapy
   4. Psychotropic drugs have a limited role

Nursing Care of Clients with Personality Disorders

A. ASSESSMENT
   1. Level of functioning with family and friends
   2. Individual's perception of problem

3. Why client is seeking treatment at this time
4. Level of anxiety
5. Pending criminal charges
6. Drug and alcohol abuse
7. History of suicidal gestures and present risk

B. ANALYSIS/NURSING DIAGNOSES
1. Anxiety related to a threat to security and self-concept, an inability to meet role expectations, and difficulty in interpersonal relationships
2. Ineffective family coping: compromised, related to abusive or destructive behavior, ambivalent family relationships, and a denial that problem exists
3. Defensive coping related to an inability to learn from experience, poorly developed or inappropriate use of defense mechanisms, and repeated manipulative behaviors
4. Impaired social interactions related to sociocultural dissonance, altered thought processes, communication barriers, and lack of interpersonal skills
5. Social isolation related to the absence of meaningful relationships
6. Risk for violence: directed toward others related to poor impulse control

C. PLANNING/IMPLEMENTATION
1. Maintain consistency and concern
2. Accept the individual as is; do not retaliate if provoked
3. Protect the individual from others while protecting others from the individual
4. Place realistic limits on behavior; make known what those limits are
5. Strive for consistency among healthcare team members
6. Initiate cognitive and behavioral strategies

D. EVALUATION/OUTCOMES
1. Demonstrates decreased episodes of acting out
2. Verbalizes decrease in anxiety
3. Accepts and continues long-term therapy
4. Recognizes and functions within limits of personality
5. Establishes and maintains positive relationships

COMMUNITY HEALTH SERVICES

Concepts

A. Purposes
1. To provide prevention, treatment, and rehabilitation services for individuals with emotional problems; also support for families
2. To maintain these individuals and families in the community
3. To provide hospital care within the community

in those instances when the individual cannot be maintained on an outpatient basis
4. Emphasis on managed care mandates shift from costly inpatient treatment to community and home health visits

B. Types of settings in which services are provided
1. Outpatient services
   a. Storefront clinics or day-care centers, mobile units
   b. Walk-in clinics in hospitals and psychiatric emergency rooms
   c. Emergency services
   d. Crisis intervention centers, including hotline phone centers and the Internet
   e. Private community practice, schools, and shelters
   f. Dual-diagnoses programs (mental health and chemical dependency)
   g. Mental health home nursing
   h. Forensic settings
2. Inpatient services
   a. Specialized psychiatric hospitals
   b. General hospital psychiatric units
3. Aftercare services
   a. Foster homes
   b. Halfway houses
   c. Sheltered workshops
   d. Day-care centers

C. Types of services
1. Observation and diagnosis
2. Assessment of the client's needs
3. Crisis intervention
4. Provide direct care services to clients, including:
   a. Individual, family, and group therapy
   b. Medications
   c. Electroconvulsive therapy
   d. Occupational therapy
   e. Recreational therapy
5. Provide a therapeutic milieu that:
   a. Supports the individual during the period of crisis
   b. Helps the individual learn new ways of coping with problems
6. Referral to proper community agencies for necessary services
7. Vocational counseling
8. Health screening
9. Provide an educational setting for various professional groups in mental health concepts

Nurse's Role

A. Case finding
B. Assessment of the individual's needs
C. Establishment of the therapeutic milieu
D. Consultation with other professionals (e.g., physicians, psychologists, social workers, school teachers,

clergy, nursing home and managed adult residential facility staff)

E. Active participation with the health team, including the individual and family

F. Involvement in individual, family, and group therapy

G. Coordination of health services for the individual and family; referral and preparation of client for scheduled appointments

H. Education of groups within the community

I. Function as client advocate

PSYCHIATRIC/MENTAL HEALTH NURSING
REVIEW QUESTIONS

Therapeutic Relationships

1. If a psychiatric nurse were to use the family systems theory in practice, the statement that would be expected when the nurse interacts with a client would be:
   1. "Describe for me in your own words what caused this situation."
   2. "You need to abide by the unit rules and attend the community meetings."
   3. "Whenever someone permanently leaves the home, the boundaries are upset."
   4. "You're doing better; let's talk to the doctor about lowering your medication dosage."

2. A nurse has been assigned to work with a depressed client on a one-to-one basis. The next morning the client refuses to get out of bed, stating, "I'm too sick to be helped and I don't want to be bothered." The nurse's best response would be:
   1. "You will feel better if you make the effort to get up and get dressed."
   2. "You sound so hopeless today. I would like to hear what you are thinking."
   3. "I know you will feel better again if you only make the attempt to help yourself."
   4. "Everyone feels this way in the beginning as they confront repressed feelings. I'll sit down with you."

3. For most nurses the most difficult part of the nurse-client relationship is:
   1. Remaining therapeutic and professional at all times
   2. Being able to understand and accept the client's behavior
   3. Developing an awareness of self and the professional role in the relationship
   4. Accepting responsibility in identifying and evaluating the real needs of the client

4. The statement that would best describe the practice of psychiatric nursing would be:
   1. Helping people with present or potential mental health problems
   2. Ensuring clients' legal and ethical rights by acting as a client advocate
   3. Focusing interpersonal skills on people with physical or emotional problems

4. Acting in a therapeutic way with people diagnosed as having a mental disorder

5. A client who works as a receptionist in a physician's office has been an inpatient on a medical unit for over 6 days. The client continues to complain of severe abdominal symptoms, is febrile, and has the primary care providers deeply concerned because there has been no response to treatment. All tests are negative. Today, the client is diagnosed with Munchausen syndrome. The primary care providers would probably experience feelings of:
   1. Pity
   2. Anger
   3. Annoyance
   4. Indifference

6. An acutely ill client with the diagnosis of schizophrenia has just been admitted to the mental health unit. When working with this client initially the nurse's most therapeutic action would be to:
   1. Use diversional activity and involve the client in occupational therapy
   2. Build trust and demonstrate acceptance by spending some time with the client
   3. Delay one-to-one interactions until medications reduce the psychotic symptoms
   4. Involve the client in multiple small group discussions to distract attention from the fantasy world

7. After several weeks of caring for a client in the terminal stage of an illness the nurse becomes increasingly aware of a need to get away from the relationship for a period of time. The best initial action by the nurse would be to:
   1. Ask to be assigned to another client
   2. Request vacation time for a few days
   3. Seek support from colleagues on the unit
   4. Withdraw emotional involvement from the client

8. In psychiatric nursing, the most important tool the nurse brings to a helping relationship is:
   1. Oneself and a desire to help
   2. Advanced communication skills
   3. Knowledge of psychopathology
   4. Years of experience in milieu management

9. The supervisor notices that the care a previously effective nurse in the ICU unit is now providing is barely adequate, that the nurse appears to be working harder although accomplishing less, and putting in at least 1 hour of overtime almost every day. The supervisor should handle this situation by stating:
   1. "I think you are trying to do too much."
   2. "What can I do to help you get finished on time?"
   3. "I've noticed you've been staying late almost every night."
   4. "I'll help you get more organized so you can leave on time."

10. A nurse asks the supervisor, "What coping strategy could I develop to prevent over-responding to stress in the future?" The supervisor could best respond:
    1. "Hone your problem-solving skills."
    2. "Improve your time management skills."
    3. "Ignore situations that you can change."
    4. "Develop a wide variety of coping strategies."

11. An elderly client has not been eating well since admission. The client repeatedly states, "No one cares." The most appropriate response by the nurse would be:
    1. "We all care about you; now please eat."
    2. "You know you have to eat to stay alive."
    3. "I care about you. What foods do you especially like?"
    4. "I care about you. Please eat some of this food for me."

12. Self-help groups such as Alcoholics Anonymous help members to learn that:
    1. They do not need a crutch
    2. Their problems are not unique
    3. They can stand stronger together
    4. Their problems are caused by alcohol

13. A male nurse is caring for a client. The client states, "You know, I've never had a male nurse before." The nurse's best reply would be:
    1. "Does it bother you to have a male nurse?
    2. "There aren't many of us; we're a minority."
    3. "How do you feel about having a male nurse?
    4. "You sound upset. Would you prefer a female nurse?"

14. As the depression begins to lift, a client is asked to join a small discussion group that meets every evening on the unit. The client is reluctant to join because, "I have nothing to talk about." The best response by the nurse would be:

1. "Maybe tomorrow you will feel more like talking."
2. "Could you start off by talking about your family?"
3. "A person like you has a great deal to offer the group."
4. "You feel you will not be accepted unless you have something to say?"

15. During a group meeting a male client tells everyone of his fear of his impending discharge from the hospital. It would be most appropriate for the group leader to respond:
    1. "You ought to be happy that you're leaving."
    2. "Maybe you're not ready to be discharged yet."
    3. "Maybe others in the group have similar feelings that they would share."
    4. "How many in the group feel that this member is ready to be discharged?"

16. The father of a 16-year-old who has just been diagnosed with Hodgkin's disease tells the nurse he does not want his child to know the diagnosis. The nurse's best response would be:
    1. "It is best if he knows the diagnosis."
    2. "The cure rate for Hodgkin's disease is high."
    3. "Let's talk about why you don't want him to know."
    4. "Would you like someone with Hodgkin's to talk to you?"

17. During individual sessions designed to help the depressed client explore alternative coping strategies, it would be most appropriate for the nurse to ask:
    1. "How have you managed your problems in the past?"
    2. "What do you feel you have learned from this suicide attempt?"
    3. "How will you manage the next time your problems start piling up?"
    4. "Were there other things going on in your life that made you want to die?"

18. To deal in a growth-promoting manner with the occasional silence that occurs during a group session, the leaders should:
    1. Be willing to sit indefinitely to wait the silence out
    2. Call on specific members to talk when silence occurs
    3. Go around the group, requiring each member to talk in turn
    4. Comment on the silence or nonverbal behavior related to the silence

19. During a special meeting to discuss the unexpected suicide of one of the female clients while on a weekend pass, the nurse overhears another client moan softly, "I'm next. Oh, my God, I'm next. They couldn't prevent hers and they can't protect me." It would be most therapeutic for the nurse to respond by saying:
   1. "You are afraid you will hurt yourself?"
   2. "The other client was a lot sicker than you are."
   3. "It's different. The other client was home; you are here."
   4. "There is no need to worry. All passes will be canceled for a while."

20. During a group discussion regarding the unexpected suicide of a young female client while on a weekend pass, one of the other clients stands up and shouts, "Oh, I know what you're all thinking; you think that I should have known that she was going to kill herself. You think I helped her plan this." The most therapeutic response by the group leader would be:
   1. "It will help if you tell us the truth."
   2. "Oh, no. We all know you liked her."
   3. "You feel we're blaming you for her death?"
   4. "Helping another person to plan a suicide would not be healthy."

21. During a group discussion, it is learned that a female group member masked her depression and suicidal urges and indeed committed suicide several days ago. The group leaders should be prepared primarily to deal with:
   1. The guilt that the group feels because they could not prevent another's suicide
   2. The lack of concern over the member's suicide expressed by some of the group
   3. The guilt, fear, and anger of the co-leaders that they failed to anticipate and prevent the suicide
   4. The fear and anxiety that some members of the group may have that their own suicidal urges may go unnoticed and unprotected

22. A client attending a mental health day-care unit is scheduled for several diagnostic studies. The client behavior that would be the best indicator that the client had received adequate preparation for these studies would be that the client:
   1. Requests that the tests be reexplained
   2. Repeatedly checks the appointment card
   3. Paces the hallway the morning before the tests
   4. Arrives early and waits quietly to be called for the tests

23. During a one-to-one interaction with a nurse, the client states, "I'm worried about going home." The nurse responds, "Tell me more about this." This response is an example of:
   1. Focusing
   2. Clarifying
   3. Reflecting
   4. Refocusing

24. The most advantageous therapy for a preschool-aged child with a history of physical and sexual abuse would be:
   1. Play therapy
   2. Psychodrama
   3. Group therapy
   4. Family therapy

25. The nurse sits with an elderly depressed client twice a day, although there is little verbal communication. One afternoon, the client asks, "Do you think they'll ever let me out of here?" The nurse's best reply would be:
   1. "Why don't you ask your doctor?"
   2. "Everyone says you're doing just fine."
   3. "Why, do you think you are ready to leave?"
   4. "You have the feeling that you might not leave?"

26. The most therapeutic nursing intervention to help the late middle-aged individual deal with the emotional aspects of aging would include:
   1. Focusing on the individual's past experiences
   2. Having the individual attend lectures on aging
   3. Assisting the individual with plans for the future
   4. Attentive listening to the what the individual is saying

27. A nurse is assigned to care for a regressed 19-year-old college student newly admitted to the psychiatric unit with a 1-month history of talking to unseen people and refusing to get out of bed, go to class, or get involved in daily grooming activities. The nurse's initial efforts should be directed toward helping the client by:
   1. Providing frequent rest periods to avoid exhaustion
   2. Facilitating the client's social relationships with a peer group
   3. Reducing environmental stimuli and maintaining dietary intake
   4. Attempting to establish a meaningful relationship with the client

28. A client with a diagnosis of major depression refuses to participate in unit activities because of being "just too tired." The nursing approach that best expresses an understanding of this client's needs would be:
    1. Planning a rest period for the client during activity time
    2. Explaining why the staff believes the activities are therapeutic
    3. Helping the client express feelings of hostility toward the activities
    4. Accepting the client's behavior calmly and, without excessive comment, setting firm limits

29. A female client on the psychiatric unit remains aloof from all other clients. The nurse with whom she has developed a friendly relationship may help her participate in some ward activity by:
    1. Finding solitary pursuits that the client can enjoy
    2. Speaking to the client about the importance of entering into activities
    3. Asking the physician to speak to the client about participating in activities
    4. Inviting another client to take part in a joint activity with the nurse and the client

30. The nurse can best reassure an elderly depressed client who is concerned about many fears that are upsetting and frightening and expresses a feeling of having committed the "unpardonable sin" by stating:
    1. "Your family loves you very much."
    2. "You know that you are not a bad person."
    3. "You know, those ideas of yours are in your imagination."
    4. "Your ideas are part of your illness and they will change as you improve."

31. A 45-year-old physician is admitted to the psychiatric unit of a community hospital. The client is restless, loud, aggressive, and resistive during the admission procedure and states, "I will take my own blood pressure." The most therapeutic response by the nurse would be:
    1. "Right now, doctor, you are just another client."
    2. "I am sorry but I cannot allow that. I must take your BP."
    3. "If you would rather, doctor. I'm sure you will do it OK."
    4. "If you do not cooperate, I will get the attendants to hold you down."

Emotional Problems Related to Physical Health and Childbearing

32. The nurse should plan to explain to the adult daughters of a dying client, whose mood changes and apparent anger at them is causing them concern, that their mother is:
    1. Frightened by her impending death
    2. Working through acceptance of her situation
    3. Attempting to reduce her family's dependence on her
    4. Hurt that the family will not take her home to die in her own bed

33. A client spontaneously delivers a healthy baby girl. Her husband expresses delight but appears anxious and tends to avoid physical contact with the baby. Later, he says to the nurse, "My wife seems so wrapped up with the baby, I hope she has time for me." The nurse's best response would be:
    1. "You seem to feel you'll have to fend for yourself."
    2. "Do you think your parents will be able to help out?"
    3. "You'll both be so busy you won't even miss her attention."
    4. "I can understand your concern about the changes you'll have to make."

34. When a continent, bedridden client with a chronic illness expresses anger through urinary incontinence, the nurse should:
    1. Limit the client's fluid intake in the evening
    2. Provide television or radio for the client when alone
    3. Frequently ask if the client needs the bedpan to void
    4. Create an environment that prevents sensory monotony

35. A client with a chronic illness who had been incontinent of urine at home has not been incontinent since being hospitalized. When discussing past and present elimination patterns, the client also tells the nurse about being angry at being bedridden and unable to go anywhere or see anyone. The nurse deduces that the client's incontinence at home may have been related to:
    1. A way of maintaining control
    2. An unconscious expression of hostility
    3. A method to determine the family's love
    4. A physiologic response expected with the elderly

36. The parents of a child who had open-heart surgery are informed that their child is in the postanesthesia care unit (PACU) and is stable. The mother is crying and extremely worried. The nurse can best help allay the mother's anxiety by:
    1. Reassuring her that their child is doing well
    2. Allowing her to continue to express her feelings
    3. Bringing her and her husband to the recovery unit for several minutes
    4. Encouraging them both to go have a cup of coffee and return in 2 hours

37. A female client who has had multiple hospital admissions for recurring congestive heart failure is returned to the hospital by her daughter. The client is admitted to the coronary care unit for observation. She states, "I know I'm sick, but I could really take care of myself at home." The nurse recognizes that the client is attempting to:
    1. Deny her illness
    2. Suppress her fears
    3. Reassure her daughter
    4. Maintain her independence

38. Clients on dialysis frequently experience the psychologic problem of:
    1. Reactive depression
    2. Postpump psychosis
    3. Depersonalization disorder
    4. Dialysis disequilibrium

Drug-Related Responses

39. A depressed client has been started on a tricyclic antidepressant. The nurse teaches the client to expect to notice a significant change in the depression within:
    1. 12 to 16 hours
    2. 4 to 6 days
    3. 1 to 4 weeks
    4. 5 to 6 weeks

40. If clients do not abide by their diet restrictions while taking a monoamine oxidase inhibitor, it is likely that they will develop:
    1. Generalized urticaria
    2. An occipital headache
    3. Severe muscle spasms
    4. Sudden, severe hypotension

41. A client is receiving lithium carbonate. While this medication is being administered, it is important that the nurse:
    1. Test the client's urine weekly
    2. Restrict the client's sodium intake

3. Monitor the client's blood level regularly
4. Withhold the client's other medications for 1 week

42. A client in the hyperactive phase of a mood disorder, bipolar type, is receiving lithium carbonate. The nurse notes that the client's lithium blood level is 1.8 mEq/L. It would be most appropriate for the nurse to:
    1. Continue the usual dose of lithium and note any adverse reactions
    2. Discontinue the drug until the lithium serum level drops to 0.5 mEq/L
    3. Notify the physician immediately, since the lithium serum level may be toxic
    4. Ask the physician to increase the dose of lithium, since the serum level is too low

43. A client on a maintenance dose of lithium therapy develops hand tremors, muscle hyperirritability, and mental confusion. The nurse should:
    1. Withhold the medication, obtain blood lithium levels, and call the physician
    2. Check for nausea, vomiting, thirst, and polyuria before administering the next dose of lithium
    3. Expect these side effects, administer the medication as ordered, and note these findings in the record
    4. Withhold the medication, check the blood pressure, and, if within normal limits, administer the correct dosage

44. Neuroleptics are the drugs of choice to relieve symptoms of:
    1. Psychosis
    2. Depression
    3. Hyperkinesis
    4. Narcotic withdrawal

45. A common manageable side effect of neuroleptics is:
    1. Ptosis
    2. Jaundice
    3. Melanocytosis
    4. Unintentional tremors

46. To actively reverse the overdose sedative effects of benzediazepines, the nurse should anticipate an order to administer:
    1. Lithium
    2. Methadone
    3. Romazicon
    4. Chlorpromazine

47. Abrupt withdrawal from barbiturate use could cause a person to experience:
1. Ataxia
2. Urticaria
3. Diarrhea
4. Seizures

48. When administered for a heroin overdose, the planned effect of naloxone hydrochloride (Narcan) is to:
1. Compete with narcotics for receptors controlling respiration
2. Decrease analgesia and the comatose state induced by heroin
3. Accelerate metabolism of heroin and stimulate respiratory centers
4. Stimulate cortical sites controlling consciousness and cardiovascular function

49. Within an hour of receiving naloxone hydrochloride (Narcan) to combat an overdose of heroin, a client is responding. Close observation of the client's status is still indicated because:
1. The drug may cause neuropathy and seizures
2. The combined action of the drug and heroin causes cardiac depression
3. The narcotic effect may cause return of symptoms after the drug is metabolized
4. Hyperexcitability and amnesia may cause the client to thrash about and become abusive

50. A 52-year-old male client with a diagnosis of schizophrenia is about to be discharged to a halfway house. This is his fifth admission in less than 1 year. He improves while in the hospital, but after discharge he forgets to take his medication, is unable to function, and must be hospitalized again. A medication that could be given IM to this client on an outpatient basis every 2 to 3 weeks would be:
1. Haldol
2. Valium
3. Lithium carbonate
4. Prolixin decanoate

51. The aspect of electroconvulsive therapy that can result in the most serious complication is the use of:
1. Positive pressure to inflate the alveoli
2. Electric voltage to induce the seizures
3. Succinylcholine chloride (Anectine) to relax muscles
4. Methohexital sodium (Brevital sodium) to induce sleep

52. The physician has ordered imipramine (Tofranil), 75 mg tid, for a client. An appropriate nursing action when giving this drug is to:
1. Avoid administration of barbiturates or steroids with this drug
2. Warn the client not to eat cheese, fermenting products, and chicken liver
3. Observe the client for increased tolerance so that the therapeutic dosage is maintained
4. Have the client checked for intraocular pressure and provide instructions to watch for symptoms of glaucoma

53. A psychiatric client is to be discharged with orders for haloperidol (Haldol) therapy. When developing a teaching plan for discharge, the nurse should include cautioning the client against:
1. Driving at night
2. Staying in the sun
3. Ingesting wines and cheeses
4. Taking medications containing aspirin

54. A client has been on an acute care psychiatric unit for 3 days and is receiving haloperidol (Haldol) tablets orally to reduce agitation and preoccupation with auditory hallucinations. There has been no decrease in the client's agitation or preoccupation with auditory hallucinations since the medication was started. The priority nursing intervention would be to:
1. Ask the psychiatrist to change the medication
2. Secure an order for prn sedation until the client calms down
3. Assess to make certain the client is swallowing the medication
4. Recognize that the therapeutic level of the drug has not been achieved

55. A client with depression is to receive fluoxetine (Prozac). A precaution that the nurse must keep in mind when initiating treatment with this drug is that:
1. Eating cheese or pickled herring or drinking wine may cause a hypertensive crisis
2. It must be given with milk and crackers to avoid hyperacidity and discomfort
3. The blood level may not be sufficient to cause noticeable improvement for 2 to 4 weeks
4. Blood levels will need to be obtained weekly for 3 months to check for appropriate levels

56. The nurse evaluates that the teaching about taking the medication amitriptyline (Elavil) has been understood when the client states:
1. "I must discontinue this medication if side effects occur."
2. "I don't need to be concerned about taking my medications."
3. "It is necessary to take each dose of my medication as ordered."
4. "I may find it necessary to adjust the dosage if side effects occur."

57. Drugs such as trihexyphenidyl (Artane), biperiden (Akineton), or benztropine (Cogentin) is often prescribed in conjunction with:
1. Barbiturates
2. Antidepressants
3. Antianxiety agents/anxiolytics
4. Antipsychotic agents/neuroleptics

58. A psychiatrist is making morning rounds, and after examining one of the adult male clients who continues to exhibit negative symptoms (flat affect, isolation, poverty of speech, and lack of motivation) of schizophrenia, the doctor writes an order to change from haloperidol (Haldol) to risperidone (Risperdal). The dosage ordered is 1 mg bid for 3 days. It is most important that the nurse:
1. Monitor the client for mood changes and suicidal tendencies especially during early therapy
2. Assess for the side effects of sedation, restlessness, and muscle spasm once the drug has been administered
3. Determine if the morning dosage of Haldol had been given and then start the initial dose of Risperdal at bedtime
4. Review the medication sheet to determine the time of the last dose of Haldol before administering the correct dosage of Risperdal at 2 PM

59. Photosensitization is a side effect associated with the use of:
1. Sertraline (Zoloft)
2. Lithium carbonate (Lithane)
3. Methylphenidate hydrochloride (Ritalin)
4. Chlorpromazine hydrochloride (Thorazine)

60. After 2 weeks of drug therapy, the nurse notices that the client has become jaundiced. The nurse continues to give the neuroleptic until the psychiatrist can be consulted. In situations such as this:

1. Jaundice is a benign side effect and has little significance
2. Jaundice is sufficient reason to discontinue the neuroleptic
3. The blood level of neuroleptics must be maintained once established
4. The psychiatrist's order for the neuroleptic should be reduced by the nurse

61. An acting-out, elderly client has been receiving fluphenazine (Prolixin) for several months. After noticing that the client sits rigidly in a chair, the nurse observes the client closely for other evidence of adverse effects of the drug, including:
1. Inability to concentrate, excess salivation
2. Uncoordinated movement of extremities, tremors
3. Minimal use of nonverbal expression, rambling speech
4. Reluctance to converse, nonverbal clues indicating fear

62. An extrapyramidal symptom that is a potentially irreversible side effect of antipsychotic drugs is:
1. Torticollis
2. Oculogyric crisis
3. Tardive dyskinesia
4. Pseudoparkinsonism

63. When monoamine oxidase inhibitors (MAOIs) are prescribed, the client should be cautioned against:
1. Prolonged exposure to the sun
2. Ingesting wines and aged cheeses
3. Engaging in active physical exercise
4. The use of medications with an elixir base

64. For the past 5 days, a client has been receiving tranylcypromine sulfate (Parnate) 10 mg po bid for treatment of a major depressive episode. This morning, the client refuses the medication, stating, "It doesn't help, so what's the use of taking it?" The response by the nurse that would best demonstrate an understanding of the action of this monamine oxidase inhibitor (MAOI) would be:
1. "Sometimes it takes 2 to 4 weeks to see an improvement."
2. "It takes 6 to 8 weeks for this medication to have an effect."
3. "You should have felt a response by now. I'll notify your physician."
4. "I'll talk to the physician about increasing the dosage, and that will help."

65. An important aspect of teaching for any client receiving a monoamine oxidase inhibitor such as tranylcypromine sulfate (Parnate) should be that:
    1. Drowsiness is an expected side effect of this medication
    2. Clients taking this type medication have special dietary restrictions
    3. The therapeutic level and the toxic level of these drugs are very close
    4. It is necessary for these clients to wear a hat outdoors and avoid the sun

66. When administering methylphenidate (Ritalin) tid to a child with an attention-deficit hyperactivity disorder, the nurse knows that the first daily dose should be given:
    1. Before breakfast
    2. Just after breakfast
    3. Immediately before lunch
    4. As soon as the child awakens

Personality Development

67. The nurse is aware that Freud's phallic stage of psychosexual development, which compares with Erikson's psychosocial phase of initiative vs. guilt, is best seen at:
    1. Adolescence
    2. 6 to 12 years
    3. Birth to 1 year
    4. 3 to $5\frac{1}{2}$ years

68. The relationship that is of extreme importance in the formation of the personality is the:
    1. Peer
    2. Sibling
    3. Parent-child
    4. Heterosexual

69. An example of displacement is:
    1. Imaginative activity to escape reality
    2. Ignoring unpleasant aspects of reality
    3. Resisting any demands made by others
    4. Pent-up emotions directed to other than the primary source

70. In the process of development the individual strives to maintain, protect, and enhance the integrity of the self. This is normally accomplished through the use of:
    1. Affective reactions
    2. Ritualistic behaviors
    3. Withdrawal patterns
    4. Defense mechanisms

71. A male college student who is smaller than average and unable to participate in sports becomes the life of the party and a stylish dresser. This is an example of the mechanism of:
    1. Introjection
    2. Sublimation
    3. Compensation
    4. Reaction formation

72. A nursing assistant complains to the nurse that an elderly female client with dementia will do things, but only when she feels like it, and wonders how one can deal with this. The nurse's response to the staff member should be based on the understanding that in addition to the dementia in this client, the elderly:
    1. Lose their coping ability
    2. Lose their ability to cooperate
    3. Have difficulty with step procedures
    4. Are ambivalent toward authority

73. A generally accepted concept of personality development is:
    1. By 2 years of age the basic personality is rather firmly set
    2. The personality is capable of change and modification throughout life
    3. The capacity for personality change decreases rapidly after adolescence
    4. By the end of the first 6 years, the personality has reached its adult parameters

74. According to psychosexual theory, the primary emergence of the personality is demonstrated around the age of:
    1. 6 months
    2. 9 months
    3. 24 months
    4. 48 months

75. Personality is unique for every individual because it is the result of the person's:
    1. Intellectual capacity, race, and socioeconomic status
    2. Genetic background, placement in family, and autoimmunity
    3. Biologic constitution, psychologic development, and cultural setting
    4. Childhood experiences, intellectual capacity, and socioeconomic status

76. Problems with dependence versus independence develop during the stage of growth and development known as:
    1. Infancy
    2. Toddler
    3. Preschool
    4. School age

77. The basic emotional task for the toddler is:
    1. Trust
    2. Industry
    3. Identification
    4. Independence

78. During the oedipal stage of growth and development, the child:
    1. Loves and hates (ambivalence) both parents
    2. Loves the parent of the same sex and the parent of the opposite sex
    3. Loves the parent of the opposite sex and hates the parent of the same sex
    4. Loves the parent of the same sex and hates the parent of the opposite sex

79. The stage of growth and development basically concerned with role identification is the:
    1. Oral stage
    2. Genital stage
    3. Oedipal stage
    4. Latency stage

80. Play for the preschool-age child is necessary for the emotional development of:
    1. Projection
    2. Introjection
    3. Competition
    4. Independence

81. Resolution of the oedipal complex takes place when the child:
    1. Rejects the parent of the same sex
    2. Introjects behaviors of both parents
    3. Identifies with the parent of the same sex
    4. Identifies with the parent of the opposite sex

82. Surgery can be a very traumatic event for a child. The nurse when performing preoperative preparation knows that according to Piaget's stages of cognitive development children will experience the greatest fear during the:
    1. Sensorimotor stage
    2. Preoperational stage
    3. Concrete operational stage
    4. Formal operational stage

83. Evidence of the existence of the unconscious is best demonstrated by:
    1. The ease of recall
    2. Slips of the tongue
    3. Déja vu experiences
    4. Free-floating anxiety

84. Mental experiences operate on different levels of awareness. The level that best portrays one's attitudes, feelings, and desires is the:
    1. Conscious
    2. Unconscious
    3. Preconscious
    4. Foreconscious

85. The ability to tolerate frustration is an example of one of the functions of the:
    1. Id
    2. Ego
    3. Superego
    4. Unconscious

86. The superego is that part of the psyche that:
    1. Contains the instinctual drives
    2. Is the source of creative energy
    3. Operates on the pleasure principle and demands immediate gratification
    4. Develops from internalizing the concepts of parents and significant others

87. Another term for the superego is:
    1. Self
    2. Ideal self
    3. Narcissism
    4. Conscience

88. The superego is that part of the self that says:
    1. I like what I want
    2. I want what I want
    3. I should not want that
    4. I can wait for what I want

89. A person has a mature personality if the:
    1. Ego responds to the demands of the superego
    2. Society sets demands to which the ego responds
    3. Superego has replaced and increased all the controls of the parents
    4. Ego acts as a balance between the pressures of the id and the superego

90. Incidents of child molestation that come out years later when the victim is an adult can best be explained by the ego defense mechanism of:
    1. Repression
    2. Regression
    3. Rationalization
    4. Reaction formation

91. A client with diabetes mellitus is able to discuss in great detail the metabolic process in diabetes while eating a piece of chocolate cake topped with butter frosting. This is an example of the defense mechanism known as:
    1. Projection
    2. Dissociation
    3. Displacement
    4. Intellectualization

92. An elderly client with a diagnosis of early dementia of the Alzheimer's type tells the nurse, "I am useless to everyone, even myself." The nurse recognizes that the client has probably failed to accomplish Erikson's developmental task of:
    1. Ego integrity versus despair
    2. Identity versus role diffusion
    3. Generativity versus stagnation
    4. Autonomy versus shame and doubt

93. The level of anxiety that best enhances an individual's power of perception is:
    1. Mild
    2. Panic
    3. Severe
    4. Moderate

94. A person seeing a design on the wallpaper perceives it as an animal. This is an example of:
    1. An illusion
    2. A delusion
    3. A hallucination
    4. An idea of reference

95. Sublimation is a defense mechanism that helps the individual:
    1. Act out in reverse something already done or thought
    2. Return to an earlier, less mature, stage of development
    3. Exclude from the conscious things that are psychologically disturbing
    4. Channel unacceptable sexual desires into socially approved behavior

Disorders First Evident Before Adulthood

96. About a month after their toddler is diagnosed as moderately retarded, the parents' discussion of the toddler's future reflects plans for their child's normal independent functioning. The nurse recognizes that the parents:
    1. Are using denial
    2. Accept the diagnosis
    3. Are using intellectualization
    4. Understand their child's limitations

97. When using behavior modification to foster toilet training efforts in a cognitively impaired child, the nurse should reinforce appropriate use of the toilet by giving the child a:
    1. Piece of fruit
    2. Piece of candy
    3. Hug and praise
    4. Choice of rewards

98. Adolescents experience a cognitive process known as a personal fable. In regard to her pregnancy, a 16-year-old's personal fable is demonstrated when she states;
    1. "Imagine me being a mother!"
    2. "I can't get pregnant if I don't want to."
    3. "My boyfriend said you can't get pregnant the first time."
    4. "My monthly cycle is still irregular, so I can't get pregnant."

99. A 7-year-old male has recently been diagnosed with an attention-deficit disorder with hyperactivity. Cylert 37.5 mg/day has been prescribed. In discussing their child's treatment with the parents, the nurse emphasizes the fact that it would be important for them to:
    1. Tutor their son in the subjects that are troublesome
    2. Monitor the effect of the medication on their son's behavior
    3. Point out to their son that he can control his behavior if he desires
    4. Avoid imposing too many rules because they would frustrate their son

100. A child scores between 55 and 68 on a standardized intelligent quotient (IQ) assessment test. The nurse is aware that this degree of intellectual impairment would be considered:
    1. Mild
    2. Severe
    3. Profound
    4. Moderate

101. A 16-year-old male has the mental age of 7 years. His nursing care plan includes provision for future ongoing care. The action that indicates the family is moving in that direction is that:
    1. He attends a sheltered workshop every day
    2. His parents are seeking his institutionalization
    3. He eats all of his meals with the rest of the family
    4. His parents are encouraging him to forget about dating

102. The problem of separation anxiety becomes most problematic for children hospitalized during the age of:
    1. 6 to 30 months
    2. 36 to 59 months
    3. 5 to $11^1/_2$ years
    4. 12 to 18 years

103. The prognosis for a normal productive life for a child diagnosed with an autistic disorder is:
    1. Dependent upon an early diagnosis
    2. Often related to the child's overall temperament
    3. Emphasized with the parents regardless of the child's level of functioning
    4. Looked upon with caution because of interference with so many parameters of functioning

104. The most common characteristic of emotionally disturbed children is that they:
    1. Respond to any stimulus
    2. Respond to little external stimulus
    3. Seem unresponsive to the environment
    4. Are totally involved with the environment

105. Autism can usually be diagnosed when the child is about:
    1. 2 years of age
    2. 6 years of age
    3. 6 months of age
    4. 1 to 3 months of age

106. The nurse should observe the autistic child for signs of:
    1. Not wanting to eat
    2. Crying for attention
    3. Catatonic-like rigidity
    4. Enjoying being with people

107. A 6-year-old child who has been diagnosed as autistic is admitted for severe dehydration. The child demonstrates frequent spinning and hand-flapping activities. Nursing intervention to limit these activities should focus on:
    1. Physically holding the child
    2. Redirecting the child's behavior
    3. Asking the child why the spinning and hand flapping is done
    4. Moving furniture to minimize the space available for these activities

108. When planning activities for a child with autism, the nurse must remember that autistic children respond best to:
    1. Large group activity
    2. Loud, cheerful music
    3. Individuals in small groups
    4. Their own self-stimulating acts

109. One of the major behavioral characteristics of children with attention-deficit disorders is their:
    1. Overreaction to stimuli
    2. Continued use of rituals
    3. Retarded speech development
    4. Inability to use abstract thought

110. Attention-deficit hyperactivity disorder in children is usually treated with:
    1. Lorazepam (Ativan)
    2. Haloperidol (Haldol)
    3. Methocarbamol (Robaxin)
    4. Methylphenidate hydrochloride (Ritalin)

111. The nursing assessment of a hyperactive 9-year-old with a history of an attention-deficit disorder, admitted for observation following a motor vehicle accident, reveals a knowledge deficit regarding personal safety. Nursing actions to meet the goal of personal safety should focus on:
    1. Requesting the child write at least 3 safety rules
    2. Asking the child to verbalize as many safety rules as possible
    3. Talking with the child about the importance of using a seat belt
    4. Encouraging the child to talk with other children about their opinions of safety rules

112. School phobia is usually treated by:
    1. Returning the child to school immediately
    2. Calmly explaining why attendance at school is necessary
    3. Allowing the parent to accompany the child to the classroom
    4. Allowing the child to enter the classroom before other children

113. The childhood problem that has legal as well as emotional aspects and cannot be ignored is:
    1. School phobias
    2. Fear of animals
    3. Fear of monsters
    4. Sleep disturbances

114. The nurse should be aware that children with attention-deficit disorder problems may be learning disabled. This means that these children:
1. Will probably not be self-sufficient as adults
2. Have intellectual deficits that interfere with learning
3. Experience perceptual difficulties that interfere with learning
4. Are usually performing two grade levels below their age norm

115. Shortly after admission, an adolescent male client falls to the floor and has tonic and clonic movements. He does not respond verbally, but the nurse notes that he is still chewing gum. The nurse should:
1. Remove the chewing gum
2. Send another client for help
3. Report and record all observation
4. Insert a tongue blade between the teeth

Eating Disorders

116. A 16-year-old, who is extremely underweight (92 pounds) for her height (5 feet, 6 inches), is admitted with the diagnosis of bulimia nervosa. The parents report that the client talks constantly about being fat and disappears into the bathroom after meals. Pills, identified as cathartics, are found in the suitcase on admission to the eating disorder unit. The most appropriate nursing diagnosis for this client at this time would be:
1. Impaired adjustment related to fear of weight gain
2. Feeding self-care deficit related to disturbed thought process
3. Altered patterns of bowel elimination related to use of laxatives
4. Altered nutrition: less than body requirements related to purging

117. The major difference between anorexia nervosa and bulimia nervosa is that the individual with bulimia nervosa:
1. Is obese and is attempting to lose weight
2. Has a distorted body image and sees the body as fat
3. Recognizes that there is a problem but is helpless to correct it
4. Is struggling with a conflict of dependence versus independence

118. A therapeutic environment for clients with bulimia nervosa would be one that is:
1. Controlling
2. Empathetic
3. Focused on food
4. Based on realistic limits

119. A young female client, age 16, is admitted to the psychiatric service with the diagnosis of anorexia nervosa. She has lost 20 pounds in 6 weeks. She is very thin but excessively concerned about being overweight. Her daily intake is 10 cups of coffee. The most important initial nursing intervention would be to:
1. Explain the value of good nutrition
2. Compliment her on her lovely figure
3. Try to establish a relationship of trust
4. Explore the reasons why she does not eat

120. An adolescent is diagnosed as having anorexia nervosa. The nurse understands that the etiology of this disorder is:
1. A low self-esteem
2. Feelings of unworthiness
3. Anger directed at the parents
4. An unconscious fear of growing up

121. An appropriate behavior modification goal for a client with anorexia nervosa would be, the client will:
1. Eat every meal for a week
2. Gain a pound of weight a week
3. Attend group therapy every day
4. Talk about food for 1 hour a day

122. During a prenatal interview in the twentieth week of gestation, the nurse becomes aware that the client has a history of pica. The most appropriate nursing action would be to:
1. Seek a psychologic referral for the client
2. Make sure the client's diet is nutritionally adequate
3. Inform the client of the danger this poses to her baby
4. Obtain an order for multivitamin supplement for the client

123. The nurse plans to discuss childhood nutrition with the mother of a 2-year-old with Down syndrome to make the mother aware that a common eating problem often encountered in children with this syndrome is:
1. Rickets
2. Anemia
3. Obesity
4. Rumination

Delirium, Dementia, and Other Cognitive Disorders

124. The nurse recognizes that dementia of the Alzheimer's type is characterized by:
1. Aggressive acting-out behavior
2. Periodic remissions and exacerbations
3. Hypoxia of selected areas of brain tissue
4. Areas of brain destruction called senile plaques

125. The approach that would be most helpful in meeting the needs of an elderly client hospitalized with the diagnosis of dementia of the Alzheimer's type is:
1. Providing a nutritious diet high in carbohydrates and proteins
2. Simplifying the environment as much as possible while eliminating need for choices
3. Providing an opportunity for many alternative choices in the daily schedule to stimulate interest
4. Developing a consistent nursing plan with fixed time schedules to provide for physical and emotional needs

126. When attempting to understand the behavior of an elderly client diagnosed with vascular dementia, the nurse recognizes that the client is probably:
1. Not capable of using any defense mechanisms
2. Using one method of defense for every situation
3. Making exaggerated use of old, familiar mechanisms
4. Attempting to develop new defense mechanisms to meet the current situation

127. The nursing plan of care for the client with vascular dementia should include:
1. An extensive reeducation program
2. Details for protective and supportive care
3. The introduction of new leisure-time activities
4. Plans to involve the client in group therapy sessions

128. When planning care for a client with delirium, dementia, or other cognitive disorders, the nurse should appropriately:
1. Teach the client new social skills to encourage participation
2. Encourage the client to talk of the past and early experiences
3. Discuss current events to keep the client in contact with reality
4. Maintain the daily routine of living with which the client is familiar

129. The best approach in helping a very confused, elderly client is to provide an environment with:
1. A specific routine
2. Group involvement
3. A trusting relationship
4. Activities that are varied

130. An elderly male client on the psychiatric unit becomes upset in the day room. When attempting to deal with the situation, the nurse should:
1. Instruct the client to be quiet
2. Allow the client to act out until he tires
3. Give directions in a firm, low-pitched voice
4. Lead the client from the room by taking him by his arm

131. An elderly, confused person with socially aggressive behavior needs an environment that:
1. Can be manipulated
2. Is mainly group oriented
3. Allows freedom of expression
4. Provides control by setting limits

132. An elderly client is admitted to a psychiatric hospital with the diagnosis of dementia. The nurse recognizes that it would be most unusual for this client to demonstrate:
1. Resistance to change
2. Preoccupation with personal appearance
3. A tendency to dwell on the past and ignore the present
4. The inability to concentrate on new activities or interests

133. The nurse is assessing a client with dementia. To effectively elicit information about the client's ability to provide self-care, the nurse should:
1. State, "I notice that your shoes do not match your dress."
2. State, "Continue to knit and I shall observe you for a while."
3. Ask, "Can you find your way from the bed to the bathroom?"
4. Ask, "Can you show me how you would open the door if you had a key?"

134. The current trend in the treatment of the older adult with delirium, dementia, or other cognitive disorders is to:
1. Provide occupational therapy
2. Maintain them in the community
3. Medicate during stressful periods
4. Encourage the assumption of responsibility

135. When answering questions from the family of a client with Alzheimer's disease, the nurse explains that this disease is:
1. A slow, relentless deterioration of the mind
2. A functional disorder that occurs in the later years
3. A disease that first emerges in the fourth decade of life
4. Easily diagnosed through laboratory and psychological tests

136. It is important for a team working with clients who have a diagnosis of dementia to adopt a common approach of care because these clients need to:
1. Relate in a consistent manner to staff
2. Learn that the staff cannot be manipulated
3. Accept external controls that are fairly applied
4. Have sameness and consistency in their environment

137. The goal of the therapeutic psychiatric environment for the confused client is to:
1. Help the staff to help the client
2. Assist the client to relate to others
3. Make the hospital atmosphere more homelike
4. Help the client become popular in a controlled setting

138. When working with clients who exhibit mild cognitive impairment, the nursing intervention considered most appropriate would be:
1. Reality orientation
2. Behavioral confrontation
3. Reflective communication
4. Reminiscence group therapy

139. An 80-year-old has been admitted with a diagnosis of dementia. The client is confused, irritable, and forgetful. An important consideration when planning care is that this client:
1. Must be closely supervised and told what to do and where to go
2. Should be allowed to function independently if therapeutically possible
3. Is more likely to remember recent experiences than past life experiences
4. Needs to be trusted to be responsible for carrying out daily self-care activities

140. A 78-year-old male has been brought to the clinic by his family because they believe he has become increasingly confused over the past week. The nurse can validate the client's orientation by asking him to:
1. Explain a proverb
2. State where he was born
3. Identify the name of the hospital
4. Recall what he had eaten for breakfast

Substance-Abuse Disorders

141. A young client is a narcotic addict who had surgery to repair a laceration of the heart caused by a bullet. The client is receiving methadone hydrochloride, which:
1. Allows symptom-free termination of narcotic addiction
2. Converts narcotic use from an illicit to a legally controlled drug
3. Provides postoperative pain control without causing narcotic dependence
4. Counteracts the depressive effects of long-term opiate use on cardiac and thoracic muscles

142. When methadone hydrochloride dosage is lowered, the surgical client who is addicted to narcotics must be observed closely for evidence of:
1. Piloerection, lack of interest in surroundings
2. Agitation, attempts to escape from the hospital
3. Skin dryness, scratching under incisional dressing
4. Lethargy, refusal to participate in therapeutic exercise

143. Following the last dose of methadone hydrochloride, withdrawal symptoms are expected to reach a peak in:
1. 8 to 24 hours
2. 24 to 48 hours
3. 48 to 72 hours
4. 72 to 96 hours

144. When caring for a drug-dependent mother and infant before discharge, the nurse should:
1. Refer the mother to a drug rehabilitation program
2. Support the mother's positive maternal responses
3. Keep the mother and the baby separated until the mother is drug free
4. Help the mother understand that the baby's problems are due to her drug intake

145. A client undergoing alcohol detoxification asks if attendance at Alcoholics Anonymous is required. The nurse's best reply would be:
1. "You'll find you'll need their support."
2. "Do you have feelings about going to these meetings?"
3. "No, it is best to wait until you feel you really need them."
4. "Yes, because you will learn how to cope with your problem."

146. A client with a long history of alcohol abuse spends 28 days in the detoxification unit. When planning for the client's discharge, the nurse should be aware that an essential component of the discharge plan would be a referral to a:
1. Halfway house
2. Family therapist
3. Psychoanalytic therapy group
4. Community based self-help group

147. The nurse is aware that a key indicator that a client with a long history of alcohol abuse is ready for treatment would be evidenced by the client's:
1. Drinking only socially
2. Not drinking for 2 weeks
3. Self-admission for detoxification
4. Verbalizing an honest desire for help

148. The nurse evaluates that a male client has accepted his drinking as a problem when he:
1. Attends scheduled inpatient group meetings
2. Takes his Antabuse each morning as ordered
3. Attends Alcoholics Anonymous meetings daily
4. Volunteers to be a sponsor for another alcoholic

149. The nurse notes that in discussing the problem of alcohol abuse with a male client, the client becomes irritable and blames his family and friends for his increased alcohol intake. The nurse recognizes that the client is using the defense mechanisms of:
1. Denial and sublimation
2. Identification and imitation
3. Suppression and repression
4. Rationalization and projection

150. Drug abuse is best defined as:
1. A physiologic need for a drug
2. A psychologic dependence on a drug
3. A compulsion to take a drug on either a continuous or periodic basis
4. An excessive drug use inconsistent with acceptable medical practice

151. The CAGE screening questionnaire is best used by the nurse with the client who is abusing:
1. Alcohol
2. Multiple drugs
3. Hallucinogens
4. Opiates/depressants

152. When teaching a group of adolescents about substance abuse, the nurse identifies a factor that might place a young person at high risk for this problem as:
1. Curiosity with a daring attitude
2. Occasional periods of depression
3. Loss of a parent through death or separation
4. Normal stresses associated with adolescence

153. When thinking about alcohol and drug abuse, the nurse should be aware that:
1. Most polydrug abusers also abuse alcohol
2. Most alcoholics become polydrug abusers
3. Addictive individuals tend to use hostile, abusive behavior
4. An unhappy childhood is a causative factor in many addictions

154. The most important factor in rehabilitation of a client addicted to alcohol is:
1. The availability of community resources
2. The accepting attitude of the client's family
3. The client's emotional or motivational readiness
4. The qualitative level of the client's physical state

155. A primary consideration for the nurse when caring for a client with a history of substance abuse is to:
1. Set firm, consistent limits and not vary from them
2. Use the same type of communication pattern that the client uses
3. Avoid upsetting the client by calling attention to the drug abuse problem
4. Realize that the client will probably need more pain medication than a nonabuser

156. Clients with a history of alcoholism with Wernicke's encephalopathy associated with Korsakoff's syndrome are treated initially by:
1. Providing a high-protein diet
2. Judicious use of neuroleptics
3. Oral administration of thorazine
4. Intramuscular injections of thiamine

157. A female client is hospitalized because of chronic alcoholism. She is irritable with the nurses and seems only to wait for a friend who visits daily. After these visits the client seems happier and more relaxed. One day the nurse sees the visitor give the client a package, which she puts away quickly. Later the client, obviously intoxicated, tells the staff that her friend has brought gin regularly. The client's husband is very upset and threatens to sue. The decision in this suit would take into consideration the fact that:
1. Clients with psychiatric problems need close supervision
2. The nurse is responsible for observing the client's behavior
3. Clients may have gifts brought to them without prior inspection
4. The client's response to her friend's visit was a clue that the nurse missed

158. A client with an alcoholic abuse problem asks if the nurse can see the bugs that are crawling on the bed. The nurse's best reply would be:
1. "No, I don't see any bugs."
2. "I will get rid of them for you."
3. "I will stay here until you are calmer."
4. "Those bugs are a part of your sickness."

159. A client with a diagnosis of alcoholic amnesic disorder resulting from chronic alcoholism is admitted to the mental health unit. When the client uses confabulation, the nurse should realize that its use is precipitated by the client's:
1. Ideas of grandeur
2. Need to get attention
3. Marked loss of memory
4. Difficulty in accepting the truth

160. A 42-year-old executive is admitted for treatment of alcoholism. The client appears suspicious of others and blames them for personal problems. The nurse understands that the client is using this behavior because of difficulties:
1. In telling the truth
2. With anxiety-reducing ego functions
3. With dependence and independence
4. In identifying who is creating problems

161. A recovering alcoholic joins Alcoholics Anonymous (AA) to help maintain sobriety. AA is classified as a:
1. Social group
2. Self-help group
3. Resocialization group
4. Psychotherapeutic group

162. Clients addicted to alcohol use denial as one of their prime defense mechanisms. The nurse understands that these clients use denial to:
1. Reduce their feelings of guilt
2. Live up to others' expectations
3. Make them seem more independent
4. Make them look better in the eyes of others

163. When a client makes up stories to fill in blank spaces of memory, it is known as:
1. Lying
2. Denying
3. Rationalizing
4. Confabulating

164. The most effective treatment of alcoholism is accomplished by:
1. Individual or group psychotherapy
2. Admission to an alcoholic unit in a hospital
3. Active membership in Alcoholics Anonymous
4. The daily administration of disulfiram (Antabuse)

165. A client with the diagnosis of AIDS and a history of substance abuse admits to having many sexual partners a night. The nurse recognizes that this behavior would be typical of a client who used:
1. Glue
2. Heroin
3. Alcohol
4. Cocaine

Schizophrenia and Other Psychotic Disorders

166. The foremost etiology of schizophrenia today is the:
1. Biologic perspective
2. Seasonal perspective
3. Immunologic perspective
4. Psychoanalytic perspective

167. A disturbed client starts to repeat phrases that others have just said. This type of speech is known as:
1. Autism
2. Echolalia
3. Neologism
4. Echopraxia

168. A male client with delusions of persecution and auditory hallucinations is admitted for psychiatric evaluation after stabbing a friend. Later, the nurse on the unit greets the client by saying, "Good evening. How are you?" The client, who has been referring to himself as "man," answers, "The man is bad." This is an example of:
1. Dissociation
2. Transference
3. Displacement
4. Reaction formation

169. Projection, rationalization, denial, and distortion by hallucinations and delusions are examples of a disturbance in:
1. Logic
2. Association
3. Reality testing
4. The thought process

170. The major reason for treating severe psychiatric disorders with neuroleptics is to:
1. Decrease neurotic symptoms
2. Decrease psychotic symptoms
3. Prevent destructiveness by the client
4. Improve social skills and poor judgment

171. The premorbid personality of a young librarian who has now been diagnosed with a schizoid personality disorder might be described as:
    1. Rigid and controlling
    2. Schizoid and introverted
    3. Dependent and immature
    4. Suspicious and socially inadequate

172. A client with schizophrenia, paranoid type, tells the nurse, "The neighbors are bugging my house; they are spying on me because they want to rob me of all my money." In the hospital, the client complains of being mistreated by the staff, of being poisoned by the food, and of being given the wrong medication. When evaluating the client's response to medications and therapy, the nurse would recognize that the client's reality testing has improved when the client:
    1. Eats food provided on the hospital tray
    2. Discusses discharge plans with the staff
    3. Questions each medication when it is administered
    4. Asks for permission to make phone calls to the hospital administration

173. Nursing interventions for a client diagnosed with a schizoid personality disorder should be appropriately directed toward:
    1. Helping the client enter into group recreational activities
    2. Convincing the client that the hospital staff is trying to help
    3. Helping the client learn to trust the staff through selected experiences
    4. Arranging the hospital environment so that the client's contact with other clients is limited

174. When caring for a client whose behavior is characterized by pathologic suspicion, the nurse should:
    1. Remove as much environmental stress as possible
    2. Help the client realize the suspicions are unrealistic
    3. Ask the client to explain the reasons for the feelings
    4. Help the client to feel accepted by the staff on the unit

175. One evening the nurse finds a client who has been experiencing persecutory delusions trying to get out the door. The client states, "Please let me go. I trust you. The Mafia are going to kill me tonight." The nurse should respond:
    1. "You are frightened. Come with me to your room and we can talk about it."

2. "Nobody here wants to harm you, you know that. I'll come with you to your room."
3. "Come with me to your room. I'll lock the door and no one will get in to harm you."
4. "Thank you for trusting me. Maybe you can trust me when I tell you no one can kill you while you're here."

176. A delusional client refuses to eat because of a belief that the food is poisoned. One of the most appropriate ways for the nurse to initially intervene is to:
    1. Taste the food in the client's presence
    2. Simply state that the food is not poisoned
    3. Suggest that food be brought in from home
    4. Tell the client that tube feedings will be started if eating does not begin

177. A client with the diagnosis of schizophrenia refuses to eat meals. The nursing action that will be the most beneficial to this client is to:
    1. Allow the client to eat whenever desired
    2. Repeatedly direct the client to eat the food
    3. Explain the importance of eating to the client
    4. Sit with the client while the meals are being eaten

178. A delusional female client has refused to eat for 36 hours. She states that the voice of her dead father has commanded her to atone for her sins by fasting for 40 days. The initial nursing intervention that might interrupt the client's delusional system is:
    1. Telling the client she has nothing for which to atone
    2. Asking the client to repeat exactly what the voice said
    3. Asking the physician to write an order for tube feedings
    4. Suggesting other means of atonement that may be less damaging

179. A client with the diagnosis of schizophrenia plans an activity schedule with the help of the treatment team. After agreement by all, a written copy is posted in the client's room. When it is time for the client to go for a walk, the nurse should approach the client by saying:
    1. "It's time for you to go for a walk now."
    2. "Do you want to take your scheduled walk now?"
    3. "When would you like to go for your walk today?"
    4. "You are supposed to be going for your walk now."

180. During the admission procedure a client appears to be responding to voices. The client cries out at intervals, "No, no, I didn't kill him. You know the truth; tell that policeman. Please help me!" The nurse should:
    1. Sit there quietly and not respond at all to the client's statements
    2. Respond to the client by asking, "Whom are they saying you killed?"
    3. Respond by saying, "I want to help you and I realize you must be very frightened."
    4. Say, "Do not become so upset. No one is talking to you; the accusing voices are part of your illness."

181. The nurse has been observing a client for some time. The client is quite delusional, talking about people who are plotting to do harm. The staff notices that the client is pacing more than usual. The nurse decides that the client is beginning to lose control. The best nursing intervention would be to:
    1. Allow the client to use a punching bag
    2. Suggest that the client sit down for a while
    3. Move the client to a quiet place on the unit
    4. Allow the client to continue pacing under supervision

182. A male client tells the nurse that he used to believe that he was God, but now he knows that this is not true. The nurse's best response would be:
    1. "You really believed that?"
    2. "You must be getting well."
    3. "Many people have this delusion."
    4. "What caused you to think you were God?"

183. Prominent symptoms of paranoid schizophrenia lasting for at least one month are:
    1. Delusions and hallucinations
    2. Poverty of speech and apathy
    3. Disturbed relationships and poor grooming
    4. Bizarre behaviors associated with drug use

184. While the nurse is talking with a client, a female client comes up and yells, "I hate you. You're talking about me again," and throws a glass of juice at the nurse. The best nursing approach would be to:
    1. Understand her behavior and say, "You hate me? Tell me about that."
    2. Ignore both the behavior and the client, clean up the juice, and talk to her when she is better

    3. Remove the client to an isolation room because she needs to have limits placed on her behavior
    4. Verbalize feelings of annoyance as an example to the client that it is more acceptable to verbalize feelings than to act out

185. As the nurse enters a room and approaches a male client with the diagnosis of schizophrenia, the client states, "Get out of here before I hit you! Go away!" The nurse recognizes that this client's aggressive behavior was probably related to the fact that he:
    1. Was hallucinating and the voices were directing his response
    2. Was afraid that he might harm the nurse if the nurse came nearer
    3. Was reminded of someone who was frightening and threatening to him
    4. Felt hemmed in and trapped when the nurse came around the bed toward him

186. A client who experiences auditory hallucinations agrees to discuss with the nurse alternative coping strategies. For the next three days when the nurse attempts to focus on alternative strategies, the client gets up and leaves the interaction. It would be most therapeutic for the nurse to state:
    1. "Come back; you agreed that you would discuss other ways to cope."
    2. "You seem very uncomfortable every time I bring up a new way to cope."
    3. "Did you agree to talk about other ways to cope because you thought that was what I wanted?"
    4. "You walk out each time I start to discuss the hallucinations; does that mean you've changed your mind?"

187. When a client openly masturbates, the nurse should most appropriately:
    1. Not react to the behavior
    2. Put the client in seclusion
    3. Restrain the client's hands
    4. State that such behavior is unacceptable

188. One of the primary goals in providing a therapeutic day-care environment for a client who is somewhat autistic, withdrawn, and seclusive is to:
    1. Foster a trusting relationship
    2. Administer medications on time
    3. Involve the client in a group with peers
    4. Remove the client from the family home

189. A client experiencing hallucinations tells the nurse, "The voices are telling me I'm no good." The client asks if the nurse hears the voices. The most appropriate response by the nurse would be:
    1. "It is the voice of your conscience, which only you can control."
    2. "No, I do not hear your voices, but I believe you can hear them."
    3. "The voices are coming from within you and only you can hear them."
    4. "The voices are a symptom of your illness; don't pay any attention to them."

190. The nurse enters a client's room and notes that the client appears preoccupied. Then, turning to the nurse the client states, "They are saying terrible things about me. Can't you hear them?" The most therapeutic response by the nurse would be:
    1. "Have you heard them before?"
    2. "Try to get control of your feelings."
    3. "There is no one here but me. I don't hear anything."
    4. "I don't hear what you say you hear, but I can see you are upset."

191. A client has delusions that the food is poisoned and therefore will not eat. The nurse tells the client that it is foolish to believe that, because the food in question comes from the same kitchen as the food for all the other clients. The nurse states, "Unless you eat, you will have to be fed by other means." This response indicates that the client has:
    1. To be reminded about needing to eat
    2. Misinterpretations that have to be corrected
    3. Created a situation the nurse cannot handle
    4. Nourishment needs and therefore has to eat

192. The nurse observes a regressed, emotionally disturbed client using the hands to eat soft foods. The nurse can handle this problem by:
    1. Placing a spoon in the client's hand and suggesting it be used
    2. Saying in a joking way, "Well, I guess fingers were made before forks."
    3. Ignore the behavior and observe several additional meals before intervening
    4. Removing the food and saying, "You can't have any more until you use your spoon."

193. A female client has been on the psychiatric unit for several days. She arouses anxiety and frustration in the staff and manipulates so well that she intimidates any nurse who comes near her. One morning, the client yells out at the nurse, "You've worked it so that I can't go out with the group today to bowl. You're as cunning as a fox—I hate you! Get out or I'll hit you." The best response by the nurse would be:
    1. "Tell me what I did to hurt you."
    2. "Go ahead and hit me if you have a need to."
    3. "I don't really like to hear your threats and insults. Can you tell me why you feel this way?"
    4. "You are being rude and I don't like it. Your behavior is stopping me from wanting to stay with you."

194. While watching TV in the day room, a female client who has demonstrated withdrawn, regressed behavior suddenly screams, bursts into tears, and runs out of the room to the far end of the hallway. The most therapeutic action for the nurse to take would be to:
    1. Walk to the end of the hallway where the client is standing
    2. Write up the incident in the client's chart while memory is fresh
    3. Accept the action as just being the impulsive behavior of a sick person
    4. Ask another client who was in the day room what made the client act as she did

195. When a regressed, emotionally disturbed client voids on the floor in the sitting room on the psychiatric unit, the nurse could best handle the problem by:
    1. Making the client mop the floor
    2. Restricting the client's fluids throughout the day
    3. More frequent toileting of the client with supervision
    4. Withholding privileges each time the client voids on the floor

196. A regressed, emotionally disturbed client who has been watching the nurse for a few days suddenly walks up and shouts, "You think you're so damned perfect and good. I think you stink!" The most appropriate response for the nurse to make would be:
    1. "You seem angry with me."
    2. "Stink? I don't understand."
    3. "Boy, you're in a bad mood."
    4. "I can't be all that bad, can I?"

197. The most appropriate way to help a withdrawn, emotionally disturbed adolescent client to accept the realities of daily living would be to:
    1. Assist the client to care for personal hygiene needs
    2. Encourage the client to keep up with school studies
    3. Encourage the client to join the other clients in group singing
    4. Leave the client alone when there appears to be a disinterest in the activities at hand

198. To encourage a withdrawn, noncommunicative client to talk, the best plan of nursing intervention would be to:
    1. Focus on nonthreatening subjects
    2. Try to get the client to discuss feelings
    3. Ask simple questions that require answers
    4. Sit and look through magazines with the client

199. When caring for clients exhibiting withdrawn patterns of behavior, an important aspect of nursing care is to:
    1. Help keep the client oriented to reality
    2. Involve the client in activities throughout the day
    3. Help the client understand that it is harmful to withdraw from situations
    4. Encourage the client to discuss why mixing with other people is avoided

200. Observation is an important aspect of nursing care. It is especially important in the care of the withdrawn client because it:
    1. Is useful in making a diagnosis
    2. Tells the staff how ill the client is
    3. Indicates the degree of depression
    4. Helps in understanding the client's behaviors

Disorders of Mood

201. A client is admitted to the mental health unit with the diagnosis of bipolar disorder, depressed. During the assessment interview when the client avoids eye contact, responds in a very low voice, and is tearful, it would be most therapeutic for the nurse to state:
    1. "You'll find that you'll get better faster if you try to help us to help you."
    2. "Hold my hand; I know you are frightened. I will not allow anyone to harm you."
    3. "I know this is difficult, but as soon as we are finished, I'll take you to your room."
    4. "I am your nurse. I'll take you to the day room as soon as I get some information."

202. A client is admitted to the mental health unit because of a progressively increasing depression over the past month. During the initial assessment, the nurse would expect the client to display:
    1. Elated affect related to reaction formation
    2. Loose associations related to thought disorder
    3. Physical exhaustion resulting from decreased physical activity
    4. Paucity of verbal expression related to slowed thought processes

203. The activity that would be the least therapeutic for severely depressed clients would be:
    1. Specific, simple instructions to be followed
    2. Simple, easily completed, short-term projects
    3. Monotonous, repetitive projects and activities
    4. Allowing the clients to plan their own activities

204. When caring for the extremely depressed client, the staff should set specific goals directed toward helping the client:
    1. Set realistic life goals
    2. Develop trust in others
    3. Express hostile feelings
    4. Get involved in activities

205. When developing a nursing care plan for a depressed client, the approach that would be most therapeutic would be:
    1. Allowing time for the client's slowness when planning activities
    2. Helping the client focus on family strengths and support systems
    3. Encouraging the client to perform menial tasks to meet the need for punishment
    4. Repeating again and again that the staff views the client as worthwhile and important

206. The statement that would be most appropriate for the nurse to use in interviewing a newly admitted, 35-year-old, depressed client whose thoughts focus on feelings of unworthiness and failure would be:
    1. "Tell me how you feel about yourself."
    2. "Tell me what has been bothering you."
    3. "Why do you feel so bad about yourself?"
    4. "What can we do to help you during your stay with us?"

207. An activity that would be most appropriate for a depressed client during the early part of hospitalization would be a:
    1. Game of Trivial Pursuit
    2. Project involving drawing
    3. Small dance-therapy group
    4. Card game with three other clients

208. A withdrawn client refuses to get out of bed and becomes upset. It would be most therapeutic for the nurse to:
1. Require the client to get out of bed at once
2. Stay with the client until the client calms down
3. Give the client the prn neuroleptic that is ordered
4. Allow the client to stay in bed for the present without company

209. Following admission, the nurse needs to evaluate a depressed client's potential for suicide. The approach that would best gain this information would be:
1. Asking the client about plans for the future
2. Asking other clients about suicide while in a group
3. Asking the family if the client has ever attempted suicide
4. Asking the client if suicide was ever or is now being considered

210. When caring for a middle-aged, female client with a major depression, who feels all her family members have been killed because she has been sinful and needs to be punished, the prime responsibility of the nurse would be to:
1. Protect the client against any suicidal impulses
2. Keep up the client's interest in the outside world
3. Help the client handle her concern for family members
4. Reassure the client that past behaviors are not being punished

211. A client is placed on suicide precautions. The most therapeutic way to provide these precautions would be to:
1. Remove all sharp or cutting objects
2. Not allow the client to leave his/her room
3. Give the client the opportunity to ventilate feelings
4. Assign a staff member to be with the client at all times

212. A client is admitted to the mental health unit after attempting suicide. When the nurse approaches, the client is tearful and silent. The nurse's best initial response would be:
1. To note the behavior, record it, and notify the attending physician
2. To sit quietly next to the client and wait until the client begins to speak

3. "You are crying; does that mean you feel badly about attempting suicide and really want to live?"
4. "I notice you are tearful and seem sad. Tell me what it's like for you and perhaps we can begin to work it out together."

213. An elderly, depressed client frequently paces the halls, becoming physically tired from the activity. To help the client reduce this activity, the nurse should:
1. Supply the client with simple, monotonous tasks
2. Request a sedative order from the client's physician
3. Restrain the client in a chair, reducing the opportunity to pace
4. Place the client in a single room, thus limiting pacing to a smaller area

214. A long-term therapy goal for a female client hospitalized for a major depressive episode should be that the client will be:
1. Able to talk about her depressed feelings
2. Able to develop new defense mechanisms
3. More realistic in accepting herself and others
4. Aware of the unconscious source of her anger

215. The action by the nurse that would be most therapeutic when a depressed client states, "I am no good. I'm better off dead." would be:
1. Stating, "I think you're good; you should think of living."
2. Stating, "I will stay with you until you are less depressed."
3. Alerting the staff to provide 24-hour observation of the client
4. Unobtrusively removing those articles that could be used in a suicide attempt

216. A positive nursing action when caring for a middle-aged, depressed client is to:
1. Play a game of chess with the client
2. Allow the client to make personal decisions
3. Sit down next to the client as often as possible
4. Provide the client with frequent periods of thinking time

217. The nurse is assigned to care for a middle-aged, depressed female client on a day when the client seems more withdrawn and depressed than usual. It would be most appropriate for the nurse to:
1. Remain visible to the client
2. Get the client involved in group activities
3. Ask the client, "May I sit down next to you for a while?"
4. Periodically spend a few minutes with the client throughout the day

218. The nurse is to discharge a client from the psychiatric unit who has been treated for a major depression. The statement by the nurse that demonstrates the most understanding at this time would be:
1. "Call the unit night or day if you have problems."
2. "I am going to miss you; we have become good friends."
3. "I know you are really going to be all right when you go home."
4. "This is my phone number; call me and let me know how you are doing."

219. A client is admitted to the hospital following a week-long period of complete inability to function and aimless activity. During the assessment, the nurse notes the client is pacing the floor, weeping, and wringing the hands. The nurse would expect the physician to order an:
1. Antimanic medication
2. Antianxiety medication
3. Antipsychotic medication
4. Antidepressive medication

220. A client admitted for suicidal ideation progresses satisfactorily and is to be discharged from the unit within a day or two. The client denies suicidal tendencies and the staff is pleased with the client's progress. One day the door to the unit is accidently left unlocked. Fifteen minutes later the client is gone and is found hanging in the bathroom. In this situation:
1. The client's actions should have been anticipated by the nurse
2. Suicidal clients should be observed until all symptoms of depression disappear
3. Determined clients almost always succeed at suicide, even with constant supervision
4. The lifting of the depression demonstrated the client's recovery, so supervision was unnecessary

221. The university health service has referred a college sophomore for admission because of an increasingly unkempt appearance and withdrawn, isolated, and depressed behavior. The referring psychiatrist notes strong suicidal tendencies. Contributing factors appear to be an abrupt ending of a romantic relationship and declining grades. The prognosis for a reasonably rapid recovery for this client is:
1. Poor, since the client has suicidal tendencies
2. Bad, since the client is failing in all sectors of life
3. Fair, since the client seems intelligent enough to pull things together
4. Good, since the onset was sudden and no previous emotional problems existed

222. On the second day after admission, a suicidal client asks the nurse, "Why am I being observed around the clock and why is my freedom to move around the unit restricted?" The nurse's most appropriate reply would be:
1. "Why do you think we are observing you?"
2. "What makes you think that we are observing you?"
3. "We are concerned that you might try to harm yourself."
4. "Your doctor has ordered it and is the one you should ask about it."

223. One day, while shaving, a male client with the diagnosis of bipolar disorder states to the nurse, "I have hidden a razor blade and tonight I am going to kill myself." The nurse's best reply would be:
1. "You're going to kill yourself?"
2. "Things can't really be that bad."
3. "I'm sure you don't really mean that."
4. "You'd better finish shaving; it's time for lunch."

224. After 4 days on the inpatient psychiatric unit, a client on suicidal precautions tells the nurse, "Hey, look! I was feeling pretty depressed for a while, but I'm certainly not going to kill myself." The nurse's best response to this statement would be:
1. "Kill yourself? I don't understand."
2. "You do seem to be feeling better."
3. "Suppose we talk some more about this."
4. "We have to observe you until your psychiatrist tells us to stop."

225. The treatment plan for a client admitted with a severe, persistent, intractable depression and suicidal ideation would probably include:
1. Electroconvulsive therapy
2. Short-term psychoanalysis
3. Nondirective psychotherapy
4. High doses of anxiolytic drugs

226. A severely depressed client is to have electroconvulsive therapy (ECT). When discussing this therapy, the nurse should tell the client that:
1. Sleep will be induced and treatment will not cause pain
2. With new methods of administration, treatment is totally safe
3. It is better not to talk about it, but you can ask any question you like
4. There may be some permanent memory loss as a result of the treatment

227. An extremely depressed client is to begin electroconvulsive therapy. The nurse, in explaining this procedure, should emphasize that:
1. Answers to any questions will be provided
2. A period of amnesia will follow the treatment
3. The treatments will make the client feel better
4. The client will not be alone during the treatment

228. A side effect of electroconvulsive therapy that a client may experience is:
1. Loss of appetite
2. Postural hypotension
3. Confusion for a time after treatment
4. Complete loss of memory for a time

229. A 46-year-old male client has just awakened from his first scheduled ECT treatment. The most appropriate nursing intervention would be to:
1. Arrange for the dietary staff to bring the client a lunch tray
2. Orient the client to time and place and tell him that he has just had a treatment
3. Get the client up and out of bed as soon as possible and back into the unit's routine
4. Take the blood pressure and pulse rate every 15 minutes until the client is fully awake

230. The premorbid personality of a 45-year-old, meticulous homemaker with no outside interests or hobbies, admitted for a major depressive disorder, could probably best be described as:
1. Suspicious, sensitive, aloof
2. Dependent, immature, insecure
3. Rigid, narrow, overly conscientious
4. Withdrawn and seclusive, with an active fantasy life

231. An extremely hyperactive client exhibiting manic behavior is admitted to the hospital. In view of the client's elated state, the nurse should arrange for the client to be in a room:
1. With another client who is very quiet
2. That will provide a great deal of stimuli
3. That has had most of the furniture removed
4. With another client exhibiting similar behavior

232. During the orientation tour for three new staff members, a young, hyperactive, manic client greets them by saying, "Welcome to the funny farm. I'm Jo-Jo, the head yo-yo." This comment might mean that the client is:
1. Trying to fill the "life-of-the-party" role
2. Looking for attention from the new staff

3. Unable to distinguish fantasy from reality
4. Anxious over the arrival of the new staff members

233. When the language of a client in the manic phase of a bipolar disorder becomes vulgar and profane, the nurse should:
1. State, "We do not like that kind of talk around here."
2. Ignore it, since the client is using it only to get attention
3. Recognize the language as part of the illness, but set limits on it
4. State, "When you can talk in an acceptable way, we will talk to you."

234. A hyperactive, manic client might be redirected therapeutically by:
1. Asking the client to guide other clients as they clean their rooms
2. Encouraging the client to tear pictures out of magazines for a scrap book
3. Suggesting the client initiate social activities on the unit for the client group
4. Providing a pencil and paper and encouraging the client to write a short story

235. The nurse is assigned to care for a 39-year-old, hyperactive, manic client who exhibits flight of ideas. The client is not eating. The nurse recognizes this may be because the client:
1. Feels undeserving of the food
2. Is too busy to take the time to eat
3. Wishes to avoid the clients in the dining room
4. Believes that at this time there is no need for food

236. A physician has been a client of the psychiatric service for the past 3 days. The client has questioned the authority of the treatment team, has advised other clients that their treatment plans are wrong, and generally has been disruptive in group therapy. The nurse's most appropriate response would be to:
1. Ignore the client and hope the disruptive behavior will stop
2. Tell the other clients that they should not pay attention to what the client says
3. Restrict the client's contact with other clients until the disruptive behavior ceases
4. Understand that the client is unable to control this behavior and that limits must be set

237. During periods of extreme mania and hyperactivity, the nursing staff should consider a client's nutritional needs by:
    1. Accepting the fact that the client will eat if hungry
    2. Following the client around the dining room with a tray
    3. Allowing the client to prepare own meals and eat when desired
    4. Providing the client with frequent, high-calorie feedings that can be handheld

238. To best help meet the nutritional needs of an extremely hyperactive client during the manic phase of a bipolar disorder, the nurse should:
    1. Provide a tray in the client's room
    2. Assure the client that the food is deserved
    3. Point out that the energy the client is burning up must be replaced
    4. Order foods that the client can hold in the hand to eat while moving around

239. A 23-year-old has been admitted to a psychiatric hospital after a month of unusual behavior that included eating and sleeping very little, talking and singing constantly, and frequent shopping sprees. In the hospital, the client is demanding, bossy, and sarcastic. The symptoms the client is exhibiting are usually found in clients with the diagnosis of:
    1. Mood disorder
    2. Major depression
    3. Personality disorder
    4. Schizophrenic disorder

240. When approaching a client during a period of great overactivity, it is essential to:
    1. Use a firm, warm, consistent approach
    2. Anticipate and physically control the client's hyperactivity
    3. Allow the client to choose the activities in which to participate
    4. Let the client know the staff will not tolerate destructive behavior

241. The plan of care for a client in the manic phase appropriately includes plans to:
    1. Arouse and focus the client's interest in reality
    2. Encourage the client to talk as much as needed
    3. Persuade the client to complete any task that has been started
    4. Provide constructive channels for redirecting the client's excess energy

242. When helping the female client with personal hygiene during the manic phase of a bipolar disorder, the nurse should:
    1. Encourage her to dress attractively and in her own clothing
    2. Allow her to apply makeup in whatever manner she chooses
    3. Suggest that she wear hospital clothing to avoid confrontations
    4. Keep makeup away from her because she will apply it too freely

Anxiety, Somatoform, and Dissociative Disorders

243. The nurse recognizes that an excellent indicator of improvement in a client with the diagnosis of generalized anxiety disorder is when the client:
    1. Learns to avoid anxiety
    2. Participates in activities
    3. Takes medication as prescribed
    4. Identifies when anxiety is developing

244. When caring for a client with a generalized anxiety disorder, the nurse should be aware that one of the best indicators of the client's present condition is the client's:
    1. Memory
    2. Behavior
    3. Judgment
    4. Responsiveness

245. An obviously distraught client arrives at the mental health clinic. The client is disheveled, is agitated, and demands that someone "do something to end this feeling." The nurse recognizes that the client has:
    1. Feelings of panic
    2. Suicidal tendencies
    3. Narcissistic ideation
    4. A demanding personality

246. The nurse is aware that as anxiety increases, one's concept of reality alters. Therefore when caring for a client with a generalized anxiety disorder, the nurse's first intervention should be to:
    1. Have the client verbalize feelings of anxiety
    2. Administer the prn medication ordered by the physician
    3. Remove as many stimuli from the client's environment as possible
    4. Have the client list the relief behaviors that are used to reduce anxiety

247. An obviously upset client comes to the mental health clinic and, after pushing ahead of the other clients, states, "I have had an argument with my daughter and I'm feeling tense, worried, and angry." After assessing this behavior, the nurse determines that the client's anxiety is at the:
    1. Mild level
    2. Moderate level
    3. Severe level
    4. Panic level

248. A client's severe anxiety and panic is often considered to be "contagious." When the nurse becomes aware that personal feelings of anxiety are increasing, the nurse should:
    1. Refocus the conversation on some pleasant topics
    2. Say to the client, "Calm down, you are making me anxious, too."
    3. Say, "I have to leave for awhile. I'll send someone in and I'll be back later."
    4. Remain quiet so that personal feelings of anxiety do not become apparent to the client

249. A phobic reaction will rarely occur unless the person:
    1. Thinks about the feared object
    2. Absolves the guilt of the feared object
    3. Introjects the feared object into the body
    4. Comes into contact with the feared object

250. The nurse, when exploring the modalities available for the treatment of phobias, should inform the client that the treatment having the highest success rate for people with phobias is:
    1. Systematic desensitization using relaxation techniques
    2. Insight therapy to determine the origin of the anxiety and fear
    3. Psychotherapy aimed at rearranging maladaptive thought processes
    4. Psychoanalytic exploration of repressed conflicts of an earlier developmental phase

251. When speaking with the client who has just experienced a panic attack, the nurse can address the client's concerns most therapeutically by stating:
    1. "You must have been really upset."
    2. "You are concerned that this might happen again."
    3. "Episodes like this can be upsetting, but they do end."
    4. "Your family was concerned that you were having a heart attack."

252. The nurse recognizes that it would be unusual for an individual with an anxiety disorder to handle the anxiety by:
    1. Acting it out with antisocial behavior
    2. Converting it into a physical symptom
    3. Regressing to earlier levels of adjustment
    4. Displacing it onto less-threatening objects

253. Physiologically, the nurse would expect a client's anxiety to be manifested by:
    1. Dilated pupils, dilated bronchioles, increased pulse rate, hyperglycemia, and peripheral vasoconstriction
    2. Constricted pupils, dilated bronchioles, increased pulse rate, hypoglycemia, and peripheral vasolidation
    3. Constricted pupils, constricted bronchioles, increased pulse rate, hypoglycemia, and peripheral vasodilation
    4. Dilated pupils, constricted bronchioles, decreased pulse rate, hypoglycemia, and peripheral vasoconstriction

254. Unsatisfied needs create anxiety that motivates an individual to action. This action is brought about mainly to:
    1. Reduce tension
    2. Deny the situation
    3. Remove the problem
    4. Relieve physical discomfort

255. The most appropriate way to decrease a client's anxiety is by:
    1. Avoiding unpleasant objects and events
    2. Prolonged exposure to fearful situations
    3. Acquiring skills with which to face stressful events
    4. Introducing an element of pleasure into fearful situations

256. A young client is admitted with a severe anxiety disorder. The client is crying, wringing the hands, and pacing. The first nursing intervention should be to:
    1. Stay physically close to the client
    2. Gently ask what is bothering the client
    3. Tell the client to sit down and try to relax
    4. Get the client involved in a nonthreatening activity

257. The nurse could most appropriately begin to help an extremely anxious client with a sleep problem, who has been assigned to a four-bed room since admission, by saying:
    1. "You seem unable to sleep at night."
    2. "I'm going to move you to a private room."
    3. "Don't worry, you'll sleep when you're tired."
    4. "I'll get you the sedative your doctor ordered."

258. The nurse can best minimize psychologic stress in an anxious client by:
1. Learning what is of particular importance to the client
2. Explaining in fine detail the procedures and therapies being used
3. Avoiding the discussion of any areas that may be emotionally charged
4. Confidently advising the client that the nurse is in charge of the situation

259. The nurse understands that in a conversion disorder pseudoneurologic symptoms such as paralysis or blindness are:
1. An unconscious method for getting attention
2. Usually necessary for the client to cope with the present situation
3. Usually solved when the client learns to deal with ongoing family conflicts
4. Reversible and will subside if the client is helped to focus on other things

260. A young man, caught in a raging conflict between his mother and his wife, complains of pain in his right arm that has progressed to the point of paralysis. An orthopedic consultation found no pathology and he is referred for a psychiatric evaluation. This client's symptoms may be an unconscious attempt to solve a conflict evolving from:
1. Hostile feelings toward his home
2. Ambivalent feelings toward his wife
3. Needs to be a dependent child and an independent adult
4. Inadequate feelings in regard to assuming the role of husband

261. A client, newly diagnosed with a conversion disorder, is manifesting paralysis of the leg. The nurse would expect this client to:
1. Demonstrate a spread of paralysis to other body parts
2. Require continuous psychiatric treatment to maintain individual functioning
3. Recover the use of the affected leg but, under stress, again develop similar symptoms
4. Follow a rather unpredictable emotional course in the future, depending on exposure to stress

262. When caring for a client who has a diagnosis of conversion disorder with paralysis of the lower extremities, it would be most therapeutic for the nurse to:
1. Encourage the client to try to walk
2. Tell the client there is nothing wrong
3. Avoid focusing on the client's physical symptoms
4. Help the client follow through with the physical therapy plan

263. For a client with a diagnosis of conversion disorder, anxiety is:
1. Diffuse and free floating
2. Consciously felt by the client
3. Projected onto the environment
4. Localized and relieved by the symptom

264. When planning care for a client with a diagnosis of conversion disorder with the chief complaint of blindness, the nurse recognizes that:
1. It is best to ignore the client's complaints
2. The client's behavior indicates a lack of willpower
3. The client's symptoms are evidence of a disturbed personality
4. If additional stress is added, the client will become permanently blind

265. A 20-year-old female client believes that doorknobs are contaminated and refuses to touch them, except with a paper tissue. When dealing with this behavior, the nurse should:
1. Supply the client with paper tissues to help her function until her anxiety is reduced
2. Explain to the client that her idea about doorknobs is part of her illness and is not necessary
3. Encourage the client to scrub the doorknobs with a strong antiseptic so she does not need to use tissues
4. Encourage the client to touch doorknobs by removing all available paper tissue until she learns to deal with the situation

266. Compulsive symptoms, such as using paper towels to open doors, develop because the clients are:
1. Consciously using this method to punish themselves
2. Listening to voices that tell them the doorknobs are unclean
3. Unconsciously controlling unacceptable impulses or feelings
4. Fulfilling a need to punish others by carrying out an annoying procedure

267. A client with a diagnosis of obsessive-compulsive disorder is frequently late for appointments because it takes so much time each day to complete a ritualistic handwashing routine. It would be most therapeutic for the nurse to:
  1. Encourage the client to speed up the ritual so that appointments can be met on time
  2. Let the client know how angry others become when the handwashing holds up activities
  3. Verbally discourage the client from washing the hands so frequently to prevent skin breakdown
  4. Accept the client's ritualistic behavior in a matter-of-fact manner without displaying amusement or criticism

268. When developing a care plan for a client with an obsessive-compulsive behavior disorder, the action that would most likely increase the client's anxiety would be:
  1. Permitting the client's ritualistic acts three times a day
  2. Having the client understand the nature of the anxiety
  3. Involving the client in establishing the therapeutic plan
  4. Providing the client with a nonjudgmental, accepting environment

269. The hospital or day-treatment center is often indicated for the treatment of the client with an obsessive-compulsive disorder because it:
  1. Prevents the client from carrying out symptomatic rituals
  2. Allows the staff to exert control over the client's activities
  3. Resolves the client's anxiety because decision making is minimal
  4. Provides the neutral environment the client needs to work through conflicts

270. The initial treatment plan for a 40-year-old client with the long-standing, obsessive-compulsive behavior of hand and body washing should include:
  1. Denying the client time for the ritualistic behavior
  2. Determining the purpose of the ritualistic behavior
  3. Providing the client with a routine schedule of activities
  4. Suggesting a symptom substitution technique to refocus the behavior

271. Before discharge, the nurse should teach the family of an anxious client that anxiety can be recognized as:
  1. A totally unique experience and feeling
  2. Consciously motivated thoughts and wishes
  3. Fears that are related to the total environment
  4. A behavior pattern observed in ourselves and others

272. A client with a history of obsessive-compulsive behaviors has been attending a psychiatric day treatment center. There has been a marked decrease in symptoms, and the client expresses a wish to obtain a part-time job. On the day of a job interview the client comes in fretful, displaying symptoms. The nurse's best response would be:
  1. "I know you're anxious, but make yourself go to the interview and conquer your fear."
  2. "If going to an interview makes you this anxious, it seems like you're not ready to work."
  3. "It must be that you really don't want that job after all. I think you should think more about it."
  4. "Going for your interview triggered some feelings in you. Perhaps you could call a friend to drive you to your appointment."

Disorders of Personality

273. To give effective nursing care to a client who is using ritualistic behavior, the nurse must first recognize that the client:
  1. Should be prevented from performing the rituals
  2. Needs to realize that the ritual serves no purpose
  3. Must immediately be diverted when performing the ritual
  4. Does not want to repeat the ritual, but feels compelled to do so

274. The nursing diagnosis that would be most appropriate for a 22-year-old client who uses ritualistic behavior would be:
  1. Ineffective coping
  2. Impaired adjustment
  3. Personal identity disturbance
  4. Sensory/perceptual alterations

275. The priority discharge criteria for a female client who has been using ritualistic behaviors would have to include that the client should be able to:
  1. Verbalize positive aspects about herself
  2. Follow the rules and regulations of the milieu
  3. Recognize that her hallucinations occur at times of extreme anxiety and can be controlled
  4. Verbalize signs and symptoms of increasing anxiety and intervene to maintain it at a manageable level

276. A psychiatrist prescribes an antiobsessional agent for a client who is using ritualistic behavior. A common antianxiety medication used for this type of client would be:
    1. Luvox (fluvoxamine)
    2. Cogentin (benztropine)
    3. Symmetrel (amantadine)
    4. Benadryl (diphenhydramine)

277. The nurse allows a client who is using ritualistic behavior ample time for the performance of the ritual because:
    1. Without consistency of limit setting, change will not occur
    2. To deny the client this activity may precipitate panic levels of anxiety
    3. This behavior is viewed as a result of anger turned inward on the self
    4. Successful performance of independent activities enhances self-esteem

278. One day a male client with the diagnoses of borderline personality disorder describes a situation that happened at work when his immediate supervisor reprimanded him for not completing an assignment. He explains that it was not his fault and states, "People get angry and take it out on me." The nurse recognizes that the client is using the defense mechanism called:
    1. Denial
    2. Projection
    3. Displacement
    4. Intellectualization

279. When working with the nurse during the orientation phase of the relationship, a client with a borderline personality disorder would probably have the most difficulty in:
    1. Controlling anxiety
    2. Terminating the session on time
    3. Accepting the psychiatric diagnosis
    4. Setting mutual goals for the relationship

280. The main personality problem for clients who need props to blur reality is usually:
    1. Mistrust
    2. Ego ideal
    3. Dependency
    4. Role blurring

281. Many people control anxiety by ritualistic behavior. When taking care of these individuals it is important for the nurse to:

1. Avoid mentioning the ritual
2. Explain the meaning of the ritual
3. Allow them time to carry out the ritual
4. Prevent them from carrying out the ritual

282. A person who habitually expresses anxiety through physical symptoms is using:
    1. Projection
    2. Regression
    3. Conversion
    4. Hypochondriasis

283. The client with an antisocial personality disorder:
    1. Suffers from a great deal of anxiety
    2. Is generally unable to postpone gratification
    3. Rapidly learns by experience and punishment
    4. Has a great sense of responsibility toward others

284. A person with an antisocial personality disorder has difficulty relating to others because of never having learned to:
    1. Count on others
    2. Empathize with others
    3. Be dependent on others
    4. Communicate with others socially

285. A young, handsome man with a diagnosis of antisocial personality disorder is being discharged from the hospital next week. He asks the nurse for her phone number so he can call her for a date. The nurse's best response would be:
    1. "We are not permitted to date clients."
    2. "No, you are a client and I am a nurse."
    3. "I like you, but our relationship is professional."
    4. "It is against my professional ethics to date clients."

286. A person who deliberately pretends an illness is usually thought to be:
    1. Neurotic
    2. Malingering
    3. Out of contact with reality
    4. Using conversion defenses

287. The basic difference between psychophysiologic disorders and somatoform disorders is that in psychophysiologic disorders there is:
    1. A feeling of illness
    2. An emotional cause
    3. A restriction of activities
    4. An actual tissue change

288. A frequent finding in clients with paraphiliac sexual disorders is that they have:
    1. Other covert or overt emotional problems
    2. Gonadal and pituitary hormone deficiencies
    3. An inadequate physical development of the sexual organs
    4. A poor adjustment due to association with society's fringe groups

289. Two 20-year-old female clients have become very much attached to one another and were recently found in bed together. They became angry and sarcastic when the nurse asked one of them to return to her own bed. The nurse can best handle this situation by:
    1. Asking the physician to transfer one of the clients to another unit
    2. Adopting a matter-of-fact, noncondemning attitude while setting limits on the behavior
    3. Restricting both their privileges for several days because their behavior is undesirable and immature
    4. Supervising them carefully and separating them when possible throughout the day and especially at night

290. Following an automobile accident involving a fatality and a subsequent arrest for speeding, a client has amnesia for the events surrounding the accident. This is an example of the defense mechanism known as:
    1. Projection
    2. Repression
    3. Dissociation
    4. Suppression

291. Although the nurse becomes tense as the client with an obsessive-compulsive personality disorder carries out a ritual, it should be recognized that a compulsive act is one which:
    1. Is purposeful but useless
    2. A person performs willingly
    3. Is performed after long urging
    4. Seems absurd but is necessary to the person

292. Therapeutic treatment of a female client with ritualistic behavior should be directed toward helping her to:
    1. Redirect her energy into activities to help others
    2. Learn that her behavior is not serving a realistic purpose
    3. Forget her fears by administering antianxiety medications
    4. Understand her behavior is caused by unconscious impulses that she fears

293. Those individuals who demonstrate obsessive-compulsive behavior can best be treated by:
    1. Restricting their movements
    2. Calling attention to their behavior
    3. Keeping them busy to distract them
    4. Supporting but limiting their behavior

294. A nurse is orienting a new client to the unit when another client rushes down the hallway and asks the nurse to sit down to talk. The client requesting the nurse's attention is extremely manipulative and uses socially acting-out behaviors when demands are unmet. The nurse should:
    1. Suggest that the client requesting attention speak with another staff member
    2. Leave the new client and talk with the other client to avoid precipitating acting out behavior
    3. Tell the interrupting client to sit down and be patient, stating, "I'll be back as soon as possible."
    4. Introduce the two clients and suggest that the client join the new client and the nurse on the tour

295. A client with a diagnosis of narcissistic personality disorder has been given a day pass from the psychiatric hospital. The client is due to return at 6 PM. At 5 PM the client telephones the nurse in charge of the unit and says, "Six o'clock is too early. I feel like coming back at 7:30." The nurse would be most therapeutic by telling the client to:
    1. Return immediately, to demonstrate control
    2. Return on time or restrictions will be imposed
    3. Come back by 6:45, as a compromise to set limits
    4. Come back as soon as possible or the police will be sent

296. An adult client with a borderline personality disorder vomits immediately after drinking 2 ounces of shampoo as a suicide gesture. The most appropriate initial response by the nurse would be to:
    1. Promptly notify the attending physician
    2. Immediately institute suicide precautions
    3. Sit quietly with the client until the vomiting subsides
    4. Assess the client's vital signs and administer syrup of ipecac

297. When teaching about child abuse, the nurse includes the fact that the defense mechanism most often used by the physically abusive individual is:
    1. Manipulation
    2. Transference
    3. Displacement
    4. Reaction formation

298. There are many common reactions noted among parents who physically abuse their children. One reaction the nurse should be aware of is that the offending parents:
1. Seldom touch or look at the child
2. Show signs of guilt about the child's injury
3. Are quick to inquire about the discharge date
4. Are very concerned about their own physical health

Crisis Situations

299. A female client, whose long-term live-in lover has just terminated their relationship, comes to the emergency service in severe crisis. After being seen by the nurse the client agrees to call the local mental health clinic for short-term counseling. The nurse evaluates that the nursing intervention was effective based on the fact that the client:
1. Is seeking out assistance in making a decision
2. Has returned to her precrisis level of functioning
3. Has learned new methods of coping with her loss
4. Is demonstrating diminished symptoms of anxiety and sadness

300. During a staff development program, the nurse educator emphasizes that nurses caring for middle-agers who are experiencing midlife crisis should be aware that this crisis is most often due to the:
1. Individual's perception of his/her life situation
2. Many role changes adults experience at this time
3. Anticipation of negative changes associated with old age
4. Lack of support from family members who are busy with their own lives

301. A 35-year-old is admitted for an amputation of the left leg. Before surgery the nurse observes that the client is diaphoretic, voiding frequently, complaining of palpitations, and having difficulty understanding what is being said. After making these assessments the nurse should first plan to:
1. Ask the client to talk about feelings
2. Have a stat ECG done on the client
3. Obtain a urine specimen for culture and sensitivity
4. Ask the physician for a stat order for an IM tranquilizer

302. During a staff development program, when discussing the reaction of middle-aged women to their children leaving home (empty nest syndrome), the nurse educator reminds the group that recent studies have demonstrated that today's women most commonly experience a feeling of:
1. Anxiety
2. Satisfaction
3. Depression
4. Hopelessness

303. A 30-year-old who has been in a gay relationship for the past 3 years comes to the emergency room in a near panic state. He tells the nurse that his lover of many years has just terminated their relationship. To help the client deal with this loss the nurse should:
1. Identify his support system
2. Explore his psychotic thoughts
3. Reinforce his current self-image
4. Suggest he attempt to use straight resources

304. The nurse is aware that the approach to be used during crisis intervention should be:
1. Passive and reflective
2. Active and goal directed
3. Interpretative and analytical
4. Future oriented and passive

305. The outcome that is unrelated to a crisis state is:
1. Learning more constructive coping skills
2. Decompensation to a lower level of functioning
3. Adaptation and a return to a prior level of functioning
4. A high level of anxiety continuing for more than 3 months

306. The most important assessment data for the nurse to gather from the client in crisis would be:
1. The client's work habits
2. Any significant physical health data
3. A history of any emotional problems in the family
4. The specific circumstances surrounding the "perceived" crisis situation

307. The best example of the nurse's use of crisis intervention would be:
1. "Tell me what you have done to help yourself."
2. "Can you tell me about what is bothering you?"
3. "I understand in the past you have had problems."
4. "I will be here for you to help you figure things out."

308. A client, admitted 5 days ago for chronic abuse of drugs and alcohol, appears to have extreme difficulty participating in an art-therapy group project. The priority assessment the nurse needs to make after the group therapy is to determine if the client is experiencing a period of:
1. Crisis
2. Disorientation
3. Confabulation
4. Hallucinations

309. When applying mental health principles to the care of any person with children, the nurse should be aware that:
1. It is easier to adjust to the first child than to later ones
2. It is pathologic to feel anger and resentment toward a child
3. Every parent has inborn feelings of love and acceptance for children
4. Many parents experience feelings of resentment toward their children

310. Strict toilet training before a child is ready will cause problems in personality development because at this age a child is learning to:
1. Satisfy own needs
2. Identify own needs
3. Satisfy parents' needs
4. Live up to society's expectations

311. A child in the first grade is murdered and counseling is planned for the children in the school. To understand a child's response to a crisis, the nurse must initially identify the:
1. Child's developmental level
2. Family communication patterns
3. Quality of the child's peer relationships
4. Child's perception of the crisis situation

312. The factor that would probably be most significant for the nurse working with the family of an infant born with a genetic disorder is their:
1. Ability to give physical care to their infant
2. Response to family's and friends' reactions to their infant
3. Understanding of the factors causing the genetic disorder
4. Ability to talk about problems their infant may have in the future

313. An infant in the newborn nursery is suspected of having cerebral palsy. When the parents are told, the mother cries, "What did we do to deserve this?" The nurse's most therapeutic response would be:
1. "Let's sit down and have a cup of coffee."
2. "Why do you feel you are being punished?"
3. "I know you must be upset, but it's too early to tell."
4. "You didn't do anything; let me tell you about this disorder."

314. A newborn boy with visible birth defects is brought to his mother for the first time. When the mother sees the baby, she becomes very disturbed, pushes him away, and states, "Oh, take him away; I never want to see him again." This reaction would indicate to the nurse that the mother is:
1. Rejecting the baby; he will have to be placed for adoption
2. Severely emotionally disturbed and in immediate need of psychiatric help
3. Responding as most normal new mothers who find it difficult to accept that their baby is less than perfect
4. Unable to cope with the situation and that arrangements will have to be made to place the baby in a foster home, at least for the first few months

315. A young, single woman delivers a child with a severe cleft palate. The nurse recognizes the fairly typical response to a baby with a visible birth defect when the woman states:
1. "I'm unhappy. I guess I'm being punished."
2. "No, you must have brought me the wrong baby."
3. "What will my parents say? What could have happened?"
4. "I shouldn't have had this baby. Now my boyfriend will never marry me."

316. When making rounds during the night, the nurse enters the room of a client who delivered a still-born baby during the evening and finds her crying. It would be most appropriate for the nurse to:
1. Pull the curtain to provide privacy for the client
2. Sit down and stay with the client, allowing her to cry
3. Explain to the client that her feelings are normal and will pass with time
4. Document on the chart that the client is having difficulty accepting the loss of her baby

317. One objective a community health nurse should have in mind when preparing to make an initial visit to a family following the loss of their infant to SIDS would be that the parents will:
1. Identify the problems that they will be facing related to the loss of the infant
2. Accept that there was nothing that they could have done to prevent the death
3. Include the infant's siblings in the events and grieving following the infant's death
4. Seek out other families who have lost infants to SIDS and receive support from them

318. A dying client gradually moves toward resolution of feelings regarding impending death. Basing care on the observations of Kübler-Ross, the nurse plans to use nonverbal interventions when assessment reveals that the client is in the:
1. Anger stage
2. Denial stage
3. Bargaining stage
4. Acceptance stage

319. The nurse is aware that a co-worker's mother died 16 months ago. The co-worker cries every time someone mentions the word "Mother" or if the mother's name is mentioned. The nurse recognizes that:
1. This person needs to seek help
2. Everyone cries when their mother dies
3. This behavior could be considered normal
4. The co-worker was extremely attached to the mother

320. The nurse stops by the room of a tearfully depressed, newly admitted client and offers to walk the client to the evening meal. The client looks intently at the nurse, saying nothing. The nurse could best respond by stating:
1. "I'll be at the desk if you need me."
2. "Tell me what you are feeling now."
3. "Pull yourself together; I'll walk you to dinner."
4. "It must be very difficult to be on a psychiatric unit."

321. A 43-year-old, well-dressed man charged with molesting a 7-year-old child is admitted for psychiatric evaluation. When the nurse asks him to come to dinner, he refuses and states, "I don't want anyone to see me. Leave me alone." The nurse's best response would be:
1. "Certainly, I respect your wishes."
2. "It will be easier to face other people right away."

3. "Only the staff members know why you are here."
4. "I hope you realize that you are the hardest judge you must face."

322. A baby born with a severe bilateral cleft lip and palate is shown to the father first. The father says, "Oh, what am I going to do? How could this happen to us? What is my wife going to do? It would have been better if she had never become pregnant." The most appropriate response by the nurse would be:
1. "This must be very hard on you. Would it help if I went with you when the doctor talks to your wife?"
2. "How can you say that? You have a lovely, healthy baby; the cleft lip can be fixed and then the baby will be fine."
3. "I know that this is very difficult for you. But you can't think of yourself now. Your wife needs you. You must be strong."
4. "I know how hard this must be for you. But believe me, you will love the baby so much, you won't even notice that there is a problem."

323. A visiting nurse is assigned to a new mother with a history of heart disease and her 6-week-old baby. When the nurse arrives, the mother appears tired and the baby is crying. The most appropriate question by the nurse would be:
1. "Is everything all right? You look tired."
2. "Tell me a little about your daily routine."
3. "When did the baby have the last bottle?"
4. "Oh, it looks like you two are having a bad day."

324. When bed rest is ordered for a multiparous client experiencing premature labor, she begins to cry and states, "I have two small children at home." The nurse should reply:
1. "Someone else will need to care for the children."
2. "You are worried about how you will be able to manage?"
3. "You'll be able to fix meals, and the children can go to nursery school."
4. "Perhaps a neighbor can help out, and your husband can do the housework in the evening."

325. The nurse is aware that the main goal in planning care for a client in crisis would be to:
1. Schedule follow-up counseling for the client
2. Restore the client's psychologic equilibrium
3. Have the client gain insight into the problems
4. Refer the client for occupational and physiotherapy

PSYCHIATRIC/MENTAL HEALTH NURSING
ANSWERS AND RATIONALES

Therapeutic Relationships

1. **3** Boundaries relate to family systems theory. (3; CJ; AN; PS; TR)
   1 This statement is reflective of crisis theory, because it addresses the client's perspective of the precipitating event.
   2 This statement is reflective of milieu theory.
   4 This statement is reflective of biologic theory.

2. **2** This statement accurately expresses the nurse's interpretation of the client's mood and presents the client with an opportunity to explore feelings. (3; CJ; IM; PS; TR)
   1 Not necessarily true; ignores the client's feelings and closes off the opportunity for further discussion of feelings.
   3 Same as answer 1.
   4 Same as answer 1.

3. **3** The nurse's major tool in psychiatric nursing is the therapeutic use of self. Psychiatric nurses must learn to be aware of their own feelings and how they affect the situation. (3; MR; EV; TC; TR)
   1 This may be true, but an awareness of self still seems the most difficult.
   2 This may be true, but is not part of the nurse-client relationship.
   4 This implies that the nurse is working alone in planning care for the client.

4. **1** An important aspect of the role of the psychiatric nurse is primary, secondary, and tertiary intervention to prevent emotional disequilibrium. (2; MR; AN; PS; TR)
   2 This is only a small part of the role of the psychiatric nurse, a role usually shared with others on the health team.
   3 Same as answer 2.
   4 This is only a part of the role of the psychiatric nurse, since psychiatry is concerned with people with varying degrees of mental and emotional disorders.

5. **2** Anger is the expected response of staff at having been duped by a client with a fictitious disorder; they feel both used and abused. (3; CJ; AN; PS; TR)

1 This is not generally seen when staff have been involved in assessing and caring for a client who has not had favorable outcomes from their interventions.
   3 Same as answer 1.
   4 Same as answer 1.

6. **2** The initial goal should be to demonstrate acceptance and work toward developing trust; spending time with the client best meets this initial goal. (1; MR; AN; PS; TR)
   1 This will increase the anxiety of the psychotic client; it would be a correct action in the working phase of the nurse-client relationship.
   3 This delays the initial stage of the nurse-client relationship and relies on antipsychotic medication to help clear communication.
   4 This would increase anxiety; it would be an acceptable action in the ongoing working phase.

7. **3** Talking to people who face the same problems and who may be able to offer constructive help is extremely important to the nurse. (2; MR; IM; PS; TR)
   1 An avoidance technique that works only for a short time, since eventually the nurse must face feelings and work through them.
   2 An avoidance technique that should only be used when seeking support and making an attempt to work through feelings.
   4 Avoids feelings and may cause client to feel rejected and nurse to become more uncomfortable.

8. **1** The nurse brings to a therapeutic relationship the understanding of self and basic principles of therapeutic communication; this is the unique aspect of the helping relationship. (2; CJ; AN; PS; TR)
   2 This supports the psychotherapeutic management model, but it is not the most important tool used by the nurse in a therapeutic relationship.
   3 Same as answer 2.
   4 Same as answer 2.

9. **3** An understanding and supportive approach to a colleague with burnout allows the individual to identify the problem. (2; MR; IM; PS; TR)
   1 This states a fact of which the individual is probably aware; it may interfere with self-identification of the problem.
   2 A lack of organizational skills may or may not be the problem; it is also an accusatory approach.
   4 This is an accusatory approach.

10. **4** This increases the individual's ability to cope with stress; different defenses can be used in various situations. (2; MR; IM; PS; TR)
   1 The nurse has identified the problem; the supervisor is not helping with a specific intervention.
   2 This may or may not be helpful.
   3 It's learning to ignore or avoid people and situations that cannot be changed that helps prevent professional burnout.

11. **3** This provides a direct response to the client's concern and allows some exploration of food choices. (2; CJ; IM; PS; TR)
   1 Focusing on several caretakers does little to meet the client's basic security needs.
   2 This does not address the client's comment that "No one cares."
   4 This encourages dependency on the nurse; the message is clearly, "Do it for me, not because it is important for you."

12. **2** Sharing problems with others who are also open and concerned because of similar problems can reduce guilt and shame and begin to increase coping abilities. (1; CJ; EV; TC; TR)
   1 AA is viewed by some as a crutch in itself.
   3 Although AA is a support group, it is a self-help support group.
   4 Their problem drinking is usually caused by how they feel about themselves.

13. **3** This statement encourages the client to express and explore feelings; also, it is open and nonjudgmental. (1; MR; IM; PS; TR)
   1 This puts the client on the defensive rather than encouraging verbalization of feelings.
   2 This does not encourage further conversation and the client will not have the opportunity to express feelings; this response focuses on the nurse rather than on the client.
   4 Same as answer 1.

14. **4** This is a reflection of feelings that allows the client to either validate or correct the nurse. (2; CJ; IM; PS; TR)

1 This delays confronting the problem and avoids exploring feelings.
2 This is a response that gives advice and does not allow the client to explore feelings.
3 This is an uncalled-for statement that does not allow the client to explore feelings.

15. **3** This permits the client to see that personal feelings are not unique but are shared by others. (1; CJ; IM; TC; TR)
   1 This statement makes the client worry about not feeling happy.
   2 This is a nonsupportive response to a realistic fear of leaving the safe hospital and going back to where problems must be confronted.
   4 How the others feel about whether the client is ready to be discharged is totally irrelevant.

16. **3** This statement does not prejudge the father; it encourages communication. (2; CJ; IM; PS; TR)
   1 This response disregards the father's feelings and cuts off further communication.
   2 This statement may stop communication and does not recognize the father's concerns.
   4 This statement is premature and does not recognize the father's concern.

17. **3** This question focuses the interaction toward the future and invites the client to explore alternative coping strategies. (3; CJ; AS; PS; TR)
   1 This question explores past coping strategies and would need to be asked as a part of the initial assessment of the client.
   2 This question attempts to explore the client's insight into present coping strategies, which should have been done before discussing the alternatives with the client.
   4 This question asks the client once more to ensure that all the precipitating stressors have been identified; this should have been done in the initial assessment.

18. **4** Commenting on the silence will encourage exploration of what is happening in the group and the members' thoughts and feelings about it. (2; MR; IM; PS; TR)
   1 Waiting indefinitely can result in increased anxiety and a power struggle between members and leaders, each determined to outwait the other.
   2 Calling on specific members limits growth potential of members; allowing the group to respond spontaneously increases growth potential.
   3 Forcing responses instead of allowing spontaneous responses will decrease thoughtful exploration of what is happening.

19. **1** This statement recognizes the importance of feelings and provides an opening so the client may talk about them. (2; CJ; EV; TC; TR)
    2 The client is not going to believe this, and it is not helping the client express feelings.
    3 The nursing goal is to help people function outside the hospital environment, not be afraid to leave it.
    4 A statement like this avoids the real issue and solves nothing.

20. **3** This puts the focus on feelings, not on a statement of what did or did not happen. (2; CJ; IM; TC; TR)
    1 This statement implies that the client may have had some part in causing another person's death.
    2 This statement does not give the client an opportunity to explore feelings.
    4 This statement closes the door to any further communication of feelings or fears.

21. **4** Ambivalence about life and death plus the introspection commonly found in clients with emotional problems would lead to increased anxiety and fear in the group members. (2; MR; PL; TC; TR)
    1 This will probably be a secondary goal of the group leader.
    2 It is not a primary goal; but this lack of concern should also be explored later on to see what is behind such apparent indifference, which may be a mask to cover feelings.
    3 These feelings must be handled within the support and supervisory systems for the staff; the other group members are the primary concern.

22. **4** The client's early arrival indicates an expected degree of anxiety; the quiet waiting indicates that the client has been told what to expect. (1; MR; EV; ED; TR)
    1 This would indicate an inadequate explanation or the inability of the client to remember the explanation that had been given.
    2 This indicates a high degree of anxiety that may denote a fear of the tests because they were not adequately explained.
    3 Same as answer 2.

23. **1** This response invited the client to explore the issue in more depth by focusing on it. (2; CJ; IM; PS; TR)
    2 Clarifying is a technique used to ask the client to give an example to better understand the nature of the client's statement.

3 Reflecting is a technique used to either reiterate the content or the feeling message; in content reflection, the nurse repeats basically the same statement; in feeling reflection, the nurse verbalizes what seems to be implied about feelings in the comment.
    4 This is incorrect; refocusing is to bring the subject back to a previous point; there is no information that this was discussed previously.

24. **1** It is the most effective method for the child to play out feelings; when feelings are allowed to surface, the child can then learn to face them by controlling, accepting, or abandoning them; through this process, the child can experience growth. (2; MR; AN; PS; TR)
    2 This is not child specific and generally is more suited for adolescents, young adults, and adults.
    3 Same as answer 2.
    4 Same as answer 2.

25. **4** The nurse's response urges the client to reflect on feelings and encourages the communication of feeling tones. (3; CJ; IM; PS; TR)
    1 This is shifting responsibility from the nurse to the doctor; it is an evasion technique.
    2 This is not what the client is asking the nurse; it closes the door to further communication.
    3 "Why" asks the client to draw a conclusion, which this client may not be able to do.

26. **3** Helping an individual to maintain an interest in future is therapeutic. (3; MR; PL; TC; TR)
    1 This would be appropriate for an older-aged adult.
    2 Lectures may or may not include emotional aspects of aging.
    4 Listening is therapeutic; however, it does not ensure the client will discuss the emotional aspects of aging.

27. **4** The first step in a plan of care should be the establishment of a meaningful relationship because it is through this relationship that the client can be helped. (2; CJ; AN; PS; TR)
    1 Encouraging this behavior would not be therapeutic.
    2 This would be a long-term goal.
    3 Reduction of stimuli may limit the hallucinations, but there is no evidence the client is not eating meals.

28. **4** The client is expressing hostility symbolically by not being cooperative. The client has a right to feel this way. If members of the staff criticize, it will only increase the client's feelings of guilt. (3; CJ; IM; PS; TR)
    1 This would allow the client to manipulate the environment.
    2 This will not change the client's mind about the activities. This response does not show an understanding of the client's needs.
    3 This will only increase feelings of guilt because the client is unaware of the hostility.

29. **4** Bringing another client into a set situation would be the most therapeutic, least threatening approach. (2; MR; IM; TC; TR)
    1 At this point in time, it would not be therapeutic to allow the client to remain with solitary pursuits.
    2 Explanations will not necessarily change behavior.
    3 This transfers nursing responsibility to the physician.

30. **4** This statement points out reality while accepting the fact that the client believes the feelings and thoughts are real. (2; CJ; IM; PS; TR)
    1 This is false reassurance that the nurse does not know as fact.
    2 The client does not know this and believes the opposite to be true.
    3 This is reality but it is not a supportive response.

31. **2** This simply states facts without getting involved in role conflict. (2; MR; IM; PS; TR)
    1 Being a doctor is a big part of this client's self-esteem, and by this remark the nurse is threatening that self-esteem.
    3 Firm, consistent limits need to be set and the nurse-client role established.
    4 Threats will only make the situation worse and set the tone for future nurse-client interactions.

Emotional Problems Related to Physical Health and Childbearing

32. **2** Understanding the stages leading to the acceptance of death may help the family to understand the client's moods and anger. (2; CJ; PL; PS; ED)
    1 This may not be true unless stated by the client; some clients welcome death as a release from pain.
    3 Untrue; anger is one of the stages of accepting death.

4 This is an assumption by the nurse unless stated by the client.

33. **4** This response lets the client know that the nurse understands adjustments will have to be made. It also is open-ended enough to let the client talk about feelings. (2; MR; IM; PS; ED)
    1 This response is not open-ended enough to foster expression of feelings about what is bothering the client.
    2 The client has not expressed his feelings enough for the nurse to offer any specific suggestions for help.
    3 This may compound his anxiety; also, it does not let him explore feelings.

34. **4** For psychologic equilibrium the client's environment must be one of novel and changing stimuli, promoting physical activity and effective interaction with others. (2; CJ; PL; PS; ED)
    1 To prevent urinary stasis and dehydration, fluid intake should be encouraged.
    2 Although stimulation is important, it should be varied and the client's preferences taken into consideration; radio and television do not promote interaction.
    3 Since the client has been able to control elimination, frequent toileting is not the problem.

35. **2** Incontinence without a physiologic basis is an act of hostility that the individual uses to deal with anxiety-producing situations. (1; CJ; AN; PS; ED)
    1 Incontinence is often seen as a symbol of regression and loss of control.
    3 Incontinence is rarely the result of conscious effort.
    4 Incontinence is not a necessary complication of age and inactivity; it can be prevented by a bladder-training program.

36. **3** This action provides the best reassurance as long as the parents know what to expect in the PACU. (2; MR; IM; PS; ED)
    1 If a PACU visit were not possible, this would be the next best action.
    2 This action might increase the mother's anxiety; seeing her child would be more therapeutic.
    4 There is an immediate need to reduce the parents' anxiety; having coffee will not meet this need.

37. **4** The client's statement is really saying, "I can manage this myself. I am capable." (3; CJ; AS; PS; ED)
 1 Nothing in the statement can be interpreted as denial; the client has stated, "I know I'm sick."
 2 None of the information given would lead to this conclusion.
 3 The statement would not be reassuring to the family member who brought the client to the hospital and who probably is more reassured having the client hospitalized.

38. **1** The potential for death is constant, which may result in depression. (2; CJ; AN; PS; ED)
 2 Although paranoia is occasionally seen in the terminal stage of the illness it is not known as "postpump psychosis."
 3 Episodes of feeling detached, numb, or unreal are not common occurrences; reactive depression is the most common.
 4 This is a physiologic problem resulting from cerebral fluid shifts that can result in seizures.

Drug-Related Responses

39. **3** It takes this long for the drug to reach therapeutic blood levels. (2; CJ; IM; TC; DR)
 1 This is much too short a time for therapeutic levels to be achieved.
 2 Same as answer 1.
 4 Improvement in depression would be demonstrated earlier than this.

40. **2** An occipital headache is the beginning of a hypertensive crisis that results from excessive tyramine. (2; CJ; EV; TC; DR)
 1 This is unrelated to the ingestion of tyramine.
 3 These are unrelated to the ingestion of tyramine.
 4 Excessive tyramine would cause a rise in blood pressure, not a drop.

41. **3** Lithium carbonate alters sodium transport in nerve and muscle cells and causes a shift toward intraneuronal metabolism of catecholamines. Since the range between therapeutic and toxic levels is very small, the client's serum lithium level should be monitored closely. (2; LE; EV; PA; DR)
 1 This is not necessary or useful.
 2 Sodium restriction may cause electrolyte imbalance and lithium toxicity.
 4 This is not necessary; it would depend on what the client was receiving.

42. **3** The lithium level should be maintained between 0.5 and 1.5 mEq/L. (2; LE; IM; TC; DR)
 1 This is unsafe.
 2 Same as answer 1.
 4 Same as answer 1.

43. **1** These are signs of advanced lithium toxicity. (2; LE; IM; PA; DR)
 2 These signs would have occurred before hand tremors, muscle hyperirritability, and confusion.
 3 Expected side effects are fine hand tremors, polyuria, and mild thirst.
 4 This nursing intervention is more appropriate for tricyclic antidepressants and antipsychotic agents.

44. **1** The neuroleptics modify the behavior of psychotic clients so they can more effectively cope with the environment and benefit from therapy. (1; CJ; AN; TC; DR)
 2 Antidepressants are used for depression.
 3 Ritalin is used to treat children with attention-deficit hyperactivity disorders; neuroleptics decrease the severity of psychotic symptoms.
 4 Neuroleptics are contraindicated during narcotic withdrawal.

45. **4** Unintentional tremors are one of the extrapyramidal side effects of the neuroleptics and are considered common and manageable. (1; CJ; EV; PA; DR)
 1 This is not a common side effect.
 2 This is a severe but not a common occurrence; periodic liver function tests should be done.
 3 This is not applicable; an excessive number of melanocytes is not a side effect.

46. **3** Flumazenil (Romazicon) is the drug of choice in the management of intentional or accidental overdose of benzodiazepines. (3; CJ; PL; TC; DR)
 1 This drug is used in the treatment of mood disorders.
 2 This drug is used for narcotic addiction withdrawal.
 4 This drug is contraindicated in the presence of central nervous system depressants.

47. **4** This is a serious side effect that may happen with abrupt withdrawal from barbiturates. (2; CJ; EV; TC; DR)
 1 This is not associated with barbiturate withdrawal.
 2 Same as answer 1.
 3 Same as answer 1.

48. 1 Narcan is used when narcotic-induced apnea occurs. It competes for CNS receptor sites, thus acting as a narcotic antagonist. (3; CJ; EV; PA; DR)
  2 This is not the specific action of this drug; it prevents respiratory arrest.
  3 Narcan does not accelerate the metabolism of heroin; it competes for CNS receptor sites.
  4 An adverse reaction is cardiovascular irritability.

49. 3 When Narcan is metabolized and its effects are diminished, the respiratory distress caused by the original drug overdose returns. (2; LE; EV; TC; DR)
  1 There is no known report of this.
  2 This combination does not cause cardiac depression.
  4 This is not a known effect after use of Narcan.

50. 4 This medication can be given IM every 2 to 3 weeks for clients who cannot be relied upon to take oral medications; it allows them to live in the community while keeping the symptoms under control. (2; CJ; PL; TC; DR)
  1 Haloperidol (Haldol) IM has an action duration of 4 to 8 hours.
  2 This drug is not given for schizophrenia.
  3 Same as answer 2.

51. 3 Succinylcholine chloride temporarily paralyzes the muscles, including those of respiration. Therefore some artificial means of respiration is necessary until the drug is metabolized and excreted. (2; CJ; AN; PA; DR)
  1 This prevents the complication of respiratory acidosis.
  2 The most significant therapeutic factor in ECT is the seizure itself.
  4 Brevital sodium decreases the occurrence of fractures; the drug is rapidly excreted with few side effects.

52. 4 The development of glaucoma is one of the side effects of imipramine (Tofranil), and the client should be alerted to the symptoms. (3; CJ; IM; TC; DR)
  1 This is true of monoamine oxidase inhibitors (MAOIs).
  2 Tofranil is not an MAOI.
  3 This would be essential for a person being treated with lithium.

53. 2 Haldol causes photosensitivity. Severe sunburn can occur on exposure to the sun. (2; CJ; PL; PA; DR)
  1 There is no known side effect that would affect night driving.
  3 This would be true if the client were taking an MAO inhibitor.
  4 Aspirin is not contraindicated.

54. 3 Since the medication is being taken orally the client may be pocketing the tablet in the buccal cavity and expelling it later; the nurse must check to ensure the administered medication is swallowed. (3; LE; EV; TC; DR)
  1 It may not be a response failure.
  2 If the client is swallowing the medication then this may be necessary; the nurse should first ensure that the medication is swallowed.
  4 This medication reaches a peak in 3 to 5 hours.

55. 3 This drug does not produce an immediate effect; nursing measures must be continued to decrease the chance of suicide. (2; CJ; IM; PA; DR)
  1 These food precautions are taken with the MAO inhibitors.
  2 These precautions are not necessary.
  4 Treatment with lithium requires close monitoring of blood levels to avoid toxicity; this is not necessary with Prozac.

56. 3 The client should be encouraged to follow the medical regimen to maximize the response to drug therapy. (2; CJ; EV; ED; DR)
  1 Client needs further teaching; the physician should be notified of side effects.
  2 Client needs further teaching; the client should be concerned.
  4 Client needs further teaching; the physician should make this decision.

57. 4 These drugs are used to control the extrapyramidal (parkinsonism-like) symptoms that often develop as a side effect of neuroleptic therapy. (2; CJ; AN; TC; DR)
  1 Barbiturates do not have extrapyramidal side effects, which would respond to these drugs.
  2 Antiparkinsonian drugs are not usually prescribed in conjunction with antidepressants because antidepressants do not cause parkinsonism-like symptoms.
  3 There is no documented use of these drugs with antianxiety agents because they do not have extrapyramidal side effects.

58. **3** It is very important that the nurse discontinue previous antipsychotic medications before starting risperidone to minimize the period of overlap to avoid a drug interaction. (3; LE; IM; PA; DR)

1 Although safety is of concern, it would be more important to monitor for mood change and suicidal tendencies once the drug titrate level has been reached, when the client will have clearer thought processes and more energy.

2 The symptoms of extrapyramidal reactions are not likely to occur with this low dosage of Risperdal.

4 This would not allow enough of a lag period between the two drugs and could precipitate a drug reaction.

59. **4** Clients taking chlorpromazine should be told to stay out of the sun. Photosensitivity makes the skin more susceptible to burning. (2; CJ; IM; TC; DR)

1 Photosensitivity is not a side effect of this drug.

2 Same as answer 1.

3 Same as answer 1.

60. **2** Liver damage is a well-documented toxic side effect of neuroleptics. By continuing to administer the drug, the nurse failed to use professional knowledge in the performance of responsibilities as outlined in the Nurse Practice Act. (2; LE; EV; PA; DR)

1 This is false; liver damage, indicated by jaundice, is a well-documented side effect.

3 This is false; blood levels must be reduced when signs of liver damage are present.

4 The neuroleptic should be stopped, not reduced; liver damage is a well-documented toxic side effect.

61. **2** Acute dystonic reactions, parkinsonian syndrome, dyskinesia, and akathisia are observable side effects of fluphenazine (Prolixin) therapy. (2; LE; EV; TC; DR)

1 After the first few days of treatment, Prolixin has no effect on concentration or other mental abilities; there would be a decrease, not an increase, in salivation.

3 These are not side effects of the drug Prolixin.

4 Same as answer 3.

62. **3** This occurs as a late and persistent extrapyramidal complication of long-term antipsychotic therapy. It can take many forms (e.g., torsion spasm, opisthotonos, oculogyric crisis, drooping of the head, protrusion of the tongue). (3; CJ; EV; TC; DR)

1 This is reversible with administration of Cogentin and Benadryl.

2 Same as answer 1.

4 Same as answer 1.

63. **2** The monoamine oxidase inhibitors can cause a hypertensive crisis if food or beverages that are high in tyramine are ingested. (2; LE; IM; TC; DR)

1 This would be important for clients taking one of the phenothiazines.

3 This is not contraindicated.

4 An elixir base, which contains alcohol, only makes the medications more palatable; alcohol does not contain tyramine.

64. **1** Improvement is usually seen within 2 to 4 weeks with this monamine oxidase inhibitor (MAOI). (2; CJ; IM; TC; DR)

2 This is not true; this medication works within 2 to 4 weeks.

3 The client may need a longer time to see an effect from this medication.

4 Same as answer 2.

65. **2** Wine, aged cheese, and other foods with a high tyramine level must be avoided. (2; LE; PL; TC; DR)

1 This is not an expected side effect but can occur as an adverse reaction.

3 This is not true for this medication.

4 No photosensitivity has been reported in clients receiving this medication.

66. **2** Ritalin is an appetite suppressant; it should be given after meals. (3; CJ; PL; PA; DR)

1 Ritalin at this time could suppress the child's appetite.

3 Same as answer 1.

4 Same as answer 1.

Personality Development

67. **4** This is the age of Freud's phallic stage and Erikson's stage of initiative versus guilt. (2; CJ; AN; PS; PD)

1 This age is Freud's genital stage and Erikson's stage of identity versus role confusion.

2 This age is Freud's latency stage and Erikson's stage of industry versus inferiority.

3 This age is Freud's oral stage and Erikson's stage of trust versus mistrust.

68. **3** Children view their own worth by the response received from their parents. This sense of worth sets the basic ego strengths and is vital to the formation of the personality. (1; CJ; AN; ED; PD)

    1 Peer groups come later in a child's development, but the parent-child relationship is still the most important.
    2 Although important, it is not as important as the parent-child relationship.
    4 This comes later in life, after the basic personality has been formed.

69. **4** When acting out against the primary source of anxiety creates even further anxiety or danger, the individual may use displacement to express feelings on a safer person or object. (1; CJ; AN; PS; PD)

    1 This would be fantasy.
    2 This is an example of denial.
    3 This shows an inability to mature and accept responsibility.

70. **4** When the individual experiences a threat to self-esteem, anxiety increases and the normal defense mechanisms are used to protect the self. (1; CJ; AN; ED; PD)

    1 Affective reactions are mood disorders.
    2 Ritualistic behaviors are not a normal aspect of the developmental process.
    3 Withdrawal patterns are an abnormal way of coping with stress; if carried to an extreme, behavior can become pathologic.

71. **3** By developing skills in one area the individual compensates or makes up for a real or imagined deficiency, thereby maintaining a positive self-image. (1; CJ; AN; PS; PD)

    1 If the student incorporated the qualities of the college athlete, that would be introjection.
    2 This would deal more with unacceptable impulses that would pose a threat.
    4 This person is not trying to make amends for unacceptable feelings (reaction formation) but rather for a felt deficiency and a poor self-image.

72. **1** Fears and anxieties about themselves and their possessions are common in the aged because of a decreased self-concept and an altered body image; these changes result in a decreased ability to cope. (2; MR; AN; ED; PD)

    2 Aging need not necessarily bring about losing one's ability to cooperate.

    3 This a behavior noted in the middle stage of Alzheimer's disease, not usually observed in the elderly client.
    4 The attitude of elderly persons about authority or others in their environment is set; indecision about life situations may be due to insecurity.

73. **2** Any behavioral therapy or learning of new methods of dealing with situations requires modifications of approach and attitudes; hence personality is always capable of change. (2; CJ; AN; ED; PD)

    1 Certain personality traits are established by age 2, but not the total personality.
    3 The capacity for change exists throughout the life cycle.
    4 Accepting this theory would close the door on all future growth and development.

74. **3** Before this age the infant has not developed enough ego strength to have an identity or personality. (3; CJ; AN; ED; PD)

    1 This is too early; the child has not developed enough ego strength to have a personality.
    2 Self-concept is nonexistent.
    4 The primary emergence of the personality has already occurred.

75. **3** The parameters set by birth, psychologic experiences, and the environment make each individual unique. Although other factors may impinge to a slight degree, these factors form the personality. (2; CJ; AN; PS; PD)

    1 These are not inclusive; they are limited to only some aspects of personality development; race plays no part.
    2 Autoimmunity plays no part in personality development.
    4 These are not inclusive; they are limited to only some aspects of personality development.

76. **2** The toddler is learning autonomy, but because of the nature of development there is still physical and emotional dependence on the parents. (1; CJ; AN; PS; PD)

    1 The major task during infancy is development of trust.
    3 This stage deals with developing a sense of initiative.
    4 This stage deals with the task of industry and developing skills for working in and relating to the world.

77. **4** Testing the self both physically and psychologically occurs during the toddler stage after trust has been achieved. (3; CJ; AN; ED; PD)
   1 Trust is the task of infancy.
   2 This task is accomplished between the ages of 6 and 12.
   3 Between the ages of 3 and 6, a child starts to identify with the parent of the same sex.

78. **3** Freud's theory is that a child develops a sexualized love for the parent of the opposite sex and becomes jealous of the parent of the same sex. These thoughts result in feelings of guilt, anxiety, fear, and hate toward the parent of the same sex, which are repressed. (1; CJ; AN; ED; PD)
   1 Ambivalence does not occur in the oedipal stage of development.
   2 The child loves the parent of the opposite sex and hates the parent of the same sex.
   4 Same as answer 2.

79. **3** The child resolves oedipal conflicts by learning to identify with the parent of the same sex and accomplishes this by mimicking the role of this parent. (2; CJ; AN; ED; PD)
   1 This is the earliest stage of development and operates solely on the pleasure principle, largely id oriented; this stage is concerned with development of trust.
   2 There is an interest shift from the anal region to the genital region, and questions about sexuality arise.
   4 There is increasing sex-role development; this stage is concerned with peer-group identification.

80. **2** Values and beliefs from parents and society are expressed through the child's play world. These values become part of the child's system through the process of internalization (introjection). (3; CJ; AN; ED; PD)
   1 If this happened, children would learn to blame others for their own faults.
   3 This would occur at a later age.
   4 The environment and others in it, rather than play, influence independence.

81. **3** The child realizes that the parent of the same sex cannot be bested in a struggle for the affection of the parent of the opposite sex. The role and behavior of the same-sex parent are therefore assumed by the child to attract the parent of the opposite sex. (2; CJ; AN; ED; PD)
   1 This would be a conflict, not a resolution.
   2 Doing this would give rise to greater conflict and leave a fragmented self.

   4 This would be in conflict with heterosexual drives.

82. **2** Children 2 to 7 years old have difficulty distinguishing reality from fantasy; this would present the greatest challenge to the nurse. (2; CJ; AN; ED, PD)
   1 Children 0 to 1 years of age focus on "in the moment" thinking; preoperative preparation would most likely not be recalled.
   3 Children 7 to 11 years of age have the ability to comprehend and visualize a series of events and can think about the past and present; would provide less of a challenge to absorb preoperative teachings.
   4 Children 12 to 16 years of age can think in the abstract and have the ability to solve complex problems; would not pose difficulty in preoperative teachings.

83. **2** Slips of the tongue, also called "Freudian slips," are material from the unconscious that slips out in unguarded moments. (1; CJ; AN; ED; PD)
   1 Material in the unconscious cannot deliberately be brought back to awareness.
   3 There is no evidence linking these experiences to the unconscious.
   4 Free-floating anxiety is linked to the unconscious, but the best evidence of the unconscious is slips of the tongue.

84. **2** The unconscious stores past experiences and the emotional feelings associated with them. These emotional feelings influence one's perceptions, attitudes, and behavior. (3; CJ; AN; PS; PD)
   1 Material in the conscious is in a state of immediate awareness.
   3 Material in the preconscious, which includes ideas and feelings, when attended to, can be made conscious.
   4 There is no such thing as the foreconscious level.

85. **2** Mediating frustration within the real world is an ego function and requires ego strengths. (2; CJ; AN; ED; PD)
   1 The id is unable to tolerate frustration because it is totally involved with gratification.
   3 The superego is involved with putting pressure on the ego because the id does not tolerate frustration.
   4 The unconscious does not deal with frustration.

86. **4** The superego incorporates all experiences and learning from external environments (society, family, etc.) into the internal environment. (2; CJ; AN; ED; PD)
1 This is the function of the id.
2 The id with its drives is a source of creative energy.
3 Same as answer 1.

87. **4** Incorporation of parental and societal values into the superego leads to the development of a sense of right and wrong. Guilt and shame are experienced when these values are broken. Thus the superego is the conscience. (2; CJ; AN; PS; PD)
1 The self is the total of the id, ego, and superego.
2 The ideal self is how a person perceives the self to be or strives to be.
3 Narcissism involves an excessive love of self with strong dependency needs that are impossible for others to meet.

88. **3** Conscience and a sense of right and wrong are expressed in the superego, which acts to counterbalance the id's desire for immediate gratification. (2; CJ; AN; ED; PD)
1 This does not reflect any part of the self.
2 This is the id seeking satisfaction.
4 A healthy ego can delay gratification and is in balance with reality.

89. **4** The mature personality does not respond to the immediate gratification demands of the id or the oppressive control of the superego because the ego is strong enough to maintain a balance between them. (1; CJ; AN; ED; PD)
1 There would be no healthy resolution of conflicts if the superego were always in control.
2 With society in control there would be chaos, rather than maturity.
3 This would create a rigid personality that makes impossible demands on the self.

90. **1** Repression is a coping mechanism in which unacceptable feelings are kept out; later, under stress or anxiety, thoughts or feelings surface and come into one's conscious awareness. (1; CJ; AN; PS; PD)
2 Regression is the use of an unconscious coping mechanism through which a person avoids anxiety by returning to an earlier, more satisfying, or comfortable time in life.
3 Rationalization does not address the delay factor; it is an attempt to falsify an experience by constructing logical or socially approved explanations.

4 Reaction formation is defined as disguising unacceptable feelings and reinforcing the opposite feelings.

91. **4** Intellectualization occurs when a painful emotion is avoided by means of a rational explanation that removes the event from any personal significance. (3; CJ; AN; PS; PD)
1 Projection is the blaming of others as a means of dealing with one's own shortcomings.
2 Dissociation is a means of handling conflict by a temporary alteration of consciousness or identity; amnesia is an example.
3 Displacement is the discharging of a pent-up feeling, generally hostility, on an object or person perceived to be weaker than the person who aroused the feelings.

92. **1** The sense of ego integrity comes from satisfaction with life and acceptance of what has been and what is. Despair is due to guilt or remorse over what might have been. (2; CJ; AS; PS; PD)
2 During puberty adolescents attempt to find themselves and integrate values with those of society; an inability to solve conflict results in confusion and hinders mastery of future roles.
3 During early and middle adulthood the individual is concerned with the ability to produce and to care for that which is produced or created; failure during this stage leads to self-absorption or stagnation.
4 Autonomy is developed during the toddler period and corresponds to the child's ability to control the body and environment; doubt can result when made to feel ashamed or embarrassed.

93. **1** Mild anxiety motivates one to action, such as learning or emotional changes. Higher levels of anxiety tend to blur the individual's perceptions and interfere with functioning. (2; CJ; AN; PS; PD)
2 Attention is severely reduced by panic.
3 The perceptual field is greatly reduced with severe anxiety.
4 The perceptual field is narrowed with moderate anxiety.

94. **1** An illusion is a misperception or misinterpretation of actual external stimuli. (2; CJ; AS; PS; PD)
2 This is a false belief that cannot be changed even by evidence; it is a fixed false belief.
3 This would deal with imaginary, not real, stimuli.
4 A belief that others are talking about the person is not a visual distortion, but rather an idea of reference.

95. **4** The individual using sublimation attempts to fulfill desires by selecting a socially acceptable activity rather than one which is socially unacceptable (e.g., pursuing a career in nursing as a means of giving and receiving love). (2; CJ; AN; PS; PD)
    1 This would be an example of reaction formation.
    2 This would be regression, not sublimation.
    3 This would be an example of repression.

Disorders First Evident Before Adulthood

96. **1** Use of denial involves failure to acknowledge the reality of a situation. (1; CJ; AS; PS; BA)
    2 Not demonstrated by this situation.
    3 Intellectualization involves discussing the child's problem in a technical manner; this is not demonstrated in the example.
    4 Same as answer 2.

97. **3** Secondary reinforcers involve the use of social approval; behaviors such as a hug meet this requirement. (2; CJ; IM; PS; BA)
    1 Food is a primary reinforcer and should not be associated with behavior modification.
    2 Same as answer 1.
    4 The child may not select an appropriate secondary reinforcer.

98. **2** Personal fable is adolescent thinking; adolescents think that they are immune to laws of nature; this thinking is reflected in this response. (3; CJ; AS; PS; BA)
    1 This is not evident of personal fable; the statement does not deny the laws of nature.
    3 This is a misunderstanding commonly held by adolescents.
    4 Same as answer 1.

99. **2** By monitoring and reporting changes in the child's behavior, the physician can determine the effectiveness of the medication. (2; MR; IM; PS; BA)
    1 Parents should not be encouraged to tutor children because there is usually too much emotional interaction.
    3 Behavior is not deliberate or controllable; this type of statement could lead to diminishing the child's self-esteem if control does not occur.
    4 Children need more structure and rules than adults.

100. **1** IQ levels between 52 and 68 are considered mild intellectual impairment. (3; CJ; AS; PA; BA)

2 IQ levels between 20 and 35 are specific to severe intellectual impairment.
3 IQ levels below 20 indicate profound intellectual impairment.
4 IQ levels between 36 and 51 are specific to moderate intellectual impairment.

101. **1** Sheltered workshops offer self-sufficiency and work skills and are evidence that the family is considering the client's future role and care. (2; MR; EV; ED; BA)
    2 Residential living is preferred to institutionalization.
    3 The client should be able to perform the task of self-feeding.
    4 Friendships with both sexes are appropriate for the client's developmental level.

102. **1** Infants and toddlers 6 to 30 months of age experience separation anxiety; it is this age group's major stressor and is most traumatic to the child and parent. (2; CJ; AN; ED; BA)
    2 Separation anxiety occurs in this age group, but it is less obvious and less serious than in the toddler.
    3 The school-age child is more accustomed to periods of separation from parents.
    4 Adolescents are often ambivalent about whether they want their parents with them when hospitalized. Peer group separation may pose more anxiety for the adolescent.

103. **4** Research studies have shown that the prognosis for normal productive functioning in autistic people is guarded, particularly if there are delays in language development. (3; MR; PL; ED; BA)
    1 Early accurate diagnosis is difficult and has not been shown to affect prognosis to any extent.
    2 While temperament may affect the child's response to treatment somewhat, it does not affect prognosis to any extent.
    3 This is false reassurance to the parents and would not be helpful.

104. **3** Poor interpersonal relationships, inappropriate behavior, and learning disabilities prevent these children from emotionally adapting or responding to the environment despite a possible high level of intelligence. (2; CJ; AS; PS; BA)
    1 It is the lack of response to stimuli that is the clue to a child's being emotionally disturbed.
    2 This is true but not most characteristic.
    4 The exact opposite is true.

105. 1 By 2 years of age the child should demonstrate an interest in others, communicate verbally, and possess the ability to learn from the environment. Before these skills develop, autism is difficult to diagnose. (2; CJ; AS; PS; BA)

 2 Autism can be diagnosed long before this age.

 3 Infantile autism can occur at this age but is difficult to diagnose.

 4 Same as answer 3.

106. 1 From infancy the child is nonresponsive. Not wanting to eat demonstrates a further withdrawal. (3; CJ; AS; TC; BA)

 2 This is not indicative of an autistic child.

 3 This would not be characteristic of autism.

 4 Children would not be diagnosed as autistic if they enjoyed being with people.

107. 2 Providing a constructive distraction will help to redirect the autistic child's behavior. (1; MR; IM; PA; BA)

 1 Physical contact is anxiety provoking for the autistic child.

 3 Since the reason is probably unknown, it is not appropriate to question such behavior.

 4 Autistic children need sameness; moving furniture will produce anxiety.

108. 4 Autistic behavior turns inward. These children do not respond to the environment but attempt to maintain emotional equilibrium by rubbing and manipulating themselves and displaying a compulsive need for behavioral repetition. (1; CJ; PL; PS; BA)

 1 Large group (or small group) activity would have little effect on the autistic child's response.

 2 These children do seem to respond to music, but not necessarily loud, cheerful music.

 3 Part of the autistic pattern is the inability to interact with others in the environment.

109. 1 A practically universal characteristic of these children is distractibility. They are highly reactive to any extraneous stimuli such as noise and movement and are unable to inhibit their responses to such stimuli. (3; CJ; AN; PS; BA)

 2 Repetition in language or movement may be seen; rituals are uncommon.

 3 Delayed development of language skills is not the major problem but may include dyslexia (reading difficulty), dysgrammatism (speaking difficulty), dysgraphia (writing difficulty), or delayed talking.

 4 Learning disabilities associated with minimal brain dysfunction are manifested in a variety of ways; loss of abstract thought is not a universal characteristic.

110. 4 This is the drug of choice in this diagnosis. It appears to act by stimulating release of norepinephrine from nerve endings in the brain-stem. (2; MR; AN; TC; BA)

 1 Ativan is a benzodiazepine used to treat anxiety and insomnia.

 2 Haldol is an antipsychotic medication.

 3 This is a muscle relaxant.

111. 3 Focusing on specifics is important for children who are easily distracted. (3; CJ; IM; TC; BA)

 1 Focusing on more than one item at a time might be difficult for an easily distracted child.

 2 Hyperactive children respond best to concrete tasks; this is not a concrete task.

 4 A child who is easily distracted would have difficulty talking to a group of children regarding a particular topic.

112. 1 The longer these children stay out, the more difficult it is to get them to return to school, because more fantasies and fears develop. (3; CJ; AN; TC; BA)

 2 The use of this approach rarely accomplishes anything.

 3 This will feed into the fear that the phobia is realistic.

 4 This would increase, not decrease, the fear.

113. 1 School phobia is a symptom that cannot legally be ignored for long because children must attend school. It requires intervention to alleviate the separation anxiety and/or to promote the child's increasing independence. (2; LE; IM; PS; BA)

 2 This symptom requires the parents to comfort, to reorient to reality, and to help the child regain self-control. Legally there are no requirements mandating treatment for this common childhood problem.

 3 Same as answer 2.

 4 Same as answer 2.

114. 3 This disorder interferes with the ability to perceive and respond to sensory stimuli, which causes a deficit in interpreting new sensory data, makes learning difficult, and results in learning disabilities. (1; CJ; AN; PS; BA)

 1 This is not necessarily true.

 2 Not true; there is no mental retardation present.

 4 Same as answer 1.

115. 3 If seizures were physiologically based, the client would not be able to continue to chew gum. This "attack" should be reported as a behavioral response, with the precipitating factors noted. (3; LE; IM; TC; BA)
1 The chewing gum is not a danger when the client is not having a true seizure.
2 This would probably not be necessary now.
4 This is unsafe; it is not even used in a true seizure.

Eating Disorders

116. 4 The client's intake is sufficient or excessive but nutrition is less than body requirements because of purging, interfering with digestion of nutrients. (3; CJ; AN; PS; ES)
1 Fear of weight gain is a response to emotional problems that have impaired the client's adjustment.
2 The client with bulimia does not have a feeding deficit problem.
3 This is not an acceptable nursing diagnosis.

117. 3 These clients hide food, eat excessively in private, and purge in secret; attempts to hide their behavior indicate that they are aware of and are ashamed of their behavior. (3; CJ; AN; PS; ES)
1 Clients with bulimia nervosa are frequently not obese.
2 This is associated with clients with anorexia nervosa.
4 Same as answer 2.

118. 4 Realistic guidelines reduce anxiety, increase feelings of security, and increase compliance with the therapeutic regimen. (3; CJ; PL; TC; ES)
1 A controlling environment would set up a power struggle between these clients and the nurse.
2 These clients need realistic rules and regulations that they recognize as helpful, not empathy.
3 This would not be therapeutic; focusing on food generally results in a power struggle between these clients and the nurse.

119. 3 The problem is psychologic. Therefore the initial approach by the nurse should be directed toward establishing trust. (1; CJ; IM; TC; ES)
1 The client is not ready for this information.
2 The client is convinced of being overweight; complimenting the client's lovely figure would not change the client's self-perception.
4 This may be a nursing intervention after trust had been established.

120. 4 Clients with anorexia nervosa are struggling between the dependency of childhood and the demands of adulthood. (2; CJ; AN; PS; ES)
1 A distortion of body image rather than a low self-esteem is the problem.
2 These clients feel fat, not unworthy.
3 These clients are not angry at anyone.

121. 2 A goal focuses on where the client should be after certain actions are taken; these clients need to gain weight. (2; CJ; AN; TC; ES)
1 This could set up a struggle between the client and the nurse; the focus of care should not be on the actual intake of food
3 Behavior modification techniques work much better than group therapy; these clients lack insight and would focus on food, not eating.
4 These clients talk freely about food; this would not be therapeutic.

122. 2 The primary concern in the practice of pica is that other intake will be nutritionally inadequate. (3; MR; PL; PS; ES)
1 Pica does not necessarily indicate a psychologic/emotional disturbance.
3 If not toxic to the mother, it is generally not fetotoxic.
4 This is not necessary if nutrition is adequate.

123. 3 Children with Down syndrome require calories based on height and weight, not age, because they are prone to obesity. (1; MR; PL; PA; ES)
1 This would be found in any child with a vitamin D deficiency; not common only to children with Down syndrome.
2 This is not found more often in children with Down syndrome.
4 This is not a typical finding in children with Down syndrome.

Delirium, Dementia, and Other Cognitive Disorders

124. 4 When an elderly person's brain atrophies, some unusual deposits of iron are scattered on nerve cells. Throughout the brain, areas of deeply staining amyloid, called senile plaques, can be found; these plaques are end stages in the destruction of brain tissue. (3; CJ; AN; PS; DD)
1 This may or may not be part of the disorder.
2 It is a chronic deterioration, not one with remissions and exacerbations.
3 This is typical of vascular dementia, not dementia of the Alzheimer's type.

125. **2** Clients with this disorder need a simple environment. Because of brain-cell destruction, they are unable to make choices. (2; MR; PL; TC; DD)
   1 A well-balanced diet is important throughout life, not just during senescence; a diet high in carbohydrates and protein may be lacking other nutrients such as fats.
   3 The client is incapable of making choices; providing many alternative choices will only increase anxiety.
   4 Physical and emotional needs must be met on a continuous basis, not just at a fixed time.

126. **3** These clients attempt to utilize defense mechanisms that have worked in the past but use them in an exaggerated manner. Because of brain-cell destruction such clients are unable to focus on one defense mechanism or develop new ones. (2; CJ; AS; PS; DD)
   1 Clients with dementia will depend on old, familiar defense mechanisms.
   2 The client is not capable of focusing on one defense mechanism.
   4 The client is incapable of developing new defense mechanisms at this time.

127. **2** Damaged brain cells do not regenerate. Care is therefore directed toward preventing further damage and providing protective and supportive care. (2; CJ; PL; TC; DD)
   1 The deterioration of the brain cells makes an extensive reeducation program unrealistic.
   3 A client with this disorder may not be able to grasp, understand, or enjoy new leisure activities.
   4 It is beyond the scope of the client's ability to function in a group therapy session.

128. **4** The client who has delirium, dementia, or another cognitive disorder will be most comfortable with the familiar and repetitive daily routine because it creates less anxiety. (2; MR; PL; TC; DD)
   1 It would be beyond the client's capabilities to develop new social skills.
   2 The memory impairment might make this impossible.
   3 Cognitive changes would make this unrealistic.

129. **3** A one-to-one trusting relationship is essential to help the client become more involved and interested in interpersonal relationships. (1; MR; PL; TC; DD)
   1 Specific routines are normally a part of any unit, for all clients.

2 A very confused individual needs to start with a one-to-one relationship before progressing to group involvement.
   4 Selected activities, rather than a large variety of activities, are best.

130. **3** Clients who are out of control are seeking control and frequently respond to simple directions stated in a firm voice. (2; MR; IM; TC; DD)
   1 "Be quiet" is an order that is nontherapeutic and is, furthermore, demeaning behavior on the part of the nurse.
   2 This would not be helping the client gain control of actions and might be frightening to other clients in the day room.
   4 This would be done only after an attempt at calming the client had failed.

131. **4** Having poor control, these individuals cannot set limits for themselves and require an environment in which appropriate limits for behavior are set for them. (1; MR; PL; TC; DD)
   1 An environment that can be manipulated teaches the client nothing; it encourages a continuation of maladjusted behavior.
   2 This would be too stimulating for a person with socially aggressive behavior.
   3 This person has too much freedom of expression and is unable to control impulses.

132. **2** The client with delirium, dementia, or another cognitive disorder rarely expresses any concern about personal appearance. The staff must meet most of the client's needs in this area. (1; CJ; AS; PS; DD)
   1 Resistance to change is a symptom of this disorder.
   3 The past is where these clients feel more comfortable rather than the threatening present.
   4 A short attention span and little or no interest in new activities is typical of dementia.

133. **4** This would provide information about the client's ability to think or use imagination, which are lost in dementia. (3; CJ; AS; PS; DD)
   1 Knowledge of the client's previous appearance is essential before an assessment of current appearance can be made.
   2 Well-practiced behavior may be repeated by the client with dementia.
   3 Same as answer 2.

134. **2** The current trend in psychiatry is to treat the clients while maintaining them in the community. This trend includes the family and community in the plan and has reduced the number of clients in institutions. (1; MR; AN; PS; DD)
1 This might be part of the overall treatment plan but not the only aspect.
3 This possibly would have the effect of masking the symptoms and should be used only in conjunction with psychotherapy.
4 This would be unrealistic for most of these clients.

135. **1** This is a true statement; clients become progressively worse over time. (2; CJ; AN; PA; DD)
2 Alzheimer's disease is an organic, not a functional, disorder.
3 Alzheimer's disease usually appears in people 60 years and older.
4 There are no diagnostic tools other than autopsy that can provide a definite confirmation of Alzheimer's disease.

136. **4** A consistent approach and consistent communication from all members of the health team help the client who has dementia remain a bit more reality oriented. (2; MR; PL; PS; DD)
1 It is the staff members who need to be consistent.
2 Clients who have this disorder do not attempt to manipulate the staff.
3 This is not needed when working with clients who have this disorder; consistency is most important.

137. **2** The therapeutic milieu is directed toward helping the client develop effective ways of dealing with interpersonal situations. (2; MR; AN; TC; DD)
1 This would be a means of achieving the goal.
3 The hospital atmosphere should be more structured and accepting than the client's home.
4 This would accomplish nothing in regard to a long-term goal of functioning in society.

138. **1** Reality orientation is generally helpful to clients exhibiting mild cognitive impairment; these clients are aware of their impairment, and orientation then reduces anxiety. (2; MR; IM; PS; DD)
2 Behavioral confrontation would not be correct, because it would cause frustration and increase psychomotor agitation in a client with cognitive impairment.
3 Reflective communication is a technique in which the nurse restates or repeats the client's statements; it can be used to clarify thoughts but can also lead to frustration when the approach is overdone.
4 Reminiscence group therapy would be helpful with severely confused, disorganized clients because it reinforces identity, acknowledges what was significant, and often compensates for the dullness of the present.

139. **2** When working with a client with dementia, the highest priority should be given to providing nursing care to maintain an optimal level of safe functioning for as long as possible. (2; MR; PL; PS; DD)
1 This does not provide for assessment of the client's level of functioning; assuming that the client needs close, constant supervision can be destructive to the remaining ego function.
3 Incorrect; there is demonstrated evidence of impairment of short-term memory in dementia.
4 Too much flexibility; does not address the nurse's responsibility for assessing client needs; independent living is hazardous, and some degree of supervision is necessary in clients with organic mental syndrome.

140. **3** Orientation to place refers to an individual's awareness of the objective world in its relation to the self; orientation to time, place, and person is part of the assessment of cerebral functioning. (1; MR; AS; PS; DD)
1 This requires abstract thinking, which involves a higher integrative function than orientation to place.
2 This would assess remote memory, not orientation.
4 This would assess recent memory, not orientation.

Substance Abuse Disorders

141. **2** Methadone can be legally dispensed; the strength of this drug is controlled and remains constant from dose to dose, which is uncertain in illicit drugs. (3; CJ; AN; TC; SA)
1 Methadone is used in the medically supervised withdrawal period to treat physical dependence on opiates; it substitutes a legal for an illegal drug.
3 Methadone is a synthetic narcotic and can cause dependence; it is only used in the treatment of heroin addiction.
4 Methadone is not known to have this action.

142. **2** When methadone is reduced, a craving for narcotics may occur. Without narcotics, anxiety will increase, agitation will occur, and the client may try to leave the hospital to secure drugs. (2; MR; EV; TC; SA)
   1 This is not related to methadone hydrochloride reduction.
   3 This is not related to reduced methadone hydrochloride dosage.
   4 This may occur with methadone hydrochloride overdose.

143. **3** The symptoms of withdrawal reach a peak on the third day. (3; CJ; EV; PA; SA)
   1 Symptoms begin within 8 hours and reach their peak on the third day.
   2 Symptoms become more severe on the third day.
   4 Symptoms begin to subside after the third day.

144. **2** The nurse should attempt to support the mother-child relationship. The mother is experiencing a developmental crisis while having to deal with drug addiction and possibly guilt. (2; MR; IM; PS; SA)
   1 The timing for this should be after adjustment to the present situation has begun.
   3 The client needs contact with her new infant to facilitate bonding.
   4 This will make the client feel guilty and not facilitate positive action at this point.

145. **2** This focuses on the client's feelings rather than the organization itself. The organization is effective only when the client is able to discuss feelings openly. (1; MR; IM; PS; SA)
   1 This may or may not be true.
   3 It may be too late by that time.
   4 This is false reassurance; AA may help clients develop insight but may not be able to help them cope with their problems.

146. **4** Referral to a community-based self-help group is an essential component of the discharge plan to provide ongoing support. (2; MR; PL; TC; SA)
   1 The client probably does not need a halfway house.
   2 Referral to a family therapist can only be made at the request of the client and/or family.
   3 Not the best possible mode of therapy and could create additional anxiety.

147. **4** When clients with alcohol problems voice a desire for help, it usually signifies they are ready for treatment because they are admitting they have a problem. (3; CJ; EV; PS; SA)
   1 Compliance with an alcohol treatment program requires abstinence.
   2 Too short a time to signal readiness for treatment.
   3 Self-admission alone is often not an indication that the client is really ready for treatment because many factors can influence admission.

148. **3** Attendance at AA meetings on a daily basis usually indicates an acceptance of the problem and a desire for help. (3; CJ; EV; PS; SA)
   1 Attendance at inpatient group meetings is helpful but is not specific to the problem of alcoholism.
   2 This drug can help maintain abstinence but may also become a crutch that fosters dependency on a pill rather than alcohol.
   4 Clients with alcohol problems should not sponsor other clients until a long period of sobriety is maintained.

149. **4** These defense mechanisms, although distorting reality, are commonly used by clients with alcohol problems, because they help make reality more acceptable. (2; CJ; AS; PS; SA)
   1 Denial is often used as a defense, but sublimation (the rechanneling of anxiety into constructive activities) is rarely used by these clients.
   2 Identification is the unconscious wish to be like another person, and imitation is the conscious copying of another person's qualities; neither is used by clients with an alcohol problem.
   3 Repression is a defense used to push uncomfortable thoughts, feelings, and wishes into the unconscious, whereas suppression keeps them in the subconscious; although repression may be used by clients with alcohol problems, suppression is rarely used.

150. **4** The drug is not taken for medical reasons but for the favorable, pleasant, unusual, or desired effects it produces. It is often taken in doses that would be fatal if the individual had not established a tolerance to it. (2; CJ; AN; PS; SA)
   1 This is true but also with psychologic dependence on the drug.
   2 This is true but also with physiologic need for the drug.
   3 It is a physiologic and psychologic need to take the drug rather than a compulsion.

151. 1 The CAGE questionnaire is one of the simplest and most reliable screening tools for alcohol abuse; CAGE is an acronym for the key words (Cut down, Annoyed, Guilty, and Eye opener) in the 4 questions asked of people suspected of abusing alcohol. (2; CJ; AS; PS; SA)
 2 The tool was not designed to screen for these substances.
 3 Same as answer 2.
 4 Same as answer 2.

152. 3 Data show a high incidence of parental loss or separation could be associated in time with the onset of addiction. (2; MR; AN; PS; SA)
 1 Curiosity may be a factor in experimenting with drugs but not abusing them.
 2 Depression would be more than occasional, in addition to other factors.
 4 The period of adolescence alone would not place a young person in a high-risk category for substance abuse.

153. 1 Polydrug users abuse a variety of drugs in their search for the ultimate "high." They usually will include alcohol in their search and frequently combine their abuses. (2; CJ; AN; PS; SA)
 2 This is not necessarily true.
 3 This is not necessarily so; some become very happy and outgoing.
 4 This has been mentioned as a possible causative factor but with no evidence to support it.

154. 3 Intrinsic motivation, stimulated from within the learner, is essential if rehabilitation is to be successful. Often clients are most emotionally ready for help when they have "hit bottom." Only then are clients motivationally ready to face reality and put forth the necessary energy and effort to change behavior. (1; CJ; AN; PS; SA)
 1 This is an important factor but not the most important one.
 2 This is an important factor and a helpful one but not the most important one.
 4 Same as answer 1.

155. 1 Setting limits gives structure and balance and demonstrates a caring attitude. (2; CJ; IM; TC; SA)
 2 The nurse serves as a role model to raise a client to a more acceptable level of behavior.

 3 The client must be helped to recognize that a problem with drugs exists.
 4 Although this may be true, it is not the priority.

156. 4 Thiamine is a coenzyme in producing energy from glucose. If thiamine is not present in adequate amounts, nerve activity is diminished and damage or degeneration of myelin sheaths occurs. (2; CJ; AN; PA; SA)
 1 A low-protein, not a high-protein, diet would be desirable.
 2 Use of these has a higher risk of toxic side effects in older or debilitated persons.
 3 Thorazine is a neuroleptic, which would not be used because it is severely toxic to the liver.

157. 2 The nurse's failure to observe what was brought in for the client constituted negligence. The nurse's knowledge of the alcoholic individual would warrant checking to see what the client was consuming. (2; LE; EV; TC; SA)
 1 This is also true, but the client has no manifestations of a severe mental illness.
 3 This is not true on a substance-abuse unit.
 4 This is true, except the nurse might have believed that the friend herself had a good effect on the client.

158. 3 This addresses the emotional impact of this hallucination. The nurse's presence can reduce anxiety and provide comfort. (3; CJ; IM; TC; SA)
 1 This is presenting reality but not offering the comfort of the nurse's presence.
 2 This would be entering into the hallucination.
 4 Same as answer 1.

159. 3 Clients have loss of memory and adapt to this by unconsciously filling in areas that cannot be remembered with false information. (2; CJ; AS; PS; SA)
 1 Ideas of grandeur do not occur in this disease.
 2 This is unrelated to confabulation.
 4 This is not true because these individuals feel they are telling the truth.

160. 2 Alcoholic clients have a low self-image and overwhelming guilt feelings. They drink to relieve these feelings, but the drinking only adds to them. (2; CJ; AN; PS; SA)
 1 There is no evidence of this.
 3 The problem is with low self-esteem, not dependence/independence.
 4 It is not with whom but with what that these clients have the difficulty.

161. **2** Alcoholics Anonymous is a self-help group of individuals who meet together to attain and maintain sobriety. (2; CJ; AN; TC; SA)
   1 A social group centers on building interpersonal relationships through participation in mutual activities.
   3 A resocialization group centers on increasing social skills that may be diminished or lacking.
   4 A psychotherapeutic group treats mental and emotional disorders by psychologic techniques and always has a member of the health care profession as its group leader.

162. **1** The client is using denial as a defense against feelings of guilt, which will reduce anxiety and protect the self. (1; CJ; AN; PS; SA)
   2 Denial would deal more with the client's own expectations.
   3 Denial would make the client seem more stable to others, not independent.
   4 This may be part of the reason, but the bigger motivating factor is to decrease guilt feelings.

163. **4** The individual is unaware of gaps in memory, so the use of stories is an unconscious attempt to deny or cover up the gaps. (1; CJ; AN; PS; SA)
   1 Lying is a deliberate attempt to deceive rather than a face-saving device for loss of memory.
   2 Denying is blocking out of conscious awareness rather than a coverup for loss of memory.
   3 Rationalizing would be used to explain and justify the behavior rather than to cover up the loss of memory.

164. **3** Members find sympathy, patience, and understanding in the group. They are able to have their dependence needs met while helping others who are even more dependent than they. (1; CJ; AN; PS; SA)
   1 This is helpful, but it does not have the success rate of AA.
   2 This is important for the detoxification stage, not for overall therapy.
   4 This is not getting at what is causing the alcohol problem.

165. **4** Cocaine is known to stimulate the sexual drive; multiple sex partners increase the risk for AIDS. (3; CJ; AS; PA; SA)
   1 Glue would not produce sexual excitation.
   2 Heroin is a less social drug than cocaine; the addicted person often uses it alone, nodding and sleeping for several hours.
   3 Whereas alcohol is a stimulant for a time, eventually the person becomes drowsy, lowering sexual excitation.

Schizophrenia and Other Psychotic Disorders

166. **1** The biologic factors including genetics, neuroanatomy, and abnormal neurotransmitter-endocrine interactions prevail as a result of studies conducted during the 20th century. (2; CJ; AN; PA; SD)
   2 Seasonal theories in some climates have been studied; this is not the prime theory.
   3 Immunologic perspective is not offered as the foremost etiology.
   4 This theory is no longer thought of as the foremost etiology.

167. **2** Echolalia is repetition of another person's remarks, words, or statements. It occurs when individuals are fearful of saying their own words and therefore just echo the words of others. (2; CJ; AS; PS; SD)
   1 This is a thought process connected with associative looseness.
   3 This is when new words are coined or old words take on private symbolic meanings.
   4 Echopraxia is the reflecting of observed movements rather than of speech.

168. **1** Talking in the third person reflects poor ego boundaries and a dissociation from the real self. (1; CJ; AN; PS; SD)
   2 Transference is the movement of emotional energy and feelings from one person to another.
   3 Displacement is the attempt to reduce anxiety by transferring the emotions associated with one object or person to another.
   4 Reaction formation is the expression of an emotion opposite the one felt.

169. **3** When individuals use these defense mechanisms they are unable to test out their feelings or differentiate the real world from their personal intrapsychic perceptions. (2; CJ; AN; PS; SD)
   1 Logic is only one part of reality testing.
   2 Association is only one part of reality testing.
   4 The thought process is only one aspect of reality testing.

170. **2** This is the major reason antipsychotic medications are used to decrease psychotic signs and symptoms, including hallucinations, delusions, and feelings of paranoia. (2; CJ; AN; PA; SD)
   1 They are not used to treat neurotic symptoms
   3 Antipsychotic drugs are used to treat psychotic symptoms, which may or may not include destructive behavior.
   4 This is not the prime reason antipsychotic drugs are used; these symptoms respond the slowest and the least.

171. **4** These clients usually display social inadequacy and suspiciousness of others. (1; CJ; AS; PS; SD)
   1 Reserve and reclusive behaviors would be manifested; therefore, this option is incorrect.
   2 These qualities are descriptive of the disorder, not the premorbid personality.
   3 The client held a responsible job before becoming sick.

172. **1** Since the client was admitted complaining that the food was poisoned, eating the food on the tray would indicate that the client feels safe. (1; CJ; EV; TC; SD)
   2 This does not provide adequate behavioral observation to evaluate reality testing.
   3 This behavior indicates that the client still does not completely trust the staff.
   4 This behavior would seem to indicate that the client still does not trust the staff and is attempting to intimidate the staff by calling the administration to complain.

173. **3** Demonstrating that the staff can be trusted is a vital initial step in the therapy program. (2; CJ; IM; TC; SD)
   1 The client is not ready to enter group activities yet and will not be until trust is established.
   2 Even proof would not convince the client with a schizoid personality that the feelings of distrust are false.
   4 This would not be realistic even if it were possible; limiting contact does not develop trust.

174. **4** Delusions are protective and can be abandoned only when the individual feels secure and adequate. This response is the only one directed at building the client's security and reducing anxiety. (2; MR; AN; PS; SD)
   1 This is helpful but almost impossible.
   2 Clients cannot be argued out of a delusion.
   3 The client is unable to explain the reason for the feelings.

175. **1** This response recognizes the client's feelings and provides assurance that the staff member will be present. (2; MR; IM; PS; SD)
   2 The client does not know this; if the client did, delusions would not be present.
   3 Locking the client in a room alone will only increase the fear and delusion.
   4 The client is not ready to accept this and really believes danger is imminent.

176. **2** Clients cannot be argued out of delusions, so the best approach is a simple statement of reality. (3; CJ; IM; TC; SD)
   1 This would be a form of entering into the client's delusions; the client would only feel that a particular part was free of poison.
   3 This may reinforce the delusion that the hospital food is poisoned.
   4 Threats are always poor nursing interventions no matter how exasperated the nurse feels.

177. **4** By this action the nurse can evaluate how much the client is eating; this encourages the client to eat and begins the building of a trusting relationship. (2; CJ; IM; TC; SD)
   1 This is unrealistic and would not ensure an adequate intake.
   2 Client would be unable to follow directions because of the nature of the illness.
   3 An explanation would be of little value to this client because of the nature of the illness.

178. **4** If clients feel a need to be punished, it is best to permit them to engage in controlled activities that expiate guilt feelings. (2; MR; IM; PS; SD)
   1 The client cannot be talked out of her delusion; she must believe within herself that she has nothing to atone for.
   2 This would do nothing to interrupt the delusional system; it would support the hallucination.
   3 A procedure such as this would reinforce her belief of the need to be punished.

179. **1** This message is concise and does not require decision making; less likely to increase anxiety. (2; MR; PL; PS; SD)
   2 Asks client to make a decision when a "no" answer would be unacceptable.
   3 Forcing the client to make a decision when acutely ill may increase anxiety; also permits unacceptable answer of "never."
   4 Somewhat accusatory; increases guilt by placing responsibility on the client.

PSYCHIATRIC/MENTAL HEALTH ANSWERS

180. **3** This response demonstrates an understanding of the client's feelings and encourages the client to share feelings, which is an immediate need. (2; CJ; IM; PS; SD)
  1 This would have the effect of only increasing the fears.
  2 The nurse is entering into the hallucination, thereby reinforcing it.
  4 This response is argumentative, making the client defensive and reinforcing the hallucination.

181. **3** Clients losing control feel frightened and threatened. They need external controls and a reduction in external stimuli. (2; MR; IM; TC; SD)
  1 This is helpful for pent-up aggressive behavior but not for agitation associated with delusions.
  2 The client would be unable, at this time, to sit in one place; agitation is building.
  4 The client may get completely out of control if allowed to continue pacing.

182. **2** This response supports reality and self-awareness while helping the client to look to the future rather than focus on the past. (3; CJ; IM; PS; SD)
  1 This may be taken as ridicule of the client; it focuses on the past.
  3 This may or may not be so; the statement dismisses an opportunity for validating how he feels at the present time.
  4 What made him have this delusion is unimportant at the moment; this focuses on the past.

183. **1** Diagnostic criteria for paranoid schizophrenia include two or more symptoms such as delusions and hallucinations; other less prominent criteria are disorganized behavior and negative symptoms. (2; CJ; AS; PS; SD)
  2 These behaviors are not prominent for paranoid schizophrenia but fit other subtypes of schizophrenia.
  3 Same as answer 2.
  4 Bizarre behavior related to drug use does not fit this diagnostic criteria.

184. **4** The nurse's response provides an example to the client that feelings can be expressed by words rather than by action. This response also demonstrates that the nurse cares enough to set limits on behavior. (2; MR; IM; TC; SD)
  1 The nurse would be accepting physical abuse, which is never done.

  2 The behavior and the client should never be ignored; the client needs limits set on behavior now.
  3 The nurse is punishing the client rather than trying to focus on what is happening at this time to cause the behavior.

185. **4** Clients acutely ill with schizophrenia frequently do not trust others; feeling hemmed in would be frightening, causing them to lash out. (3; CJ; AN; PS; SD)
  1 There is no indication that voices are speaking to the client in this instance.
  2 Clients acutely ill with schizophrenia are usually more concerned with what is happening to them and are not able to be concerned with others.
  3 Although this may be true, it is not the primary motivation for this behavior.

186. **2** This response focuses on a feeling that the client may be experiencing and provides an opportunity to validate the nurse's observation. (1; CJ; IM; PS; SD)
  1 This response demands that the client stay in an uncomfortable situation without offering any support.
  3 This response provides an explanation for the client's behavior that fails to recognize the part anxiety plays in changing behavior.
  4 This response comes across as an attack on the client and offers an explanation for the behavior, but fails to convey an understanding that changing behavior is anxiety producing.

187. **4** The nurse sets limits on behavior; accepts the client but rejects the behavior. (3; CJ; IM; TC; SD)
  1 The nurse has a responsibility to the other clients to limit the behavior.
  2 This is a punishment rather than a setting of limits.
  3 This is unrealistic and would violate the client's rights.

188. **1** An interpersonal relationship based on trust must be established before clients can be helped back to reality. (1; CJ; PL; PS; SD)
  2 This is an important part of the treatment and care, but of lesser importance than a trusting relationship.
  3 Socialization would come at a later time in therapy.
  4 There is nothing to indicate an urgency to remove the client from the home.

189. **2** The nurse, demonstrating knowledge and understanding, accepts the client's perceptions even though they are hallucinatory. (2; CJ; IM; PS; SD)
  1 This would increase the client's guilt and fear.
  3 The client would be unable to accept this; it would only increase fear.
  4 This presents reality but negates the client's feelings and asks for unrealistic responses.

190. **4** This is the most therapeutic option; it interjects reality and focuses on the client's behavior. (1; CJ; IM; PS; SD)
  1 This response elicits a yes or no answer and is a closed question.
  2 This is a directive response by the nurse and it will be perceived as threatening by a disturbed client experiencing hallucinations.
  3 Although this interjects reality, it is not the most therapeutic response.

191. **3** A client cannot be argued out of a delusion. Statements made by the nurse show a lack of knowledge and constitute a threat, which is a form of assault. (3; LE; EV; PS; SD)
  1 There is no indication that the client needed a reminder to eat.
  2 A person cannot be argued out of a delusion.
  4 Everyone needs nourishment, but threats accomplish little.

192. **1** The client needs limits set. This response by the nurse sets limits and rejects the behavior but accepts the client. (2; CJ; IM; PS; SD)
  2 This does not help raise the client to a functioning level.
  3 This serves no useful purpose; inappropriate behavior should be dealt with when first noted.
  4 This is a punishing action; it shows no support or acceptance of the client.

193. **3** This shows acceptance for the client yet sets firm limits on the behavior. (2; CJ; IM; TC; SD)
  1 This puts the focus on the nurse rather than on what is behind the outburst.
  2 The nurse accepts the client but should not accept physical abuse from the client.
  4 This statement not only rejects the behavior but also attacks the client.

194. **1** This lets the client know the nurse is available. It also demonstrates an acceptance of the client. (2; CJ; IM; TC; SD)

2 Although it is important to note the incident on the chart, it does not take precedence over letting the client know the nurse is there if needed.
  3 This is an avoidance technique; it shows a lack of acceptance of the client as a person.
  4 Another client's perception of the incident may or may not be valid.

195. **3** The client is voiding on the floor not to express hostility but because of confusion. Taking the client to the toilet frequently limits voiding in inappropriate places. (2; CJ; PL; TC; SD)
  1 This is a form of punishment for something the client cannot control.
  2 This is not realistic; it will have no effect on the problem.
  4 If the client were doing this to express hostility, such action would be useful; but not when the client is unable to control the behavior.

196. **1** This response reflects on the client's feelings rather than focusing on the verbalization. (2; CJ; EV; TC; SD)
  2 This response focuses on the statement rather than on the feeling behind it.
  3 This response dismisses the client and the client's feelings.
  4 This response puts the client on the defensive and asks for verification that the nurse is indeed a good person; it fails to focus on the feeling behind the statement.

197. **1** Assisting clients with grooming keeps them in contact with reality and allows them to see that staff members care enough to help. It also places value on appearance. (1; CJ; IM; PS; SD)
  2 This would be a long-term goal.
  3 A one-to-one relationship would be best initially.
  4 The client may withdraw even more.

198. **1** Nursing care involves a steady attempt to draw the client into some response. This can best be accomplished by focusing on non-threatening subjects that do not demand a specific response. (2; CJ; IM; TC; SD)
  2 The client is not ready yet to discuss feelings, so the first step is to focus on nonthreatening subjects.
  3 Questions like these do not encourage a person to speak.
  4 By doing this, the nurse is showing acceptance of the client but is doing nothing to encourage communication.

199. **1** Keeping the withdrawn client oriented to reality prevents the client from withdrawing even further into a private world. (1; CJ; PL; TC; SD)
  2 A gradual involvement in selected activities would be best.
  3 This would be futile at this time.
  4 The client would be unable to tell anyone why this is so.

200. **4** By observing the client, the nurse is better able to understand the client's behavior, which can be an indication of feelings. (2; CJ; AS; TC; SD)
  1 It is only one of the many aspects that are part of making a diagnosis; this is true in the care of all clients, not just the withdrawn individual.
  2 Observation alone is insufficient to make this judgment; however, it would allow the staff to individualize the plan of care to suit the client's needs.
  3 It is more important to have insight into what the person may be feeling rather than the degree of depression.

Disorders of Mood

201. **3** This recognizes feelings and tells what is expected. (2; CJ; IM; PS; MO)
  1 This is threatening and gives false reassurance; puts the responsibility on the client and does not allow for expression of feelings.
  2 Could lead the client to think that the environment is unsafe, which would increase insecurity and anxiety.
  4 Being with other people in a strange situation will add more stress to the new and already frightening experience of hospitalization.

202. **4** As depression increases, thought processes become more slowed and verbal expression decreases. (3; CJ; AN; PS; MO)
  1 The affect of the depressed person is usually one of sadness, or it may be blank.
  2 Loose associations are seen most often in clients with schizophrenia, not depressed clients.
  3 Decreased physical activity would not produce physical exhaustion.

203. **4** Severely depressed clients are not motivated to take action or to plan ahead. They are unable to direct their energy on the environment. (3; CJ; PL; PS; MO)
  1 This would be helpful to a severely depressed client, whose attention span is limited.
  2 This would be helpful to a severely depressed client because it requires little thought and provides gratification and satisfaction.

  3 This would be helpful for a person with depression as well as for the cognitively impaired.

204. **3** Depressed clients find it difficult to express anger and hostility because they have internalized these feelings and turned them on themselves. (2; CJ; AN; PS; MO)
  1 There is nothing to indicate that the client has unrealistic goals.
  2 This would develop in time; it is not really a goal of therapy.
  4 This would be part of the intervention, not a goal.

205. **1** Routines should be kept simple and no demands should be made that the client cannot meet. The client is depressed, and all reactions will be slow. Putting pressure on the client will only increase anxiety and feelings of worthlessness. (3; MR; PL; TC; MO)
  2 The client will have to focus on personal strengths, not on family strengths.
  3 This would feed into the client's feelings of unworthiness and frustration.
  4 Feelings of worth must come from within the individual; the nurse must reassure the client through actions, not words.

206. **1** The nurse must base nursing intervention on a client's problems. Since major depression is due to the client's feelings of self-rejection, it is important for the nurse to have the client identify these feelings before a plan of action can be taken. (2; CJ; AS; PS; MO)
  2 This is asking the client to draw a conclusion; the client may be unable to do so at this time.
  3 Asking why does not let a client explore feelings; it usually elicits an "I don't know" response.
  4 This is beyond the scope of the client's abilities now; clients would rather have the nurse tell them how staff can help them than help themselves.

207. **2** An art-type project that could be worked on successfully at one's own pace would be important. (2; CJ; IM; PS; MO)
  1 This would require too much concentration and increase the client's feelings of despair.
  3 This is used mostly for severely regressed clients, and at this point it may not be appropriate for this client.
  4 Same as answer 1.

208. **2** This provides support and security without rejecting the client or placing value judgments on behavior. (3; MR; IM; PS; MO)

1 Limits will have to be set in giving care, but staying with the client and showing acceptance are immediate nursing actions.

3 This would only calm the client down; it does not try to deal with the problem.

4 This would be ignoring the problem; isolation would imply punishment.

209. **4** Directness is the best approach at the first interview, because this sets the focus and concern and lets the nurse know what the client is feeling now. (2; LE; EV; TC; MO)

1 At this point the client is most likely unable to think past the present, much less deal with future plans; too general a question.

2 This may be helpful during the course of treatment, but initially the direct approach with the client is best.

3 This would be one resource for input; but regarding suicide, it is best to approach the client directly.

210. **1** Suicidal impulses take priority, and the client must be stopped from acting on them while treatment is in progress. (2; LE; AN; TC; MO)

2 This has a very low order of priority.

3 Safety is the primary responsibility.

4 Reassurance will not necessarily decrease the client's feeling; safety is the priority.

211. **4** Emotional support and close surveillance can demonstrate the staff's caring and their attempt to prevent acting out of suicidal ideation. (2; MR; IM; TC; MO)

1 This would be routinely done; by itself it is not necessarily therapeutic.

2 This would be punishment for a client who still may find a way to carry out a suicide attempt in the room.

3 This is not a suicide precaution.

212. **4** Recognizes feelings and behavior and encourages the client to share feelings; it also promotes trust, which is essential to a therapeutic relationship. (2; CJ; IM; PS; MO)

1 While it is important to record behavior and notify the physician, it is not enough and does not meet the client's needs.

2 This will not meet the depressed client's needs.

3 Assumes too much and may be inaccurate.

213. **1** These clients can usually be fairly easily distracted by planned involvement in repetitious, simple tasks. (2; CJ; IM; TC; MO)

2 This should be employed only if the client's restlessness cannot be controlled with other measures and physical exhaustion creates a danger for the client.

3 This would be abusive treatment for a client with a need to pace and would reinforce the client's belief that punishment was required for redemption.

4 The client may perceive this isolation as a punishment, and it would not allow for observation by the staff.

214. **3** A major part of depression involves an inability to accept the self as it is, which leads to making demands on others to meet unrealistic needs. (3; CJ; PL; TC; MO)

1 A short-term goal would be to talk about the client's depressed feelings; a long-term goal would be to look at what is causing those feelings.

2 Developing new defense mechanisms is not the priority because they tend to help the client avoid reality.

4 This is not important or crucial to the client's recovery.

215. **3** This is the most therapeutic approach. The staff member also provides special attention to help the client meet dependency needs and reduce a self-defeating attitude. (3; CJ; PL; TC; MO)

1 This response negates client's feelings and cuts off further communication.

2 This is unrealistic because the nurse cannot be with the client constantly until the depression lifts.

4 The priority is 24-hour observation of the client; removing articles that could provide a means for suicide would also be done.

216. **3** This gives the client the nonverbal message that someone cares and views the client as being worthy of attention and concern. (2; CJ; IM; PS; MO)

1 The concentration required for chess is too much for the client at this time.

2 The client is incapable of making decisions at this time.

4 Depressed clients often have too much thinking time.

217. **4** Spending extra time with the client demonstrates that the client is worthy of the nurse's time and that the nurse cares. (3; CJ; IM; PS; MO)

1 This does not show the acceptance and care that sitting with the client would.

2 The client may be unable, at this point, to expend energy on anything outside the self.

3 It is unlikely that the client would respond to the nurse because of feeling unworthy and depressed.

218. **1** This response demonstrates an understanding that the newly discharged client needs to have the support of the therapeutic unit when discharged. The client needs to feel that in a crisis the staff will be there for support. (2; MR; IM; TC; MO)

2 The role of the nurse was not to become a good friend but to aid the client in becoming a functioning being again.

3 This response provides false reassurance; the nurse could not know this.

4 This is unprofessional and blurs the roles of nurse and client.

219. **4** These behaviors are signs of clinical depression and need to be treated with antidepressives such as SSRIs, tricyclic antidepressants, or monamine oxidase inhibitors, which stimulate purposeful activity. (3, CJ; PL; PA; MO)

1 These behaviors indicate agitated depression, not mania.

2 These behaviors are signs of agitated depression, not anxiety.

3 Antipsychotic medications such as the phenothiazine group, haloperidol, and clozapine are used to treat the manic phase of bipolar disorder, not for any depression.

220. **1** The nurse failed to use knowledge regarding suicidal clients and did not protect the client from this ever present danger. This failure could be legally defined as negligence. (2; LE; EV; TC; MO)

2 Clients need observation even after the depression has lifted, especially when plans for discharge are pending.

3 Constant supervision would help prevent suicide; the unit was left unlocked and the client was not under constant supervision.

4 Clients are in greater danger of suicide when they are coming out of depression.

221. **4** Past level of success demonstrates ego strengths that can be built on. (2; CJ; AN; PS; MO)

1 This constitutes only a crisis situation, not necessarily a poor prognosis.

2 The client's premorbid personality must be fairly sound because the client is in the second year of college and thus has achieved some success.

3 Intelligence has little to do with recovery, but the client's ego strengths play a big part.

222. **3** This statement helps the client realize that staff members care and feel that the client is worthy of care. (2; MR; IM; PS; MO)

1 This is a response that places the client on the defensive.

2 This is an inappropriate response to a rather obvious situation.

4 This is an evasive tactic by the nurse.

223. **1** The client is asking for help to prevent suicide. This response focuses on feelings and does not challenge or deny them. (1; CJ; IM; PS; MO)

2 This response negates the client's feelings and interprets the situation for the client.

3 This response denies the client's feelings and does not follow through on what the client is saying.

4 This response ignores the client's cry for help and does not follow through on what the client is expressing.

224. **3** This encourages the client to talk about feelings without really setting the focus for the discussion. (2; CJ; EV; TC; MO)

1 This would make the client wonder where the nurse had been for 4 days.

2 This cuts off any further communication of feelings; it ignores what the client has expressed to the nurse.

4 This shifts the responsibility of care to the psychiatrist rather than dealing with it directly.

225. **1** Electroconvulsive therapy, which interrupts established patterns of behavior, helps relieve symptoms and limits possible suicide attempts in clients with severe, intractable depressions that do not respond to antidepressant medication. (2; MR; AN; PS; MO)

2 The client's depressed mood would greatly limit participation in psychotherapy; feelings precipitated by therapy may lead to suicidal acting out.

3 Psychotherapy is directed toward helping the person learn new coping mechanisms and better ways of dealing with problems; the depressed client needs direction to accomplish this.

4 These are antianxiety medications that would not ordinarily be used for clients with depression.

226. **1** Clients fear this therapy because of the expected pain. If they are reassured that they will be asleep and have no pain, there will be less anxiety and more cooperation. (2; CJ; IM; PS; MO)
    2 No treatment requiring anesthesia is totally safe.
    3 Clients may not realize their own fears and not know what questions to ask; this statement cuts off future communication.
    4 Temporary, not permanent, loss occurs.

227. **4** The staff's presence provides continued emotional support and helps relieve anxiety. (2; MR; IM; PS; MO)
    1 This will be part of explaining the treatments; the focus should be not on fear but on having someone present.
    2 Not all clients experience amnesia, and the amnesia passes; placing emphasis on amnesia will increase fear.
    3 They may not make the client better; this would be false reassurance.

228. **3** The electrical energy passing through the cerebral cortex during ECT results in a temporary state of confusion after treatment. (2; CJ; EV; PA; MO)
    1 This is not a usual or expected side effect.
    2 Same as answer 1.
    4 Same as answer 1.

229. **2** Clients are confused when they awaken after electroconvulsive therapy. They have a loss of recent memory, so it is important to orient them to time, place, and situation. (2; CJ; IM; TC; MO)
    1 This would be a later action, if the client asked for food.
    3 This would not be appropriate for a client who has just awakened after a treatment.
    4 This is not necessary.

230. **3** From the history the nurse can determine that the client's contacts were limited, schedule fixed, and demands on self quite rigid. (2; CJ; AS; PS; MO)
    1 The symptoms described are not characteristically noted in this disorder.
    2 Same as answer 1.
    4 Same as answer 1.

231. **3** Overactive individuals are stimulated by environmental factors. A responsibility of the nurse is to simplify their surroundings as much as possible. (1; MR; IM; PS; MO)
    1 The quiet client may become the target of this client's overactivity.
    2 During this phase the client needs a decrease in stimuli.
    4 During this phase the client needs a decrease in stimuli; two overactive clients together would produce excessive stimuli.

232. **4** The client's behavior demonstrates increased anxiety. Since it was directed toward the new staff, it was probably precipitated by their arrival. (2; CJ; AN; PS; MO)
    1 The client is not filling the "life-of-the-party" role; the client is resorting to previous coping behavior in the face of extreme stress.
    2 This is possible, but the remark is more indicative of increased anxiety.
    3 The client is aware of what is going on and who everyone is at this time.

233. **3** Recognizing the language as part of the illness makes it easier to tolerate, but limits must be set for the benefit of the staff and other clients. Setting limits also shows the client that the nurse cares enough to stop the behavior. (2; MR; IM; TC; MO)
    1 This statement shows little understanding or tolerance of the illness.
    2 Ignoring the behavior is a form of rejection; the client is not using the behavior for attention.
    4 This statement demonstrates a rejection of the client and little understanding of the illness.

234. **2** Physical activity will help utilize some of the excess energy without requiring the client to make decisions or forcing other clients to deal with the behavior. (3; MR; IM; TC; MO)
    1 The client needs guidance and would not be able to guide others.
    3 The client would greatly disrupt the unit because of the excess activity and bossiness associated with this disorder.
    4 The client's extreme activity would limit concentration or task completion.

235. **2** Hyperactive clients frequently will not take the time to eat because they are overinvolved in everything that is going on. (2; CJ; AN; TC; MO)
    1 This is indicative of a depressive episode.
    3 The client is unable to sit long enough with the other clients to eat a meal; this is not conscious avoidance.
    4 The client probably gives no thought to food because of overinvolvement with the activities in the environment.

236. **4** Clients out of control need controls set for them. The staff must understand that the client is not deliberately trying to disrupt the unit. (3; MR; PL; TC; MO)
   1 Ignoring the client will not stop the disruptive behavior; the nurse has a responsibility to the other clients.
   2 This is demeaning the client in the eyes of the other clients, and does not deal with the problem directly.
   3 This may be a last resort taken to solve the problem but should not be used until other alternatives are explored.

237. **4** Hyperactive clients burn up large quantities of calories, which must be replenished. Since these clients will not take the time to sit down to eat, providing them with food they can carry with them sometimes helps. (2; MR; PL; PA; MO)
   1 The client will probably not be aware of any hunger and could go without food for a dangerously long time.
   2 This is an exercise in futility for the nurse.
   3 The client is not presently capable of preparing food.

238. **4** The hyperactive client will frequently eat hand foods that do not require sitting down to eat. (2; MR; IM; TC; MO)
   1 The client will most likely ignore the tray.
   2 Unworthy feelings are part of a depressive episode.
   3 It is unlikely that the client would understand or care about this information.

239. **1** Hyperactive behavior in individuals such as this is typical of the manic flight into reality associated with mood disorders. (1; CJ; AS; PS; MO)
   2 Depression, loss of interest in usual activities, and poor appetite are more indicative of a major depression.
   3 The symptoms are more indicative of a mood than a personality disorder.
   4 A flat affect and apathy are more indicative of a schizophrenic disorder.

240. **1** This will help reduce the client's anxiety, thereby reducing hyperactivity. (2; MR; PL; TC; MO)
   2 It is not possible physically to control hyperactivity.
   3 The client is not capable of choosing activities at this time.
   4 The client is not capable of controlling overactive behavior; setting verbal limits will not be effective.

241. **4** The hyperactive client is usually rather easily distracted, so the excess energy can be redirected into constructive channels. (1; CJ; PL; TC; MO)
   1 There is nothing to indicate at this time that the client is not in touch with reality.
   2 The client will talk a great deal with no encouragement.
   3 The client will not be able to stay long enough with one thing to finish it.

242. **1** Having these clients wear personal clothing helps keep them more in touch with reality. (2; MR; IM; PS; MO)
   2 This may set the client up as a target of ridicule by the other clients.
   3 This is not helping the client learn new and better ways to deal with situations.
   4 The client will need help with makeup, since these clients usually go to extremes with it.

Anxiety, Somatoform, and Dissociative Disorders

243. **4** Recognition of anxiety or symptoms of increasing anxiety are an indication that the client is improving. (3; CJ; EV; PS; AX)
   1 Avoidance of anxiety is not a good indication of improvement; there is no guarantee that anxiety can always be avoided.
   2 This does not indicate improvement or recognition of feelings; the client may just be doing what others expect.
   3 Same as answer 2.

244. **2** The client's current behavior is the best indicator of the client's current level of functioning; all behavior has meaning. (3; CJ; AS; PS; AX)
   1 This is important and should be assessed, but it is not the best indicator of current level of functioning.
   3 Same as answer 1.
   4 Same as answer 1.

245. **1** The client can no longer control or tolerate feelings and attempts to disregard reality as a means of avoiding it. (3; CJ; AS; PS; AX)
   2 The client has not indicated plans for self-harm; the client is asking others to do something to help relieve the feeling.
   3 The client is experiencing panic and is crying for help; this behavior is not typical of a narcissistic personality.
   4 The client is in a state of panic and is crying for help; this behavior does not indicate a demanding personality.

246. 3 Removing as many external stimuli as possible helps reduce the client's anxiety by limiting the factors that must be dealt with; decreasing stimuli usually decreases anxiety. (3; CJ; AN; PS; AX)
1 This would not decrease anxiety and may in fact increase it.
2 This may or may not be necessary; not the first intervention until an assessment is completed.
4 The anxiety level must be decreased before this intervention can be implemented.

247. 2 The client is focused on one part of reality but is unable to grasp the total picture; this situation defines the moderate level of anxiety. (3; MR; AS; PS; AX)
1 Mild anxiety is the level where the individual is cognizant of all aspects of reality but has a "jumpy feeling" and "butterflies."
3 Severe anxiety is the level where individuals lose touch with reality and have a feeling of impending doom, which tends to immobilize them.
4 Panic is the level where the individual is no longer in contact with reality, is unable to make decisions, has impaired judgment, and is really dysfunctional.

248. 3 The nurse who is anxious should leave the situation after providing for continuity of care; the client will be aware of the nurse's anxiety, and the nurse's staying would be nonproductive and nontherapeutic. (3; MR; AS; PS; AX)
1 This meets the nurse's need; this response could make the client feel guilty that something was said that upset the nurse; the client will be aware of the nurse's anxiety, which will increase the client's own anxiety.
2 Same as answer 1.
4 The client will probably sense the nurse's anxiety through nonverbal channels, if not through verbal responses.

249. 4 In phobias the individual transfers anxiety to a rather safe inanimate object. Therefore the anxiety and resulting feelings will only be precipitated when in direct contact with the object. (2; CJ; AN; PS; AX)
1 It is not thinking about the feared object that causes anxiety; it is the possibility of having to come into contact with it.
2 It is the guilt or fear within the person, not the object, that must be dealt with.
3 It is not possible to introject the feared object into the body.

250. 1 The most successful therapy for clients with phobias involves behavior modification techniques using desensitization. (2; CJ; IM; ED; AX)
2 Insight into the origin of the phobia will not necessarily help the client overcome the problem.
3 May increase understanding of the phobia but may not help the client to deal with the fear; there is no maladaptive thought process associated with phobias.
4 Psychoanalysis may increase understanding of the phobia, but may not help the client deal successfully with the unreasonable fear.

251. 2 Recurrence of attacks is a common concern. (3; MR; IM; PS; AX)
1 This is not therapeutic.
3 Although this response initially focuses on feelings it then cuts off communication.
4 The client will be focused on own needs, not what the family says.

252. 1 Acting out anxiety with antisocial behavior is most commonly found in individuals with personality rather than anxiety disorders. (3; CJ; AS; TC; AX)
2 This is an example of a conversion disorder.
3 Regression is an attempt during periods of stress to return to behavior that has been satisfying and is appropriate at an earlier stage of development.
4 This is an example of a phobic disorder.

253. 1 The "fight or flight" responses of the autonomic nervous system would be stimulated and result in these findings. (2; CJ; EV; PA; AX)
2 The pupils would dilate, not constrict, and the blood glucose would increase, not decrease.
3 The "fight or flight" response is not characterized by constricted pupils, constricted bronchioles, and hypoglycemia.
4 The pulse rate would be increased, and the blood glucose would increase, not decrease.

254. 1 When tension is reduced, anxiety diminishes and the person feels more comfortable, safe, and secure. (2; CJ; AN; PA; AX)
2 There would be less anxiety if the person were able to deny the situation.
3 When anxiety is high the client is unable to focus on the problem.
4 This action would have an effect on psychologic rather than physical discomfort.

255. **3** Learning a variety of coping mechanisms helps reduce anxiety in stressful situations. (1; CJ; PL; PS; AX)
1 A person must learn to cope with unpleasant objects and events.
2 Prolonged exposure would increase anxiety to possibly uncontrollable levels.
4 Fearful situations can never be viewed as pleasurable.

256. **1** By staying physically close, the nurse conveys to the client the message that someone cares enough to be there and that the client is a person worth caring for. (3; CJ; IM; PS; AX)
2 The client is incapable of telling anyone what the problem is.
3 Sitting still will increase the tension the client is experiencing.
4 This would not be an initial nursing intervention.

257. **2** The client is too anxious to sleep in a four-bed room and should simply be moved to a private room. (3; MR; IM; PS; AX)
1 Just talking about the problem will not improve it; quietly moving the client to a private room would be better intervention at this time.
3 This is false reassurance.
4 This probably would not help since it would not relieve the client's anxiety.

258. **1** Providing support, understanding, and acceptance of feelings that the client is experiencing is essential for reducing stress. (2; CJ; IM; PS; AX)
2 This would most likely have the effect of increasing anxiety.
3 The hospital provides the client with a safe, accepting environment in which to face problems and discuss emotionally charged areas.
4 This is unrealistic; the nurse cannot be present at all times. Concerns about the nurse's absence would increase anxiety.

259. **2** The client is caught between two equally compelling needs, and movement or sight is impossible. Paralysis or blindness justifies to the client the inability to move in any direction. (2; CJ; AS; PS; AX)
1 It is an unconscious method of solving a conflict.
3 It is more important that the client learn how to deal with personal feelings before dealing with family conflicts.
4 It is necessary for the client to focus on the problem causing the disorder, not on other things.

260. **3** Needing to be dependent while wanting to be independent creates a struggle that makes all movement psychologically difficult. Symptoms develop and remove psychologic choice, making movement physically impossible. (2; CJ; AS; PS; AX)
1 It is unlikely the feelings would involve the home; rather the people in it.
2 This is a part of the picture but not the total picture.
4 Same as answer 2.

261. **3** The conversion type of defense tends to be a learned behavioral response that the individual will use when put under stress. (2; CJ; AN; PS; AX)
1 This is not a likely occurrence if the client learns to deal with problems.
2 Psychiatric treatment may be needed at different times throughout life but usually not on a continuous basis.
4 Based on studies of this disorder, it usually returns when the client is under severe stress.

262. **3** The physical symptoms are not the client's major problem and therefore should not be the focus for care. This is a psychologic problem, and the focus should be on this level. (2; CJ; PL; PS; AX)
1 This would be focusing on the physical symptoms of the conflict; the client is not ready to give up the symptom.
2 The disorder operates on an unconscious level but is very real to the client; this response denies feelings.
4 Psychotherapy would have to come before physical therapy.

263. **4** The client's anxiety results from being unable to choose psychologically between two conflicting actions. The conversion to a physical disability removes the choice and therefore reduces the anxiety. (3; CJ; AN; PS; AX)
1 The anxiety is put under control by the conversion to a physical disability.
2 The anxiety is decreased, and the conversion disorder operates on an unconscious level.
3 The anxiety is internalized into a physical symptom.

264. **3** The symptoms are problematic to the client and thus have caused emotional pain that is beyond conscious control. (1; CJ; PL; PS; AX)

1 Ignoring the client's complaints will increase anxiety.
2 Willpower does not enter into it; a conversion disorder operates on an unconscious level.
4 There is no evidence that this will occur.

265. **1** The client is using this compulsive behavior to control anxiety and needs to continue with it until the anxiety is reduced and more acceptable methods are developed to handle it. (2; MR; IM; TC; AX)

2 This would not reduce the client's anxiety since she is aware that doorknobs are not contaminated but cannot stop the compulsive act.
3 Same as answer 2.
4 This would greatly increase anxiety; compulsive behavior is a defense that cannot be interrupted until new defenses are learned.

266. **3** By carrying out the compulsive ritual, the client unconsciously tries to control the situation so that unacceptable impulses and feelings will not be acted on. (2; CJ; AN; PS; AX)

1 This mechanism does not operate on a conscious level.
2 Hallucinations are not part of a phobic disorder.
4 They feel no need to punish others.

267. **4** Responding to the behavior in a matter-of-fact way avoids reinforcing the behavior; allowing time for rituals avoids increasing anxiety. (3; CJ; IM; TC; AX)

1 Attempts to speed up ritualistic behavior will only increase anxiety.
2 Disparaging the client will decrease self-esteem, increase anxiety and guilt, and may increase symptoms.
3 Attempts to discourage ritualistic behavior often increase anxiety and symptoms.

268. **1** This sets an unrealistic limit that would increase anxiety by removing a defense the client needs. (3; CJ; AN; PS; AX)

2 This is done in therapy as the client's condition improves. Insight is slowly developed to minimize anxiety.
3 This would increase self-esteem and self-control, not increase anxiety.

4 This would reduce, not increase, anxiety, because the client would feel free to express feelings.

269. **4** These clients can better work through their underlying conflicts when demands are reduced and the routine is simple. (1; MR; AN; PS; AX)

1 Preventing these clients from carrying out rituals can precipitate panic reactions.
2 The intent of therapy should be to help the client gain control, not to enable others to do the controlling.
3 Since anxiety stems from unconscious conflicts, a controlled environment alone is not enough to effect resolution.

270. **3** The initial action is to avoid hurrying the client because this increases anxiety and the performance of the ritual. (3; MR; PL; PS; AX)

1 Taking away all of the client's ritualistic behaviors would be ineffective and serve to increase anxiety.
2 This is one of the goals to be accomplished during the client's hospitalization, not in the initial phase.
4 This action is an appropriate intervention during the working phase of the nurse-client intervention, not the initial phase.

271. **4** Anxiety is a normal human response, causing both physical and emotional changes that everyone experiences when faced with stressful situations. (2; MR; IM; PS; AX)

1 Anxiety is experienced to a greater or lesser degree by every person.
2 Anxiety does not operate from the conscious level.
3 The fear may be related to a specific aspect of, rather than the total, environment.

272. **4** The symptoms are a defense against anxiety resulting from decision making, which triggers old fears; the client needs support. (2; CJ; IM; PS; AX)

1 This denies the client's overwhelming anxiety and lacks realistic support.
2 This is judgmental; the client should be encouraged to work through symptoms, not avoid risk.
3 This is judgmental; an increase in anxiety does not necessarily mean the client does not want to attain the goal.

Disorders of Personality

273. 4 The repeated thought or act defends the client against even higher, more severe levels of anxiety. (3; CJ; PL; PS; PR)
1 To deny the client the ritual may precipitate panic levels of anxiety.
2 The client already recognizes that the ritual serves little purpose.
3 Same as answer 1.

274. 1 Ineffective coping is the impairment of a person's adaptive behaviors and problem-solving abilities in meeting life's demands; ritualistic behavior fits under this category as a defining characteristic. (3; CJ; AN; PS; PR)
2 Not enough information is available to use this nursing diagnosis in this situation.
3 Same as answer 1.
4 Same as answer 1.

275. 4 This outcome would result from teaching the client to recognize situations that provoke ritualistic behavior and the client's learning how to interrupt the pattern. (3; MR; EV; PS; PR)
1 Not a priority; the client probably had little difficulty in this area.
2 Same as answer 1.
3 No evidence was presented to indicate the client was hallucinating.

276. 1 This drug blocks the uptake of serotonin. (2; CJ; AN; PS; PR)
2 This is an antiparkinsonian agent, not an antidepressant.
3 Same as answer 2.
4 This is an antihistamine, not an antianxiety agent.

277. 2 The repeated thought or act defends the client against severe anxiety; the client does not want to perform the ritual but feels compelled to do so to keep anxiety at a controllable level. (2; CJ; AN; PS; PR)
1 No limits are being set by the nurse's action.
3 This causes depression and is unrelated to ritualistic behavior.
4 Rituals are not activities that enhance self-esteem; they control anxiety.

278. 2 Attributing unacceptable feelings or attributes to others is the mechanism known as projection; the data demonstrate use of this defense mechanism. (2; CJ; AS; PS; PR)
1 Denial is the unconscious refusal to recognize the reality of an anxiety-producing situation; the data do not demonstrate use of this defense mechanism.
3 Displacement is the shifting of feelings from an emotionally charged situation to a substitute person or object; the data do not demonstrate use of this defense mechanism.
4 Intellectualization is the use of reasoning to avoid confronting an objectionable impulse; the data do not demonstrate use of this defense mechanism.

279. 4 Clients with borderline personality disorders frequently demonstrate a pattern of unstable interpersonal relationships, impulsiveness, affective instability, and frantic efforts to avoid abandonment; these behaviors usually create great difficulty in establishing mutual goals. (2; CJ; AS; PS; PR)
1 The client with a borderline personality disorder usually would not have difficulty in this area.
2 Same as answer 1.
3 Same as answer 1.

280. 3 When props are needed to blur reality, the individual is not able to rely on the self to test out situations, and therefore dependence on others or props increases. (3; CJ; AN; PS; PR)
1 The person who mistrusts has not learned to trust the environment; however, the person does not necessarily need props.
2 The person with an ego ideal would not need props to blur reality.
4 Role blurring is not a problem requiring a prop.

281. 3 Clients prevented from using ritualistic behavior to control anxiety will be deprived of a defense and have no way of relieving tension. (1; MR; PL; TC; PR)
1 The client's behavior should never be ignored; it is important to accept and support these clients during this time.
2 This would not decrease the ritualistic behavior.
4 Preventing ritualistic behavior will only increase anxiety.

282. **3** The development of physical symptoms without a physical cause is an anxiety-reducing mechanism known as conversion. (2; CJ; AN; PS; PR)
  1 Blaming others in the environment for failure and mistakes is not converting anxiety into physical symptoms.
  2 Going back to an earlier state when one felt safer and more secure is not converting anxiety into physical symptoms.
  4 This is a continued concern about health characterized by anxiety and an unrealistic interpretation of real or imaginary symptoms as indication of serious illness.

283. **2** Individuals with this personality disorder tend to be self-centered and impulsive. They lack judgment and self-control and do not profit from their mistakes. (3; CJ; AN; PS; PR)
  1 Generally, just the opposite is true.
  3 These people never learn from their mistakes, experiences, and punishment.
  4 These people are too self-centered to have a sense of responsibility to anyone.

284. **2** The lack of superego control allows the ego and the id to control the behavior. Self-motivation and self-satisfaction are of paramount concern. (3; CJ; AN; PS; PR)
  1 They count on others to extricate them from the problems they find themselves faced with.
  3 These people are extremely dependent on others.
  4 These people are usually charming on the surface and can easily "con" people into doing what they want.

285. **3** Accepts the client as a person of worth rather than being cold or implying rejection. However, the nurse maintains a professional rather than a social role. (1; MR; IM; TC; PR)
  1 This is shifting responsibility from the issue at hand to the institution.
  2 This does not respond to the statement; the client is aware of their roles.
  4 This avoids the real issue and elevates the nurse to a higher social order.

286. **2** When the individual consciously pretends an illness with no physical basis, it is called malingering. (3; CJ; AS; PS; PR)
  1 People using neurotic defenses really believe they are sick.

  3 A person out of contact with reality is unable to pretend an illness.
  4 The use of conversion defenses is not a conscious act.

287. **4** The psychophysiologic response (hyperfunction or hypofunction) creates actual tissue change. Somatoform disorders are unrelated to organic changes. (2; CJ; AN; PS; PR)
  1 There is a feeling of illness in both instances.
  2 There is an emotional component in both instances.
  3 There may be a restriction of activities in both instances.

288. **1** Clients with these sexual disorders usually have many other emotional problems that may be overt or covert in nature. (2; CJ; AS; PS; PR)
  2 There is no proof of a deficiency of these hormones.
  3 There is normal development of sexual organs in individuals with paraphiliac sexual disorders.
  4 This has no basis in fact.

289. **2** Everyone has the right to personal sexual preference, but limits must be set on acting-out behavior within the hospital. (3; MR; IM; TC; PR)
  1 This would be a punishing attitude, especially for the client who would be transferred.
  3 Limits would need to be set; punishment is inappropriate.
  4 This approach does not address the immediate situation; helping the clients deal with their sexuality in a more appropriate manner is more therapeutic than continuous separation by staff.

290. **3** Dissociation is defined as handling emotional conflicts, or internal or external stressors, by a temporary alteration of consciousness or identity. (1; CJ; AN; PS; PR)
  1 Projection is attributing one's own unacceptable feelings and thoughts to others.
  2 Repression is unconsciously keeping unacceptable feelings out of awareness.
  4 Suppression is consciously keeping unacceptable feelings and thoughts out of awareness.

291. 4 The client's exact compliance in carrying out the compulsive ritual relieves anxiety, at least temporarily. Furthermore, it meets a need and is necessary to the client. (1; CJ; AN; PS; PR)
1 The compulsive act is purposeless repetition and useful only in that it decreases anxiety for the client.
2 The person cannot stop the activity; it is not under voluntary control.
3 Urging has no effect on trying to have the client start or stop the ritualistic behavior.

292. 4 Helping clients understand that a behavior is being used to control impulses usually makes them more amenable to psychotherapy. (2; MR; IM; TC; PR)
1 Part of treatment may include activities to help the client, not others.
2 The client usually understands this already.
3 This would only mask symptoms and would not get at the root of what is bothering the client.

293. 4 Accepting these clients and their symptomatic behavior sets the foundation for the nurse-client relationship. Setting limits provides external controls and helps lower anxiety. (3; MR; PL; TC; PR)
1 Restricting movements would have no effect other than to increase anxiety.
2 This will only increase their anxiety and increase their use of the behavior.
3 This is unrealistic.

294. 3 Sets realistic limits on behavior without rejecting the client. (2; MR; IM; PS; PR)
1 This would constitute a rejection of the person rather than the behavior.
2 This would encourage further manipulation of the staff by the client.
4 The other client is entitled to a special time with the nurse; this is inconsistent limit setting on the part of the nurse.

295. 2 This sets limits, points out reality, and places responsibility for behavior on the client. (2; MR; IM; PS; PR)
1 This is a punishing response and endangers the trust relationship.
3 Clients such as this need limits set; changing the time shows inconsistency.
4 The nurse using this response is showing inconsistency, endangering the trust relationship, and using a threat to gain control.

296. 3 This intervention demonstrates the nurse's caring presence which is vital for this client. (3; MR; PL; TC; PR)
1 While the treatment team does need to know about the event, notification is not the immediate concern.
2 This is premature and it reinforces the client's predisposition to manipulative behavior.
4 This medication is inappropriate in this situation; vomiting would be expected after the ingestion of shampoo.

297. 3 Displacement is a defense mechanism in which one's pent-up feelings toward threatening others are discharged on less-threatening others. (2; MR; AN; PS; PR)
1 Manipulation is a mechanism by which individuals attempt to manage, control, or use others to suit their own purpose or to gain an advantage; unrelated to child abuse.
2 Transference is a mechanism by which affects or emotional tones are shifted from one individual to another; unrelated to child abuse.
4 Reaction formation is a mechanism by which unacceptable feelings are repressed while the exact opposite feelings are expressed; unrelated to child abuse.

298. 1 Typically, the abusing parent has difficulty showing concern for the child. The parent is unable to comfort the child, such as through touch, and gives little indication of realizing how the child feels. (3; CJ; AS; PS; PR)
2 Rather than guilt, battering parents tend to feel angry at the child for the injury.
3 Battering parents rarely show concern about the child's care or progress.
4 This is not particularly a characteristic reaction of abusive parents.

Crisis Situations

299. 1 Going for counseling demonstrates the client's recognition that assistance is needed. (2; MR; EV; PS; CS)
2 There are no data to support this conclusion.
3 Same as answer 1.
4 Same as answer 1.

300. 1 It is not the events but how the individual perceives them that is most significant in either precipitating or avoiding crisis. (2; MR; AN; PS; CS)

2 Changes in role may occur but again, the individual's perception of these changes is most influential.

3 This may be a factor, but perception is most important.

4 This is not a significant factor; the family may provide support and a crisis can still occur.

301. 1 The symptoms presented are indicative of a severe anxiety reaction related to a crisis; the client has a need to vent feelings. (1; CJ; PL; PS; CS)

2 A premature action that requires a physician's order.

3 The symptoms presented are not indicative of a urinary tract infection.

4 An order for a mild tranquilizer may be necessary later; this would be too soon.

302. 2 Studies demonstrate that as more women enter the work force they experience fewer negative responses to the empty nest created by children leaving home. (2; MR; AN; PS; CS)

1 This may occur for some women but not many.

3 Same as answer 1.

4 Same as answer 1.

303. 1 A client in crisis needs to rely on available support systems for assistance; therefore it is vital for the nurse to identify the client's support system. (3; CJ; IM; PS; CS)

2 Nothing in the history demonstrates psychotic thoughts are present.

3 The client's self-image would be fairly negative at this time and should not be reinforced.

4 This would add to the client's anxiety and not help the client deal with the loss.

304. 2 During crisis intervention the nurse should be goal directive and active in assessing the current situation and handle the interview with authority. (3; CJ; PL; PS; CS)

1 These are not appropriate; the client cannot move without direction.

3 This approach might be more appropriate for long-term therapy.

4 These are not appropriate to crisis intervention.

305. 4 This is not an expected outcome of a crisis because by definition a crisis would be resolved in 6 weeks. (2; CJ; EV; PS; CS)

1 This is a desirable outcome of a crisis situation.

2 Although this is not the most ideal outcome for a crisis situation, it is a possible outcome.

3 This is a desirable outcome of a crisis situation.

306. 4 This assessment assists the nurse in determining what the situation means to the client. (2; MR; AS; TC; CS)

1 This is not as important but should be included in a later assessment.

2 Same as answer 1.

3 Same as answer 1.

307. 4 Clients in crisis need assistance with coping; the nurse must be involved with problem solving. (3; CJ; IM; TC; CS)

1 Although a positive interview statement, it does not focus on the nurse's involvement with problem solving.

2 Same as answer 1.

3 Same as answer 1.

308. 1 The client's behavior indicates that a problem is occurring in response to the therapy group. The nurse should assess whether participating in the group is creating a crisis for the client. (2; CJ; AS; TC; CS)

2 There are no data to suggest the client is disoriented.

3 There are no data to suggest the client is using confabulation.

4 There are no data to suggest the client is hallucinating.

309. 4 Feelings of resentment toward children by parents is a normal response. To relieve feelings of guilt and shame, it is vital to help parents realize this. (1; CJ; IM; PS; CS)

1 The first child causes the greatest amount of adjustment in one's life.

2 These are normal feelings.

3 This is an untrue generalization.

310. **2** Toddlers struggle to identify their own needs. Too early and too strict toilet training results in ambivalence because toddlers' needs and physical abilities are in conflict with parental demands. Toddlers are faced with giving up these needs or risking parental disapproval. (2; CJ; AN; PS; CS)

1 Children are involved from birth in satisfying their own needs.

3 Children are involved from birth in satisfying their parents' needs, but toilet training is really the first time a conflict develops.

4 A child has no interest in society's expectations.

311. **1** Developmental level is essential to understanding a child's response to a crisis situation. (2; CJ; AS; ED; CS)

2 This is not an initial assessment.

3 Same as answer 2.

4 This is important to assess after the developmental level has been ascertained.

312. **4** When the parents can verbalize a recognition that their infant may have present or future problems, it usually signifies that they are beginning to face reality. (1; MR; EV; PS; CS)

1 This is not a problem specifically related to an infant with a genetic disorder. It is therefore not the most significant factor for the nurse working with this particular family.

2 Although this may have an effect on the parents' reaction to their infant, it is probably not critically significant to the nurse at this time.

3 This would be after the fact for this infant; it is not the most significant factor to be considered by the nurse at this time.

313. **1** Sitting down shows the client that the nurse cares enough to spend time. It also opens up channels of communication. (2; MR; IM; PS; CS)

2 The nurse sets dimensions on the mother's feelings; this does not promote free expression of feelings.

3 This statement provides false hope; the possibility of the diagnosis has been introduced.

4 This statement ignores the mother's need to express feelings; it takes a cognitive approach to the problem.

314. **3** The usual initial response to a crisis situation such as this is denial that it could occur and that she and her husband could produce a less than normal child. The mother's response is her way of dealing with the reality of the situation. (1; CJ; EV; PS; CS)

1 Although the mother initially rejected her baby, time and coping may help her accept the anomaly.

2 The mother's reaction is a normal part of the grief response.

4 First reactions to a child with a congenital anomaly cannot be judged as final.

315. **2** Denial or disbelief and shock are considered initial responses of grieving. There is a feeling of guilt and inadequacy when a child is born with a defect or abnormality. (2; CJ; AS; PS; CS)

1 It would be unusual for a client initially to verbalize feelings of punishment or guilt so directly.

3 A sense of shame and guilt is voiced later; after denial, disbelief, and shock.

4 It would be unusual for a client to use rationalization and voice it so obviously.

316. **2** This action demonstrates recognition of the client's behavior as a normal response to the situation. (1; MR; IM; PS; CS)

1 This may make the client feel that the behavior is wrong or is annoying others.

3 This closes off communication and does not allow the client to talk about feelings.

4 This may be done later; the need to respond to the client's feelings is the priority at this time.

317. **3** The other children need to remain with their parents and work through their own grief. (3; MR; PL; TC; CS)

1 The initial visit is too early for this to occur.

2 Same as answer 1.

4 Same as answer 1.

318. **4** Communication and intervention during this stage are mainly nonverbal, as when a client gestures to hold the nurse's hand. (3; CJ; PL; PS; CS)

1 Kübler-Ross' studies have shown that this stage usually needs verbal interventions and communication.

2 Same as answer 1.

3 Same as answer 1.

319. **1** Crying is a release but the grieving process should be resolved by this time. (2; CJ; AN; PS; CS)

2 Not necessarily; people express grief in a variety of ways.

3 Generally the grieving process is resolved by this time.

4 This is an assumption and is not a valid assessment.

320. 4 This statement lets the client know the nurse realizes the client is having difficulty without asking direct questions or focusing on specific behavior. (1; CJ; IM; TC; CS)
1 This is an avoidance technique.
2 This response is stated more like an order than an offering of an opportunity to express feelings.
3 This would be negating the client's feelings.

321. 4 The client is in the hospital for treatment and evaluation, not judgment of behavior. Because the client feels people are judging, it is important to point out that at this time the only one filling this role is the client. (3; CJ; IM; TC; CS)
1 This statement ignores feelings and does not help the client deal with the situation.
2 This may or may not be true and could be false reassurance.
3 The nurse does not know this to be a fact.

322. 1 Identifying feelings and providing support during stressful times are both ways of demonstrating concern during a crisis. (1; MR; IM; PS; CS)
2 This is not a supportive or insightful reply.
3 This is an inappropriate reply that may instill guilt feelings; the father as well as the mother needs support through this crisis.
4 Same as answer 2.

323. 2 This provides for collection of more data. (2; MR; AS; PS; CS)
1 This implies that things are not well, and the mother may be to blame.
3 This could make the mother feel guilty about not meeting her baby's needs.
4 This is a negative comment that closes communication.

324. 1 The therapeutic regimen includes bed rest; peace of mind can best be achieved if the children are adequately cared for. (3; MR; IM; PS; CS)
2 This explores feelings without including the therapeutic regimen.
3 Complete bed rest has been prescribed.
4 This is giving specific solutions rather than exploring the situation with the client.

325. 2 Crisis intervention is short-term therapy with the major goal of restoring clients to their precrisis state. (2; MR; PL; PS; CS)
1 This is not the goal of crisis intervention, although it may be necessary if psychologic equilibrium cannot be restored.
3 This is not always necessary for clients to be able to function effectively.
4 This is not a goal but an action to help achieve a goal; not part of crisis intervention.

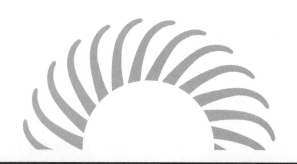

CHAPTER 4

Childbearing and Women's Health Nursing

PUBERTY

A period during which the organs of reproduction mature and are prepared for their reproductive function

A. Physical and physiologic changes
   1. Males
      a. Occur between 10 and 14 years of age; less dramatic than in females
      b. Deepening voice and growth of body hair on the face, axillae, and genitalia
      c. Spermatogenesis occurs in second year after onset: increased activity of sweat glands, with periodic erections and emissions of mature sperm
      d. Dramatic body growth spurt
      e. Ejaculation is beginning of fertility and end of puberty
   2. Females
      a. Occur between 9 and 17 years of age
      b. First sign of puberty is an acceleration of body growth
      c. Thelarche: breast budding
      d. Adrenarche: growth of pubic and axillary hair
      e. Menarche: onset of menses; a late pubertal event, occurring after peak of growth has passed–ovaries produce estrogen
      f. For the first year menstrual cycles are often anovulatory and irregular
B. Psychologic changes
   1. Maturational changes according to age
   2. Heterosexual interests: girls earlier than boys, girls interested in older boys
   3. Emancipation struggles with parents: independence versus dependence
   4. Need for belonging to a peer group

MENSTRUAL CYCLE

A. Menstrual cycle refers mainly to changes in the uterus and ovaries, which recur cyclically from the time of the menarche to the menopause
B. Length of cycle measured from the onset of a period of uterine bleeding to the onset of the next period of bleeding; mean cycle length is 28 days with a range of 21 to 45 days
C. During each cycle several follicles begin the maturation process, but usually only one reaches full maturity and expels its contained ovum into the abdominal cavity and then to a fallopian tube
D. The menstrual cycle may be divided into phases of ovarian and/or endometrial activity that are correlated with concentration fluctuations in hypothalamic, hypophyseal, and ovarian hormones

1. First phase (menstrual or ischemic stage): characterized by shedding of the spongiosum endometrium with the discharge exiting through the vagina; the prostaglandin content of the endometrium reaches its highest levels at this time; the vasoconstriction and myometrial contractions associated with menstrual events are believed mediated by prostaglandins; estrogen and progesterone levels are relatively low, which stimulates the release of follicle-stimulating hormone (FSH). Combined with a steady low level of luteinizing hormone (LH) secretion, ovarian estrogen secretion begins.
2. Second phase (follicular [ovary] or proliferative [endometrium]): endometrium regenerates and thickens in preparation for possible implantation. At the same time, a single dominant follicle develops from a cohort of maturing follicles, and approaches full maturation under the influence of estradiol (the principal estrogenic hormone), which is being produced by the ovarian follicles. Rising blood levels of estradiol exert negative feedback on FSH secretion and positive feedback on LH secretion. Estradiol's feedback effects are exerted on the hypothalamic secretion of FSH-releasing hormone and LH-releasing hormone, which control the hypophyseal secretion of FSH and LH. As a result of a surge in the LH level, ovulation occurs. Ovulation usually takes place 14 days before menstruation. The ovum remains viable for 24 to 36 hours.
3. Third phase (luteal [ovary] and secretory [endometrium]): begins after ovulation and is a relatively finite time period of about 12 to 14 days. Under continuing LH secretion, a temporary endocrine gland is formed (corpus luteum) from the ruptured follicle. Granulosa and thecal cells of the follicle enlarge, divide into and occupy the cavity of the follicle and secrete progesterone and estrogen; progesterone stimulates the already proliferated endometrium to become glandular with a high glycogen-secreting potential (prepared for implantation); if fertilization does not occur, the corpus luteum becomes nonfunctional 10 to 12 days after ovulation; progesterone and estrogen blood levels drop, the negative feedback effect of estrogen on FSH ceases, and the first phase begins again.
E. Clinical applications
   1. Synthetic preparations of estrogen-like and/or progesterone-like compounds are contained in oral and parenteral contraceptive agents
   2. These agents prevent pregnancy by inhibiting gonadotropin (FSH and LH) secretion by affecting both pituitary and hypothalamic cen-

ters. The progestational agent primarily suppresses LH secretion whereas the estrogenic agent suppresses FSH secretion

3. Premenstrual syndrome may occur from ovulation to menstruation; symptoms include bloating, breast tenderness, constipation/diarrhea, acne, moodiness, fatigue, insomnia, backache, cramping
   a. Dietary modifications include reduction of salt and refined carbohydrates, reduction of alcohol and caffeine
   b. Stress management, exercise, and rest
   c. Nonsteroidal inflammatory inhibiting agents (because of their antiprostaglandin action) have proven effective in relieving abdominal cramping associated with the ischemic or menstrual phase of the cycle; diuretics, progesterone, oral contraceptives may also be used

CLIMACTERIC

A. The period in a woman's life when there is gradual cessation of ovarian function and menstrual cycles is known as the climacteric
B. The cessation of the menstrual period for 12 months is known as the menopause
C. Menopause may occur between 40 and 60 years of age with an average age of 51
D. Physiologic changes
   1. Ovaries lose their ability to respond to gonadotropic hormones
   2. Dramatic decrease in levels of circulating estradiol and progesterone because ovaries have ceased functioning
   3. Increased FSH gonadotropin level in the blood, since production is no longer inhibited by the ovaries; false-positive pregnancy test may occur
E. Clinical applications
   1. The woman needs to understand changes and have an opportunity to discuss feelings
   2. Atrophic changes in reproductive organs or hormonal stimulation of the sympathetic nervous system may result in dyspareunia, weight gain, facial hair growth, cardiac palpitations, hot flashes, profuse diaphoresis, constipation, pruritus, faintness, headache; long-range problems may include osteoporosis and cardiovascular disease
   3. Emotional/behavioral responses may include irritability and anxiety about loss of reproductive function, sexual feelings, and feelings of womanliness
   4. Hormonal replacement therapy (HRT) may be used to ease transition through climacteric (control vasomotor instability, reduce atrophic genitourinary changes), reduce the risk of cardiovascular disease, and prevent osteoporosis; used judiciously because of cancer-causing potential
   5. Herbal therapy, diet management, and relaxation modalities are useful in easing the transition

PREGNANCY CYCLE

▼ PRENATAL PERIOD

Development of the Embryo
A. Formation of gametes
   1. The ovum and spermatozoon each have one set of 23 chromosomes; this is in contrast to other cells of the body, which have two sets, or 46 chromosomes (23 pairs)
   2. The production of ova and spermatozoa requires a special type of nuclear division (meiosis) in which the chromosome number is reduced from two sets (46 chromosomes) to one set (23 chromosomes)
B. Chromosomes
   1. Humans have 23 pairs of homologous chromosomes
   2. In males the sex chromosomes (the X and Y) are not equal in size
   3. Homologous chromosomes carry sets of matching genes (alleles); one may be dominant and the other recessive, or they may have blending expressions
C. Sex determination in humans
   1. Genetic females have two sets of autosomes (nonsex chromosomes) and two X chromosomes, whereas genetic males have two sets of autosomes and one X chromosome and one Y chromosome
   2. All ova produced by females have one set of autosomes and one X chromosome; spermatozoa produced by a male have a set of autosomes and either an X or a Y chromosome
   3. If an X-bearing spermatozoon fertilizes an ovum, a female will result; if a Y-bearing spermatozoon fertilizes an ovum, a male will result
D. Genes
   1. Sex-linked genes: genes carried on the X chromosome are called sex-linked genes and are always expressed in the male, even though they may be recessive; examples of such genes cause hemophilia and colorblindness
   2. Multiple genes: many different genes may combine to produce cumulative effects, such as the degree of pigmentation or height

3. Multiple alleles: an example of human traits controlled by multiple alleles are the genes controlling blood types; the genes for type O are dominated by the genes for type A or type B; the genes for A and B are both expressed

Genes	Blood type
OO	O
AO	A
AA	A
BO	B
BB	B
AB	AB

4. Following are some other obvious human traits controlled by genes:

Dominant	Recessive
Brown eyes	Blue eyes
Normal blood clotting	Hemophilia (sex-linked)
Normal color vision	Colorblind (sex-linked)
Normal pigmentation	Albinism
Rh positive (multiple alleles)	Rh negative
Normal red blood cell development	Sickle cell trait

E. Chromosomal alterations
   1. In rare cases additional sex chromosomes may appear and produce abnormal individuals
      a. X chromosome and no Y chromosome: Turner's syndrome
      b. Two or more X chromosomes and a Y chromosome: Klinefelter's syndrome
   2. Translocation of chromosome: a cytogenetic abnormality such as trisomy 21 (Down syndrome)
   3. Mutations
      a. Changes in DNA are mutations; there may also be chromosomal changes
      b. The frequency of mutations may be increased by certain agents such as ultraviolet radiation, x-rays, radioactive radiation, and chemical substances
F. Fertilization
   1. Spermatozoa are deposited in the vagina
   2. Fertilization usually occurs in the fallopian tube when the ovum is about one third of the way down the tube; usually this is about 24 hours after ovulation
   3. Sperm must be in the genital tract 4 to 6 hours before they are able to fertilize an ovum; during this period the enzyme hyaluronidase is activated; this enzyme is able to dissolve the cement substance (hyaluronic acid), which holds together the cells that surround the ovum
   4. Male nucleus enters the cytoplasm of the ovum and several events follow

a. Fertilization membrane forms around the ovum to prevent the entrance of other sperm
b. Sperm tail is lost and the male nucleus (male pronucleus) moves toward the female nucleus (female pronucleus)
5. Fertilization proper occurs when the male pronucleus unites with the female pronucleus, restoring the chromosome number to two sets (46 chromosomes)
G. Cleavage
   1. In a short time after fertilization, the zygote undergoes rapid mitotic division to produce a mass of cells (morula) that descends in the fallopian tube
   2. As it descends, it also divides to form a hollow ball called the blastocyst
H. Implantation
   1. The blastocyst implants in the uterine wall
      a. The blastocyst is differentiated into an inner cell mass, a blastocoele (internal cavity)
      b. An outer covering of cells, the trophectoderm, becomes the trophoderm and will form the fetal portion of the placenta, the vehicle for exchange of nutrients, gases, and wastes
      c. Implantation occurs 7 to 8 days after fertilization, generally in the upper fundal portion of the uterus
      d. Increased maternal hormonal action is necessary to sustain implantation of the embryo
   2. Placenta and umbilical cord development
      a. Placenta
         (1) Organ of dual origin (maternal and embryonic portions) serving as the site for interchange of food, gases, and wastes between mother and embryo (or fetus) during pregnancy
         (2) Formed from villous portion of chorion (chorion frondosum) and the portion of uterine endometrium (called the decidua during pregnancy) directly underlying the implanted embryo (decidua basalis); chorionic villi project into placental sinuses (in decidua basalis) filled with maternal blood
         (3) Functions as the fetal digestive tract and also as fetal lungs, kidneys, and as a major endocrine gland (producing estrogens, progesterone, adrenocorticotropic hormone [ACTH], growth hormone, and the gonadotropic hormones, human chorionic gonadotropin [hCG] and human placental lactogen [hPL])
         (4) Serves as a protective barrier against harmful effects of some drugs and microorganisms
      b. Umbilical cord

(1) Inserted close to central portion of placenta and attached to fetus

(2) Cord has one vein (which transports nourishment) and two arteries (which transport wastes) between the mother and infant

(3) Wharton's jelly, a protective covering, surrounds the entire cord

I. Embryonic period

1. First 2 months conceptus is termed embryo; after this period called a fetus

2. The inner cell mass differentiates into germ layers

   a. Ectoderm: outer layer of skin and mouth cavity and nervous tissue

   b. Mesoderm: connective tissue, including blood and muscle tissue; cardiovascular system and major organs

   c. Endoderm: linings of the alimentary tract, respiratory system, and several glands

3. About 12 days after fertilization, a fetal membrane, the amnion, forms around the embryo; another membrane, the yolk sac, develops beneath the embryo

   a. Amnion is fluid filled (amniotic fluid)

   b. Yolk sac serves as an initial embryonic source of erythrocytes

4. Later an allantois develops that will supply the placental blood vessels

5. A chorion surrounds the embryo; this will eventually form the major part of the placenta; fingerlike projections of the chorion, called chorionic villi, grow into the decidua (endometrium); chorionic villi project into placental blood sinuses; the combination of chorionic villi, placental blood sinuses, and placental blood constitutes the placenta

6. Embryonic development–differentiation of cells occurs

   a. At 14 days: heart begins to beat; brain, early spinal cord, and muscle segments present

   b. At 26 days: tiny buds for arms appear

   c. At 28 days: tiny buds for legs appear

   d. At 30 days: embryo $^1/_4$ to $^1/_2$ inch (0.6 to 1.2 cm) in length, definite form, beginning of umbilical cord is visible

   e. At 31 days: arm buds develop into hands, arms, and shoulders

   f. At 33 days: finger outlines present

   g. At 46 to 48 days: cartilage in upper arms replaced by first bone cells, amniotic fluid surrounds the embryo (amniotic fluid is a protective cushion, equalizes pressures, maintains temperature, and facilitates the infant's movements for adequate growth and development)

   h. The first 8 weeks, known as the period of organogenesis, is a time of rapid growth and development. Any interference with maternal physiology may cause irreparable damage; no drugs should be taken during the first trimester unless absolutely necessary

J. Fetal development

1. Genitalia well differentiated

2. By 12 weeks: fetus moves body parts, swallows, practices inhaling and exhaling, weighs 28 g (1 oz); fetal heart audible with Doptone; rapid rate of 120 to 160 beats per minute

3. At 16 to 20 weeks: fetal movements felt by mother (known as quickening), weighs 170 g (6 oz), is 20 to 25 cm (8 to 10 inches) in length; 200 ml of amniotic fluid present; amniocentesis is possible by 14 to 16 weeks; vernix and lanugo cover and protect the fetus

4. At 20 to 24 weeks: hair growth on head, eyelashes and brow, skeleton hardens, eyelids closed, weighs 0.45 kg (1 lb), is 30.5 cm (12 inches) in length, fetal heart audible with fetoscope; respiratory movements become more regular

5. At 24 to 28 weeks eyelids open, amniotic fluid increases to 1 quart with a daily exchange of 6 gallons, weighs 0.5 kg ($1^1/_4$ lb); alveolar cells of lungs produce pulmonary surfactants that minimize surface tension

6. At 28 to 32 weeks: many fat deposits, weighs 0.5 to 0.7 kg (1 to $1^1/_2$ lb)

7. At 32 to 36 weeks: stores protein for extrauterine life, gains 1.8 kg (4 lb)

8. Fetal circulation: contains mixed blood with less than maximal O_2 concentration; the only exception is in the umbilical vein upon its immediate entrance into liver

   a. Foramen ovale is an opening between the right and left atria during fetal life, bypassing fetal lungs

   b. Ductus arteriosus is a connection between pulmonary trunk and aorta, also bypassing fetal lungs

   c. Ductus venosus is a connection between umbilical vein and ascending vena cava, bypassing fetal liver

Physical and Physiologic Changes in Mother During Pregnancy

Pregnancy is a normal physiologic process that affects all body systems and results in both objective and subjective changes; it is a stressful time requiring many adaptations and may lead to minor discomforts

A. Endocrine

1. During pregnancy the chorion of the placenta secretes a hormone, hCG, that maintains the

corpus luteum; the continuation of progesterone and estrogen secretion from the corpus luteum maintains the pregnancy during the early weeks of development; presence of hCG hormone is an indicator of pregnancy; hCG, which plays a role in morning sickness, reaches a peak in the third month and then drops; high hCG levels are found in the presence of a hydatidiform mole

2. Estrogen and progesterone increase and continue to be secreted from the placenta during the last 6 months of pregnancy; progesterone acts to inhibit uterine contractions, which might occur as the result of the uterus stretching as the fetus grows; increase in these hormones leads to sodium and water retention and muscle relaxation, which leads to fatigue

3. Thyroid activity is increased; normal pregnancy may mimic a mild hyperthyroid state

4. Parathyroid glands and the production of their hormone increase during pregnancy

5. Human placental lactogen (hPL), sometimes called human chorionic somatomammotropin (hCS), is increased. It is a diabetogenic hormone (diminished insulin efficiency) that decreases maternal use of glucose, leaving it available for fetal use; it also affects lipid and protein metabolism

6. Estriol levels increased; sometimes used as indicator of fetal well-being

7. The posterior pituitary secretion of oxytocin, which stimulates uterine contractions, coupled with the drop in progesterone and the increase in estrogen and prostaglandins, brings about labor; uterine contractions increase in frequency and intensity, culminating in fetal expulsion (birth); following birth oxytocin contracts the uterus and stimulates the milk ejection reflex

8. The pancreas increases the production of insulin early in pregnancy; in addition, the mother's body becomes increasingly sensitive to insulin during the first half of pregnancy

B. Reproductive
1. Amenorrhea occurs because the corpus luteum persists, and ovulation is inhibited by the high levels of circulating estrogen and progesterone; low circulating levels of these hormones stimulate ovulation

2. Breast changes such as fullness, tingling, soreness, and darkening of the areolae and nipples occur along with an increase in hormonal levels

3. Leukorrhea is increased as hormonal levels rise, and the increased acidity is a protection from bacterial invasion

4. Changes in the uterus are circulatory, hormonal, and related to fetal growth

a. Softening of the cervix: Goodell's sign
b. Softening of the lower uterine segment: Hegar's sign
c. Purplish hue to the cervix and vaginal mucosa: Chadwick's sign
d. Uterus enlarges in size
e. Changes in position of the uterus: first trimester uterus is in pelvic cavity, second and third trimester uterus is in abdominal cavity

C. Gastrointestinal
1. Reduction in gastric motility and relaxation of esophageal sphincter result from hormonal changes causing nausea and vomiting (morning sickness) and pyrosis (heartburn)

2. Elevated estrogen levels cause excessive salivation (ptyalism)

3. Hyperemia and softening of gums with accompanying hyperacidity of oral secretions result in nonspecific gingivitis; increased vitamin C intake and regular oral hygiene are indicated

4. Decreased emptying time of gallbladder may precipitate gallstones

5. Food cravings may occur; only significant if substance craved is unusual (pica); for example, clay, starch, dirt

6. Heartburn (pyrosis) occurs because of delayed emptying time of stomach and reflux of gastric acid contents into esophagus; gastric irritants such as coffee, tea, and chocolate should be avoided; sodium antacids should be avoided

7. Hiatal hernia is a complication that may occur in older or obese women or in those with multiple fetuses

8. Constipation is caused by hypoperistalsis, lack of fluids, poor dietary habits, pressure of the enlarged uterus on internal organs, effects of progesterone on muscle, and hemorrhoids

D. Excretory
1. Weight of uterus on bladder in early and late pregnancy causes urinary frequency

2. Bladder tone is reduced by effects of hormones on smooth muscle

3. Asymptomatic bacteriuria can occur and must be treated aggressively; if ascending infections occur they can cause premature labor

4. Bladder capacity up to 1500 ml in second trimester

5. Increased urinary output results in lowered specific gravity

6. Increased excretion of sugar caused by lowered renal threshold

7. Pressure of enlarging uterus causes dilation of right ureter and kidney

8. Compensatory increase in the excretion of bicarbonate, which may counteract respiratory alkalosis resulting from hyperventilation at term

E. Circulatory
   1. Physiologic anemia occurs as a result of hemo-dilution of the blood; there is a 45% to 50% increase in blood volume expansion, which is about 75% plasma and 25% red blood cells (RBCs); the imbalance between the plasma and RBCs leads to a reduced hematocrit. Blood volume is increased to meet the needs of the mother and developing fetus
   2. Cardiac output increases 30% to 50%, peaking at 28 to 32 weeks
   3. Heart rate increases 10 to 15 beats per minute in the latter half of pregnancy
   4. Palpitations occur in early months from sympathetic nervous stimulation and in later months from increased thoracic pressure because of enlarged uterus
   5. Blood pressure may drop slightly in second trimester; note maternal position when recording
   6. Supine hypotension syndrome (vena caval syndrome): in supine position weight of enlarged uterus obstructs vena cava, which decreases blood return to heart; decreased cardiac output ensues with hypotension, lightheadedness, faintness, and palpitations
   7. White blood cells, fibrinogen, and other clotting factors increase; WBC from 5000 to 12,000
   8. Varicose veins of legs, vulva, and perianal area may occur
   9. Edema of extremities common in the last 6 weeks of pregnancy because of stasis of blood
   10. If thrombophlebitis occurs heparin may be administered because it does not cross the placental barrier
F. Respiratory
   1. During the third trimester, pressure of the enlarged uterus on the diaphragm and lungs may cause dyspnea that subsides when lightening occurs at about 38 weeks
   2. Oxygen consumption is increased by about 15% between the 16th and 40th weeks, although there may be only a slight increase in vital capacity during pregnancy; tidal volume increases because of an expansion of thoracic cavity up to 40%
   3. Hyperventilation occurs because of mother's need to blow off increased CO_2 transferred to her from fetus
   4. Nasal congestion and epistaxis occurs as a response to increased estrogen levels
G. Integumentary
   1. Excretion of wastes through the skin causes diaphoresis
   2. Skin changes: darkening of the areolae, darkening patches on the face (melasma, formerly chloasma), linea alba becomes nigra on the abdomen, related to increased melanin; striae on the abdomen and legs caused by skin stretching as pregnancy advances; erythematous changes on the palms and face in some women
H. Skeletal
   1. Softening of all ligaments and joints, especially symphysis and sacroiliac joint, caused by increased hormonal action of estrogens and relaxin
   2. Leg cramps may occur from an imbalance of calcium (hypocalcemia) in the body and from pressure of the gravid uterus on nerves supplying lower extremities
I. Emotional
   1. Ambivalence about pregnancy and parenting
   2. Acceptance of biologic fact of pregnancy; usually occurs during first trimester
   3. Acceptance of growing fetus as distinct from self; usually occurs during second trimester
   4. Preparation for birth; usually occurs during third trimester
   5. Mood swings
   6. Increase or decrease in sexual desire
   7. Anxiety related to birth and adult responsibilities
J. Affirmation and confirmation of pregnancy
   1. Presumptive signs: mostly subjective; may be indicative of other illnesses: amenorrhea; fatigue; nausea and vomiting; breast changes; urinary frequency; darkening of pigmentation on face, breasts, and abdomen; quickening (feeling of movement about 15 to 20 weeks)
   2. Probable signs: objective but still not definite confirmations of pregnancy
      a. Uterine changes: Chadwick's sign, Hegar's sign, Goodell's sign, enlargement of the uterus
      b. Fetal outline; ballottement
      c. Pregnancy tests: urine and blood of woman tested to detect hCG (human chorionic gonadotropin)
      d. Braxton Hicks contractions
   3. Positive signs: confirm pregnancy
      a. Fetal heart beat
      b. Fetal outline and movement as felt by examiner
      c. Ultrasonography revealing movement of fetal heart
      d. Roentgenography of fetal skeleton (rarely used because x-ray may be damaging to fetus)
   4. Early determination of more than one fetus is vital; multiple gestation contributes to perinatal mortality
   5. Estimating date of birth (EDB) and duration of pregnancy

a. Nägele's rule: count back 3 months from first day of last menstrual period and add 7 days (9 calendar months, 270 days or 10 lunar months, 280 days) and 1 year

b. Fundal height: measurement from symphysis pubis to top of fundus; the fundus rises about 1 cm per week; at 20 weeks it should be at the umbilicus and at 36 weeks at the xiphoid process

c. Ultrasonography: establishes fetal age from head measurements (term pregnancy: biparietal diameter is 9.8 cm or more); early in pregnancy, done when woman has full bladder (women instructed to drink before test)

K. Nutritional needs during pregnancy

1. Consideration of preconceptional nutritional status; obesity or underweight; age and parity of mother; biologic interactions between mother, fetus, and placenta; and individual needs, such as in times of stress

2. Weight gain should be evaluated with regard to quality of gain; most of weight gain is related to size of fetus

3. Severe caloric restriction during pregnancy is contraindicated because it is a potential hazard to the mother and fetus, especially during organogenesis

4. Weight reduction should never be started as a regimen during pregnancy

5. Restriction of sodium and administration of diuretics are potentially dangerous to mother and fetus during pregnancy; they may limit interstitial fluid reserve, which may be needed if the blood volume decreases

6. Nausea and vomiting: limited fluids with meals, small frequent feedings, restricted fat, high carbohydrate; protein snacks at bedtime

7. Constipation: increased fluids and residue or fiber; appropriate activity level

8. Consideration of demands of pregnancy related to growth and development of fetus during various trimesters; provide adequate nutrition to meet increased maternal and fetal nutrient demands

a. Increased calories to meet increased basal metabolic needs (300 additional calories during 2nd and 3rd trimesters), spare protein for growth, and promote weight gain to support pregnancy

b. Average weight gain should be 14.4 to 16 kg, or 25 to 35 lbs, but is individual according to needs; underweight women should gain more, overweight women should gain less, about 15 to 25 lbs; women carrying more than one fetus should gain more than the recommended weight

c. Increased protein to provide for growth demands

d. Increased vitamins, especially folic acid to prevent anemia and neural tube defects

e. Increased minerals with supplement of iron to prevent anemia

f. Iodized salt to provide needed sodium and iodine

g. Increased calcium from milk and cheese to prevent hypocalcemia

9. Dietary assessment and counseling should be an integral part of prenatal care for every pregnant woman; assess for adequate weight gain, about 4 lbs every month after an initial 3- to 4-lb gain in first trimester

10. Dietary assessment should consider cultural, economic, and psychologic needs

11. Food intake should be based on a balanced diet

a. Additional calories, protein, and fluids during pregnancy

b. Daily minimum food intake during pregnancy should include 4 dairy products, which provide calcium, protein, vitamins A and D, and riboflavin; 3 (2 oz) servings of protein foods; 6 or more servings of bread and cereal; 5 servings of fruits or vegetables containing vitamin C; 1 serving of leafy, dark-green or deep-yellow vegetables; 1 serving of yellow fruit or vegetables; and 2 servings of other vegetables or fruits

c. Minerals such as iron, calcium, phosphorus, iodine, zinc, and sodium are needed in the diet

d. At least 6 to 8 glasses of fluid per day

12. Adolescent nutritional needs

a. Weight gain for normal pregnancy and expected weight gain for maternal growth are added together

b. Iron needs higher to support enlarging muscle mass and increasing blood volume

c. Calcium intake increased by 400 mg— requires a 1- to 2-g calcium diet

L. Health monitoring during pregnancy

1. History, including medical, surgical, gynecologic, and obstetric data; family history of hereditary and transmittable diseases such as diabetes, tuberculosis, heart disease

2. Physical examination of the skin, thyroid, teeth, lungs, heart, and breasts; abdominal palpation; auscultation; height of fundus; vaginal examination; and pelvic evaluation (before last 4 weeks of pregnancy)

3. Cervical smears for gonorrhea and chlamydia; Papanicolaou test for cancer; wet prep for bacterial vaginosis since this is linked to preterm labor

4. Blood pressure; weight; and urinalysis for acetone, albumin, and glucose done at all visits
5. Blood specimens taken for typing, crossmatching, Rh factor, hematocrit, hemoglobin, serologic test for syphilis (repeated at 32 weeks), and rubella titer
6. Screening tests
   a. Tine testing for tuberculosis
   b. Tay-Sachs screening, particularly for Jewish women
   c. Sickle cell screening, particularly for black women
   d. Alpha-fetoprotein (AFP) testing for neural tube defects
   e. Serum glucose for gestational diabetes mellitus
   f. Group beta streptococcus culture after 36 weeks
   g. Blood type and count
   h. Screening to determine the presence of cytomegalovirus, hepatitis B, HIV, parvovirus 19, rubella, toxoplasmosis, varicella-zoster virus
   i. Herpes cultures at first visit and at 36 weeks if woman or partner has a history of genital herpes
7. Weight is monitored and compared with prepregnant levels
8. Routine sonogram is scheduled to confirm dates, assess placenta, fetus, and amniotic fluid
9. Amniocentesis for women who are 35 or older to determine chromosomal abnormalities

General Nursing Care During the Prenatal Period

A. ASSESSMENT
1. Initial visit
   a. Date of last menstrual period
   b. Personal, gynecologic, obstetric, and family medical history
   c. Physical examination: including baseline vital signs and weight
   d. Current nutritional status
   e. Pelvic examination: vaginal and rectal
   f. Understanding of pregnancy and related care
   g. Presence of multiple gestation
2. Monthly and final weekly visits
   a. Weight, blood pressure, pulse, respirations; signs of supine hypotension
   b. Signs of facial or digital edema
   c. Fundal height and size
   d. Fetal heart rate and fetal activity
   e. Testing for glucose, albumin, ketones, acetone in urine

B. ANALYSIS/NURSING DIAGNOSES
1. Disturbed body image related to physical changes of pregnancy
2. Decreased cardiac output related to pressure on vena cava by gravid uterus when in supine position
3. Constipation related to slowed peristalsis and pressure from gravid uterus
4. Family coping: potential for growth related to acceptance of pregnancy and fulfillment of parental tasks
5. Risk for fluid volume excess related to increasing demands of pregnancy
6. Imbalanced nutrition: less than body requirements related to increased needs of pregnancy or nausea and vomiting
7. Impaired urinary elimination related to pressure of gravid uterus

C. PLANNING/IMPLEMENTATION
1. Assist the parents in understanding the anatomy and physiology of pregnancy, labor, and birth
2. Teach mother to monitor for:
   a. Visual disturbances; edema of face, fingers, or feet; persistent, severe headaches; seizures
   b. Epigastric pain; persistent, severe vomiting
   c. Signs of infection; burning on urination
   d. Any vaginal discharge, including blood
   e. Abdominal pain
   f. Absence of or decrease in fetal movements after initial presence
   g. Signs and symptoms of premature labor
3. Teach mother about physiologic changes and related discomforts that occur during pregnancy (nausea, vomiting, backaches, varicosities, hemorrhoids, constipation, leg pain, etc.)
4. Respond to mother's questions about bathing, douching, work, sex, exercise, etc.
5. Help parents discuss and explore feelings related to childbearing and rearing
6. Prepare mother for physical work of labor through the use of relaxation and breathing exercises for the various phases of labor
7. Identify parents' situational support systems
8. Prepare the father for a coaching and supporting role during pregnancy, labor, and birth
9. Introduce families to health facilities available for continued health care
10. Teach mother to avoid alcohol, tobacco, contact with second-hand smoke, and certain herbs
11. Discuss various childbirth preparation techniques such as Lamaze, Read, and Bradley
12. Teach the mother to avoid over-the-counter or prescription drugs without checking with her care provider because many drugs considered harmless may be teratogenic to the developing fetus

13. Teach mother the importance of adequate fluid intake and moderate exercise to promote circulation and prevent stasis
14. Teach mother the importance of continuing breast self-examination throughout pregnancy
15. Ask mother about domestic violence and follow up findings to prevent damage to woman and fetus

D. EVALUATION/OUTCOMES

Mother

1. Keeps weight gain within recommended limits
2. Abstains from alcohol, drugs, and tobacco
3. Adjusts to physiologic changes associated with pregnancy
4. Identifies signs of complications
5. Attends childbirth classes with partner

Fetus

1. Survives interuterine period
2. Growth and development within acceptable parameters

▼ INTRAPARTAL PERIOD (PERIOD OF BIRTH)

A. Labor: an involuntary physiologic process whereby the contents of the gravid uterus are expelled through the birth canal into the external environment
B. Anatomy of the bony pelvis
   1. Parts: ischium, ilium, sacrum, coccyx
   2. Joints: sacroiliac, sacrococcygeal, symphysis pubis (all soften during pregnancy)
   3. Divisions: false pelvis supports the enlarged uterus in the abdominal cavity; true pelvis is the bony inner pelvis through which the infant must pass
   4. Diameters: at inlet: true conjugate (anterior/posterior diameter), transverse (widest diameter at inlet), right and left oblique diameters; at outlet: conjugate diagonal (anterior/posterior is widest diameter), transverse (one ischial tuberosity to the other)
   5. Classification of pelvis: gynecoid (normal female pelvis), android (male pelvis), anthropoid, and platypelloid
   6. Normal female pelvis has an ample pubic arch, curved sacrum, curved side walls, blunt ischial spines, and a movable coccyx
C. Attitude: relationship of fetal parts to each other
D. Lie: relationship of the long axis of the fetus to the long axis of the mother
E. Presentation: fetus' body part that engages in the true pelvis
   1. Cephalic (head): vertex, brow, or face
   2. Breech: frank, complete, single, or double footling

3. Shoulder: cannot be delivered vaginally
F. Position: relationship of presenting parts to four quadrants of the mother's pelvis (the letters L and R are used for left or right; A and P for anterior or posterior; O for occiput; M for mentum or face; S for sacrum)
   1. Vertex: occiput, LOA, LOP, ROA, ROP
   2. Face: chin (mentum), LMA, LMP, RMA, RMP
   3. Breech: sacrum, LSA, LSP, RSA, RSP
G. Station: relationship of presenting part to the false and true pelves
   1. Floating: presenting part movable above the true pelvic inlet
   2. Engaged: suboccipitobregmatic diameter fixed into the pelvic inlet
   3. Station O: presenting part at level of the ischial spines: levels below spines +1, +2, +3; levels above spines −1, −2, −3
H. Amniotic fluid: about 1000 ml of fluid enclosed in membranes (amniotic sac) is present at term
   1. Spontaneous rupture of membranes (SROM or SRM): usually occurs in mid or late labor but can occur before labor begins
   2. Artificial rupture of membranes (amniotomy, AROM, or ARM): expedites labor; should not be done until presenting part is at 0 or lower (+1, +2) station
   3. Nitrazine paper: may be used to confirm the presence of amniotic fluid; turns dark blue because of the alkaline nature of the fluid
   4. Assessment of amniotic fluid
      a. Color: normally strawlike and clear; may contain small particles of vernix caseosa; greenish color indicates meconium staining
      b. Odor: normally musky smelling but nonoffensive; foul smelling indicates infection (chorioamnionitis)
      c. Amount: 1 L of fluid at term; excessive amount is called polyhydramnios; scant amount is called oligohydramnios; scant or excessive fluid may be associated with congenital anomalies
I. Clinical findings before labor
   1. Physiologic
      a. Lightening: fetus drops down into the true pelvis
      b. Braxton Hicks contractions: usually painless contractions in preparation for true labor
      c. Increased vaginal secretions
      d. Softening of cervix (ripening)
      e. Spontaneous rupture of membranes (SROM) may occur
      f. Bloody show; softening and effacement of cervix causes mucous plug to be expelled; this is accompanied by small blood loss

2. Psychologic: mother shows signs of nesting (increased activity) caused by sudden rise in energy level

J. Clinical findings of true labor
1. Uterine contractions that increase in frequency, strength, and duration and do not disappear when lying down or walking around
2. Effacement (shortening or thinning of the cervix) and dilation of the cervix

K. Mechanisms of labor: rotation and descent of vertex presentation through true pelvis
1. Engagement, descent with flexion: at onset of labor, head descends and chin flexes on the chest
2. Internal rotation: as labor contractions and uterine forces move the fetus downward, the head internally rotates to pass through the ischial spines
3. Extension: occiput emerges under the symphysis pubis and the head is delivered by extension
4. External rotation: allows for rotation of shoulders to an anterior/posterior position
5. Expulsion: rest of infant is delivered

L. Stages of labor and maternal changes
1. First stage: from onset of true labor to complete effacement and dilation of cervix
   a. Latent phase: mild, short contractions, cervix dilated 0 to 3 cm; mother excited and happy that labor has started, some apprehension; follows directions readily; walking assists labor process
   b. Active phase: moderate to strong contractions 5 minutes apart, cervix dilates from 4 to 7 cm, bloody show, membranes may rupture; slow, deep breathing techniques help in relaxing; medication may be necessary for discomfort; supportive measures help (e.g., encouragement, praise, reassurance, back pressure or back rubs, keeping the mother informed of progress, providing rest between contractions, presence of a supporting person); has difficulty in following directions
   c. Transition phase: strong contractions 1 to 2 minutes apart (lasting 45 to 60 seconds or more with little rest in between); cervix dilates from 7 to 10 cm with a bloody show; mother becomes irritable, restless, agitated, highly emotional, belches, has leg tremors, perspires, pale white ring around mouth (circumoral pallor), flushed face, sudden nausea, and vomiting; feels need to have a bowel movement because of pressure on anus; unable to communicate or follow directions

2. Second stage: beginning with full dilation of the cervix and ending with birth of the infant; perineum bulges, pushing with contractions, grunting sounds, behavior changes from great irritability to great involvement and work, sleep and relaxation occur between contractions, leg cramps are common

3. Third stage: following birth of the infant through expulsion of the placenta; placental separation (5 to 30 minutes) after birth heralded by globular formation of uterus, lengthening of umbilical cord, and gush of blood; may have alteration in perineal structure either from episiotomy (prophylactic incision into perineum to allow for birth of head) or laceration from rapid expulsion of presenting part

4. Fourth stage: following expulsion of placenta to 1 to 2 hours after birth; fundus firm in the midline and at or slightly above the umbilicus; moderate, bloody vaginal discharge (lochia rubra); fatigue, thirst, chills, nausea; excitement and intermittent dozing

M. Oxytocics
1. Description
   a. Drugs that stimulate the uterus to contract
   b. Used in the pregnant female to initiate labor; given slowly and in small doses during labor
   c. Used to augment contractions that have already begun
   d. Capable of inducing contraction of the lacteal glands, which aids in let-down reflex for nursing
   e. Exert vasopressor and antidiuretic effects
   f. Used to control postpartum uterine atony; may be given rapidly
   g. Oxytocics are available in parenteral (IM, IV), oral, and nasal preparations

2. Example: oxytocin (Pitocin, Syntocinon)

3. Major side effects
   a. Maternal
      (1) Hypertension (contracture of smooth muscles of blood vessels)
      (2) Dysrhythmias; tachycardia (vasoconstriction)
      (3) Hypertonic uterus; uterine rupture
      (4) Water intoxication (antidiuretic effect)
      (5) Seizures and coma (water intoxication)
   b. Fetal
      (1) Anoxia; asphyxia (vasoconstriction)
      (2) Dysrhythmias (premature ventricular beats [PVBs], bradycardia)
      (3) Hyperbilirubinemia (hepatic dysfunction)

4. Nursing care of clients receiving oxytocics
   a. Monitor client continuously
   b. Have O_2 and emergency resuscitative equipment available

c. Use infusion-control device for IV administration; always given by secondary line
d. Monitor uterine contractions; discontinue infusion if prolonged uterine contractions occur
e. Assess blood pressure and pulse every 15 minutes
f. Maintain fetal monitoring

N. Maternal analgesia and anesthesia
  1. Analgesia
    a. Meperidine hydrochloride (Demerol) IV, IM, epidural, or intrathecal during active labor; administration timed to allow metabolism and excretion of drug before birth to avoid respiratory depression in the newborn; Naloxone (Narcan) used to counteract this respiratory depression
    b. Butorphanol (Stadol) IM; 30 to 40 times more potent than meperidine; does not interfere with labor; less neonatal depression
    c. Nalbuphine (Nubain) IV or IM
    d. Fentanyl (Sublimaze) IV, IM, epidural, or intrathecal; 100 times more potent than meperidine; minimal respiratory depression in the newborn
  2. Regional analgesia and anesthesia
    a. Epidural: may be used during labor, for anesthesia during a cesarean birth, and postcesarean anesthesia when abdomen is being closed
    b. Spinal: may be used during labor or for anesthesia during a cesarean birth; placed in the subarachnoid space; given in a single dose; may wear off before procedure is complete
    c. Pudendal: may be used during the second stage of labor
    d. Local infiltration: most frequently used to repair episiotomy
  3. Nursing care of clients receiving anesthetic/analgesic agents
    a. Observe mother and newborn for respiratory depression if narcotic analgesic is given; monitor mother for hypotension
    b. After epidural: monitor for maternal hypotension; if hypotension occurs, position client on left side, increase IV infusion, and administer oxygen

General Nursing Care During the Intrapartal Period

A. ASSESSMENT (ON ADMISSION)
  1. Age, weight, height, vital signs, allergies
  2. Obstetric history; expected date of birth; intent to breastfeed or bottlefeed; prenatal care
  3. Time and type of last meal
  4. Time of onset of contractions and their frequency, duration, and intensity
  5. Presence of bloody show; status of amniotic membrane
  6. Fetal heart rate and pattern
  7. Leopold's maneuvers to determine fetal presentation, position, and station
  8. Factors that influence labor (the four Ps)
    a. Power—contraction's expulsive effect
    b. Passenger—the newborn's size, position, and presentation
    c. Passage—the maternal pelvis
    d. Psyche—the emotional energy and anxiety level of the mother
  9. Emotional response to labor; presence of support persons

B. ANALYSIS/NURSING DIAGNOSES
Mother
  1. Risk for ineffective tissue perfusion related to weight of uterus on vena cava
  2. Ineffective coping related to exhaustion and unfamiliarity with the labor process
  3. Risk for injury related to lack of control, position during birth, and anesthesia
  4. Pain related to labor process and perineal trauma
  5. Situational low self-esteem related to inability to live up to behavioral expectations of self or others
  6. Impaired urinary elimination related to pressure of enlarged uterus, use of oxytocics, analgesia or anesthesia, and trauma of labor and birth

Newborn
  1. Risk for altered tissue perfusion related to maternal position, patterns of uterine contractions, or cord compression
  2. Ineffective airway clearance related to excessive mucus, aspiration of meconium, or inability to clear airway
  3. Risk for injury related to trauma of birth or maternal infection
  4. Ineffective thermoregulation related to immature heat regulation, inability to shiver, and lack of brown fat

C. PLANNING/IMPLEMENTATION
First stage
  1. Orient to unit
  2. Time and assess contractions
  3. Assist with or perform vaginal examination
  4. Test urine for protein, glucose, and ketones
  5. Assess bladder and bowel function
  6. Collect blood for complete blood count (CBC) and crossmatch
  7. Provide emotional support to mother and labor coach

8. Monitor frequency, duration, and strength of contractions
   a. Interpret data on maternal uterine monitor
   b. Observe for prolonged contractions if oxytocin is being administered
9. Monitor fetal heart rate (FHR) by Doppler or internal or external fetal monitor
10. Interpret data of fetal monitoring
    a. Baseline FHR: FHR between uterine contractions is usually 120 to 160 beats per minute
    b. Tachycardia: FHR above 160 beats per minute lasting over 10 minutes
       (1) May result from maternal fever or dehydration and drugs such as atropine, Vistaril, ritodrine, terbutaline
       (2) Reduce underlying cause: lower maternal fever; increase maternal fluids; monitor for amnionitis
    c. Accelerations: transient tachycardia may occur with fetal activity
    d. Bradycardia: FHR below 110 beats per minute lasting longer than 10 minutes
       (1) May be caused by fetal hypoxia as a result of anesthetics, maternal hypotension, prolonged umbilical cord compression, or analgesics
       (2) Reduce underlying cause (reposition mother on side, assess for prolapsed cord, position mother to relieve pressure on cord, elevate mother's lower extremities, administer oxygen)
    e. Variability: normal irregularity of cardiac rhythm (balance between sympathetic and parasympathetic divisions of autonomic nervous system); manifested by cyclic fluctuations and beat-to-beat changes of FHR; absence of these fluctuations is indicative of fetal central nervous system depression; associated with narcotics and barbiturates, and with fetal hypoxia, acidosis, and immaturity; reduce underlying cause (administer oxygen, reposition mother on side)
    f. Early decelerations: FHR decreases, but usually not below 100 beats per minute
       (1) Occur early in contraction phase, before peak, and end before uterus returns to resting tone
       (2) Indicates head compression; no nursing intervention needed
    g. Late decelerations: FHR decreases below 100 beats per minute but, if severe, may decrease to 60 beats per minute
       (1) Occur as contraction peaks; lowest rate after peak; has long recovery time; FHR may not return to baseline until well after contraction ends
       (2) May be accompanied by bradycardia or tachycardia; often associated with loss of variability and is ominous if persistent or related to decreased variability
       (3) Indicates uteroplacental insufficiency caused by uterine tetany from oxytocin administration; postterm pregnancy; maternal supine hypotension; regional anesthesia; hypertensive disorders; diabetes mellitus; or other chronic disorders
       (4) Nursing intervention includes discontinuing oxytocin if being administered, positioning mother on left side, administering oxygen by mask at 8 to 10 L per minute, increasing rate of intravenous fluids, assisting with fetal blood sampling; preparing for birth if there is no improvement
    h. Variable decelerations: abrupt transitory decrease in FHR that is variable in duration, intensity, and time in relation to contractions; FHR may decrease as low as 70 beats per minute for as long as 30 seconds with a relatively rapid return to baseline
       (1) Usually observed late in labor with fetal descent and pushing and is related to umbilical cord compression; occur in about 50% of labors; usually transient, correctable, and is unrelated to low Apgar scores
       (2) Nursing intervention: see Late decelerations and attempt to relieve pressure of descending part on cord if it is prolapsed
11. Prevent supine hypotension by positioning mother on side to keep gravid uterus from compressing vena cava
12. Assist the mother with breathing techniques throughout labor by teaching and encouraging appropriate breathing patterns in varying phases of labor and rebreathing techniques to correct and prevent hyperventilation
13. Use measures to promote comfort and rest by explaining procedures and equipment; providing warmth, administering analgesics or anesthesia; may use opioid analgesics such as butorphanol (Stadol) and nalbuphine (Nubain); epidural or intrathecal narcotic as ordered, except in late phase of labor (less than 2 hours before birth) to prevent fetal depression
    a. Encourage use of relaxation techniques and positions learned in childbirth classes; recognize maternal movements will be restricted with external fetal monitor; support and encourage mother and coach
    b. Carefully monitor vital signs during administration of regional anesthetics

c. Have a narcotic agonist such as Narcan readily available

14. Observe perineum for bloody show and appearance of amniotic fluid (indicates ruptured membranes); note: amount; color (if greenish, check for breech position and obtain fetal heart rate); odor (if foul may indicate amnionitis)

15. FHR following spontaneous rupture of membranes or amniotomy (AROM); assess for presence of prolapsed cord

16. Monitor for:
    a. Prolonged strong contractions; may indicate tetanic uterus
    b. Taut, boardlike abdomen; may indicate abruptio placentae
    c. Increase in pulse and temperature; may indicate infection
    d. Hypertension; may indicate preeclampsia
    e. Hypotension; may occur following epidural or spinal anesthesia
    f. Bright red vaginal bleeding; may indicate placenta previa
    g. Meconium-stained amniotic fluid; may indicate breech position or may be a late sign of fetal distress
    h. Abnormal variations in FHR patterns; may indicate fetal distress

17. Keep mother NPO approaching second stage of labor

Second stage

1. Assist mother with pushing; transfer to delivery room or prepare birthing bed when perineum bulges with contractions

2. Make certain mother's legs are positioned simultaneously to avoid trauma to uterine ligaments

3. Monitor FHR

4. Assist with anesthesia at this time, which could include pudendal block, saddle block, or local infiltration

Third stage

1. Care of infant
    a. Clear airway of mucus
    b. Use Apgar scoring to determine respiratory effort and physical status
    c. Maintain body heat
    d. Assess the newborn for visible anomalies
    e. Place in parent's arms or view to begin bonding process
    f. Administer antibiotic ophthalmic medication into each eye after bonding to prevent ophthalmia neonatorum
    g. Identify the mother and infant before leaving delivery room according to institutional protocol

2. Assist with delivery of placenta

3. Promote attachment

4. Provide support for parents if infant has an abnormality

5. Record birth and accompanying events

Fourth stage

1. Palpate the fundus q 15 minutes for firmness and height in relation to umbilicus; if relaxed and/or dextroverted, check for bladder fullness

2. Check for bladder distention; determine voiding pattern; uterus is unable to contract in the presence of a full bladder; the client may hemorrhage

3. Check the perineum for vaginal and suture line bleeding; count vaginal pads; assess for concurrent uterine relaxation; massage uterus

4. Monitor temperature, BP, and pulse; report fluctuations

5. Administer oxytocic medication as ordered; after birth an oxytocic may be administered immediately to enhance uterine contractions

6. Check episiotomy or laceration site for hematoma, bleeding, or edema; apply icebag to perineum immediately after birth to reduce edema

7. Shivering is common after birth; exact cause unknown; keeping the client warm diminishes the sensation of chilling, which is most likely caused by air-conditioned birthing room

8. Provide fluid and food as tolerated

D. EVALUATION/OUTCOMES

Mother

1. Progresses through labor that culminates in safe delivery

2. Remains free of infection

3. Maintains hemostasis

Newborn

1. Establishes airway, and respiratory effort sustains life without assistance

2. Achieves an Apgar score of 7 or above at 5 minutes after birth

---

▼ POSTPARTAL PERIOD

A. Puerperium: 6-week period following birth in which the reproductive organs undergo physical and physiologic changes, a process called involution; because of the many physiologic and psychologic stresses of the postpartum period, there is a trend to increase this period to 3 months following birth and call it the fourth trimester of pregnancy

B. Systemic changes during the puerperium
   1. Reproductive system
      a. Uterus: intermittent contractions bring about involution, afterpains may cause discomfort, necessitating analgesics; oxy-

tocin release during breastfeeding speeds up involution; involution normally follows a one-fingerbreadth descent daily, by the 7th to 9th day fundus cannot be felt

b. Lochia: vaginal flow following birth changes from rubra to serosa, then becomes alba

c. Vagina practically returns to its prepregnant state through a healing of soft tissue and cicatrization

d. Menstruation occurs about 6 weeks after birth in nonnursing mothers and up to 24 weeks in nursing mothers

e. Abdominal wall soft and flabby but eventually regains tone

f. Breasts

(1) As placenta is delivered, there is activation of luteinizing hormone in the anterior pituitary; secretion of prolactin stimulates milk production

(2) In breastfeeding mothers, the posterior pituitary secretes oxytocin that initiates the let-down reflex with milk ejection as infant suckles

(3) Absence of suckling at breast in nonnursing mothers inhibits oxytocin and prolactin secretion; the let-down reflex does not occur, and milk production is inhibited

(4) Breast engorgement occurs in both nursing and nonnursing mothers on the second or third day because of vasodilation before lactation

2. Digestive system

a. Following birth clients are hungry and thirsty; if general anesthesia was not administered during birth, clients can be given oral nourishment

b. Added proteins and calories to replenish those lost with the process of involution

c. Fiber, fluid, and exercise relieve constipation and distention

d. Bowel movements usually do not occur for a few days, probably because of fear of pain from hemorrhoids and/or episiotomy and decreased food intake during labor; stool softeners may be prescribed and, if unsuccessful, suppositories or an enema may be used

3. Circulatory system

a. Blood volume usually back to normal by the third week after birth

b. Blood fibrinogen levels and platelets increase during the first week; this may lead to thrombus formation

c. Increase in leukocytes; may go as high as 30,000/mm³ if labor was lengthy

d. Drop in hemoglobin and red blood cell count on the fourth postpartal day

4. Excretory system

a. Increased urinary output (diuresis), second to fifth postpartal day

b. Bladder tone altered during pregnancy; retention with overflow may occur

c. Activation of lactogenic hormone may result in lactose in the urine

d. Excretion of nitrogen as involution occurs

5. Integumentary system

a. Profuse diaphoresis as wastes are being excreted

b. Pigmentational changes such as striae, linea nigra, and darkened areolae begin to fade but do not completely return to nulliparous state

6. Vital signs

a. Temperature elevation (not above 100.4° F) up to 24 hours after birth as result of exertion and dehydration

b. Blood pressure returns to baseline; drop suggests hemorrhage; elevation suggests pregnancy-induced hypertension

c. Pulse drops slightly because of decreased cardiac effort; blood volume is decreased

7. Emotional needs

a. Mother may experience "infant blues/ postpartum blues" following "crisis" of birth; may occur on the third day with periods of irritability, restlessness, and anxiety

b. An emotional disorder associated with pregnancy may occur within 6 months with exaggerated signs and symptoms of postpartum blues

General Nursing Care During the Postpartal Period

A. ASSESSMENT

1. Breasts, abdomen, and fundus

2. Perineum: lochia; episiotomy; signs of hematoma; hemorrhoids

3. Vital signs

4. Hydration status; voiding; bowel movements

5. Signs of interaction with or attachment to infant

6. Signs of thrombophlebitis

B. ANALYSIS/NURSING DIAGNOSES

1. Anxiety related to insecurities about parental role and parenting activities

2. Impaired urinary elimination related to effects of anesthesia, use of oxytocics, and edema of perineal area

3. Constipation related to pain on defecation and decreased peristalsis

4. Risk for infection related to inadequate perineal care and perineal trauma

5. Pain related to perineal trauma, perineal edema, breast engorgement, hemorrhoids, or uterine involution
6. Disturbed sleep pattern related to discomfort, parenting activities, and anxiety

C. **PLANNING/IMPLEMENTATION**
1. Use standard precautions and aseptic technique when giving perineal care
2. Teach mother and assist mother with self-care
3. Teach mother breast care; inspect breasts for tissue and nipple breakdown, palpate to rule out growths (teach breast self-examination for continued health), support breasts with well-fitted brassiere
4. Teach the importance of hand washing when caring for self and infant
5. Observe vital signs: a temperature above 100.4° F (38° C) for 2 consecutive days (excluding first 24 hours after birth) considered sign of beginning puerperal infection, which can occur following hemorrhage or trauma; bradycardia is a normal phenomenon following birth
6. Palpate fundus for firmness and descent below the umbilical level; a boggy fundus indicates poor contractile power of uterus and results in bleeding; check for full bladder, which displaces the fundus upward and to the right
7. Administer oxytocic medication as ordered to promote involution
   a. Methylergonovine maleate (Methergine)
   b. Ergonovine maleate (Ergotrate)
   c. Maintains the uterus in a slightly contracted state that controls bleeding from intrauterine sites and maintains tone, rate, and amplitude of rhythmic contractions required for involution; may cause hypertension, especially ergonovine maleate, if uterus is boggy
8. Check lochia for color, amount, clots, odor (foul odor indicates beginning infection); observe episiotomy suture line if present for redness, ecchymosis, edema, discharge, and approximation (REEDA)
9. Assess for pain; afterpains are more common in multiparas; for pain in perineal suture line, apply cold applications for first 24 hours and then sitz baths
10. Promote bladder and bowel function; secure catheterization order if the client is unable to void; profuse diaphoresis should not affect voiding
11. Encourage Kegel exercises to strengthen pubococcygeal muscles
12. Provide or instruct about a diet adequate in proteins and calories to restore body tissues
13. Encourage early ambulation to prevent blood stasis
14. Monitor laboratory reports for hemoglobin (Hgb), hematocrit (Hct), and white blood cell count (WBC)
15. Observe for "postpartal blues," which may be caused by a drop in hormonal levels; if discharged early, mother and support persons should be alerted to signs and symptoms
16. Meet the mother's needs to enable her to meet the infant's needs
17. Assist the mother with care of the infant as needed
18. Provide for group discussion on breastfeeding, infant care, etc.
19. Discuss resumption of intercourse and family planning; include information about when to expect menses
20. If Rh-negative mother, assess need for administration of RhoGAM
21. Give rubella vaccine if indicated
22. Provide instructions to contact personnel when questions arise
23. Involve the family in care and teaching

D. **EVALUATION/OUTCOMES**
1. Progresses through process of involution
2. Remains free from hemorrhage, infection, and pain
3. Maintains bowel function
4. Initiates voiding and empties bladder
5. Performs perineal care after each voiding and defecation, as taught
6. Successfully feeds and cares for infant

VARIATIONS IN PREGNANCY

▼ ADOLESCENT PREGNANCY

A. High-risk pregnancy because:
1. Physical development is not yet completed; bone growth may be incomplete and increased levels of estrogen may close epiphysis
2. PIH is a prevalent complication because of poorly developed vascular system of placenta and possible inadequate adolescent nutrition
3. Developmental tasks of adolescence have not been fulfilled
4. Emotional maturity has not been achieved

B. Factors contributing to the incidence of adolescent pregnancy
1. Inadequate coping mechanisms
2. Need to enhance self-concept
3. Belief in own invulnerability
4. Need for immediate gratification; the present, not the future, is the focus; lack of concern for long-term consequences
5. Immature search for attention, closeness, and/

or idealized or idolized love
6. Lack of knowledge about conception or contraception
7. Sexual acting out; indulgence in risk-taking behavior
8. Increase in dysfunctional families; change in morality and family life

Nursing Care of Pregnant Adolescents
A. ASSESSMENT
1. Personal and family health; menstrual history
2. Developmental level
3. Support system; financial status
4. Potential role of infant's father
5. Understanding of responsibility of pregnancy
B. ANALYSIS/NURSING DIAGNOSES
1. Disturbed body image related to altered appearance
2. Decisional conflict related to immature problem-solving abilities
3. Ineffective health maintenance related to lack of knowledge about the changes and responsibilities associated with pregnancy
4. Imbalanced nutrition: more than or less than body requirements related to food preferences, fast food, or food fads common in the adolescent
5. Risk for impaired parenting related to age, lack of knowledge, lack of support system
C. PLANNING/IMPLEMENTATION
1. Gain trust of adolescent
2. Refer to appropriate agencies and resources
3. Promote problem-solving abilities
4. Involve father, if desired by the mother
5. Provide prenatal education; encourage consistent prenatal care
6. See Pregnancy Cycle
D. EVALUATION/OUTCOMES
1. Arrives at decisions regarding the pregnancy
2. Keeps prenatal appointments and attends child-care classes
3. Involves significant others in planning concerning pregnancy

▼ DELAYED PREGNANCY

A. Occurs in first-time pregnant women over 35 years of age
B. High risk because:
1. Increased chance of chromosomal abnormalities
2. Preexisting medical conditions
3. Increased chance of multiple gestation secondary to fertility drug use
4. Emotional concerns related to changes in role, job, income, and child-care issues
5. Bleeding in the first trimester may be due to spontaneous abortions, or trophoblastic or ectopic pregnancies

Nursing Care of Women Older than 35 Years of Age Who Are Pregnant for the First Time
A. ASSESSMENT
1. Personal and family health
2. Genetic history, counseling, and testing
3. Nutritional status
4. Use of medications and drugs
5. History of fibroids
B. ANALYSIS/NURSING DIAGNOSES
1. Body image disturbance related to altered body appearance
2. Family coping: potential for growth related to readiness and desire to assume parenting roles
C. PLANNING/IMPLEMENTATION
1. Refer for genetic counseling
2. Provide prenatal care with an emphasis on preexisting conditions and immunizations
3. Allow for verbalizations of plans regarding work, changing responsibilities, and altered lifestyle
D. EVALUATION/OUTCOMES
1. Expresses feelings regarding expectations of body changes
2. Uses appropriate agencies for risk assessment
3. Makes appropriate plans for role change during pregnancy and following delivery

▼ MULTIPLE GESTATION

A. Twin births account for 1 in 80 births in the United States; the number is increasing because of higher incidence of fertility drug use
B. Elective fetal reduction is sometimes suggested when the risk of fetal death is great
C. Women with multiple gestation are at high risk for developing preterm labor, pregnancy-induced hypertension, hyperemesis gravidarum, iron or folate anemia
D. Fetuses are at high risk for congenital anomalies and intrauterine growth retardation

Nursing Care of Clients with Multiple Gestation
See Nursing Care Related to High-Risk Conditions under Complications of Labor and Birth

THE NEWBORN

▼ FAMILY AND PRENATAL HISTORY

A. Chronic illness in the mother's or father's family
B. Previous medical-surgical illnesses of the mother and father

C. Age and present health status of the mother and father
D. History of previous pregnancies
E. Prenatal history
   1. Medical supervision during pregnancy
   2. Nutrition during pregnancy
   3. Course of pregnancy: illnesses, medications taken, or treatments required
   4. Duration of gestation
   5. Course and amount of sedation and anesthesia required
   6. Type of birth and significant events during the immediate period after birth
   7. Immediate response of newborn (Apgar score at 1 and 5 minutes following birth)
   8. Presence of maternal infections during pregnancy
   9. History of alcohol or drug use, sexually transmitted diseases, or smoking during pregnancy

▼ PARENT-CHILD RELATIONSHIPS

A. Concepts basic to parent-infant relationships
   1. Early and frequent parent-infant contact is essential for survival (bonding)
   2. Childbearing is a developmental crisis; parenting abilities can be fostered and developed
   3. Biologic changes that occur at puberty and during pregnancy influence the development of nurturance
   4. Interaction between mother and child begins from the moment of conception and can be shared with the father
   5. Love for the infant grows as the parents interact and give care
   6. As the parent gives to the infant and the infant receives, the parent in turn receives satisfaction from parenting tasks
   7. Any disturbance in give-and-take cycle sets up frustrations in parents and infant
   8. Parental behavior is learned and frequent parent-infant contact enhances development of parenting abilities; ambivalence is a natural phenomenon as are feelings of resentment
B. Infant's basic needs
   1. Physiologic—food, clothing, bathing, and protection from environment
   2. Emotional—security, comfort, fondling, caressing, rocking, being spoken to, and contact with one person on a consistent basis
C. Mothering and fathering are:
   1. Based on a biologic inborn desire to reproduce
   2. Role concepts that begin with own childhood experiences

3. Primitive emotional relationships
4. Maturing processes
5. Fostered by the parent-infant interaction that constantly reinforces gratification as needs are met and security develops
6. Abilities that are learned rather than innate
D. Parent-child relationships are affected by:
   1. Readiness for pregnancy
      a. Planned or unplanned
      b. Health status prior to pregnancy
      c. Determinants such as age, cultural backgrounds, number in family unit, financial status
   2. Nature of the pregnancy
      a. Health status during pregnancy
      b. Preparation for parenthood
      c. Support from family members and members of the health care team
   3. Character of the labor and birth
      a. Length and pattern of labor, type of birth
      b. Type and amount of analgesia/anesthesia received
      c. Support from family and health team
   4. Factors that impede bonding
      a. Physical status of newborn or mother
      b. Medical therapies that interfere with bonding
      c. Disturbance of idealized image of infant
E. Significant phases of maternal adjustment
   1. Taking-in phase: mother's needs have to be met before she can meet infant's needs; talks about self rather than infant; may not touch infant, cries easily, integrates birth experience into reality
   2. Taking-hold phase: characterized by mother's starting to assume responsibility for her own baby; lasts from day 2 to day 10; concerned about infant, interested in learning; teachable, reachable, and referable time
   3. Letting-go phase: mother lets go of her idealized notion of childbirth; at this time there may be periods of guilt or grief over the childbirth experience
F. Supportive care to promote bonding/attachment
   1. Give parents ample time to inspect and begin to identify with infant; allow the parents to touch, fondle, and hold infant
   2. Encourage give-and-take between parents and infant; support these beginning relationships
   3. Teach parents about their newborn; showing by example helps parents to learn care necessary to meet infant's needs and their own
   4. Evaluate parents' and infant's response and revise plan as necessary; identify beginning of disturbed relationships
   5. Provide therapeutic environment for various family life-style types: single parent, gay, blended

▼ ADAPTATION TO EXTRAUTERINE LIFE

A. Immediate needs at the time of birth
1. Aspiration of mucus to provide an open airway
2. Evaluation by use of Apgar score 1 and 5 minutes following birth; score determined by points for heart rate, respiration, muscle tone, reflex irritability, and color (Table 4-1); scores: 7 to 10, good condition; 3 to 6, moderately depressed; 0 to 2, severely depressed
3. Maintenance of body temperature by drying infant and placing next to mother or under radiant warmer
4. Promotion of interaction between parents and newborn
5. Constant observation of physical condition
6. Identification of infant by applying an identification band to infant and mother
7. Eye care: prophylactic instillation of ordered medicine (e.g., erythromycin) in each eye to prevent ophthalmia neonatorum
8. Assessment of behavioral characteristics during transition period: first period of reactivity, period of inactivity, second period of reactivity

B. Characteristics of and changes in the newborn during the first week of life
1. Circulatory
   a. Clamping of cord at birth brings changes in fetal circulation: closure of foramen ovale and ductus arteriosus and obliteration of umbilical arteries produce an adultlike circulation within 1 hour after birth
   b. Heart rate regular: 120 to 160, but variable depending on infant's activity; soft heart murmur common for first month of life
   c. Clotting mechanism poor because intestinal flora is absent; vitamin K is given IM in the United States and orally in Canada
   d. Liver immature (although large): cannot destroy excessive red cells in newborn, resulting in physiologic jaundice by third day
   e. Hemoglobin level high: 14 to 20 g per 100 ml of blood
   f. White blood cell count high: 6000 to 22,000 mm^3

2. Respiratory: respirations diaphragmatic, irregular, abdominal; 30 to 50 per minute, quiet with periods of apnea
3. Temperature: temperature maintained at 97.8° F or 98° F (36.2° C or 36.6° C); environmental factors may affect temperature
4. Excretory
   a. Stools: first stool, black-green and tenacious, called meconium; by third day, becomes mixed with light yellow, called transitional
   b. Kidneys immature: newborn should void during first 24 hours (at 2 weeks of age voids 20 times daily), albumin and urates (brick-red staining on diaper) common during first week because of dehydration
5. Integumentary
   a. Lanugo: fine, downy hair growth over the entire body; preterm infants have increased lanugo
   b. Milia: small, whitish, pinpoint spots over the nose caused by retained sebaceous secretions
   c. Mongolian spots: blue-black discolorations on back, buttocks, and sacral region that disappear by first year
   d. Telangiectatic nevi or "stork bites" are pink or red areas caused by capillary dilation
6. Digestive
   a. Has stores of nutrients from intrauterine existence, therefore needs very little nourishment first few days
   b. Roots and sucks when anything is brought to mouth
   c. Digests simple carbohydrates, fats, and proteins readily
   d. Cardiac sphincter of stomach not well developed, therefore regurgitates if stomach is overfull
   e. Needs to be bubbled frequently to get rid of air bubbles in stomach
   f. Gastric acidity remains low for 2 to 3 months
7. Metabolic
   a. All newborns normally lose 5% to 10% of body weight by first week of life

TABLE 4-1 APGAR score chart			
Adaptation	**0**	**1**	**2**
Heart rate	Absent	Slow, below 100	Over 100
Respiratory effort	Absent	Weak cry	Strong cry
Muscle tone	Limp	Some flexion of extremities	Active motion
Reflex irritability	No response	Grimace	Cry
Color	Cyanotic, pale	Body pink, extremities cyanotic	Completely pink

b. Screening for inborn errors of metabolism (IEM)
   (1) Phenylketonuria (PKU) testing done 24 hours after first feeding; some hospitals test earlier because of early discharge and repeat test at first visit; infants with absence of phenylalanine will need special diet to prevent retardation
   (2) T4 screening; inadequate thyroxine may lead to cretinism
   (3) Lactose intolerance; eliminate milk products

8. Endocrine
   a. Enlargement of breasts in males (gynecomastia) and females is normal as a result of hormones transmitted to infant by mother
   b. Female infants may have blood in the vagina (pseudomenstruation) because of withdrawal of maternal hormones

9. Neural
   a. CNS and brain not well developed: infant needs constant supply of oxygen
   b. Breathing, sucking, and crying are early neural activities necessary for the infant's survival

10. Sleep
    a. Lowers body metabolism
    b. Helps restore energy and assimilate nutrients for growth

C. Nutrition
   1. Initial weight loss of 5% to 10% of birth weight is normal and usually regained by tenth day of life
   2. Infant feeding: put to breast or bottlefeed immediately after birth
   3. Newborn needs to ingest simple proteins, carbohydrates, fats, vitamins, and minerals for continued cell growth
   4. Fluid (130 to 200 ml per kilogram or 2 to 3 oz fluid per pound of body weight)
   5. Calories (110 to 130 calories per kilogram or 50 to 60 calories per pound of body weight)
   6. Protein (2.0 to 2.2 g per kilogram of body weight from birth to 6 months of age; 1.8 g per kilogram of body weight from 6 to 12 months of age)
   7. Self-regulation schedule
      a. Each infant born with different degree of maturity and rhythm of needs
      b. Superior to rigid schedule; should be modified to meet needs of infant and parents
      c. Bottlefed infants fed on demand or about every 4 hours
      d. Breastfed infants fed on demand
      e. Feeding behavior and degree of satisfaction reflect psychologic development of child

f. Close mother-infant relationship in feeding process meets basic need of trust (Erikson's stage of trust)

General Nursing Care of the Newborn

A. **ASSESSMENT (INCLUDING APPRAISAL OF THE NEWBORN AFTER BIRTH)**
   1. Gestational age
      a. Preterm (premature): birth at less than 37 weeks' gestation, regardless of weight
      b. Term: birth between the thirty-eighth and forty-second week of gestation
      c. Postterm: birth after 42 weeks' gestation
      d. Postmature: birth after 42 weeks' gestation; subjected to the effects of progressive placental insufficiency
   2. Birth weight
      a. Appropriate for gestational age (AGA): weight falls between 10th and 19th percentile for age
      b. Large for gestational age (LGA): weight is above 19th percentile for age
      c. Small for gestational age (SGA): weight is below 10th percentile for age
      d. Low birth weight (LBW): weight of 2500 g or less at birth
      e. Intrauterine growth retardation (IUGR): fetal growth rate does not meet expected norms
   3. Skin
      a. Body is normally pink with slight cyanosis of hands and feet (acrocyanosis); jaundice is abnormal during the first 24 hours of life
      b. Check for abrasions, rashes, crackling, and elasticity, which indicate the status of tissue hydration; at times, milia (white, pinpoint spots over the nose caused by retained sebaceous secretions), birthmarks, forceps marks, ecchymosis, or papules are present
      c. Skin turgor
   4. Vital signs: first monitor respirations, then heart rate, then temperature; heart rate is rapid; respirations are abdominal and irregular, with a rate of 30 to 60 per minute (retractions with depression of the sternum are abnormal)
   5. Head and sensory organs
      a. Head and chest circumference nearly equal with chest slightly smaller than head; if reversed the infant should be assessed for microcephaly
      b. Fontanels should be flat; bulging when baby cries could indicate increased ICP; sunken fontanels indicate dehydration
      c. Symmetry of face: as infant cries, sides of the face move equally
      d. Head for molding, abrasions, or skin breakdown; observe for caput succedaneum: edema of soft tissue of scalp; cephalhe-

matoma: edema of scalp caused by effusion of blood between the bone and periosteum; extend the head fully in all directions for adequacy in range of motion; infant's head will lag as infant is raised

e. Observe eyes for discharge or irritation; check pupils for reaction to light, equality of eye movements (there is usually some ocular incoordination); check the sclerae for clarity, jaundice, or hemorrhage

f. Nose: observe for patency of both nostrils; sneezing commonly occurs in an attempt to clear mucus from nose

g. Mouth: observe and palpate the gums and hard and soft palates for any openings; mucosa of mouth usually clear (white patches that bleed on rubbing indicate thrush, a monilial infection)

h. Ears: auricles open; vernix covers tympanic membrane, making otoscopic examination useless (ring bell close to ear—infant should stir); both eyes should be same level as ears; upper earlobes normally curved (flatness indicative of kidney anomaly)

6. Chest and abdomen
  a. Chest auscultation: only respiratory sounds should be audible (noisy crackling sounds unexpected); heart rate: regular 120 to 160 beats per minute (rubbing or unusual sounds unexpected); may increase to 180 if active
  b. Abdomen
    (1) Listen to bowel sounds over the abdomen
    (2) Palpate the spleen with fingertips under the left costal margin: tip should be palpable
    (3) Palpate liver on the right side: normally 1 cm below the costal margin
    (4) Observe umbilical cord for redness, odor, or discharge; number of vessels present (normally one vein and two arteries; the presence of only 2 vessels is frequently associated with congenital abnormalities)
    (5) Observe for umbilical hernia when newborn cries
    (6) Palpate the femoral pulses gently at inner aspect of the groin: indicate intact circulation to extremities

7. Genitalia
  a. Males
    (1) Palpate the scrotum for testes: at times undescended at birth, which is normal (must descend by puberty or sperm will be destroyed by high temperature within the abdominal cavity)
    (2) Enlargement of scrotum: indicates hydrocele (diagnosis affirmed by transparent

appearance of the scrotum when a flashlight is held close to the scrotal sac; known as translumination)
    (3) Observe tip of penis for the urinary meatus: epispadias, meatus on upper surface of penis; hypospadias, meatus on lower surface; voiding
  b. Females
    (1) Observe the genitalia for labia, urinary meatus, and vaginal opening
    (2) Discharge from nipples, edema of labia and bloody mucoid discharge is expected; these findings result from transfer of maternal hormones
    (3) Check for voiding
  c. Ambiguous genitalia
    (1) External genitalia do not allow for clear identification of gender
    (2) Further studies to determine gender are performed with surgical intervention as required

8. Extremities
  a. Hands and arms: thumbs clenched in fist; wrist angle is 0
    (1) Check for number and variation of fingers
    (2) Check the clavicles and scapulae while putting arms through normal range of motion; clicking or resistance indicates dislocation or fracture
    (3) Palpate for fractures; crepitation is indicative
  b. Feet and legs
    (1) Check toes: appearance and number
    (2) Adduct and abduct feet through range of motion; there should be no resistance or tightness
    (3) Flex both legs onto lower abdomen; there should be no resistance or tightness; abduct knees and listen for click (Ortolani's sign—indicates developmental dysplasia of hip)
    (4) Place both feet on a flat surface and bend the knees; knees should be at the same height (when unequal, known as Allis' sign—indicates developmental dysplasia of the hip)
    (5) Observe gluteal folds for symmetry; asymmetry indicates developmental dysplasia of the hip

9. Back: turn the infant on the abdomen, run a finger along the vertebral column; any dimples, separations, or swellings indicative of spina bifida

10. Anus: patency confirmed with passage of meconium; imperforate anus is ruled out by digital examination

11. Neuromuscular development: check reflexes
    a. Rooting: touch the infant's cheek; infant should search for finger; may persist for up to 1 year
    b. Sucking: place an object close to the infant's mouth; infant should make an attempt to suck; persists throughout infancy
    c. Gag: stimulation of posterior pharynx causes choking; persists through life
    d. Grasp: place fingers in palm of infant's hand (palmar) or on sole of foot below toes (plantar); fingers and toes flex in a grasping motion; lessen by 3 and 8 months, respectively
    e. Babinski: run thumb up middle undersurface of infant's foot; toes will separate and flare out; disappears after 1 year
    f. Moro: sudden jar or change in equilibrium causes extension and abduction of extremities followed by flexion and adduction; disappears by 3 to 4 months
    g. Startle: make a loud, sharp noise close to the infant; will result in the infant's bringing both arms and legs close to the body as if in an embrace; disappears by 4 months of age
    h. Crawl: when the infant is on a firm surface and turned on its abdomen, crawling movements will follow; disappears at about 6 weeks
    i. Step or dance: while the infant is supported under both arms, stepping movements will occur when feet are placed on a firm surface; disappears after 3 to 4 weeks
    j. Tonic neck or fencing: extension of the arm and/or leg on the side to which the head is turned quickly with flexion of the contralateral limbs; usually disappears by 3 to 4 months

B. **ANALYSIS/NURSING DIAGNOSES**
    1. Ineffective airway clearance related to mucus obstruction
    2. Imbalanced nutrition: less than body requirements related to limited sucking ability
    3. Pain related to circumcision and heel sticks for testing
    4. Altered parenting related to change in family structure
    5. Ineffective thermoregulation related to immaturity of nervous system
    6. Risk for trauma related to immature blood-clotting mechanisms

C. **PLANNING/IMPLEMENTATION**
    1. Monitor and maintain a patent airway
       a. Suction mucus as needed to maintain an open airway
       b. Position: side-lying position to facilitate drainage of mucus
       c. Observe for signs of respiratory distress: grunting, flaring of nostrils, sternal retractions

2. Provide warmth
    a. Keep in heated crib until body temperature is stabilized to prevent chilling; infant is unable to shiver and breaks down brown fat to produce energy for warmth; premature or small-for-gestational-age infants can be compromised by chilling because of a small amount of brown fat available for breakdown
    b. Clothing should be loose, soft
    c. Environment should be warm and free from drafts
    d. Skin should be kept clean and dry
3. Monitor vital signs; weigh daily
4. Provide daily sponge bath; change diaper frequently
5. Care for cord
6. Administer Vitamin K to prevent hemorrhagic disease of the newborn; absence of bacteria in sterile gut of newborn prevents synthesis of clotting factors
7. Administer hepatitis B vaccine
    a. Centers for Disease Control mandate that newborns receive vaccine regardless of mother's status
    b. Vaccine must be administered within the first 12 hours of life
8. Provide for feeding (See Breastfeeding and Bottlefeeding)
9. Teach care of infant to parents
10. Care for circumcision: observe for bleeding, monitor urination, apply diaper loosely, change dressing as ordered
11. Provide for human contact: touching, talking, rocking, singing

D. **EVALUATION/OUTCOMES**
    1. Maintains patency of the airway
    2. Stabilizes body temperature within acceptable range
    3. Urinates amounts commensurate with fluid intake
    4. Passes stool
    5. Maintains 90% of birth weight
    6. Remains free from complications associated with the perinatal period

▼ BREASTFEEDING

A. Advantages
    1. Psychologic value of closeness and satisfaction in beginning mother-child relationship
    2. Optimum nutritional value for infant
    3. Economic and readily accessible
    4. Infant is less likely to be allergic to mother's milk

5. Develops facial muscles, jaw, and nasal passages of infant because stronger sucking is necessary
6. Assists in involution of uterus
7. Reduces chances of infection because of maternal antibodies present in colostrum and milk
B. Prerequisites
   1. Psychologic readiness of mother is a major factor in successful breastfeeding
   2. Adequate diet to ensure high-quality milk; extra milk, protein, calories, and noncaffeinated fluids are necessary
   3. Suitable rest and exercise
   4. Infant's sucking at the breast stimulates the maternal posterior pituitary to produce oxytocin, the properties of which, in the blood system, constrict the lactiferous sinuses to move the milk down through the nipple ducts: known as the let-down reflex; a poor sucking reflex of the child will inhibit the let-down of milk; sucking also stimulates prolactin secretion
   5. Family support and absence of emotional stress in the mother, because anxiety inhibits the let-down reflex
C. Contraindications
   1. In mother: active tuberculosis; acute contagious disease; HIV positive; chronic disease such as cancer, advanced nephritis, cardiac disease; extensive surgery; narcotic addiction
   2. In infant: cleft lip or palate or any other condition that interferes with or prevents grasp of the nipple is the only real contraindication
   3. Many drugs are excreted in breast milk and have harmful effects on the developing infant; these drugs must be avoided or taken with care if they must be taken by the mother; careful monitoring of the infant is required

Nursing Care of the Breastfeeding Mother and Infant

A. **ASSESSMENT**
   1. Condition of nipples
   2. Desire to breastfeed
   3. Level of anxiety regarding breastfeeding
   4. Knowledge of breastfeeding and breast care
   5. Family support
B. **ANALYSIS/NURSING DIAGNOSES**
   1. Risk for infection related to cracked nipples
   2. Ineffective/interrupted breastfeeding related to improper breastfeeding techniques, condition of nipples, and infant's sucking ability
C. **PLANNING/IMPLEMENTATION**
   1. Teach feeding schedule
      a. Self-demand schedule is desirable; usually 2 to 3 hours
      b. Length of feeding time is usually 20 minutes,

with greatest quantity of milk consumed in first 5 to 10 minutes
   2. Teach feeding techniques
      a. Mother and infant in comfortable position, such as semireclining or in comfortable chair
      b. Entire body of infant should be turned toward mother's breast; alternate starting breast and use both breasts at each feeding
      c. Initiate feeding by stimulating rooting reflex and direct nipple straight into infant's mouth (stroking cheek toward breast, being careful not to stroke other cheek, because this will confuse infant)
      d. Burp or bubble infant during and after feeding to allow for escape of air: sit infant on lap, flexed forward; rub or pat back (avoid jarring infant)
      e. Breast milk intake similar to formula intake: 130 to 200 ml of milk per kilogram (2 to 3 oz of milk per pound) of infant's weight; from one sixth to one seventh of infant's weight per day
      f. After lactation has been established, occasional bottlefeeding can be substituted
      g. Length of time for continuing breastfeeding is variable (may be discontinued when teeth erupt, because this can be uncomfortable for mother)
   3. Teach care of breasts
      a. Cleanse with plain water once daily (soap or alcohol can cause irritation and dryness)
      b. Support breasts day and night with properly fitting brassiere
      c. Nursing pads should be placed inside bra cup to absorb any milk leaking between feedings; allow nipples to air dry at intervals
      d. Plastic bra liners should be avoided because they increase heat and perspiration and decrease air circulation necessary for drying of the nipple
      e. If breasts are engorged, teach mother to take warm showers and put infant to breast more frequently
D. **EVALUATION/OUTCOMES**
   1. Mother demonstrates effective breastfeeding techniques
   2. Mother remains free from nipple cracking and infection
   3. Infant produces six or more wet diapers daily
   4. Infant gains weight

▼ BOTTLEFEEDING

A. Advantages
   1. Provides an alternative to breastfeeding

2. Less restrictive than breastfeeding; may meet needs of working mothers
3. Allows a more accurate assessment of intake
4. May be indicated in the presence of a congenital anomaly such as cleft palate
5. May be necessary for infants who require special formulas because of allergies or inborn errors of metabolism

B. Types of formulas
1. Commercial liquid or powdered formulas
2. Special formulas
3. Unmodified regular cow's milk, liquid or reconstituted; not appropriate for infants before 12 months of age; cow's milk contains more protein and calcium and less vitamin C, iron, and carbohydrate than breast milk

C. Contraindications
1. Deficient knowledge of formula preparation
2. Poor storage and refrigeration practices
3. Contaminated water supply
4. Cost of formula and equipment
5. Lack of equipment to adequately prepare bottles

Nursing Care of the Bottlefeeding Mother and Infant

A. **ASSESSMENT**
1. Desire to bottlefeed
2. Sucking ability of infant
3. Knowledge of formulas and formula preparation

B. **ANALYSIS/NURSING DIAGNOSES**
1. Ineffective infant feeding pattern related to infant sucking difficulties
2. Infant's imbalanced nutrition: less than body requirements related to formula that does not meet infant's needs

C. **PLANNING/IMPLEMENTATION**
1. Teach preparation of formula
   a. Calculation of formula to yield 110 to 130 calories and 130 to 200 ml of fluid per kilogram of body weight; caution regarding dangers of overdilution (water intoxication) and underdilution (excess weight gain)
   b. Proper sterilization of formula by terminal heat method
   c. Teach about commercial formulas
   d. Proper refrigeration of formula
2. Teach feeding techniques
   a. Always hold infant during feeding to provide warm body contact (bottle propping may contribute to aspiration of formula)
   b. Hold bottle so nipple is always filled with milk to prevent excessive air ingestion
   c. Adjust size of nipple hole to needs of infant (a premature infant needs a larger hole that requires less sucking)
   d. Burp during and after feeding; place infant on side to aid digestion and prevent aspiration
   e. Feeding should be offered on demand to meet the infant's needs

D. **EVALUATION/OUTCOMES**
1. Mother demonstrates effective bottlefeeding techniques
2. Infant produces six or more wet diapers daily
3. Infant gains weight

COMPLICATIONS OF PREGNANCY

▼ IDENTIFYING AND/OR MONITORING HIGH RISK PREGNANCY

A. Alpha-fetoprotein (AFP) enzyme blood test: elevated levels may identify the pregnant woman carrying a baby with neural tube defects (spina bifida and anencephaly); may also indicate twins; if the AFP is elevated for two samples, it is followed by ultrasonography and amniocentesis for further confirmation; done at 14 to 16 weeks' gestation

B. Ultrasonography: high-frequency sound-wave testing; discerns multiple pregnancy, placental location, and gestational age by measurement of biparietal diameters
1. Visualization during first 20 weeks of gestation is improved if the bladder is full; a full bladder is not necessary after 20 weeks' gestation
2. A level II sonogram may be performed to assess formation of organs
3. Nursing care: encourage fluids and refrain from voiding before the test

C. Chorionic villi sampling (CVS): supplies same data as amniocentesis but can be done after 10 weeks
1. Aspiration of villi done during the eighth to twelfth week of pregnancy
2. Nursing care: instruct to drink fluid so that bladder is full; after test monitor for uterine contractions, vaginal discharge, and teach to observe for signs of infection

D. Amniocentesis: aspiration of amniotic fluid used to detect sex, chromosomal or biochemical defects, fetal age, L/S ratio (2/1 ratio indicates lung maturity), increased bilirubin level associated with Rh disease, and phosphatidylglycerol (PG), which appears in amniotic fluid after thirty-fifth week, indicating fetal lung maturity
1. Test done with sonogram; usually after 12 to 15 weeks of gestation
2. Nursing care: have client void; after test monitor for uterine contractions, vaginal discharge; teach to observe for signs of infection; encourage rest

E. Nonstress test (NST): to observe for accelerations of FHR in response to fetal movement over a 30- to 40-minute period
   1. Classification of results
      a. A test is negative or reactive if
         (1) Baseline FHR is 120 to 160
         (2) There are two accelerations in 10 minutes, each increasing the FHR by 15 and lasting 15 seconds
         (3) The tracing shows variability of 10 or more beats per minute
      b. Test is positive or nonreactive if the three criteria are not met
      c. Unsatisfactory: recording uninterpretable; repeat test in 24 hours
   2. Nursing care: fasting is not necessary; observe the fetal monitor; explain test to decrease anxiety; evaluate response to procedure
F. Contraction stress test (CST): to demonstrate whether a healthy fetus can withstand a decreased oxygen supply during the stress of a contraction produced by exogenous oxytocin (Pitocin) or stimulation of nipples manually or by moist heat; if late decelerations appear, the fetus may be compromised because of uteroplacental insufficiency
   1. Classification of results
      a. Negative: no late decelerations with a minimum of three contractions in 10 minutes; indicates that the fetus has good chance of surviving labor
      b. Positive: persistent and late decelerations occurring with more than half the contractions; indicates need for considering premature intervention
      c. Suspicious: late decelerations occurring in less than half of uterine contractions; test should be repeated in 24 hours
   2. Nursing care: void before test; monitor fetal heart rate for 30 minutes before test; monitor mother after test to observe for possible initiation of labor; evaluate response to procedure
G. Biophysical profile (BPP): assesses breathing movements, body movements, tone, amniotic fluid volume, and FHR reactivity (NST); a score of 2 is assigned to each finding, with a score of 8 to 10 indicating a healthy fetus
   1. Used for fetus that may have intrauterine compromise
   2. Nursing care: provide emotional support; evaluate response to procedure
H. Maternal assessment of fetal activity: need to contact physician or nurse midwife when there are fewer than 10 fetal movements in a 12-hour period, fewer than three fetal movements in an 8-hour period, or no fetal movements in the morning
   1. Used to determine vitality of fetus
   2. Nursing care: teach how to record and report movements
I. Fetal scalp pH sampling: may be done during labor when fetal heart patterns begin to indicate distress; capillary blood samples are taken from fetal scalp in utero
   1. Results: if acidosis present, immediate birth of infant is indicated
   2. Nursing care: cleanse vaginal area to avoid contamination during test
J. Fetal Acoustic Stimulation Test (FAST) and Vibroacoustic Stimulation Test (VST): fetal heart baseline is measured; a buzzing (FAST) or vibration (VST) is created over the head of fetus for 5 seconds and 1-minute intervals for 5 minutes
   1. A reactive test occurs when there are two accelerations of 15 beats/min lasting 15 seconds within 10 minutes
   2. Test is noninvasive

▼ PREGNANCY-INDUCED HYPERTENSION (GESTATIONAL HYPERTENSION, PREECLAMPSIA, ECLAMPSIA, HELLP SYNDROME)

Data Base
A. Characterized by a triad of symptoms: edema, hypertension, and proteinuria occurring after the twentieth to twenty-fourth week of gestation and disappearing 6 weeks after birth
B. Occurs primarily in primiparas below 17 years of age and above 35 years of age and women with numerous pregnancies, chronic hypertension, diabetes mellitus, severe nutritional deficiencies, multiple pregnancy, or trophoblastic disease
C. Clinical findings
   1. Gestational hypertension
      a. Increased blood pressure during pregnancy that resolves within 6 weeks after birth
      b. No edema or proteinuria is present; blood changes rarely occur in uncomplicated gestational hypertension
   2. Preeclampsia
      a. Mild: systolic pressure increased 30 mm Hg or more above normal; diastolic pressure increased 15 mm Hg or more above normal; proteinuria +1; edema manifested by excessive weekly weight gain and upper-body edema
      b. Severe: BP is 160/110 or above on two readings taken 6 hours apart after bed rest; proteinuria 3+ to 4+; extensive edema (puffiness of hands and face); hyperreflexia
   3. Eclampsia: seizures and/or coma associated with hypertension, proteinuria, and edema

4. HELLP syndrome (H, hemolysis; EL, elevated liver enzymes; LP, low platelet count)
   a. Occurs with little warning and often with no previous signs of PIH
   b. Right upper-quadrant pain occurs in 90% of affected women; proteinuria may occur
   c. Liver enzymes are elevated; platelets and RBCs are low
   d. Blood smear reveals broken red blood cells (schistocytes or burr cells)
   e. Occurs after 28 weeks' gestation or 48 to 72 hours after birth
5. Blood chemistry: rise in hematocrit, uric acid, liver enzymes, and blood urea nitrogen concentrations and decrease in RBCs, platelets, and CO_2 combining power indicate worsening preeclampsia
6. Qualitative urinalysis: increase in albumin output (proteinuria) and/or decreased urinary output indicates worsening preeclampsia

D. Guidelines for prevention of pregnancy-induced hypertension
1. Sound nutrition counseling during pregnancy and lactation
2. Increase protein to 60 g daily in the second and third trimesters
3. Infant aspirin or Motrin may be used daily
4. Caloric intake should be increased 10% during pregnancy; severe calorie restriction is harmful during pregnancy
5. Restriction of sodium is harmful during pregnancy and can result in electrolyte imbalance and elimination of essential nutritional components; may contribute to reduced circulatory volume
6. Diuretics are contraindicated during pregnancy because they cause hypovolemia and deplete essential nutrients for mother and fetus

E. Therapeutic interventions
1. Gestational hypertension
   a. Frequent rest periods
   b. Dietary management with increased fluid intake
   c. Treat symptoms
2. Mild preeclampsia
   a. High-protein diet
   b. Ambulatory care; frequent visits to obstetrician
   c. Frequent rest periods with feet elevated; side-lying position to enhance renal and placental perfusion
3. Severe preeclampsia or eclampsia
   a. Hospitalization and complete bed rest
   b. Magnesium sulfate given IV by infusion pump to prevent or limit seizures
   c. Albumin concentrate to increase renal flow and correct the hypovolemia

d. Antihypertensives: hydralazine (Apresoline), labetalol hydrochloride (Adalat), methyldopa (Aldomet)
e. Foley catheter
f. Labor induction or cesarean birth once symptoms are under control
g. Calcium gluconate for the mother and levallorphan (Lorfan) for the newborn if respiratory depression occurs from magnesium sulfate
h. If fetus is less than 34 weeks' gestation, stimulation of surfactant production with betamethasone is attempted
4. HELLP syndrome
   a. Same as severe preeclampsia or eclampsia
   b. Blood or blood products may be administered if necessary

Nursing Care of Clients with Pregnancy-Induced Hypertension (Preeclampsia, Eclampsia, HELLP Syndrome)

A. **ASSESSMENT**
1. Blood pressure elevation
2. Presence of edema; excessive weight gain; puffiness of hands, feet, or face
3. Albumin in urine; oliguria
4. Hyperreflexia; persistent headache; blurred vision
5. Epigastric pain

B. **ANALYSIS/NURSING DIAGNOSES**
1. Anxiety related to course of pregnancy and possible death of fetus
2. Deficient fluid volume related to fluid shift out of intravascular compartment
3. Risk for injury to mother related to sedation, seizures, magnesium toxicity
4. Risk for injury to fetus related to hypoxic episodes during maternal seizures

C. **PLANNING/IMPLEMENTATION**
1. Monitor blood pressure: every 15 minutes during critical phase; every 1 to 4 hours as condition improves
2. Insert Foley catheter; monitor urine for output and albumin
3. Assess edema: daily weights, intake and output
4. Maintain high-protein diet with normal salt intake
5. Monitor hyperreflexia
6. Administer magnesium sulfate as ordered (check for sufficient urinary output before starting)
7. Monitor for magnesium toxicity
   a. Assess for depressed patellar reflexes
   b. Assess for depressed respirations, below 12 to 14 breaths per minute
   c. Magnesium blood levels every 6 hours; therapeutic range is 4 to 8 mg/dl

d. Have calcium gluconate available if magnesium sulfate toxicity is present
8. Observe for indications of a seizure; maintain seizure precautions; monitor vital signs and fetal heart rate following a seizure
9. Maintain on bed rest in left side-lying position; maintain quiet environment; limit visitors
10. Monitor FHR
11. Observe for signs of labor and bleeding
12. Monitor hematologic studies related to HELLP syndrome
13. Assess anxieties and concerns
14. Be prepared for an induced or emergency cesarean birth
15. Continue to monitor for related complications for 48 hours after birth

D. EVALUATION/OUTCOMES
1. Maintains (mother and fetus) vital signs within acceptable range
2. Remains free from seizures
3. Maintains fluid balance

▼ ABORTION

Data Base
A. Definition
1. A spontaneous or planned interruption of pregnancy in which there is complete expulsion or partial expulsion (incomplete) of the products of conception before the period of viability (see Induced Abortion)
2. Period of gestation is 20 weeks or less, the conceptus will weigh below 500 g and will be less than 16.5 cm long
3. May be caused by the presence of embryonic defects, external mechanical force, or trauma
B. Types/clinical findings
1. Threatened abortion: cervix closed, but bleeding, cramping and backache occur; pregnancy may continue uninterrupted
2. Imminent or inevitable abortion: bleeding and cramping become more severe, cervix dilates, and membranes may rupture
3. Incomplete abortion: all the products of conception are not expelled after dilation of cervical os
4. Complete abortion: all products of conception expelled within 24 to 48 hours
5. Missed abortion: fetus dies in utero but not expelled; client must be monitored for disseminated intravascular coagulopathy (DIC)
6. Habitual abortions: three consecutive pregnancies that end in abortion
C. Therapeutic interventions

1. Complete bed rest
2. Diagnostic/therapeutic blood studies: blood cell count, blood typing, Rh incompatibility, and cross-matching with availability of blood
3. Assessment of serum progesterone or serial beta-hCG
4. Dilation and curettage or vacuum aspiration performed if the products of conception are retained

Nursing Care of Clients Experiencing Abortion
A. ASSESSMENT
1. Vital signs; amount of bleeding
2. Pain
3. Emotional response to loss
B. ANALYSIS/NURSING DIAGNOSES
1. Anticipatory grieving related to loss of expected infant
2. Pain related to uterine contractions
3. Situational low self-esteem related to inability to carry pregnancy to term
C. PLANNING/IMPLEMENTATION
1. Institute measures to alleviate fear and anxiety; assist with grieving process
2. Point out physiologic reality, but encourage client to work through feelings; grieving may last up to 24 months
3. Encourage participation with thanatology services and bereavement groups when appropriate
4. Monitor amount and type of bleeding: save and count number of pads; distinguish between dark clotted blood and frank bleeding, which is bright red; monitor fundus for firmness after products of conception are expelled
5. Monitor vital signs for signs of hypovolemia, shock, and infection; monitor CBC, hemoglobin, and hematocrit; prepare for administration of blood; administer oxygen if necessary
6. Maintain fluid and electrolyte balance
7. Administer RhoGAM to Rh-negative client after abortion
8. Educate about necessity for follow-up care and support groups
D. EVALUATION/OUTCOMES
1. Remains free from complications such as hemorrhage and infection
2. Expresses feelings

▼ ECTOPIC PREGNANCY

Data Base
A. Pregnancy in which implantation occurs outside the uterus (most frequent site is middle portion of fallopian tube, other sites are abdomen, ovaries, or cervix)

B. Early signs and symptoms are usually concealed; may be diagnosed by ultrasonography and radioimmunoassay for B-hCG
C. Pattern in tubal pregnancy: spotting after one or two missed menstrual periods; sudden, sharp, knife-like lower right or left abdominal pain radiating to shoulder; concealed bleeding from site of rupture leads to sudden shock
D. Clients who have had pelvic inflammatory disease (PID) or tubal surgery are predisposed to ectopic pregnancies
E. Therapeutic interventions
1. Diagnosis confirmed by ultrasound examination, laparoscopy, or culdocentesis
2. Immediate blood replacement if blood loss is severe
3. Surgical repair or removal of ruptured fallopian tube may be attempted
4. Chemical therapies to salvage fallopian tube (e.g., methotrexate) or therapies to inhibit cell division if fetus is less than 4 cm by ultrasound

Nursing Care of Clients with an Ectopic Pregnancy

A. ASSESSMENT
1. Vital signs; signs of shock
2. Bleeding; rigid tender abdomen
3. Character and location of pain
4. Level of anxiety
B. ANALYSIS/NURSING DIAGNOSES
1. Ineffective cardiopulmonary tissue perfusion related to hemorrhage
2. Fear related to potential disturbance in future childbearing ability
3. Anticipatory grieving related to loss of expected infant
4. Pain related to tubal rupture
C. PLANNING/IMPLEMENTATION
1. Assess continuously for signs of shock; administer blood transfusion if ordered for excessive blood loss
2. Administer analgesics as ordered for pain
3. Provide emotional support
4. Provide preoperative and postoperative care
5. Administer RhoGAM to Rh-negative client
D. EVALUATION/OUTCOMES
1. Maintains hemostasis
2. States implications for future childbearing
3. Expresses feelings

▼ TROPHOBLASTIC DISEASE

Data Base

A. Definition
1. A group of disorders in which there is an abnormal proliferation of tissues and high hGC levels

2. These disorders include hydatidiform mole, invasive mole, and choriocarcinoma
B. Clinical findings
1. Types include:
   a. Molar pregnancy—no fetus or amnion
   b. Partial molar pregnancy—a fetus or amniotic sac present
   c. Invasive mole—locally invasive to surrounding tissues
   d. Choriocarcinoma—may occur years after a hydatidiform mole
2. Uterus is generally larger for period of gestation and fetal parts are not palpable; doughlike consistency
3. Symptoms of pregnancy-induced hypertension and hyperemesis are common
4. Potential for uterine perforation, hemorrhage, passing of "grapelike" substance, and infection
5. Confirmation by ultrasonography
C. Therapeutic interventions
1. If spontaneous evacuation does not occur, evacuation by dilation and curettage or hysterotomy is performed
2. Continued follow-up of serum gonadotropin levels is imperative for 1 year to rule out metastasis from chorionic carcinoma (increased gonadotropin levels require chemotherapy); metastasis to lungs is common
3. Preventing a new pregnancy is essential for 1 year
4. Chemotherapy when malignant

Nursing Care of Clients with Hydatidiform Mole or Trophoblastic Disease

A. ASSESSMENT
1. Vaginal bleeding (brownish, prune juice) containing grapelike tissue
2. Uterine enlargement; fundal height greater than expected for length of pregnancy
3. Vomiting
4. Elevated blood pressure earlier than 24 weeks' gestation
5. Absence of fetal heart tones or activity
B. ANALYSIS/NURSING DIAGNOSES
1. Ineffective coping related to loss of expected infant, uncertainty of continuing a future pregnancy
2. Fear related to the possible development of cancer
3. Situational low self-esteem related to carrying an abnormal pregnancy
C. PLANNING/IMPLEMENTATION
1. See Nursing Care of Clients Experiencing Abortion
2. Teach about importance of follow-up care
D. EVALUATION/OUTCOMES
1. Continues follow-up care
2. Uses measures to prevent pregnancy for 1 year

▼ INCOMPETENT CERVIX

Data Base
A. Definition
1. Cervical effacement and dilation in early second trimester resulting in expulsion of products of conception
2. Usually results from previous forceful dilation and curettage, difficult birth, or congenitally short cervix
B. Clinical findings
1. Painless contractions in midtrimester
2. Birth of dead or nonviable fetus
C. Therapeutic interventions
1. Cerclage procedure during 14th to 16th week of gestation; suture or ribbon placed beneath cervical mucosa to close cervix
2. At end of pregnancy, cesarean birth or cutting of suture for vaginal birth
3. Bed rest

Nursing Care of Clients with an Incompetent Cervix
A. **ASSESSMENT**
1. Weeks of gestation
2. Obstetric history
3. Knowledge of the cerclage procedure
B. **ANALYSIS/NURSING DIAGNOSES**
1. Anticipatory grieving related to potential loss of expected infant
2. Situational low self-esteem related to inability to complete pregnancy without intervention
3. Risk for infection related to invasive procedure
C. **PLANNING/IMPLEMENTATION**
1. Maintain bed rest for 24 hours after cerclage
2. Monitor for rupture of membranes or bleeding
3. Monitor FHR
D. **EVALUATION/OUTCOMES**
1. Describes signs of labor and need to seek immediate medical care when labor begins
2. Continues pregnancy to term

▼ PLACENTA PREVIA

Data Base
A. Definition: abnormal implantation of the placenta in the lower uterine segment
B. Types
1. Type I–Low-lying: placenta is at lower uterine segment next to os; as uterus stretches with gestation, placenta moves away from os
2. Type II–Marginal: placental edge is at the os, but does not cover it
3. Type III–Partial: placental edge partially covers the os
4. Type IV–Complete: placenta is centered over the cervical os
C. Clinical findings
1. Painless, bright-red bleeding; hemorrhage in the third trimester
2. Soft uterus in the latter part of pregnancy
3. Signs of infection may be present
D. Therapeutic interventions
1. Ultrasonography to confirm the presence of placenta previa
2. Depends on location of placenta, amount of bleeding, and status of the fetus
3. Home monitoring with repeated ultrasounds may be possible with type I–low-lying
4. Control bleeding
5. Replace blood loss if excessive
6. Cesarean birth, if necessary
7. Betamethasone is indicated to increase fetal lung maturity

Nursing Care of Clients with Placenta Previa
A. **ASSESSMENT**
1. Presence of bright-red blood with absence of pain
2. Vital signs indicating shock (hypovolemic)
3. Changes in or absence of FHR
4. Level of anxiety (usually increases)
B. **ANALYSIS/NURSING DIAGNOSES**
1. Ineffective cardiopulmonary tissue perfusion in mother and fetus related to hemorrhage and interruption of placental oxygen supply
2. Fear related to acuteness of physical status and possible death of fetus and/or mother
3. Anticipatory grieving related to outcome of pregnancy and threat of termination of childbearing ability
C. **PLANNING/IMPLEMENTATION**
1. No admission vaginal examination; if a vaginal examination is to be performed, double setups (vaginal and cesarean) must be provided
2. Maintain bed rest in semi-Fowler's position
3. Monitor FHR continuously; will be normal if placenta is functioning
4. Monitor maternal vital signs continuously; assess color for pallor or cyanosis; administer oxygen
5. Assess perineal pads to determine blood loss; monitor Hgb and Hct; prepare for cesarean birth if bleeding persists
6. Administer intravenous therapy and/or blood replacement
D. **EVALUATION/OUTCOMES**
1. Delivers viable, stable newborn
2. Demonstrates hemodynamic stability

▼ ABRUPTIO PLACENTAE

Data Base

A. Definition: partial, marginal, or complete premature separation of a normally implanted placenta in the third trimester; degree of separation may be mild, moderate, or severe (Grade 1, 2, or 3)
B. Clinical findings
    1. Concealed bleeding if center of the placenta separates and margins are intact
    2. Dark-red blood may not be evident with partially detached placenta at margins
    3. Moderate to agonizing abdominal pain
    4. Persistent uterine contraction; normal to board-like abdomen
    5. Hyperactivity and then cessation of fetal movements
    6. Frequently associated with pregnancy-induced or chronic hypertension, maternal cocaine use, previous history of abruptio placentae, trauma, and aggressive Pitocin induction
    7. Predisposes client to hemorrhage, disseminated intravascular coagulopathy (DIC), and hypofibrinogenemia
C. Therapeutic interventions
    1. Replacement of blood loss
    2. With moderate or severe separation or maternal or fetal distress: emergency cesarean birth
    3. With mild separation without fetal distress and in the presence of some cervical effacement and dilation: induction of labor may be attempted
    4. Oxygen if necessary
    5. Maintenance of fluid and electrolyte balance

Nursing Care of Clients with Abruptio Placentae

A. **ASSESSMENT**
    1. Presence of pain with or without dark-red bleeding
    2. Increased tonicity of abdominal wall
    3. Vital signs indicating shock
    4. Changes in or absence of FHR
    5. Level of anxiety usually increases
B. **ANALYSIS/NURSING DIAGNOSES**
    1. Ineffective cardiopulmonary tissue perfusion in both mother and fetus related to hemorrhage and interruption of placental oxygen supply
    2. Fear related to acuteness of physical status and possible death of fetus and/or mother
    3. Anticipatory grieving related to outcome of pregnancy and threat of termination of childbearing ability
C. **PLANNING/IMPLEMENTATION**
    1. Maintain bed rest in left-lateral recumbent position
    2. Monitor FHR continuously

    3. Monitor maternal vital signs continuously; assess color for pallor or cyanosis; administer oxygen
    4. Type and crossmatch, coagulation studies, hemoglobin, and hematocrit
    5. Kleihauer-Betke test to assess fetal cells in maternal circulation
    6. Assess abdominal pain, tonicity of abdomen, perineal pads if bleeding is evident, and hemoglobin and hematocrit levels; prepare for cesarean birth if abruptio is moderate or severe
    7. Administer intravenous therapy and/or blood replacement
    8. Observe for signs of DIC such as seepage of blood from IV site or incisional areas
D. **EVALUATION/OUTCOMES**
    1. Delivers viable, stable newborn
    2. Demonstrates hemodynamic stability

▼ INDUCED ABORTION

Data Base

A. Menstrual extraction or minisuction: vacuum of uterine contents with a 50-ml syringe; done 5 to 7 weeks after last menstrual period
B. Vacuum aspiration: done under local paracervical, epidural, or general anesthesia in first 12 weeks of pregnancy; the cervix is dilated and products of conception are suctioned by a small, hollow tube; the uterus is then curettaged to remove all fetal tissue
C. Dilation and curettage: performed during the first 12 to 14 weeks of pregnancy under local paracervical or general anesthesia; the cervix is dilated and uterus is curettaged
D. Saline injection
    1. Labor is induced when a pregnancy is 14 to 24 weeks in duration by injecting a sterile saline solution into the uterus by amniocentesis; labor usually begins within 8 to 24 hours after instillation of saline; produces a macerated fetus
    2. Adverse effect: headache caused by hypernatremia
E. Prostaglandin
    1. Used during second trimester to trigger vasoconstriction and uterine contractions that interfere with endocrine function of placenta (examples: carboprost tromethamine (Prostin/15 m), dinoprostone (Prostin E2)
    2. Adverse effects: nausea, vomiting, diarrhea, pain at extrauterine sites, allergic reactions (not administered to clients with history of asthma)
F. Hysterotomy: performed after 16 weeks of pregnancy by surgically removing the fetus and placenta abdominally

Nursing Care of Clients Undergoing Induced Abortion

A. ASSESSMENT
1. History and physical examination
2. Specimens for laboratory tests
3. Rh status
4. Length of pregnancy
5. Level of anxiety
6. Understanding of procedure and postprocedure care

B. ANALYSIS/NURSING DIAGNOSES
1. Decisional conflict related to termination of pregnancy and the diversity of options
2. Risk for infection related to introduction of foreign objects or substances into the body
3. Risk for injury related to mechanical termination of pregnancy
4. Pain related to induced labor

C. PLANNING/IMPLEMENTATION
1. Be aware of own feelings about abortion; essential if the nurse is to intervene therapeutically with women having abortions; nurses with strong feelings about abortion should not counsel clients
2. Encourage the client's expression of feelings
3. Obtain informed consent
4. Be objective and support the client's decision about abortion
5. Make certain that a complete history and physical examination, complete laboratory workup, pelvic examination and Papanicolaou test, and a pregnancy test are done before induced abortion
6. Counsel concerning contraceptive methods if requested
7. Administer RhoGAM when client is Rh negative and negative for antibodies

D. EVALUATION/OUTCOMES
1. Expels products of conception
2. Remains free from complications
3. Returns for health supervision
4. Express feelings

COMPLICATIONS OF LABOR AND BIRTH

▼ INDUCTION OR STIMULATION OF LABOR

Data Base
A. Elective induction: initiation of labor contractions by:
1. Pharmacologic means
   a. Vaginal insertion of prostaglandin E2 gel or suppository to promote cervical softening and effacement (ripening)
   b. Eight to 12 hours after prostaglandin E2 administration, pump infusion of oxytocin (Pitocin) to stimulate contractions
2. Mechanical means
   a. Artificial rupture of membranes (amniotomy)
   b. Insertion of *Laminaria* tent (dried seaweed that swells in presence of moisture) to promote cervical ripening, and then induction begins; *Laminaria* is also used to dilate the cervix in elective abortions
   c. Stimulation of breasts to bring about neural stimulation of posterior pituitary and secretion of oxytocin
3. Medical or obstetric reasons: diabetes; pyelonephritis; PIH; Rh incompatibility; polyhydramnios; placental insufficiency; premature rupture of membranes at term without onset of labor; postterm gestation; history of precipitate birth, fetal jeopardy
B. Augmentation of labor: assisting client when labor process is not progressing normally (prolonged labor) by pharmacologic or mechanical means
C. Induction or augmentation of labor is not done with cephalopelvic disproportion, malpresentation of fetus, fetal distress, placenta previa, or active genital herpes

Nursing Care of Clients During Induction or Stimulation of Labor

A. ASSESSMENT
1. Obstetric history, including expected date of birth
2. Maternal status: parity; contractions; status of membranes; status of cervix; ultrasonographic findings; level of anxiety
3. Fetal status: gestational age; absence of cephalopelvic disproportion; position; results of fetal monitoring and nonstress test

B. ANALYSIS/NURSING DIAGNOSES
1. Anxiety related to uncertainty about the labor and birth process
2. Risk for infection related to ruptured membranes
3. Pain related to use of oxytocics
4. Risk for trauma related to possibility of sustained contractions from oxytocin or fetal cord prolapse following amniotomy

C. PLANNING/IMPLEMENTATION
1. Prepare mother and labor coach for induction: explain all procedures; obtain informed consent whenever necessary
2. Obtain and record baseline information such as maternal vital signs, FHR, contractions for later comparison; continue to monitor all vital indices
3. Monitor Pitocin administration
   a. Typically oxytocin is piggybacked through an infusion device at 0.5 to 2 mU/min; titrated according to contraction pattern and fetal response

b. Discontinue Pitocin drip if a sustained uterine contraction occurs; fetal accelerations/decelerations persist; urinary flow decreases to 30 ml per hour (related to water intoxication); signs of placenta previa or abruptio placentae develop

4. Monitor effect of prostaglandin: if hypertonic contractions occur, discontinue infusion; if they persist, prepare for tocolytic therapy

5. Assist with artificial rupture of membranes (amniotomy)
   a. Maintain asepsis
   b. Immediately after rupture, monitor FHR
   c. Note color and amount of amniotic fluid
   d. Record time of rupture; prolonged rupture may predispose client to sepsis

6. Maintain hydration

7. Provide for blood typing, Rh compatibility, cross-matching

8. Have oxygen, suction, and resuscitation equipment readily available

9. Prepare for emergency cesarean birth if necessary

D. EVALUATION/OUTCOMES
1. Progresses through labor to safe delivery of newborn
2. Remains free from complications

▼ PREMATURE RUPTURE OF MEMBRANES (PROM)

Data Base
A. Definition: spontaneous rupture of membranes before onset of labor
B. Maternal implication: ascending infection
C. Fetal implications
   1. Prolapsed cord
   2. FHR decelerations caused by cord compression from lack of amniotic fluid
   3. Sepsis from ascending infection
D. Therapeutic interventions
   1. Hospitalization with bed rest after 37 weeks of gestation
   2. Amnioinfusion of isotonic saline in some cases to allow for fetal movement and lessen danger of cord compression
   3. Prophylactic antibiotics

Nursing Care of Clients with Premature Rupture of Membranes
A. ASSESSMENT
1. Time of rupture of membranes
2. Fetal heart rate and maternal vital signs
3. Perineum for prolapsed cord
4. Confirmation of rupture of membranes by fern

test: microscopic examination reveals fernlike crystals of sodium chloride

5. Confirmation of presence of amniotic fluid by nitrazine test; paper turns blue when touched by alkaline solution (7.0 to 7.5) rather than acidic vaginal secretions

6. Characteristics of leaking amniotic fluid: odor and color

B. ANALYSIS/NURSING DIAGNOSES
1. Anxiety related to outcome of pregnancy
2. Risk for ineffective fetal tissue perfusion related to prolapsed cord
3. Risk for infection related to premature rupture of membranes

C. PLANNING/IMPLEMENTATION
1. Monitor FHR and maternal vital signs; temperature and pulse every 2 hours
2. Monitor uterine activity
3. Avoid unnecessary vaginal examinations
4. Ensure adequate hydration
5. Educate parents: amniotic fluid is still being produced
6. Provide perineal hygiene
7. Administer antibiotics as ordered

D. EVALUATION/OUTCOMES
1. Remains free from infection
2. Progresses through labor to safe delivery of newborn

▼ PRETERM LABOR

Data Base
A. Contractions begin after the twentieth week but before the thirty-eighth week of gestation, causing effacement and dilation of the cervix
   1. A fetus of 20 or more weeks' gestation who dies before or during delivery is classified as stillborn
   2. Preterm births account for 75% to 85% of neonatal morbidity and mortality
B. Contributing factors include history, risky lifestyle, multiple gestation, maternal illness with fever, heroin and opiate use, bacterial vaginitis, multiple abortions, pyelonephritis, and asymptomatic bacteriuria
C. Diagnostic studies
   1. Transvaginal cervical sonography
   2. Immunoassay for fetal fibronectin
D. Therapeutic interventions
   1. Bed rest; side-lying position, preferably left side
   2. Tocolytic therapy directed toward postponing labor
      a. Betasympathomimetics such as ritodrine (Yutopar) and terbutaline sulfate (Brethine)
      b. Magnesium sulfate
      c. Prostaglandin inhibitors

d. Calcium channel blockers such as nifedipine
3. Glucocorticoid therapy
   a. Betamethasone (Celestone)
   b. Administered 24 to 48 hours before birth if birth appears inevitable
   c. Reduces incidence and severity of respiratory distress syndrome (RDS) in preterm infants; enhances formation of surfactant
4. Home uterine monitoring

Nursing Care of Clients During Preterm Labor

A. ASSESSMENT
1. Number of weeks of gestation
2. Presence of live and viable fetus
3. Presence of labor: two contractions lasting 30 seconds within 15 minutes; cervical dilation less than 4 cm; effacement 50% or less
4. No signs of hemorrhage or infection
5. Presence of severe pregnancy-induced hypertension
6. Prolonged rupture of membranes
7. Emotional status of mother

B. ANALYSIS/NURSING DIAGNOSES
1. Situational low self-esteem related to failure to carry pregnancy to full term
2. Fear related to acute status of infant and potential for death
3. Compromised family coping related to need for specialized care and continued hospitalization of the newborn

C. PLANNING/IMPLEMENTATION
1. Prevention by decreasing risk factors when possible
   a. Teach regarding drug use and lifestyle risks
   b. Teach the importance of early reporting of temperature elevations
   c. Assess prenatal vaginal cultures
   d. Monitor for urinary tract infections; asymptomatic bacteriuria (ASB) shows a positive culture above 100,000/mm^3
2. Monitor vital signs, FHR, contractions, and progression of labor
3. Maintain bed rest
4. Inform client about medication; obtain consent; explain that the use of pain medications will be limited to avoid their depressive effects on the fetus
5. Provide emotional support: reduce anxiety and prepare for possible loss of infant
6. Provide special care related to the administration of tocolytic medications
   a. Obtain baseline blood data and electrocardiographic (ECG) readings
   b. Monitor vital signs; hypotension can occur with all tocolytics; tachycardia can occur with terbutaline and ritodrine

c. Maintain hydration but monitor for pulmonary edema
   d. Monitor for signs of hypokalemia and hyperglycemia
   e. Monitor intake and output and neurologic reflexes
7. Prepare for use of glucocorticoid therapy for fetus
8. Prepare for preterm birth if labor continues
9. Provide home instruction for halting preterm labor
   a. Assessments by home health nurse should include vital signs, FHR, breath sounds, fetal activity, cervical status, blood and urine glucose levels, fundal height, maternal weight, urine evaluation, presence of edema
   b. Rest periods in lateral position; avoidance of vigorous activity
   c. Increased fluid intake
   d. No sexual intercourse or sexual activity that leads to orgasm
   e. No nipple stimulation
   f. Avoidance of stressful events
   g. Empty bladder regularly and if contractions occur

D. EVALUATION/OUTCOMES
1. Mother demonstrates cessation of labor
2. Fetus remains in utero with acceptable fetal heart rate and fetal movements
3. Mother and partner state recurring signs of preterm labor

▼ POSTTERM LABOR

Data Base
A. Extends beyond the forty-first week of gestation or 2 weeks beyond expected date of birth; 38 to 42 weeks' gestation is considered full term
B. Fetal risk
   1. Decreased amniotic fluid may lead to cord compression during labor
   2. Decreased placental function because placental aging lowers oxygen and nutritional transport; fetus becomes compromised during labor (may become asphyxic or hypoglycemic)
   3. Increasing size (mainly length) and hardening of skull may contribute to cephalopelvic disproportion
C. Maternal risk present only if infant is excessively large
D. Therapeutic intervention: induction of labor

Nursing Care of Clients During Postterm Labor
A. ASSESSMENT
1. Number of weeks of gestation; date of last menstrual period; EDB

2. Biophysical profile, particularly amount of amniotic fluid
3. Fetal heart rate; results of stress and nonstress tests
4. Presence of meconium
5. Level of anxiety related to delayed date of birth
6. Newborn will have little vernix, long nails and hair, peeling wrinkled skin, reduced subcutaneous fat, meconium staining

B. ANALYSIS/NURSING DIAGNOSES
1. Fear related to fetal well-being because of aging placenta and decreased amniotic fluid
2. Risk for injury to mother and neonate related to large size of neonate

C. PLANNING/IMPLEMENTATION
See Planning/Implementation under Induction of Labor

D. EVALUATION/OUTCOMES
1. Progresses through labor to safe delivery of neonate
2. Remains free from complications

▼ DYSTOCIA

Data Base

A. Mechanical factors: cephalopelvic disproportion; contracted pelvis; malpresentation or position; multiple gestation
B. Faulty uterine contractions
   1. Hypertonic: increased frequency of contractions with decreased intensity; usually occurs in early labor; cervix does not dilate and mother becomes exhausted; increased fetal molding (caput succedaneum or cephalhematoma) may occur in older primigravidas or very anxious women
   2. Hypotonic: slowing of rate and intensity of contractions in latter part of labor
C. Maternal complications include cervical trauma, postpartal hemorrhage, infection, and exhaustion
D. Therapeutic interventions
   1. Deciding factors are length of labor, condition of mother and fetus, amount of cervical effacement and dilation, and fetal presentation, position, and station
   2. Oxytocics to stimulate labor
   3. Cesarean birth

Nursing Care of Clients with Dystocia

A. ASSSESSMENT
1. Progress of labor
2. Status of mother
3. Status of fetus; FHR
4. Ultrasonographic or x-ray examination to determine fetal and pelvic size

B. ANALYSIS/NURSING DIAGNOSES
1. Anxiety related to the uncertainty and length of labor process
2. Fatigue related to prolonged labor
3. Pain related to prolonged unproductive contractions and administration of oxytocics
4. Risk for trauma related to failure of cervix to amply dilate and/or mechanical problems

C. PLANNING/IMPLEMENTATION
1. Relieve back pain, caused by prolonged posterior pressure from fetus in occiput posterior position, by applying sacral pressure during contraction
2. Observe for signs of maternal exhaustion such as dehydration and acidosis/alkalosis
3. Monitor for signs of fetal distress
4. Have oxygen, suction, and resuscitation equipment readily available
5. Constantly monitor contractions, FHR, and vital signs when client is receiving oxytocic stimulation
6. Provide emotional support; keep client and family informed about progress
7. Administer fluids as ordered
8. Administer sedatives as ordered

D. EVALUATION/OUTCOMES
1. Rests/sleeps between contractions and after delivery
2. Progresses through labor to safe delivery of newborn
3. Remains free from complications

▼ PRECIPITATE LABOR

Data Base

A. Rapid labor and birth of less than 3-hour duration
B. Hazards to mother are perineal laceration and postpartum hemorrhage
C. Hazards to infant are anoxia and intracranial hemorrhage

Nursing Care of Clients During Precipitate Labor

A. ASSESSMENT
1. Rapid cervical dilation
2. Accelerated fetal descent
3. History of rapid labor
4. Rapid uterine contractions with decreased periods of relaxation between contractions

B. ANALYSIS/NURSING DIAGNOSES
1. Risk for maternal injury related to rapid expulsion of fetus resulting in lacerations and hemorrhage
2. Risk for fetal trauma related to cranial battering during rapid birth

C. PLANNING/IMPLEMENTATION
1. Remain with mother and monitor closely
2. Keep emergency birth pack at bedside
3. Keep mother and partner informed throughout process of labor and birth
4. Support and guide fetal head through birth canal when birth occurs

D. EVALUATION/OUTCOMES
1. Mother remains injury free
2. Neonate remains injury free

▼ BREECH BIRTH

Data Base

A. Position of fetus in which buttocks alone (frank breech), buttocks and feet (complete breech), or one or both feet (footling) descend through the birth canal first
B. Maternal implication: cesarean birth may be required, especially in primigravida
C. Fetal implications
1. Increased mortality
2. Occurrence of prolapsed cord leading to asphyxia
3. Birth trauma such as brachial palsy and fracture of the upper extremities

Nursing Care of Clients During Breech Birth

A. ASSESSMENT
1. Recognition of breech presentation on performing Leopold's maneuvers and vaginal examination
2. Auscultation of fetal heart tones above umbilicus
3. Presence of meconium without signs of fetal distress

B. ANALYSIS/NURSING DIAGNOSES
1. Pain related to prolonged posterior pressure of fetal buttocks
2. Risk for maternal or neonatal injury related to difficult birth
3. Risk for suffocation of fetus related to interruption in umbilical blood flow because of umbilical cord compression

C. PLANNING/IMPLEMENTATION
1. Use measures to promote comfort
2. Monitor the FHR in upper quadrants
3. Watch for prolapsed cord; if it occurs:
   a. With a sterile gloved hand push the presenting part off the cord
   b. Place the client in the Trendelenburg position to keep presenting part away from the cord
   c. Keep prolapsed cord moist with sterile saline
4. Observe for frank meconium; results from con-

traction of the uterus on lower colon of the fetus; not significant in breech birth
5. Add Piper forceps to the delivery set-up if vaginal birth is anticipated
6. Prepare client for cesarean birth; usually done in primigravidas
7. Teach mother and partner about the process of breech birth

D. EVALUATION/OUTCOMES
1. Mother remains free from injury
2. Neonate remains free from injury

▼ ABDOMINAL DELIVERY

Data Base

A. Birth of infant via transabdominal incision: transverse incision; lower uterine vertical incision
B. Indicated in cephalopelvic disproportion, dystocia, placenta previa and abruptio placentae, postmaturity, growths within the birth canal, multiple births, diabetes, PIH, Rh incompatibility, fetal distress, active herpes, and malpresentations such as breech birth
C. Vaginal birth after cesarean (VBAC) is an alternative for a woman who has had a horizontal uterine incision for an abdominal delivery
1. Each pregnancy may have different variables that make this attempt possible or impossible
2. Multiple uterine incisions may cause uterine rupture during labor

Nursing Care of Clients Following Abdominal Delivery

A. ASSESSMENT
1. Vital signs
2. Abdominal dressing: intact; presence of bleeding
3. Fundus and lochia; lochia may be less than that with vaginal birth
4. Urinary output: amount; specific gravity; presence of blood
5. Neurovascular status following regional anesthesia
6. Presence of pain
7. Response to neonate

B. ANALYSIS/NURSING DIAGNOSES
1. Ineffective breathing pattern related to pain on inhalation
2. Risk for infection related to surgical incision
3. Pain related to incision and/or flatus
4. Situational low self-esteem related to inability to deliver vaginally

C. PLANNING/IMPLEMENTATION
1. Assist with bonding; offer emotional support; encourage touching; include father in process
2. Encourage early ambulation to prevent blood stasis and promote peristalsis

3. Check vital signs, fundus, and abdominal incision; maintain IV infusion of oxytocin if ordered
4. Encourage eating of solids to promote peristalsis (prevents distention) when bowel sounds have returned
5. Administer analgesics as ordered
6. Promote lung aeration: deep breathing and coughing; incentive spirometer
7. Maintain fluid and electrolyte balance; monitor intake and output
8. Monitor urinary output

D. EVALUATION/OUTCOMES
1. States relief from pain
2. Maintains urinary and fecal elimination
3. Remains free from complications
4. Demonstrates bonding with newborn

▼ ASSISTED BIRTH

Data Base

A. Forceps: instrument used to shorten the second stage of labor; applied to head or presenting part to allow physician to control traction on infant's head; indicated in ineffective pushing, malposition, and large infants
B. Vacuum extraction: safer option than forceps; a cup is placed on the presenting part through which suction is applied to pull infant down; infant may develop succedaneum but is otherwise unharmed

Nursing Care of Clients During and Following Assisted Births

See Nursing Care During the Intrapartal Period and Nursing Care During the Postpartal Period

▼ POSTPARTAL BLEEDING

Data Base

A. Definition: bleeding in excess of 500 ml within the first 24 hours following birth; usually associated with uterine atony; vaginal, cervical, and perineal lacerations; hematomas; and retained placental fragments
1. Uterine atony may be influenced by overextension of uterus or increased tension on fibers
2. Lacerations are classified as
   a. First degree: superficial, extends through skin
   b. Second degree: extends through muscles of the perineum
   c. Third degree: extends through the anal sphincter
   d. Fourth degree: extends through all these structures and the anterior rectal wall

3. Hematomas may occur in the vagina, uterus, or perineum; they result from increased fundal pressure from fetus, forceps, or manipulation
4. Placental abnormalities can cause life-threatening hemorrhage
   a. Placenta accreta occurs when chorionic villi adhere to the uterine myometrium
   b. Placenta increta occurs when chorionic villi invade the myometrium
   c. Placenta percreta occurs when chorionic villi invade and pass through the myometrium to the peritoneal covering
B. Clinical findings
1. Large amount of frank, red bleeding
2. Boggy uterus
3. Signs of hypotension
4. Signs of disseminated intravascular coagulopathy (DIC)
   a. Profuse, uncontrollable bleeding from uterus
   b. Oozing of blood from episiotomy, laceration, or IV site
   c. Fragmented or distorted red blood cells
   d. Decreased coagulation factors (pathologic form of clotting)
C. Therapeutic interventions
1. Emptying bladder
2. Massaging of fundal portion of uterus
3. Administration of oxytocics
4. Blood replacement with severe blood loss
5. Surgical repair of vaginal and cervical lacerations
6. Removal of retained placental fragments
7. Cryoprecipitate, fresh frozen plasma for DIC

Nursing Care of Clients with Postpartal Bleeding

A. ASSESSMENT
1. Risk factors: multiparity; prolonged labor; analgesia; multiple gestation; abruptio placentae or placenta previa; PIH, especially HELLP
2. Vaginal bleeding and clots
3. Uterus for lack of tone (boggy)
4. Urinary output for decrease
5. Vital signs for signs of shock; pallor and fatigue
6. Level of anxiety

B. ANALYSIS/NURSING DIAGNOSES
1. Ineffective cardiopulmonary tissue perfusion related to hemorrhage
2. Fear related to uncontrollable bleeding and possible death
3. Risk for ineffective cerebral or peripheral tissue perfusion related to pathologic clotting

C. PLANNING/IMPLEMENTATION
1. Monitor vital signs and review laboratory results of blood studies

2. Assess fundus for height and firmness every 15 minutes; massage if boggy
3. Keep bladder from distending so that the uterus can contract; insert Foley catheter as ordered if voiding is insufficient; monitor intake and output
4. Ultrasonography for retained placental fragments
5. Monitor for bleeding: perineal pads, presence of clots
6. Administer oxytocin as ordered
7. Prepare for transfusions or emergency surgery if condition worsens

D. EVALUATION/OUTCOMES
1. Demonstrates hemodynamic stability
2. Remains free from complications

MATERNAL INJURIES RESULTING FROM BIRTH

▼ EPISIOTOMY

Data Base
A. Incision into perineum to facilitate birth and prevent lacerations and overstretching of the pelvic floor; it is usually made between the vaginal introitus and the rectum
B. Closed surgically; usually performed under regional anesthesia

Nursing Care of Clients After an Episiotomy
A. ASSESSMENT
1. Assess "REEDA": Redness; Edema; Ecchymosis; Discharge or drainage; Approximation of wound edges
2. Extent of pain
3. Signs of hematoma

B. ANALYSIS/NURSING DIAGNOSES
1. Risk for infection related to location of site near anal orifice and lack of knowledge of perineal care
2. Pain related to trauma to perineum

C. PLANNING/IMPLEMENTATION
1. Apply cold to limit edema during the first 12 to 24 hours if ordered
2. Provide and teach perineal care including when to change pads
3. Administer analgesics as ordered; may be systemic and/or local
4. Provide sitz baths if ordered
5. Teach perineal exercises (Kegel)

D. EVALUATION/OUTCOMES
1. States relief from pain
2. Remains free from infection

PREEXISTING HEALTH PROBLEMS THAT AFFECT PREGNANCY

▼ HEART DISEASE

Data Base
A. Origin: 90% rheumatic (incidence expected to decrease as incidence of rheumatic fever decreases); 10% congenital lesions or syphilis
B. Normal hemodynamics of pregnancy that adversely affect the client with heart disease
1. Oxygen consumption increased 10% to 20%; related to needs of growing fetus
2. Plasma level and blood volume increase; RBCs remain the same (physiologic anemia)
C. Functional or therapeutic classification of heart disease during pregnancy
1. Class I: no limitation of physical activity; no symptoms of cardiac insufficiency or angina
2. Class II: slight limitation of physical activity; may experience excessive fatigue, palpitation, angina, or dyspnea; slight limitations as indicated
3. Class III: moderate to marked limitation of physical activity; dyspnea, angina, and fatigue occur with slight activity, and bed rest is indicated during most of pregnancy
4. Class IV: marked limitation of physical activity; angina, dyspnea, and discomfort occur at rest; pregnancy should be avoided; indication for termination of pregnancy

Nursing Care of Pregnant Clients with Heart Disease
A. ASSESSMENT
1. Prenatal period: vital signs; weight gain; dietary patterns; emotional outlook; knowledge about self-care; signs of heart failure; stress factors such as work, household duties
2. Intrapartal period: vital signs (heart rate will increase); respiratory changes (dyspnea, coughing, or crackles); FHR patterns
3. Postpartal period: signs of heart failure or hemorrhage related to fluid shifts; intake and output

B. ANALYSIS/NURSING DIAGNOSES
1. Activity intolerance related to increased cardiac workload
2. Anxiety related to unknown course of pregnancy, possible loss of fetus, and inability to perform role responsibilities
3. Decreased cardiac output related to stress of pregnancy and pathology associated with heart disease

4. Fear related to possible death
5. Excess fluid volume related to fluid shifts resulting from a decrease in intraabdominal pressure following birth and/or a decrease in vascular space resulting from cessation of need for fetal circulation and uterine blood flow following birth
6. Risk for impaired parenting related to increased responsibility of caring for a neonate

C. PLANNING/IMPLEMENTATION
1. Prenatal period
   a. Teach importance of rest and avoidance of stress
   b. Instruct regarding use of elastic stockings and periodic elevation of legs
   c. Teach importance of continued medical supervision by cardiologist
   d. Teach appropriate dietary intake: adequate calories to ensure appropriate, but not excessive, weight gain; limited, not restricted, salt intake
   e. Administer medications as ordered: heparin, furosemide (Lasix), digitalis, betablockers (Inderal); antidysrhythmics (quinidine), disopyramide phosphate (Norpace)
   f. Monitor for signs of heart failure, such as respiratory distress and tachycardia; may be precipitated by severe anemia of pregnancy
2. Intrapartal period
   a. Encourage mother to remain in semi-Fowler's or left lateral position
   b. Provide continuous cardiac monitoring
   c. Provide electronic fetal monitoring
   d. Assist mother to cope with discomfort; minimal analgesia and anesthesia are used
   e. Assist with forceps birth in second stage of labor to avoid work of pushing
   f. Monitor for signs of heart failure, such as respiratory distress and tachycardia
3. Postpartal period: most critical time because of increased circulating blood volume after birth of placenta
   a. Institute early ambulation schedule; apply elastic stockings
   b. Monitor for signs of heart failure, such as respiratory distress and tachycardia
   c. Monitor heart rate; accelerated heart rate of mother in latter half of pregnancy puts extra workload on her heart
   d. Provide for adequate rest; the increase in oxygen consumption with contractions during labor makes length of labor a significant factor
   e. Provide close supervision; sudden tachycardia during birth or sudden bradycardia and normal increase in cardiac output following birth may cause cardiac arrest

   f. Administer prescribed prophylactic antibiotics to mother with history of rheumatic fever
   g. Refer to various agencies for family support, if necessary, on discharge
   h. Newborn risks include intrauterine growth retardation, prematurity, and hypoxia; fetal demise may occur

D. EVALUATION/OUTCOMES
1. Delivers healthy infant
2. Maintains cardiac status within acceptable limits
3. Uses resources to obtain help in the home

▼ DIABETES MELLITUS

Data Base
A. Normal physiology of pregnancy that affects woman with diabetes
   1. Vomiting during pregnancy, especially in the first trimester, decreases carbohydrate intake with resulting acidosis and insulin dosage adjustment
   2. Human placental lactogen decreases insulin response in pregnant diabetics; maternal sparing of glucose, and more oxidation of fats occurs to provide fetal nourishment; this leads to a greater need for insulin; although insulin increases, resistance to insulin also increases because of the presence of placental lactogen; thus more exogenous insulin is required to maintain normal serum glucose, especially in the latter part of pregnancy
   3. Elevated basal metabolic rate and decrease in carbon dioxide combining power increase tendency toward acidosis
   4. Normal lowered renal threshold for glucose can result in glucosuria
   5. Muscular activity during labor depletes glycogen; therefore carbohydrate intake must be increased
   6. During puerperium insulin antagonists are removed, hypoglycemia is common as involution and lactation occur and thus insulin needs decrease
B. Diabetes mellitus during pregnancy may be:
   1. Pregestational
      a. Type 1 diabetes
         Complications include retinopathy, neuropathy, and coronary artery disease
      b. Type II diabetes
         Complications include retinopathy, neuropathy, and coronary artery disease
   2. Gestational
      a. Diet controlled
      b. Insulin required

C. Hazards of diabetes during pregnancy
1. Often there is a history of anomalies, stillbirths, and fetal deaths
2. Babies are excessively large, weighing over 4000 g (macrosomia)
3. Neonatal deaths occur as a result of hypoxia, hypoglycemia, congenital anomalies, and preterm labor
4. Pregnancy-induced hypertension and hydramnios are common
5. Insulin therapy instituted; oral hypoglycemics contraindicated
6. Frequent hospitalization may be necessary during prenatal period
7. Cesarean birth may be necessary

Nursing Care of Pregnant Clients with Diabetes Mellitus

A. ASSESSMENT
1. Length of time client has had diabetes mellitus
2. Dietary patterns
3. Signs of infection
4. Blood glucose level; glucose tolerence test results; hemoglobin A_{1c} level
5. Understanding of disease in relation to pregnancy
6. Presence of support persons

B. ANALYSIS/NURSING DIAGNOSES
1. Fear related to health of newborn
2. Deficient fluid volume related to osmotic diuresis
3. Ineffective health maintenance related to lack of knowledge of newly diagnosed diabetes mellitus or management of previously diagnosed diabetes mellitus during pregnancy
4. Imbalanced nutrition: less than body requirements related to fetal growth and increased maternal metabolism
5. Risk for trauma related to large size of neonate

C. PLANNING/IMPLEMENTATION
1. Care of mother
   a. Encourage preconception counseling and early medical and prenatal supervision
   b. Teach and encourage adherence to dietary and insulin regimens
   c. Teach signs and symptoms of hyperglycemia (acidosis) and hypoglycemia (insulin reaction)
   d. Teach serum glucose testing, insulin administration, and record keeping
   e. Reinforce need for various tests for fetal well-being, such as ultrasound, stress and non-stress tests, amniocentesis for phosphatidylglycerol levels and L/S ratio
   f. Prepare client for induction of labor or cesarean birth if indicated
   g. Continue monitoring for fluid and electrolyte balance and ketoacidosis during intrapartal and postpartal periods
   h. Monitor glucose levels of all diabetic mothers

for the first 48 hours; postpartum women who were not insulin dependent before pregnancy will most likely not require it after delivery
2. Care of neonate
   a. Admit infant to neonatal intensive care unit if necessary
   b. Keep the infant warm because of poor temperature control mechanisms
   c. Observe respiration (stomach aspiration performed at time of birth, because hydramnios inflates stomach, which pushes up and interferes with diaphragm)
   d. Observe for signs of hypoglycemia and hypocalcemia such as lethargy, poor sucking reflex, cyanosis, or muscular twitching; decreased blood glucose (30 to 45 mg/dl)
   e. Provide glucose water feeding to prevent acidosis (with poor sucking reflex, glucose should be given parenterally)
   f. Observe for congenital anomalies; there is an increased incidence in babies of diabetic mothers
   g. Promote early mother-child interaction

D. EVALUATION/OUTCOMES
1. Maintains serum glucose levels within acceptable limits
2. Delivers a healthy newborn
3. Remains free from injury

▼ RESPIRATORY DISEASES

Data Base
A. Asthma is a lower respiratory tract disorder characterized by reversible hyperreactivity and bronchoconstriction; condition preexists and may worsen during pregnancy
1. May experience nonproductive cough, chest tightness, wheezing, and shortness of breath
2. Occurrence of an upper respiratory tract infection exacerbates symptoms, as does elevation of the uterus in the abdominal cavity
B. Tuberculosis is an infectious disease caused by the mycobacterium tuberculosis; populations at risk are those frequently immunocompromised or live under substandard conditions
1. May experience lethargy, systemic infections, cough, night sweats, weight loss, and fever
2. Occurrence of an upper respiratory tract infection exacerbates symptoms, as does elevation of uterus in the abdominal cavity
3. PPD is used for screening
C. Therapeutic interventions
1. Asthma
   a. Identify woman's triggers for attacks and prevent respiratory tract infection

b. Allergy desensitization (may be safely done during pregnancy if necessary)

c. Yearly influenza vaccination recommended by CDC (may be administered during pregnancy because it does not contain a live organism)

d. Inhaled bronchodilators are indicated during exacerbations; albuterol and metaproterenol are indicated

e. When bronchodilators are ineffective, glucocorticoids may be used to decrease inflammation and mucus secretions

2. Tuberculosis

a. Administration of isoniazid and rifampin unless the woman demonstrates resistance to isoniazid; treatment should continue for full 9 months

b. Ethambutol may be substituted for isoniazid

c. Pyridoxine (B_6) 50 mg/day is indicated

d. No other pharmacologic treatment may be substituted during pregnancy

e. Babies of untreated mothers are at risk when cared for by the mother after birth; transmission rate is 50%

f. Uninfected infants may receive BCG vaccine

Nursing Care of Pregnant Clients with Respiratory Disease

A. ASSESSMENT

1. Health history during initial prenatal visit to identify history of respiratory disease/exposure to tuberculosis

2. History of symptoms of tuberculosis

3. PPD test and follow-up cultures and chest x-ray if findings indicate possible infection

4. Case finding to limit spread of infection to family/community

5. History of predisposing factors/triggers to asthma attacks

B. ANALYSIS/NURSING DIAGNOSES

1. Fear related to impact of health problem on the newborn

2. Ineffective breathing pattern related to pressure of enlarging uterus on compromised lungs

3. Impaired fetal gas exchange related to maternal hypoxia

C. PLANNING/IMPLEMENTATION

1. Collaboration between pulmonary specialist and obstetric practitioners

2. Encourage mother to follow up on therapies and tests

3. Teach importance of adhering to pharmacologic protocols and maintaining hydration

4. Teach importance of continued prenatal evaluations to monitor fetal heart rate and activity

D. EVALUATION/OUTCOMES

1. Maintains pharmacologic regimen throughout pregnancy

2. Modifies activities to maintain optimal oxygenation

3. Maintains oxygenation so fetus remains well oxygenated and exhibits normal growth and reactivity

▼ CANCER

Data Base

A. Cancer risks increase with age and as women postpone pregnancy

B. Cancer of the breast is most common; cervical cancer, ovarian cancer, melanoma, leukemia, and lymphomas also occur

C. Cancer during this time creates a moral dilemma for the woman, the family, and the health team

D. Laparoscopic approach may be used for node sampling; surgical procedures increase risk for premature delivery, IUGR, and fetal demise

E. Chemotherapy is generally contraindicated because almost all drugs are teratogenic, especially in the first trimester

F. Radiotherapy is contraindicated because it puts the fetus at risk for abnormalities, low birth weight, cancer later in life, possible genetic effects on future generations of that fetus

Nursing Care of Pregnant Clients with Cancer

A. ASSESSMENT

1. Staging of cancer without exposing the fetus to radiation; ultrasound and magnetic resonance studies are preferred

2. Blood studies related to organ functioning are helpful; tumor markers may be influenced by oncofetal proteins found in maternal blood

B. ANALYSIS/NURSING DIAGNOSES

1. Anxiety related to threatened death of self/fetus

2. Fatigue related to overwhelming emotional and physiologic demands

3. Ineffective coping related to threat of loss of mother/fetus

C. PLANNING/IMPLEMENTATION

1. Explain treatment choices and plan

2. Assess woman's understanding of her condition and its effects on her and the pregnancy

3. Allow woman and family to express emotions; refer to appropriate practitioners, agencies, and clergy as needed

D. EVALUATION/OUTCOMES

1. Maintains emotional and physiologic well-being

2. Verbalizes fears

3. Arrives at decisions through problem solving
4. Uses appropriate support systems

PROBLEMS IN THE NEWBORN

▼ ASSESSMENT OF THE NEWBORN

Data Base

A. First stage of transition to extrauterine life (period of reactivity)
   1. Lasts 0 to 30 minutes
   2. Alert and moving
   3. Gustatory movements
   4. Heart rate increases to 160 to 180 beats per minutes for 15 minutes and then declines to 100 to 120 beats per minute
   5. Respirations are 60 to 80 per minute and irregular; grunting, flaring, and retractions may occur

B. Second stage of transition to extrauterine life (period of decreased responsiveness)
   1. Lasts 30 minutes to 2 hours
   2. Relaxation and rest occurs as baby settles down
   3. Heart rate between 100 and 120 beats per minute
   4. Respirations are fast (as high as 60 per minute), shallow, and synchronous; chest gradually changes shape to increase anterior-posterior diameter
   5. Bowel sounds begin to be heard

C. Third stage of transition to extrauterine life (second period of reactivity)
   1. Lasts 2 to 8 hours
   2. Increased responsiveness to stimuli
   3. Cardiac and respiratory cycles may increase
   4. Changes in color and muscle tone may occur
   5. Bowel sounds increase; may pass meconium

Nursing Care of the Newborn

A. ASSESSMENT
   1. Respiratory rate, heart rate, temperature, and cry
   2. Reflexes
   3. Weight, length, and head and chest circumference
   4. Head to toe assessment for structural deformities, color, molding, vernix, lanugo
   5. Glucose screening for presence of hypoglycemia

B. ANALYSIS/NURSING DIAGNOSES
   1. Ineffective airway clearance related to excessive secretions in respiratory passages
   2. Risk for ineffective thermoregulation related to immature compensation to change in the environment

C. PLANNING/IMPLEMENTATION
   1. Monitor respiratory and cardiac status; suction as needed; observe color; maintain temperature
   2. Wash baby after inspection; prevent chilling; swaddle after dressing
   3. Support mother's choice for feeding infant; assist with feeding techniques
   4. Support family in baby care choices
   5. Teach and monitor baby care related to safety issues; holding and carrying infant, sleeping with infant, bubbling infant, diaper changes, bathing, use of car seat, etc.

D. EVALUATION/OUTCOMES
   1. Maintains respiratory functioning free of respiratory distress
   2. Maintains temperature within normal limits

▼ PRETERM OR LOW–BIRTH-WEIGHT INFANT

Data Base

A. Prevention
   1. Prevention of preterm birth is vital because this is the cause of more than half of the neonatal deaths in the United States
   2. Prevention of malnutrition and underweight in the mother because these are associated with higher preterm birth rates, intrauterine growth retardation, and low–birth-weight babies
   3. Education about nutrition and general hygiene before planning a family
   4. Education about the hazards of drug use and smoking
   5. Adequate and early prenatal health supervision
   6. Referrals to community agencies to facilitate services to persons in need

B. Classification
   1. Classification of newborn infants is made on the basis of gestational age as well as birth weight; full-term infant may be of low birth weight, preterm infant need not be
   2. Preterm infant: born before term (36 weeks or less)
   3. Low–birth-weight infant: weighs 2500 g ($5\frac{1}{2}$ pounds) or less at birth

C. Therapeutic interventions for the low–birth-weight infant (LBW) immediately after birth
   1. Suctioning of mucus to maintain an open airway
   2. Direct laryngoscopy, tracheal suctioning, intubation, and mouth-to-tube resuscitation in the absence of respirations
   3. Suctioning of stomach contents at birth facilitates respirations

4. Heated Isolette; maintenance of body temperature is difficult because of heat loss by skin evaporation and limited subcutaneous fat
5. Readily available oxygen and resuscitation equipment at all times

D. Characteristics of preterm infant
1. Less subcutaneous fat, therefore the skin is wrinkled and blood vessels and bony structures are visible; lanugo present on face; eyebrows are absent; ears are poorly supported by cartilage; breast bud size is small with underdeveloped nipples; square window sign present
2. Circumference of the head is large in comparison with the chest; the fontanels are small and bones are soft
3. Skin color changes when infant is moved; upper half or one side of the body pale and lower half or one side of the body red (harlequin sign)
4. Posture is one of complete relaxation with marked extension of the legs and abduction of the hips; random movements are common with slightest stimulus
5. Heat regulation poorly developed because of immaturity of CNS; heat loss caused by large skin surface area and lack of subcutaneous and brown fat; poorly developed respiratory center with diminished oxygen consumption causing asphyxia; weak heart action, therefore slower circulation and poor oxygenation; insufficient heat production caused by inadequate metabolism
6. Respirations are not efficient because of muscular weakness of lungs and rib cage and limited surfactant production; retraction at xiphoid is evidence of air hunger; infant should be stimulated if apnea occurs
7. Atelectasis can occur; manifested by: cyanosis that decreases with crying; rapid, irregular respirations; flaring of nostrils; intercostal or suprasternal retractions; grunting on expiration
8. Greater tendency toward capillary fragility; red and white blood cell counts are low; anemia during first few months of life
9. Higher incidence of intracranial hemorrhage; manifested by muscle twitching, convulsions, cyanosis, abnormal respirations, and a short, shrill cry
10. Weak sucking and swallowing reflexes; small capacity of stomach; low gastric acidity; slow emptying time of the stomach; the usual caloric intake of 110 to 130 calories per kilogram (50 to 60 calories per pound) of body weight may need to be increased to 200 to 220 calories per kilogram (100 calories per pound) for adequate growth and development

11. Reduced glomerular filtration rate results in decreased ability to concentrate urine and conserve fluid

Nursing Care of Preterm Infants

A. ASSESSMENT
1. Respiratory rate and effort; heart rate; temperature; blood pressure
2. Oxygen concentrations via oximeter
3. Skin color and integrity
4. Daily weight; fluid and electrolyte status
5. Ability of infant to suck; nutritional status
6. Parents' ability to cope with preterm birth

B. ANALYSIS/NURSING DIAGNOSES
1. Risk for aspiration related to weak or absent gag reflex and/or administration of tube feedings
2. Impaired gas exchange related to interference with respiratory stimulation, lung immaturity, or airway obstruction
3. Impaired spontaneous ventilation related to respiratory muscle fatigue, cerebral immaturity, or damage to the cerebral respiratory center
4. Hypothermia related to lack of subcutaneous and brown fat deposits, inadequate shiver response, immature thermoregulation center, large body surface area in relation to body weight, and/or lack of flexion of extremities toward the body
5. Risk for infection related to immature immune response, stasis of respiratory secretions, and/or aspiration
6. Imbalanced nutrition: less than body requirements related to lack of energy to suck and/or weak or absent sucking reflex

C. PLANNING/IMPLEMENTATION
1. Maintain airway; check ventilator function if used; position to promote ventilation; suction when necessary; maintain temperature of environment
2. Observe for changes in respirations, color, and vital signs
3. Check efficacy of Isolette: maintain heat, humidity, and oxygen concentration; administer oxygen only if necessary; monitor oxygen carefully to prevent retinopathy of the newborn
4. Maintain aseptic technique to prevent infection
5. Adhere to the techniques of gavage feeding for safety of infant
6. Observe weight-gain patterns
7. Determine blood gases frequently to prevent acidosis
8. Institute phototherapy should hyperbilirubinemia occur
9. Refer parents to support group
10. Support parents by letting them verbalize and ask questions to relieve anxiety

11. Provide liberal visiting hours for parents, allow them to participate in care
12. Arrange follow-up before and after discharge by a visiting nurse

D. EVALUATION/OUTCOMES
1. Maintains respiratory functioning
2. Maintains body temperature within acceptable limits
3. Remains free from infection
4. Gains weight

▼ ASPHYXIA NEONATORUM

Data Base

A. Occurs when respirations are not well established within 60 seconds after birth as a result of anoxia, cerebral damage, or narcosis
B. Therapeutic interventions
   1. Preventive interventions: early prenatal care; prenatal education; early management of deviations from a normal pregnancy
   2. Medical management during labor and birth; resuscitative measures at birth

Nursing Care of Infants with Asphyxia Neonatorum

A. ASSESSMENT
1. Asphyxia livida: persistent generalized cyanosis and good muscle tone
2. Asphyxia pallida: marked pallor, poor muscle tone

B. ANALYSIS/NURSING DIAGNOSES
1. Impaired gas exchange related to respiratory depression secondary to narcosis
2. Impaired spontaneous ventilation related to respiratory or cerebral pathology

C. PLANNING/IMPLEMENTATION
1. Resuscitate immediately
2. Keep under close observation for first 24 hours
3. Keep equipment for intubation and oxygen administration readily available

D. EVALUATION/OUTCOMES
1. Breathes on own
2. Maintains adequate oxygen saturation

▼ RESPIRATORY DISTRESS SYNDROME (RDS)

Data Base

A. A deficiency in surface-active (detergent-like) lipoproteins (surfactant) results in inadequate lung inflation and ventilation
B. Can occur in preterm and low–birth-weight infants, and in infants following cesarean birth

C. Therapeutic intervention: surfactant replacement given to preterm infants through endotracheal tube

Nursing Care of Infants with Respiratory Distress Syndrome (RDS)

A. ASSESSMENT
1. Cyanosis
2. Tachypnea; dyspnea; sternal retractions; nasal flaring; grunting
3. Respiratory and metabolic acidosis

B. ANALYSIS/NURSING DIAGNOSES
1. Impaired gas exchange related to inadequate lung expansion
2. Impaired spontaneous ventilation related to immaturity of lung
3. Imbalanced nutrition: less than body requirements related to difficulty feeding

C. PLANNING/IMPLEMENTATION
1. Admit to neonatal intensive care unit
2. Keep the airway patent
3. Keep in an Isolette with oxygen and high humidity; prevent chilling
4. Administer surfactant by aerosol as ordered
5. Administer antibiotics as ordered
6. Maintain function of mechanical ventilation if employed
7. Monitor for signs of respiratory and metabolic acidosis
8. Administer feedings as ordered; prevent exhaustion

D. EVALUATION/OUTCOMES
1. Remains free from respiratory distress
2. Maintains fluid and electrolyte balance
3. Gains weight

▼ MECONIUM ASPIRATION SYNDROME (MAS)

Data Base

A. A hypoxic insult to fetus that causes increased intestinal peristalsis with passage of meconium into the amniotic fluid; the meconium-stained fluid is aspirated by the infant during the first few breaths after birth, causing an obstruction in the lung that results in chemical pneumonitis
B. Therapeutic interventions
   1. Suctioning after head is delivered
   2. Oxygenation and ventilation
   3. Prophylactic antibiotic therapy
   4. Bicarbonate for acidosis

Nursing Care for Infants with Meconium Aspiration Syndrome

A. ASSESSMENT
1. Signs of fetal hypoxia and meconium-stained amniotic fluid during intrapartum

2. Respiratory distress after birth
3. Signs of sepsis
4. Altered neurologic status (seizures)

B. ANALYSIS/NURSING DIAGNOSES
1. Impaired gas exchange related to aspiration of meconium and amniotic fluid into lungs
2. Risk for infection related to aspiration of meconium and amniotic fluid into lungs
3. Imbalanced nutrition: less than body requirements related to difficulty feeding

C. PLANNING/IMPLEMENTATION
1. Remove meconium and amniotic fluid from infant's nasopharynx and oropharynx immediately after birth
2. See Planning/Implementation under Respiratory Distress Syndrome (RDS)

D. EVALUATION/OUTCOMES
1. Maintains respiratory functioning
2. Remains free from infection
3. Feeds without difficulty

▼ CRANIAL BIRTH INJURIES

Data Base
A. Caput succedaneum: edema with extravasation of serum into scalp tissues caused by molding during the birth process; crosses the suture lines of the bony plates of the skull; no treatment is necessary; it subsides in a few days
B. Cephalhematoma: edema of the scalp with effusion of blood between the bone and periosteum; stops at the suture line; no treatment is necessary; it disappears within a few weeks to a few months after birth; resolution of hematoma can lead to hyperbilirubinemia
C. Intracranial hemorrhage: bleeding into cerebellum, pons, and medulla oblongata caused by a tearing of the tentorium cerebelli; occurs in preterm infants and following prolonged labor, difficult forceps birth, precipitate birth, version, or breech extraction

Nursing Care of Infants with Cranial Birth Injuries
A. ASSESSMENT
1. Abnormal respirations; cyanosis
2. Shrill or weak cry
3. Flaccidity or spasticity; seizures
4. Restlessness; wakefulness
5. Impaired sucking reflex

B. ANALYSIS/NURSING DIAGNOSES
1. Ineffective cerebral tissue perfusion related to intracranial hemorrhage
2. Risk for trauma related to edema

C. PLANNING/IMPLEMENTATION
1. Keep in Isolette with oxygen

2. Maintain in high-Fowler's position
3. Administer prescribed vitamins C and K to control and prevent further hemorrhage
4. Institute ordered gavage feedings when sucking reflex is impaired
5. Support parents because of guarded prognosis

D. EVALUATION/OUTCOMES
1. Remains free from neurologic damage
2. Gains weight

▼ NEUROMUSCULOSKELETAL BIRTH INJURIES

Data Base
A. Facial paralysis: asymmetry of face caused by damage to facial nerves from a difficult forceps birth
B. Erb-Duchenne paralysis (brachial palsy): caused by a difficult forceps or breech extraction birth; manifested by a flaccid arm with elbows extended; treatment depends on severity of paralysis
C. Dislocations and fractures are diagnosed by crepitation, immobility, and variations in range of motion; treatment depends on the site of fracture

Nursing Care of Infants with Neuromusculoskeletal Birth Injuries
A. ASSESSMENT
1. Variation in range of movement; immobility
2. Crepitation

B. ANALYSIS/NURSING DIAGNOSES
1. Pain related to injury
2. Impaired physical mobility related to injury, prescribed restrictions, and/or pain
3. Risk for impaired skin integrity related to impaired mobility and/or use of immobilizing devices
4. Risk for disuse syndrome related to injury

C. PLANNING/IMPLEMENTATION
1. Facial paralysis: no treatment is necessary because it usually disappears in a few days
2. Erb-Duchenne paralysis
   a. Massage and exercise arm as ordered to prevent contractures
   b. Place in "traffic cop" or "maitre d" position
   c. Apply ordered splints and braces, which are used when paralysis is severe
3. Dislocations and fractures: position as ordered; swaddling, splints, slings, or casts are used
4. Reassure parents and teach necessary care and positioning

D. EVALUATION/OUTCOMES
1. Maintains correct alignment of limb
2. Achieves movement in affected part

▼ CONGENITAL ABNORMALITIES

Structural or metabolic problems that may be genetically determined or a result of environmental interference during intrauterine life (See Pediatric Nursing for specific congenital problems)

▼ HEMOLYTIC DISEASE

Data Base

A. Rh incompatibility occurs when an Rh-negative woman is sensitized to Rh-positive blood from an Rh-positive fetus or other sources and develops antibodies against the Rh-positive blood
   1. In subsequent pregnancies these antibodies are transferred through the placental barrier to the fetus, with a resulting agglutination and destruction of red cells (erythroblastosis fetalis); rarely a problem in first pregnancy
   2. Prevention: RhoGAM, a preparation of Rho (D antigen) immune globulin, is now given intramuscularly to the Rh-negative mother about the twenty-eighth week of pregnancy and within 72 hours after birth or abortion to prevent the development of antibodies in this and future pregnancies; mother must be negative for Rh antibodies to receive RhoGAM
B. ABO incompatibility occurs when the fetal blood type is A, B, or AB and the mother is type O; mother's anti-A or anti-B antibodies are transferred through the placental barrier to the fetus, causing hemolysis and resulting in fetal anemia, jaundice, and kernicterus (excessively high bilirubin levels); ABO incompatibility is more common but less severe than Rh incompatibility; previous exposures to A, B, or AB blood does not increase the formation of anti-A or anti-B antibodies, so first pregnancy can be affected
C. Therapeutic interventions
   1. During pregnancy, amniotic fluid determinations are done by chemical and spectrophotometric analysis; elevated readings warrant either intrauterine transfusion or induction of labor, depending on the weeks of gestation
   2. Phototherapy is used in an attempt to reduce mild to moderate kernicterus
   3. Exchange transfusions are done on severely affected infants to decrease the antibody level and increase infant red blood cells and hemoglobin levels

Nursing Care of Infants with Hemolytic Disease

A. **ASSESSMENT**
   1. Blood incompatibility (ABO, Rh) between mother and fetus
   2. Jaundice and increasing bilirubin levels during first 24 hours
   3. Bilirubin, hematocrit, and hemoglobin levels
   4. Lethargy or irritability
   5. Poor feeding pattern; vomiting
   6. Enlargement of the liver and spleen
   7. Signs of kernicterus develop without exchange transfusion: absence of Moro reflex; apnea; high-pitched cry; opisthotonos; tremors; seizures
B. **ANALYSIS/NURSING DIAGNOSES**
   1. Risk for injury (agglutination and destruction of red blood cells) related to maternal antibody formation and (brain cell damage) related to high bilirubin levels
   2. Risk for deficient fluid volume related to phototherapy
C. **PLANNING/IMPLEMENTATION**
   1. Monitor maternal antibody titers
   2. Administer RhoGAM within 72 hours after birth if mother is Rh negative and neonate is Rh positive; teach why RhoGAM is necessary
   3. Teach mother why an exchange transfusion for the newborn may be necessary if the bilirubin level rises over 20 mg/dl
   4. Care for the neonate receiving phototherapy: protect eyes from light; monitor for signs of dehydration
D. **EVALUATION/OUTCOMES**
   1. Mother remains free from Rh isoimmunization
   2. Neonate remains free from injury

▼ THRUSH

Data Base

A. A mouth infection caused by *Candida albicans*
B. Organism may be transmitted as the neonate passes through the vaginal canal, by unclean feeding utensils, breasts that are improperly cleansed before breastfeeding, or by ineffective handwashing techniques

Nursing Care of Infants with Thrush

A. **ASSESSMENT**
   1. White patches on tongue, palate, and inner cheeks that bleed when touched
   2. Difficulty in sucking
B. **ANALYSIS/NURSING DIAGNOSES**
   1. Pain related to oral lesions
   2. Imbalanced nutrition: less than body requirements related to impaired sucking and oral pain
C. **PLANNING/IMPLEMENTATION**
   1. Teach how to cleanse breasts or feeding equipment before feeding
   2. Teach how to apply oral topical agents such as nystatin (Mycostatin)

D. EVALUATION/OUTCOMES
   1. Achieves infection-free status
   2. Gains weight

▼ OPHTHALMIA NEONATORUM

Data Base

A. An eye infection caused by *Neisseria gonorrhoeae* and *Chlamydia trachomatis*
B. Organism is transmitted from the genital tract of an infected mother during birth or by infected hands
C. Chlamydial infections can also cause pneumonia
D. Prevention: ophthalmic antibiotic (0.5% erythromycin ophthalmic ointment or 1% tetracycline ointment) instilled at birth after providing for initial bonding

Nursing Care of Infants with Ophthalmia Neonatorum

A. ASSESSMENT
   1. Perinatal history of maternal infection
   2. Purulent conjunctivitis if prophylactic treatment is not used; manifested 3 to 4 days after birth
   3. Respiratory status with chlamydial infection
B. ANALYSIS/NURSING DIAGNOSES
   1. Risk for infection related to transmission during gestation, passage through infected birth canal, and/or contamination by caregiver
   2. Risk for injury (corneal ulceration, blindness) related to infectious process
C. PLANNING/IMPLEMENTATION
   1. Cleanse the eyes with normal saline by wiping from inner to outer canthus
   2. Treat with prescribed antibiotics as ordered
   3. Refer for ophthalmic evaluation
   4. Monitor vital signs and administer oxygen with chlamydial infection
D. EVALUATION/OUTCOMES
   1. Maintains or achieves infection-free status
   2. Remains free from sequelae of infection

▼ SYPHILIS

Data Base

A. A congenital systemic infection caused by *Treponema pallidum*
B. Prenatal syphilis transmitted to fetus by the mother
C. Incidence of fetal infection varies with stage of the disease in the mother at the time of pregnancy; newborn of infected mother should be screened for syphilis
D. Before fourth month fetus seldom infected; Langhans' cells in chorion are protective barrier

E. The longer the infection goes untreated the greater the damage to the fetus; pregnant women are treated with penicillin when diagnosed
F. Adequate treatment of pregnant woman treats the fetus

Nursing Care of Infants with Syphilis

A. ASSESSMENT
   1. Perinatal history of maternal infection
   2. Maculopapular lesions of the palms of the hands and soles of the feet
   3. Restlessness
   4. Rhinitis; hoarse cry
   5. Enlargement of the spleen; palpable lymph nodes
   6. Enlarged ends of long bones on x-ray examination
B. ANALYSIS/NURSING DIAGNOSES
   1. Risk for infection related to transmission during gestation, passage through infected birth canal, and/or cross contamination by caregiver
   2. Delayed growth and development related to microbial invasion of cardiac and/or cerebral tissue
C. PLANNNING/IMPLEMENTATION
   1. Administer ordered antibiotics, usually penicillin
   2. Teach the importance of continued medical supervision
D. EVALUATION/OUTCOMES
   1. Maintains or achieves infection free status
   2. Remains free from sequelae of infection

▼ ACQUIRED IMMUNODEFICIENCY SYNDROME (AIDS)

Data Base

A. Generalized invasion of T cells by the human immunodeficiency virus (HIV)
B. Gynecologic manifestations occur first
   1. Recurrent vulvovaginal candidiasis
   2. Bacterial vaginosis
   3. Recurrent genital herpes simplex
   4. Human papillomavirus
   5. Pelvic inflammatory disease
   6. Cervical dysplasia and neoplasms
C. Transmitted by mother who is HIV positive
D. Infant should be screened for HIV infection when either parent is at high risk for or diagnosed as HIV positive.
E. Symptoms are usually not present at birth
F. If zidovudine (AZT) is taken by pregnant woman, transmission of HIV infection to the fetus is greatly reduced

Nursing Care of Infants with Acquired Immunodeficiency Syndrome

A. ASSESSMENT
   1. Signs of prematurity or small for gestational age
   2. Failure to thrive
   3. Enlarged spleen and liver
   4. Diarrhea; weight loss
   5. Neurologic deficits
   6. Frequent and debilitating infections as the child ages

B. ANALYSIS/NURSING DIAGNOSES
   1. Risk for infection related to transmission during gestation, passage through infected birth canal, and/or cross-contamination by care-giver
   2. Delayed growth and development related to microbial invasion of cardiac and/or cerebral tissue

C. PLANNING/IMPLEMENTATION
   1. Obtain blood specimen for HIV testing
   2. Institute and teach parents standard (blood and body fluid) precautions
   3. Inform parents that the virus may be transmitted via breast milk and that infant should be bottlefed
   4. Stress the importance of continued medical supervision
   5. Provide human contact to meet emotional needs

D. EVALUATION/OUTCOMES
   1. Infant remains free from opportunistic infections
   2. Caregiver maintains standard precautions

▼ NECROTIZING ENTEROCOLITIS (NEC)

Data Base

A. Necrotic lesions in intestines resulting from three factors: intestinal ischemia; presence of pathologic bacteria colonies; excess formula in intestines
B. More common in preterm infants and formula-fed infants; occurs several weeks after birth
C. Prevention: encouragement of breastfeeding
D. Therapeutic intervention: surgical excision often required, which may lead to short bowel syndrome

Nursing Care of Infants with Necrotizing Enterocolitis

A. ASSESSMENT
   1. Abdominal distention; diminished or absent bowel sounds
   2. Impaired sucking; vomiting; loss of weight
   3. Gastrointestinal bleeding

B. ANALYSIS/NURSING DIAGNOSES
   1. Deficient fluid volume related to diarrhea
   2. Impaired nutrition: less than body requirements related to impaired sucking, oral discomfort, diarrhea, and/or increased basal metabolic rate

C. PLANNING/IMPLEMENTATION
   1. Maintain NPO and nasogastric decompression
   2. Administer IV therapy and total parenteral nutrition as ordered
   3. Monitor fluid and electrolyte balance
   4. Provide ileostomy or colostomy care if ostomy has been created

D. EVALUATION/OUTCOMES
   1. Maintains fluid and electrolyte balance
   2. Gains weight

▼ SEPSIS

Data Base

A. A generalized bacterial infection
B. Precipitated by infected amniotic fluid, an infected birth canal, or a break in aseptic technique

Nursing Care of Infants with Sepsis

A. ASSESSMENT
   1. Poor feeding; vomiting
   2. High temperature
   3. Lethargy; increasing irritability
   4. Signs of anemia; pallor
   5. Increased number of stools

B. ANALYSIS/NURSING DIAGNOSES
   1. Risk for infection related to transmission during gestation, passage through infected birth canal, and/or cross-contamination by caregiver
   2. Hyperthermia related to microbial toxins
   3. Diarrhea related to pathogenic infection
   4. Deficient fluid volume related to diarrhea

C. PLANNING/IMPLEMENTATION
   1. Monitor intravenous fluid administration
   2. Administer oxygen as ordered
   3. Administer IV antibiotic therapy as ordered

D. EVALUATION/OUTCOME
   1. Maintains fluid and electrolyte status
   2. Achieves infection free status

▼ TORCHS

Data Base

A. An acronym for the following infections:
   1. **T**—Toxoplasmosis (*Toxoplasma gondii*): can be acquired by eating raw or undercooked meat or contacting cat feces; organism crosses the placenta; severity of infection related to gestational age; can cause hydrocephalus, intracranial calcifications, or chorioretinitis in the infant

2. **O**—Others (HIV, gonorrhea [*Neisseria gonorrhoeae*], human papillomavirus, varicella zoster, group B streptococcus, hepatitis B, measles, mumps)
3. **R**—Rubella (rubella virus): greatest risk to the fetus when maternal infection occurs in first 12 weeks of gestation; baby may be born with encephalitis, ocular abnormalities, cardiac maldevelopment, and other defects; these infants may have active viral infection and should be isolated until pharyngeal mucus and urine are free of virus; for mothers who have not had rubella or who are serologically negative, rubella vaccine should be given in the immediate postbirth period, not during pregnancy
4. **C**—Cytomegalic inclusion disease (cytomegalovirus): pregnant women usually asymptomatic; this sexually transmitted infection may cause hemolytic anemia, hydrocephalus, microcephalus, intrauterine growth retardation, or neonatal death
5. **H**—Herpes genitalis (herpesvirus): contracted by the mother during sexual relations; characterized by periods of exacerbations and remissions; first attack most severe; intercourse must be avoided during last 4 to 6 weeks of pregnancy; during active stage the infant must be delivered by cesarean birth; if delivered vaginally, neonatal infection can be disseminated and result in death; surviving infants suffer CNS involvement
6. **S**—Syphilis
B. Therapeutic interventions: care is directed toward prevention and early treatment in the pregnant woman to eliminate or reduce risk to the fetus

▼ SUBSTANCE DEPENDENCE (NEONATAL ABSTINENCE SYNDROME)

Data Base
A. Infant born with physiologic dependence on alcohol or drugs as a result of maternal drug use and/or abuse
B. Dependence: many preparations, including alcohol, methadone, heroin, cocaine
C. Perinatal mortality: 6 to 8 times higher than in nonusing control group
D. Alcohol abuse in the mother can result in fetal alcohol syndrome, producing congenital defects and retardation
E. Clinical findings
   1. Infant may exhibit signs of respiratory distress, jaundice, congenital anomalies, and behavioral aberrations

   2. Withdrawal symptoms appear soon after birth; severity depends on the length of maternal addiction, the type of drug used, the amount of drug taken, the concurrent use of other drugs, and the time the drug was taken before birth; may persist for up to 4 months

Nursing Care of Infants Who Are Dependent on Alcohol or Drugs
A. ASSESSMENT
   1. Maternal intake of drug, including type, time, and amount
   2. Signs of withdrawal in the infant
      a. Facial scratches; hyperactivity; tremors; seizures
      b. Yawning; disturbed sleep
      c. Tachypnea; sneezing; stuffy nose
      d. Shrill cry
      e. Poor sucking; drooling; vomiting
      f. Diarrhea; excoriated buttocks
B. ANALYSIS/NURSING DIAGNOSES
   1. Ineffective breathing pattern related to respiratory depression because of presence of narcotic
   2. Delayed growth and development related to addiction to narcotics, congenital anomalies, and/or mental retardation associated with fetal alcohol syndrome
   3. Imbalanced nutrition: less than body requirements related to hyperactivity, lethargy, and/or uncoordinated sucking
   4. Pain related to withdrawal
   5. Sleep pattern disturbance related to withdrawal and/or use of sedatives
C. PLANNING/IMPLEMENTATION
   1. Monitor infant's neuromuscular status
   2. Monitor vital signs; support respiratory functioning
   3. Provide small, frequent feedings
   4. Administer sedatives or narcotics as ordered
   5. Keep environmental stimuli to a minimum; maintain seizure precautions
   6. Promote mother-infant bonding when possible; provide a constant caregiver
   7. Hold and cuddle frequently but provide for periods of uninterrupted rest
   8. Swaddle infant when in crib
   9. Use soft nipple to reduce sucking effort; administer supplemental methods of nutritional support as ordered
   10 Encourage continued medical supervision
   11. Refer to appropriate community-service agencies for family support and supervision
D. EVALUATION/OUTCOMES
   1. Maintains respiratory functioning
   2. Survives withdrawal from drug
   3. Establishes a sleeping pattern
   4. Gains weight

FAMILY PLANNING

▼ CONTRACEPTIVE METHODS

Data Base

A. Oral contraceptives: used to prevent conception by inhibiting ovulation; causing atrophic changes in the endometrium to prevent implantation; and causing a thickening of cervical mucus to inhibit sperm travel
1. Combined form: inhibits hypothalamus, pituitary, and various hormone production
   a. Monophasic: synthetic estrogen in each pill that is taken for 21 days; package usually contains 28 pills, seven of which are free of estrogen; withdrawal bleeding occurs during the 7 days when the nonmedication pills are taken
   b. Biphasic: small amounts of estrogen are taken throughout the cycle; in a 21-day package, the first 10 pills contain small amounts of synthetic estrogen and the next 11 pills contain an increased amount of estrogen
   c. Triphasic: small doses of combined hormones that alter levels of estrogen and progesterone throughout the cycle
   d. Advantages of combined oral contraceptives: 100% effective if taken correctly; coitus independence because they are not taken in relation to intercourse; bleeding days are predictable; pills may alleviate symptoms of premenstrual syndrome (PMS), endometriosis, and dysmenorrhea
   e. Examples of estrogen-progestin products (combined form): Demulen; Loestrin; Ortho-Novum
2. Minipills: a low dose of progesterone is given alone; inhibits ovulation; regimen makes uterine environment hostile to sperm
   a. Advantages of minipills: fewer side effects; can be used by lactating women; may be used by women over 35 and those with a history of headaches and mild hypertension
   b. Examples of progestin products (minipills): Micronor; Ovrette
3. Major side effects
   a. Thrombophlebitis (increased platelets and clotting factors, intimal thickening, and vein dilation)
   b. Hypertension; breast tenderness (fluid retention)
   c. Libido changes (hormonal effect)
   d. Hyperglycemia (decreased carbohydrate tolerance)
   e. CNS disturbances (hormonal effects and fluid retention)
   f. Breakthrough bleeding (estrogen effect)
4. Contraindications for the use of oral contraceptives: advanced maternal age; smoking; hypertension; thrombophlebitis; breast malignancy; cerebral vascular accident; breastfeeding mothers, depending on the form of drug

B. Intrauterine devices (IUD): device inserted into the uterus preventing fertilization or implantation; copper IUD damages sperm and few reach ovum; progesterone IUD affects cervical mucus and endometrial maturation; may cause uterine irritability, increased bleeding, and risk for infection
C. Diaphragm: mechanical device that fits over cervix and prevents sperm from entering cervical os; use with spermicide
D. Cervical cap: a rubber thimblelike device that fits over the cervix after it is filled with a spermicide; may provide protection for up to 48 hours after insertion
E. Female condom: latex vaginal sheath that is an elongated pouch with a ring at each end; one ring covers the cervix and the other covers the labia; available without a prescription
F. Male condom: latex sheath that covers penis and prevents semen from entering cervical os
G. Creams, jellies, foam tablets, and vaginal suppositories: spermicidal (generally low pH) preparations inserted into vaginal canal by applicator immediately before coitus (used in conjunction with the diaphragm and condom for added protection); method of choice with health problems such as diabetes mellitus
H. Coitus interruptus: withdrawal during sexual intercourse before ejaculation; least effective method
I. Fertility awareness methods: the plotting of the basal body temperature to determine fertile period so that abstinence from coitus is practiced; the basal body temperature dips slightly 24 hours before ovulation, then rises sharply; stress and infection can falsely elevate temperature; used in conjunction with cervical mucus changes (Billings method)
J. Norplant system (implantable progestin): placement of six flexible rods of levonorgestrel under the skin of the upper arm; effective for 5 years; removal restores fertility; irregular periods may occur
K. Depo-Provera (injectable progestin): IM injection of medroxyprogesterone acetate that lasts 3 months; suppresses FSH and LH
L. Postcoital contraception: used after unprotected intercourse ("morning after pill"); pharmacologic management of high dose of estrogen, progesterone, or testosterone; mechanical technique is insertion of an IUD
M. Surgical sterilization

1. Bilateral vasectomy: small incision made into the scrotum and the vas deferens is ligated, producing sterilization in the male by preventing ejaculation of sperm; usually performed on an outpatient basis
2. Tubal ligation: interruption in the continuity of fallopian tubes by surgical transection, electric cautery, or compression with soft clamp, preventing impregnation of ovum by sperm; accomplished by laparotomy, laparoscopy, or culdoscopy

Nursing Care of Clients Concerned with Family Planning

A. ASSESSMENT
1. Medical and family history of woman
2. Clients' beliefs about sexuality, pregnancy, contraception, and abortion
3. Clients' understanding of family planning
4. Clients' readiness to learn

B. ANALYSIS/NURSING DIAGNOSES
1. Health-seeking behaviors related to desire to control future pregnancies
2. Decisional conflict related to lack of relevant information, uncertainty about alternative contraceptive methods, lack of experience with contraceptives, and/or challenge to a personal value
3. Anxiety related to potential irreversibility of some methods and potential side effects

C. PLANNING/IMPLEMENTATION
1. Help couples to expand their knowledge about human sexuality
2. Maintain optimum emotional and physical health of the family
3. Inform the couple of available methods; include both in planning
4. Provide an accepting atmosphere; give them the freedom of choice
5. Review specific medication/administration schedule with client and review procedure to follow if doses are missed when oral contraceptives are being used
6. Teach side effects of oral contraceptives and instruct client to inform the physician if they should occur
7. Encourage periodic physical examination for all women using any contraceptive method; should include breast and pelvic examination, Papanicolaou test, and mammography
8. Teach couples electing surgical sterilization that in the female sterility is immediately achieved, whereas in the male sterility is not achieved until semen is free of sperm; use an additional method of birth control until semen is free of sperm

D. EVALUATION/OUTCOMES
1. Couple delays pregnancy until desired
2. Returns for follow-up health care

▼ INFERTILITY AND STERILITY

Data Base

A. Sterility: presence of an absolute factor that makes a person unable to produce offspring
B. Infertility: inability on the part of a couple to conceive after consistent attempts for a 1-year period; woman has never conceived; man has never impregnated a woman
   1. Primary infertility occurs when the couple has never had a child
   2. Secondary infertility occurs when the couple has conceived but the woman is unable to sustain pregnancy or conceive again
C. Male infertility and sterility
   1. Coital difficulties: chordee (painful, downward-curving erection) or marked obesity
   2. Spermatozoal abnormalities: small ejaculatory volume, low sperm count, increased viscosity, reduced motility of spermatozoa, and/or more than 30% abnormal sperm forms
   3. Testicular abnormalities: agenesis or degenesis of testes, cryptorchidism; poor maturation of the spermatozoa; physical injury caused by trauma, mumps, irradiation, or increased temperature for prolonged periods
   4. Varicocele: a swollen vein in the testicle
   5. Abnormalities of the penis or urethra: hypospadias or urethral stricture
   6. Prostate and seminal vesicle abnormalities: chronic prostatitis or seminal vesiculitis
   7. Abnormalities of the epididymis and vas deferens: inflammation or closure
   8. Severe nutritional deficiencies
   9. Other factors such as radiation to testicles, excessive smoking and alcohol intake, smoking of marijuana, and in utero, exposure to diethylstilbestrol (DES)
D. Female infertility and sterility
   1. Endocrine disorders: pituitary, thyroid, or adrenal
   2. Vaginal disorders: absence or stenosis of vagina, imperforate hymen, vaginitis, chronic infections
   3. Cervical abnormalities: cervical obstruction by cervical polyps or tumors
   4. Uterine abnormalities: hypoplasia, endometriosis, uterine neoplasms
   5. Tubal disorders: obstruction (generally the result of infections such as chlamydia or gonorrhea), perisalpingeal adhesions

6. Ovarian abnormalities: congenital abnormalities such as ovarian dysgenesis or agenesis, infections, tumors; hormonal imbalances
7. Emotional problems: severe psychoneurosis or psychosis may cause anovulatory cycles
8. Coital factors: feminine hygiene preparations (including douches) that decrease vaginal pH may inactivate or destroy spermatozoa; sodium bicarbonate douches may be used to raise vaginal pH
9. Chronic disease states
10. Immunologic reactions to sperm
11. Nutritional factors such as malnutrition, anorexia nervosa

E. Combined factors
   1. Lack of coital success
   2. Female antibodies to male sperm

F. Diagnostic measures
   1. Male: history, physical examination, semen analysis
   2. Female: history, physical examination, CBC, sedimentation rate, serologic tests, urinalysis, T3, T4, TSH, x-ray films of the chest, basal metabolic rate determination, postcoital (Sims-Huhner) test, endometrial biopsy, tubal insufflation, hysterosalpingography, culdoscopy, urine lutenizing hormone predictor kits (measure the LH in the urine to predict ovulation to time intercourse or artificial insemination), laparoscopy, chlamydia test

G. Therapeutic interventions
   1. Education about the menstrual cycle and timing of intercourse
   2. Surgery, depending on the cause
   3. Pharmacologic management
   4. Intrauterine insemination (IUI) and ovulation-inducing drugs
   5. In vitro fertilization
   6. IVF with intracytoplasmic sperm injection for severe male infertility
   7. Stress management
   8. Adoption
   9. Surrogate motherhood

H. Drugs that affect gonadal function and fertility
   1. Androgens (testosterone derivatives)
      a. Used to replace deficient hormones in males after puberty and before the climacteric to improve development of secondary sex characteristics
      b. Adverse effects: adolescent males may have premature epiphyseal closure (decreased skeletal development, height stops increasing)
   2. Estrogens
      a. Primarily used to replace deficient hormones to control hormonal balance in menopausal or postmenopausal women or to maintain menses and fertility during reproductive years
      b. Adverse effects of estrogen: anorexia (depression of appetite center); nausea and vomiting (gastrointestinal irritation); tissue fluid accumulation (altered tissue hydrostatic pressure)
   3. Conception enhancers
      a. Ovulatory stimulants
         (1) Clomiphene citrate (Clomid) is a follicle-maturing agent used during the fifth to tenth day of the menstrual cycle
         (2) Bromocriptine (Parlodel) inhibits the release of prolactin, which can cause anovulation
         (3) Human menopausal gonadotropin (Pergonal) acts similarly to FSH or LH to stimulate growth and maturation of ovarian follicles
         (4) Gonadotropin-releasing hormone (GnRH) is used when clomiphene is ineffective
      b. Hormone replacement therapy with conjugated estrogens and medroxyprogesterone
      c. For hyperplasia defects
         (1) Danazol (Danocrine and Cyclomen) reduces endometrial hyperplasia; acts on estrogen receptors to inhibit estrogen defects
         (2) Prednisone reduces adrenal hyperplasia
         (3) These drugs have an androgenic effect that can cause weight gain, hirsutism, decreased breast size, and oiliness of the skin
      d. Adverse effects of conception enhancers
         (1) Multiple births (increases ovulation)
         (2) Visual changes (direct toxic effect)
         (3) Dizziness, lightheadedness (CNS depression)

WOMEN'S HEALTH

THE FEMALE REPRODUCTIVE SYSTEM
Ovaries: Female Gonads
A. Location: behind and below uterine tubes, anchored to uterus and broad ligaments
B. Size and shape of large almonds
C. Microscopic structure: each ovary of the newborn female consists of several hundred thousand graafian follicles embedded in connective tissues; follicles are epithelial sacs in which ova develop; usually, between the years of menarche and menopause, one follicle matures each month, ruptures the surface of the ovary, and expels its ovum into the pelvic cavity

D. Functions
   1. Oogenesis: formation of a mature ovum in a graafian follicle
   2. Ovulation: expulsion of the ovum from follicle into the pelvic cavity
   3. Secretion of ovarian hormones: maturing follicle secretes estrogens (estradiol, estrone, and estriol) and corpus luteum secretes progesterone and estrogens
      a. Estrogens: stimulate development of secondary sexual characteristics, thickening of endometrium, development of breasts, contractions of the pregnant uterus; mildly accelerate sodium and water reabsorption by kidney tubules; increase water content of uterus; accelerate protein anabolism; stimulate long bone calcification
      b. Progesterone: prepares endometrium for implantation of fertilized ovum; inhibits uterine contractions during pregnancy; promotes development of alveoli of estrogen-primed breasts; necessary for lactation; inhibits oxytocin release by neurohypophysis; oxytocin is otherwise released in response to vaginal distention

Uterine Tubes (Fallopian Tubes, Oviducts)

A. Location: attached to upper, outer angles of uterus
B. Structure: same three coats as uterus; distal ends fimbriated and open into pelvic cavity; mucosal lining of tubes and peritoneal lining of pelvis in direct contact here (permits spread of infection from tubes to peritoneum)
C. Function: serve as ducts through which ova travel from ovaries to uterus; fertilization normally occurs in tube

Uterus

A. Location: in pelvic cavity between the bladder and rectum
B. Structure
   1. Shape and size: pear-shaped organ approximately the size of a clenched fist
   2. Divisions.
      a. Body: upper and main part of the uterus; fundus, the bulging upper surface of the body
      b. Cervix: narrow, lower part of the uterus; projects into the vagina
   3. Walls: composed of smooth muscle (myometrium) lined with mucosa (endometrium)
   4. Cavities
      a. Body cavity: small and triangular with three openings into it; two from uterine tubes, one into cervical canal

      b. Cervical cavity: canal with constricted opening, internal os into body cavity and another, external os, into vagina
   5. Blood supply: uterine and ovarian arteries
C. Position: flexed between body and cervix with the body portion lying over the bladder, pointing forward and slightly upward; cervix joins the vagina at right angles; ligaments hold the uterus in position (broad ligaments, uterosacral ligaments, posterior ligament, anterior ligament, round ligaments)
D. Functions: menstruation; pregnancy; labor

Vagina

A. Location: between rectum and urethra
B. Structure: collapsible, musculomembranous tube, capable of great distention; outlet to exterior covered by fold of mucous membrane called hymen
C. Functions
   1. Receives semen from the male
   2. Constitutes lower part of birth canal
   3. Acts as excretory duct for uterine secretions and menstrual flow

Vulva

Consists of numerous structures that together constitute external genitals
A. Mons veneris: hairy, skin-covered pad of fat over the symphysis pubis
B. Labia majora: hairy, skin-covered folds
C. Labia minora: small folds covered with modified skin
D. Clitoris: small mound of erectile tissue, below junction of two labia minora
E. Urinary meatus: just below clitoris; opening into urethra
F. Vaginal orifice: below urinary meatus; opening into vagina; hymen, fold of mucosa, partially closes orifice
G. Skene's glands: small mucous glands; ducts open on each side of the urinary meatus
H. Bartholin's glands: two small, bean-shaped glands; duct from each gland opens on side of the vaginal orifice; both Bartholin's glands and Skene's glands frequently become infected (especially by gonococci)

Breasts (Mammary Glands)

A. Location: just under skin, over the pectoralis major muscles
B. Size: depends on deposits of adipose tissue rather than on amount of glandular tissue (which is approximately same in all females)
C. Structure: divided into lobes and lobules that, in turn, are composed of racemose glands; excretory

duct leads from each lobe to opening in nipple; circular pigmented area, the areola, borders nipples
D. Function: secrete milk (lactation)
   1. Shedding of placenta causes marked decrease in blood levels of estrogens and progesterone, which in turn stimulates anterior pituitary to increase prolactin secretion; high blood level of prolactin stimulates alveoli of breast to secrete milk
   2. Suckling controls lactation in two ways: by acting in some way to stimulate anterior pituitary secretion of prolactin and to stimulate posterior pituitary secretion of oxytocin, which stimulates release of milk out of alveoli into ducts (let-down reflex) from which infant can remove it by suckling

 RELATED PHARMACOLOGY

Estrogens

(See Drugs that affect gonadal function and fertility under Infertility and Sterility)
A. Description
   1. Organic compounds secreted by ovarian follicles in females; exert effect during the proliferative phase of the menstrual cycle
   2. Used to regulate menstrual disorders, uterine bleeding, menopausal and postmenopausal problems, and as a contraceptive; also used as hormonal therapy for men with certain cancers of the reproductive/urinary system; used judiciously because of cancer-causing potential
   3. Available in oral, parenteral (IM, IV), intravaginal, and topical, including transdermal, preparations
B. Examples
   1. Diethylstilbestrol (DES)
   2. Estradiol preparations (Estrace, Estraderm)
   3. Estrogenic substances, conjugated (Premarin)
C. Major side effects
   1. Thrombophlebitis (increased clot formation)
   2. Nausea (irritation of gastric mucosa)
   3. Breast tenderness (promotion of sodium and water retention)
   4. Hyperglycemia (decreased carbohydrate tolerance)
   5. Males: gynecomastia, loss of libido, and testicular atrophy (hormonal imbalance related to estrogen antagonism)
   6. Deficiency of one or more of the B complex vitamins may be induced with prolonged use
D. Nursing care
   1. Obtain history to assess for medical problems that may contraindicate use
   2. Assess for edema
   3. Instruct client to:

      a. Use proper procedure for application of topical or intravaginal preparations
      b. Report unusual vaginal bleeding to physician immediately
      c. Avoid smoking during therapy to decrease risk of serious cardiovascular side effects
      d. Eat foods rich in B complex vitamins daily; B complex vitamin supplements should also be considered
   4. Monitor blood glucose in diabetics during therapy
   5. Reassure male clients that feminizing side effects will subside when therapy is completed

Progestins

A. Description
   1. Female ovarian hormones that prepare the uterus for implantation of a fertilized ovum; essential for the maintenance of pregnancy
   2. Used in the treatment of endometriosis, infertility, dysmenorrhea, secondary amenorrhea, and to suppress ovulation
   3. Available in oral and parenteral (IM) preparations
B. Examples
   1. Hydroxyprogesterone caproate (Hylutin)
   2. Medroxyprogesterone acetate (Provera, Depo-Provera)
   3. Megestrol acetate (Megace)
   4. Norethindrone (Norlutin)
   5. Progesterone (Progestaject)
C. Major side effects
   1. Initial use may cause profuse vaginal flow (shedding of accumulations of endometrial tissue), spotting, irregular bleeding, nausea, lethargy, jaundice
   2. Edema (promotion of sodium and water retention)
   3. GU disturbances (renal dysfunction aggravated by fluid retention)
   4. Visual disturbances (possibility of blood clots or neuroocular lesions)
   5. Scleral jaundice (hepatic alterations)
   6. Thrombophlebitis (increased clot formation)
   7. Depression (CNS effect)
   8. Deficiency of one or more B complex vitamins may result from prolonged use
D. Nursing care
   1. Obtain client history to assess for medical problems that may contraindicate use
   2. Assess client for edema during therapy
   3. Inform significant others regarding potential for development of depression
   4. Instruct client to eat foods rich in the B complex vitamins daily; B complex vitamin supplements should also be considered

RELATED PROCEDURES
Pelvic Examination
A. Definition
1. Examination of female reproductive structures
2. Consists of:
   a. Abdominal examination
   b. Inspection and palpation of external genitalia
   c. Vaginal examination bimanually and with a speculum to inspect cervix and vaginal walls
3. As indicated or ordered, obtain specimen for:
   a. Gonorrheal culture from endocervical canal
   b. *Chlamydia trachomatis* smear from urethra and cervix (fluorescien-monoclonal antibody test)
   c. Herpes simplex 1 and 2 viral culture of a smear from the lesion
   d. Cytologic examination (Papanicolaou test) of cells from endocervical canal and cervix
B. Nursing care
1. Explain examination and collection of specimens to client
2. Teach to avoid douching 24 hours before examination
3. Request client to empty bladder before examination
4. Help to relax by asking client to:
   a. Breathe slowly and deeply, exhaling with mouth open and lips in "O" shape
   b. Avoid squeezing eyes closed or clenching fists
5. Instruct to bear down when speculum is introduced
6. If client is pregnant, observe for signs of hypotension, such as pallor, dizziness, tachycardia, nausea, and diaphoresis; if symptoms occur position client on side until symptoms subside and vital signs are within normal limits

Mammography
A. Definition
1. An x-ray study of the soft tissue of the breast
2. Technique allows detection of nonpalpable masses
3. Women between the ages of 35 and 40 should have a baseline mamography; between the ages of 40 and 50 a mamography should be performed yearly
B. Nursing care
1. Instruct client to avoid use of deodorants or powders before test
2. Maintain privacy
3. Explain that stretching and compression of breast tissue may be uncomfortable
4. Stress importance of regular breast self-examinations (BSE) for early detection; schedule examination after menstrual period when breast density and tenderness are decreased

Breast Biopsy
A. Definition
1. Excision: removal of mass for cytologic study
2. Incision: removal of tissue from mass for cytologic study
3. Needle (aspiration, stereotactic): removal of tissue or fluid from mass through needle for cytologic study
B. Nursing care
1. Explain procedure to client
2. Allow ample time to express feelings
3. Instruct to assess site for bleeding or edema
4. Stress importance of continued health-care supervision

MAJOR DISORDERS AFFECTING WOMEN'S HEALTH

▼ CANCER OF THE CERVIX

Data Base
A. Etiology and pathophysiology
1. Slow, malignant change in the tissue forming the neck of the uterus at the squamocolumnar junction
2. Multiple sexual partners and sexually transmitted diseases are considered risk factors
3. High cure rate when diagnosed early
4. Tends to spread by direct invasion of surrounding tissues and metastases to the lungs, bones, and liver
5. Females exposed to diethylstilbestrol (DES) in utero have an increased risk of vaginal cancer
6. Females with viral exposure to HPV, HIV, or HSV are at increased risk
7. Erosions of cervix often result from changes in pH and can be precursors of cancer
B. Clinical findings
1. Subjective (when invasive): back and leg pain
2. Objective
   a. Spotting between menstrual periods and after intercourse
   b. Vaginal discharge
   c. Lengthening of the menstrual period
   d. Papanicolaou cytologic finding of cellular changes consistent with precancerous or cancerous conditions
C. Therapeutic interventions
1. Type of surgical intervention depends on extent of lesion and physical condition of client:
   a. Stage I—confined to the cervix
   b. Stage II—extends beyond the cervix but not to the pelvic sidewall

c. Stage III—extends to the pelvic sidewall and lower vagina

d. Stage IV—extends beyond the pelvis to the bladder or rectum

2. Hysterosalpingo-oophorectomy (panhysterectomy) to remove uterus, fallopian tubes, and ovaries; menstruation and ovarian function ceases; in advanced lesions parametrial tissue and lymph nodes may also be removed

3. Hysterectomy to remove uterus; menstruation ceases but ovarian function continues

4. Internal or external radiation therapy alone or in conjunction with surgery may be ordered to reduce the lesion and limit metastases

5. Laser therapy

6. Cryosurgery—freezing technique

7. Conization to remove cone-shaped area of cervix while preserving reproductive functions

8. Loop electrode excision

Nursing Care of Clients with Cancer of the Cervix

A. ASSESSMENT

1. Risk factors from history

2. Description of onset and progression of symptoms

3. Cervical specimen for Papanicolaou smear

B. ANALYSIS/NURSING DIAGNOSES

1. Disturbed body image related to alteration in structure

2. Anticipatory grieving related to loss of body part and concerns about dying

3. Ineffective sexuality patterns related to alteration in structure and function of reproductive system

C. PLANNING/IMPLEMENTATION

1. Assist the client and family in dealing with the diagnosis of cancer

2. Allow and encourage the client to express feelings and concerns about change in self-image and sexual functioning

3. Support the client's feminine image

4. Provide care for the client receiving internal radiation

a. Explain the procedures involved and the side effects that may occur

b. Instruct the client in maintaining proper positioning (supine with head of bed flat or only slightly elevated)

c. Inspect the implant for proper position

d. Provide low-residue diet and antidiarrheal agents to prevent bowel movements; urinary catheterization to avoid displacement of radioactive substance and irradiation of adjacent tissues

e. Explain the need for isolation; explain to client and visitors that the amount of time they can spend in the room will be limited to avoid overexposure to radiation; pregnant women and children should be restricted from visiting

f. Utilize principles of time, distance, and shielding to minimize staff exposure

g. See Radiation in Medical-Surgical Nursing

5. Provide care following surgery

a. Maintain patency of the urinary catheter that was inserted before surgery to decompress the bladder and reduce stress on the operative site

b. Observe for reestablishment of bowel sounds

c. Maintain accurate intake and output

d. After removal of the urinary catheter, note the amount of output and pattern of voiding; catheterize for residual urine if ordered and whenever necessary for urinary retention

e. See Nursing Care of Clients with a Hysterectomy under Uterine Neoplasms

D. EVALUATION/OUTCOMES

1. Verbalizes feelings to family and health care providers

2. Maintains satisfying sexual expression

3. Copes with effects of treatment and potential prognosis

4. Continues health supervision

▼ UTERINE NEOPLASMS

Data Base

A. Etiology and pathophysiology

1. Endometrial polyps

a. Localized overgrowths of endometrial glands and stroma that occur on cervix and more frequently in the fundus of the uterus; usually benign

b. Stimulated by estrogen

c. Occur more frequently in premenopausal women who are anovulatory

2. Uterine fibroids (leiomyomas, myomas, fibromas, and fibromyomas)

a. Benign tumors of the uterine muscle

b. Occur more frequently in black women and women who have not been pregnant

c. Stimulated by estrogen

d. Diminish after menopause

e. Rarely become malignant

3. Endometrial cancer (adenocarcinoma, adenoacanthoma, and adenosquamous carcinoma)

a. Malignant overgrowth of the lining of the uterus

b. Risk factors include hormone replacement therapy (HRT), unopposed estrogen therapy, pelvic radiation, obesity, and family history

c. Most common malignancy of the female reproductive system

d. Occurs more frequently with hormone imbalance, obesity, nulliparity, late menopause, dysfunctional bleeding, anovulation, uninterrupted estrogen stimulation, diabetes mellitus, and early menarche

e. Occurs twice as often in white women as in black women

f. Spreads by direct extension or metastasis

g. Direct extension to myometrium, vagina, and paracervical tissue

h. Metastasizes to abdominal cavity, liver, lung, brain, and bone; progression is slow and metastasis occurs late

B. Clinical findings
1. Endometrial polyps
   a. Frequently asymptomatic
   b. Intermenstrual bleeding (metrorrhagia)
2. Leiomyomas
   a. Frequently asymptomatic
   b. Excessive menstrual bleeding (menorrhagia)
   c. Signs of pressure from an enlarging mass such as low abdominal discomfort, backache, visceral displacement, and constipation
   d. Painful menstruation (dysmenorrhea)
   e. Problems with pregnancy such as preterm labor, abortion, and dystocia
3. Endometrial cancer
   a. Premenopausal recurrent metrorrhagia
   b. Postmenopausal bleeding
   c. FIGO classification system of endometrial cancer extends from stage IA G123, where tumors are limited to endometrium, to stage IVB, where there are distant metastases to the intraabdominal area or inguinal lymph nodes

C. Therapeutic interventions
1. Intervention depends on the type and extent of the lesion, the physical condition of the client, and the stage of the endometrial carcinoma
2. Dilation and curettage (D&C) for polyps
3. Myomectomy or hysterectomy for benign neoplasms; when surgery is not advisable, radiation therapy is employed
4. Total hysterectomy with bilateral salpingo-oophorectomy for endometrial neoplasms
5. Intracavitary radiation may be done before or after surgery, depending on the stage of endometrial cancer
6. Hormonal therapy with progestins for endometrial cancer
7. Combination chemotherapy with antineoplastic drugs such as cyclophosphamide (Cytoxan), doxorubicin (Adriamycin), and cisplatin (Platinol) for endometrial neoplasms

Nursing Care of Clients with a Hysterectomy

A. **ASSESSMENT**
1. Gynecological history
2. Description of onset and progression of symptoms if present
3. Feelings regarding loss of uterus

B. **ANALYSIS/NURSING DIAGNOSES**
1. Pain related to surgical procedure
2. Anticipatory grieving related to loss of uterus, concerns about dying, loss of childbearing ability
3. Ineffective sexuality pattern related to loss of uterus
4. Ineffective tissue perfusion (peripheral) related to pelvic vascularity

C. **PLANNING/IMPLEMENTATION**
1. Encourage healthy lifestyle, weight reduction if overweight, use of combined HRT, and routine pelvic examinations
2. Monitor fluid and electrolyte balance
3. Maintain patency of urinary catheter; assess output while catheter is in place and after it is removed
4. Encourage coughing and deep breathing at frequent intervals
5. Assess bowel sounds and gas pains; insert a rectal tube or administer a Harris flush as ordered
6. Encourage frequent ambulation and elevation of extremities when sitting to prevent thrombophlebitis; apply antiembolism stockings if ordered
7. Provide emotional support; encourage ventilation of feelings
8. Teach to postpone driving for several weeks and to avoid sexual intercourse, strenuous exercise, and heavy lifting for 6 to 8 weeks
9. Care for the client receiving chemotherapy or radiation (see General Nursing Care of Clients Receiving Either Chemotherapy or Radiation Therapy)
10. Emphasize the importance of continuing health supervision

D. **EVALUATION/OUTCOMES**
1. Verbalizes concerns
2. Adjusts to loss of reproductive organs
3. Establishes bowel and bladder patterns
4. Continues health supervision

▼ CANCER OF THE OVARY

Data Base

A. Etiology and pathophysiology
1. Histologic cell types influenced by age
   a. Malignant germ cell tumors more frequent between 20 to 40 years of age

b. Epithelial cell tumors more frequent in perimenopausal women
2. More common in white women than in black women; rare in Asian women
3. Incidence influenced by hormonal factors; environmental factors have been implicated but not proven
4. Risk factors: ovarian dysfunction; irregular menses; infertility; genetic predisposition (BRCA 1 or BRCA 2 genes are observed in families); endometriosis; early menopause; nulliparity
5. Rarely diagnosed early because the abdominal cavity can accommodate an enlarging ovary without causing symptoms; poor prognosis because of the advanced stage at initial diagnosis, which is usually stage II to IV
6. Metastasizes to the peritoneum, omentum, and bowel surfaces
B. Clinical findings
1. Subjective: vague, lower abdominal discomfort or pain; feeling of fullness; rapid satiation; dyspepsia; nausea
2. Objective
a. Increasing abdominal girth (ovarian enlargement or ascites)
b. Constipation; anemia; vomiting; cachexia
c. Change in weight
d. Urinary frequency and urgency
e. Enlarged ovary on palpation
f. Elevated CA 125 antigen
g. Pleural effusion
C. Therapeutic interventions
1. Depend on the stage of disease
2. Surgical removal of the tumor via oophorectomy, salpingo-oophorectomy, panhysterectomy, and removal of any involved structures; oophorectomy causes surgical menopause
3. Cytoreductive surgery to debulk poorly vascularized large tumors; the smaller the remaining tumor the better the response to adjuvant therapy
4. Adjuvant therapy after tumor debulking
a. Chemotherapy with antineoplastic drugs such as cyclophosphamide (Cytoxan), cisplatin (Platinol), and doxorubicin (Adriamycin) for epithelial carcinoma
b. Intraperitoneal instillation of radioactive phosphorus (^{32}P)
c. External radiation therapy
d. Paclitaxel (Taxol) for ovarian cancer that has been unresponsive to first line or other therapy

Nursing Care of Clients with Ovarian Cancer
See Nursing Care Of Clients with A Hysterectomy under Uterine Neoplasms and General Nursing Care of Clients Receiving Either Chemotherapy or Radiation Therapy

▼ VAGINITIS
Data Base
A. Etiology and pathophysiology
1. Trichomoniasis: infection with *Trichomonas vaginalis,* a protozoan
2. Candidiasis (moniliasis): caused by *Candida albicans,* a fungus; incidence is high in clients with diabetes mellitus and those receiving antibiotic therapy because of change in normal flora
3. Bacterial vaginosis: caused by overgrowth of normal vaginal flora
4. Atrophic vaginitis: common in the postmenopausal period
5. May occur because of oral contraceptive use, sexually transmitted diseases, or allergic reactions
B. Clinical findings
1. Subjective: pruritus; burning; dysuria; dyspareunia (pain with intercourse)
2. Objective
a. Vaginal discharge
(1) Malodorous, thin, yellow discharge (trichomoniasis)
(2) White "cheesy" discharge (moniliasis)
(3) Grayish-white discharge; malodorous (bacterial vaginosis)
b. Vaginal smear can indicate *Trichomonas vaginalis, Candida albicans,* or other microorganisms
C. Therapeutic interventions
1. Antifungal preparations for candidiasis: terconazole (Terazol), over-the-counter antifungal creams; yogurt may also be used
2. Antiprotozoan preparation for trichomoniasis: metronidazole (Flagyl) tablets taken orally; clotrimazole cream vaginally
3. For bacterial vaginosis clindamycin (Cleocin) cream or oral administration, metronidazole (Flagyl) cream or tablets
4. Estrogen therapy prescribed for atrophic vaginitis

Nursing Care of Clients with Vaginitis
A. ASSESSMENT
1. History of onset and progression of symptoms
2. Presence of risk factors: improper use of tampons or douches; antibiotic use; multiple sexual partners; diabetes mellitus
3. Appearance and color of vaginal discharge
4. Pelvic examination and specimen for culture
B. ANALYSIS/NURSING DIAGNOSES
1. Risk for infection related to lack of information

2. Pain related to inflammation
3. Ineffective sexuality patterns related to fear of transmission, restriction of intercourse until infection resolves

C. PLANNING/IMPLEMENTATION
1. Advise the client to have sexual partner use a condom during coitus until vaginitis is resolved; sexual partner may also require treatment
2. Explain that frequent douching will alter the normal pH environment of the vagina, predisposing to vaginitis
3. Teach the importance of wearing loose-fitting clothing and cotton underwear and to avoid wearing pantyhose and tight pants
4. Administer a douche if ordered
   a. Explain procedure to the client; provide privacy
   b. Assemble equipment, including douche bag, catheter tip, bedpan, gloves, waterproof pads, and solution at 110° F (45° C) (30 ml of vinegar may be added to a liter of solution for acetic solution; alkaline solutions should never be utilized for vaginitis)
   c. Have the client assume the dorsal recumbent position on a bedpan
   d. Wearing gloves, separate the labia and insert the tip into the vagina toward the sacrum
   e. Rotate the douche tip gently so the solution reaches all vaginal folds
   f. When all solution is used, instruct the client to bear down to expel as much remaining solution as possible; solution returns during the entire procedure
   g. Dry the perineal area gently
5. Instruct the client who is receiving antibiotics or having recurrent vaginal infections to include yogurt or food supplements containing *Lactobacillus acidophilus* in the diet to maintain the normal vaginal flora

D. EVALUATION/OUTCOMES
1. Expresses relief of pruritus and pain
2. Discusses need for diagnostic screening and precautions with sexual partner
3. Achieves resolution of infection

▼ ENDOMETRIOSIS

Data Base

A. Etiology and pathophysiology
1. Growth of endometrial tissue in areas outside the uterus, such as ovaries, ligaments, or any abdominal organ
2. May be linked to retrograde menstruation or vascular and lymphatic system dissemination of endometrial tissue relocation

3. Generally affects young, nulliparous women; unrelated to menopause
4. Endometrial cells are stimulated by the ovarian hormones; will cause bleeding during normal menstrual cycle (if located in ovary, a pseudocyst or chocolate cyst is formed)
5. Adhesions are common and may result in sterility and pain
6. Adenomyosis is a similar condition affecting women 40 to 50 years old in which the endometrial cells invade the muscles of the uterus

B. Clinical findings
1. Subjective
   a. Chronic lower abdominal pain and backache beginning 2 to 7 days before menstruation, becoming progressively worse, and then diminishing as the menstrual flow decreases
   b. Dyspareunia
   c. Pain associated with defecation
2. Objective
   a. Abnormal uterine bleeding (metrorrhagia, menorrhagia)
   b. Infertility

C. Therapeutic interventions
1. Hormone therapy to suppress ovulation; young married women are advised not to delay pregnancy if children are desired; breastfeeding delays return of symptoms
   a. Oral contraceptives and/or progesterone to cause tissue to slough off
   b. Synthetic analog of gonadotropin-releasing hormone, such as nafarelin (Synarel) may be administered intranasally to reduce lesions because they are sensitive to ovarian hormones
   c. Gonadotropin inhibitors such as danazol (Cyclomen)
2. Surgical intervention
   a. Laparoscopic evaluation to confirm diagnosis
   b. Resection of lesions
   c. Oophorectomy, salpingectomy, and total hysterectomy if condition is severe
3. Laser ablation

Nursing Care of Clients with Endometriosis

A. ASSESSMENT
1. Description of onset and progression of symptoms
2. Pelvic examination
3. Concerns about childbearing

B. ANALYSIS/NURSING DIAGNOSES
1. Pain related to disease process, surgical procedures
2. Anticipatory grieving related to loss of body part, potential for infertility
3. Ineffective role performance related to infertility

C. **PLANNING/IMPLEMENTATION**
1. Provide time for client to talk about feelings
2. Administer analgesics as ordered
3. Review contraindications, side effects, and administration of prescribed hormones (see Related Pharmacology in Women's Health)
4. Discuss alternatives if pregnancy does not occur
5. Provide care following surgery (see Nursing Care of Clients with a Hysterectomy under Uterine Neoplasms)
6. Provide referrals to Endometriosis Society and other community-based support groups

D. **EVALUATION/OUTCOMES**
1. Experiences relief from pain
2. Verbalizes concerns about altered body image and infertility

▼ PELVIC INFLAMMATORY DISEASE (PID)

Data Base
A. Etiology and pathophysiology
1. Occurs within female pelvic cavity; can affect the uterus (endometriosis), fallopian tubes (salpingitis), ovaries (oophoritis), peritoneum, surrounding connective tissue, and pelvic veins
2. May be acute or chronic, bilateral or unilateral
3. Caused most often by the introduction of bacteria (usually through the cervical opening), such as gonococci and chlamydia, or tubercle bacilli that are transported by the blood from the lungs
4. If untreated, can lead to adhesions, sterility, ectopic pregnancy, and peritonitis
5. Risk factors include multiple sex partners, history of sexually transmitted diseases, IUD insertion, douching, sexual activity during menses, and nulliparity
B. Clinical findings
1. Subjective: severe cramping pain in lower abdomen; nausea; malaise; dysmenorrhea; dyspareunia
2. Objective
   a. Elevated temperature; increased WBC
   b. Foul-smelling, purulent vaginal discharge
   c. Cultures of vaginal discharge reveal causative organism
C. Therapeutic interventions
1. Medication to control pain and fever
2. Antibiotics depending on the organism
3. Identification and notification of sexual contacts and the state department of health if sexually transmitted disease is present

Nursing Care of Clients with Pelvic Inflammatory Disease (PID)
A. **ASSESSMENT**
1. Description of onset and progression of symptoms
2. Potential source of infection
3. Pelvic examination and specimens for culture
4. Characteristics of discharge
5. Vital signs and white blood cell count for baseline data
B. **ANALYSIS/NURSING DIAGNOSES**
1. Pain related to inflammation
2. Anticipatory grieving related to loss of body part, potential for infertility
3. Ineffective sexuality patterns related to fear of transmission of infection
C. **PLANNING/IMPLEMENTATION**
1. Monitor temperature, white blood cell count, and culture reports
2. Explain the importance of completing prescribed antibiotic therapy; advise client of side effects; follow up 72 hours after treatment is begun to assess response to therapy
3. Maintain the client on bed rest in a semi-Fowler's position to localize the infection and prevent the formation of abscesses within the abdominal cavity
4. Apply heat if ordered to the abdomen or via a douche to improve circulation
5. Observe and record the amount and character of vaginal discharge
6. Change perineal pads frequently using gloves; tampons should not be used
7. Explain safety measures to prevent reinfection of the client or others; during the treatment phase the client should abstain from intercourse
8. Allow time for client to verbalize feelings about illness and/or possible complication of infertility
9. Explain importance of prenatal care if pregnancy occurs
10. Teach signs of ectopic pregnancy because of increased risk
D. **EVALUATION/OUTCOMES**
1. Expresses relief from pain
2. Discusses need for diagnostic screening and precautions with sexual partner
3. Achieves resolution of infection
4. Verbalizes concerns

▼ CYSTOCELE AND/OR RECTOCELE

Data Base
A. Etiology and pathophysiology
1. Cystocele: herniation of the bladder into the vagina

2. Rectocele: herniation of the rectum into the vagina
3. Both conditions may be present at the same time and are generally associated with relaxation or injury of the pelvic muscles during childbirth
4. Fistulas may occur
   a. Rectovaginal: opening between rectum and vagina
   b. Vesicovaginal: opening between bladder and vagina
   c. Ureterovaginal: opening between a ureter and vagina

B. Clinical findings
   1. Subjective: feeling of fullness in vagina; back pain; constant urge to urinate or defecate; dysuria
   2. Objective
      a. Soft, reducible mass evident during vaginal examination that increases when client is asked to bear down
      b. Stress incontinence; frequency; urgency
      c. Residual urine (60 ml or more after voiding)
      d. Constipation

C. Therapeutic interventions
   1. Anterior colporrhaphy to correct a cystocele
   2. Posterior colporrhaphy to correct a rectocele
   3. Insertion of a pessary for mild symptoms

Nursing Care of Clients with a Cystocele and/or Rectocele

A. **ASSESSMENT**
   1. Description of onset and progression of symptoms
   2. Pelvic examination
   3. Presence and extent of urinary retention
   4. Impact of symptoms on client's lifestyle

B. **ANALYSIS/NURSING DIAGNOSES**
   1. Constipation related to pressure on the colon
   2. Impaired urinary elimination related to obstruction
   3. Incontinence (stress, urge) related to disease process
   4. Situational low self-esteem related to incontinence

C. **PLANNING/IMPLEMENTATION**
   1. Teach client care related to use of a pessary (e.g., cleaning, removing, or having it done periodically)
   2. Encourage the client to perform Kegel exercises to strengthen perineal muscles
   3. Instruct client about preventing constipation (e.g., high-fiber diet, fluids, exercise, and stool softeners as prescribed)
   4. Provide time for client to verbalize fears and ask questions

5. Provide postoperative care
   a. Maintain patency of urinary catheter; when catheter is removed assess for signs of retention
   b. Encourage voiding every 4 hours to prevent strain on the suture line from a distended bladder; perform residual urines as ordered (no more than 150 ml should accumulate)
   c. After each bowel movement and voiding, cleanse perineum with warm soap and water and flush with warm water using a peri-bottle; always cleanse away from vagina and toward anus; sitz baths can also be used
   d. Administer douches if ordered; include client instruction
   e. Apply anesthetic spray, or ice packs if ordered to relieve discomfort
   f. Administer ordered stool softeners to limit straining at stool and pressure on the suture line
   g. Encourage intake of liquids on first postoperative day and a regular diet on the second day

D. **EVALUATION/OUTCOMES**
   1. Establishes a regular pattern of bowel elimination
   2. Remains free from episodes of urinary incontinence

▼ PROLAPSED UTERUS

Data Base
A. Etiology and pathophysiology
   1. As a result of weakness of the pelvic floor, the uterus descends into the vagina; most often associated with childbirth injury or increased intraabdominal pressure (classified first to fourth degree)
   2. If severe, the entire uterus may protrude outside the vaginal orifice; in this case, the vagina is actually inverted; referred to as procidentia
   3. Ulcerations in procidentia increase risk of cancer

B. Clinical findings
   1. Subjective: heaviness within the pelvis; low back pain
   2. Objective
      a. Mass in the lower vagina or outside the orifice
      b. Elongated cervix
      c. Urinary retention and/or incontinence

C. Therapeutic interventions
   1. Vaginal pessary to maintain the uterus in correct position
   2. Surgical intervention

a. Suspension of the uterus and correction of retroversion

b. Pelvic floor exercises

c. Pelvic surgery to resuspend the uterus and resupport the musculature

d. Vaginal hysterectomy (if postmenopausal or if future pregnancy is not desired)

Nursing Care of Clients with a Prolapsed Uterus

A. ASSESSMENT

1. Description of onset and progression of symptoms

2. Pelvic examination; note degree (grade) of prolapse and presence of cystocele or rectocele

3. Degree of interference with urinary and bowel elimination

4. Presence of ulcerations on skin or mucous membranes

B. ANALYSIS/NURSING DIAGNOSES

1. Urinary retention related to physical obstruction of the urethra

2. Incontinence (stress, urge) related to disease process

3. Constipation related to pressure on the colon

4. Ineffective role performance related to interference with sexual functioning

C. PLANNING/IMPLEMENTATION

1. If procidentia is present, observe for ulcerations; apply warm saline compresses or protective ointment to prevent ulceration

2. Explain that if pessary is used, it must be taken out periodically and cleaned

3. Monitor the color, amount, and frequency of urination

4. Monitor the consistency, amount, and frequency of bowel movements

5. Provide postoperative care (see Nursing Care of Clients with Cancer of the Cervix)

D. EVALUATION/OUTCOMES

1. Maintains integrity of skin and mucous membranes

2. Establishes a regular pattern of bowel elimination

3. Establishes a regular pattern of urinary elimination

4. Reestablishes a satisfying sexual relationship

▼ BENIGN BREAST DISEASE

Data Base

A. Etiology and pathophysiology

1. Fibrocystic breast condition is characterized by fluid-filled cysts in the breast; linked to hormonal imbalance and caffeine consumption; may feel soft or hard on palpation; pain is common; it is a risk factor for breast cancer

2. Papillomas are intraductal lesions within the terminal duct; occur in women older than 40 years; may cause bloody nipple discharge; multiple growths may be cancerous

3. Ductal ectasia occurs in the subareolar area of aging breasts (seen in perimenopausal or postmenopausal women); duct is palpable with burning, pain, sticky nipple discharge; not generally associated with cancer

B. Clinical findings

1. Subjective: painful tender breasts (mastalgia)

2. Objective

a. Palpable lesions that may be hard or soft

b. Nipple discharge may be bloody with papilloma or sticky with ductal ectasia

3. Mammography identifies location and shape of lesion

4. Biopsy determines pathology of lesions

C. Therapeutic interventions

1. Interventions depend on the extent of the disorder

2. Aspiration of cysts for cytology studies; biopsies of suspicious findings

3. Mammographies and breast self-examination on a regular basis

4. Dietary modification to decrease the intake of caffeine and fat

Nursing Care of Clients with Benign Breast Disease

A. ASSESSMENT

1. Breast-oriented history that includes menstrual history, mammographies, hormone therapy, and breast cancer

2. Breast examination

B. ANALYSIS/NURSING DIAGNOSES

1. Disturbed body image related to fear of disfiguring procedures

2. Fear related to possible diagnosis of cancer

3. Ineffective therapeutic regimen management related to fear of finding another mass

C. PLANNING/IMPLEMENTATION

1. Instruct client regarding importance of monthly breast self-examination and yearly mammography studies

2. Explain importance of dietary restrictions of caffeine and fat

3. Listen to client's feelings and concerns regarding fear of findings; do not minimize concerns

D. EVALUATION/OUTCOMES

1. Discusses feelings and concerns with health team members

2. Expresses decreased pain in the breasts

3. Continues planned follow-up with breast self-examination and yearly mammographies

▼ CANCER OF THE BREAST

Data Base

A. Etiology and pathophysiology
1. Frequently begins as a hard, nontender, relatively fixed nodule; found most often in the upper, outer quadrant of the breast
2. Most breast cancers are adenocarcinomas originating in the ducts and lobes
3. Incidence increases with age and longer exposure to estrogen; influenced by heredity, the number of menstrual cycles (menarche before age 12, menopause after age 55), nulliparity or parity after age 35; multiparas and women with early menopause have a lower incidence
4. History of first-degree relative with breast cancer or presence of BRCA genes greatly increases risk
5. Recent studies have implicated a high-fat, selenium-deficient diet; estrogen-replacement therapy; obesity; and alcohol as contributing factors
6. Most common sites of metastasis are bone, bone marrow, soft tissue, lungs, liver, and brain
7. Extent of disease reflected by staging; nodal involvement most important prognostic factor; tumors may be estrogen- or progesterone-receptor positive

B. Clinical findings
1. Subjective: lesion generally nontender; malaise in later stages
2. Objective
   a. Palpable, irregularly shaped, fixed mass; most often in upper, outer quadrant
   b. Asymmetry of breasts; inversion and discharge from nipple
   c. Dimpling and change of color of skin over lesion; in late stages skin has orange-peel (peau d'orange) appearance
   d. Enlarged axillary lymph nodes
   e. Positive findings in following tests
      (1) Mammography: baseline between 35 and 40 years of age; q 1 to 2 years after 40 years of age; every year after 50 years of age
      (2) Thermography: heat-sensing device to evaluate abnormal circulatory signs
      (3) Sonography
      (4) Biopsy for cytologic evaluation (see Biopsy in Related Procedures)
      (5) Estrogen receptor assay: if positive, indicates need for alteration of the hormonal environment by surgical or chemical means
      (6) Tumor markers: Ca 15-3 and Ca 125; carcinoembryonic antigen (CEA) in serum, plasma, or cerebrospinal fluid: indicative of progression of cancer, particularly of the breast, ovaries, and gastrointestinal tract

C. Therapeutic interventions
1. Intervention depends on the extent of the TNM assessment and the physical status of the client
2. Surgical intervention
   a. Partial mastectomy (lumpectomy, wide excision, segmental resection, or quadrantectomy): removal of the lump and surrounding breast tissue
   b. Simple mastectomy: removal of the breast only
   c. Radical mastectomy: removal of the breast, pectoral muscles, pectoral fascia, and nodes (pectoral, subclavicular, apical, and axillary); this procedure may be modified; rarely performed today
   d. Modified radical mastectomy: similar to a radical mastectomy but pectoral muscles are not removed
   e. Sentinel node biopsy or lymphectomy to determine the status of regional lymph node involvement and risk for metastasis
   f. Breast reconstruction (tissue expanders, saline implants, muscle flaps)
   g. Oophorectomy, adrenalectomy, and/or hypophysectomy to control metastases by altering endocrine environment
3. Radiation therapy through an external beam or an interstitial implant using iridium 192 (^{192}Ir)
4. Chemotherapy
   a. Alkylating agents: cyclophosphamide (Cytoxan); chlorambucil (Leukeran); triethylenethiophosphoramide (Thiotepa)
   b. Antimetabolites: 5-fluorouracil (5-FU, Fluorouracil); methotrexate (Amethopterin, MTX)
   c. Plant alkaloids: paclitaxel (Taxol); vincristine (Oncovin)
   d. Antitumor antibiotic: doxorubicin (Adriamycin)
   e. Hormones: androgens; estrogens
   f. Corticosteroid: prednisone
   g. Antiestrogen: tamoxifen citrate (Nolvadex)
5. Bone marrow transplant (BMT) adjuvant to chemotherapy and radiation

Nursing Care of Clients with Cancer of the Breast

A. ASSESSMENT
1. Personal and family history of breast cancer
2. Age at menarche, menopause, and birth of first child

3. Regularity of breast self-examinations and mammograms
4. Breast tissue, noting characteristics of lesion and skin surface
5. Enlargement of lymph nodes
6. Client's coping skills and availability of support system

B. ANALYSIS/NURSING DIAGNOSES
1. Disturbed body image related to alteration in breast structure, lymphedema
2. Fear related to diagnosis of cancer, potential for death
3. Pain related to surgical incision
4. Impaired physical mobility related to pain, inflammation, lymphedema, limited range of motion
5. Risk for injury (lymphedema) related to surgery
6. Ineffective sexuality patterns related to loss of breast
7. Ineffective therapeutic regimen management related to lack of knowledge about breast self-examination, fear of finding another mass

C. PLANNING/IMPLEMENTATION
1. Encourage and instruct the client concerning monthly breast self-examination
   a. Perform exam 7 days after the start of menstruation if premenopausal or the same time every month if postmenopausal
   b. Inspect while standing with hands at sides, overhead, and then on the hips for asymmetry, retraction of the nipple, dimpling of skin, color change
   c. Palpate the axillary and supraclavicular nodes
   d. Palpate the breast tissue using a systematic pattern when standing and lying down with the arm abducted
   e. Squeeze the nipple of each breast to check for discharge
2. Assist the client and family to cope with the diagnosis of cancer and altered body image by encouraging them to talk with staff and each other
3. Listen to and accept the client's feelings, and do not attempt to minimize them
4. Support the client's feminine image
5. Care for the client after a mastectomy
   a. Observe for hemorrhage by checking all areas of the dressing underneath the client, the drainage unit, and vital signs
   b. Maintain functioning of portable wound drainage system by ensuring patency of tube, emptying before half full, and supporting to avoid tension at site of insertion; drainage should not exceed 200 ml in 8 hours
   c. Encourage correct posture and provide assistance with ambulation until the client adjusts to altered balance

d. Prevent or reduce lymphedema by elevating and supporting the client's hand above the elbow and the elbow above the shoulder; inflatable or elastic sleeve may also be ordered
   e. Instruct the client to avoid carrying heavy articles and to avoid cuts or bruises, having blood drawn, injections, or blood pressure readings in the arm on the affected side
   f. Encourage exercises of the affected arm, beginning gradually the day after surgery if approved by the physician; exercises include squeezing a ball, brushing hair, wall hand climbing, turning rope
   g. Instruct the client as to the types of prostheses and where to obtain them; cotton covered by gauze may be used to fill a client's bra until she is seen by a professional fitter
   h. Use programs such as Reach for Recovery to help the client with physical and emotional readjustment
6. Support natural defense mechanisms of client; encourage intake of foods rich in the immune-stimulating nutrients, especially vitamins A, C, and E, and the mineral selenium; encourage low-fat diet
7. See Nursing Care of Clients Receiving Either Chemotherapy or Radiation

D. EVALUATION/OUTCOMES
1. Expresses improvement in body image
2. Identifies precautions necessary to prevent injury to the arm on the affected side after a mastectomy
3. Maintains strength and mobility of arm on affected side
4. Discusses feelings with health care providers, family, and sexual partner
5. Demonstrates and continues to perform monthly BSE

▼ OSTEOPOROSIS

Data Base
A. Etiology and pathophysiology
1. Systemic skeletal disease characterized by microarchitectural deterioration of bone tissue and low bone mass
2. Bone fragility predisposes to fractures; most commonly affects the vertebrae, pelvis, and femur
3. Risk factors include heredity (60% to 80%), low body weight (less than 127 pounds), prolonged premenopausal amenorrhea, early menopause, low physical activity, low levels of dietary calcium, low serum vitamin D, smoking, and alcohol use; also, long-term steroid therapy

B. Clinical findings
   1. Subjective: back pain that increases with activity and decreases with rest; difficulty maintaining balance
   2. Objective
      a. Decreased height resulting from compression of the vertebrae; kyphosis
      b. Bone mass measurements (e.g., x-ray examinations, dual-energy densitometry [absorptiometry])
      c. Pathologic fractures
C. Therapeutic interventions
   1. Planned program of weight-bearing exercise to increase calcium deposition in bone
   2. Estrogen replacement therapy (ERT); estrogen decreases bone reabsorption
   3. Biophosphate therapy, such as alendronate (Fosamax) and calcitonin (Miacalein), to inhibit osteoclasts and reduce bone resorption
   4. High-protein, high-calcium diet with vitamin D supplement
   5. Support for the spine (e.g., corset, Philadelphia collar, Taylor brace)
   6. Treatment of modifiable related factors

Nursing Care of Clients with Osteoporosis

A. ASSESSMENT
   1. Factors that may have contributed to development of osteoporosis
   2. Usual dietary pattern and use of over-the-counter medications
   3. History of loss of balance, falls, pain, fractures
   4. Integrity of vertebral column

B. ANALYSIS/NURSING DIAGNOSES
   1. Disturbed body image related to alteration in structure and function
   2. Impaired physical mobility related to pain
   3. Risk for injury (falls, fractures) related to bone fragility

C. PLANNING/IMPLEMENTATION
   1. Encourage active weight-bearing and range-of-motion exercises
   2. Instruct the client about proper body mechanics
   3. Encourage use of assistive devices such as walker or cane to promote stability
   4. Encourage diet that will supply nutrients needed for mineralization of bone (vitamins A, C, and D, and the minerals calcium, magnesium, and phosphorus)
   5. Advise client to avoid caffeine, alcohol, and sodium because they increase calcium excretion
   6. Encourage use of orthotic devices if ordered

D. EVALUATION/OUTCOMES
   1. Reports a reduction in pain
   2. Complies with dietary and drug regimens
   3. Participates in weight-bearing exercises
   4. Remains free from injury

CHILDBEARING AND WOMEN'S HEALTH NURSING

REVIEW QUESTIONS

Emotional Needs Related to Childbearing and Women's Health

1. A 16-year-old comes to the prenatal clinic because she has missed three menstrual periods. Before her physical examination, the client says, "I don't know what the problem is, but I can't be pregnant." The nurse's most therapeutic response to this statement would be:
   1. "The doctor will let you know shortly."
   2. "What brought you to the prenatal clinic then?"
   3. "Many young women are irregular at your age."
   4. "If you have had intercourse, you are probably pregnant."

2. A newly delivered mother, with three young children at home, comments to the nursery nurse that she cannot hold the baby for feedings once she gets home. She has just too much to do, and anyhow, it spoils the baby. The best response for the nurse to make is:
   1. "You seem concerned about time. Let's talk about it."
   2. "That's entirely up to you; you have to do what works for you."
   3. "Holding the baby when feeding is important for development."
   4. "It is most unsafe to prop a bottle. The baby could aspirate the fluid."

3. After a client has a spontaneous abortion, the nurse notes that the involved couple are visibly upset. The husband has tears in his eyes and the wife has her face turned toward the wall and is sobbing quietly. The nurse's best approach would be to go over to the woman and say:
   1. "I know that you are upset now, but hopefully you will become pregnant again very soon."
   2. "I see that both of you are very upset. I brought you a glass of juice and will be here if you want to talk."
   3. "I know how you feel, but you should not be so upset now; it will make it more difficult for you to get well quickly."
   4. "I can understand that you are upset, but be glad it happened early in your pregnancy and not after you carried the baby for the full time."

4. After delivery, a 37-week primigravida is transferred to the postpartum unit. The nursing action that best promotes the attachment process between the mother and baby is:
   1. Teaching the client to breastfeed the baby
   2. Allowing the client extra visiting privileges in the newborn nursery
   3. Encouraging the client to room in with her infant on a 24-hour basis
   4. Arranging staffing so that one nurse is assigned to care for the client and her baby

5. A client suspects that she is pregnant, but because she is the only wage earner in her family, she is ambivalent about continuing the pregnancy. The nurse recognizes that the client is in crisis and also remembers that pregnancy and birth are called crises because:
   1. There are mood changes during pregnancy
   2. They are periods of change and adjustment to change
   3. There are hormonal and physiologic changes in the mother
   4. Narcissism in the mother affects the husband-wife relationship

6. A young couple attend the prenatal clinic. The wife is 8 weeks' pregnant and asks the clinic nurse for information about an abortion. The nurse expresses the opinion that abortion is immoral and that many women have long-term guilt feelings after an abortion. The couple leave the clinic in a very disturbed state. Legally, the:
   1. Client had a right to correct, unbiased information
   2. Nurse's statements need not be based on scientific knowledge
   3. Physician should have been called in, since nurses should not discuss abortion
   4. Nurse had a right to state feelings as long as they were identified as the nurse's own

7. An amniocentesis done on a client, 16 weeks' gestation, reveals a Down syndrome infant. The client and her husband elect to have the pregnancy terminated. The nurse giving care to a client whose pregnancy is surgically terminated should be aware that:
   1. The risk of postoperative infection is high
   2. The client is emotionally unstable at this time
   3. Contraceptive counseling should be deferred to a later time
   4. The client needs to express her feelings of guilt, anger, and frustration

8. Research concerning the emotional factors of pregnancy indicates:
   1. A rejected pregnancy will result in a rejected infant
   2. Ambivalence and anxiety about mothering are common
   3. Maternal love is fully developed within the first week after birth
   4. A good mother experiences neither ambivalence nor anxiety about mothering

9. A 26-year-old multigravida of Asian descent weighs 104 pounds, having gained only 14 pounds during this pregnancy. On her second postpartum day the client's temperature spikes to 102.8° F. She seems to have a poor appetite and rarely gets out of bed. The nurse should:
   1. Refer this problem to the nursing supervisor to discuss with the physician
   2. Encourage the family to bring in special foods and drinks preferred in their culture
   3. Order a high-protein milkshake as a between meal snack to stimulate her appetite
   4. Explain to the family that the dietitian plans nutritious meals that the client must eat

10. A client with severe abdominal pain and heavy bleeding is prepared for delivery. Nursing care should include:
    1. Teaching coughing and deep-breathing techniques
    2. An abdominal prep and administration of a Fleet enema
    3. Obtaining an informed consent and assessment for drug allergies
    4. Inserting a Foley catheter and administering a tap-water enema

11. When caring for a client who is having a prolonged labor, the nurse must be aware that the client is very concerned when her labor deviates from what she sees as the norm. A response conveying acceptance of the client's expressions of frustration and hostility would be:
    1. "I'll rub your back; tell me if it helps."
    2. "I'll leave so you can talk to your husband."
    3. "All women get weary and frustrated during labor."
    4. "Would you like to talk about what's bothering you?"

12. The husband of a client who is in the transitional phase of labor becomes very tense and nervous during this period and asks the nurse, "Do you think it is best for me to leave, since I don't seem to do my wife much good?" The most appropriate response by the nurse would be:
    1. "This is the time your wife needs you. Don't run out on her now."
    2. "This is hard for you. Let me try to help you coach her during this difficult phase."
    3. "I know this is hard for you. Why don't you go have a cup of coffee and relax and come back later if you feel like it?"
    4. "If you feel that way, you'd best go out and sit in the father's waiting room for a while because you may transmit your anxiety to your wife."

13. After an 8-hour, uneventful labor a client delivers a baby boy spontaneously under epidural block anesthesia. As the nurse places the baby in the mother's arms immediately following delivery, the mother asks, "Is he normal?" The most appropriate response by the nurse would be:
    1. "Most babies are normal; of course he is."
    2. "He must be all right, he has such a good strong cry."
    3. "Yes, because your pregnancy and labor were so normal."
    4. "Shall we unwrap him so you can look him over for yourself?"

14. Supportive nursing care in the beginning mother-infant relationship should include:
    1. Requiring the mother to assist with simple aspects of her infant's care
    2. Encouraging the mother to decide between breastfeeding and bottlefeeding
    3. Allowing the mother ample time to undress and to carefully inspect her infant
    4. Unobtrusive observation of the mother and her infant to pick up a disturbed relationship

15. While holding her baby, a primipara calls the nurse and worriedly comments that the baby seems to sneeze a lot and breathes very rapidly and irregularly. She expresses fear that her baby may be sick like her neighbor's baby was and will have to be taken back to the hospital after being home for a few days. The nurse should:
    1. Pick up the baby and tell the mother that the nurses will watch the baby closely
    2. Look the baby over and tell the mother that the baby is fine and nothing is wrong
    3. Look the baby over and explain to the mother that sneezing is normal and helps the baby to get rid of mucus, and that a baby normally has rapid, shallow, irregular respirations
    4. Assess the baby, take the baby to the nursery immediately, and return to the mother to tell her that the physician has been called, since the baby is obviously in respiratory distress

16. During the taking-hold phase, the nurse would expect the new mother to:
    1. Talk about the baby
    2. Call the baby by name
    3. Touch the baby with her fingertips
    4. Be passively involved with the baby

17. Following delivery, while considering nursing measures to help parent-child relationships, the nurse should be aware that the most important factor at this time is the:
    1. Anesthesia during labor
    2. Duration and difficulty of labor
    3. Physical condition of the infant
    4. Health status during pregnancy

18. When caring for a family on a postpartum unit, the nurse must be aware that all the tasks, responsibilities, and attitudes that make up child care can be called parenting, and that either parent can exhibit these qualities. A person is able to perform parenting because of:
    1. A marriage with flexible roles
    2. An inborn ability based on instinct
    3. Positive childhood roles and concepts
    4. A good education in growth and development

19. At 9 PM the visiting hours are officially over but the relatives of one postpartum client remain at the bedside. The nurse's most appropriate response would be to:
    1. Firmly remind the client and visitors that visiting hours are over
    2. Call the evening nursing supervisor to tactfully handle the situation
    3. Encourage the family members to participate in care as much as the client wishes
    4. Get written permission from the client's husband for the family members to remain

20. A decision to withhold "extraordinary care" for a newborn with severe abnormalities is actually:
    1. A decision to let the newborn die
    2. The same as pediatric euthanasia
    3. Presuming that the newborn has no rights
    4. Unethical and illegal medical and nursing practice

21. It is important for the nurse to support the parents' decision to abort a fetus with a birth defect because:
    1. Supporting them will eliminate feelings of guilt
    2. It is essential for maintenance of family equilibrium
    3. The parents are legally responsible for the decision
    4. The nurse's support will relieve the pressure associated with decision making

Drug-Related Responses

22. In the 12th week of gestation a client completely expels the products of conception. Because the client is Rh negative, the nurse must:
    1. Administer RhoGAM within 72 hours
    2. Make certain she receives RhoGAM on her first clinic visit
    3. Not give RhoGAM, since it is not used with the birth of a stillborn
    4. Make certain the client does not receive RhoGAM, since the gestation was only 12 weeks

23. A pregnant client develops thrombophlebitis of the left leg and is admitted to the hospital for bed rest and anticoagulant therapy. The anticoagulant the nurse should expect to administer is:
    1. Heparin
    2. Dicumarol
    3. Diphenadione (Dipaxin)
    4. Warfarin (Coumadin sodium)

24. A client, undergoing treatment for infertility, is diagnosed as having endometriosis. The nurse is aware that one of the drugs that may be used to treat this condition is:
    1. Relaxin (Releasin)
    2. Leuprolide (Lupron)
    3. Ergonovine (Ergotrate)
    4. Esterified estrogen (Climestrone)

25. During labor a client who has been receiving epidural anesthesia has a sudden episode of severe nausea, and her skin becomes pale and clammy. The nurse's immediate reaction is to:
    1. Notify the physician
    2. Elevate the client's legs
    3. Check for vaginal bleeding
    4. Monitor the FHR every 3 minutes

26. A client at 6 weeks' gestation is receiving antibiotic therapy for pyelonephritis. The nurse is aware that the safest antibiotic for administration during pregnancy is:
    1. Gantrisin
    2. Ampicillin
    3. Tetracycline
    4. Nitrofurantoin

27. A client who was admitted in active labor has only progressed from 2 cm to 3 cm in 8 hours. She is diagnosed as having hypotonic dystocia and is given oxytocin (Pitocin) to augment her contractions. The most important aspect of nursing at this time is:
    1. Monitoring the FHR
    2. Checking perineum for bulging
    3. Timing and recording length of contractions
    4. Preparing for an emergency cesarean delivery

28. A client, 38 weeks' gestation, is admitted for induction of labor. She has a history of ruptured membranes for the past 12 hours. She has no other symptoms of labor. The nurse is aware that if the proper conditions exist, the physician will prescribe:
    1. Progesterone
    2. Oxytocin (Pitocin)
    3. Lututrin (Lutrexin)
    4. Ergonovine maleate

29. At about 5 cm, a laboring client receives medication for pain. The nurse is aware that one of the medications given to women in labor that could cause respiratory depression of the newborn is:
    1. Scopolamine
    2. Promazine (Sparine)
    3. Meperidine (Demerol)
    4. Promethazine (Phenergan)

30. A client in the midphase of labor becomes very uncomfortable and asks for medication. Meperidine (Demerol) 50 mg is ordered. This medication:
    1. Acts to produce amnesia
    2. Acts as preliminary anesthetics
    3. Induces sleep until the time of delivery
    4. Increases the client's pain threshold, resulting in pain reduction

31. A client begins preterm labor and the physician orders terbutaline sulfate (Brethine). After its administration, the nurse assesses the client for the therapeutic effect of:
    1. Reduction of pain in the perineal area
    2. Decrease in blood pressure from 120/80 to 90/60
    3. Decrease in frequency and duration of contractions
    4. Dilation of the cervix from 1 to 1.5 cm for every hour of labor

32. A client is on magnesium sulfate therapy for severe preeclampsia. The nurse must be alert for the first sign of an excessive blood magnesium level, which is:
    1. Disturbance in sensorium
    2. Increase in respiratory rate
    3. Development of cardiac dysrhythmia
    4. Disappearance of the knee-jerk reflex

33. A 16-year-old who is 30 weeks' pregnant, begins to experience contractions every 5 to 7 minutes. She is admitted to the hospital with suspected preterm labor. It is determined that the client's baby would be at severe risk if delivered because of lung immaturity. The client is receiving terbutaline sulfate (Brethine) to halt labor, without adequate response. The nurse should expect the health care provider to order:
    1. Ringer's lactate
    2. Ritodrine Hcl (Yutopar)
    3. Progest-50 (progesterone)
    4. Theophylline (aminophylline)

34. Despite medication, a client's preterm labor continues, her cervix dilates, and delivery appears to be inevitable. The nurse understands the baby's chance of extrauterine survival may improve if the physician orders:
    1. Ampicillin by piggyback
    2. Dexamethasone by infusion
    3. An immediate cesarean delivery
    4. An intrauterine exchange transfusion

Reproductive Choices

35. Following delivery, a cardiac client with type 2 diabetes asks the nurse, "Which contraceptives will I be able to use to prevent pregnancy in the near future?" The nurse's best response would be:
    1. "You may use oral contraceptives. They are almost 100% effective in preventing a pregnancy."
    2. "You may want to use a foam and a condom to prevent pregnancy until you consult with your doctor at your postpartum visit."
    3. "The intrauterine device is best for you because it does not allow a fertilized ovum to become implanted in the uterine lining."
    4. "You do not need to worry about becoming pregnant in the near future. Clients with cardiac conditions usually become infertile."

36. The nurse teaches that the most frequent side effect associated with the use of IUDs is:
    1. Ectopic pregnancy
    2. Expulsion of the IUD
    3. Rupture of the uterus
    4. Excessive menstrual flow

37. The nurse should explain that a common problem that has been associated with IUDs when they are used is:
    1. Perforation of the uterus
    2. Discomfort associated with coitus
    3. Development of vaginal infections
    4. Spontaneous expulsion of the device

38. A client seeking advice about contraception asks the nurse about an IUD. The nurse explains that the IUD provides contraception by:
    1. Blocking the cervical os
    2. Increasing the mobility of the uterus
    3. Preventing the sperm from reaching the vagina
    4. IUDs interfere with either fertilization or implantation, promoting contraception

39. In a lecture on sexual functioning, the nurse plans to include the fact that ovulation occurs when the:
    1. Oxytocin level is high
    2. Blood level of LH is high
    3. Progesterone level is high
    4. Endometrial wall is sloughed off

40. After ovulation has occurred, the ovum is believed to remain viable for:

1. 1 to 6 hours
2. 12 to 18 hours
3. 24 to 36 hours
4. 48 to 72 hours

41. The time of ovulation can be determined by taking the basal temperature. During ovulation the basal temperature:
    1. Drops markedly
    2. Drops slightly and then rises
    3. Rises suddenly and then falls
    4. Rises markedly and remains high

42. When oral contraceptives are prescribed for a client the nurse should teach the client about the potential of developing:
    1. Cervicitis
    2. Ovarian cysts
    3. Fibrocystic disease
    4. Breakthrough bleeding

43. A young couple has been using oral contraceptives to delay pregnancy. When the wife misses her regular menstrual period, she decides to find out if she is pregnant. She tells the nurse that pregnancy may have occurred because she missed taking her contraceptive pills for 1 week because of the flu. The nurse's best response would be:
    1. "Contraceptive pills are very unpredictable anyhow. You probably would have become pregnant even if you had taken them regularly as prescribed."
    2. "Don't think about that now. It's too late to worry anyhow. First find out whether you really are pregnant. If you are, you may want to consider having an abortion."
    3. "You may well be correct; one of the reasons for prescribing an exact schedule is that the effect of contraceptive drugs depends on the regularity with which they are taken."
    4. "That's the trouble with using contraceptive pills. People become too careless and don't use proper restraint. If you had used the rhythm method, this probably would not have happened."

44. The nurse explains that the efficiency of the basal body temperature (BBT) method of contraception depends on fluctuation of the basal body temperature. A factor that will alter its effectiveness is:
    1. Presence of stress
    2. Length of abstinence
    3. Age of those involved
    4. Frequency of intercourse

45. A biphasic antiovulatory medication of combined progestin and estrogen is prescribed for a female client. The nurse, instructing the client about the medication, should include the need to:
1. Have bimonthly Pap smears
2. Increase her intake of calcium
3. Temporarily restrict sexual activity
4. Report any irregular vaginal bleeding

46. During the salinization method of elective abortion, the nurse should be alert for side effects of hypernatremia such as:
1. Edema
2. Oliguria
3. Headache
4. Bradycardia

47. Following a salinization procedure for an elective abortion of a 20-week pregnancy, the client is told that labor will probably begin within:
1. Two hours after the procedure
2. Four hours following the procedure
3. Eight to 24 hours after the procedure
4. Several minutes following the procedure

48. In the dilation and suction evacuation method of elective abortion, *Laminaria* is used in the dilation stage of the procedure because:
1. Dilation occurs within 2 hours
2. They are hygroscopic and expand
3. They are stronger in action than instruments
4. Less anesthesia is necessary with this method

49. A couple indicate that they do not want any more children. The wife is scheduled for a bilateral tubal ligation. Preoperative teaching should include the statement:
1. "Your family can drive you home within an hour after surgery."
2. "You will need to use birth control until you return in 6 weeks."
3. "You must avoid lifting and strenuous exercise for a few weeks."
4. "If you decide you want children, the operation is easily reversible."

50. One day the family planning clinic is very busy, and the supervisor asks a nurse from the pediatric clinic who is strongly opposed to any chemical or mechanical method of birth control to work in the family planning clinic. The most professional response that this nurse could give to the supervisor would be:

1. "I will go, but it is against my beliefs."
2. "I won't do it. I do not believe in birth control."
3. "Is there another assignment not contrary to my beliefs?"
4. "I will have to reinforce that the rhythm method is the method of choice."

Reproductive Problems

51. One of the responsibilities of a nurse in a fertility specialist's office is to provide health teaching to the client in relation to timing of intercourse. Instructions to the client should include the information that the best time to achieve a pregnancy would be:
1. Midway between periods
2. Immediately after menses end
3. Fourteen days before the next period is expected
4. Fourteen days after the beginning of the last period

52. A factor in infertility may be related to the pH of the vaginal canal. A medication that is ordered to alter the vaginal pH is:
1. Estrogen therapy
2. Sulfur insufflations
3. Lactic acid douches
4. Sodium bicarbonate douches

53. A diagnostic test used to evaluate fertility is the postcoital test. It is best timed:
1. 1 week after ovulation
2. Immediately after menses
3. Just before the next menstrual period
4. Within 1 to 2 days of presumed ovulation

54. A tubal insufflation test is done to determine whether there is a tubal obstruction. Infertility caused by a defect in the tube is most often related to a:
1. Past infection
2. Fibroid tumor
3. Congenital anomaly
4. Previous injury to a tube

55. In dealing with a couple who have been identified as having an infertility problem, the nurse should know that:
1. Infertility is usually psychologic in origin
2. Infertility and sterility are essentially the same problem
3. The couple has been unable to have a child after trying for a year
4. One partner has a problem that makes that person unable to have children

56. A high concentration of estrogen in the blood:
1. Causes ovulation
2. Stimulates lactation
3. Inhibits secretion of FSH
4. Is one cause of osteoporosis

57. A test commonly used to determine the number, motility, and activity of sperm is the:
1. Rubin test
2. Postcoital test
3. Friedman test
4. Papanicolaou test

58. In the female, evaluation of the pelvic organs of reproduction is accomplished by:
1. Biopsy
2. Cystoscopy
3. Culdoscopy
4. Hysterosalpingogram

59. When assessing a client with a tentative diagnosis of hydatidiform mole, the nurse should be alert for:
1. Hypotension
2. Decreased FHR
3. Unusual uterine enlargement
4. Painless, heavy vaginal bleeding

60. When obtaining the nursing history from a client with a diagnosis of a ruptured tubal pregnancy, the nurse should expect the client to indicate that her symptoms of pain in the lower abdomen and vaginal bleeding started:
1. About the sixth week of pregnancy
2. At the beginning of the last trimester
3. Midway through the second trimester
4. Immediately after implantation occurred

61. The nurse would suspect an ectopic pregnancy if the client complained of:
1. An adherent painful ovarian mass
2. Lower abdominal cramping for a long period of time
3. Leukorrhea and dysuria a few days after the first missed period
4. Sharp lower right or left abdominal pain radiating to the shoulder

62. The most common type of ectopic pregnancy is tubal. Within a few weeks after conception the tube may rupture suddenly, causing:
1. Painless vaginal bleeding
2. Intermittent abdominal contractions
3. Continuous dull, upper-quadrant abdominal pain
4. Sudden knifelike, lower-quadrant abdominal pain

63. A client who has missed two menstrual periods comes to the prenatal clinic complaining of vaginal bleeding and one-sided lower-quadrant pain. The nurse suspects that this client has:
1. Abruptio placentae
2. An ectopic pregnancy
3. An incomplete abortion
4. A rupture of a graafian follicle

64. A couple who recently immigrated from Israel are concerned about a genetic disease that is prevalent among Jewish people and speak to the clinic nurse. The nurse recommends that they go for a genetic blood test to determine the possibility of any of their children being born with:
1. PKU
2. Cystic fibrosis
3. Cooley's anemia
4. Tay-Sachs disease

65. After a spontaneous abortion the nurse should observe the client for:
1. Hemorrhage and infection
2. Dehydration and hemorrhage
3. Subinvolution and dehydration
4. Signs of pregnancy-induced hypertension

66. Most spontaneous abortions are caused by:
1. Physical trauma
2. Unresolved stress
3. Congenital defects
4. Germ plasm defects

67. A client whose husband is overseas in the military is admitted to the hospital with vaginal staining but no pain. The client's history reveals amenorrhea for the last 2 months and pregnancy confirmation by her physician after her first missed period. She is admitted for observation with a possible diagnosis of:
1. Missed abortion
2. Inevitable abortion
3. Ectopic pregnancy
4. Threatened abortion

68. A few hours after being admitted with a diagnosis of inevitable abortion, a client begins to experience bearing-down sensations and suddenly expels the products of conception in bed. To give safe nursing care, the nurse should first:
    1. Check the fundus for firmness
    2. Give her the sedation ordered
    3. Immediately notify the physician
    4. Take her immediately to the delivery room

69. After an incomplete abortion, a client tells the nurse that although her doctor explained what an incomplete abortion was, she did not understand. The nurse could best respond:
    1. "I really don't think you should focus on what happened right now."
    2. "This is when the fetus dies but is retained in the uterus for 8 weeks or more."
    3. "I think it would be best if you asked your doctor for the answer to that question."
    4. "An incomplete abortion is when the fetus is expelled but part of the placenta and membranes are not."

Healthy Childbearing

70. The inner membrane that encloses the fluid medium for the embryo is the:
    1. Funis
    2. Amnion
    3. Chorion
    4. Yolk sac

71. The chief function of progesterone is the:
    1. Stimulation of follicles for ovulation to occur
    2. Development of female reproductive organs
    3. Preparation of the uterus to receive a fertilized ovum
    4. Establishment of the secondary male sex characteristics

72. During the process of gametogenesis, the male and female sex cells divide, and each mature sex cell contains:
    1. Twenty-two pairs of autosomes in their nuclei
    2. Forty-six pairs of chromosomes in their nuclei
    3. A diploid number of chromosomes in their nuclei
    4. A haploid number of chromosomes in their nuclei

73. The placenta does not produce:
    1. Somatotropin
    2. Chorionic gonadotropin
    3. Follicle-stimulating hormone
    4. Progesterone precursor substances

74. The developing cells are called a fetus from the:
    1. Time the fetal heart is heard
    2. Eighth week to the time of birth
    3. Implantation of the fertilized ovum
    4. End of the second week to the onset of labor

75. During pregnancy the volume of tidal air increases because there is:
    1. An increase in total blood volume
    2. Increased expansion of the lower ribs
    3. Upward displacement of the diaphragm
    4. A relative increase in the height of the rib cage

76. The uterus rises out of the pelvis and becomes an abdominal organ at about the:
    1. Tenth week of pregnancy
    2. Eighth week of pregnancy
    3. Twelfth week of pregnancy
    4. Eighteenth week of pregnancy

77. First fetal movements felt by the mother are known as:
    1. Lightening
    2. Quickening
    3. Ballottement
    4. Engagement

78. In prenatal development, fetal weight gain is greatest in the:
    1. First trimester
    2. Third trimester
    3. Second trimester
    4. Implantation period

79. After the first 3 months of pregnancy the chief source of estrogen and progesterone is the:
    1. Placenta
    2. Adrenal cortex
    3. Corpus luteum
    4. Anterior hypophysis

80. In fetal blood vessels the oxygen content is highest in the:
    1. Umbilical artery
    2. Ductus venosus
    3. Pulmonary artery
    4. Ductus arteriosus

81. A client relates that the first day of her last menstrual period was July 22. The estimated date of birth would be:
    1. May 5
    2. May 14
    3. April 15
    4. April 29

82. A client visits the prenatal clinic to confirm her suspicions that she is pregnant and, if so, to begin prenatal care. The client states her last menstrual period began June 10. According to Nägele's rule, her expected date of delivery (EDD) would be:
    1. March 17
    2. April 17
    3. March 10
    4. April 10

83. Anticipatory guidance during the first trimester of pregnancy is primarily directed toward increasing the pregnant woman's knowledge of:
    1. Labor and delivery
    2. Signs of complications
    3. Role transition into parenthood
    4. Physical changes resulting from pregnancy

84. The anterior/posterior diameter of the pelvic inlet is an important measurement of the pelvis and is known as the:
    1. Conjugate vera
    2. Diagonal conjugate
    3. Transverse diameter
    4. Transverse conjugate

85. During pregnancy, the uterine musculature hypertrophies and is greatly stretched as the fetus grows. This stretching:
    1. By itself inhibits uterine contraction until oxytocin stimulates the birth process
    2. Is prevented from stimulating uterine contraction by high levels of estrogen during late pregnancy
    3. Inhibits uterine contraction along with the combined inhibitory effects of estrogen and progesterone
    4. Would ordinarily stimulate uterine contraction but is prevented by high levels of progesterone during pregnancy

86. The nurse recognizes that a normal, expected change in the hematologic system that occurs during the second trimester of pregnancy is:
    1. A decrease in WBCs
    2. An increase in hematocrit
    3. An increase in blood volume
    4. A decrease in sedimentation rate

87. The nurse is aware that a normal adaptation of pregnancy is an increased blood supply to the pelvic region that results in a purplish discoloration of the vaginal mucosa, which is known as:

    1. Ladin's sign
    2. Hegar's sign
    3. Goodell's sign
    4. Chadwick's sign

88. Physiologic anemia during pregnancy is a result of:
    1. Decreased dietary intake of iron
    2. Increased plasma volume of the mother
    3. Decreased erythropoiesis after the first trimester
    4. Increased detoxification demands on the mother's liver

89. On a first prenatal visit, a client asks the nurse, "Is it true the doctor will do an internal examination today?" The nurse should respond:
    1. "Yes, an internal is done on all mothers on the first visit."
    2. "Are you fearful of having an internal examination done?"
    3. "Yes. Have you ever had an internal examination done before?"
    4. "Yes, an internal is done on all mothers, but it is only slightly uncomfortable."

90. A normal cardiopulmonary symptom experienced by most pregnant women is:
    1. Tachycardia
    2. Dyspnea at rest
    3. Progressive dependent edema
    4. Shortness of breath on exertion

91. A client asks the nurse why menstruation ceases once pregnancy occurs. The nurse's best response would be that this occurs because of the:
    1. "Reduction in the secretion of hormones by the ovaries."
    2. "Production of estrogen and progesterone by the ovaries."
    3. "Secretion of luteinizing hormone produced by the pituitary."
    4. "Secretion of follicle-stimulating hormone produced by the pituitary."

92. The nurse is aware that the nausea and vomiting commonly experienced by many women during the first trimester of pregnancy is an adaptation to the increased level of:
    1. Estrogen
    2. Progesterone
    3. Luteinizing hormone
    4. Chorionic gonadotropin

93. A pregnant client works as a keypunch operator. This would necessarily have implications for her plan of care during pregnancy. The nurse should recommend that the client:
1. Try to walk about every few hours during the workday
2. Ask for time in the morning and afternoon to elevate her legs
3. Tell her employer she cannot work beyond the second trimester
4. Ask for time in the morning and afternoon to obtain nourishment

94. The nurse in the prenatal clinic should provide nutritional counseling to all newly pregnant women because:
1. Most weight gain during pregnancy is fluid retention
2. Dietary allowances should not increase during pregnancy
3. Pregnant women must adhere to a specific pregnancy diet
4. Different sources of essential nutrients are favored by different cultural groups

95. A primigravida in her tenth week of gestation is concerned because she has read that nutrition during pregnancy is important for proper growth and development of the baby. She wants to know something about the foods she should eat. The nurse should:
1. Instruct her to continue eating a normal diet
2. Assess what she eats by taking a diet history
3. Give her a list of foods so she can better plan her meals
4. Emphasize the importance of limiting salt and highly seasoned food

96. A client, in her eighth week of pregnancy complains of having to go to the bathroom often to urinate. The nurse explains to the client that urinary frequency often occurs because the capacity of the bladder during pregnancy is diminished by:
1. Atony of the detrusor muscle
2. Compression by the enlarging uterus
3. Compromise of the autonomic reflexes
4. Constriction of the ureteral entrance at the trigone

97. A client who is 10 weeks pregnant calls the clinic and complains of morning sickness. To promote relief, the nurse should suggest:
1. Eating dry crackers before arising
2. Increasing her fat intake before bedtime
3. Having two small meals daily and a snack at noon

4. Drinking more high-carbohydrate fluids with her meals

98. When attending the prenatal clinic, a newly pregnant client, having her first child, expresses concern about her "dark nipples" and a "dark line" from her navel to the pubis. The nurse explains that these adaptations are due to hyperactivity of the:
1. Ovaries
2. Thyroid gland
3. Adrenal gland
4. Pituitary gland

99. The nurse can try to help a pregnant client overcome first-trimester morning sickness by suggesting that the client:
1. Eat protein before sleep
2. Take an antacid before bedtime
3. Eat nothing until the nausea subsides
4. Request her care provider to prescribe an antiemetic

100. Nutritional planning for a newly pregnant woman of average height weighing 130 pounds should include:
1. A decrease to 1000 calories per day
2. A decrease in fat and protein consumption
3. An increase to 1800 to 2000 calories per day
4. An increase in caloric intake to 2800 calories per day

101. A client is concerned about gaining weight during pregnancy. The nurse explains that the largest part of weight gain during pregnancy is because of:
1. The fetus
2. Fluid retention
3. Metabolic alterations
4. Increased blood volume

102. A client who is pregnant for the first time attends the prenatal clinic. She tells the nurse, "I'm worried about gaining too much weight because I have heard that it is bad for me." The nurse's best response would be:
1. "Yes, weight gain causes complications during pregnancy."
2. "If you gain over 15 pounds, you'll have to follow a low-calorie diet."
3. "Don't worry about gaining weight. We are more concerned if you don't gain enough weight to ensure proper growth of your baby."
4. "A 25-pound weight gain is recommended; however, the pattern of your weight gain will be of more importance than the total amount."

103. A client, 7 weeks pregnant, confides to the nurse in the prenatal clinic that she is very sick every morning with nausea and vomiting and is sure that she is being punished for having initially thought of aborting the pregnancy. The nurse assures her that this is not punishment but a common occurrence in early pregnancy and will probably disappear by the end of the:
1. 5th month
2. 4th month
3. 3rd month
4. 2nd month

104. A client who is pregnant is being prepared for a pelvic examination. The client complains of feeling very tired and sick to her stomach, especially in the morning. The best response for the nurse to make is:
1. "This is common. There is no need to worry."
2. "Can you tell me how you feel in the morning?"
3. "Perhaps you might ask the nurse midwife about it."
4. "Let's discuss some ways to deal with these common problems."

105. During a prenatal examination the nurse draws blood from a young client and explains that the determination of Rh is routinely performed on expectant mothers to predict whether the fetus is at risk for developing:
1. Acute hemolytic anemia
2. Protein metabolism deficiency
3. Physiologic hyperbilirubinemia
4. Respiratory distress syndrome

106. The best advice the nurse can give to a pregnant woman in her first trimester is to:
1. Cut down on drugs, alcohol, and cigarettes
2. Avoid all drugs and refrain from smoking and ingesting alcohol
3. Avoid smoking, limit alcohol consumption, and do not take any aspirin
4. Take only prescription drugs, especially in the second and third trimesters

107. A client is in her fourth month of pregnancy. When she comes for her monthly examination, the nurse asks if she would like to listen to the baby's heartbeat. The woman, commenting on how rapid it is, appears frightened and asks if this is normal. The nurse should respond:
1. "The baby's heart rate is usually twice the mother's pulse rate."
2. "The baby's heartbeat is rapid to accommodate the nutritional needs."
3. "A baby's heart rate is rapid, and your baby's is within the normal range."
4. "It is far better that the heart rate is rapid; when it is slow, there is need to worry."

108. A client who is pregnant asks the nurse if she can continue to have sexual relations. The nurse's response is based on the knowledge that coitus during pregnancy would be contraindicated in the presence of:
1. Leukorrhea
2. Increased FHR
3. Gestation of 30 weeks or more
4. Premature rupture of membranes

109. When involved in prenatal teaching, the nurse should inform clients that an increase in vaginal secretions during pregnancy is called leukorrhea caused by increased:
1. Metabolic rates
2. Production of estrogen
3. Functioning of the Bartholin glands
4. Supply of sodium chloride to the cells of the vagina

110. A primigravida, unsure of the date of her last menstrual period, is told by the obstetrician that she appears to be about 20 weeks pregnant. The nurse explains that this is because the fundus:
1. Is 18 cm, and the baby has just started to move
2. Is 28 cm, and the fetal heart can be heard with a Doppler
3. Is just over the symphysis, and the fetal heart cannot be heard
4. Is at the umbilicus, and the fetal heart can be heard with a fetoscope

111. A 21-year-old client who is 6 months into her second pregnancy is experiencing increasing edema in the lower extremities. Besides advising rest with the legs elevated, the nurse discusses and gives instructions concerning the diet. In this instance:
1. The nutritionist should be brought in to plan a diet
2. The foods selected should have a normal salt content
3. Dietary preferences must influence the food that is eaten
4. The client should be advised to see the physician at the prenatal clinic

112. The nurse explains the treatment for fluid retention during pregnancy, which is:
    1. Adequate fluid and a low-salt diet
    2. A low-salt diet and elevation of the lower extremities
    3. Adequate fluid and elevation of the lower extremities
    4. Judicious use of diuretics and elevation of the lower extremities

113. In the thirty-seventh week of gestation a client is scheduled for a nonstress test. The nurse, after explaining the procedure, evaluates that the client understands the teaching when she says:
    1. "I hope this test does not cause my labor to begin early."
    2. "I hope the baby doesn't get too restless after this procedure."
    3. "I hate having needles in my arm, but now I understand why it is necessary."
    4. "If my baby's heart reacts normally during the test, he should do okay during delivery."

114. A client in the thirty-second week of pregnancy is scheduled for ultrasonography. The nurse explains the procedure and informs the client that for this test she will have to:
    1. Be given an enema the night before the examination
    2. Refrain from voiding for at least 3 hours before the test
    3. Be monitored closely afterward for signs of precipitate labor
    4. Be kept NPO for 12 hours to minimize the possibility of vomiting

115. At a prenatal visit at 36 weeks' gestation, a client complains of discomfort with Braxton Hicks contractions. The nurse instructs the client to:
    1. Lie down until they stop
    2. Walk around until they subside
    3. Time the contractions for $1/2$ hour
    4. Take 10 grains of aspirin for the discomfort

116. When teaching a young primigravida about labor, the nurse should tell her to come to the hospital when:
    1. Contractions are 10 to 15 minutes apart
    2. She has a bloody show and back pressure
    3. Membranes rupture or contractions are 5 to 8 minutes apart
    4. Contractions are 2 to 3 minutes apart and she cannot walk about

117. True labor can be differentiated from false labor because in true labor contractions will:
    1. Bring about progressive cervical dilation
    2. Occur immediately after membrane rupture
    3. Stop when the client is encouraged to walk around
    4. Be less uncomfortable if client is in a side-lying position

118. The nurse teaches a pregnant woman to avoid lying on her back during labor. The nurse has based this statement on the knowledge that the supine position can:
    1. Unduly prolong labor
    2. Cause decreased placental perfusion
    3. Interfere with free movement of the coccyx
    4. Lead to transient episodes of hypertension

119. The nurse should teach pregnant women the importance of conserving the "spurt of energy" before labor because:
    1. Fatigue may influence need for pain medication
    2. Energy helps to increase the progesterone level
    3. Energy is needed to push during the first stage of labor
    4. This energy will decrease the intensity of the uterine contractions

120. A client is admitted to the labor room in early active labor. The priority nursing intervention on admission of this laboring client would be:
    1. Auscultating the fetal heart
    2. Taking an obstetric history
    3. Asking the client when she ate last
    4. Ascertaining if the membranes are ruptured

121. A client who is a gravida 1, para 0, is admitted in labor. Her cervix is 100% effaced and she is dilated 3 cm. Her fetus is at a +1 station. The nurse is aware the fetus' head is:
    1. Not yet engaged
    2. Entering the pelvic inlet
    3. Below the ischial spines
    4. Visible at the vaginal opening

122. After doing Leopold's maneuvers on a laboring client, the nurse determines that the fetus is in the ROP position. To best auscultate the fetal heart tones, the Doppler is placed:
    1. Above the umbilicus in the midline
    2. Above the umbilicus on the left side
    3. Below the umbilicus on the right side
    4. Below the umbilicus near the left groin

123. A client in active labor begins to tremble, becomes very tense with contractions, and is quite irritable. She frequently states, "I cannot stand this a minute longer." This kind of behavior may be indicative of the fact that the client:
    1. Is entering the transition phase of labor
    2. Needs immediate administration of an analgesic or anesthetic
    3. Has been very poorly prepared for labor in the parents' classes
    4. Is developing some abnormality in terms of uterine contractions

124. The physician asks the nurse the frequency of a laboring client's contractions. The nurse assesses the client's contractions by timing from the beginning of one contraction:
    1. Until the time it is completely over
    2. To the end of a second contraction
    3. To the beginning of the next contraction
    4. Until the time that the uterus becomes very firm

125. The nurse observes the client's amniotic fluid and decides that it appears normal, because it is:
    1. Clear and dark-amber colored
    2. Milky, greenish yellow, containing shreds of mucus
    3. Clear, almost colorless, containing little white specks
    4. Cloudy, greenish-yellow, containing little white specks

126. A multigravida has a normal spontaneous vaginal delivery of a healthy infant. Five minutes after delivery of the infant the placenta is expressed. The nurse upon assessing the fundus at this time would expect the fundus to be:
    1. Difficult to find
    2. Just below the xiphoid process
    3. At the umbilicus in the upper right quadrant
    4. Halfway between the symphysis pubis and the umbilicus

127. One problem that confronts the client when an external fetal monitor is being used is the:
    1. Restriction of movement
    2. Inability to take sedatives
    3. Interference with Lamaze techniques
    4. Increased frequency of vaginal examinations

128. A laboring client is placed on an external fetal monitor. The nurse notes that fetal heart decelerates in a uniform wave shape reflecting the shape of the contraction. The nurse should:
    1. Notify the physician because there may be head compression
    2. Place the client in a knee-chest position to avoid cord compression
    3. Continue to observe for return of fetal heart rate to baseline when contraction ends
    4. Put the client in a dorsal recumbent position to prevent compression of the vena cava

129. When examining the fetal monitor strip following rupture of the membranes in a laboring client, the nurse notes decelerations in the fetal heart rate. The nurse should:
    1. Stop the oxytocin infusion
    2. Change the client's position
    3. Prepare for immediate delivery
    4. Take the client's blood pressure

130. A client in active labor spontaneously ruptures membranes. The nurse should first:
    1. Monitor the FHR
    2. Call the physician
    3. Check BP and pulse
    4. Time the contractions

131. The membranes of a client who is 39 weeks pregnant have ruptured spontaneously. She comes to the hospital accompanied by her husband. Her cervix is 4 cm dilated and 75% effaced. The fetal heart rate is 136. The nurse should:
    1. Place the mother in bed and attach an external fetal monitor
    2. Let the mother undress while the nurse takes the history from the father
    3. Introduce the staff nurses to the couple and try to make them feel welcome
    4. Have them wait in the examining room while the nurse notifies the physician that they have arrived

132. A primigravida, 40 weeks' gestation, is admitted with q 3 to 5 min contractions, a bloody show, and intact membranes. Vaginal examination reveals that the cervix is fully effaced, 6 cm dilated, and the head is at +1 station. The nurse is aware that according to these data the client is in the:
    1. Latent phase of labor
    2. Active phase of labor
    3. Transition phase of labor
    4. Accelerated phase of labor

133. A client, 41 weeks' gestation, comes to the labor suite with a bloody show and no contractions. A vaginal exam reveals that the baby's head is at +1 station. To induce labor the nurse should expect an order for:
    1. A tap-water enema
    2. An IM injection of oxytocin
    3. Artificial rupture of membranes
    4. Administration of prostaglandins

134. A client is admitted to the hospital in active labor. After an amniotomy the nurse would expect:
    1. Diminished bloody show
    2. Increased fetal heart rate
    3. Less discomfort with contractions
    4. Progressive dilation and effacement

135. A primigravida, 40 weeks' gestation, arrives at the birthing center with abdominal cramping and a bloody show. Her membranes ruptured 30 minutes before arrival. A vaginal examination reveals 1 cm dilation and presenting part at –1 station. After obtaining the fetal heart rate and maternal vital signs, the nurse should:
    1. Teach the client how to push
    2. Review Lamaze breathing techniques with the client
    3. Provide the client with comfort measures used for women in labor
    4. Prepare to type and cross-match the client's blood for a possible transfusion

136. A primigravida at term is admitted with contractions q 5 to 8 minutes and a bloody show. She and her husband attended childbirth preparation classes. Vaginal examination reveals 3 cm dilation and 75% effacement, +1 station with occiput anterior, and intact membranes. The client is cheerful and relaxed and asks the nurse if it is all right for her to walk around. Based on the observations of the client's contractions and knowledge of the physiology and mechanism of labor, the nurse could best respond:
    1. "I can't make a decision on that; you will have to ask the doctor."
    2. "Please stay in bed; walking may interfere with proper uterine contractions."
    3. "It is quite all right for you to be up and about as long as you feel comfortable and your membranes are intact."
    4. "You will have to stay in bed; otherwise your contractions cannot be timed and no one can listen to the fetal heart."

137. A client and her husband are working together during the wife's labor. The client is now 7 cm dilated and the presenting part is low in the mid-pelvis. To alleviate discomfort during contractions, the nurse should instruct the husband to encourage his wife to:
    1. Pant
    2. Pelvic rock
    3. Deep breathe slowly
    4. Athletic chest breathe

138. The expectant couple asks the nurse about the cause of low back pain in labor. The nurse replies that this pain occurs most when the position of the fetus is:
    1. Breech
    2. Transverse
    3. Occiput anterior
    4. Occiput posterior

139. A laboring client complains of low back pain. To increase the client's comfort the nurse should recommend that the client's husband:
    1. Instruct her to flex her knees
    2. Place her in the supine position
    3. Apply back pressure during contractions
    4. Help her perform neuromuscular control exercises

140. To promote comfort during back labor, the nurse teaches the client to avoid the:
    1. Sitting position
    2. Supine position
    3. Side-lying position
    4. Knee-chest position

141. The nurse withholds foods and limits fluids as a laboring client approaches the second stage of labor because:
    1. The mechanical and chemical digestive process requires energy that is needed for labor
    2. Undigested food and fluid may cause nausea and vomiting and limit the choice of anesthesia
    3. Food will further aggravate gastric peristalsis, which is already increased because of the stress of labor
    4. The gastric phase of digestion stimulates the release of hydrochloric acid and may cause dyspepsia

142. The management of a client in the transition phase of labor is primarily directed toward:
    1. Helping the client maintain control
    2. Decreasing the intravenous fluid intake
    3. Reducing the client's discomfort with medications
    4. Having the client breathe simple breathing patterns during contractions

143. The breathing technique that the mother should be instructed to use during delivery as the fetus' head is crowning is:
    1. Blowing
    2. Slow chest
    3. Shallow breaths
    4. Accelerated-decelerated

144. When a client is positioned for delivery, both legs should be positioned simultaneously to prevent:
    1. Venous stasis in the legs
    2. Pressure on the perineum
    3. Excessive pull on the fascia
    4. Trauma to the uterine ligaments

145. A laboring primipara should be prepared for delivery when the nurse observes:
    1. The client becoming irritable and not following instructions
    2. That the perineum is beginning to bulge with each contraction
    3. An increase in the amount of bloody discharge from the vagina
    4. The contractions are occurring every 2 to 3 minutes and lasting 60 seconds

146. During the period of induction of labor, a client should be observed carefully for signs of:
    1. Severe pain
    2. Uterine tetany
    3. Hypoglycemia
    4. Prolapse of the umbilical cord

147. A client in labor is fully dilated, totally effaced, and the head is at +2. During each contraction the nurse should encourage her to:
    1. Push with glottis open
    2. Blow so as not to grunt
    3. Relax by closing her eyes
    4. Pant to prevent cervical edema

148. During labor, station +1 indicates that the presenting part is:
    1. On the perineum
    2. High in the false pelvis
    3. Slightly below the ischial spines
    4. Slightly above the ischial spines

149. A client is admitted in active labor; the baby's head is crowning, the client is bearing down, and delivery appears imminent. The nurse should:
    1. Transfer her immediately by stretcher to the delivery room
    2. Tell her to breathe through her mouth and not to bear down
    3. Instruct the client to pant during contractions and to breathe through her mouth
    4. Support the perineum with the hand to prevent tearing and tell the client to pant

150. A laboring client is to have a pudendal block. The nurse plans to tell the client that once the block is working she:
    1. Will not feel the episiotomy
    2. May lose the ability to push
    3. May lose bladder sensation
    4. Will no longer feel contractions

151. During delivery the physician performs an episiotomy. The nurse reminds the client that this is most commonly done to:
    1. Stretch the perineum
    2. Limit postpartal discomfort
    3. Reduce trauma to the fetus
    4. Prevent lacerations during birth

152. Following delivery the nurse teaches a client to cleanse her episiotomy to prevent infection. The nurse determines that the teaching was effective when the client:
    1. Changes her perineal pad at least twice daily
    2. Rinses with water after applying an analgesic spray
    3. Washes her hands before and after changing her perineal pads
    4. Cleanses her perineum from the anus toward the symphysis pubis

153. Several hours after delivery when assessing a client's episiotomy, the nurse finds there is edema with severe ecchymosis, and the client is complaining of severe perineal and rectal pressure. The fundus is firm and there is no lochia. The vital signs are T 99° F, P 108, R 20, BP 105/60. This assessment most likely indicates:
    1. An urinary infection
    2. An uterine infection
    3. A vaginal hematoma
    4. A postpartal hemorrhage

154. A client delivers a healthy baby girl. An indication to the nurse that the placenta is beginning to separate from the uterus and is about ready to be delivered would be the:
    1. Descent of the uterus in the abdomen
    2. Relaxation and softening of the uterus
    3. Appearance of a sudden gush of blood
    4. Retraction of the umbilical cord into the vagina

155. The two most important predisposing causes of puerperal or postpartal infection are:
    1. Hemorrhage and trauma during labor
    2. Preeclampsia and retention of placenta
    3. Malnutrition and anemia during pregnancy
    4. Organisms present in the birth canal and trauma during labor

156. Eight hours after delivery the nurse notices that a client is voiding frequently in small amounts. Intake and output are important in the early postpartal period because small amounts of output:
    1. May indicate retention of urine with overflow
    2. Are commonly voided and should cause no alarm
    3. May be indicative of beginning glomerulonephritis
    4. Are common because less fluid is excreted following delivery

157. When checking a client's fundus on the second postpartum day, the nurse observes that the fundus is above the umbilicus and displaced to the right. The nurse evaluates that the client probably has:
    1. A slow rate of involution
    2. A full, overdistended bladder
    3. Retained placental fragments
    4. Overstretched uterine ligaments

158. During the postpartum period following a cesarean birth, the nurse examines the client and identifies the presence of lochia serosa and feels the fundus four fingerbreadths below the umbilicus. This indicates that the time elapsed is:
    1. 1 to 3 days postpartum
    2. 4 to 5 days postpartum
    3. 6 to 7 days postpartum
    4. 8 to 9 days postpartum

159. The pituitary hormone that stimulates the secretion of milk from the mammary glands is:
    1. Prolactin
    2. Oxytocin
    3. Estrogen
    4. Progesterone

160. The nurse is aware that one of the factors influencing the availability of milk in the lactating woman is the:
    1. Amount of erectile tissue in the nipples
    2. Age of the woman at the time of delivery
    3. Attitude of the woman's family toward breastfeeding
    4. Amount of milk and milk products consumed during pregnancy

161. When caring for a client with an episiotomy during the postpartum period, the nurse encourages sitz baths three times a day for 15 minutes. Sitz baths primarily aid the healing process by:
    1. Promoting vasodilation
    2. Softening the incision site
    3. Cleansing the perineal area
    4. Tightening the rectal sphincter

162. The postpartum nurse should encourage newly delivered clients to ambulate early in order to:
    1. Promote respiration
    2. Increase the tone of the bladder
    3. Maintain tone of abdominal muscles
    4. Increase peripheral vasomotor activity

163. When performing a discharge teaching for a postpartum client, the nurse should inform her that:
    1. She may not have any bowel movements for up to a week after delivery
    2. The episiotomy sutures will be removed at the first postpartum checkup
    3. She has to schedule a postpartum checkup as soon as her menses returns
    4. The perineal tightening exercises started after delivery should be continued indefinitely

164. When teaching a prenatal class about infant feeding, the nurse is asked a question about the relationship between the size of breasts and breastfeeding. The nurse's best response would be:
    1. "Everybody can be successful at breastfeeding."
    2. "You seem to have some concern about breastfeeding."
    3. "The size of your breasts has nothing to do with the production of milk."
    4. "The amount of fat and glandular tissue in the breasts determines the amount of milk produced."

165. A woman in a class on infant feedings asks how anyone who is breastfeeding gets anything done with a baby on demand feedings. The nurse's best response would be:
    1. "Most mothers find that feeding the baby whenever the baby cries works out fine."
    2. "Perhaps a schedule might be better because the baby is already accustomed to the hospital routine."
    3. "Most mothers find babies on breast do better on demand feeding because the amount of milk ingested varies at each feeding."
    4. "Although the baby is on demand feedings, the baby will eventually set a schedule, so there will be time for your household chores."

166. The nurse should teach the client that breastfeeding is always contraindicated with:
    1. Mastitis
    2. Hepatitis C
    3. Inverted nipples
    4. Herpes genitalis

167. A client asks about the difference between cow's milk and the milk from her breasts. The nurse should respond that cow's milk differs from human milk in that it contains:
    1. More protein, less calcium, and less carbohydrate
    2. Less protein, less calcium, and more carbohydrate
    3. More protein, more calcium, and less carbohydrate
    4. Less protein, more calcium, and more carbohydrate

168. The client response that indicates correct understanding of teaching regarding breast care in the mother who is breastfeeding would be, "I will:
    1. Use a mild soap for washing."
    2. Remove my brassiere at night."
    3. Air dry my nipples after feeding."
    4. Line my breast pads with plastic."

169. A client who is breastfeeding is being discharged. The client tells the nurse that she is worried because her neighbor's breasts dried up when she got home and she had to discontinue breastfeeding. The nurse would best reply:
    1. "This is not true; once lactation is established, this rarely happens."

2. "You have little to worry about because you already have a good milk supply."
    3. "This commonly happens with the excitement of going home. Putting the baby to breast more frequently will reestablish lactation."
    4. "This commonly happens; however, we will give you a formula to take home so the baby won't go hungry until your milk supply returns."

170. When teaching breastfeeding the nurse should recognize the client needs further instructions when she states, "I will:
    1. Try to empty my breasts at each feeding."
    2. Use an alternate breast at each feeding."
    3. Wash my breasts with water before each feeding."
    4. Wash my breasts with soap and water before feeding."

171. The nurse should plan to teach a recently delivered client who is bottlefeeding her infant to minimize breast discomfort by:
    1. Gently applying cocoa butter
    2. Manually expressing colostrum
    3. Applying covered ice packs to her breasts
    4. Placing warm, wet washcloths on her nipples

172. Since having a baby by cesarean delivery a client has walked to the nursery numerous times to see her baby each day. Two days postpartum the client complains of pain in the right leg. The nurse's initial response should be to:
    1. Apply hot soaks
    2. Massage the affected area
    3. Encourage ambulation and exercise
    4. Maintain bed rest and notify the physician

173. A 38-year-old becomes pregnant and attends the prenatal clinic. The nurse tells her that a serum alphafetoprotein test will probably be done to detect the presence of:
    1. Trisomy 21
    2. Turner's syndrome
    3. Open neural tube defects
    4. Chromosomal aberrations

174. A nurse, planning an initial home care visit following delivery of a newborn, recognizes that the visit will be more productive if scheduled when the:
    1. Mother is feeding the infant
    2. Husband is out of the home
    3. Time is convenient for the family
    4. Nurse has time to spend with the family

175. During a postpartal visit, a client whose infant is now 4 weeks old complains of leg cramps. The nurse suspects:
    1. Hypercalcemia and tells her to increase her activity
    2. Hypocalcemia and tells her to increase her intake of milk
    3. Hyperkalemia and tells her to see a physician immediately
    4. Hypokalemia and tells her to increase her intake of green, leafy vegetables

176. During the postpartum period a client tells the nurse she is having leg cramps. The nurse should suggest that the client increase her intake of:
    1. Eggs and bacon
    2. Liver and onions
    3. Juices and water
    4. Cheese and broccoli

177. The nurse teaches a multipara who has just delivered a large baby what to do to maintain a contracted uterus. The nurse recognizes that teaching has been effective when the client states:
    1. "If I start to bleed I will call for help."
    2. "I will gently massage my uterus to keep it firm."
    3. "If I urinate frequently, my uterus will stay contracted."
    4. "I will call you every 15 minutes to massage my uterus."

Normal Newborn

178. Immunity transferred to the fetus from an immune mother through the placenta is:
    1. Active natural immunity
    2. Active artificial immunity
    3. Passive natural immunity
    4. Passive artificial immunity

179. A baby is delivered precipitously in the labor room. The nurse's initial action should be to:
    1. Establish an airway for the baby
    2. Ascertain the condition of the fundus
    3. Quickly tie and cut the umbilical cord
    4. Move mother and baby to the delivery room

180. Closure of the foramen ovale after birth is caused by:
    1. A decrease in the aortic blood flow
    2. A decrease in pressure in the left atrium
    3. An increase in the pulmonary blood flow
    4. An increase in the pressure in the right atrium

181. After birth, in a normal neonate, the ductus arteriosus becomes the:
    1. Venous ligament
    2. Ligamentum teres
    3. Superior vesical artery
    4. Ligamentum arteriosum

182. A client delivers a 6-pound baby girl. She decides to room in with her baby, and both are transferred to the postpartum unit. The baby is lying quietly in the bassinet with her eyes wide open. In response to this infant behavior the nurse:
    1. Turns up the lights in the room
    2. Instructs the mother to talk to her baby
    3. Begins the baby's physical examination
    4. Wraps her snugly and turns her on her side

183. The primary critical observation for Apgar scoring is the:
    1. Heart rate
    2. Respiratory rate
    3. Presence of meconium
    4. Evaluation of Moro reflex

184. When performing a newborn assessment, the nurse should measure the vital signs in the following sequence:
    1. Pulse, respirations, temperature
    2. Temperature, pulse, respirations
    3. Respirations, temperature, pulse
    4. Respirations, pulse, temperature

185. Within 3 minutes after birth the normal heart rate of the infant may range between:
    1. 100 and 180
    2. 130 and 170
    3. 120 and 160
    4. 100 and 130

186. In a noisy room, the newborn is noted to startle and have rapid movements initially, but soon goes to sleep. The most appropriate nursing action would be to:
    1. Test the infant's hearing
    2. Allow the infant to sleep
    3. Assess the infant's vital signs
    4. Stimulate the infant's respirations

187. The normal respiratory rate of an infant within 3 minutes after birth may be as high as:
    1. 50
    2. 60
    3. 80
    4. 100

188. The nurse is aware that a normal newborn's respirations are:
   1. Regular, abdominal, 40 to 50 per minute, deep
   2. Irregular, abdominal, 30 to 60 per minute, shallow
   3. Irregular, initiated by chest wall, 30 to 60 per minute, deep
   4. Regular, initiated by the chest wall, 40 to 60 per minute, shallow

189. Just after beginning the first feeding with glucose water a newborn begins to cough and choke, and the lips turn cyanotic. Immediate nursing action should be to:
   1. Stimulate crying to help clear the airway
   2. Change to plain sterile water for the feeding
   3. Attempt to suction the infant and provide oxygen
   4. Allow the infant to rest before continuing the feeding

190. At 10 hours of age an infant has a large amount of mucus and becomes slightly cyanotic. The nurse should first:
   1. Insert a Levin tube
   2. Give the infant oxygen
   3. Suction the mucus as needed
   4. Note the incident on the chart

191. To help limit the development of hyperbilirubinemia in the neonate, the nursing care plan should include:
   1. Monitoring for the passage of meconium each shift
   2. Instituting phototherapy for 30 minutes every 6 hours
   3. Substituting breastfeeding for formula during the second day after birth
   4. Supplementing breastfeeding with glucose water during the first 24 hours

192. The Moro reflex response is marked by:
   1. Extension of the arms
   2. Adduction of the arms
   3. Abduction and then adduction of the arms
   4. Extension of the legs and fanning of the toes

193. Asymmetric Moro reflexes are frequently associated with:
   1. Down syndrome
   2. Cranial nerve damage
   3. Cerebral or cerebellar injuries
   4. Brachial plexus, clavicle, or humerus injuries

194. A newborn has small, whitish, pinpoint spots over the nose, which the nurse knows are caused by retained sebaceous secretions. When charting this observation, the nurse identifies it as:
   1. Milia
   2. Lanugo
   3. Whiteheads
   4. Mongolian spots

195. The nurse observes a normal newborn lying in a supine position with the head turned to the side, legs and arms extended on the same side and flexed on the opposite side. This is:
   1. The Moro reflex
   2. The Landau reflex
   3. A tonic neck reflex
   4. An abnormal reflex

196. An infant's intestines are sterile at birth, therefore lacking the bacteria necessary for the synthesis of:
   1. Bilirubin
   2. Bile salts
   3. Prothrombin
   4. Intrinsic factor

197. When newborns have been on formula for 36 to 48 hours they should have a:
   1. Vitamin K injection
   2. Screening for PKU
   3. Test for necrotizing enterocolitis
   4. Heel stick for blood glucose level

198. The nurse teaches a group of postpartal clients that all their newborns will be screened for PKU to:
   1. Detect possible retardation
   2. Test for thyroid insufficiency
   3. Measure protein metabolism
   4. Identify chromosomal damage

199. The practice of separating parents and child immediately after birth and limiting their time with the newborn in the first few days would appear to contradict studies based on:
   1. Bonding
   2. Rooming in
   3. Taking-in behaviors
   4. Taking-hold behaviors

200. After delivery, when inspecting her newborn baby girl, the mother notices a discharge from the nipples of both breasts of the baby. The nurse should explain that this is evidence of:
   1. Monilia contracted during birth
   2. An infection contracted in utero
   3. Congenital hormonal imbalance
   4. The influence of the mother's hormones

201. The nurse decides on a teaching plan for a new mother and her infant. The plan should include:
     1. Discussing the matter with her in a nonthreatening manner
     2. Setting up a schedule for teaching the mother how to care for her baby
     3. Showing by example how to care for the infant and explain her needs
     4. Supplying emotional support to the mother and encouraging her dependence

202. A client asks the nurse what advantage breastfeeding has over bottlefeeding. The nurse replies that one major group of substances in human milk that is of special importance to the newborn and cannot be reproduced in any bottle formula is:
     1. Amino acids
     2. Complex carbohydrates
     3. Essential ions (electrolytes)
     4. Gamma globulins (antibodies)

203. A new mother is breastfeeding her 2-day-old infant and tells the home health nurse that she cannot believe her newborn wants to breastfeed again, since she just fed him $2^1/_2$ hours ago. The nurse should plan to teach the client that a newborn usually should be nursed:
     1. Hourly
     2. On demand
     3. Every 4 hours
     4. At 5-hour intervals

204. A client asks the nurse why sugar was added to the baby's formula. The nurse's response would depend on the following understanding:
     1. Sugar in cow's milk is a disaccharide
     2. Sugar in cow's milk is not assimilated well
     3. Cow's milk contains fewer calories than breast milk
     4. Diluted cow's milk provides less sugar than the baby needs

205. A 2-day old infant who weighs 2722 g (6 lb) is fed formula every 4 hours. Newborns need about 73 ml (2 to 3 oz) of fluid per pound of body weight each day. Based on this information the nurse knows that at each feeding the infant should be fed at least:
     1. 2 to 3 oz
     2. 1 to 2 oz
     3. 3 to 4 oz
     4. 4 to 5 oz

206. A new mother notices that her infant often regurgitates after the feedings and asks the nurse if her baby is ill. The nurse explains to the mother that this is normal and due to:
     1. Intake of air while sucking
     2. A spasm at the pyloric valve
     3. An underdeveloped cardiac sphincter
     4. The position that the baby is in after feeding

High-Risk Pregnancy

207. A 42-year-old client has an amniocentesis during the sixteenth week of gestation because of concern about Down syndrome. Examination of the amniotic fluid will also provide information regarding:
     1. Fetal diabetes
     2. Fetal lung maturity
     3. Cardiac anomalies
     4. Presence of neural tube defects

208. The fetus is most likely to be structurally damaged by the pregnant woman's ingestion of drugs during the:
     1. First trimester
     2. Second trimester
     3. Third trimester
     4. Entire pregnancy

209. More than half the neonatal deaths in the United States are caused by:
     1. Atelectasis
     2. Prematurity
     3. Congenital heart disease
     4. Respiratory distress syndrome

210. A pregnant client asks the clinic nurse how smoking will affect the baby. The nurse's answer reflects the following knowledge:
     1. The placenta is permeable to specific substances
     2. Smoking relieves tension and the fetus responds accordingly
     3. Vasoconstriction will affect both fetal and maternal blood vessels
     4. Fetal and maternal circulation are separated by the placental barrier

211. A client, 12 weeks' gestation, comes to the prenatal clinic complaining of severe nausea and frequent vomiting. The nurse suspects that this client has hyperemesis gravidarum and knows that this is frequently associated with:
     1. Excessive amniotic fluid
     2. A GI history of cholecystitis
     3. High levels of chorionic gonadotropin
     4. Slowed secretion of free hydrochloric acid

212. Contraindications for an oxytocin challenge test (CST) would include:
1. Prematurity
2. Hypertension
3. Drug addiction
4. Uterine activity

213. When caring for a woman with a positive contraction stress test, the nurse should be chiefly concerned with observing her for signs and symptoms of:
1. Preeclampsia
2. Placenta previa
3. Uteroplacental insufficiency
4. Imminent premature delivery

214. The nurse's initial responsibility in teaching the pregnant adolescent client is:
1. Informing her of the benefits of breastfeeding
2. Advising her about the proper care of an infant
3. Instructing her to watch for danger signs of preeclampsia
4. Impressing her with the importance of consistent prenatal care

215. The major concern about pregnant, unmarried teenagers is that they are often:
1. Diabetogenic
2. Socially ostracized
3. Financially dependent
4. Prone to pregnancy-induced hypertension

216. The presence of multiple gestation should be detected as early as possible and the pregnancy managed with high risk in mind because:
1. Postpartum hemorrhage is an expected complication
2. Perinatal mortality is two to three times greater than in single births
3. Maternal mortality is much higher during the prenatal period in multiple gestation
4. The mother needs time to adjust psychologically and physiologically after delivery

217. One of the most common causes of hypotonic uterine dystocia is:
1. Twin gestation
2. Maternal anemia
3. Pelvic contracture
4. Pregnancy-induced hypertension

218. The nurse teaches the warning signs that should be reported throughout pregnancy. The nurse is aware that the client understands the instructions when the client states that she would call the prenatal clinic to report:

1. Abdominal pain
2. A whitish vaginal discharge
3. Puffiness of her ankles every night
4. Mild intermittent painless contractions

219. In the fifth month of pregnancy, ultrasonography is performed on a client. The results indicate that the fetus is small for gestational age and there is evidence of a low-lying placenta. The nurse would use this information in the last trimester of pregnancy by assessing the client for signs of possible:
1. Placenta previa
2. Premature labor
3. Abruptio placentae
4. Precipitate delivery

220. A client who is 6 months pregnant comes to the prenatal clinic complaining of painful urination, flank tenderness, and hematuria. A diagnosis of pyelonephritis is made. An important nursing intervention for this client during the attack is:
1. Limiting fluid intake
2. Examining the urine for albumin
3. Maintaining her on a low-salt diet
4. Observing for signs of premature labor

221. The nurse encourages continued health care supervision for the pregnant woman with pyelonephritis because:
1. Preeclampsia frequently occurs following pyelonephritis
2. A low-protein diet is given until the pregnancy is terminated
3. Antibiotic therapy should be administered until the urine is sterile
4. Pelvic inflammatory disease occurs with untreated pyelonephritis

222. A client in the thirty-third week of pregnancy begins to experience contractions. She is to be treated at home with bed rest. The teaching plan for this client should include the information that the client:
1. Needs to have the foot of the bed raised on blocks
2. Needs to sit in bed with several large pillows supporting her back
3. Should be placed on her side with her head raised on a small pillow
4. Should assume the knee-chest position every 2 hours for 10 minutes while awake

223. A client comes to the clinic for a sonography at 36 weeks' gestation. Before the test begins, the client complains of severe abdominal pain. Heavy vaginal bleeding is noted and the client's BP drops while her pulse rate increases. The nurse should suspect that the client has a:
    1. Hydatidiform mole
    2. Vena caval syndrome
    3. Marginal placenta previa
    4. Complete abruptio placentae

224. The nurse realizes that the abdominal pain associated with abruptio placentae initially may be caused by:
    1. Hemorrhagic shock
    2. Inflammatory reactions
    3. Concealed hemorrhage
    4. Blood in the uterine muscle

225. The nurse is aware that the bleeding following severe abruptio placentae is usually caused by:
    1. Polycythemia
    2. Hyperglobulinemia
    3. Thrombocytopenia
    4. Hypofibrinogenemia

226. Abruptio placentae is most likely to occur in a woman with:
    1. Cardiac disease
    2. Hyperthyroidism
    3. Cephalopelvic disproportion
    4. Pregnancy-induced hypertension

227. A client experiences an episode of painless vaginal bleeding during the last trimester. The nurse realizes that this may be caused by:
    1. Placenta previa
    2. Abruptio placentae
    3. Frequent intercourse
    4. Excessive alcohol ingestion

228. The care of a client with placenta previa includes:
    1. Vital signs at least once per shift
    2. A tap-water enema before delivery
    3. Observation and recording of the bleeding
    4. Limited ambulation until the bleeding stops

229. Nursing care of women in premature labor includes:
    1. Encouraging them not to bear down
    2. Reassuring them that the situation is under control
    3. Keeping them NPO to prevent abdominal distention
    4. Explaining why pain medication is kept at a minimum

230. The nurse should explain to a client who is experiencing premature contractions in the thirty-fifth week of gestation with the cervix dilated 2 cm that coitus:
    1. Need not be restricted in any way
    2. Is prohibited, as it may stimulate labor
    3. Should be restricted to the side-lying position
    4. Is permitted as long as penile penetration is shallow

231. Following a delivery of twins a client may be predisposed to experiencing a postpartum hemorrhage. The nurse understands that the reason for this is:
    1. Atony of the uterus
    2. A secondary infection
    3. A laceration of the cervix
    4. Retained placental fragments

232. When assessing clients after delivery, the nurse should be aware that postpartal hemorrhage rarely occurs as a complication of:
    1. Retained placenta
    2. Overdistended bladder
    3. Delivery of twins or hydramnios
    4. Uncomplicated gestational hypertension

233. During the postpartal period it is not uncommon for a new mother to have an increased cardiac output with tachycardia. Because of this, the nurse should carefully observe the postpartum client with known cardiac problems for signs of:
    1. Irregular pulse
    2. Hypovolemic shock
    3. Respiratory distress
    4. Increased vaginal bleeding

234. The nurse notifies the physician that a client has been admitted in her thirty-sixth week of pregnancy. The client is bleeding, has severe abdominal pain, a hard fundus, and is demonstrating signs of shock. In addition to notifying the physician, the nurse also prepares for:
    1. A high forceps delivery
    2. The insertion of a fetal monitor
    3. An immediate cesarean delivery
    4. The administration of oxytocin (Pitocin)

235. A client is being prepared for an emergency cesarean delivery because of fetal distress. The most important thing for the nurse to assess before surgery is that:
    1. A signed consent is on the chart
    2. A Foley catheter has been inserted
    3. An IV of Ringer's lactate has been started
    4. The abdomen has been shaved and prepared

236 During the first hour after a cesarean delivery, the nurse notes that the client's lochia has saturated one peripad. Based on the knowledge of normal lochial flow, the nurse concludes that this indicates:
1. Scant lochial flow
2. Postpartum hemorrhage
3. Retained placental fragments
4. Lochial flow within normal limits

237. A client undergoes a cesarean delivery because of cephalopelvic disproportion. In addition to the routine care given to all postpartum clients during the first 24 hours, the nurse should:
1. Encourage early ambulation
2. Maintain IV infusion of oxytocin
3. Check the fundus gently but firmly
4. Check vital signs for evidence of shock

238. When taking the health history the nurse recognizes that a client would be at risk for developing pregnancy-induced hypertension if it is determined that she:
1. Is 31 years old
2. Is an obese primigravida
3. Has had six previous pregnancies
4. Has been on oral contraceptives within 3 months of conception

239. The nurse knows that along with elevated blood pressure readings another sign that may be indicative of a diagnosis of pregnancy-induced hypertension would be a:
1. Positive HCG test
2. Positive urine glucose
3. Fetal heart rate of 110 beats/min
4. Weight gain of 6 pounds in 1 month

240. When assessing a client with pregnancy-induced hypertension, the nurse should expect the client's blood pressure to be:
1. 150/100 mm Hg while standing and sitting
2. Elevated and accompanied by a headache
3. Above the baseline and fluctuating at each reading
4. 30/15 mm Hg over the baseline on two occasions 6 hours apart

241. When a client is admitted to the labor suite with a blood pressure of 130/90, 2+ proteinuria, and edema of the hands and face, the nurse should ask the client about the presence of:
1. Constipation, edema, visual problems, headache
2. Leakage of fluid, bleeding, edema, pain in the abdomen
3. Visual disturbances, headaches, constipation, bleeding
4. Headache, visual disturbances, edema, pain in the abdomen

242. The first assessable objective sign of a seizure in a client with eclampsia is frequently:
1. Epigastric pain, nausea, and vomiting
2. Persistent headache and blurred vision
3. Spots or flashes of light before the eyes
4. Rolling of the eyes to one side with a fixed stare

243. The nurse evaluates that the danger of a seizure in a woman with eclampsia ends:
1. After labor begins
2. After delivery occurs
3. 24 hours postpartum
4. 48 hours postpartum

244. In the immediate postpartal period, the most critical assessment of a client with pregnancy-induced hypertension would be:
1. Obtaining the client's vital signs
2. Observing for signs of hemorrhage
3. Evaluating the client's emotional status
4. Monitoring for hypovolemic shock resulting from fluid shifts

245. A birth hazard associated with breech delivery may be:
1. Abruptio placentae
2. Cephalhematoma
3. Pathologic jaundice
4. Compression of cord

246. During an emergency delivery, the nurse notes the baby's head crowning on the perineum. The nurse's priority action is to support the head by:
1. Applying suprapubic pressure over it
2. Distributing the fingers evenly around it
3. Placing a hand firmly against the perineum
4. Maintaining firm pressure against the anterior fontanel

247. The safest position for a woman in labor when the nurse notes a prolapsed cord is:
1. Prone
2. Fowler's
3. Lithotomy
4. Trendelenburg

248. The normal hemodynamics of pregnancy that affect the pregnant cardiac client include the:
1. Gradually increasing size of the uterus
2. Decrease in the number of red blood cells
3. Rise in cardiac output after the thirty-fourth week
4. Cardiac acceleration in the last half of pregnancy

249. A pregnant client with a class II cardiac condition is concerned that her pregnancy will be an added burden on her already compromised heart. The nurse explains to this client that during pregnancy the cardiac system is most compromised during the:
1. First trimester
2. Third trimester
3. Transitional phase of delivery
4. First forty-eight hours after delivery

250. A pregnant client with a history of rheumatic heart disease since childhood is concerned about the delivery of her baby and asks what to expect. The nurse should mention that at term her care will probably include:
1. An elective cesarean delivery
2. Induction of labor to reduce stress
3. General anesthesia and forceps-assisted delivery
4. Regional anesthesia and forceps-assisted delivery

251. A client with a history of rheumatic fever and class I cardiac disease is admitted to the labor suite in active labor. Proper positioning for this client would be:
1. Supine; high-Fowler's
2. Supine; semi-Fowler's
3. Left lateral; semi-Fowler's
4. Lying on right side; head elevated 30°

252. A cardiac client goes into labor. To prevent the client from developing cardiac decompensation during labor, the nurse should:
1. Administer an IV infusion of isotonic saline
2. Maintain an IV infusion of potassium chloride
3. Administer oxytocin to accelerate contractions
4. Position her on her side with shoulders elevated

253. A specific nursing intervention for laboring clients with cardiac problems is:
1. Monitoring BP every hour
2. Encouraging frequent voiding
3. Auscultating for crackles q 30 minutes
4. Turning from side to side at 15-minute intervals

254. The nurse understands that the diabetic mother's metabolism is significantly altered during pregnancy as a result of:
1. The lower renal threshold for glucose
2. The increased effect of insulin during pregnancy
3. An increase in the glucose tolerance level of the blood
4. The effect of hormones produced in pregnancy on carbohydrate and lipid metabolism

255. A pregnant client with diabetes is referred to the clinic nutritionist for nutritional assessment and counseling. The dietary program worked out for this client would be:
1. A diet high in protein of good biologic value and decreased calories
2. A balanced diet to meet increased dietary needs with insulin adjusted as necessary
3. Adequate balance of carbohydrate and fat to meet energy demands and prevent ketosis
4. A low-carbohydrate, low-calorie diet to stay within her present insulin coverage and avoid hyperglycemia

256. The nurse is aware that in the second half of pregnancy women who are diabetic require:
1. Decreased caloric intake
2. Increased dosage of insulin
3. Administration of pancreatic enzymes
4. Administration of estrogenic hormones

257. The nurse should anticipate that on the first postpartal day, the insulin requirements of a client with diabetes mellitus will:
1. Rapidly increase
2. Remain unchanged
3. Demonstrate a slow decrease
4. Decrease sharply and suddenly

258. At 38 weeks' gestation a client begins active labor and is placed on a fetal monitor. Late decelerations in the FHR begin to appear when she is 6 cm dilated, with q 4-minute contractions lasting 45 seconds. Late decelerations may signify:
1. Imminent vaginal delivery
2. Uteroplacental insufficiency
3. A pattern of nonprogressive labor
4. A reassuring response to contractions

259. Following delivery of the placenta in a client who has six living children, an infusion of lactated Ringer's with 10 units of Pitocin is ordered. The nurse understands that this is indicated for this client because:
    1. Multigravidas are at increased risk for uterine atony
    2. Retained placental fragments must be expelled
    3. This was an extramural delivery
    4. She had a precipitate delivery

260. The nurse notes a new mother has type B negative blood. Her baby's blood type is AB positive. The nurse is aware that the mother's plan of care should include:
    1. Obtaining an order for RhoGAM
    2. Observing for ABO incompatibility
    3. Determining the father's blood type
    4. Immediate typing and crossmatching of her blood

High-Risk Newborn

261. A laboring client begins to experience contractions 2 to 3 minutes apart that last about 45 seconds. Between contractions the nurse records a fetal heart rate of 100 beats per minute. The nurse should:
    1. Notify the physician immediately
    2. Continue to monitor the fetal heart
    3. Closely monitor the maternal vital signs
    4. Chart the rate as a normal response to contractions

262. The finding that would probably necessitate prolonged follow-up care of a newborn would be:
    1. A birth weight of 3500 g
    2. An initial Apgar score of 5
    3. An umbilical cord that contained only two vessels
    4. The aspiration of 20 ml of milky-colored fluid from the newborn's stomach

263. The nurse suspects that a newly admitted infant is showing signs of drug withdrawal when assessment of the infant demonstrates:
    1. Lethargy and constipation
    2. Grunting and a low-pitched cry
    3. Irritability and nasal congestion
    4. Watery eyes and elevated respirations

264. Typical signs of drug dependence in babies result from withdrawal and usually begin within 24 hours after birth. The nurse should observe the babies of suspected or known drug users for:
    1. Hyperactivity
    2. Hypotonicity of muscles
    3. Prolonged periods of sleep
    4. Dehydration and constipation

265. A low Apgar score at 5 minutes after birth correlates with the occurrence of:
    1. Cerebral palsy
    2. Genetic defects
    3. Mental retardation
    4. Neonatal morbidity

266. An infant born in the thirty-sixth week of gestation weighs 4 lb, 9 oz (2062 g) and has an Apgar of 7/9. Upon admission to the nursery, it would be unnecessary for the nurse to:
    1. Record vital signs
    2. Administer oxygen
    3. Support body temperature
    4. Evaluate the newborn's status

267. On a home visit to a known drug abuser who delivered 4 days ago, the visiting nurse assesses that the baby has a purulent discharge from the eyes. The nurse suspects that the infant has:
    1. Symptoms of *Chlamydia trachomatis* infection
    2. Retinopathy of prematurity (retrolental fibroplasia)
    3. Signs of acquired immunodeficiency syndrome (AIDS)
    4. Developed a reaction to the ophthalmic antibiotic ointment instilled after birth

268. An infant develops purulent conjunctivitis on the fourth day of life and is brought to the emergency department. The nurse should:
    1. Teach the mother about hand washing
    2. Assess the infant for signs of pneumonia
    3. Secure an order for allergy testing of the infant
    4. Bathe the infant's eyes with tepid boric acid solution

269. When caring for preterm infants, the precautions that should be taken against retinopathy of prematurity (retrolental fibroplasia) include:
    1. Carefully controlling temperature and humidity
    2. Using phototherapy to prevent jaundice and retinopathy
    3. Keeping oxygen at reduced concentrations and discontinuing it as soon as feasible
    4. Maintaining a high concentration of oxygen (above 75%) together with high humidity

270. The care of a newborn infant whose mother has had untreated syphilis since the second trimester of the pregnancy would be:
    1. Assessing for a cleft palate
    2. Eliciting hypotonicity of skeletal muscles
    3. Observing for maculopapular lesions of the soles
    4. Having the baby immediately screened for syphilis

271. A newborn has asymmetric gluteal folds. The nurse suspects:
    1. CNS damage
    2. Dysplasia of hip
    3. An inguinal hernia
    4. Peripheral nervous system damage

272. An infant is born in the breech position. Because Erb's palsy may be seen as the result of a difficult forceps or breech delivery, the nurse should assess the infant for:
    1. A flaccid arm with the elbow extended
    2. Loss of grasp reflex on the affected side
    3. Inability to turn the head to the affected side
    4. A negative Moro reflex on the unaffected side

273. Immediate nursing care for the affected arm of an infant born with Erb's palsy should include:
    1. Constant immobilization of the affected arm
    2. Teaching the parents to manipulate the muscle
    3. Immediate active ROM exercises to the affected arm
    4. Daily measurement of girth and length of the affected arm

274. When determining the difference between cephalhematoma and caput succedaneum, the nurse understands that with caput succedaneum the:
    1. Affected area will be tender
    2. Swelling crosses the suture line
    3. Swelling increases within 24 hours
    4. Scalp over the swelling becomes ecchymotic

275. The nurse should be aware that the chief hazard to an infant during a precipitate delivery is:
    1. Brachial palsy
    2. Dislocated hip
    3. Fractured clavicle
    4. Intracranial hemorrhage

276. An infant in the newborn nursery has cyanosis of the hands and feet and circumoral pallor when crying. The nurse should:
    1. Report this circumoral pallor to the physician because it could signal a cardiac problem
    2. Take no specific action because both signs are normal for a newborn until 2 weeks of age.
    3. Take no specific action because circumoral pallor is a normal finding for the first 72 to 96 hours
    4. Notify the physician because cyanosis and pallor usually accompany increased intracranial pressure

277. A preterm neonate admitted to the neonatal intensive care nursery has muscle twitching, convulsions, cyanosis, abnormal respirations, and a short shrill cry. The nurse suspects that this infant may have:
    1. Tetany
    2. Spina bifida
    3. Hyperkalemia
    4. Intracranial hemorrhage

278. Shortly following birth, a newborn is diagnosed as having Erb's palsy. The nurse is aware that this problem is caused by:
    1. A disease acquired in utero
    2. An X-linked inheritance pattern
    3. A tumor arising from muscle tissue
    4. An injury to the brachial plexus during birth

279. The nurse observes a yellowish color of the skin of a baby in the newborn nursery. The immediate nursing action should be to:
    1. Ascertain the age of the infant
    2. Notify the physician of the development
    3. Take a heel blood sample and send it to the laboratory
    4. Cover the baby's eyes with a blindfold and put the baby under the ultraviolet light

280. When observing a newborn for signs of pathologic jaundice, the nurse should be alert for:
    1. Muscular irritability at birth
    2. Neurologic signs during the first 24 hours
    3. The appearance of jaundice during the first 24 hours
    4. Jaundice developing between the second and fourth day of life

281. The nurse is aware that Isolettes are used for preterm infants to maintain body temperature at a constant level, because the heat-regulation mechanism of preterm babies is one of the least developed functions. This is related to the fact that these babies:
    1. Have a smaller surface area than full-term newborns
    2. Perspire a great deal, thus losing heat almost constantly
    3. Lack subcutaneous fat, which would furnish some insulation
    4. Have a limited ability to produce antibodies against infections

282. The nurse must continuously monitor a pretem infant's temperature and provide appropriate nursing care because the preterm infant:
    1. Has an inability to break down glycogen to glucose
    2. Has a limited ability to use shivering to produce heat
    3. Has a limited supply of brown fat available to provide heat
    4. Has an underdeveloped pituitary system to control internal heat

283. When meeting a preterm infant's hydration needs, the nurse should know that urinary function in the preterm baby:
    1. Is the same as in a full-term newborn
    2. Results in the loss of large amounts of urine
    3. Leads to urine with an elevated specific gravity
    4. Adequately maintains an acid-base and electrolyte balance

284. The nurse must continuously monitor preterm infants for the most common preterm complication of:
    1. Hemorrhage
    2. Brain damage
    3. Aspiration of mucus
    4. Respiratory distress

285. When caring for preterm infants with respiratory distress, the nurse should keep:
    1. Them prone to prevent aspiration
    2. Them in a high-humidity environment
    3. Their caloric intake low to decrease metabolic rate
    4. Their oxygen concentration low to prevent eye damage

286. The newly delivered newborn of a diabetic mother will be screened for hypoglycemia by the nurse's:

1. Scheduling a fasting blood sugar
2. Drawing blood for serum glucose
3. Beginning a glucose tolerance test
4. Doing a heel stick using a glucose-oxidase strip

287. In the nursery, the newborn of a mother with a history of long-standing diabetes should be provided with:
    1. Fast-acting insulin
    2. Special high-risk care
    3. Routine newborn care
    4. A decreased glucose intake

288. The nurse understands that following delivery, infants of diabetic mothers often have tremors, periods of apnea, cyanosis, and poor sucking ability. These symptoms are associated with:
    1. Hypoglycemia
    2. Hyperglycemia
    3. Central nervous system edema
    4. Congenital depression of the islets of Langerhans

289. The nurse is aware that infants of diabetic mothers are larger than other newborns because of:
    1. Increased somatotropin and lowered glucose utilization
    2. Increased somatotropin and increased glucose utilization
    3. Decreased somatotropin and increased glucose utilization
    4. Decreased somatotropin and decreased glucose utilization

290. A nursing diagnosis that should have priority for an infant born with exstrophy of the bladder is:
    1. Urinary retention
    2. Risk for infection
    3. Deficient fluid volume
    4. Risk for sexual dysfunction

Women's Health

291. The large amount of progesterone secreted during the secretory phase of the menstrual cycle is responsible for:
    1. The onset of ovulation
    2. The regulation of menstruation
    3. The incidence of capillary fragility
    4. Sustaining the thick endometrium of the uterus

292. The hormones responsible for the proliferation phase of menstruation are:
    1. Luteinizing hormone and estrogen
    2. Luteinizing hormone and progesterone
    3. Lactogenic hormone and progesterone
    4. Follicle-stimulating hormone and estrogen

293. The main blood supply to the uterus is directly from the:
1. Uterine and ovarian arteries
2. Ovarian arteries and the aorta
3. Uterine and hypogastric arteries
4. Aorta and the hypogastric arteries

294. A woman menstruates regularly every 30 days. Her last menses started on January 1. She will most probably ovulate again on:
1. January 5
2. January 15
3. January 17
4. January 28

295. A 15-year-old client complains of persistent dysmenorrhea. The nurse should encourage her to:
1. Maintain daily activities
2. Have a gynecologic exam
3. Eat a nutritious diet containing iron
4. Practice relaxation of abdominal muscles

296. Endometriosis is characterized by:
1. Amenorrhea and insomnia
2. Ecchymoses and petechiae
3. Painful menstruation and backache
4. Early osteoporosis and pelvic inflammation

297. Overstretching of perineal supporting tissues as a result of childbirth can bring about a rectocele. The most common symptom is:
1. Crampy abdominal pain
2. A bearing-down sensation
3. Urinary stress incontinence
4. Recurrent urinary tract infections

298. When taking the health history of a client who is admitted for repair of a cystocele and rectocele, the nurse would expect the client to report the occurrence of:
1. Heavy leukorrhea, pruritus
2. Sporadic bleeding accompanied by abdominal pain
3. Stress incontinence, feeling of low abdominal pressure
4. Change in acidity level of the vagina, leukorrhea, spotting

299. A client has an anterior and posterior colporrhaphy and returns from the postanesthesia unit with an indwelling catheter in place. The primary reason for the catheter is to prevent:
1. Retention
2. Discomfort
3. Loss of bladder tone
4. Pressure on the suture line

300. After an anterior-posterior colporrhaphy in a client past menopause the nurse should teach the client how to prevent:
1. Pregnancy
2. Constipation
3. Incontinence
4. Rectovaginal fistulas

301. The physician informs the nurse that a client has severe procidentia (prolapse of the uterus). The nurse plans to assess the client for:
1. Exudate
2. Swelling
3. Ulcerations
4. Vaginal discharge

302. A client with a prolapsed uterus is scheduled for a vaginoplasty. Preoperatively the nurse may expect to:
1. Encourage ambulation
2. Apply moist compresses
3. Elevate the foot of the bed
4. Manipulate the procidentia

303. The most therapeutic position for a client with pelvic inflammatory disease would be the:
1. Sims' position
2. Fowler's position
3. Lithotomy position
4. Supine position with knees flexed

304. Early treatment of cervical erosion is performed specifically to prevent:
1. Metrorrhagia
2. Cancer of the cervix
3. Further erosions from occurring
4. Infections of the reproductive system

305. The nurse knows that cervical polyps:
1. Do not cause bleeding until they are malignant
2. Are frequently the precursors of uterine cancer
3. Are usually malignant, and curettage is always done
4. Are usually benign, but curettage of the uterus is always done

306. A manifestation of cancer of the cervix that should have brought the client to the gynecologist is:
1. Abdominal heaviness
2. Foul-smelling discharge
3. Pressure on the bladder
4. Bloody spotting after intercourse

307. The most common site for cancer cell growth in the cervix is at the:
    1. External os and the regional nodes
    2. Internal os and the endocervical glands
    3. Junction of the cervix and lower uterine segment
    4. Columnosquamous junction of the internal and external ossa

308. Following a biopsy for suspected cervical cancer, the laboratory report reveals a stage 0 lesion. According to the International Federation of Gynecology and Obstetrics, stage 0 is indicative of:
    1. Carcinoma in situ
    2. Early stromal invasion
    3. Parametrial involvement
    4. Carcinoma strictly confined to the cervix

309. To elicit information about a client's risk for exposure to DES, the nurse, doing the medical history on a young woman in the prenatal clinic, should first ask:
    1. "Were you born before 1963?"
    2. "Have you ever taken oral contraceptives?"
    3. "Have you noticed any lesions in your perineal area?"
    4. "Did your mother take hormones during her pregnancy?"

310. A 35-year-old client is scheduled for a conization of the cervix to remove dysplasic cervical cells and determine the extent of involvement. The nurse would determine that the client understands the postoperative course if the client:
    1. States she will resume sexual intercourse within 48 hours
    2. Demonstrates the ability to change sterile surgical dressings
    3. Makes a positive adjustment to the loss of reproductive function
    4. Verbalizes expectations of a vaginal discharge for 3 to 5 days and altered menstrual periods

311. A client who is scheduled to have an abdominal panhysterectomy asks how the surgery will affect her periods. The nurse should respond:
    1. "You will no longer menstruate."
    2. "Initially your periods will increase."
    3. "Your monthly periods will be lighter."
    4. "Your monthly periods will be more regular."

312. A client expresses concern about having a hysterectomy at age 45 because she has heard from friends that she will undergo severe symptoms of menopause after surgery. The most appropriate response for the nurse would be:
    1. "This is something that does occur in older women on occasion, but you don't have to worry about it."
    2. "It's too bad you did not discuss this with your doctor. I really can't give you any kind of information about this."
    3. "You are correct. This happens following this type of surgery. Your friend probably had a similar diagnosis."
    4. "Some women occasionally experience exaggerated symptoms of menopause if in addition to their uterus, their ovaries are removed."

313. After a hysterosalpingo-oophorectomy a client wants to know if it would be wise for her to take hormones right away to prevent symptoms of menopause. The most appropriate response by the nurse would be:
    1. "It is best to wait; you may not have any symptoms at all."
    2. "You have to wait until symptoms are severe; otherwise, hormones will have no effect."
    3. "Isn't it comforting to know that hormones are available if you should really need them?"
    4. "This is something you should discuss with your physician, because it is important for the physician to know how you feel and what your concerns are."

314. Following an abdominal hysterectomy, the nurse notes that the urine in the client's Foley bag has become increasingly sanguinous. The nurse suspects that the client may have:
    1. An incisional nick in the bladder
    2. A urinary infection from the catheter
    3. Uterine relaxation with increased lochia
    4. Disseminated intravascular coagulopathy

315. The day following a hysterectomy, the client asks for sanitary pads because she feels she is going to menstruate. The nurse should base a response on the fact that:
    1. The client will not menstruate because the uterus has been removed
    2. It will take several weeks before normal menstruation is reestablished
    3. The client is probably showing signs of developing an anxiety response
    4. The appearance of frank vaginal bleeding is expected following this type of surgery

316. A client's pathology report shows metastatic adenocarcinoma of the breast. The client is to receive doxorubicin (Adriamycin), as part of the drug protocol. This drug modifies the growth of cancer cells by:
    1. Preventing folic acid synthesis
    2. Changing the osmotic gradient in the cell
    3. Inhibiting RNA synthesis by binding DNA
    4. Increasing the permeability of the cell wall

317. A client who had a mastectomy asks about the term ERP-positive. The nurse explains that tumor cells are evaluated for estrogen receptor protein to determine:
    1. If breast reconstruction is feasible
    2. The need for supplemental estrogen
    3. Potential response to hormone therapy
    4. The degree of metastasis that has occurred

318. Following a mastectomy, the nurse should position the client's arm on the affected side:
    1. In adduction supported by sandbags
    2. In abduction surrounded by sandbags
    3. With the hand higher than the arm on pillows
    4. Lower than the level of the right atrium on pillows

319. When encouraging a client to cough and deep breathe following a bilateral mastectomy, the client says, "Leave me alone, don't you know I'm in pain!" The nurse's most therapeutic response would be:
    1. "I'm sure you are in pain, rest now and I'll come back later."
    2. "Your pain is to be expected, but you must exercise your lungs."
    3. "I'll give you something for your pain; we'll start exercising tomorrow."
    4. "If you are unable to cough, I understand, but try to take five or six deep breaths."

320. When writing a teaching plan about osteoporosis, the nurse should recall that osteoporosis is best described as:
    1. Avascular necrosis
    2. Pathologic fractures
    3. Hyperplasia of osteoblasts
    4. A decrease in bone substance

321. The plan of care for a client with osteoporosis includes active and passive exercises, calcium supplements, and daily vitamins. The desired effect of therapy would be noted by the nurse if the client:
    1. Increased mobility
    2. Experienced fewer muscular spasms
    3. Had fewer bruises than on admission
    4. Developed fewer cardiac irregularities

322. The operative procedure that would result in surgical menopause would be a:
    1. Tubal ligation
    2. Simple hysterectomy
    3. Bilateral oophorectomy
    4. Bilateral salpingectomy

323. A nurse teaches a women's group that hot flashes are caused by the:
    1. Accumulation of acetylcholine
    2. Cessation of pituitary gonadotropins
    3. Overstimulation of the adrenal medulla
    4. Hormonal stimulation of the sympathetic system

324. Menopause is the cessation of menstrual function. One of the reasons given for the cessation of menses is:
    1. A decrease in gonadotropin in the blood
    2. A decrease in the production of prostaglandins
    3. The inability of the ovary to respond to gonadotropic hormones
    4. An increase in the secretion of progesterone from the follicles in the ovary

325. A female client is very upset with her diagnosis of gonorrhea and asks the nurse, "What can I do to prevent getting another infection in the future?" The nurse is aware that the teaching for this client has been understood when the client states, "My best protection is to:
    1. Douche after every intercourse."
    2. Avoid engaging in sexual behavior."
    3. Insist that my partner use a condom."
    4. Use a spermicidal cream with intercourse."

CHILDBEARING AND WOMEN'S HEALTH NURSING
ANSWERS AND RATIONALES

Emotional Needs Related to Childbearing and Women's Health

1. **2** This response points out reality and allows the client to elaborate. (2; CJ; AS; PS; EC)
   1 This response would close off any future communication with the client.
   3 This may be a true statement, but it does not allow for much discussion to follow.
   4 This response sounds rather critical or judgmental and would probably cut off further discussion with the client.

2. **1** This opens up an area of communication to get at what really is troubling the mother about feeding the baby. (1; MR; IM; PS; EC)
   2 Because the nurse is aware that this is not the best method, the problem of time should be explored with the mother.
   3 Holding can be accomplished at times other than feeding periods; it does not explore the client's feelings.
   4 This is true, but the mother should not be frightened; a more gentle explanation should be used.

3. **2** This allows the husband and wife to comfort each other while letting them know the nurse is available; it also allows them to recognize and accept their feelings of loss. (2; MR; IM; PS; EC)
   1 This makes an assumption that another pregnancy will ensue; it also cuts off further communication.
   3 Telling the client not to be upset cuts off communication and wrongly implies that it prolongs recovery.
   4 Grieving for the unborn child will and should occur during any period of pregnancy.

4. **3** Rooming in provides time for the mother and infant to be together; the mother can become acquainted with the infant more quickly. (2; CJ; PL; PS; EC)
   1 It is possible that the client does not want to breastfeed; attachment can be furthered by rooming in.
   2 This may not be a judicious action; rooming in is far more preferable.
   4 This will not promote bonding and attachment.

5. **2** Normal periods of marked change and adjustment are called developmental crises and predispose the woman to a situational crisis. (1; CJ; AN; PS; EC)
   1 These are transient; they are similar to previous mood changes and should not affect the mother's ability to cope.
   3 These occur throughout the life cycle of a mature woman and should not now be classified as a crisis.
   4 It becomes a crisis only if the husband withdraws support.

6. **1** Nurses with positive attitudes toward abortion should counsel women who are thinking of undergoing the procedure; they should know what services are available and the various methods that are used to induce abortion. (2; LE; EV; ED; EC)
   2 Nursing practice necessitates scientific knowledge; statements must be based on fact, not personal feelings or beliefs.
   3 The nurse is capable of giving information about abortion and need not defer to the physician.
   4 The nurse should give the client only the information requested and should not state personal feelings.

7. **4** The client must feel comfortable enough to verbalize her feelings of guilt if she is to be able to complete the grieving process. (2; CJ; AN; PS; EC)
   1 This is a sterile procedure and should not predispose the client to postoperative infection.
   2 This is a false assumption.
   3 Studies show that contraceptive counseling at this time is most important, because the client may not return after the abortion.

8. **2** Because mothering is not an inborn instinct, almost all mothers, including multiparas, report some ambivalence and anxiety about their ability to be good mothers. (1; MR; AS; PS; EC)
   1 This is untrue; very often the maternal instinct is nurtured by the sight of the infant.
   3 This is untrue; it may take a much longer time.
   4 This is untrue; ambivalent feelings are universal in response to the infant.

9. **2** Family-centered childbearing should adapt needs to the cultural system whenever possible. (2; MR; PL; TC; EC)
    1 Unnecessary; the primary nurse can handle this problem.
    3 This may be useful, but the primary intervention here is to address the client's cultural needs.
    4 Forcing the issue does not address the underlying problem; the nurse must address the client's cultural needs.

10. **3** In an emergency surgical situation when invasive techniques are necessary, it is important to have a consent signed as well as a history of the client's known allergies. (3; LE; IM; TC; EC)
    1 This is not a priority item in an emergency such as this.
    2 An enema is not given to a bleeding client; it may stimulate contractions and further bleeding.
    4 Same as answer 2.

11. **1** This response provides the client with a comfort measure while giving her an opportunity to verbalize her fears about having an abnormal labor. (2; MR; IM; PS; EC)
    2 This closes off communication with the client.
    3 This is of no help to the client; she is concerned with what is happening to her.
    4 This can be answered "yes" or "no" and leaves no further avenue for discussion.

12. **2** Both the father and the mother need additional support during the transitional stage of labor. (2; MR; IM; PS; EC)
    1 This statement is judgmental; this approach suggests that he will be failing his wife.
    3 The husband should be present throughout labor to support his wife; he should be assisted in this role.
    4 This does not encourage him to fulfill his role in supporting the mother during labor.

13. **4** Mothers need to explore their infants visually and tactilely to assure themselves that the infants are normal in all respects. (1; MR; AS; ED; EC)
    1 This is false reassurance; this comment closes off communication with the mother at a very opportune moment.
    2 Crying is not indicative of congenital defects; a strong cry does not ensure "normalcy."
    3 The "normalcy" of the mother's pregnancy and labor does not always have a relationship to the "normalcy" of the infant.

14. **3** Allowing the mother time to inspect the child permits viewing, touching, and holding, promoting bonding. (2; MR; PL; PS; EC)
    1 The client will proceed at her own rate; requiring her to do things is not supportive.
    2 The mother should have made this decision before delivery.
    4 This can be done only by allowing the mother ample time to interact with her baby.

15. **3** Sneezing is the way in which the newborn clears mucus from the nose; breathing is normally rapid and irregular. (1; MR; IM; PS; EC)
    1 This would discourage the mother from taking responsibility and slow the mothering process; it also implies that something could be wrong.
    2 More explanation is needed, and it also shuts off communication; the mother needs to express her feelings of anxiety.
    4 These are normal newborn responses and indicate no respiratory distress.

16. **2** The mother has completed the taking-in phase (the mother's needs predominate) and has moved into the taking-hold phase (active maternal involvement with self and infant) when she calls the baby by name. (3; MR; AS; PS; EC)
    1 This may occur in either phase.
    3 This is the initial early action of the taking-in phase.
    4 This is part of the taking-in phase.

17. **3** Bonding between parent and baby is most successful when interaction is possible right after birth; if the child is ill, contact is limited. (3; CJ; PL; ED; EC)
    1 Though the effect of anesthesia is certainly a factor, the most important factor is the physical condition of the infant.
    2 Though the duration and difficulty of labor is certainly a factor, the most important factor is the physical condition of the infant.
    4 Health status during pregnancy may be a factor, but the most important factor is the physical condition of the infant.

18. **3** Parenting is not an inborn instinct but rather a learned behavior based on past experiences or current instruction. (3; MR; AN; PS; EC)
    1 Marriage is not essential for good parenting.
    2 This is untrue; parenting is learned, not inborn.
    4 This knowledge does not ensure the ability to parent.

19. **3** Family-centered maternity care focuses on the whole family; including the relatives in the care will be most therapeutic for the client. (2; MR; IM; PS; EC)
    1 This would be poor intervention; family-centered maternity care focuses on the whole family, and the relatives should be permitted to take part in the care of the client.
    2 The primary nurse should be able to handle this situation.
    4 The husband's permission is not required.

20. **1** Based on the family's decision, extraordinary care does not have to be employed; the child's basic needs are met, and nature is allowed to take its course. (2; LE; PL; PS; EC)
    2 Euthanasia is a deliberate intervention to cause death.
    3 If the child's physical needs are met and comfort is provided, the child's rights are not ignored; "extraordinary," not "all," care is being withheld.
    4 It is neither unethical nor illegal to withhold extraordinary treatment; once such treatment is started, it becomes a legal issue.

21. **2** Although support will help minimize guilt, it will not eliminate it; however, support will sustain family cohesion and unity. (1; LE; IM; PS; EC)
    1 Support may help, but in no way does it completely alleviate guilt feelings.
    3 Support does not affect the legal responsibility of the parents.
    4 This may help, but cannot completely relieve pressure.

Drug-Related Responses

22. **1** This is correct; it is given within 72 hours postpartum. (2; LE; PL; TC; DR)
    2 It would be useless at this time.
    3 RhoGAM is always indicated at the termination of a pregnancy, even with fetal demise.
    4 RhoGAM is always indicated at the termination of a pregnancy, even with a short-term pregnancy.

23. **1** Heparin is used because its molecular size is too large to pass the placental barrier. (1; CJ; PL; PA; DR)
    2 This drug can pass the placental barrier and cause hemorrhage in the fetus.
    3 Same as answer 2.
    4 Same as answer 2.

24. **2** Lupron decreases LH and FSH and hormone-dependent tissue. (3; CJ; AN; PA; DR)
    1 Relaxin is used for dysmenorrhea; it causes relaxation of the symphysis pubis.
    3 Ergotrate is used to contract the uterus.
    4 This is an estrogen that affects release of pituitary gonadotropins and inhibits ovulation.

25. **2** Maternal hypotension is a common complication of this anesthesia for labor, and nausea is one of the first clues that this has occurred. Elevating the extremities restores blood to the central circulation. (3; LE; EV; TC; DR)
    1 If signs and symptoms do not abate after elevation of the legs, the physician should be notified.
    3 This is not a specific observation after caudal anesthesia; it is part of the general nursing care during labor.
    4 If the FHR is being monitored, it is a constant process; if not, the FHR should be monitored every 15 minutes.

26. **2** There is no known teratogenic effect associated with penicillin. (2; CJ; AN; TC; DR)
    1 Sulfonamides may cause hemolysis in the fetus.
    3 Tetracycline causes permanent yellow staining of teeth in children whose mothers receive the drug during pregnancy.
    4 This drug is contraindicated in severe renal disease.

27. **3** The oxytocic effect of Pitocin increases the intensity and durations of contractions; prolonged contractions will jeopardize the safety of the fetus and necessitate discontinuing the drug. (3; LE; IM; TC; DR)
    1 This is important throughout labor.
    2 Because she is only 2 to 3 cm, there will be no bulging.
    4 There is no indication at this time that a cesarean delivery is necessary.

28. **2** Oxytocin is a small polypeptide hormone normally synthesized in the hypothalamus and secreted from the neurohypophysis during parturition or suckling; the synthetic form promotes powerful uterine (smooth muscle) contractions and thus is used to induce labor. (3; CJ; AN; PA; DR)
    1 Progesterone builds up the endometrium; it does not initiate uterine contractions.
    3 There is no drug by this name for this purpose.
    4 Ergonovine can lead to sustained contractions, which would be undesirable in labor.

29. 3 Respiratory depression occurs with the use of meperidine (Demerol) and produces significant depression of the infant at birth if circulating levels are high at delivery. (1; LE; EV; TC; DR)
 1 Scopolamine induces amnesia and forgetfulness in the mother but does not cause respiratory depression; this medication is not presently used.
 2 Promazine (Sparine), an anxiolytic, augments the effects of Demerol, thereby lessening the amount of drug needed.
 4 Promethazine (Phenergan), an antihistamine, does not cause respiratory depression.

30. 4 Meperidine (Demerol) is classified as a narcotic analgesic drug and is effective for the relief of pain. (1; CJ; EV; TC; DR)
 1 These medications do not induce amnesia.
 2 These medications act as analgesics, not anesthetics.
 3 This is an undesirable effect because the mother could not participate in the delivery process.

31. 3 Terbutaline sulfate (Brethine) is a beta-mimetic drug that acts on the smooth muscles of the uterus to reduce contractility, which in turn inhibits dilation and contractions. (1; MR; EV; PA; DR)
 1 Terbutaline sulfate (Brethine) has no analgesic effects.
 2 Terbutaline sulfate (Brethine) does not act to decrease blood pressure.
 4 Terbutaline sulfate (Brethine) acts to arrest preterm labor by relaxing the uterus; this would result in stopping cervical dilation rather than increasing it.

32. 4 Magnesium sulfate has a CNS depressant effect; therefore toxic levels will be reflected in decreased respiration and the absence of the knee-jerk reflex. (3; LE; EV; TC; DR)
 1 This may happen from sedation, not from magnesium sulfate.
 2 There is a decrease in respirations with excessive magnesium sulfate.
 3 This may be caused by increased potassium, not magnesium sulfate.

33. 2 This is a tocolytic agent that stops uterine contractions and halts labor. (2; LE; PL; TC; DR)
 1 This fluid is given to hydrate the client; it will do nothing to stop labor.

 3 This is a hormone that maintains pregnancy; it will do nothing to halt labor.
 4 Aminophylline is not used as a tocolytic agent; however, terbutaline sulfate (Brethine), another smooth muscle relaxant, is sometimes used.

34. 2 Steroids are given for a short period before delivery; by some obscure mechanism they help to mature the fetus' lungs. (3; MR; AN; TC; DR)
 1 Antibiotics would not be indicated if there were no signs of infection.
 3 This will not improve the chance of survival; because the fetus is only 30 weeks' gestation, steroids may be ordered first to enhance lung maturity.
 4 This would be indicated if an Rh incompatibility were present in the fetus.

Reproductive Choices

35. 2 Some type of a barrier contraceptive (condom with foam or jelly or a diaphragm) is usually recommended for the client with diabetes mellitus and a cardiac condition. (2; MR; IM; ED; RC)
 1 Oral contraceptives are not recommended for this client because of their tendency to alter glucose tolerance.
 3 An IUD is not recommended because it may predispose this client to infection.
 4 This is untrue; clients with a cardiac condition can become pregnant again in the future.

36. 4 Subsequent to IUD insertion, there may be an excessive menstrual flow for several cycles; this is because of an increase in the blood supply resulting from the inflammatory process because the IUD is really a foreign body. (3; CJ; EV; ED; RC)
 1 There is no documentation of this.
 2 This may occur but is not classified as a side effect.
 3 This may occur upon insertion but is fairly uncommon.

37. 4 The IUD may cause irritability of the myometrium, inducing contraction of the uterus and expulsion of the device. (3; MR; IM; ED; RC)
 1 This is a rare rather than a common occurrence.
 2 Clients do not complain of discomfort during coitus when an IUD is in place.
 3 Increased vaginal infections are not reported with the use of an IUD.

38. 4 Sperm are damaged by copper IUDs, while progesterone IUDs interfere with endometrial maturation. (3; MR; AN; PA; RC)
  1 A diaphragm blocks the cervical os.
  2 Mobility of the uterus is not related to contraception.
  3 This is the function of a condom.

39. 2 It is the surge of LH secretion in midcycle that is responsible for ovulation. (1; CJ; PL; ED; RC)
  1 This is not related; this stimulates ejection of milk into the mammary ducts.
  3 This occurs when the progesterone level is low.
  4 This occurs when the endometrial wall is built up.

40. 3 The ovum is capable of being fertilized for only 24 to 36 hours following ovulation; after this time it travels a variable distance between the fallopian tube and uterus, disintegrates, and is phagocytized by leukocytes. (2; CJ; PL; PA; RC)
  1 The ovum is viable for 24 to 36 hours.
  2 The ovum is viable a longer time.
  4 The ovum is not fertilizable after 36 hours.

41. 2 As ovulation approaches, there may be a drop in the basal temperature because of an increased production of estrogen; when ovulation occurs, there will be a rise in the basal temperature because of an increased production of progesterone. (2; MR; AN; PA; RC)
  1 At ovulation the temperature drop is slight, not marked.
  3 At ovulation the temperature rises after a slight drop.
  4 At ovulation the temperature drops slightly and then rises.

42. 4 This commonly occurs when clients first start on oral contraceptives; it is midcycle bleeding and if it persists, pill dosage is changed. (2; LE; IM; ED; RC)
  1 Cervicitis is unrelated to pill use.
  2 At this time there is no evidence that ovarian cysts are related to pill use.
  3 Fibrocystic breast disease is unrelated to pill use.

43. 3 There are monophasic, biphasic, and triphasic oral contraceptives; regardless of which is prescribed, the regimen should be followed exactly. Interruption permits release of luteinizing hormone, resulting in ovulation and possible pregnancy. (2; MR; IM; PA; RC)

  1 This is untrue; there is a very high rate of success if the oral contraceptive is taken regularly and correctly.
  2 This is too much information at this time; also, telling the client not to worry may close off communication.
  4 This is judgmental and a value statement on the part of the nurse. Contraceptive practice is the client's choice.

44. 1 Stress or infection alters the body's metabolism, causing an elevation in temperature; a rise in temperature from these causes may be misinterpreted as ovulation. (2; MR; AN; PA; RC)
  2 This may increase sperm volume but does not affect the female's basal temperature.
  3 Age is not a factor concerning efficiency of the rhythm method.
  4 Frequency of intercourse may affect the volume of sperm but does not alter the female's basal temperature.

45. 4 Antiovulatory drugs suppress menstruation. Breakthrough bleeding is abnormal with biphasic drugs. The drug is given for only 21 days and a menstrual flow does not occur during this time. (2; MR; IM; ED; RC)
  1 There is no indication for increased Papanicolaou smears; once a year is sufficient.
  2 Increased calcium to counteract osteoporosis from menopause is not indicated for this client.
  3 No restriction of sexual activity is indicated when one is taking oral contraceptives.

46. 3 A headache is a symptom of hypernatremia, which can occur with the salinization method of elective abortion. (3; CJ; EV; TC; RC)
  1 Edema may occur as a result of water intoxication and is not a sign of hypernatremia associated with saline abortion.
  2 This is a serious manifestation of water intoxication.
  4 Bradycardia may occur with the use of spinal or regional anesthesia, not salinization.

47. 3 The saline causes puffing of the placenta, fetal death, placental separation, release of fibrin, and then labor and paradoxical hemorrhaging. This takes at least 8 to 24 hours in most cases. (3; CJ; IM; ED; RC)
  1 This is too quick; normally labor starts 8 to 24 hours after the procedure.
  2 Same as answer 1.
  4 Same as answer 1.

48. 2 *Laminaria* is a seaweed that expands in a moist environment. It is a natural and safe method of dilating the cervix. (2; CJ; AN; TC; RC)

    1 It takes 24 hours for the *Laminaria* to expand.

    3 This is untrue; they may not be as strong but are certainly less traumatic.

    4 Anesthesia is not used in the dilation phase of abortion.

49. 3 This is necessary to protect the incisional area because sutures may slip with pulling or stretching. (2; CJ; PL; TC; RC)

    1 Unrealistic; recovery from procedure takes more than 1 hour.

    2 Sterility is immediate; no waiting period is required as in a vasectomy.

    4 Untrue; microsurgery to reverse the procedure is not guaranteed or easily accomplished.

50. 3 This response is a positive negotiation to be reassigned to an area not against the nurse's personal values. (2; MR; IM; PS; RC)

    1 This is a poor way to resolve value conflict; undoubtedly any client would sense this conflict.

    2 The nurse may not have the legal, ethical, or professional right to refuse this assignment if employed by the facility.

    4 Imposing this kind of advice would be unethical and unprofessional.

Reproductive Problems

51. 3 Ovulation occurs 14 days before the onset of menses. (3; MR; IM; ED; RP)

    1 Midway between her cycles would be appropriate only if the client had a 28-day cycle.

    2 This would mean that ovulation would occur on approximately day 5 of the menstrual cycle.

    4 Variations in the cycle occur in the preovulation period; thus this is wrong information.

52. 4 Sperm motility is increased at pH values near neutral or slightly alkaline; a sodium bicarbonate douche will reduce the acidity of fluids in the vagina and help optimize the pH. (3; MR; IM; PA; RP)

    1 Estrogen does not alter the pH.

    2 Sulfur does not change the pH in any way.

    3 This would increase the acid content and kill the sperm.

53. 4 At this time, because of increased estrogen levels, the cervical mucus is abundant, and its quality changes in such a way as to optimize sperm survival time. (2; CJ; PL; PA; RP)

    1 Cervical mucus at this time is still thick and not yet receptive to spermatozoa.

    2 The cervical mucus at this time is not receptive to spermatozoa.

    3 Cervical mucus is destructive to spermatozoa at this time, and sperm penetration cannot occur.

54. 1 Past infections may cause tubal occlusions, most of which are caused by postinfection adhesions. (3; CJ; AN; PA; RP)

    2 This is a tumor of the uterus and does not affect the tube.

    3 This is rare; anomalies of the uterus are more common than those of a tube.

    4 This is possible, but infections in the tube are more common.

55. 3 Infertility is the inability of a couple to conceive after at least 1 year of adequate exposure to the possibility of pregnancy. (2; CJ; AS; ED; RP)

    1 Infertility may be psychogenic; however, statistics show that physiologic problems are more often the cause.

    2 This is untrue; infertility may be corrected, but sterility is irreversible.

    4 This may or may not be true; it is possible that there is a problem with both.

56. 3 High levels of plasma estrogen inhibit pituitary secretion of FSH; this effect appears to be mediated by the hypothalamus and its releasing factors. (3; CJ; AN; PA; RP)

    1 LH (luteinizing hormone) causes ovulation.

    2 Lactogenic hormone (prolactin) stimulates lactation.

    4 Low concentrations of estrogen may precipitate demineralization of bone.

57. 2 This test determines the number and condition of sperm aspirated from the cervix within 2 hours after coitus. (2; CJ; AS; PA; RP)

    1 The Rubin test determines the patency of the fallopian tubes.

    3 The Friedman test was a test done to establish the diagnosis of pregnancy; it has been replaced by more sophisticated tests.

    4 The Papanicolaou test is used for the early diagnosis of cervical cancer.

58. **4** This test enables the examiner to visualize the uterus and fallopian tubes and the pelvic organs for reproduction. (1; CJ; AS; PA; RP)
    1 A biopsy is the surgical excision of tissue for diagnostic purposes.
    2 A cystoscopy is used to evaluate the urinary bladder.
    3 A culdoscopy is the direct examination of female pelvic viscera using an endoscope introduced through a perforation in the vagina.

59. **3** The proliferation of trophoblastic tissue filled with fluid causes the uterus to enlarge more quickly than it would with a normally growing fetus. (2; CJ; AS; TC; RP)
    1 Hypertension, not hypotension, often occurs with molar pregnancy.
    2 There is generally no living fetus with a hydatidiform mole.
    2 There may be slight vaginal bleeding without pain.

60. **1** At this time the products of conception are too large for the tube to accommodate and rupture occurs. (1; CJ; AS; PA; RP)
    2 Tubal pregnancies cannot advance to this stage because of the tube's inability to expand to accommodate a pregnancy of this size.
    3 Tubal pregnancies cannot advance to this stage because the tube cannot expand to accommodate a pregnancy of this size.
    4 The size of the fertilized egg at this time is miniscule and will cause no problem.

61. **4** A fallopian tube is unable to contain and sustain a pregnancy to term; as the fertilized ovum grows, there is excessive stretching or rupture of the fallopian tube, causing pain. (3; CJ; AS; TC; RP)
    1 This would be difficult for the client to identify correctly.
    2 The pain is sudden, intense, knifelike, and usually located on one side.
    3 Leukorrhea and dysuria may be indicative of a vaginal or bladder infection.

62. **4** A symptom of sudden rupture of a fallopian tube is pain on the affected side, usually sudden, excruciating, and radiating over the lower abdomen and to the shoulder; sometimes the pain is associated with nausea, vomiting, and diarrhea. (1; CJ; AS; TC; RP)
    1 There may be some vaginal bleeding with a ruptured tubal pregnancy; usually severe pain is present.

2 There are no contractions since the pregnancy is not uterine.
3 The pain is exquisite, sharp, and sudden in the lower abdomen.

63. **2** Ectopic pregnancy is one of the leading causes of first-trimester bleeding; unless an embryo and placenta happen to be located in the abdominal cavity, they cannot grow outside the uterus for more than 10 to 12 weeks without showing the classic signs of pressure and bleeding. (2; CJ; AN; TC; RP)
    1 Abruptio placentae is accompanied by sharp abdominal pain with or without bleeding.
    3 Abdominal cramping pain is present with an incomplete abortion.
    4 This occurs monthly during ovulation without pain or vaginal bleeding; occasionally pain occurs when the follicle ruptures (mittelschmerz), but bleeding does not.

64. **4** This is a genetic disorder transmitted as an autosomal recessive trait that occurs primarily among Ashkenazi Jews. (2; CJ; IM; ED; RP)
    1 This disease does not have a higher prevalence in the Jewish population.
    2 Same as answer 1.
    3 Same as answer 1.

65. **1** Hemorrhage may result from retained placental tissue or uterine atony; infection may occur from the introduction of organisms into the warm, moist environment, which is favorable to microbial growth. (1; MR; PL; TC; RP)
    2 There is no indication at this time that the client has been deprived of fluids or has lost large amounts of blood.
    3 Subinvolution usually occurs after a full-term delivery and there is no indication of dehydration.
    4 An abortion would occur too early for pregnancy-induced hypertension to be present.

66. **4** About 75% of all spontaneous abortions take place between 8 and 12 weeks of gestation and show embryonic defects. (2; CJ; AS; PA; RP)
    1 Though possible, physical trauma rarely causes an abortion.
    2 Unresolved stress may lead to congenital defects but is rarely associated with abortion.
    3 Congenital defects are asymptomatic during pregnancy and do not usually cause an abortion.

67. **4** Spotting in the first trimester may indicate that the client may be having a threatened abortion; any client with the possibility of hemorrhage should not be left alone; therefore, admitting this client for observation is safe medical practice; abortion is usually inevitable if accompanied by pain and cervical dilation. (1; CJ; AN; PA; RP)

 1 This may not cause any outward symptoms; only the signs of pregnancy disappearing.
 2 This can be confirmed only if vaginal examination reveals cervical dilation.
 3 This is usually accompanied by severe pain radiating to the shoulder on the affected side.

68. **1** After a spontaneous abortion the fundus should be checked for firmness, which would indicate effective uterine tone; if the uterus is not firm or appears to be hypotonic, hemorrhage may occur; a soft or boggy uterus may also indicate retained placental tissue. (1; MR; IM; TC; RP)

 2 The nurse would do this if necessary after checking for fundal firmness.
 3 The priority action is to check for firmness of the fundus and possible bleeding.
 4 This is unnecessary; fetal and placental contents are small and expelled easily in bed.

69. **4** A correct and simple definition answers the question and fulfills the client's need to know. (2; MR; IM; ED; RP)

 1 This denies the client's right to know.
 2 This is the definition of a missed abortion.
 3 The nurse can independently reinforce and clear misconceptions.

Healthy Childbearing

70. **2** The amnion encloses the embryo and the shock-protective amniotic fluid in which the embryo floats. (1; CJ; AN; PA; HC)

 1 This is another name for the umbilical cord.
 3 The chorion is the outermost membrane; it does not secrete fluid.
 4 The yolk sac contains the stored nutrients of the ovum.

71. **3** Progesterone stimulates differentiation of the endometrium into a secretory type of tissue. (2; CJ; AN; PA; HC)

 1 This is influenced by high levels of luteinizing hormone.
 2 This is influenced by estrogen.
 4 Secondary male characteristics are influenced by testosterone.

72. **4** This is the result of a reduced chromosome number, from 46 to 23, readying the sex cells for fertilization. (3; CJ; AN; ED; HC)

 1 They each have one set of chromosomes (23).
 2 There are only 23 pairs of chromosomes in the nuclei.
 3 The diploid number (46 chromosomes) is reached when fertilization occurs.

73. **3** Follicle-stimulating hormone is secreted from the anterior pituitary gland. (3; CJ; AN; PA; HC)

 1 This is produced by syncytiotrophoblastic tissue, a preplacental tissue.
 2 Chorionic gonadotropin is secreted by the trophoblastic tissue, which makes up part of the placenta.
 4 Chorionic gonadotropin is a precursor of progesterone and is secreted by the trophoblastic tissue.

74. **2** In the first 7 to 14 days the developing ovum is known as a blastocyst; it is called an embryo until the eighth week; the developing cells are then called a fetus until birth. (2; CJ; AN; PA; HC)

 1 The fetal heart is heard between the twelfth and twentieth weeks; the developing cells are known as a fetus at the end of the eighth week.
 3 At the time of implantation the group of developing cells is called a blastocyst.
 4 The developing cells are known as a fetus from the eighth week until birth.

75. **2** To allow for the larger intake of air, the normal adaptation is to increase the size of the thoracic cavity. (3; CJ; AN; PA; HC)

 1 Blood volume is not related to tidal air volume.
 3 Upward displacement would decrease tidal air volume.
 4 There is no change in the height of the rib cage.

76. **3** By this time the fetus and placenta have grown, expanding the size of the uterus. The extended uterus expands into the abdominal cavity. (2; CJ; AN; PA; HC)

 1 The uterus is still within the pelvic area.
 2 The uterus is still within the pelvic area at this time.
 4 The uterus has already risen out of the pelvis and is expanding farther into the abdominal area.

77. **2** The word originates from the Middle English word *quik,* which means alive. (3; CJ; AS; PA; HC)
1 Lightening is the descent of the fetus into the birth canal.
3 Ballottement is the bouncing of the fetus in the amniotic fluid against the examiner's hand.
4 Engagement occurs when the presenting part is at the level of the ischial spines.

78. **2** This is the period in which the fetus stores deposits of fat. (2; CJ; AN; PA; HC)
1 The first trimester is the period of organogenesis, when cells differentiate into major organ systems.
3 Growth is occurring, but fat deposition does not occur in this period.
4 This is the period of the blastocyst, when initial cell division takes place.

79. **1** When placental formation is complete, around the twelfth week of pregnancy, it produces progesterone and estrogen. (2; CJ; AN; PA; HC)
2 This is not the chief source of progesterone and estrogen; only small amounts are secreted.
3 The corpus luteum supplies the estrogen and progesterone needed to sustain the pregnancy until the placenta is ready to take over.
4 FSH is secreted by the anterior hypophysis, but it is not secreted during pregnancy.

80. **2** The umbilical vein carries blood high in oxygen from the placenta and empties it into the fetal vena cava by way of the ductus venosus. (1; CJ; AN; PA; HC)
1 The blood in the umbilical artery is more deoxygenated.
3 The pulmonary artery carries only a small amount of oxygenated blood, since the lungs are not functioning.
4 This contains a mixture of arterial and venous blood.

81. **4** Nägele's rule is an indirect, noninvasive method for estimating the date of birth: EDB = LMP + 7 days – 3 months + 1 year (2; CJ; AN; ED; HC)
1 This is a miscalculation.
2 Same as answer 1
3 Same as answer 1.

82. **1** Using Nägele's rule, subtract 3 months add 1 year and 7 days to the first day of the last menstrual period. (2; CJ; AN; PA; HC)
2 Incorrect calculation; this date is too late.
3 Incorrect calculation; this date is too early.
4 Same as answer 2.

83. **4** Increasing the client's knowledge of physical and psychologic changes resulting from pregnancy is done during the first trimester. (2; MR; PL; ED; HC)
1 This is too early; this would be done in the last trimester.
2 The client should be alerted to danger signs; however, primary teaching is directed toward increasing her knowledge of normal physiologic changes.
3 Concerns about role transition to parenthood should be addressed in the third trimester.

84. **2** The diagonal conjugate is an estimation of the true conjugate with the lower edge of the symphysis pubis used as its anterior point and the sacral promontory posteriorly; the true conjugate uses the upper ridge of the symphysis pubis anteriorly but cannot be measured on a living woman. (3; CJ; AN; PA; HC)
1 This is the distance from the upper margin of the symphysis to the sacral promontory.
3 This is the widest diameter at the inlet.
4 This is the diameter between the ischial tuberosities.

85. **4** Progesterone acts to reduce contractility of the uterine musculature and to maintain the decidual bed. (2; CJ; AN; PA; HC)
1 Elevated progesterone levels would inhibit contractility of the uterine musculature.
2 Progesterone, not estrogen, inhibits contractions.
3 This would tend to stimulate contractions but is inhibited by progesterone, not estrogen.

86. **3** The blood volume increases by approximately 50% during pregnancy. Peak blood volume occurs between 30 and 34 weeks of gestation. (2; CJ; AN; PA; HC)
1 White blood cell values remain stable during the antepartum period.
2 The hematocrit decreases as a result of hemodilution.
4 The sedimentation rate increases because of a decrease in plasma proteins.

87. **4** A purplish color results from the increased vascularity and blood vessel engorgement of the vagina. (1; CJ; AS; PA; HC)
    1 This is increased vascularity and cervical softening.
    2 This is softening of the lower uterine segment.
    3 This is softening of the cervix.

88. **2** There is a 30% to 50% increase in maternal plasma volume at the end of the first trimester, leading to a decrease in the concentration of hemoglobin and erythrocytes. (2; CJ; AS; TC; HC)
    1 Dietary intake of iron is unrelated to the development of physiologic anemia of pregnancy.
    3 Erythropoiesis is increased after the first trimester.
    4 Detoxification demands are unchanged during pregnancy.

89. **3** Before health teaching is instituted, the nurse should ascertain the client's past experiences; they will influence the teaching plan. (2; MR; AS; ED; HC)
    1 This answer does not give the client a chance to discuss her feelings about the examination.
    2 This response presupposes a "yes" or "no" answer and does not really give the client an opportunity to discuss it further.
    4 This answer does not give the client a chance to discuss her feelings about the examination; the nurse can only assume that the client's concerns are related to discomfort.

90. **4** A normal cardiopulmonary symptom in pregnancy; caused by increased ventricular rate and elevated diaphragm. (2; CJ; AS; PA; HC)
    1 This is pathologic, a sign of impending cardiac decompensation.
    2 Same as answer 1.
    3 Same as answer 1.

91. **1** Menstruation during pregnancy is interrupted because secretion of the ovarian hormones ceases. This response answers the client's question in understandable terms. (2; MR; IM; ED; HC)
    2 These hormones are needed to rebuild the layers of cells lining the uterus that are sloughed off during menstruation.
    3 LH stimulates the maturation of a primitive follicle into a vesicular graafian follicle; also promotes secretion of estrogen by the ovary.
    4 This brings about the development of the ova.

92. **4** Chorionic gonadotropin, secreted in large amounts by the placenta during gestation, and the metabolic changes associated with pregnancy can precipitate nausea and vomiting in early pregnancy. (2; CJ; AN; PA; HC)
    1 Estrogen is elevated throughout pregnancy; symptoms of morning sickness disappear after the first trimester.
    2 Progesterone is elevated throughout pregnancy; symptoms of morning sickness disappear after the first trimester.
    3 The luteinizing hormone is present only during ovulation.

93. **1** Maintaining the sitting position for prolonged periods may constrict the vessels of the legs, particularly in the popliteal spaces, as well as diminish venous return. Walking contracts the muscles of the legs, which apply gentle pressure to the veins in the legs, thus promoting venous return. (2; MR; AN; PA; HC)
    2 A better means of improving circulation would be to walk about several times each morning and afternoon; she could also keep her legs elevated while sitting at her desk.
    3 If the client is feeling well, there are no contraindications to working until her due date.
    4 Adequate nourishment can be obtained during mealtimes; the client does not require extra nutrition breaks.

94. **4** The nurse should become informed about the cultural eating patterns of clients so that foods containing the essential nutrients, which are part of these dietary patterns, will be included in the diet. (3; MR; AN; PS; HC)
    1 Fluid retention is only one component of weight gain; growth of the baby, placenta, breasts, etc., also contribute to weight gain.
    2 Calories and nutrients are increased during pregnancy.
    3 Pregnancy diets are not specific; they are merely composed of the essential nutrients.

95. **2** By taking a diet history, the nurse can assess the woman's level of nutritional knowledge and gain clues for appropriate methods of counseling. (1; MR; AS; ED; HC)
    1 "Normal" is too vague a term; the client will need increased protein and caloric intake.
    3 These foods may be too expensive and different from her normal choices, leading to noncompliance.
    4 Salt is no longer limited in healthy pregnancy.

96. 2 The uterus and bladder occupy the pelvic cavity and lie very closely together; as the uterus enlarges with the growing fetus, it impinges on the space normally occupied by the bladder and thereby diminishes bladder capacity. (1; MR; IM; ED; HC)

1 Atony would not cause frequency; more likely it would lead to retention.

3 This would lead to incontinence rather than frequency.

4 This is an unlikely occurrence; the uterus would not impinge on that area.

97. 1 Nausea and vomiting in the morning occur in almost 50% of all pregnancies. Eating dry crackers before getting out of bed in the morning is a simple remedy that may provide relief. (1; MR; IM; ED; HC)

2 Increasing fat intake does not relieve the nausea.

3 Two small meals and a snack at noon would not meet the nutritional needs of a pregnant woman, nor would it relieve nausea. Some women find that eating five or six small meals daily instead of three large ones is helpful.

4 This is not helpful; separating fluids from solids at mealtime is more advisable.

98. 4 This pigmentation is caused by the anterior pituitary hormone, melanotropin, which increases during pregnancy. (3; MR; IM; ED; HC)

1 During pregnancy, ovarian activity is very quiet because of the feedback mechanism.

2 Hyperthyroidism is manifested by increased temperature, pulse, and respirations and a fine hand tremor.

3 Hyperactivity of the adrenal glands is manifested by symptoms of Cushing's syndrome.

99. 1 Nausea and vomiting of pregnancy can be relieved with small snacks of protein before bedtime to slow digestion; presently SeaBands (used for seasickness) are being used successfully on some women. (1; MR; IM; TC; HC)

2 An antacid may affect electrolyte balance; also this will not help morning sickness.

3 This is unsound advice, because both fetus and mother need nourishment.

4 Medications in the first trimester are contraindicated; this is the period of organogenesis, and congenital anomalies could result.

100. 3 This is the recommended caloric intake for adult women during pregnancy. (2; CJ; PL; PA; HC)

1 This is a caloric intake that will produce weight reduction; not recommended during pregnancy.

2 A decrease in these nutrients is not recommended during pregnancy.

4 This is the recommended caloric intake for breastfeeding mothers.

101. 1 The average weight gain during pregnancy is 25 to 35 lbs (11.9 to 15.8 kg); of this, the fetus accounts for 7 to 8 lbs (3.18 to 3.6 kg), or approximately 30% of weight gain. (3; MR; IM; ED; HC)

2 Fluid retention accounts for about 20% to 25% of weight gain.

3 Metabolic alterations do not cause a weight gain.

4 Increased blood volume accounts for about 12% to 16% of weight gain.

102. 4 A sudden sharp increase in weight may indicate water retention and the beginning of pregnancy-induced hypertension. (2; MR; IM; TC; HC)

1 This is untrue; weight gain is necessary to ensure adequate nutrition for the fetus.

2 There is no hard-and-fast number of pounds that the client should gain, and low-calorie diets may be harmful.

3 This closes off communication; it does not allow the client to ask more questions about weight gain.

103. 3 Because of changes in the hormone levels, morning sickness seldom persists beyond the first trimester. (1; MR; IM; ED; HC)

1 It usually ends at the end of the third month, when the chorionic gonadotropin level falls.

2 Same as answer 1.

4 It is still present at this time; it is related to the high level of chorionic gonadotropin.

104. 4 This allows the client to discuss her feelings and participate in her care. (2; MR; IM; ED; HC)

1 This cuts off communication; this also may cause the client to worry that something is seriously wrong.

2 The client has already told the nurse how she feels.

3 This statement cuts off communication and does not address the totality of the client's concern.

CHILDBEARING/WOMEN'S HEALTH   ANSWERS

105. **1** When an Rh-negative mother carries an Rh-positive fetus there is a risk of maternal antibodies against Rh-positive blood; antibodies cross the placenta and destroy the fetal RBCs. (2; MR; IM; PA; HC)

2 Testing for Rh factor will not provide information about protein metabolism deficiency.

3 Physiologic bilirubinemia is a common occurrence in newborns; it is not associated with the Rh factor.

4 Determination of the lecithin-sphingomyelin ratio, not the Rh factor, may provide information about the risk of developing RDS.

106. **2** The first trimester is the period when all major organs are being laid down; drugs, alcohol, and tobacco may cause major defects. (1; MR; IM; ED; HC)

1 Cutting down is insufficient; these teratogens should be eliminated.

3 Even 1 oz of alcohol is considered harmful; baby aspirin is now given to some women who are considered at risk for pregnancy-induced hypertension.

4 Drugs, unless absolutely necessary, should be avoided throughout pregnancy; but the first trimester is most significant.

107. **3** The FHR is usually between 120 and 160 beats per minute. This is to be expected normally, and the mother should be made aware of this fact. (1; MR; IM; ED; HC)

1 This is too variable; the normal heart rate for a fetus is 120 to 160 beats per minute.

2 To accommodate the metabolic needs of the fetus, the heart rate is rapid.

4 This is unnecessary information; the mother should be informed only of that which is normal.

108. **4** Intact membranes act as a barrier against organisms that may cause an intrauterine infection. (2; CJ; IM; TC; HC)

1 This is common because of increased production of mucus containing exfoliated vaginal epithelial cells; intercourse is not contraindicated.

2 This may occur during sex but there is no literature indicating that it is harmful for the fetus.

3 Intercourse is not contraindicated if membranes are intact; modification of sexual positions may be needed because of an enlarged abdomen after the thirtieth week.

109. **2** The increase of estrogen during pregnancy causes hyperplasia of the vaginal mucosa, which leads to increased production of mucus by the endocervical glands. The mucus contains exfoliated epithelial cells. (2; MR; IM; ED; HC)

1 Increased metabolism leads to many systemic changes but does not increase vaginal discharge.

3 Normal functioning of the glands, which lubricate the vagina during intercourse, remains unchanged during pregnancy.

4 There is no additional supply of sodium chloride to the cells during pregnancy.

110. **4** These are the parameters that can be used to diagnose a 20-week pregnancy. (2; MR; IM; ED; HC)

1 These parameters suggest a 16- to 18-week pregnancy.

2 This indicates that the client is about 28 weeks pregnant.

3 These parameters are indicative of a 10-week pregnancy.

111. **2** The nurse fulfills the expectation set forth in the Nurse Practice Act, which includes teaching. In this case the nurse has knowledge of dietary needs and their relation to the client's well-being during pregnancy. (2; LE; EV; ED; HC)

1 Immediate planning based on the nurse's knowledge of proper diet is better intervention.

3 Not all preferences can be included; the diet should contain normal sodium, high protein, and sufficient calories.

4 Unless the nurse thought there was a need for medical intervention, the nurse could supervise prenatal care.

112. **3** Fluids, proteins, and salt should not be restricted, for they are necessary to the well-being of the mother and fetus; elevation of the extremities several times daily is recommended to decrease the edema. (2; MR; IM; ED; HC)

1 Salt is not limited during pregnancy.

2 Same as answer 1.

4 Diuretics can be harmful and are not used during pregnancy.

113. **4** This is a correct statement; the nonstress test evaluates the response of the infant to movement and activity. (3; MR; EV; ED; HC)
    1 This is highly unlikely because Pitocin is not used in nonstress tests.
    2 This test will not influence the fetus' activity because no exogenous stimulus like Pitocin is used.
    3 No injections of any kind are used during a nonstress test; this test involves only the use of a fetal monitor to record the fetal heart rate during periods of activity.

114. **2** A full bladder is required for effective visualization in early pregnancy. (2; MR; PL; TC; HC)
    1 This is unnecessary because the procedure is not done via the colon and will not cause fecal contamination.
    3 This procedure is noninvasive; in no way can it irritate the uterus and initiate labor.
    4 For this noninvasive procedure nothing is passed through the alimentary tract. Also, fasting is contraindicated during pregnancy.

115. **2** Ambulation relieves Braxton Hicks contractions. (2; MR; IM; ED; HC)
    1 Braxton Hicks contractions increase when the client is resting.
    3 These contractions are not indicative of true labor and need not be timed.
    4 Aspirin may be harmful to the fetus because it can hemolyze red blood cells.

116. **3** When the membranes rupture, the potential for infection is increased, and when the contractions are 5 to 8 minutes apart, they are usually of sufficient force to warrant medical supervision. Therefore, for the safety of the mother and fetus, the mother should go to the hospital. (2; MR; PL; PA; HC)
    1 This is too early; the client still has a great deal of time and would be better off with her family and moving about at home.
    2 These may be early signs of labor or signs of posterior fetal position.
    4 This is indicative of advanced labor, and the client may have difficulty getting to the hospital at this time.

117. **1** Progressive dilation of the cervix is the most accurate indication of true labor. (3; CJ; AS; PA; HC)
    2 Contractions may not begin until 24 to 48 hours later.

3 With true labor contractions will increase with activity.
    4 Contractions of true labor persist in any position.

118. **2** This is because of impedance of venous return by the gravid uterus, which causes hypotension and decreased systemic perfusion. (2; MR; AN; PA; HC)
    1 This may be partially true, but more significantly, it is the least comfortable position and may cause hypotension.
    3 Even if true, this is not significant as a factor of labor.
    4 This is false; it can lead to supine hypotension.

119. **1** Fatigue will influence other coping strategies, such as distraction. (2; MR; IM; PA; HC)
    2 Progesterone is decreased at this time.
    3 The client does not push during the first stage of labor; pushing is done during the second stage.
    4 This energy will enhance the quality of contractions.

120. **1** Determining fetal well-being supercedes all other measures; if the fetal heart rate (FHR) is absent or persistently decelerating, immediate intervention is required. (2; CJ; AS; PA; HC)
    2 Important, but the determination of fetal well-being is the priority.
    3 Same as answer 2.
    4 Same as answer 2.

121. **3** A station of +1 indicates that the fetal head is 1 cm below the ischial spines. (2; CJ; AS; PA; HC)
    1 This would be designated as 0 station.
    2 The head is now past the points of engagement, which are the ischial spines.
    4 The head must be at +3 to +5 to be visible at the vaginal opening.

122. **3** Fetal heart tones are best auscultated through the fetal back; because the position is ROP (right occiput presenting), the back would be below the umbilicus and on the right side. (2; CJ; AS; ED; HC)
    1 This could be used when the fetus is lying in the midline in a breech position.
    2 This would be appropriate for an LSA position.
    4 This would be appropriate for LOA or LOP position.

123. 1 The contractions become stronger, last longer, and are erratic during this stage; the intervals during the contractions are shorter than the contractions themselves; much concentration and effort are needed by the mother to pace herself with each contraction. (2; CJ; AS; PA; HC)

2 This is not true; administration of an analgesic or anesthetic at this point could reduce the effectiveness of labor and depress the fetus.

3 Even clients who have been adequately prepared will experience these behaviors during the transition stage.

4 There is no indication that any abnormality is developing.

124. 3 This is the way to determine the frequency of the contractions. (1; CJ; AN; PA; HC)

1 This is the duration of a contraction.

2 This assessment does not give any valid data.

4 This assessment will determine the intensity of a contraction.

125. 3 By 36 weeks' gestation, normal amniotic fluid is colorless with small particles of vernix caseosa present. (1; CJ; AS; PA; HC)

1 Dark-amber fluid suggests the presence of bilirubin, an ominous sign.

2 Greenish-yellow fluid may indicate the presence of meconium and suggests fetal distress.

4 Cloudy fluid suggests the presence of purulent material, and greenish-yellow may indicate the presence of meconium.

126. 4 Immediately following delivery the fundus is found midway between the symphysis pubis and the umbilicus. (2; CJ; AS; PA; HC)

1 This is untrue; the fundus is easily palpable midway between the symphysis pubis and the umbilicus.

2 The fundus never gets this high.

3 The fundus is not this high until 1 hour after delivery; if the uterus is deviated to the right, it usually indicates bladder distention.

127. 1 Because the client is attached to a machine and movement may alter the tracings, movement is discouraged. (2; CJ; AN; PA; HC)

2 Placement of the monitor leads does not interfere with the administration of sedatives.

3 Lamaze techniques work well with a monitor.

4 An external monitor does not necessitate more frequent vaginal examinations.

128. 3 This may occur with head compression but is perfectly normal if the FHR returns to baseline at the end of the contraction. (3; CJ; AS; PA; HC)

1 Needs no medical intervention; this is a normal occurrence as long as the FHR returns to baseline at the end of the contraction.

2 Cord compression is a common occurrence; no intervention is necessary if the FHR returns to normal baseline at the end of the contraction.

4 This position would increase pressure on the vena cava.

129. 2 Variable decelerations are often seen as a result of cord compression; a change of position will relieve the pressure on the cord. (3; CJ; IM; TC; HC)

1 Variable decelerations are not oxytocin related.

3 This is premature; in addition, delivering the client is a medical, not a nursing decision.

4 Blood pressure readings in the mother will not be affected by variable decelerations.

130. 1 When the membranes rupture, there is always the possibility of a prolapsed cord leading to fetal distress, which would manifest itself in a slowed fetal heartbeat. (2; CJ; IM; TC; HC)

2 This is unnecessary unless there is a marked change in the FHR.

3 This is done routinely throughout the entire labor process; at this point, fetal status takes priority.

4 This is regularly done before and after the membranes rupture; however, fetal status takes priority.

131. 3 The client is in the first stage of labor, and the first priority of care is to establish a trusting relationship with her and her husband. This will help to allay their anxiety. (1; CJ; IM; PS; HC)

1 This may be necessary later; however, it is not the first priority.

2 The history should be taken from the client as long as she is capable of providing it.

4 This is not an initial priority; the physician probably knows the mother is on her way.

132. **2** Characteristics of the midphase of labor for the primiparous client include regular contractions 30 to 45 seconds long and 3 to 5 minutes apart, station of the presenting part at +1 to +2, and pink to bloody show in moderate amount. (3; CJ; AN; PA; HC)
   1 Contractions are less frequent in the latent phase, and dilation is not so advanced.
   3 In this phase, dilation is 8 to 10 cm, and contractions are more frequent.
   4 This terminology is not appropriate for a phase of labor.

133. **3** Transcervical amniotomy (artificial rupture of the membranes) requires that the cervix be soft, partially effaced, and slightly dilated with the presenting part engaged or engaging; this client would meet these criteria, as demonstrated by the bloody show and the head at +1. (3; MR; PL; PA; HC)
   1 A tap-water enema would be ineffective for inducing labor.
   2 IM injection of oxytocin is extremely dangerous because of the physician's inability to control the effects of the drug; oxytocin by intravenous infusion is considered safe as long as maternal and fetal monitoring is continuous.
   4 Prostaglandins are used to soften and ripen the cervix. This client has a bloody show indicating that her cervical plug has already been passed and the cervix is no longer hard; in addition prostaglandins are an expensive and uncomfortable way of inducing labor.

134. **4** Artificial rupture of the membranes (amniotomy) allows for more effective pressure of the fetal head on the cervix, enhancing dilation and effacement. (3; CJ; EV; PA; HC)
   1 Vaginal bleeding may increase because of the progression of labor.
   2 This does not directly affect the fetal heart rate.
   3 Discomfort may become greater because contractions usually increase after an amniotomy.

135. **3** The client is experiencing the expected discomforts of labor; the nurse should initiate measures that will promote relaxation. (2; MR; IM; PA; HC)
   1 During the last phase of labor, pushing is unavoidable; the client is in early labor, and should not push at this time.
   2 The client is not receptive to teaching at this time; all energy is being directed inward.
   4 There is no evidence at this time that the client is losing excessive blood (hemorrhage).

136. **3** Contractions are stronger and more regular when the woman is standing; also, during walking the diameter of the pelvic inlet increases and allows for easier entrance of the head into the pelvis. (2; MR; IM; PA; HC)
   1 This denies the nurse's understanding of the physiology of labor.
   2 This is untrue; contractions of true labor are enhanced when the mother walks about.
   4 Timing can continue even if the client walks around.

137. **3** This slow, deep breathing expands the spaces between the ribs and raises the abdominal muscles, allowing room for the uterus to expand and preventing painful pressure of the uterus against the abdominal wall. (1; MR; IM; ED; HC)
   1 Panting is used to halt or delay the pushing out of the baby's head before complete dilation.
   2 Pelvic rocking is used to relieve pressure from back labor.
   4 Athletic chest breathing is not one of the exercises used in this stage of labor.

138. **4** A persistent occiput-posterior position causes intense back pain because of fetal compression of the sacral nerves. (2; CJ; IM; PA; HC)
   1 Breech positions are not associated with back pain.
   2 The transverse position usually does not cause back pain.
   3 This is the most common fetal position and does not cause back pain.

139. **3** The application of back pressure combined with frequent positional changes will help alleviate the discomfort. (1; MR; IM; PA; HC)
   1 Although this may be comfortable for some individuals, rubbing the back and alternating positions are more universally effective.
   2 The supine position places increased pressure on the back and often aggravates the pain.
   4 Neuromuscular control exercises are used to teach selective relaxation in childbirth classes; they will not relieve back pain.

140. **2** Low back pain is aggravated when the mother is in the supine position because of increased pressure from the fetus. (2; MR; IM; ED; HC)
   1 This position relieves back pain.
   3 This position relieves back pain.
   4 The knee-chest position may help to relieve back pain.

141. **2** Gastric peristalsis often ceases during periods of stress. Abdominal contractions put pressure on the stomach and can cause nausea and vomiting, increasing the risk of aspiration. (1; CJ; IM; TC; HC)
    1 Gastric activity and digestion cease during periods of stress.
    3 Same as answer 1.
    4 Although food may cause dyspepsia, the primary reason for withholding it is to prevent aspiration.

142. **1** This is the most difficult part of labor, and the client needs encouragement and support to cope. (2; MR; PL; PS; HC)
    2 Fluids should be increased because of the increase in metabolism.
    3 Medication at this time will depress the infant and is contraindicated.
    4 Breathing patterns should be complex and require a high level of concentration to distract the client.

143. **1** Blowing forcefully through the mouth controls the strong urge to push and allows for a more controlled delivery of the head. (2; MR; IM; ED; HC)
    2 This is used during the latent phase of the first stage of labor; it is not helpful in overcoming the urge to push.
    3 This breathing pattern does not help to control expulsion.
    4 This is used during active labor when the cervix is 3 to 7 cm dilated; it is not helpful in overcoming the urge to push.

144. **4** As the uterus rises into the abdominal cavity, the uterine ligaments become elongated and hypertrophied; raising both legs at the same time limits the tension placed on these ligaments. (2; MR; IM; TC; HC)
    1 Lifting the legs simultaneously does not negatively affect circulation in the legs.
    2 There is already pressure on the perineum from the baby's head; this maneuver places tension on the uterine ligaments.
    3 There is no effect on the fascia with this maneuver.

145. **2** The bulging perineum indicates that the fetal head is on the pelvic floor and birth is imminent. (1; MR; EV; PA; HC)
    1 This is a sign that occurs during transition or the beginning of the second stage; the second stage lasts approximately 1 hour in a primipara.
    3 Same as answer 1.
    4 Same as answer 1.

146. **2** Uterine tetany would result from the use of oxytocin to induce labor. Because oxytocin promotes powerful uterine contractions, exogenous administration of this hormone may induce uterine tetany, which does not optimize progression of labor and may restrict fetal blood flow. (2; MR; EV; TC; HC)
    1 Severe pain is associated with intense contractions.
    3 This is unrelated to uterine contractions.
    4 This is not likely to occur unless the baby is in the breech position.

147. **1** The contractions in this phase of labor are expulsive in nature; having the client push or bear down with the glottis open will hasten expulsion. (1; MR; IM; PA; HC)
    2 Blowing is encouraged to slow down pushing; she should be encouraged to push.
    3 Contractions are now frequent and intense; the client is anxious to complete the labor process; she will be unable to relax.
    4 The client should be pushing; panting will prevent this.

148. **3** In reporting progress in the descent of the presenting part, the level of the tip of the ischial spines is considered to be zero, and the position of the bony prominence of the fetal head is described in centimeters—minus (above the spines) or plus (below the spines). (2; CJ; EV; PA; HC)
    1 This would be referred to as crowning and would be designated as +5.
    2 This is designated by the term *floating*, meaning that the presenting part has not yet engaged.
    4 Minus one (−1) would indicate that the head is above the ischial spines.

149. **4** Gentle pressure is applied against the baby's head as it emerges so it is not delivered too rapidly. The head is never held back, and it should be supported as it emerges so there will be no vaginal lacerations. (2; MR; IM; TC; HC)
    1 Unless she pants to slow the pushing, she will deliver on the stretcher.
    2 Unless she pants and blows breath out, she will push involuntarily.
    3 It is impossible to push and pant at the same time.

150. **1** A pudendal block provides anesthesia to the perineum. (3; MR; PL; PA; HC)
    2 This does not affect muscle control.
    3 This affects only the perineum, not the bladder.
    4 This anesthetizes only the perineum, not the cervix or body of uterus.

151. **4** A neat surgical incision is usually easier to repair and quicker to heal than an irregular laceration. (1; MR; IM; TC; HC)
   1 Contrariwise; upon healing it will tighten up the perineum.
   2 An episiotomy will contribute to rather than limit postpartal discomfort.
   3 This may or may not influence birth trauma to the fetus; it usually reduces trauma to the mother.

152. **3** This action prevents the transfer of microorganisms from the hands to the genital tract or from the genital tract to the hands. (1; MR; EV; TC; HC)
   1 This is an inadequate number of changes; soiled pads promote the growth of microorganisms because they are warm and moist and provide a medium for growth.
   2 This action interferes with analgesic action and does not prevent infection.
   4 This action promotes contamination of the vagina and urethra by organisms from the perianal area.

153. **3** These are the classic symptoms of a vaginal hematoma. (2; CJ; AS; PA; HC)
   1 The symptoms do not indicate this infection; the temperature would be elevated in the presence of infection.
   2 Same as answer 1.
   4 Not enough information; this condition would reveal persistent vaginal bleeding with a dropping blood pressure.

154. **3** When the placenta separates from the uterine wall, it tears blood vessels and results in a gush of blood from the vagina. (2; CJ; AS; PA; HC)
   1 When the placenta separates, the fundus rises into the abdomen.
   2 This is not a desired outcome; the uterus should become tense and firm.
   4 The reverse occurs; as the placenta separates it falls into the vaginal introitus and the umbilical cord appears longer and protrudes from the vagina.

155. **1** Blood loss depletes the normal cellular response to infection; trauma provides an excellent avenue for bacteria to enter. (3; CJ; AS; TC; HC)
   2 Preeclampsia is generally not a predisposing cause of postpartum infection.

3 These may create problems if hemorrhage occurs because the hemoglobin and hematocrit are already low.
4 Endogenous infection is rare; infection is usually caused by outside contamination; trauma and the denuded placental site do contribute to the development of infection.

156. **1** Retention of urine with overflow will be manifested in small, frequent voidings. The bladder should be palpated for distention. (1; CJ; AN; PA; HC)
   2 There should be large amounts of urine voided because of the increased fluid volume at this time.
   3 An elevated temperature with urinary symptoms would indicate impending infection.
   4 This is untrue; more circulating fluid is present, causing an increased output.

157. **2** A distended bladder will easily displace the fundus upward and laterally. (1; CJ; AN; PA; HC)
   1 This would be manifested by a slow contraction and uterine descent into the pelvis.
   3 If this were true, in addition to being displaced, the uterus would be soft and boggy and vaginal bleeding would be heavy.
   4 From this assessment the nurse cannot make a judgment about overstretched uterine ligaments.

158. **2** The fundus descends one fingerbreadth per day from the day after delivery; lochia serosa begins to flow on the fifth day. (2; CJ; AN; PA; HC)
   1 The fundus would be one to three fingers below the umbilicus (one fingerbreadth per day).
   3 The fundus would be descending into the pelvis at this time.
   4 The fundus would be within the pelvis and indiscernible at this time.

159. **1** Prolactin is the hormone from the anterior pituitary that stimulates mammary gland secretion. Progesterone and estrogen are ovarian hormones that influence breast development and other female sexual characteristics. (1; CJ; AN; PA; HC)
   2 Oxytocin, a posterior pituitary hormone, stimulates the uterine musculature to contract and causes the let-down reflex.
   3 Estrogen is not a pituitary hormone; it is secreted by the ovaries and placenta.
   4 Progesterone is not a pituitary hormone; it is secreted by the corpus luteum of the ovary.

160. **3** If the woman perceives a negative attitude from others, she may be tense and let-down may not occur; a positive attitude of others toward breastfeeding promotes relaxation and let-down. (2; CJ; AN; PA; HC)
    1 This has no influence on lactation.
    2 Same as answer 1.
    4 Milk or milk product intake during pregnancy has little influence on lactation.

161. **1** Heat causes vasodilation and an increased blood supply to the area. (1; CJ; IM; TC; HC)
    2 Sitz baths do not soften the incision site.
    3 Cleansing is done with a perineal bottle and cleansing solution immediately after voiding and defecating.
    4 Neither relaxation nor tightening of the rectal sphincter will increase healing of an episiotomy.

162. **4** There is extensive activation of the blood clotting factor after delivery; this, together with immobility, trauma, or sepsis, encourages thromboembolization, which can be limited through activity. (2; MR; IM; TC; HC)
    1 This can be accomplished by turning the client from side to side and encouraging her to deep breathe and cough.
    2 Tone would be improved by regular emptying and filling of the bladder.
    3 Abdominal muscle tone will be improved with exercise over the next 6 weeks.

163. **4** Kegel exercises can be resumed immediately and should be done for the rest of her life. (2; MR; IM; ED; HC)
    1 Bowel movements spontaneously return in 2 to 3 days after delivery; delaying bowel movements promotes constipation, perineal discomfort, and trauma.
    2 Episiotomy sutures do not have to be removed.
    3 The usual postpartal examination is 6 weeks after delivery; menses can return earlier or later than this time period and should not be a factor in scheduling an examination.

164. **2** Some mothers will respond to mores and pressures by trying to breastfeed in spite of the fact that they would prefer to give the baby a bottle. The nurse should elicit more information before responding. (2; MR; IM; PS; HC)
    1 This is untrue; successful breastfeeding requires mastery, and some women are unable to do this.
    3 Although this is true, the mother's statement indicates some concerns about breastfeeding and should be further explored.
    4 The baby's sucking and emptying the breasts will determine the amount of milk.

165. **4** Most average-sized babies regulate themselves on an approximate 3- to 4-hour schedule. However, wide variations do exist. (2; MR; IM; ED; HC)
    1 Some of the episodes of crying do not indicate that the baby is hungry; the mother will learn the difference.
    2 It is best to allow the baby to set the schedule; usually close to the hospital routine.
    3 Although this is true, this does not answer the mother's question concerning the time for doing things.

166. **2** Breastfeeding with hepatitis C is contraindicated to limit the transmission of infection (3; MR; AN; PA; HC)
    1 Breastfeeding with mastititis is not always contraindicated; the baby already has the organism in the mouth, and nursing will decrease the mother's discomfort.
    3 Breastfeeding is not contraindicated with inverted nipples, because a breast shield can provide mild suction to help pull out a nipple.
    4 Breastfeeding is not always contraindicated with this disorder.

167. **3** Cow's milk is diluted with water and has sugar added to make it resemble human milk. (3; CJ; IM; ED; HC)
    1 Cow's milk contains more calcium.
    2 Cow's milk contains more protein and more calcium.
    4 Cow's milk contains more protein and less carbohydrate.

168. **3** Air drying nipples after feedings limits irritation and disruption of skin integrity. (2; MR; EV; PA; HC)
    1 Application of soap to breast tissue may result in drying and cracking of tissue.
    2 Wearing a brassiere continuously except for bathing is recommended for 2 to 3 weeks postpartum to provide support to breast tissue structures.
    4 Plastic liners trap moisture against tissue and may increase skin breakdown.

169. **3** Frequently the emotional excitement of going home will diminish lactation and/or the let-down reflex for a brief period. When the mother knows that this may happen and how to cope with it, the problem is apt to be a minor one and easily overcome. (2; MR; IM; ED; HC)
   1 Many factors (stress) inhibit lactation, and the client should be aware of this; false reassurance.
   2 This supply may diminish or stop under stress factors; false reassurance.
   4 This response lacks an explanation of why it happens as well as concrete instructions for remedying the situation.

170. **4** Soap irritates, cracks, and dries breasts and nipples, making it painful for the mother when the baby sucks. (2; MR; EV; ED; HC)
   1 The client should empty the breasts at each feeding to keep milk flowing.
   2 This is a permissible and often-used technique of breastfeeding.
   3 The breasts should be washed before feeding to remove encrustations and microorganisms.

171. **3** Covered ice packs promote comfort by decreasing vasocongestion. (2; MR; PL; PA; HC)
   1 Nipple stimulation precipitates the release of prolactin, which leads to more milk production and further engorgement and discomfort.
   2 Emptying the breasts stimulates lactation, leading to further engorgement and discomfort.
   4 Same as answer 1.

172. **4** Although thrombophlebitis is suspected, before a definitive diagnosis the client should be confined to bed so that further complications will be avoided. (2; LE; EV; TC; HC)
   1 This may cause extreme vasodilation, which would allow a thrombus to dislodge and circulate freely.
   2 If a thrombus is present, massage may dislodge it and lead to pulmonary embolism.
   3 Assessment of the leg may indicate thrombophlebitis; the client should be put to bed.

173. **3** Elevated levels of AFP, a fetal serum protein, have been found to reflect open neural tube defects such as spina bifida and anencephaly. (2; MR; AS; PA; HC)
   1 Genetic testing, not AFP testing, will reveal chromosomal aberrations.
   2 This is revealed by genetic testing of fetal cells in the amniotic fluid.
   4 Genetic studies after birth will reveal the presence of just one X chromosome in a female child.

174. **3** Forcing the family to be involved at the nurse's convenience would interfere with development of a productive relationship and affect cooperation of the family. (1; MR; PL; ED; HC)
   1 This would be an inconvenient time for the mother and interfere with productivity.
   2 The father should be included in the visit if at all possible.
   4 This may be at a time that would be inconvenient for the family and thus interfere with productivity.

175. **2** The most likely cause is a disturbance in the ratio of calcium to phosphorus, with the amount of serum calcium reduced and the serum phosphorus increased; milk is an excellent source of calcium. (1; CJ; IM; PA; HC)
   1 Leg cramps are usually related to low calcium intake, not hypercalcemia.
   3 Elevated potassium levels are very serious; they are not manifested by leg cramps.
   4 A low potassium level is not a usual occurrence; it is not improved by ingestion of leafy vegetables.

176. **4** The leg cramps may be related to low calcium intake; cheese and broccoli both have high calcium content. (3; MR; IM; ED; HC)
   1 These are poor sources of calcium.
   2 Same as answer 1.
   3 Same as answer 1.

177. **2** The uterus responds rapidly to touch and this involves the mother in her care. (1; MR; EV; ED; HC)
   1 The uterus must be massaged before there are signs of bleeding.
   3 Although this would be beneficial, the client should be taught to massage the uterus to cause it to contract.
   4 This does not actively involve the mother in her own care and could be unsafe if the uterus becomes boggy between the 15-minute time periods.

Normal Newborn

178. **3** This immunity is developed from an antigen-antibody response in the mother that is passed to the fetus. (2; CJ; AN; PA; NN)
   1 This is acquired by an individual in response to a disease or an infection.
   2 This is acquired by an individual in response to small amounts of antigenic material (e.g., vaccination).
   4 This is conferred by the injection of antibodies already prepared in another host.

179. **1** Position the baby with head lower than chest and rub the infant's back to stimulate crying so he or she can oxygenate the lungs. (1; MR; IM; PA; NN)
  2 This is not the priority at the present moment; the uterus still contains placenta and will not contract.
  3 There is no need for haste in cutting the cord; a clear airway is the priority.
  4 There is no time, and the mother will not be able to cooperate with a move to the stretcher.

180. **3** The increased pulmonary blood flow raises the pressure in the left atrium functionally forcing the septum to close the foramen ovale. (3; CJ; AN; PA; NN)
  1 There is an increased aortic blood flow.
  2 This is caused by increased pressure in the left atrium.
  4 There is decreased pressure in the right atrium.

181. **4** There is anatomic obliteration of the lumen by fibrous proliferation, leading to the term ligamentum arteriosum. (2; CJ; AN; PA; NN)
  1 This refers to the ductus venosus after it closes.
  2 This is a descriptive term meaning a long and round ligament.
  3 There is no such vessel.

182. **2** A quiet, alert state is an optimum time for infant stimulation. (3; MR; IM; PA; NN)
  1 Bright lights are disturbing to newborns and may impede mother-child interaction.
  3 A good time for mother-infant interaction; physical examination can be delayed.
  4 This position does not increase stimulation; the infant cannot see anything.

183. **1** Heart rate is vital and is the most critical observation in Apgar scoring at birth. (3; CJ; AS; PA; NN)
  2 Respiratory effort rather than rate is included in the Apgar score; the rate is very erratic.
  3 This may or may not be present at this time and is not a part of Apgar scoring.
  4 This should be assessed later, but is not a part of Apgar scoring.

184. **4** This sequence is least disturbing. Touching with the stethoscope and inserting the thermometer increase anxiety and elevate vital signs. (1; CJ; AS; ED; NN)

  1 Measuring the respirations should precede the heart rate because the vital signs will change when the baby is touched.
  2 Temperature should be measured last.
  3 Respirations should be measured first, but temperature should be measured after the heart rate.

185. **3** The heart rate varies with activity; crying will increase the rate, whereas deep sleep will lower it; a rate between 120 and 160 is within normal range. (2; CJ; AS; PA; NN)
  1 Heart rates below 120 are considered bradycardia; above 180, tachycardia.
  2 The normal heart rate is between 120 and 160.
  4 A heart rate below 120 is considered bradycardia.

186. **2** This response by the neonate is called habituation and is normal. (1; MR; IM; PA; NN)
  1 The infant is responding to noise and therefore hears.
  3 This is not necessary because the neonate's response is normal.
  4 Same as answer 3.

187. **2** The respiratory rate is associated with activity and can be as rapid as 60 breaths per minute; over 60 breaths per minute is considered tachypneic in the infant. (2; CJ; AS; PA; NN)
  1 Respirations may go up to 60 with activity.
  3 Any respiratory rate above 60 is considered to be tachypneic.
  4 This respiratory rate is considered to be tachypneic in the newborn.

188. **2** Normally the newborn's breathing is abdominal and irregular in depth and rhythm; the rate ranges from 30 to 60 breaths per minute. (2; CJ; AS; PA; NN)
  1 Newborns' respirations are usually irregular.
  3 Newborns' respirations are abdominal.
  4 Newborns' respirations are irregular and abdominal in origin.

189. **3** Cyanosis, choking, and coughing denote aspiration and hypoxia, for which suctioning and oxygenation are needed. (3; MR; IM; PA; NN)
  1 Crying could add to the infant's distress.
  2 The water could be aspirated and intensify the infant's problems.
  4 The infant is showing signs of a blocked airway; priority action is to suction and oxygenate the infant.

190. 3 To maintain a patent airway and promote respiration and gaseous exchange, mucus must be removed. (2; MR; CW; IM; TC)

1 This is for aspirating the stomach contents, not for airway clearance.

2 If the airway is obstructed, oxygen will be of no use; therefore suctioning is a priority.

4 Documentation is important, but secondary to clearing a passageway for air.

191. 1 Bilirubin is excreted via the gastrointestinal tract; if meconium is retained, the bilirubin is reabsorbed. (3; MR; PL; PA; NN)

2 This is treatment for hyperbilirubinemia; it does not prevent its development.

3 Early feeding, whether by breast or formula, tends to keep the bilirubin level low by stimulating gastrointestinal activity.

4 Maintaining an adequate fluid volume does not affect the development of hyperbilirubinemia.

192. 3 The Moro reflex is a sudden extension and abduction of the arms at the shoulders and spreading of the fingers, with the index finger and thumb forming the letter "C"; this is followed by flexion and adduction; the legs may weakly flex, and the infant may cry vigorously. (2; CJ; EV; ED; NN)

1 This is only part of the normal Moro response; it should be accompanied by abduction and spreading of the fingers, followed by flexion.

2 The reflex is abduction, followed by adduction.

4 The legs generally flex weakly.

193. 4 Injury to the brachial plexus, clavicle, or humerus prevents the abductive and adductive movements of an upper extremity. (2; CJ; AN; ED; NN)

1 Children with Down syndrome exhibit a normal Moro reflex.

2 This is not usually associated; however, if the cochlea is undeveloped or the eighth cranial (vestibulocochlear) nerve were injured, it would affect equilibrium and response to the test.

3 These injuries usually cause a symmetric loss of the Moro reflex.

194. 1 Milia occur commonly, are not indicative of any illness, and eventually disappear. (1; CJ; AN; ED; NN)

2 Lanugo is fine, downy hair.

3 This is a lay term for milia; it would not be used in charting.

4 These are bluish-black spots on the buttocks that present on darkly pigmented infants.

195. 3 The tonic neck reflex (fencing position) is a spontaneous postural reflex of the newborn that may or may not be present during the first days of life; once apparent, it persists until the third month. (1; CJ; AS; PA; NN)

1 This is the startle reflex.

2 This is a demonstration of muscle tone while held prone and suspended in midair.

4 This is a normal, expected reflex in the neonate.

196. 3 Bacteria, especially *Escherichia coli*, produce substances necessary to synthesize prothrombin. (3; CJ; AN; PA; NN)

1 This is an orange bile pigment produced by the breakdown of hemoglobin.

2 Bile salts are manufactured in the liver, not synthesized by bacteria.

4 This is secreted by the gastric glands, not synthesized by bacteria.

197. 2 By now the newborn will have ingested an ample amount of the amino acid phenylalanine, which, if not metabolized because of a lack of the liver enzyme, can deposit injurious metabolites in the bloodstream and brain; early detection can determine if the liver enzyme is absent; PKU can be treated with Lofenalac formula and retardation can be prevented. (3; CJ; PL; TC; NN)

1 The baby will have a vitamin K injection immediately upon admission to the nursery to prevent any bleeding problems.

3 The infant will demonstrate clinical symptoms that suggest necrotizing enterocolitis; they can occur at any time and are not related to a 36-hour intake of formula.

4 Heel sticks are done on admission to the nursery to rule out hypoglycemia; heel sticks are not related to a 36- to 48-hour formula intake.

198. 3 Phenylalanine is an essential amino acid necessary for growth that may be absent in infants with PKU; testing is done on all newborns. (2; CJ; IM; ED; NN)

1 Untreated PKU can lead to retardation; the test will not identify retardation.

2 Done at the same time as PKU testing, but thyroid deficiency does not lead to PKU.

4 PKU is a genetic, not a chromosomal, disorder.

199. **1** There is a sensitive period in the first minutes or hours after birth during which it is important, for later interpersonal development, that the mother and father have close contact with their new infant. (2; CJ; IM; ED; NN)

2 Rooming-in is not usually immediate; it occurs once the mother is in the postpartal unit.

3 Taking-in is a psychologic behavior described by Reva Rubin that occurs during the first 2 postpartal days.

4 Taking-hold is a psychologic behavior described by Reva Rubin that occurs after the third postpartal day.

200. **4** Some maternal oxytocin crosses the placenta and induces the secretion of fluids that have accumulated in the fetal breasts (sometimes called witch's milk). (1; CJ; IM; ED; NN)

1 This is usually manifested in the oral mucosa as thrush (white, adherent patches).

2 Evidence of infection would not appear so rapidly after birth.

3 This is uncommon and usually undetectable in the newborn period.

201. **3** Teaching the mother by example is a nonthreatening approach that allows her to proceed at her own pace. (2; MR; PL; ED; NN)

1 Mothers need demonstration of appropriate mothering skills, not just a discussion.

2 Learning does not occur by schedule; questions must be answered as they arise.

4 Satisfying the mother's needs will allow her to develop reserves to give the child; plan should promote security in her role and facilitate more independent caregiving.

202. **4** The antibodies in human milk provide the newborn infant with immunity against all or most of the pathogens that the mother has encountered. (2; CJ; IM; ED; NN)

1 These are present in commercial formulas.

2 Complex carbohydrates are not required by the infant.

3 Same as answer 1.

203. **2** Breast milk is digested faster than formula. Breastfed infants therefore become hungry sooner. (1; CJ; PL; ED; NN)

1 An infant may want to nurse hourly if irritable, but this is not a usual feeding pattern.

3 A breastfed newborn must be fed more often than this.

4 All infants must be fed more often than this.

204. **4** Human milk contains 42% carbohydrate, and cow's milk 30% carbohydrate; the carbohydrate in cow's milk is further diluted when water is added to the formula, so additional sugar is required to supplement it. (2; CJ; IM; ED; NN)

1 The sugar in cow's milk is lactose, a simple sugar.

2 The sugar in cow's milk is assimilated well.

3 The calorie content is about the same, 20 calories/ounce.

205. **1** Infants require about 73 ml (2 to 3 oz) of fluid per pound and 60 calories a day per pound for growth. (2; CJ; PL; PA; NN)

2 This is too little; infants require 2 to 3 oz of fluid per pound, 18 oz/24 hr.

3 This is too much; 18 oz/24 hr is required, or about 3 oz every 4 hours.

4 Same as answer 3.

206. **3** The cardiac sphincter in the newborn is poorly developed; if the stomach is too full, formula backs up through the sphincter and the infant regurgitates. (2; MR; IM; ED; NN)

1 This may cause cramping or colic; it usually does not cause regurgitation.

2 This would be manifested by projectile vomiting, not regurgitation.

4 This is a nondescriptive answer; the position is not described; it might happen if the baby were upside down.

High-Risk Pregnancy

207. **4** AFP in amniotic fluid is elevated in the presence of neural tube defects. (2; CJ; AS; PA; HP)

1 Fetal diabetes cannot be detected.

2 Fetal lung maturity cannot be determined until after 35 weeks' gestation.

3 Cardiac disorders cannot be detected.

208. **1** The greatest danger of drug-induced malformation is during the first trimester of pregnancy, because this is the period of organogenesis. (2; CJ; AN; TC; HP)

2 This may cause problems, but organogenesis has already taken place by the second trimester.

3 The fetus is totally formed at this time, and damage from drugs would not be likely.

4 Drugs should be avoided, but the first trimester (period of organogenesis) is the most critical.

209. 2 About two thirds of neonatal deaths are caused by prematurity; there appears to be a correlation with teenage pregnancy, lack of prenatal care, nonwhite mothers, and chronic health problems. (3; CJ; AS; PA; HP)
  1 Atelectasis may occur from respiratory distress, which in turn is associated with prematurity, the leading cause of death.
  3 Most babies who die from congenital heart disease die after the neonatal period.
  4 This usually occurs as a result of prematurity, the leading cause of death.

210. 3 Heavy cigarette smoking or continued exposure to a smoke-filled environment causes both maternal and fetal vasoconstriction, resulting in fetal growth retardation and increased fetal and infant mortality. (1; CJ; IM; ED; HP)
  1 Smoking causes vasoconstriction; permeability of the placenta to smoke is irrelevant.
  2 There is no concrete evidence that smoking relieves tension; this is not a factor in the situation described.
  4 The fetal and maternal circulations are separate; the answer is not related to the question.

211. 3 High levels of chorionic gonadotropin frequently are associated with severe vomiting of pregnancy, especially in the presence of hydatidiform mole and often in twin pregnancy. (2; CJ; AN; PA; HP)
  1 Polyhydramnios (excessive amniotic fluid) is associated with multiple gestation; maternal dehydration is generally associated with hyperemesis gravidarum.
  2 Cholecystitis is unrelated to this problem; hyperemesis gravidarum is due to HCG.
  4 This is associated with vomiting; undigested food remains in the stomach, which leads to a reflexive action and vomiting; this is common but not severe in early pregnancy.

212. 1 Threatened premature labor, a history of premature births, nipple stimulation, or administration of oxytocin too early in pregnancy can cause uterine contractions and premature delivery. (3; CJ; AN; TC; HP)
  2 The contraction stress test would be indicated because of the influence of hypertension on the placental circulation.
  3 The contraction stress test would be indicated to determine the fetus' response to labor.
  4 Same as answer 3.

213. 3 A positive contraction stress test (CST) indicates a compromised fetal heart rate during contractions, which is associated with uteroplacental insufficiency. (2; MR; AS; TC; HP)
  1 Preeclampsia does not cause a positive CST.
  2 Contraction stress tests are contraindicated in women with suspected placenta previa, because oxytocin may stimulate contractions.
  4 A contraction stress test is contraindicated in women with a suspected premature fetus or a pregnancy of less than 33 weeks' gestation because oxytocin may induce labor.

214. 4 It is not uncommon for adolescents to avoid prenatal care; many do not recognize the deleterious effect that lack of prenatal care can have on them and their babies. (3; MR; IM; ED; HP)
  1 This should come later in pregnancy, but not before ascertaining the client's feelings about breastfeeding.
  2 This can be done in the later part of pregnancy and reinforced during the postpartal period.
  3 This will have to be done, but it is not the priority intervention.

215. 4 The pregnant teenager is generally more prone to pregnancy-induced hypertension because of age, inadequate diet, and lack of prenatal care. (3; CJ; AN; PA; HP)
  1 This is unrelated; there is no proof that teenagers are more diabetogenic than other pregnant women.
  2 This is a false assumption; societal mores vary, and the pregnancy of an unmarried female may be acceptable.
  3 This may or may not be true.

216. 2 Perinatal morbidity and mortality are greatly increased in multiple pregnancy because the high metabolic demands and the possibility of malpositioning of one or both fetuses may increase the potential for medical and obstetric complications. (2; MR; AS; PA; HP)
  1 Although postpartum hemorrhage does occur more frequently after multiple births, it is not a routine occurrence.
  3 Maternal mortality during the prenatal period is not increased in the presence of multiple gestation.
  4 Multiple gestation is usually identified before delivery; the mother would have this time for adjustment.

217. **1** Multiple pregnancy thins the uterine wall by over-stretching; thus the efficiency of contractions is reduced. (2; CJ; AN; TC; HP)

   2 Anemia may cause fatigue in the mother; it does not affect uterine contractility.

   3 A pelvic contracture may lead to a difficult delivery because of cephalopelvic disproportion; it does not affect uterine contractions.

   4 PIH may bring about premature labor; it does not cause hypotonic uterine dysfunction.

218. **1** Abdominal pain should be reported immediately because it may indicate abruptio placentae or the epigastric discomfort of severe preeclampsia. (3; MR; EV; ED; HP)

   2 Leukorrhea normally occurs during pregnancy as a result of increased estrogen and progesterone levels.

   3 This is normal physiological edema of pregnancy caused by a gravid uterus and will disappear with elevation of the legs.

   4 These are Braxton Hicks contractions, which are normal and help prepare the uterus for labor.

219. **1** Placenta previa is defined as an abnormally implanted placenta (i.e., low-lying or covering the cervical os). (1; MR; PL; PA; HP)

   2 This can occur at any time; it is not specific to low-lying placentas.

   3 Premature separation of the placenta can occur with normally implanted placentas.

   4 This can occur without a low-lying placenta; factors such as poor muscular tone of the uterus and excessive oxytocin during induction may cause this to occur.

220. **4** Pyelonephritis often causes premature labor, leading to increased neonatal morbidity and mortality. (2; MR; IM; TC; HP)

   1 Fluids should be increased; the inflammatory process may lead to fever, dehydration, and an accumulation of toxins.

   2 Albuminuria occurs with pregnancy-induced hypertension and is not accompanied by pain or flank tenderness; the client's symptoms are indicative of a kidney infection.

   3 An inflammatory, not a degenerative, kidney process is present.

221. **3** Health care supervision requires treatment with an appropriate antibiotic for 2 to 3 weeks until two negative cultures are obtained; retreatment may be necessary if there is a recurrence; recurring pyelonephritis often leads to preterm birth. (3; MR; PL; PA; HP)

   1 Signs of preeclampsia occur spontaneously; it is not preceded by specific infections.

   2 A low-protein diet inhibits fetal development and is contraindicated in pregnancy.

   4 Pelvic inflammatory disease is associated with infections of the genital, not the urinary, tract.

222. **3** Bed rest keeps the pressure of the fetus off the cervix, minimizing cervical dilation; the side-lying position enhances uterine perfusion. (2; MR; PL; ED; HP)

   1 This position is used only when the cord is prolapsed.

   2 Sitting in bed will increase pressure on the cervix; this may lead to further dilation.

   4 This may aid in relieving pressure of the fetus on the cervix, but it will not enhance uterine perfusion.

223. **4** Severe pain accompanied by bleeding at term or close to it is symptomatic of complete premature detachment of the placenta (abruptio placentae). (2; MR; AS; TC; HP)

   1 A hydatidiform mole does not usually last until 36 weeks; no severe pain accompanies it.

   2 There is no bleeding with vena caval syndrome.

   3 Bleeding caused by marginal placenta previa should not be painful.

224. **3** The blood cannot escape from behind the placenta, thus the abdomen becomes board-like and painful because of the entrapment. (2; CJ; AN; PA; HP)

   1 Symptoms of hemorrhagic shock do not include pain.

   2 This is not an immediate response; it may occur later if the client's resistance is lessened.

   4 Blood at the site of placental separation may seep into the uterine muscle (Couvelaire uterus).

225. **4** Clotting defects are common in moderate and severe abruptio placentae because of the loss of fibrinogen from severe internal bleeding. (2; CJ; AN; PA; HP)

   1 An excessive amount of red blood cells is not related to the depletion of fibrinogen.

   2 Excessive globulin in the blood is unrelated to clotting.

   3 This is a decrease in the number of platelets; bleeding of abruptio placentae is caused by depletion of fibrinogen, not platelets.

226. **4** Hypertension in PIH leads to vasospasms; this in turn causes the placenta to tear away from the uterine wall (abruptio placentae). (3; CJ; AS; TC; HP)
  1 Generally cardiac disease does not cause abruptio placentae.
  2 This may cause endocrine disturbance in the infant but does not affect the blood supply to the uterus.
  3 This may affect the delivery of the fetus but does not affect the placenta.

227. **1** As the lower uterus contracts and dilates, the edge of the low-lying placenta separates from the walls of the uterus, opening placental sinuses and allowing blood to escape. (2; CJ; AN; TC; HP)
  2 Abruptio placentae is usually accompanied by intense pain.
  3 This is highly unlikely unless placenta previa is present.
  4 Placenta previa, a low-implanted placenta, causes painless vaginal bleeding; alcohol ingestion does not.

228. **3** Observation and record keeping of bleeding are independent nursing functions and necessary for implementing safe care, because hemorrhage and shock can be life threatening. (1; CJ; PL; TC; HP)
  1 Vital signs should be checked more often if bleeding persists.
  2 This is absolutely forbidden, because it may cause further separation of the placenta.
  4 The client should be restricted to complete bed rest until bleeding stops.

229. **4** Any medication that might further depress a premature infant is given with extreme caution. (2; CJ; IM; ED; HP)
  1 At the proper time the client is encouraged to bear down.
  2 This would be false reassurance; there is no absolute control of premature labor.
  3 If the client is kept NPO, it is done to lessen the risk of aspiration should anesthesia become necessary.

230. **2** Prostaglandins in semen may stimulate labor, and penile contact with the cervix may increase myometrial contractility. (1; MR; PL; TC; HP)
  1 Sexual intercourse may cause labor to progress; it is not advised.

3 The position is irrelevant; sexual intercourse is not advised in week 35 of pregnancy with 2 cm dilation.
  4 Sexual intercourse may cause labor to progress; it is not advised in week 35 of pregnancy with 2 cm dilation.

231. **1** Atony often results from an overdistended uterus; uterine contraction does not occur readily. (2; CJ; AN; PA; HP)
  2 This would cause systemic responses other than hemorrhage.
  3 This is unusual and may occur with improper use of forceps; it is not indicated in this situation.
  4 This can occur in any delivery (not just twins) if careful inspection of the placenta is not done.

232. **4** Uncomplicated gestational hypertension does not interfere with uterine involution, return of uterine tone, or constriction of vessels at the placental site. (3; CJ; AS; TC; HP)
  1 Retained placenta inhibits uterine myometrial contractions; also manual removal of placenta may cause uterine trauma.
  2 This may inhibit myometrial contraction of the uterus at the placental site.
  3 Overdistention of the uterus may lead to delayed or poor uterine myometrial contraction at the placental site after delivery.

233. **3** A symptom of heart failure is respiratory distress. (3; MR; AS; TC; HP)
  1 Although pulse is important, the primary observation should be for respiratory distress, which suggests heart failure.
  2 Signs of heart failure, not hypovolemic shock, might develop.
  4 Increased vaginal bleeding is not caused by alterations in cardiac status.

234. **3** Immediate cesarean delivery is the treatment of choice for complete placental separation. The risk of fetal death is too high to delay. (1; MR; IM; TC; HP)
  1 This is too time consuming; a high forceps delivery is rarely used because the forceps may further complicate the situation by tearing the cervix.
  2 The fetus would probably expire if this course of action were taken.
  4 Same as answer 2.

235. **1** It is imperative that a consent be obtained before anesthesia is induced. (2; LE; IM; TC; HP)
   2 This can be done later, even after anesthesia.
   3 Same as answer 2.
   4 Same as answer 2.

236. **4** Up to two peripads can be saturated normally in the first hour. (3; CJ; AS; PA; HP)
   1 A scant flow would be less and would probably not even saturate one pad.
   2 Hemorrhage would saturate more than two pads in 1 hour.
   3 This would be accompanied by heavy bleeding and require more than two pads in the first hour.

237. **2** IV oxytocin (Pitocin) is used to enhance postpartum uterine contractions after cesarean delivery, because massage of the fundus is difficult and painful after surgery; the drug produces effective clamping down on the vessels. (3; MR; IM; PA; HP)
   1 This is done for all postoperative clients.
   3 This may be difficult because of the new incision.
   4 This is done routinely for all postoperative clients.

238. **2** First pregnancy and obesity are both documented risk factors. (3; MR; AS; PA; HP)
   1 The risk age for PIH is under 20 and over 35 years of age.
   3 This is not a documented risk factor.
   4 This is not a documented risk factor.

239. **4** Rapid weight gain indicates fluid retention, another sign of PIH. (2; CJ; AS; ED; HP)
   1 HCG levels are positive throughout pregnancy.
   2 This would be indicative of gestational diabetes.
   3 Slow fetal heart tones may indicate the baby is sleeping.

240. **4** Blood pressure increases of 30 mm Hg systolic and 15 mm Hg diastolic on two occasions at least 6 hours apart may indicate preeclampsia. (2; CJ; AS; PA; HP)
   1 Incomplete data; many women have low baseline blood pressures and could be hypertensive at 120/75.
   2 Hypertension is not always accompanied by headaches.
   3 This can occur at any time, not specifically in clients with pregnancy-induced hypertension.

241. **4** To ascertain the severity of preeclampsia, these are the signs that must be assessed. (3; MR; AS; PA; HP)
   1 Constipation is not related to preeclampsia.
   2 Leakage of fluid and bleeding are not related to preeclampsia.
   3 Constipation and bleeding are not associated with preeclampsia.

242. **4** This is a sign of CNS involvement that the nurse can observe without obtaining subjective data from the client. (3; CJ; AS; TC; HP)
   1 Pain and nausea are subjective symptoms and are not directly observable.
   2 These are subjective symptoms; the client must indicate their presence.
   3 These are subjective symptoms and are not obvious to the nurse.

243. **4** The danger of seizure in a woman with eclampsia ends when postpartum diuresis has occurred, usually 48 hours after delivery. (3; CJ; EV; TC; HP)
   1 This is untrue; the danger of seizure in eclampsia ends when postpartum diuresis occurs about 48 hours after delivery.
   2 Same as answer 1.
   3 Same as answer 1.

244. **1** Clients with pregnancy-induced hypertension are at high risk for compromised cardiovascular and renal function and are still at risk for convulsions in the immediate postpartal period; frequent monitoring is vital in the first 48 hours. (2; CJ; AS; TC; HP)
   2 This client is at no higher risk for hemorrhage than any other pregnant client
   3 Although an integral part of care, it is not life threatening.
   4 This is not the priority assessment in PIH; hypervolemia may initially occur from fluid shifts from the extravascular to the vascular compartment.

245. **4** The cord may prolapse, and pressure of the baby's head on the cord may compress the cord causing fetal hypoxia. (2; CJ; AS; TC; HP)
   1 This is associated with PIH; it is not attributable to a breech delivery.
   2 In a breech delivery the head is not the presenting part bearing the brunt of pressure against the pelvic floor.
   3 This is generally caused by Rh disease; it is not associated with a breech delivery.

246. **2** Distribution of the fingers around the head will prevent a rapid change in intracranial pressure while the head is being delivered. (3; MR; AN; TC; HP)

1 This will not assist with the delivery of the head.

3 Placing a hand firmly over the perineum may interfere with the delivery and harm the baby.

4 The application of firm pressure over the anterior fontanel may injure the baby.

247. **4** A position in which the mother's head is below the level of the hips helps decrease compression of the cord and therefore maintains the blood supply to the infant. (1; CJ; EV; TC; HP)

1 This does not relieve the pressure of the oncoming head on the cord.

2 This may increase the pressure of the presenting part on the cord.

3 The pressure of the presenting part on the cord is not relieved in this position.

248. **4** The heart rate increases by about 10 beats per minute in the last half of pregnancy; this increase plus the increase in total blood volume can strain a damaged heart beyond the point at which it can efficiently compensate. (3; CJ; AN; PA; HP)

1 The increased size of the uterus is related to the growth of the fetus, not to any hemodynamic change.

2 The number of RBCs does not decrease during pregnancy; plasma volume increases, simulating lowered hemoglobin.

3 Cardiac output begins to decrease by the thirty-fourth week of gestation.

249. **4** This is the most critical period because of the rapid fluid shift as extravascular fluid returns to the bloodstream; this mobilization of fluid can place a strain on the heart and lead to cardiac decompensation. (3; MR; IM; ED; HP)

1 During the first trimester the increased amount of circulating blood volume is minimal and occurs gradually; thus it does not usually place a large burden on the heart.

2 The risk of cardiac decompensation increases as pregnancy progresses; however, the increase in blood volume occurs gradually and the mother is monitored closely.

3 There is an increased risk of stress on the heart during delivery; however, close monitoring and the use of agents to provide rest and pain relief have decreased these risks.

250. **4** Forceps reduce the mother's need to push, conserving energy; regional anesthesia will relieve the stress of pain, and it does not compromise cardiovascular function. (2; MR; PL; TC; HP)

1 Major abdominal surgery is performed on clients with cardiac problems only when absolutely necessary.

2 Induced labor is often more stressful and painful than natural labor.

3 Forceps reduce the mother's need to push, conserving energy; however, general anesthesia would compromise cardiovascular function.

251. **3** The semi-Fowler's position facilitates easier oxygen exchange, and side lying promotes better venous return. (2; MR; IM; PA; HP)

1 This is too straight and uncomfortable; the gravid uterus will impede venous return from the legs.

2 The supine gravid uterus may inhibit venous return and result in placental congestion and supine hypotension.

4 At full term, clients are placed in the left side-lying position to enhance venous return.

252. **4** The side-lying position takes the weight off large blood vessels, and blood flow to the heart is increased; elevating the shoulders relieves pressure on the diaphragm. (3; MR; IM; TC; HP)

1 Sodium leads to increased fluid retention; it is contraindicated in the cardiac client.

2 Potassium chloride is contraindicated unless lowered potassium levels indicate the need.

3 This is contraindicated unless some uterine inertia occurs.

253. **3** Clients with cardiac problems are prone to heart failure in this stage of labor. (2; MR; PL; TC; HP)

1 This is done for all laboring clients; with cardiac problems, the priority is monitoring for heart failure.

2 Same as answer 1.

4 This is not necessary; clients are maintained on the side to facilitate venous return.

254. **4** The pregnant woman's increased hormones, metabolic rate, and increased blood volume place additional demands on the pancreas, thus altering carbohydrate and lipid metabolism. (2; CJ; AN; PA; HP)
   1 Pregnancy lowers the renal threshold for glucose in nondiabetics as well; it does not affect metabolism.
   2 The hormones of pregnancy act as antagonists to insulin, thus reducing its effect.
   3 The diabetic mother's glucose tolerance does not differ from that in her prepregnant state.

255. **2** Increased metabolic demands on the body during pregnancy require an increased ingestion of glucose; appropriate levels of insulin must be provided to permit normal glucose utilization by the body. (3; MR; PL; PA; HP)
   1 The caloric content is increased, not decreased, during pregnancy.
   3 This diet would not be sufficient to prevent ketosis; insulin would be necessary to cover carbohydrate intake.
   4 This type of diet is contraindicated; it would not meet the demands of pregnancy and the growing fetus.

256. **2** Usually, as pregnancy progresses, there are alterations in glucose tolerance and in the metabolism and utilization of insulin. The result is an increased need for exogenous insulin. (1; CJ; PL; PA; HP)
   1 Caloric intake is increased to meet demands of the growing fetus.
   3 Pancreatic enzymes or hormones other than insulin are not taken by diabetics.
   4 Estrogenic hormones are not administered during pregnancy.

257. **4** Insulin requirements may fall suddenly during the first 24 to 48 hours postpartum because the endocrine changes of pregnancy are reversed. (3; CJ; AN; TC; HP)
   1 Insulin requirements do not suddenly rise at this time.
   2 Insulin requirements do not remain unchanged at this time.
   3 Insulin requirements do not slowly decrease at this time.

258. **2** Late decelerations are indicative of uteroplacental insufficiency and if left uncorrected, leads to fetal hypoxia and/or myocardial depression. (3; MR; AN; PA; HP)
   1 This cannot be determined from the fetal heart rate, only from cervical dilation.
   3 This cannot be determined from the fetal heart rate, only from cervical dilation.
   4 Late decelerations are not expected and must not be ignored.

259. **1** Multiple pregnancies and deliveries result in overstretched uterine muscles that do not contract efficiently, and bleeding may ensue. (3; MR; AN; TC; HP)
   2 The placenta should be expelled intact; the attendant at the delivery should check for this.
   3 Delivering outside the labor and delivery room area does not necessarily predispose the client to postpartal hemorrhage.
   4 The client is being given Pitocin because her grand multiparity, not precipitate delivery, may predispose her to postpartum hemorrhage.

260. **1** RhoGAM will prevent sensitization from Rh incompatibility that may arise between an Rh-negative mother and an Rh-positive infant. (2; MR; PL; PA; HP)
   2 No incompatibility exists; it could if the mother were O positive and the infant had type AB blood.
   3 Unnecessary; only the mother and the infant's Rh factors are relevant now.
   4 Blood types of the infant and mother are not compatible; however, it is very doubtful that the infant will need a transfusion.

High-Risk Newborn

261. **1** Bradycardia (baseline FHR below 120 beats per minute) indicates fetal distress and requires medical intervention. (3; MR; EV; TC; HN)
   2 This would be dangerous; the fetus is in distress, and time should not be spent on monitoring.
   3 This is not an indication of maternal distress.
   4 The normal FHR is 120 to 160 beats per minute.

262. **3** The congenital absence of a vessel in the umbilical cord is often associated with life-threatening congenital anomalies. (2; CJ; EV; TC; HN)
   1 This is the average weight for a full-term newborn.
   2 If the Apgar score 5 minutes later showed marked improvement, there would be no need for placing the infant in the ICU.
   4 The fetus may have swallowed some amniotic fluid; this is not unusual or dangerous.

263. **3** Withdrawal affects the central nervous system and respiratory system. (2; MR; AS; PA; HN)
   1 These symptoms may occur in a newborn with thyroid deficiency.
   2 These symptoms may indicate that the newborn is experiencing cold or respiratory distress.
   4 These symptoms may occur in a child affected with syphilis.

264. **1** Drug dependence in the newborn is physiologic. As the drug is cleared from the body, symptoms of drug withdrawal become evident. Tremors, irritability, difficulty sleeping, twitching, and convulsions may result. (2; MR; EV; PA; HN)
   2 Hypertonicity of muscles would be seen.
   3 Symptoms of drug withdrawal involve signs of excessive stimulation.
   4 Dehydration is secondary to poor feeding; it is not a result of withdrawal per se.

265. **4** This is related to neonatal morbidity and mortality; by 5 minutes the healthy neonate is relatively stable and requires minimal care. (3; MR; AS; PA; HN)
   1 The diagnosis of cerebral palsy is not related to the Apgar score.
   2 Genetic defects may or may not be apparent at this time. They are not related to the Apgar score.
   3 This has not been proven, although research continues in this area.

266. **2** This is unnecessary; the baby's Apgar (7/9) does not indicate a need for oxygen. (2; MR; IM; PA; HN)
   1 This is an important part of record keeping on all newborns.
   3 Poor thermoregulation necessitates keeping the baby warm to stabilize body temperature.
   4 All newborns are evaluated immediately.

267. **1** This conjunctivitis occurs about 3 to 4 days after birth; if it is not treated with tetracycline, chronic follicular conjunctivitis with conjunctival scarring will occur. (2; CJ; AN; TC; HN)
   2 High oxygen concentrations cause vasoconstriction of retinal capillaries, which can lead to blindness.
   3 AIDS in the newborn does not manifest itself in any type of conjunctivitis.
   4 This chemical conjunctivitis occurs within the first 48 hours and is not purulent in nature.

268. **2** *Chlamydia trachomatis* is associated with the development of pneumonia in the newborn infant. (3; MR; AS; TC; HN)
   1 This is done at all times; the first priority here is to monitor for pneumonia, which is often associated with chlamydial infections.
   3 Purulent conjunctivitis at this time suggests a chlamydial infection, not an allergic response.
   4 Physician's order is required; bathing the eyes with solution will not stem the infection; the infant will be put on intensive systemic antibiotic therapy.

269. **3** Prolonged oxygen administration at relatively high concentrations in a premature infant whose retina is incompletely differentiated and/or vascularized may result in retinopathy of prematurity (retrolental fibroplasia); when oxygen therapy is discontinued, capillary overgrowth in the retina and vitreous body may result and include capillary hemorrhage, fibrosis, and retinal detachment. (2; MR; PL; TC; HN)
   1 Though true, temperature and humidity are not factors in the development of retinopathy of prematurity.
   2 Phototherapy is used to decrease hyperbilirubinemia; it is unrelated to retrolental fibroplasia; however, the eyes are covered to prevent injury for all infants receiving phototherapy.
   4 High oxygen concentration is dangerous and a factor in the development of retinopathy of prematurity.

270. **4** Because physical symptoms of congenital syphilis are difficult to detect at birth, the infant should be screened immediately to determine if treatment is necessary. (3; CJ; AS; TC; HN)
   1 This defect occurs in the first trimester; *Treponema pallidum* does not affect a fetus before the sixteenth week of gestation.
   2 This is found in children with Down syndrome, not congenital syphilis.
   3 This does not become manifest in the syphilitic infant until about 3 months of age.

271. 2 Asymmetry of the gluteal dorsal surface of the thighs and inguinal folds indicates developmental dysplasia of the hip; folds on the affected side appear higher than those on the unaffected side. (1; CJ; AS; PA; HN)
  1 Impaired reflex behavior and a shrill cry, etc., would indicate CNS damage.
  3 An inguinal hernia is evidenced by protrusion of the intestine into the inguinal sac.
  4 Peripheral nervous system damage would be manifested by limpness or flaccidity of extremities.

272. 1 In Erb-Duchenne paralysis there is damage to spinal nerves C5 and C6, which causes paralysis of the arm. (3; MR; EV; TC; HN)
  2 The grasp reflex is intact because the fingers usually are not affected; if C8 is injured, paralysis of the hand results (Klumpke's paralysis).
  3 There is no interference with turning of the head; injury usually results from excessive lateral flexion of the head during delivery of the shoulder.
  4 There would be a negative Moro reflex on the affected side only.

273. 2 Gentle massage and manipulation of the muscles help prevent contractures. (3; MR; PL; PA; HN)
  1 This would be dangerous because it would lead to permanent contractures.
  3 Active ROM is impossible because of injury; gentle passive ROM is delayed for 10 days to prevent additional injury to the brachial plexus.
  4 The length of the arm will not change on a daily basis.

274. 2 This is the sign that differentiates between these two conditions; cephalhematoma does not extend beyond the suture line. (2; CJ; AS; PA; HN)
  1 Pain is not usually associated with either condition.
  3 This is unusual; it usually decreases in size.
  4 Bruising can occur with either condition.

275. 4 A rapid delivery does not give the fetal head adequate time for molding, so pressure against the head is increased. (3; CJ; AN; PA; HN)
  1 This results from excessive pulling on the head and shoulders during delivery; it is not incurred in precipitous delivery.
  2 This is more likely to occur in a footling breech delivery.

  3 This may occur with a pull on the shoulders during delivery; it is not likely to occur with precipitous delivery.

276. 1 Cardiac pathology can be assessed at an early age and circumoral pallor may be a symptom. (2; MR; AN; TC; HN)
  2 Circumoral pallor is not a normal sign for a newborn.
  3 This is not a normal sign at any age.
  4 These symptoms do not indicate increased intracranial pressure.

277. 4 Intracranial bleeding may occur in the subdural, subarachnoid, or intraventricular spaces of the brain, causing pressure on vital centers; clinical signs are related to the area and degree of cerebral involvement. (1; CJ; AN; PA; HN)
  1 This is caused by hypocalcemia; it is manifested by exaggerated muscular twitching.
  2 This is an obvious defect of the spinal column; it is easily recognized.
  3 Elevated potassium causes cardiac irregularities.

278. 4 The brachial plexus is injured by excessive pressure during a difficult delivery requiring the use of forceps or during a breech delivery; it is considered a birth injury and is not related to genetic factors or disease. (2; CJ; AN; ED; HN)
  1 Erb's palsy is a birth injury, not a disease.
  2 Erb's palsy is a birth injury, not a genetic problem.
  3 Erb's palsy is a birth injury to nervous tissue, not a tumor arising from muscle tissue.

279. 1 Development of jaundice before 24 to 48 hours after birth may indicate a blood dyscrasia, requiring immediate medical investigation. Jaundice occurring between 48 and 72 hours after birth is a consequence of the normal physiologic breakdown of fetal red cells and immaturity of the liver. (3; MR; EV; ED; HN)
  2 Unless the jaundice was pathologic (occurring in the first 24 hours of life), this is not necessary.
  3 First, the age of the infant must be ascertained to see whether this is physiologic jaundice; then, the nurse can do a "heel-stick" to determine the amount of bilirubin.
  4 Bilirubin studies would be done first to determine whether the amount of bilirubin present warranted phototherapy.

280. 3 Development of jaundice in the first 24 hours indicates hemolytic disease of the newborn. (3; MR; AS; TC; HN)

1 May or may not be present during first 24 hours; it usually develops later.

2 These may or may not be present in first 24 hours; they are dependent on the bilirubin level.

4 This is normal; serum bilirubin normally accumulates in the neonatal period because of the short life span of fetal erythrocytes, reaching levels of 7 mg/100 ml the second to third day, when jaundice appears.

281. 3 Much of a full-term infant's birth weight is gained during the last month of pregnancy (almost a third), and most of this final spurt is subcutaneous fat, which serves as insulation; the preterm infant has not had the time to grow in the uterus and has little of this insulating layer. (1; CJ; AN; ED; HN)

1 There is a relatively larger surface area per body weight.

2 There is an extremely limited shivering and sweating response in the preterm infant.

4 This is unrelated to the maintenance of body temperature.

282. 3 Neonates are unable to shiver; they use the breakdown of brown fat to supply body heat; the preterm baby has a limited supply of brown fat available for this breakdown. (3; MR; AN; ED; HN)

1 The breakdown of glycogen into glucose does not supply body heat.

2 Newborns are unable to use shivering to supply body heat.

4 The pituitary gland does not supply body heat.

283. 2 The preterm infant has a reduced glomerular filtration rate and reduced ability to concentrate urine or conserve water. (3; CJ; AN; ED; HN)

1 This is untrue; all systems of the preterm baby are less developed than in the full-term infant.

3 The opposite occurs; urine is very dilute.

4 The fluid and electrolyte balance of preterm infants is easily upset.

284. 4 Immaturity of the respiratory tract in preterm infants can be evidenced by a lack of functional alveoli, smaller lumina with increased possibility of collapse of the respiratory passages, weakness of respiratory musculature, and insufficient calcification of the bony thorax leading to respiratory distress. (1; MR; PL; TC; HN)

1 This is not a common occurrence at the time of birth unless trauma has occurred.

2 This is not a primary concern unless severe hypoxia occurred during labor; it is difficult to diagnose at this time.

3 This may be a problem, but generally the air passageway is well suctioned at birth.

285. 2 The moisture provided by the humidity liquifies the tenacious secretions, making gas exchange possible. (2; MR; PL; PA; HN)

1 They should be side lying rather than prone; the prone position is associated with apnea and SIDS.

3 Actually the caloric intake will be increased; the amount, number, and type of feedings will be related to the metabolic rate.

4 This is not a routine action; oxygen concentration will depend on the babies' blood gases.

286. 4 Glucose oxidase strips are used by nurses to screen infants for hypoglycemia. (1; MR; AS; TC; HN)

1 Fasting blood sugar levels are not routinely used to screen newborns for hypoglycemia; fasting may reduce glucose levels further.

2 This test is not used to screen for hypoglycemia.

3 This test is not used as a screening tool.

287. 2 The infant of a diabetic mother is a newborn at risk because of the interplay between the maternal disease and the developing fetus. (2; MR; IM; TC; HN)

1 A baby of a diabetic mother is generally hypoglycemic because of oversecretion of insulin by the baby's hypertrophied pancreas.

3 Infants of diabetic mothers are at high risk and require intensive monitoring.

4 The baby may be prone to hypoglycemia and will need increased glucose.

288. **1** In diabetic mothers the fetal pancreas responds to the mother's hyperglycemia by secreting more than normal amounts of insulin; this leads to infant hypoglycemia after birth. (2; CJ; AN; TC; HN)

2 Increased insulin production by the fetus diminishes the glucose content of the blood; babies are most often hypoglycemic.

3 There may be a generalized edema, but not specific to the central nervous system.

4 In response to the increased glucose received from the mother, the islets of Langerhans in the fetus may have become hypertrophied; they are not congenitally depressed.

289. **2** The higher-than-normal glucose level in a fetus of a diabetic mother leads to increased fat synthesis and deposition; increased glucose utilization is also promoted by the combined presence of the pituitary growth hormone and placental somatotropin. (3; CJ; AN; TC; HN)

1 This is false; glucose utilization is increased, with resultant macrosomia.

3 This is false; somatotropin concentration is increased during pregnancy.

4 This is false; somatotropin concentration is increased and glucose utilization is increased.

290. **2** The greatest problem facing this infant is infection of the bladder mucosa and excoriation of the surrounding tissue; meticulous hygiene is necessary both preoperatively and postoperatively. (2; MR; PL; TC; HN)

1 Urinary retention is not a problem because the urine drains continuously.

3 Deficient fluid volume is not a problem because intake and output are not affected.

4 Although sexual dysfunction is a problem, it is not a priority problem at this time.

Women's Health

291. **4** The function of progesterone is to relax the uterus and maintain a succulent endometrium to foster implantation of the fertilized ovum. (3; CJ; AN; PA; WH)

1 Ovulation is stimulated by increases in the levels of luteinizing hormone (LH) and estrogen.

2 Menstruation is controlled by regulating factors from the hypothalamus and pituitary (FSH-RH, FSH, LH-RH, LH); these hormones stimulate the production of ovarian follicles, ovulation, estrogen, and progesterone by the ovarian cells.

3 Capillary fragility is often associated with deficiency of vitamin C (ascorbic acid); progesterone is not responsible.

292. **4** Estrogen is found in the follicular fluid of the ovaries and aids in the growth of the endometrium. (2; CJ; AN; PA; WH)

1 The luteinizing hormone promotes the development of ovarian follicles as well as stimulating ovulation and the production of estrogen and progesterone by the ovarian cells.

2 The luteinizing hormone promotes the development of ovarian follicles as well as stimulating ovulation and the production of estrogen and progesterone; progesterone prepares the endometrium for implantation and the breasts for lactation.

3 These hormones prepare the breasts for milk secretion (lactation).

293. **1** A generous supply of blood is carried by the uterine arteries (branches of the internal iliac arteries). The vaginal and ovarian arteries also supply the uterus with blood by anastomosing with the uterine vessels. (2; CJ; AN; PA; WH)

2 The aorta does not supply the uterus directly.

3 The hypogastric or internal iliac arteries supply the pelvic wall and viscera.

4 The hypogastric arteries (internal iliac) supply the pelvic wall and gluteal area, and the external branches (called uterine arteries) supply the uterus and genitalia; the aorta does not supply the uterus directly.

294. **3** The time between ovulation and the next menstruation is relatively constant. Within a 30-day cycle the first 15 days are preovulatory, ovulation occurs on day 16, and the next 14 days are postovulatory. Ovulation therefore occurs on January 17. (2; CJ; AS; PA; WH)

1 This is within the first 15 days and is the preovulatory phase.

2 Same as answer 1.

4 This is within the last 14 days of the cycle and is postovulatory.

295. **2** Persistent pain of any kind is usually a symptom, and the client should seek medical attention (2; MR; IM; ED; WH)

1 Although diversion is a method to alter pain perception, the presence of pain requires investigation of possible causes.

3 Although a nutritious diet is beneficial, iron does not prevent the pain of dysmenorrhea.

4 Voluntary relaxation of the abdominal muscles does not cause cessation of uterine contractions.

296. 3 Endometriosis is the presence of aberrant endometrial tissue outside the uterus. The tissue responds to ovarian stimulation, bleeds during menstruation, and causes severe pain. (1; CJ; AS; PA; WH)

1 These are not symptoms of endometriosis.
2 Ecchymoses and petechiae are not characteristic of this disorder.
4 Osteoporosis may be a complication of menopause because of decreased estrogen levels; pelvic inflammation usually results from infection.

297. 2 The posterior vaginal wall is pushed forward by the herniation of the rectum; this protrusion increases rectal pressure and causes the bearing-down sensation. (3; CJ; AS; PA; WH)

1 A rectocele is not accompanied by abdominal pain.
3 This is the primary symptom of a cystocele.
4 A cystocele is associated with urinary tract infections.

298. 3 As the uterus drops, the vaginal wall relaxes. When the bladder herniates into the vagina (cystocele) and the rectal wall herniates into the vagina (rectocele), the individual feels pressure or pain in the lower back and/or pelvis. When there is an increase in intraabdominal pressure in the presence of a cystocele, incontinence results. (2; CJ; AS; PA; WH)

1 These do not indicate cystocele and rectocele; they are common with infection.
2 These do not indicate cystocele and rectocele.
4 Same as answer 2.

299. 1 The effects of anesthesia and the inflammatory process may impede voiding, leading to urinary retention; an indwelling catheter empties the bladder continuously, preventing retention. (3; CJ; AN; TC; WH)

2 Distention causes discomfort; this is avoided by preventing retention.
3 Because the bladder is continually empty when an indwelling catheter is in place, it loses tone. This is an expected but undesirable effect.
4 Distention places pressure on the suture line; this is avoided by preventing retention.

300. 2 Following this type of surgery, pain is associated with bearing down; to prevent constipation the client should be instructed to increase fluid, fiber, and activity. (3; MR; IM; ED; WH)

1 The client is past childbearing age.
3 The anterior colporrhaphy is expected to reduce incontinence.
4 The colporrhaphy involves only the vaginal wall, the rectum should not be involved.

301. 3 Ulcerations may occur when the vagina and uterus are inverted. (2; CJ; AS; PA; WH)

1 Exudate would not be present with procidentia.
2 Development of ulcerations, not edema, is usually the problem.
4 The vagina would be everted, and therefore discharge would not be present.

302. 2 Moist compresses may be indicated to prevent ulcerations. (2; CJ; IM; TC; WH)

1 Ambulation would encourage the development of ulcerations.
3 This would be ineffective; gravity alone does not correct the procidentia.
4 The tissue should be protected, and manipulation, which causes irritation, should be avoided.

303. 2 The Fowler's position facilitates localization of the infection by pooling pelvic drainage. (2; CJ; IM; TC; WH)

1 This position does not make use of gravity to promote drainage of exudate.
3 This position does not make use of gravity to promote pelvic drainage.
4 Same as answer 3.

304. 2 Erosion of the cervix frequently occurs at the squamocolumnar junction, the most common site for carcinoma of the cervix. (1; CJ; PL; TC; WH)

1 This may be present as erosion develops into carcinoma; however, spotting may be the earliest sign and will be eliminated when the cancer is treated; treatment of the erosion is done to prevent the cancer from progressing.
3 Even though a cervical erosion is treated, another may occur and repeat treatment may be necessary.
4 Infection may occur in the cancerous area accompanied by profuse, malodorous discharge; treatment of the erosion is done to prevent cancer, not the secondary infection.

CHILDBEARING/WOMEN'S HEALTH ANSWERS

305. 4 Polyps are usually benign but should undergo biopsy because epidermoid cancer occasionally arises from cervical polyps. (1; CJ; AS; TC; WH)

1 Bleeding may occur whether they are malignant or not.

2 This is untrue; polyps are rarely the precursors of uterine cancer.

3 This is untrue; polyps are usually benign.

306. 4 Any sign of abnormal vaginal bleeding may indicate cervical cancer and must be checked by a physician. (3; CJ; AS; PA; WH)

1 There are few nerve endings; discomfort is a late sign.

2 Discharge becomes foul smelling only after there is necrosis and infection; it is not an early sign.

3 If pressure occurs, it is not an early symptom because the cancer must be extensive to cause pressure.

307. 4 The endocervical surface is frequently altered by metaplasia or covered by a variant of squamous epithelium. It is thus called the transitional zone. This area is often distorted by eversion and laceration, especially in pregnancy. Therefore it is a frequent site for carcinoma. Erosion in this area most frequently leads to squamous cell carcinoma, accounting for 95% of cervical cancer. (3; CJ; AS; PA; WH)

1 Extension to lymph nodes is a later stage.

2 Adenocarcinoma, accounting for only 5% of cervical cancers, may be found in the endocervical glands.

3 The cervix is the lower portion of the uterus; the juncture of the uterine body with the cervical canal is called the internal os; erosion most frequently occurs distal to this point, between the external and internal ossa, closer to the external.

308. 1 When the cancerous cells are completely confined within the epithelium of the cervix without stromal invasion, it is stage 0 and called carcinoma in situ or preinvasive carcinoma. (3; CJ; AN; PA; WH)

2 This is Stage I A; there is minimal stromal invasion.

3 This is Stage II B and involves the area around the broad ligaments but not the pelvic wall; there is extension to the corpus of the uterus.

4 This is Stage I.

309. 4 Rare cell adenoma of daughters is associated with mothers who took DES or DES-type drugs during pregnancy. (3; CJ; AS; PA; WH)

1 DES was prescribed between 1941 and 1971 to reduce the risk of spontaneous abortion in high-risk women.

2 Use of oral contraceptives is not associated with DES exposure.

3 The client with DES-related problems may exhibit abnormal bleeding or a heavy mucoid vaginal discharge, not lesions on the perineum.

310. 4 After conization there will be a blood-tinged vaginal discharge for several days and menstrual periods may be heavy for 2 to 3 cycles. (2; MR; EV; PA; WH)

1 Vaginal packing will be in place for two to three days; intercourse and tampon use should be delayed until total healing occurs.

2 Conization does not involve any external incision or dressing.

3 Conization affects only the cervix and does not alter reproductive ability.

311. 1 An abdominal panhysterectomy in the premenopausal woman produces artificial onset of menopause. (1; MR; IM; ED; WH)

2 This is untrue; because the uterus was removed, there will be no uterine endometrial proliferation and no desquamation.

3 Same as answer 2.

4 Same as answer 2.

312. 4 A hysterectomy involves only removal of the uterus. The ovaries, which secrete estrogen and progesterone, are not removed. Therefore menopause will not be precipitated but will occur naturally. (2; MR; IM; ED; WH)

1 If the ovaries were being removed, older women might have less severe symptoms than younger women; however, in this instance there would be no symptoms.

2 The nurse should serve as a resource person; the comment does not answer the question.

3 This is incorrect; there is a difference between a hysterectomy and a hysterosalpingo-oophorectomy.

313. **4** The prescribing of medications is the legal responsibility of the physician. In addition, the use of hormones is still somewhat controversial and depends on the physician's beliefs and the client's needs. (2; MR; IM; ED; WH)
   1 This is an evasive response; the client is left without direction.
   2 Hormones may be used to prevent the development of severe symptoms.
   3 This is an evasive response; it does not answer the client's question.

314. **1** During an abdominal hysterectomy, the urinary bladder may be nicked. (2; CJ; AN; PA; WH)
   2 The client is not likely to develop an infection with bleeding so soon.
   3 Increased lochia will not appear in the Foley bag because it is coming from the vagina, not the bladder.
   4 Bleeding would be present from other sites such as the incision and IV as well as in the Foley bag.

315. **1** Menstruation is the shedding of the endometrial lining of the uterus. A woman who has undergone a hysterectomy has had her uterus removed and will no longer menstruate. (2; MR; AN; PA; WH)
   2 After a hysterectomy there is no endometrial lining to shed.
   3 This is not an anxiety response; additional symptoms would be necessary before this diagnosis would be appropriate.
   4 Frank bleeding is not expected postoperatively.

316. **3** Doxorubicin hydrochloride (Adriamycin) is a chemotherapeutic agent classified as an antibiotic. It achieves its therapeutic effect by inhibiting the synthesis of RNA. This blocks protein synthesis and cell division. (3; CJ; AN; TC; WH)
   1 This is not a physiologic action of Adriamycin.
   2 Same as answer 1.
   4 Same as answer 1.

317. **3** Estrogen receptor protein-positive tumors have a more dramatic response to hormonal therapies that reduce estrogen. (3: CJ; IM; ED; WH)
   1 This does not influence breast reconstruction.
   2 Estrogen contributes to tumor growth; supplements are not indicated.
   4 This is unrelated to metastasis.

318. **3** Postoperatively the arm on the operated side is elevated on pillows with the hand higher than the arm to prevent muscle strain and edema. (2; MR; IM; PA; WH)
   1 Total immobilization should be avoided, and adduction may put undue pressure on the operative site.
   2 Although the arm is slightly abducted, sandbags are not utilized because complete immobility should be prevented.
   4 This would impair venous return and increase edema.

319. **4** Deep breathing aids in fully expanding lung tissue and prevents stasis of pulmonary secretions. (2; MR; IM; TC; WH)
   1 This may result in atelectasis and retained respiratory secretions.
   2 Does not deal directly with the problem; only states a fact and gives the client no sense of control.
   3 Although empathetic, it could compromise respiratory status.

320. **4** This defect in the bone matrix formation weakens the bones, making them unable to withstand normal stresses. (1; CJ; AN; ED; WH)
   1 Avascular necrosis is death of bone tissue that results from reduced circulation to bone.
   2 Pathologic fractures occur during normal activity or after minimal injury in bones weakened by disease.
   3 This is incorrect; hyperplasia of osteoblasts is not related to osteoporosis. This occurs during bone healing.

321. **1** This regimen limits bone demineralization. It also reduces osteoporotic pain, which promotes increased activity. (3; CJ; EV; PA; WH)
   2 This is unrelated to osteoporosis; it would be an expected outcome if the client were receiving calcium for hypocalcemia.
   3 This is unrelated to osteoporosis; it would be expected if the client were receiving vitamin C for capillary fragility.
   4 This is unrelated to osteoporosis or the rationale for therapy.

CHILDBEARING/WOMEN'S HEALTH ANSWERS

322. **3** The ovaries are responsible for producing the female sex hormones, estrogen and progesterone; a bilateral oophorectomy causes an abrupt cessation in the production of most of these hormones (the adrenal cortex produces small quantities of female sex hormones) and results in surgical menopause. (2; CJ; EV; PA; WH)

1 A tubal ligation is the surgical severing of the fallopian tubes to produce sterility, and ovarian function is unaffected.
2 A hysterectomy is the removal of the uterus, and ovarian function is unaffected.
4 A salpingectomy is the removal of the fallopian tubes, and ovarian function is unaffected.

323. **4** Alteration of ovarian hormones causes vasomotor instability; periodic systemic vasodilation is then triggered by the sympathetic nervous system, causing the feeling of warmth. (3; CJ; IM; ED; WH)

1 Acetylcholine does not cause hot flashes; it is the chemical mediator of cholinergic nerve impulses.
2 Gonadotropins do not cause hot flashes; they stimulate the function of the testes and ovaries.
3 Hot flashes may be associated with understimulation of the adrenals.

324. **3** The lack of utilization of gonadotropin by the ovaries causes an elevation of gonadotropin in the blood; ovarian function is diminished; there is little or no follicular activity. (3; CJ; AN; PA; WH)

1 There would be an increase in gonadotropin in the blood, for it is not used by the ovaries.
2 There would be an increase in prostaglandins.
4 There would be a decrease in secretion of progesterone.

325. **3** The nurse's best response is one that is realistic; once people become sexually active they usually remain sexually active; a condom, although not 100% effective, is the best protection against gonorrhea in a sexually active person. (3; CJ; EV; TC; WH)

1 Douching has no proven protective effect against sexually transmitted disease; excessive douching can actually alter the natural environment of the vagina and may even promote an ascending infection.
2 Although this is the best way to prevent a sexually transmitted disease, it is not the most realistic response to a sexually active person.
4 Spermicidal cream has no protective effect against sexually transmitted diseases; spermicidals kill sperm and limit the risk of pregnancy.

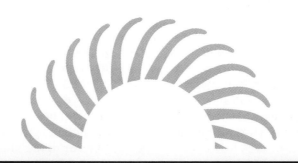

CHAPTER 5

Pediatric Nursing

HUMAN GROWTH AND DEVELOPMENT

PRINCIPLES OF GROWTH

A. Children are individuals, not little adults, who must be seen as part of a family
B. Children are influenced by genetic factors, home and environment, and parental attitudes
C. Chronologic and developmental ages of children are the most important contributing factors influencing their care
D. Play is a natural medium for expression, communication, and growth in children
E. Growth is complex, with all aspects closely related
F. Growth is measured both quantitatively and qualitatively over a period of time
G. Although the rate is uneven, growth is a continuous and orderly process
   1. Infancy: most rapid period of growth
   2. Preschool to puberty: slow and uniform rate of growth
   3. Puberty: (growth spurt) second most rapid growth period
   4. After puberty: decline in growth rate till death
H. There are regular patterns in the direction of growth and development, such as the cephalocaudal law (from head to toe) and the proximodistal law (from center of body to periphery)
I. Different parts of the body grow at different rates
   1. Prenatally: head grows the fastest
   2. During the first year: elongation of trunk dominates
J. Both rate and pattern of growth can be modified, most obviously by nutrition
K. There are critical or sensitive periods in growth and development, such as brain growth during uterine life and infancy
L. Although there are specified sequences for achieving growth and development, each individual proceeds at own rate
M. Development is closely related to the maturation of the nervous system; as primitive reflexes disappear, they are replaced by a voluntary activity

CHARACTERISTICS OF GROWTH

Circulatory System

A. Heart rate decreases with increasing age
   1. Infancy: 120 beats per minute (bpm)
   2. One year: 80 to 120 bpm
   3. Childhood: 70 to 110 bpm
   4. Adolescence to adulthood: 55 to 90 bpm
B. Blood pressure increases with age
   1. The 50th percentile ranges from 55 to 70 mm Hg diastolic to 100 to 110 mm Hg systolic
   2. These levels increase about 2 to 3 mm Hg per year starting at age 7 years
   3. Systolic pressure in adolescence: higher in males than in females
C. Hemoglobin
   1. Highest at birth, 17 g per 100 ml of blood; then decreases to 10 to 15 g per 100 ml by 1 year
   2. Fetal hemoglobin (60% to 90% of total hemoglobin) gradually decreases during the first year to less than 5%
   3. Gradual increase in hemoglobin level to 14.5 g per 100 ml between 1 and 12 years of age
   4. Level higher in males than in females

Respiratory System

A. Rate decreases with increase in age
   1. Infancy: 30 to 40 per minute
   2. Childhood: 20 to 24 per minute
   3. Adolescence and adulthood: 16 to 18 per minute
B. Vital capacity
   1. Gradual increase throughout childhood and adolescence, with a decrease in later life
   2. Capacity in males exceeds that in females
C. Basal metabolism
   1. Highest rate is found in the newborn
   2. Rate declines with increase in age; higher in males than in females

Urinary System

1. Premature and full-term newborns have some inability to concentrate urine
   a. Specific gravity (newborn): 1.001 to 1.02
   b. Specific gravity (others): 1.002 to 1.03
2. Glomerular filtration rate greatly increased by 6 months of age; reaches adult values between 1 and 2 years; gradually decreases after 20 years

Digestive System

1. Stomach size is small at birth; rapidly increases during infancy and childhood
2. Peristaltic activity decreases with advancing age
3. Blood glucose levels gradually rise from 75 to 80 mg per 100 ml of blood in infancy to 95 to 100 mg during adolescence
4. Premature infants have lower blood glucose levels than do full-term infants
5. Enzymes are present at birth to digest proteins and a moderate amount of fat but only simple sugars (amylase is produced as starch is introduced)
6. Secretion of hydrochloric acid and salivary enzymes increases with age until adolescence; then decreases with advancing age

Nervous System

1. Brain reaches 90% of total size by 2 years of age
2. All brain cells are present by the end of the first year, although their size and complexity will increase
3. Maturation of the brainstem and spinal cord follows cephalocaudal and proximodistal laws

PLAY

FUNCTIONS OF PLAY

A. Educational: learn about physical world and associate names with objects
B. Recreational: release surplus energy
C. Sensorimotor: muscle development and tactile, auditory, visual, and kinesthetic stimulation
D. Social and emotional adjustment: learn moral values; develop the idea of sharing
E. Therapeutic: release of tension and stress; manipulation of syringe and other equipment allows control over threatening events

TYPES OF PLAY

A. Active, physical: push-and-pull toys; riding toys; sports and gym equipment
B. Manipulative, constructive, creative, or scientific: blocks; construction toys such as erector sets; drawing sets; microscope and chemistry sets; books; computer programs
C. Imitative, imaginative, and dramatic: dolls; dress-up costumes; puppets
D. Competitive and social: games; role playing

Criteria for Judging the Suitability of Toys

A. Safety
B. Compatibility: child's age; level of development; experience
C. Usefulness
1. Challenge to development of the child; assist child to achieve mastery
2. Enhance social and personality development; increase motor and sensory skills; develop creativity; express emotions
3. Implement therapeutic procedures

Criteria for Judging the Nonsuitability of Toys

A. Unsafe
B. Beyond the child's level of growth and development; overstimulating; frustrating
C. Foster isolation from peer group

THE FAMILY

STRUCTURE OF THE FAMILY

A. The basic unit of a society
B. Composition varies, although one member is usually recognized as head
C. Usually share common goals and beliefs
D. Roles change within the group and reflect both individual's and group's needs
E. Status of members determined by position in family in conjunction with views of society

FUNCTIONS OF THE FAMILY

A. Reproduction: group developed to reproduce and rear members of a society
B. Maintenance to provide
1. Clothing, housing, food, and medical care
2. Social, psychologic, and emotional support for family members
3. Protection, because immaturity of young children necessitates that care be given by adults
4. Status: child is a member of a family that is also a part of the larger community
C. Socialization
1. Child is "acculturated" by introduction to social situations and instruction in appropriate social behaviors
2. Self-identity develops through relationships with other family members
3. Child learns appropriate sex roles and responsibilities
D. Growth of individual members toward maturity and independence

THE FAMILY OF A CHILD WITH SPECIAL NEEDS

MEETING THE NEEDS OF THE FAMILY

A. Recognize that members of the family will exhibit a variety of responses, such as grief and mourning, chronic grief, and excessive use of defense mechanisms
B. Understand the stages of chronic grief
1. Shock and denial: parents tend to:
   a. Learn about the deformity but deny the facts
   b. Feel inadequate and guilty
   c. Feel insecure in their ability to care for the child
   d. "Doctor shop" in hope of finding solutions
2. Adjustment to special needs: parents tend to:
   a. Feel guilty and self-accuse
   b. Envy well children: closely related to bitterness and anger

c. Search for clues or reasons why this happened to them

d. Have feelings toward child: overprotectiveness, rejection, denial, gradual acceptance

3. Reintegration and acknowledgment: parents tend to:

a. See the child's special needs in proper perspective

b. Function more effectively and realistically

c. Socially and emotionally accept the child

d. Reintegrate family life without centering it around the child

C. Help parents and siblings gain awareness of the child's special needs

1. Learning cannot take place until awareness of the problem exists

2. Help the parents develop an awareness through their own realization of the problem rather than identifying problem for them

D. Help the family understand the child's potential ability and assist them in setting realistic goals

1. Help family feel a sense of adequacy in parenting by emphasizing appropriate care, identifying small steps in child's learning process

2. Teach family how to stimulate the child's learning of new skills (e.g., sitting, walking, talking, toileting)

3. Teach parents how to help the child deal with frustration

E. Encourage the parents to treat the child as normally as possible

1. Encourage them to avoid overprotection and to use consistent, simple discipline

2. Help them become aware of the effects of this child on siblings, who may resent the excessive attention given to this child

F. Provide the family with an outlet for own emotional tensions and needs

1. Be a listener, not a preacher

2. Acquaint them with organizations, especially groups of parents who have children with similar problems

3. Assist siblings who may fear having children with similar problems

G. Teach parents the importance of continued health supervision

H. Evaluate clients' responses and revise plan as necessary

GENERAL NURSING DIAGNOSES FOR THE FAMILY OF A CHILD WITH SPECIAL NEEDS

A. Risk for impaired parenting related to loss of image of ideal child, child's physical condition that limits handling or fondling, inability of parents to meet child's special needs

B. Risk for caregiver role strain related to care requirements of child with special needs

C. Compromised family coping related to child's needs and care

D. Decisional conflict related to need for medical therapies

E. Risk for disorganized infant behavior related to pain, oral/motor problems, invasive procedures

F. Deficient diversional activity deficit related to inadequate support systems to provide respite

G. Anticipatory grieving related to loss of image of ideal child, possible death of child

H. Impaired parenting related to unrealistic expectations of child, knowledge deficit

I. Situational low self-esteem related to loss of image of ideal child

J. Spiritual distress related to decisions regarding conflicts over the cessation or continuation of treatment

K. Chronic sorrow related to loss of perfect child

PAIN ASSESSMENT

INFANT

A. Total body response; arms and legs may tremor

B. Facial expressions: grimace, surprise, frowns, facial flinching

C. Tense, harsh cry

D. Increase in blood pressure and heart rate, decrease in oxygen saturation

TODDLER

A. Generalized restlessness; guards or rubs painful area

B. Loud crying; uses words to describe pain (e.g., boo-boo, ouch)

C. Tries to delay painful situations

PRESCHOOLER

A. Crying; can describe pain location

B. Regression to earlier stage of development; withdrawal

C. May believe pain is punishment for bad behavior

D. May have been told to be brave and deny pain; fear of injections may contribute to denial of pain

E. May hit or kick caregiver

SCHOOL AGE

A. Stiff body posture; withdrawal

B. Able to describe pain

C. Afraid of bodily harm; may delay or bargain to avoid painful situations
D. Recognizes that death exists

ADOLESCENT

A. Increased muscle tension; decreased activity; withdrawal
B. Describes location and intensity of pain
C. Understands cause and effect
D. Perceives pain at physical, emotional, and mental levels

PEDIATRIC MEDICATIONS

A. Pediatric dosages differ from adult medication dosages as a result of differences in physiology
  1. Immature liver and kidney function
  2. Changing metabolic rate
  3. Decreased plasma protein concentration
  4. Altered body composition: decreased fat; increased water
B. The most reliable method to calculate dosage is based on body surface area (m²) to ensure that the child receives the correct drug dosage within a safe therapeutic range
C. The dosage prescribed by the physician is very often ordered based on kg of body weight; using the manufacturer's recommended daily dose (mg per kg of body weight) in the formula the nurse is able to determine the amount the child should receive and whether this amount is within safe limits for this medication
D. Child must be closely monitored for signs and symptoms of effectiveness and toxicity
E. Childrens' pain is real and must be addressed

THE INFANT

GROWTH AND DEVELOPMENT
Developmental Timetable
1 Month
A. Physical
  1. Weight: gains about 150 to 210 g (5 to 7 oz) weekly during the first 6 months of life
  2. Height: grows about 2.5 cm (1 inch) a month for the first 6 months of fife
  3. Head circumference: grows about 1.5 cm (½ inch) a month for the first 6 months
B. Motor
  1. Assumes flexed position with pelvis high, but knees not under abdomen, when prone

  2. Holds the head parallel with the body when suspended in prone position
  3. Can turn head from side to side when prone; lifts head momentarily from bed
  4. Asymmetric posture dominates, such as tonic neck reflex
  5. Primitive reflexes still present
C. Sensory
  1. Eye movements coordinated most of the time; follows a light to midline
  2. Visual acuity 20/100
D. Socialization and vocalization
  1. Watches face intently while being spoken to
  2. Utters small, throaty sounds

2 to 3 Months
A. Physical: posterior fontanel closed
B. Motor
  1. Holds the head erect for a short time and can raise chest supported on forearms
  2. Bears some weight on legs when held in standing position
  3. Actively holds rattle but will not reach for it
  4. Grasp, tonic neck, and Moro reflexes are fading; step or dance reflex disappears
  5. Plays with fingers and hands
C. Sensory
  1. Follows a light to the periphery
  2. Has binocular coordination (vertical and horizontal vision)
  3. Listens to sounds
D. Socialization and vocalization
  1. Smiles in response to a person or object; cries less
  2. Laughs aloud and shows pleasure in making sounds

4 to 5 Months
A. Physical
  1. Birth-weight doubles
  2. Drools because salivary glands are functioning but child does not have sufficient coordination to swallow saliva
B. Motor
  1. Can sit when the back is supported; knees will be flexed and back rounded; balances the head well
  2. Symmetric body position predominates
  3. Can sustain a portion of own weight when held in a standing position
  4. Reaches for and grasps an object with the whole hand but misjudges distances
  5. Can carry hand or an object to the mouth at will
  6. Can roll over from abdomen to back
  7. Lifts head and shoulders at a 90° angle when prone
  8. Primitive reflexes (e.g., grasp, tonic neck, and Moro) have disappeared

C. Sensory
   1. Recognizes familiar objects and people
   2. Has coupled eye movements; accommodation is developing
D. Socialization and vocalization
   1. Coos and gurgles when talked to; enjoys social interaction
   2. Vocalizes displeasure when an object is taken away

6 to 7 Months

A. Physical
   1. Weight: gains about 90 to 150 g (3 to 5 oz) weekly during second 6 months of life
   2. Height: grows about 1.25 cm ($^1/_2$ inch) a month
   3. Head circumference: grows about 0.5 cm ($^1/_5$ inch) a month
   4. Teething may begin with eruption of two lower central incisors, followed by upper incisors
B. Motor
   1. Can turn over equally well from stomach or back
   2. Sits fairly well unsupported, especially if placed in a forward-leaning position
   3. Lifts head off table when supine; when lying down, lifts head as if trying to sit up
   4. Can approach a toy and grasp it with one hand; can transfer a toy from one hand to the other and from hand to mouth
   5. Plays with feet and puts them in mouth
   6. Neurologic reflexes
     a. Landau (from 6 to 8 months to 12 to 24 months): when suspended in a horizontal prone position, the head is raised, legs and spine are extended
     b. Parachute (7 to 9 months, persists indefinitely): when the infant is suspended in a horizontal prone position and suddenly thrust forward, hands and fingers extend forward as if to protect from falling
C. Sensory
   1. Has taste preferences; will spit out disliked food
   2. Begins to recognize that things are still present even though they cannot be seen
D. Socialization and vocalization
   1. Begins to differentiate between strange and familiar faces and shows "stranger anxiety"
   2. Makes polysyllabic vowel sounds
   3. Vocalizes "m-m-m-m" when crying; cries easily on slightest provocation but laughs just as quickly

8 to 9 Months

A. Motor
   1. Sits steadily alone; pulls self to standing position; stands holding onto furniture

   2. Has good hand-to-mouth coordination
   3. Developing pincer grasp, with preference for use of one hand over the other
   4. Crawls, may go backward at first
B. Sensory
   1. Depth perception is increasing
   2. Displays interest in small objects
C. Socialization and vocalization
   1. Definite social attachment is evident (e.g., stretches out arms to loved ones); shows anxiety with strangers (e.g., turns or pushes away and cries)
   2. Responds to own name; is separating self from mother by desire to act on own
   3. Reacts to adult anger; cries when scolded
   4. Has imitative and repetitive speech, using vowels and consonants such as "Dada"; no true words as yet, but comprehends words such as "bye-bye"

10 to 12 Months

A. Physical
   1. Weight: birth-weight triples
   2. Height: birth-length increases by 50%
   3. Head and chest circumference are equal
   4. Upper and lower lateral incisors usually have erupted, for total of 6 to 8 teeth
   5. Hematocrit: 29% to 41%
B. Motor
   1. Creeps (creeping is more advanced than crawling because abdomen is supported off floor)
   2. Stands alone for short times; walks with help; moves around by holding onto furniture
   3. Can sit down from a standing position without help
   4. Can eat from a spoon and a cup but needs help; prefers using fingers
   5. Can play pat-a-cake and peek-a-boo; holds a crayon to make a mark on paper
   6. Helps in dressing, such as putting arm through sleeve
C. Sensory
   1. Visual acuity 20/50+; amblyopia (lazy eye) may develop with lack of binocularity
   2. Discriminates simple geometric forms
D. Socialization and vocalization
   1. Shows emotions such as jealousy, affection, anger
   2. Enjoys familiar surroundings and will explore away from mother
   3. Fearful in strange situations or with strangers; clings to mother
   4. May develop habit of "security" blanket
   5. Can say two words besides Dada or Mama with meaning; understands simple verbal requests, such as, "Give it to me."

Play During Infancy (Solitary Play)

A. Safety is chief determinant in choosing toys (aspirating small objects is one cause of accidental death)
B. Mostly used for physical development
C. Toys need to be simple because of short attention span
D. Visual and auditory stimulation is important
E. Suggested toys: rattles; soft, stuffed toys; mobiles; push-pull toys; simple musical toys; strings of big beads and large snap toys; unbreakable mirrors; weighted or suction toys; squeeze toys; teething toys; books with textures; activity boxes; nested boxes and fitting forms

HEALTH PROMOTION DURING INFANCY

Feeding Milestones

A. At birth the full-term infant has sucking, rooting, and swallowing reflexes
B. Newborn feels hunger and indicates desire for food by crying; expresses satiety by contentedly falling asleep
C. At 1 month has strong extrusion reflex
D. By 5 to 6 months can use fingers to eat teething cracker or toast
E. By 6 to 7 months is developmentally ready to chew solids
F. By 8 to 9 months can hold a spoon and play with it during feeding
G. By 9 months can hold own bottle
H. By 12 months usually can drink from a cup, although fluid may spill and bottle may be preferred at times

Infant Nutrition

A. Nutrition as it affects growth
 1. Birth weight usually doubled by 5 months of age and tripled by 1 year
 2. Growth during the first year should be charted to observe for comparable gain in length, weight, and head circumference
 3. Generally, growth charts demonstrate the percentile of the child's growth rate (below the fifth and above the ninety-fifth percentile are considered abnormal)
 4. Percentiles of growth curves must be seen in relation to: deviation from a steady rate of growth; hereditary factors of parents (size and body shape); height and weight
 5. Satisfactory rate of growth judged by:
  a. Weight and length (overweight and underweight constitute malnutrition)
  b. General appearance; muscular development; tissue tone and turgor
  c. Activity level; amount of crying and needed sleep
  d. Mental status and behavior in relation to norms for the age
  e. Presence or absence of illness
B. Proper feeding essential to growth and development
 1. Diet that promotes growth but prevents overweight, nutritional deficiencies, and gastrointestinal disturbances such as vomiting or constipation
 2. Establishment of appropriate eating habits
 3. Consistency of foods should progress from liquid to semisoft to soft to solids as the dentition and jaw develop

Guidelines for infant feedings

A. Breast milk is the most complete diet for the first 6 months but requires supplements of fluoride, iron by 6 months, and vitamin D if the mother's supply is deficient or the infant is not exposed to frequent sunlight
B. Iron-fortified commercial formula is an acceptable alternative to breastfeeding; requires fluoride supplements in areas where the fluoride content of drinking water is below 0.3 ppm
C. Breast milk or iron-fortified commercial formula is recommended for the first year of life
D. Solids can be introduced by about 6 months; the first food is often commercially prepared iron-fortified infant cereals; rice cereal is usually introduced first because of its low allergenic potential; infant cereals should be continued until 18 months of age
E. With the exception of infant cereals, the order of introducing other foods is variable; recommended sequence is weekly introduction of one food; fruits and vegetables, and then meats
F. First solid foods are strained, puréed, or mashed
G. Finger foods such as toast, teething cracker, or raw fruit are introduced at 6 to 7 months
H. Chopped table food or commercially prepared junior foods can be started by 9 to 12 months
I. Fruit juices should be offered as early as possible from a cup, to reduce development of nursing bottle caries
J. Method
 1. Feed when the baby is hungry, after a few sucks of breast milk or formula
 2. Introduce one food at a time, usually at intervals of 4 to 7 days, to allow for identification of food allergies
 3. Begin spoonfeeding by placing food on back of the tongue, because of the infant's natural tendency to thrust tongue forward
 4. Use a small spoon with straight handle; begin with 1 or 2 teaspoons of food; gradually increase to a couple of tablespoons per feeding

5. As the amount of solid food increases, milk needs to be decreased to approximately 900 ml (30 oz) daily to prevent overfeeding
6. Never introduce foods by mixing them with the formula in the bottle

K. Weaning
1. Giving up the bottle or breast for a cup is psychologically significant because it requires the relinquishing of a major source of pleasure
2. Usually, readiness develops during second half of the first year because of pleasure from receiving food by a spoon and desire for more freedom and control over body and the environment
3. Gradually replace one bottle at a time with a cup and finally end with the nighttime bottle
4. If breastfeeding must be terminated before 5 or 6 months of age, a bottle should be used to allow for continued sucking needs; after about 6 months wean directly to a cup

Immunizations

A. Types of immunizations
1. Diphtheria, pertussis, and tetanus (DTP)
   a. Tripedia diphtheria, tetanus, and attenuated pertussis (DTaP): given at 2, 4 and 6 months; boosters given at 15 months and 5 years of age
   b. Diphtheria toxoid: effective for about 10 years; febrile reaction more commonly seen in older children, so the adult type tetanus and diphtheria (Td) toxoid is recommended every 10 years after the last booster at 5 years of age; Td is also used for any children over the age of 7 who have not been previously immunized
   c. Tetanus toxoid: nearly 100% effective; induces immunity for about 10 years; given at 5-year intervals in the event of a possibly contaminated wound; tetanus is characterized by severe muscle spasms and is potentially fatal
   d. Pertussis vaccine; started early because no passive immunity from mother exists, as with diphtheria and tetanus; not given after seventh birthday because risk of disease is less than vaccine's side effects
2. Measles, mumps, and rubella vaccine (MMR)
   a. MMR vaccine (live attenuated vaccine): generally given at 12 months of age because of the presence of natural immunity from mother; a second dose should be administered at 4 to 6 years of age
   b. Not given to any unimmunized pregnant woman or if pregnancy is suspected because of potential infection of the fetus; pregnancy

must be prevented until 3 months after immunization to eliminate danger to fetus
   c. Rubella vaccine given to prevent occurrence of rubella (German measles; a disease with a maculopapular rash) in women during the first trimester of pregnancy; mumps vaccine is given because mumps (swelling of the parotid glands) may cause sterility in postpubescent males
   d. If respiratory symptoms, a fever, Koplik's spots on the buccal mucosa, or a skin rash on the trunk and extremities are present, measles cannot be prevented by the administration of MMR
3. Inactivated polio vaccine (IPV)
   a. Recommended for all children younger than 18 years of age
   b. Infants receive 3 doses (given at 2, 4 and 6 months); fourth dose given at 4 to 6 years of age
   c. Infants/children who are asymptomatic HIV positive or those with immune deficiencies and their siblings should receive inactivated polio vaccine (IPV)
4. *Haemophilus influenzae* type B vaccine (Hib)
   a. Polysaccharide vaccine given at 2, 4, 6, and 15 months of age (can be given sooner if child is in high-risk category; e.g., child who attends day-care center, is asplenic, or has sickle cell anemia)
   b. DTP can be given at same visit, but a different site should be used
5. Hepatitis-B vaccine (HEP-B)
   a. Infants receive 3 doses (given at birth to 1 month, 4 months, and 9 months); should be considered for all adolescents not immunized
   b. Must be given by IM injection; can be given at same time as DTP but separate sites must be used
6. Chickenpox vaccine (Varivax)
   a. Children under 12 receive 1 dose; teenagers and adults need 2 doses
   b. Vaccine is 70% to 90% effective in preventing chickenpox and its sequelae, such as encephalitis and thrombocytopenia

B. Factors influencing administration of immunizations
1. The benefit from being protected by the immunization is believed to greatly outweigh the risk from the disease
2. Presence of maternal antibodies
3. Administration of blood transfusion or immune serum globulin within 3 months
4. High fever, serious illness (common cold is not a contraindication)
5. Impaired immune system or immunosuppressive therapy in child or family member

6. Generalized malignancy such as leukemia
7. Neurologic problems such as convulsions after administration of pertussis vaccine
8. Allergic reaction to a previously administered vaccine or anaphylactic reaction to egg protein

Injury Prevention (Age-Related Specifics)

A. Accidents are one of the leading causes of death during infancy
   1. Mechanical suffocation causes most accidental deaths in children under 1 year of age
   2. Aspiration of small objects and ingestion of poisonous substances occur most often during second half of the first year and into early childhood
   3. Trauma from rolling off a bed or falling down stairs can occur at any time
B. Teaching is an essential aspect of prevention
   1. Birth to 4 months
      a. Sudden infant death: place infant to sleep on side or back; do not use soft, moldable bedding such as pillows and quilts
      b. Aspiration: not as great a danger to this age group but should begin practicing safeguards early (see 4 to 7 months); inform parents of dangers from baby powder and encourage its proper use and storage if used
      c. Suffocation
         (1) Keep plastic bags away; do not cover mattress or pillows with soft plastic
         (2) Use a firm mattress; do not use pillows and loose blankets
         (3) Make sure crib design follows regulations and mattress fits snugly
         (4) Keep crib away from other furniture and cords from window blinds
         (5) Do not tie pacifier on string around infant's neck; remove bibs after use
         (6) Drowning: never leave infant alone in bath
      d. Falls
         (1) Always raise crib rails; tie rails to crib if malfunctioning
         (2) Never leave infant on a raised, unguarded surface; when in doubt, use the floor
         (3) Restrain child in the infant seat and never leave unattended while the seat is resting on a raised surface
         (4) Avoid using a high chair until child is old enough to sit well
      e. Poisoning: not as great a danger to this age group but should begin practicing safeguards early (see 4 to 7 months)
      f. Burns
         (1) Check bath water and warmed formula and food

         (2) Do not pour hot liquids when infant is close by, such as sitting on lap
         (3) Keep cigarettes and their ashes away from infant
         (4) Do not leave in the sun for more than a few minutes; use hats and sunscreens
         (5) Wash flame-retardant clothes according to label directions
         (6) Check surface heat of car restraint; do not keep child in parked car
      g. Motor vehicles
         (1) Transport infant in a specially constructed rear-facing car seat with appropriate restraints; do not place infant on the seat or in the lap
         (2) Do not place a carriage or stroller behind a parked car
      h. Bodily damage: avoid sharp, jagged-edged objects; keep diaper pins closed and away from infant
   2. 4 to 7 months
      a. Aspiration
         (1) Keep buttons, beads, and other small objects out of infant's reach; keep floor free of small objects; inspect toys for removable parts
         (2) Use pacifier with one-piece construction and loop handle
         (3) Do not feed infant hard candy, nuts, food with pits or seeds, or whole hot dogs
         (4) Avoid balloons as playthings
      b. Suffocation: begin to teach swimming as part of water safety
      c. Falls: restrain in high chair; keep crib rails raised to full height
      d. Poisoning
         (1) Make sure that paint for furniture or toys does not contain lead
         (2) Place toxic substances on a high shelf and/or locked cabinet; do not store toxic substances in food containers; avoid storing large quantities of cleaning fluids, paints, pesticides, and other toxic substances; discard used containers of poisonous substances
         (3) Hang plants or place on a high surface rather than on floor
         (4) Know telephone number of local poison control center
      e. Burns
         (1) Always check bath water and adjust household hot-water temperature to 120° F (49° C) or lower
         (2) Place hot objects (cigarettes, candles, incense) on high surfaces

f. Motor vehicles: see birth to 4 months
g. Bodily damage: avoid long, pointed objects as toys; give toys that are smooth and rounded, made of wood or plastic

3. 8 to 12 months
a. Aspiration: see 4 to 7 months
b. Suffocation
   (1) Keep doors of bathrooms, ovens, dishwashers, refrigerators, and front-loading clothes washers and dryers closed at all times
   (2) If storing or discarding an appliance, such as a refrigerator, remove door
   (3) Fence swimming pools; always supervise when near any source of water, including toilets and cleaning buckets
c. Falls: fence stairways at top and bottom if child has access to either end
d. Poisoning
   (1) Administer medications as a drug, not as a candy
   (2) Do not administer adult medications unless prescribed by a physician
   (3) Replace caps to medications and poisons immediately after use; use child protector caps
e. Burns
   (1) Place guards in front of any heating appliance, fireplace, or furnace
   (2) Keep electrical wires hidden or out of reach; do not allow child to play with electrical appliances
   (3) Use plastic guards in electrical outlets; place furniture in front of outlets
   (4) Avoid use of overhanging tablecloths
f. Motor vehicles
   (1) Do not use adult seat or shoulder belt without infant car seat
   (2) Do not allow infant to crawl behind a parked car
   (3) If infant plays in a yard, have the yard fenced or use a playpen
g. Bodily damage
   (1) Do not allow infant to use a fork for self-feeding; use plastic cups or dishes
   (2) Check safety of toys and toy box
   (3) Protect from animals, especially dogs

HEALTH PROBLEMS FIRST NOTED DURING INFANCY

Hospitalization
A. Reactions to parental separation (begins later in infancy: refer to the Toddler)
B. Infant recognizes pain but is not emotionally traumatized by intrusive procedures
C. Procedures, such as urinary catheterization, that

may have a sexual connotation to older children usually are not emotionally traumatic for infants

▼ CHROMOSOMAL ABERRATIONS

General Nursing Care of Children with Chromosomal Aberrations
A. **ASSESSMENT**
   1. Presence of chromosomal abnormality
   2. Parental perceptions of child
   3. Child's health status; functional limitations; and presence of other congenital abnormalities such as cardiac malformation
B. **ANALYSIS/NURSING DIAGNOSES**
   1. Ineffective airway clearance related to nasal obstruction, excessive thick secretions, impaired musculature
   2. Risk for aspiration related to impaired swallowing, nasogastric tube feedings, impaired gag reflex
   3. Disturbed body image related to unrealistic self-expectations, sterility, and lack of pubertal changes (Turner's and Klinefelter's syndromes)
   4. Impaired verbal communication related to cognitive impairment
   5. Fear related to hospitalization
   6. Chronic low self-esteem related to unrealistic self-expectations, sterility, and lack of pubertal changes (Turner's and Klinefelter's syndromes)
   7. See Analysis/Nursing Diagnoses under Nursing Care of Children Who Are Cognitively Impaired
   8. See General Nursing Diagnoses for the Family of a Child with Special Needs
C. **PLANNING/IMPLEMENTATION**
   1. Provide emotional support to parents
   2. Encourage genetic counseling appropriate for type of problem
   3. Assist parents in setting realistic expectations and goals for the child
   4. Refer for careful testing of intellectual functioning for guidance to parents
   5. See Planning/Implementation under Nursing Care of Children Who Are Cognitively Impaired
D. **EVALUATION/OUTCOMES**
   1. Breathes without difficulty
   2. Communicates needs, feelings, and concerns
   3. Demonstrates behavior indicative of positive self-esteem

▼ TRISOMY 21 (DOWN SYNDROME)

Data Base
A. Types
   1. Trisomy 21: frequently associated with advanced

parental age (40 to 44 years of age—1%; over 45 years of age—2%); can occur in all age groups

2. Translocation 15/21: translocated chromosome transmitted most often by the mother, who is a carrier; age not a factor

3. Mosaicism: mixture of normal cells and cells that are trisomic for 21 (usually leads to a less severe phenotype)

B. Clinical findings

1. Small, rounded skull with a flat occiput; small nose with a depressed bridge (saddle nose)

2. Inner epicanthic folds and oblique palpebral fissures; speckling of the iris (Brushfield's spots)

3. Small, sometimes low-set, ears; short, thick neck

4. Protruding, sometimes fissured, tongue; respiratory problems

5. Hypotonic musculature (protruding abdomen, umbilical hernia); hyperflexible and lax joints

6. Broad, short, and stubby hands and feet; simian line (transverse crease on the palmar side of the hand)

7. Delayed or incomplete sexual development (men with Down syndrome usually are infertile)

Nursing Care of Children with Trisomy 21

A. Prevent infection, especially respiratory

B. Provide activity consistent with abilities and limits

C. Provide physical supervision and habilitation

D. See General Nursing Care of Children with Chromosomal Aberrations

▼ TRISOMY 18

Data Base

A. Types: trisomy; translocation; mosaicism

B. Clinical findings

1. Deformed and low-set ears; abnormal smallness of the jaws, especially the lower jaw (micrognathia); rocker-bottom feet; prominent occiput; webbed neck; short digits

2. Failure to thrive and short survival; if surviving, severe mental retardation

Nursing Care of Children with Trisomy 18

A. Because of short survival, prepare the parents for loss of their child

B. See General Nursing Care of Children with Chromosomal Aberrations

▼ TURNER'S SYNDROME (GONADAL DYSGENESIS)

Data Base

A. Chromosome monosomy (XO karyotype) in females

B. Clinical findings

1. Congenital malformations such as short stature, webbed neck, infantile genitalia, and developmental failure of secondary sex characteristics at puberty

2. Usually normal intelligence; problems in directional sense and space-form recognition

Nursing Care of Children with Turner's Syndrome

A. Prepare child for lack of pubertal changes and need for hormonal replacement

B. Counsel with emphasis on adoption rather than on the person's inability to conceive

C. See General Nursing Care of Children with Chromosomal Aberrations

▼ KLINEFELTER'S SYNDROME

Data Base

A. Sex-chromosomal abnormality of XXY in males

B. Clinical findings

1. Physical characteristics: tall; skinny; long legs and arms; small, firm testes; gynecomastia; and poorly developed secondary sex characteristics at puberty

2. Behavioral disorders and mental defects often present

Nursing Care of Children with Klinefelter's Syndrome

A. Counsel with emphasis on positive aspects such as adoption or donor insemination of mate

B. Recognize that emotional problems may require lifelong counseling

C. See General Nursing Care of Children with Chromosomal Aberrations

DEFECT CAUSED BY MATERNAL INGESTION OF ALCOHOL

▼ FETAL ALCOHOL SYNDROME

Data Base

A. Predictable abnormal patterns of fetal and neonatal morphogenesis attributed to severe, chronic alcoholism in women who continue to drink heavily during pregnancy; exact amount of alcohol needed to produce teratogenic effect is unknown

B. Leading cause of preventable mental retardation
   1. Occurs in approximately 2 per 1000 live births
   2. Women with a history of heavy drinking should be informed of risks
   3. Women who drink should be made aware of sources for treatment to decrease or eliminate alcohol ingestion
C. Clinical findings
   1. Diagnosis based on minimum criteria of signs in each of three categories: growth restriction, CNS malfunctions, and craniofacial features
   2. Growth: prenatal growth retardation, persistent postnatal growth lag
   3. Neurologic: includes mental retardation, motor retardation, microcephaly, hypotonia, hearing disorders
   4. Facial features: includes hypoplastic maxilla, micrognathia, hypoplastic philtrum, short palpebral features
   5. Behavior: includes irritability, sleeplessness, inconsolable crying, and feeding difficulties in infants; hyperactivity in children
   6. Gender: Two thirds of newborns affected with FAS are female
   7. Speech or language problems, learning disabilities, and behavioral problems evidenced in some children
D. Therapeutic interventions
   1. Pharmacologic management depending on the severity of central nervous system dysfunction and withdrawal symptoms
   2. Phenobarbital and diazepam for seizures
   3. Intravenous fluids and nutrients until able to maintain feedings
   4. Therapy specific to the individualized needs of infant; may be similar to needs of preterm infants

Nursing Care of Infants with Fetal Alcohol Syndrome

A. ASSESSMENT
   1. Mother's prenatal record indicating alcohol abuse
   2. Growth deficiencies
   3. Central nervous system adaptations associated with FAS
   4. Distinctive craniofacial characteristics related to FAS
   5. Behaviors related to withdrawal

B. ANALYSIS/NURSING DIAGNOSES
   1. Delayed growth and development related to effects of maternal substance abuse
   2. Disturbed sleep pattern related to withdrawal
   3. Imbalanced nutrition: less than body requirements related to difficulty feeding and vomiting
   4. Disorganized infant behavior related to effects of maternal substance abuse

   5. Risk for injury related to seizure activity
C. PLANNING/IMPLEMENTATION
   1. Monitor vital signs
   2. Maintain a protective environment
      a. Limit environmental stimuli; quiet, dimly lit room
      b. Monitor for seizure activity (withdrawal begins 6 to 12 hours after birth and persists for about 3 days); protect from injury during a seizure; seizures after the newborn period are rare
      c. Provide a warm physical environment
      d. Touch gently and avoid sudden postural changes
      e. Position on side
      f. Have suctioning equipment available to maintain patent airway
   3. Console infant
      a. Encourage parent to engage in "Kangaroo care"
      b. Use containment devices or swaddle with extremities in a flexed position
      c. Allow hand to mouth activity to promote self-soothing
      d. Provide opportunities for nonnutritive sucking with a pacifier
      e. Provide safe objects for infant to grasp
   4. Provide fluid and nutrients as ordered; breastfeeding is not contraindicated but excessive alcohol consumption may intoxicate the newborn and inhibit the let-down reflex
      a. Provide time for and patience during feedings
      b. Provide frequent, small feedings
      c. Burp infant often during the feedings
      d. Elevate head of mattress after feedings
      e. Monitor intake and output and weigh daily
   5. Reinforce positive parenting activities
D. EVALUATION/OUTCOMES
   1. Remains free from injury
   2. Exhibits resolution of withdrawal
   3. Demonstrates ingestion and retention of adequate nutrients
   4. Maintains or gains weight
   5. Parents demonstrate effective infant care

GASTROINTESTINAL MALFORMATIONS

▼ CLEFT LIP

Data Base
A. Failure of union of embryonic structure of face
   1. Fusion of maxillary and premaxillary processes
   2. Occurs between 5 and 8 weeks of fetal life
B. Cause unknown; evidence of hereditary influence

1. Incidence in general population is 1 in 800 births; more common in males
2. Multifactorial inheritance; increased frequency in relatives; higher incidence in monozygotic twins than in dizygotic twins

C. Classification
   1. Bilateral or unilateral; if unilateral, more common on the left side
   2. Can be of several degrees; complete cleft usually continuous with cleft palate

D. Clinical findings
   1. Difficulty feeding because infant cannot form a vacuum with the mouth to suck; may be able to breastfeed (breast may fill the cleft, making sucking easier)
   2. Mouth breathing results in: increased swallowed air, causing a distended abdomen and pressure against the diaphragm; mucous membranes of the oropharynx become dried and cracked with increased risk of infection

E. Therapeutic intervention: surgical repair; performed 6 to 12 weeks after birth; further modification may be necessary; multidisciplinary team approach used; aids infant's ability to suck; helps parents with the visible aspects of the defect

Nursing Care of Children with a Cleft Lip

A. ASSESSMENT
   1. Feeding behaviors; does infant consume adequate calories for growth without excessive energy expenditure
   2. Mucous membranes for dryness, signs of infection
   3. Parent/infant interaction and the effect of facial defect on bonding

B. ANALYSIS/NURSING DIAGNOSES
   1. Risk for disorganized infant behavior related to pain and discomfort and need to restrict sucking
   2. Imbalanced nutrition: less than body requirements related to feeding difficulties
   3. Risk for impaired parenting related to visible physical defect
   4. Disturbed sensory perception related to inability to suck

C. PLANNING/IMPLEMENTATION
   1. Preoperative nursing care
      a. Feed in an upright position with a soft large-holed nipple or rubber-tipped syringe or cleft lip or palate nurser
      b. Burp frequently because of swallowed air
      c. Prevent infection from irritation of the lip; restrain infant's arms, if needed
   2. Postoperative nursing care
      a. Maintain a patent airway because of edema and infant's habit of mouth breathing; keep

laryngoscope, endotracheal tube, and suction nearby
      b. Cleanse the suture line to prevent crust formation and eventual scarring
      c. Prevent crying, because of pressure on suture line; encourage a parent to stay
      d. Place the infant in supine position with arm or elbow restraints; change position to the side or sitting up to prevent hypostatic pneumonia; remove restraints only when supervised
      e. Feed (same as before surgery)
      f. Support the parents and accept the infant's appearance

D. EVALUATION/OUTCOMES
   1. Maintains integrity of suture line
   2. Experiences no trauma
   3. Experiences minimal or no pain
   4. Consumes adequate calories for growth and development
   5. Demonstrates ability to be comforted by means other than sucking
   6. Family members accept infant despite altered appearance

▼ CLEFT PALATE

Data Base

A. Failure of union of embryonic structure of face; fusion of palatal structures between 9 and 12 weeks; may involve the soft or hard palate and may extend into the nose, forming an oronasal passageway
B. Cause unknown; evidence of hereditary influence similar to cleft lip
C. More common in females
D. Clinical findings
   1. Infection, especially aspiration pneumonia
   2. Altered speech; palate is needed to trap air in the mouth
   3. Dental development; excessive dental caries; malocclusion from displacement of the maxillary arch
   4. Hearing problems caused by recurrent otitis media (eustachian tube connects the nasopharynx and middle ear and transports pathogens to ear)
E. Therapeutic interventions
   1. Speech appliance to help prevent guttural sounds if repair is delayed beyond speech development
   2. Surgical repair usually after the child has grown but before speech is well developed; between 12 and 18 months; tonsils usually not removed because they help to trap air
   3. Multidisciplinary-team approach, including speech therapist

Nursing Care of Children with a Cleft Palate

A. **ASSESSMENT**
1. Feeding behaviors; oral hygiene
2. Respiratory status
3. Hearing ability
4. Parent/child interaction

B. **ANALYSIS/NURSING DIAGNOSES**
1. Risk for disorganized infant behavior related to pain, discomfort, need to restrict sucking
2. Risk for impaired parenting related to having a child with a physical defect
3. Risk for infection related to possible aspiration, otitis media
4. Imbalanced nutrition: less than body requirements related to feeding difficulties
5. Impaired verbal communication related to altered oropharyngeal structures

C. **PLANNING/IMPLEMENTATION**
1. Preoperative nursing care: same as for infants with cleft lip except:
   a. Feed upright to prevent aspiration; gavage may be ordered
   b. Encourage early use of spoon and cup
   c. Teach parents the need for dental hygiene and regular dental supervision
2. Postoperative nursing care: same as for infants with cleft lip except:
   a. Avoid traumatizing the operative site; tell child who can follow directions not to rub tongue on roof of mouth; avoid the use of straw, spoon, toothbrush
   b. May be placed on abdomen immediately after surgery
   c. Provide liquid or blenderized diet
   d. Provide emotional support for parents; recovery is long and the prognosis uncertain
3. See Meeting the Needs of the Family of a Child with Special Needs

D. **EVALUATION/OUTCOMES**
1. Demonstrates ability to be comforted by means other than sucking
2. Maintains integrity of suture line
3. Experiences no trauma
4. Experiences minimal pain
5. Consumes adequate calories for growth and development
6. Family members accept infant despite altered appearance

▼ NASOPHARYNGEAL AND TRACHEOESOPHAGEAL ANOMALIES

Data Base

A. May be associated with low birth weight and other anomalies

B. Chalasia: an incompetent cardiac sphincter
C. Choanal atresia: a nasopharyngeal anomaly; the lack of an opening between one or both of the nasal passages and the nasopharynx
D. Tracheopharyngeal anomalies
1. Absence of the esophagus
2. Atresia of the esophagus without a tracheal fistula
3. Tracheoesophageal fistula
4. The most common type of anomaly is proximal esophageal atresia combined with distal tracheoesophageal fistula
E. Clinical findings
1. Excessive salivation and drooling
2. Choking, sneezing, and coughing during feeding, with regurgitation of formula through the mouth and nose
3. Inability to pass a catheter into the stomach
4. Abdominal distention
F. Therapeutic intervention: surgical repair, which can be done in one procedure or several, depending on infant's condition and severity of defect

Nursing Care of Children with Nasopharyngeal and Tracheoesophageal Anomalies

A. **ASSESSMENT**
1. Three Cs of tracheoesophageal fistula: coughing; choking; cyanosis
2. Signs of respiratory distress
3. Parent/infant interaction

B. **ANALYSIS/NURSING DIAGNOSES**
1. Risk for aspiration related to excessive secretions, regurgitation, incompetent cardiac sphincter
2. Impaired swallowing related to physical defect
3. Risk for disorganized infant behavior related to pain, difficulty breathing
4. Imbalanced nutrition: less than body requirements related to alteration in structure or function

C. **PLANNING/IMPLEMENTATION**
1. Preoperative nursing care
   a. Keep NPO; monitor intake and output; change position to prevent pneumonia
   b. Maintain in upright position
   c. Observe for signs of respiratory distress; suction oropharynx to remove accumulated secretions
2. Postoperative nursing care
   a. Maintain body temperature
   b. Maintain gastrostomy tube to drainage
   c. Change position to prevent pneumonia
   d. Perform proper care of chest tubes if used
   e. Maintain nutrition by oral, parenteral, or gastrostomy route
   f. Provide comfort and physical contact; provide a pacifier if oral feedings are contraindicated

D. EVALUATION/OUTCOMES
  1. Maintains patent airway
  2. Receives adequate calories for growth and development

▼ INTESTINAL OBSTRUCTION

Data Base

A. Congenital life-threatening obstruction of the intestines
  1. Mechanical: constricted or occluded lumen
  2. Muscular: interference with normal muscular contraction
B. Clinical findings
  1. Abdominal distention; paroxysmal pain
  2. Absence of stools, especially meconium in the newborn (meconium ileus)
  3. Vomiting of bile-stained material; may be projectile
  4. Weak, thready pulse; cyanosis; and weak, grunting respirations from abdominal distention, causing the diaphragm to compress the lungs
C. Therapeutic interventions
  1. Surgical repair: either by single-staged or multistaged procedures if defect is severe
  2. Prevention of pneumonia
  3. Supportive nutritional therapy

Nursing Care of Children with an Intestinal Obstruction

A. ASSESSMENT
  1. Abdomen for distention and visible peristaltic waves
  2. Absence of bowel movements
B. ANALYSIS/NURSING DIAGNOSES
  1. Risk for disorganized infant behavior related to pain, discomfort, need to restrict oral intake
  2. Constipation related to obstruction of intestinal lumen, decreased intestinal peristalsis
  3. Risk for deficient fluid volume related to fluid shifts
C. PLANNING/IMPLEMENTATION
  1. Preoperative nursing care
    a. Keep NPO; provide a pacifier; observe for signs of dehydration and shock
    b. Maintain nasogastric suction; monitor intake and output
  2. Postoperative nursing care: depends on type of surgery performed
    a. Keep operative sites clean and dry, especially after passage of stool
    b. Position on side rather than abdomen to prevent pulling legs up under chest

  c. Care of colostomy: prevent excoriation of skin by frequent cleansing and use of a diaper held on by a belly binder
  d. Instruct the parents about colostomy care (include avoidance of tight diapers and clothes around the abdomen)
D. EVALUATION/OUTCOMES
  1. Establishes a regular pattern of bowel elimination
  2. Maintains fluid and electrolyte balance
  3. Rests comfortably

▼ ANORECTAL ANOMALIES (IMPERFORATE ANUS)

Data Base

A. Failure of the membrane separating the rectum from the anus to absorb during eighth week of fetal life; fistulas within the vagina, urinary tract, or scrotum are common; most frequent intestinal anomaly
B. Low anomalies: puborectalis muscle, internal and external sphincter present and well developed with normal function
C. Intermediate anomalies: rectum at or below puborectalis muscle; rectal opening anterior in perineum; may be persistent opening to genitourinary tract
D. High anomalies: rectum ends above puborectalis muscle; absence of internal and external sphincters
E. Clinical findings: failure to pass meconium stool; abdominal distention
F. Therapeutic interventions: immediate surgical correction unless fistula is present; possible colostomy with multistaged surgical repair

Nursing Care of Children with Anorectal Anomalies

A. ASSESSMENT
  1. Rectum for opening, passage of meconium
  2. Abdomen for distention
B. ANALYSIS/NURSING DIAGNOSES
  1. Risk for disorganized infant behavior related to discomfort, need to restrict oral intake
  2. Constipation related to obstruction of intestinal lumen
  3. Compromised family coping related to lack of knowledge about colostomy care
C. PLANNING/IMPLEMENTATION
  See Planning/Implementation under Intestinal Obstruction
D. EVALUATION/OUTCOMES
  1. Rests comfortably
  2. Achieves pattern of regular bowel elimination
  3. Family demonstrates ability to care for child

▼ HYPERTROPHIC PYLORIC STENOSIS (HPS)

Data Base

A. Congenital hypertrophy of muscular tissue of the pyloric sphincter; usually presents 1 to 10 weeks after birth
   1. Grossly enlarged circular muscle of pylorus
   2. Narrowed opening between stomach and duodenum
   3. Inflammation and edema can result in total obstruction
B. Five times more common in males than females
C. Clinical findings
   1. Vomiting, progressively projectile; non–bile-stained vomitus
   2. Leads to complete obstruction within 4 to 6 weeks
   3. Constipation; distention of the epigastrium
   4. Visible peristalsis; palpable olive-shaped mass in the right upper quadrant
   5. Dehydration and weight loss
D. Therapeutic intervention: surgical repair

Nursing Care of Children with Pyloric Stenosis

A. ASSESSMENT
   1. Feeding history and type of vomiting; failure to gain weight
   2. Upper abdomen for distention and the epigastrium just to the right of umbilicus for a palpable olive-shaped mass
   3. Visible peristaltic waves; no evidence of pain or discomfort

B. ANALYSIS/NURSING DIAGNOSES
   1. Imbalanced nutrition: less than body requirements related to vomiting
   2. Deficient fluid volume related to vomiting
   3. Acute pain related to surgical incision

C. PLANNING/IMPLEMENTATION
   1. Preoperative nursing care: keep NPO; monitor intake and output; monitor for signs of dehydration
   2. Postoperative nursing care is the same as for any abdominal surgery
   3. Teach parents the specific feeding method
      a. Give small, frequent feedings and feed slowly
      b. Hold the infant in a high-Fowler's position during feeding and place on the right side after feeding with head of bed slightly elevated
      c. Bubble frequently during feeding and avoid handling afterward

D. EVALUATION/OUTCOMES
   1. Maintains fluid and electrolyte balance
   2. Rests comfortably
   3. Consumes adequate calories for growth and development

▼ MEGACOLON (HIRSCHSPRUNG'S DISEASE)

Data Base

A. Absence of parasympathetic ganglion cells in a portion of the bowel, which causes enlargement of the bowel proximal to the defect
   1. Length of involved bowel varies from only internal sphincter to entire colon
   2. Rectosigmoid colon the most commonly affected site
B. Four times more common in males than females
C. Clinical findings
   1. Symptoms may occur gradually
   2. Constipation or passage of ribbonlike or pellet-like, foul-smelling stool; intestinal obstruction
   3. Refusal of food; vomiting; abdominal distention
D. Therapeutic intervention
   1. Regimen of enemas
   2. Surgical intervention usually in 2 stages; removal of aganglionic portion of the bowel and a temporary colostomy followed later by anastomosis

Nursing Care of Children with Megacolon

A. ASSESSMENT
   1. Elimination history; characteristics of stools; onset of constipation
   2. Abdomen for distention
   3. Nutrition and hydration status; poor feeding
   4. Behavior for fussiness; irritability

B. ANALYSIS/NURSING DIAGNOSES
   1. Constipation related to defective bowel motility
   2. Acute pain related to trauma of surgery
   3. Compromised family coping related to lack of knowledge about procedures for enema, colostomy care

C. PLANNING/IMPLEMENTATION
   1. Teach parents the correct procedure for enemas if indicated; use only isotonic solutions; point out danger of water intoxication
   2. Use the following suggested amounts of fluid for enemas:

Age	Amount (ml)
Infant	120 to 240
2 to 4 years	240 to 360
4 to 10 years	360 to 480
11 years	480 to 720

   3. Postoperative nursing care depends on type of surgery performed (see Planning/Implementation under Intestinal Obstruction)

D. EVALUATION/OUTCOMES
   1. Rests comfortably
   2. Achieves pattern of regular bowel evacuation
   3. Family demonstrates ability to care for child

CARDIAC MALFORMATIONS

Data Base

A. Circulatory changes that occur at or shortly after birth are disrupted including: the rapid increase in pulmonary circulation and the closure of the foramen ovale, ductus arteriosus, and ductus venosus resulting from decreased oxygen concentration
B. Classification of cardiac defects
   1. Defects with increased pulmonary blood flow
      a. Intracardiac communication along the septum or between the great arteries allows blood to flow from high pressure left side to lower pressure right side
      b. Increased blood pressure on right side of heart increases pulmonary flow and decreases systemic circulation
      c. Children have signs and symptoms of heart failure
      d. Atrial and ventricular septal defects and patent ductus arteriosus are examples
   2. Defects with decreased pulmonary blood flow
      a. An obstruction of pulmonary blood flow exists and an anatomic defect (atrial septal defect or ventricular septal defect) between the right and left side of the heart
      b. Blood cannot exit the right side of the heart because of the obstruction that raises the pressure on the right side of the heart, exceeding the pressure on the left
      c. Desaturated, oxygen-poor blood shunts from right to left causing desaturation in the left side of the heart and systemic circulation
      d. Children are hypoxemic and appear cyanotic
      e. Tetralogy of Fallot, transposition of great vessels, truncus arteriosus, and tricuspid atresia are examples
   3. Obstructive defects
      a. Blood exiting the heart meets an area of anatomic narrowing or stenosis causing an obstruction to blood flow
      b. The pressure in the ventricle and the great artery before the obstruction is increased
      c. The pressure beyond the obstruction is decreased
      d. Usually located near a valve
      e. There is an increased pressure load on the ventricle and decreased cardiac output. Children with significant obstruction exhibit signs of HF
      f. Coarctation of the aorta, aortic stenosis, and pulmonic stenosis are examples

C. General clinical findings
   1. Dypsnea, especially on exertion
   2. Feeding difficulty and failure to thrive, often first signs noted by the parent
   3. Stridor or choking spells
   4. Heart rate over 200, respiratory rate about 60 in the infant
   5. Recurrent respiratory tract infections
   6. In the older child, poor physical development, delayed milestones, and decreased exercise tolerance
   7. Cyanosis and clubbing of fingers and toes
   8. Squatting or knee-chest position is assumed because it decreases venous return by constricting the femoral veins
   9. Heart murmurs
   10. Excessive perspiration
   11. Signs of heart failure
      a. Tachycardia and hypotension progressing to extreme pallor or duskiness
      b. Tachypnea, dyspnea, and costal retractions progressing to grunting respirations
      c. Weight gain, ascites, and pleural effusions progressing to peripheral edema
D. General therapeutic interventions
   1. Surgical intervention
   2. Pharmacologic approach: cardiac glycosides to increase the efficiency of heart action
      a. Positive inotropic effect is achieved by increasing the permeability of muscle membranes to the calcium and sodium ions required for contraction of muscle fibrils
         (1) Forceful contraction during systole improves peripheral tissue perfusion
         (2) Chamber emptying allows additional venous blood to enter the cardiac chambers during diastole
      b. Negative chronotropic effect is achieved through an action mediated by the vagus nerve that slows firing of the sinoatrial (SA) node and impulse transmission through the atrioventricular (AV) node
      c. Drug preparations have the same qualitative effect on heart action but differ in potency, rate of absorption, amount absorbed, onset of action, and speed of elimination
         (1) Digitalis: longer onset, peak action, and half-life
         (2) Digoxin (Lanoxin): rapid onset and peak action and short half-life; drug of choice in children, especially because the risk of toxicity is lessened by the shorter half-life
      d. Digitalization
         (1) Provides an initial loading dose for acute effect on the enlarged heart

(2) After desired effect is achieved, the dosage is lowered to maintenance level, replacing the drug metabolized and excreted each day

e. Adverse effects

(1) Most frequent: nausea, vomiting, headache, drowsiness, insomnia, vertigo, confusion; all attributable to drug action at central nervous system (CNS) sites; oral forms also cause nausea and vomiting by irritation of the gastric mucosa

(2) Bradycardia attributable to drug-induced slowing of SA node firing

(3) Dysrhythmias are first evidence of toxicity in one third of clients; premature nodal or ventricular impulses; varying degrees of heart block caused by drug action that slows transmission of impulses through the AV node

(4) Xanthopsia (yellow vision) caused by drug effect on the visual cones

(5) Gynecomastia (mammary enlargement) in males resulting from the estrogen-like steroid portion of digitalis glycosides

f. Considerations during therapy

(1) Premature contractions elevate the audible apical rate and mask the pacemaker conduction rate; apical pulse is taken before administration and drug is withheld when pulse rate drops to 110 to 90 in infants and below 70 in older children

(2) Immaturity of hepatic and renal systems in premature and newborn infants or depressed hepatic or renal function in children may result in cumulation

(3) Because potassium ions are required for interaction of digitalis glycosides with sodium-potassium–dependent membranes, the lowering of serum potassium ions may foster digitalis toxicity

(4) Because calcium ions act synergistically with digitalis on myocardial membranes, an elevation of serum calcium ion levels may increase sensitivity of cardiac muscle to digitalis action

g. Drug interactions

(1) Phenobarbital, phenytoin, and phenylbutazone accelerate metabolism of digitalis glycosides by induction of hepatic microsomal enzymes; serum levels are lower when drugs are used concomitantly

(2) Diuretics that cause hypokalemia may contribute to the incidence of serious dysrhythmias when administered concurrently with digitalis glycosides; sup-

plemental potassium may be used for replacement of losses, or potassium-sparing diuretics may be prescribed to prevent potassium ion losses

h. Prophylactic antibiotic therapy may be necessary before invasive procedures and surgery; may be necessary throughout life

▼ DEFECTS WITH INCREASED PULMONARY BLOOD FLOW

Ventricular Septal Defect (VSD)

A. Abnormal opening between the two ventricles

B. Severity of the defect depends on size of the opening

C. Higher pressure in the right ventricle causes hypertrophy, with development of pulmonary hypertension

D. Low, harsh murmur heard throughout systole

E. Specific therapeutic intervention: closure of the opening at the septum

F. Prognosis: a single membranous defect has less than a 5% mortality rate; multiple muscular defects can have a mortality risk of 20%

Atrial Septal Defect (ASD)

A. Types

1. Ostium primum defect (ASD1): opening at lower end of septum; may be associated with mitral valve abnormalities

2. Ostium secundum defect (ASD2): opening is near the center of the septum

3. Sinus venosus defect, in which the superior portion of the atrial septum fails to form near the junction of the atrial wall with the superior vena cava

B. Murmur heard high on the chest, with fixed splitting of the second heart sound

C. Specific therapeutic intervention: closure of the opening at the septum

D. Prognosis: this defect has less than a 1% operative mortality

Patent Ductus Arteriosus (PDA)

A. Failure of the fetal connection between the aorta and pulmonary artery to close

B. Blood shunted from the aorta back to the pulmonary artery; may progress to pulmonary hypertension and cardiomegaly

C. Machinery-type murmur heard throughout the heartbeat in the left second or third interspace

D. Specific therapeutic intervention: closure of the opening between the aorta and the pulmonary artery; in critically ill newborns, pharmacologic closure may be attempted with a prostaglandin inhibitor (e.g., indomethacin)

E. Prognosis: this defect has less than a 1% mortality

▼ DEFECTS WITH DECREASED PULMONARY BLOOD FLOW

Tetralogy of Fallot

A. Four associated defects
   1. Pulmonary valve stenosis
   2. Ventricular septal defect, usually high on the septum
   3. Overriding aorta, receiving blood from both ventricles, or an aorta arising from the right ventricle
   4. Right ventricular hypertrophy
B. Specific therapeutic interventions
   1. Palliative treatment: surgery performed to increase pulmonary blood flow; anastomosis of subclavian and pulmonary artery (Blalock-Taussig procedure)
   2. Complete repair: closure of the ventricular septal defect and resection of the infundibular stenosis, possibly with a pericardial patch to enlarge the right ventricular outflow tract
C. Prognosis: this defect has less than a 5% surgical repair mortality

Transposition of the Great Vessels

A. Aorta exits from the right ventricle and pulmonary artery leaves the left ventricle
B. Incompatible with life unless there is a communication between the two sides of the heart, such as an atrial septal defect, ventricular septal defect, or patent ductus arteriosus
C. Specific therapeutic interventions
   1. Palliative procedures performed to prevent pulmonary vascular resistance and heart failure until child is able to tolerate complete repair
      a. Rashkind procedure: enlargement of an existing atrial septal defect by pulling a balloon through the defect (balloon septostomy) during a cardiac catheterization
      b. Pulmonary artery banding if a ventricular septal defect is present to decrease blood flow to the lungs and increase shunting of oxygenated blood intraventricularly to the aorta
      c. Pharmacologic dilation of patent ductus arteriosus with use of prostaglandins (e.g., Prostin VR)
      d. Blalock-Hanlon operation: surgical creation of an atrial septal defect
   2. Complete repair
      a. Rastelli's procedure: closure of ventricular septal defect (VSD) (directing left ventricular blood through VSD into aorta, pulmonic valve closed and conduit made from right ventricle to pulmonary artery) results in physiologic normal circulation but requires revision as child grows; procedure of choice for infants with transposition of the great vessels, VSD, and severe pulmonic stenosis
      b. Mustard or Senning procedure: removing the entire atrial septum and creating a new atrial septum from existing pericardium or a prosthesis that tunnels or baffles blood for more effective oxygenation, with creation of two new functionally correct atrial chambers
      c. Jatene operation: transposing the great vessels to their correct anatomic placement with reimplantation of the coronary arteries
D. Prognosis: this defect has a 5% to 10% surgical mortality

Tricuspid Atresia

A. Absence of the tricuspid valve
B. Incompatible with life unless there is a communication between the right and left sides of the heart, such as atrial septal defect, ventricular septal defect, or patent ductus arteriosus
C. Specific therapeutic interventions
   1. Palliative treatment procedures: same as for tetralogy of Fallot
   2. Complete repair: modified Fontan procedure—conversion of the right atrium into an outlet for the pulmonary artery, which involves placing a tubular conduit with a valve between the two and closing the atrial septal defect; physiologically corrects tricuspid atresia by preventing any mixing of systemic blood in the left atrium and shunting the entire venous blood to the lungs for oxygenation
D. Prognosis: this defect has a surgical mortality greater than 10%

Truncus Arteriosus

A. Single great vessel arising from the base of the heart, serving as a pulmonary artery and aorta
B. Systolic murmur is heard, and a single semilunar valve produces a loud second heart sound that is not split
C. Specific therapeutic intervention:
   Complete repair: Rastelli's operation: excising pulmonary arteries from aorta and attaching them to the right ventricle by means of a prosthetic valve conduit; septal defects also repaired
D. Prognosis: this defect requires complex repair and has a mortality of 10%

▼ OBSTRUCTIVE DEFECTS

Pulmonary Stenosis

A. Narrowing of the pulmonary valve
B. Causes decreased blood flow to lungs and increased pressure to right ventricle

C. Specific therapeutic intervention: valvotomy or balloon angioplasty

D. Prognosis: this defect has less than a 2% mortality

Aortic Stenosis

A. Narrowing of the aortic valve

B. Causes increased workload on the left ventricle, and the lowered pressure in the aorta reduces coronary artery flow

C. Specific therapeutic intervention: division of the stenotic valves of the aorta

D. Prognosis: this defect has a significant (greater than 20%) mortality in critically ill newborns; older children have a lower mortality risk

Coarctation of the Aorta

A. Localized narrowing of aorta near the insertion of the ductus arteriosus

B. Increased systemic circulation above the stricture: bounding radial and carotid pulses, headache, dizziness, epistaxis

C. Decreased systemic circulation below the stricture: absent femoral pulses, cool lower extremities

D. Increased pressure in aorta above the defect causes left ventricular hypertrophy

E. Murmur may or may not be heard

F. Specific therapeutic intervention: angioplasty; resection of the defect and anastomosis of ends of the aorta

G. Prognosis: this defect has less than a 5% mortality in children with isolated coarctation

General Nursing Care of Children with Cardiac Malformations

A. **ASSESSMENT**
1. Color: cyanosis, pallor
2. Apical pulse, peripheral pulses, presence of murmurs
3. Respirations, dyspnea, frequency of colds
4. Blood pressure
5. Chest abnormalities

B. **ANALYSIS/NURSING DIAGNOSES**
1. Activity intolerance related to imbalance between oxygen supply and demand
2. Risk for disorganized infant behavior related to pain and discomfort
3. Disturbed body image related to having a physical defect
4. Risk for caregiver role strain related to caring for ill child
5. Decreased cardiac output related to structural defect
6. Interrupted family processes related to having a child with a heart condition
7. Delayed growth and development related to inadequate oxygen and nutrients to tissues and limited socialization with peers
8. Risk for infection related to debilitated physical status
9. Risk for injury (complications) related to cardiac condition and therapies
10. Social isolation related to inability to participate in active play

C. **PLANNING/IMPLEMENTATION**
1. Correctly calculate the dosage of digoxin; usually prescribed in micrograms (1000 µg = 1 mg)
2. Take apical pulse before administering the drug; withhold if below age norm
3. Observe for signs of digitalis toxicity
4. Teach the parents home administration of digoxin
   a. Give digoxin at regular intervals, usually every 12 hours
   b. Plan the times so that drug is given 1 hour before or 2 hours after feedings
   c. Use a calendar to mark off each dose that is given or post a reminder, such as a sign on the refrigerator
   d. Have the prescription refilled before the medication is completely used
   e. Administer the drug carefully by slowly squirting it in the side and back of the mouth
   f. Do not mix it with other foods or fluids because refusal to consume these results in inaccurate intake of the drug
   g. If the child has teeth, give water after administering the drug; whenever possible, brush the teeth to prevent tooth decay from the sweetened liquid
   h. If a dose is missed and more than 4 hours has elapsed, withhold the dose and give the next dose at the regular time; if less than 4 hours has elapsed, give the missed dose
   i. If child vomits within 15 minutes of receiving the digoxin, repeat the dose once; if more than 15 minutes has elapsed, do not give a second dose
   j. If more than two consecutive doses have been missed, notify the practitioner
   k. Do not increase or double the dose for missed doses
   l. If the child becomes ill, notify the practitioner immediately
   m. Keep digoxin in a safe place, preferably a locked cabinet
   n. In case of accidental overdose of digoxin, call the nearest poison control center immediately
5. Help the parents cope with symptoms of the disease

a. During dyspenic/cyanotic spell, place the child in a side-lying knee-chest position, with the head and chest elevated

b. Keep the child warm; encourage rest and sleep

c. Decrease the child's anxiety by remaining calm

d. Feed the child slowly; allow frequent burping; gavage feedings may be ordered

e. Administer small, frequent meals

f. Introduce solids and spoonfeeding early

g. Encourage the anorexic child to eat

h. Encourage parents to include others in child's care to prevent exhaustion

6. Foster growth-promoting family relationships

a. Encourage family members to discuss their feelings about each other and the child's defect

b. Maintain expectations from all siblings as equally as possible

c. Provide consistent discipline, especially from infancy, to prevent behavioral problems

d. Encourage acceptable pursuits for the child

e. Discuss school entry with the teacher and school nurse

f. Guide parents to the eventual hazards of fostering overdependency

g. Help the parents feel adequate in their maternal-paternal roles by emphasizing growth and developmental progress of the child

h. Help the parents foster the child's development by stimulating the child to age-appropriate goals consistent with the child's activity tolerance

i. Provide social experiences for the child

7. Preoperative assessment areas necessary for planning postoperative care

a. Keep a sleep record so care can be organized around the child's usual rest pattern

b. Avoid constipation and straining after surgery: assess the child's elimination pattern; know words the child uses; have the child practice using a bedpan

c. Record the level of activity and list favorite toys or games that require gradually increased exertion

d. Determine the child's fluid preferences for postoperative maintenance

e. When recording vital signs, always indicate the child's activity at the time of measurement

f. Observe the child's verbal and nonverbal responses to pain

8. Prepare the child physically and emotionally for surgery

a. Main assessment factor in preparation of the child is the developmental and chronologic age

(1) Explanation of the heart differs according to age of the child

(2) Children 4 to 6 years of age know that the heart is in the chest, describe it as valentine shaped, and characterize its function by the sound of "tick tock"

(3) Children 7 to 10 years of age do not see the heart as valentine shaped, know it has veins, have an idea of its function (e.g., "It makes you live"), but do not understand the concept of pumping

(4) Children over 10 years of age have a concept of veins, valves, circulation, and why death occurs when the heart stops

b. Preparation is based on the principle that fear of the unknown increases anxiety

c. The same nurse should participate in preoperative and postoperative preparation as a source of support for the child and parents

d. Nurses must know what equipment is usual after open or closed heart surgery

e. Let the child play with equipment such as stethoscope, blood pressure machine, oxygen mask, suction, and syringes

f. For the young child, especially the preschooler, use dolls and puppets to describe procedures

g. Preparation for cardiac catheterization before surgery is essential as well

h. For the young child, talk about the size of the bandage; for the older child, discuss the actual incision

i. Familiarize the child with the postoperative environment, such as the postanesthesia unit and intensive care unit, stressing the strange noises

j. Have the child practice coughing and breathing with an incentive spirometer

k. Explain to the child why coughing and moving are necessary even though they may be uncomfortable

l. Explain to the child what tubes may be used and what they will look like

9. Specifics of postoperative care are similar to those for any major surgery

10. Help the child and family adjust to correction of the cardiac defect

a. Improved physical status is often difficult for the child who has become accustomed to the sick role and its secondary gains

b. Improved physical status of the child is also difficult for the parents, because it reduces child's dependency

c. The child may have difficulty learning to relate to peers and siblings on a competitive basis

d. The child can no longer use the disability as a crutch for educational and social short-comings

e. Parental expectations must be adjusted to accommodate the child's new physical vigor and search for independence

D. EVALUATION/OUTCOMES

1. Chooses and participates in appropriate activities for age, energy, and developmental levels
2. Consumes sufficient nutrients for growth and development
3. Family and child discuss fears and feelings about disorder and limitations
4. Family demonstrates home care for child

NEUROLOGIC MALFORMATIONS

▼ SPINA BIFIDA

Data Base

A. Malformation of the spine in which the posterior portion of the laminae of the vertebrae fails to close; most common site is the lumbosacral area

B. Associated defects include weakness or paralysis below the defect, bowel and bladder dysfunction, clubfeet, dislocated hip, and hydrocephalus

C. Arnold-Chiari syndrome: defect of the occipitocervical region with swelling and displacement of the medulla into the spinal cord

D. Classifications

1. Spina bifida occulta: defect only of the vertebrae; spinal cord and meninges are intact
2. Spina bifida cystica
   a. Meningocele: meninges, but no neural elements, protrude through the defect; spinal fluid exits through the defect
   b. Meningomyelocele: meninges and spinal nerves protrude through the defect; spinal fluid exits through the defect; the most serious type

E. Clinical findings

1. Degree of neurologic dysfunction directly related to level of defect
2. Defective nerve supply to bladder affects sphincter and muscle tone
3. Frequently poor anal sphincter control

F. Therapeutic management

1. Multidisciplinary approach including rehabilitation
2. Surgical repair of the sac to maintain neurologic function and prevent infection

Nursing Care of Children with Spina Bifida

A. ASSESSMENT

1. Condition of the myelomeningocele sac
2. Level of neurologic involvement
3. Neurologic impairment of elimination
4. Head circumference and fontanels at least daily

B. ANALYSIS/NURSING DIAGNOSES

1. Interrupted family processes related to the birth of a child with a physical defect
2. Risk for infection related to exposed myelomeningocele sac
3. Risk for impaired skin integrity related to paralysis, incontinence
4. Risk for trauma related to spinal cord lesion

C. PLANNING/IMPLEMENTATION

1. Protect against infection because breakdown of the sac leaves the spinal cord open to the environment
   a. Keep area clean from urine and feces
   b. Apply a sterile, moist, nonadherent dressing over the sac to keep it from drying; diapers are not used
   c. Change dressing every 2 to 4 hours; inspect sac for leaks, abrasions, irritation, or signs of infection
   d. Avoid pressure on sac
2. Maintain function through proper position: place in prone position, hips slightly flexed and abducted, feet hanging free of mattress, and a slight Trendelenburg slope to reduce spinal fluid pressure
3. Because of restriction in position, feed child in prone position; establish eye contact and encourage parents to visit and feed the child
4. Foster elimination in the infant with a neurogenic bladder:
   a. Use the Credé method or slight pressure against the abdomen for complete emptying of the bladder; may need intermittent straight catheterization
   b. While the infant is prone, apply pressure to the abdomen above symphysis pubis with the sides of the fingers and counterpressure with the thumbs against the buttocks
5. Postoperative nursing care
   a. Measure head size to determine whether hydrocephalus is developing
   b. Monitor for signs of increased intracranial pressure

D. EVALUATION/OUTCOMES

1. Remains free of infection
2. Maintains intact meningeal sac
3. Maintains skin integrity
4. Family demonstrates ability to care for child

▼ HYDROCEPHALUS

Data Base

A. Abnormal accumulation of cerebrospinal fluid within the ventricular system
B. Classifications
   1. Noncommunicating: obstruction within the ventricles such as congenital malformation, neoplasm, or hematoma
   2. Communicating: inadequate absorption of cerebrospinal fluid (CSF) resulting from infection, trauma, or obstruction by thick arachnoid membrane or meninges
C. Clinical findings
   1. Increasing head size in the infant because of open sutures and bulging fontanels
   2. Prominent scalp veins and taut, shiny skin
   3. "Sunset" eyes (sclera visible above iris), bulging eyes, and papilledema of retina
   4. Head lag, especially important after 4 to 6 months
   5. Increased intracranial pressure: projectile vomiting not associated with feeding, irritability, anorexia, high shrill cry, seizures
   6. Damage to the brain because increased pressure decreases blood flow to the cells, causing necrosis
D. Therapeutic interventions
   1. Relief of hydrocephalus
      a. Removal of the obstruction if that is the cause
      b. Mechanical shunting of fluid to another area of the body–ventricular peritoneal shunt: catheter passed subcutaneously to the peritoneal cavity; revised as necessary
   2. Treatment of complications
   3. Management of problems that cause psychomotor problems

Nursing Care of Children with Hydrocephalus

A. **ASSESSMENT**
   1. Head circumference/fontanels
   2. Signs of increased intracranial pressure
B. **ANALYSIS/NURSING DIAGNOSES**
   1. Interrupted family process related to having a seriously ill child
   2. Risk for infection related to shunt
   3. Risk for injury related to increased intracranial pressure
   4. Risk for impaired skin integrity related to immobility
C. **PLANNING/IMPLEMENTATION**
   1. Prevent breakdown of scalp, infection, and damage to spinal cord
      a. Place the infant in a Fowler's position to facilitate draining of fluid; infant should be positioned flat postoperatively with no pressure on shunted side
      b. Support the neck and head when holding the infant
      c. Observe shunt site (abdominal site in peritoneal procedure) for infection
   2. Monitor for increasing intracranial pressure
      a. Monitor neurologic signs
      b. Measure head circumference
      c. Control pain with acetaminophen with or without codeine for mild to moderate pain and opioids for severe pain
      d. Check the valve frequently for patency
   3. Promote adequate nutrition
      a. Monitor for vomiting, irritability, lethargy, and anorexia because these will decrease the intake of nutrients
      b. Perform all care before feeding to prevent vomiting; hold infant if possible
      c. Observe for signs of dehydration
   4. Keep eyes moist and free of irritation if eyelids incompletely cover corneas
   5. Postoperative: place the infant or child on bed rest after surgery, with minimal handling to prevent damage to shunt
   6. Support parents because continued shunt revisions are necessary as growth occurs and they are usually very concerned about developmental delays; teach parents how to observe and record developmental milestones
   7. Teach parents: to pump the shunt, if indicated to maintain patency; signs of increasing intracranial pressure, infection, and dehydration
D. **EVALUATION/OUTCOMES**
   1. Remains free of signs of increased intracranial pressure
   2. Remains free from infection
   3. Maintains skin integrity
   4. Family demonstrates ability to care for child

GENITOURINARY MALFORMATIONS

▼ EXSTROPHY OF THE BLADDER

Data Base

A. Absence of portion of abdominal wall and bladder wall, causing the bladder to appear to be turned inside out and outside the abdominal cavity
B. May be accompanied by defects such as pubic bone malformations, inguinal hernia, epispadias, undescended testes, or short penis in boys and a cleft clitoris or absent vagina in girls
C. Occurs three times more frequently in males than females
D. Clinical findings
   1. Bladder is exposed and appears to be turned inside out

2. Constant seepage of urine leading to skin breakdown and infection
3. Progressive renal failure may result from infection and obstruction

E. Therapeutic interventions
1. Plastic surgery
2. Closure of the bladder within 48 hours if possible; final repair attempted before school age
3. Ileal conduit (also called ureteroileal cutaneous ureterostomy); the child wears an ileostomy appliance over the stoma, which collects the continuously flowing urine
4. Cutaneous ureterostomy: the ureters are attached directly to the abdominal wall, usually at a site proximal to the level of the kidneys; two collecting appliances are worn over the bilateral openings

Nursing Care of Children with Exstrophy of Bladder

A. **ASSESSMENT**
1. Condition of skin
2. Renal function; urine output
3. Parental interaction with child

B. **ANALYSIS/NURSING DIAGNOSES**
1. Interrupted family processes related to loss of image of ideal child
2. Risk for infection related to structural alterations
3. Risk for impaired skin integrity related to presence of urine

C. **PLANNING/IMPLEMENTATION**
1. Help the parents to accept the disorder and the long-term sequelae
2. Scrupulously clean the area around the bladder and apply sterile petrolatum gauze
3. Use loose clothing to avoid pressure over the area
4. Change clothing frequently because of odor
5. Care for the urine-collecting appliance; change frequently

D. **EVALUATION/OUTCOMES**
1. Maintains skin integrity
2. Remains free from infection
3. Maintains renal function within acceptable limits
4. Family demonstrates ability to care for child

▼ DISPLACED URETHRAL OPENINGS

Data Base

A. Urethral opening is abnormally located
B. In males severity varies, depending on distance from the tip of the penis and involvement of additional penile deformities

C. Classification
1. Hypospadias
   a. In males the urethra opens on the lower surface of the penis from just behind the glans to the perineum (placement varies)
   b. In females the urethra opens into the vagina
2. Epispadias
   a. Occurs only in males
   b. Urethra opens on dorsal surface of the penis; often associated with exstrophy of the bladder
3. Defect can be a sign of ambiguous genitalia

D. Clinical findings
1. Procreation may be interfered with in severe cases
2. Increased risk of urinary tract infection

E. Therapeutic interventions
1. Circumcision, if desired, is delayed until surgical repair of the defect
2. Surgical repair of the detect
3. Surgical repair may be performed in several stages

Nursing Care of Children with a Displaced Urethral Opening

A. **ASSESSMENT**
1. Parental knowledge of defect
2. Origin of urinary stream

B. **ANALYSIS/NURSING DIAGNOSES**
1. Risk for disorganized infant behavior related to pain and discomfort
2. Disturbed body image related to perception of physical defect
3. Acute pain related surgical trauma
4. Social isolation related to frequent hospitalization; concern about appearance

C. **PLANNING/IMPLEMENTATION**
1. Provide the parents with an explanation of child's future functioning
2. Prepare child for surgery; the boy needs help in coping with anatomic difference from peers and the adjustments to voiding in the sitting position

D. **EVALUATION/OUTCOMES**
1. Remains free from pain
2. Maintains peer interactions
3. Child and parents will verbalize effects of the defect

SKELETAL MALFORMATIONS

▼ CLUBFOOT

Data Base

A. Foot has been twisted out of normal shape or position

B. Most common type: talipes equinovarus: foot is fixed in plantar flexion (downward) and deviated medially (inward)

C. Clinical findings
   1. Deformity is readily apparent at birth
   2. Deformity may be rigid or flexible

D. Therapeutic interventions
   1. Treatment is most successful when started early in infancy because delay causes muscles and bones of legs to develop abnormally, with shortening of tendons
   2. Nonsurgical treatment: gentle, repeated manipulation of the foot with casting; done every few days for 1 to 2 weeks then at 1- to 2-week intervals
   3. Surgical treatment: done if nonsurgical treatment not effective
      a. Tight ligaments released
      b. Tendons lengthened or transplanted
   4. Follow-up care of the client
      a. Extended medical supervision is required because there is a tendency for this deformity to recur (considered cured when the child is able to wear regular shoes and walk properly)
      b. Care emphasizes muscle reeducation (by manipulation) and proper walking
      c. Heels and soles of braces or shoes prescribed following correction must be kept in repair
      d. Corrective shoes may have sole and heel lifts on lateral border to maintain proper position

Nursing Care of Children with Clubfoot

A. ASSESSMENT
   1. Parental understanding of treatment regimen
   2. Skin and circulation of affected limb

B. ANALYSIS/NURSING DIAGNOSES
   1. Risk for injury related to use of corrective devices
   2. Risk for impaired skin integrity related to use of corrective devices
   3. Risk for peripheral neurovascular dysfunction related to use of corrective devices

C. PLANNING/IMPLEMENTATION
   1. Observe toes for signs of circulatory impairment; make sure toes are visible at the end of the cast
   2. Watch for signs of weakness and wear of the cast, especially if the child is allowed to walk on it
   3. Teach parents all the necessary care and emphasize the need for follow-up, which may be prolonged
   4. For other areas of cast care see Developmental Dysplasia of the Hip

D. EVALUATION/OUTCOMES
   1. Remains free from complications
   2. Parents demonstrate ability to care for child

▼ DEVELOPMENTAL DYSPLASIA OF THE HIP

Data Base
A. Imperfect development of hip—can affect femoral head, acetabulum, or both
B. Head of the femur does not lie deep enough within the acetabulum and slips out on movement
C. Occurs in females seven times more often than in males
D. Classification
   1. Acetabular dysplasia: mildest form; femoral head remains in acetabulum
   2. Subluxation: most common form; femoral head partially displaced
   3. Dislocation: femoral head not in contact with acetabulum; displaced posteriorly and superiorly
E. Clinical findings
   1. Limitation in abduction of leg on the affected side
   2. Asymmetry of gluteal, popliteal, and thigh folds
   3. Audible click when abducting and externally rotating the hip on the affected side (Ortolani's sign)
   4. Apparent shortening of the femur (Galeazzi's sign)
   5. Waddling gait and lordosis when the child begins to walk
F. Therapeutic interventions
   1. Directed toward enlarging and deepening the acetabulum by placing the head of the femur within the acetabulum and applying constant pressure
   2. Positioning with legs slightly flexed and abducted: Pavlik harness; spica cast from the waist to below the knees; brace
   3. Surgical intervention (e.g., open reduction with casting)

Nursing Care of Children with Developmental Dysplasia of the Hip

A. ASSESSMENT
   1. Limb shorter on affected side
   2. Positive Ortolani's test (hip click)
   3. Restricted abduction of hip on affected side

B. ANALYSIS/NURSING DIAGNOSES
   1. Delayed growth and development related to immobilization
   2. Impaired physical mobility related to immobilizing device
   3. Risk for injury related to corrective device; immobility

C. PLANNING/IMPLEMENTATION
1. Respiratory problems: hypostatic pneumonia
   a. Change position frequently; raise head of mattress rather than head to prevent flexion of the neck
   b. Teach parents postural drainage and exercises for child, such as blowing bubbles to increase lung expansion
   c. Encourage parents to seek immediate medical care if the child develops congestion or cough
2. Infection and excoriation of skin
   a. Observe for circulation to toes, pedal pulses, and blanching
   b. Do not let the child put small toys or food inside cast
   c. Use gauze strips inside cast as a scratcher
   d. Alert parents to signs of infection, such as odor
   e. Protect cast edges with adhesive tape or waterproof material, especially around perineum
   f. Use diapers and plastic lining to minimize soiling of cast by feces and urine
3. Constipation from immobility
   a. Teach parents to observe for straining on defecation and constipation
   b. Increase fluids and fiber to prevent constipation
4. Nutrition
   a. Provide small, frequent meals because of inflexibility of cast around waist (a window may be made over the abdominal area to allow for expansion with meals)
   b. Adjust calorie intake, because less energy expenditure can lead to obesity
5. Transportation and positioning
   a. Use wagon or stroller with back flat or mechanic's creeper
   b. Protect child from falling when positioned
   c. Never pick up child by the bar between the legs of the cast (use two people to provide adequate body support if necessary)
6. Meet emotional needs
   a. Use touch as much as possible; small children can be picked up and cuddled
   b. Stimulate and provide for play activities appropriate to age
7. Provide parents with help and support
   a. Give written instructions
   b. Schedule routine home visits with telephone counseling available
   c. Stress need for follow-up care because treatment may be prolonged
   d. Prepare parents for the possible use of an abduction brace after the cast is removed

8. When a spica cast is applied see Fractures in Medical-Surgical Nursing for care of the client with a cast

D. EVALUATION/OUTCOMES
1. Moves about and controls environment
2. Remains free of injury
3. Regains earlier movement (crawling/walking) when device is removed
4. Parents demonstrate ability to care for child

INBORN ERRORS OF METABOLISM

Inherited autosomal recessive trait disorders caused by absence of substances essential to cellular metabolism. Characterized by abnormal fat, protein, or carbohydrate metabolism.

▼ PHENYLKETONURIA (PKU)

Data Base
A. Lack of the enzyme phenylalanine hydroxylase, which changes phenylalanine (essential amino acid) into tyrosine
B. Clinical findings
   1. Mental retardation from damage to the nervous system by buildup of phenylalanine if untreated
      a. Often noticed by 4 months of age
      b. IQ is usually below 50 and most frequently under 20
   2. Strong musty odor in urine from phenylacetic acid
   3. Absence of tyrosine reduces the production of melanin and results in blond hair and blue eyes
   4. Fair skin is susceptible to eczema
C. Therapeutic interventions
   1. Early detection is essential
   2. Guthrie blood test: testing should be done after protein ingestion; if testing is done during initial 24 hours, it should be repeated by the third week of life
   3. Dietary: low-phenylalanine: use of Lofenalac or PKU-1 as a milk substitute and restriction of foods to those low in this amino acid
      a. Use of phenylalanine-free formulas such as PKU-2 or Phenyl-Free for children over 3
      b. Dietary restrictions of phenylalanine through adolescence and possibly life
      c. Individuals with phenylketonuria who become pregnant must consume a low-phenylalanine diet
      d. Use of the artificial sweetener aspartame is prohibited
   4. Treat eczema; see Atopic Dermatitis (Eczema)

▼ GALACTOSEMIA

Data Base

A. Missing enzyme that converts galactose to glucose
B. Clinical findings
   1. Weight loss/vomiting
   2. Hepatosplenomegaly; jaundice
   3. Cataracts
C. Therapeutic interventions
   1. Early detection: test for galactosemia at birth; Beutler test (method similar to Guthrie test for PKU) mandatory in many states
   2. Dietary reduction of lactose: use a soy-based formula as a milk substitute and restrict foods to those low in lactose (usually continued until the child is 7 to 8 years of age), followed by a dietary modification throughout life

▼ CONGENITAL HYPOTHYROIDISM

Data Base

A. Failure of embryonic development of the thyroid gland or inborn enzyme defect in the formation of thyroxine
B. Clinical findings
   1. Prolonged physiologic jaundice, feeding difficulties, inactivity (excessive sleeping, little crying), anemia, problems resulting from hypotonic abdominal muscles (constipation, protruding abdomen, and umbilical hernia)
   2. Appears at 3 to 6 months of age in formula-fed babies; may be delayed in breastfed babies
   3. Impaired development of nervous system leads to mental retardation; level depends on degree of hypothyroidism and interval before therapy is begun
   4. Decreased growth and decreased metabolic rate resulting in increased weight
   5. Characteristic infant facies: short forehead; wide, puffy eyes; wrinkled eyelids; broad, short, upturned nose; large, protruding tongue; hair is dry, brittle, and lusterless with low hairline
   6. Skin is mottled because of decreased heart rate and circulation
   7. Skin is yellowish from carotenemia resulting from decreased conversion of carotene to vitamin A
C. Therapeutic interventions
   1. Detection: neonatal screening for thyroxine (T4) and thyroid-stimulating hormone (TSH)
      a. Test is routine and mandatory in many areas
      b. Performed by heel-stick blood test at the same time as other neonatal metabolic tests
   2. Treatment: replacement therapy with thyroid hormone; if therapy is begun before 3 months

of age, chances for normal growth and normal IQ are increased

General Nursing Care of Children with Inborn Errors of Metabolism

A. **ASSESSMENT**
   1. Verification of test results
   2. Parents' understanding of disorder
   3. Growth and development
B. **ANALYSIS/NURSING DIAGNOSES**
   1. Interrupted family processes related to situational crisis; genetic illness
   2. Anticipatory grieving related to loss of perfect child
   3. Delayed growth and development related to changes in metabolism
   4. Imbalanced nutrition: less than body requirements related to restrictive diet
C. **PLANNING/IMPLEMENTATION**
   1. Help parents to understand the disease and the role of diet
   2. Refer parents for genetic counseling
   3. Specific nursing care for children with hypothyroidism
      a. Instruct parents regarding administration of thyroid replacement and signs of overdose (rapid pulse, dyspnea, insomnia, irritability, sweating, fever, and weight loss)
      b. Teach parents to take pulse
D. **EVALUATION/OUTCOMES**
   1. Achieves satisfactory growth and development
   2. Consumes adequate nutrients for growth
   3. Child and family verbalize necessity of diet and acceptable modifications
   4. Child and family verbalize and demonstrate prescribed diet/medications

HEALTH PROBLEMS THAT DEVELOP DURING INFANCY

(Problems may continue past infancy)

▼ INTUSSUSCEPTION

Data Base

A. Telescoping of one portion of the intestine into another; occurs most frequently at the ileocecal valve
B. Males affected two times more frequently than females
C. Usually occurs between 3 to 12 months of age
D. Clinical findings
   1. Healthy, well-nourished infant or child who wakes up with severe paroxysmal abdominal pain, evidenced by kicking and drawing legs up to the abdomen

2. One or two normal stools, then bloody mucus stool ("currant jelly–like" stool)
3. Palpation of sausage-shaped mass
4. Other signs of intestinal obstruction usually present
E. Therapeutic interventions
   1. Medical reduction by hydrostatic pressure (barium enema)
   2. Surgical reduction; sometimes with intestinal resection

Nursing Care of Children with Intussusception

A. ASSESSMENT
   1. Sudden, acute, intermittent abdominal pain
   2. Red "currant jelly–like" stools
   3. Tender, distended abdomen; vomiting
B. ANALYSIS/NURSING DIAGNOSES
   1. Acute pain related to invaginating bowel
   2. Interrupted family processes related to having a child with life-threatening illness
   3. Imbalanced nutrition: less than body requirements related to decreased intake; increased peristalsis
   4. Risk for deficient fluid volume related to vomiting; diarrhea
C. PLANNING/IMPLEMENTATION
   1. Same as for any abdominal surgery
   2. Make provisions for frequent parental visits because the problem usually occurs when the child is 6 to 8 months of age and separation anxiety is acute
D. EVALUATION/OUTCOMES
   1. Remains free from pain
   2. Consumes sufficient nutrients for growth
   3. Maintains fluid balance
   4. Family can verbalize feelings about the illness

▼ FAILURE TO THRIVE (FTT)

Data Base

A. The term used to describe infants and children whose weight and sometimes height fall below the fifth percentile for their age
B. Persistent deviation from established growth curve
C. Classification
   1. Organic (OFTT): result of a physical cause, such as congenital heart defects, neurologic lesions, microcephaly, chronic urinary tract infection, malabsorption syndrome, gastroesophageal reflux, renal insufficiency, endocrine dysfunction, or cystic fibrosis; syndrome is often called marasmus
   2. Nonorganic (NFTT): caused by psychosocial factors, problem being between the child and the primary caregiver; in this situation the lack

of physical growth is secondary to the lack of emotional and sensory stimulation
   3. Idiopathic (IFTT): unexplained by the usual organic or environmental etiologies but usually classified as NFTT
   4. Nonorganic and idiopathic failure to thrive account for the majority of FTT
D. Clinical findings
   1. Organic: identifiable physical cause of the growth failure
   2. Nonorganic
      a. Characteristics of nonorganic FTT in children
         (1) Growth failure: below the fifth percentile in weight only or height and weight
         (2) Developmental retardation: social, motor, adaptive, language; hearing not affected
         (3) Apathy; difficulty forming meaningful relationships; withdrawn behavior
         (4) Inadequate hygiene
         (5) Feeding or eating disorders, such as vomiting, anorexia, voracious appetite, pica, rumination
         (6) No fear of strangers at the age when stranger anxiety is expected
         (7) Avoidance of eye-to-eye contact; wide-eyed gaze and continual scan of the environment ("radar gaze")
         (8) Stiff and unyielding or flaccid and unresponsive; minimal smiling
      b. Characteristics of the individual providing care
         (1) Difficulty perceiving and assessing the infant's needs
         (2) Frustrated and angered at the infant's dissatisfied response
         (3) Frequently under stress and in crisis, with emotional, social, and financial problems
E. Therapeutic interventions
   1. Provide sufficient nutrients to achieve a rate of growth greater than expected for age
   2. Treat underlying cause: coexisting medical problems; parent-child relationship

Nursing Care of Children with Failure to Thrive

A. ASSESSMENT
   1. Accurate baseline height and weight and daily weight
   2. Feeding behavior
   3. Parent-child behavior/interactions
   4. Developmental level
B. ANALYSIS/NURSING DIAGNOSES
   1. Delayed growth and development related to physiologic factors; physical neglect; social neglect
   2. Imbalanced nutrition: less than body requirements related to feeding or eating disorders

3. Impaired parenting related to knowledge deficit; poverty; infant's failure to develop

C. PLANNING/IMPLEMENTATION

1. Provide a consistent caregiver who can begin to satisfy routine needs
2. Provide optimum nutrients
   a. Make feeding a priority intervention
   b. Keep an accurate record of intake to determine daily calories
   c. Weigh daily and record to ascertain weight gain
3. Introduce a positive feeding environment
   a. Establish a structured routine and follow it consistently; assign one nurse for feeding; follow the child's rhythm of feeding; be persistent
   b. Hold the young child for feeding; maintain eye-to-eye contact; maintain a calm, even temperament; provide a quiet, unstimulating environment
   c. Talk to the child by giving appropriate directions and praise for eating
4. Increase stimulation appropriate to the child's present developmental level
5. Provide the parent an opportunity to talk
6. When necessary, relieve the parent of childrearing responsibilities until able and ready emotionally to support the child
7. Demonstrate proper infant care by example, not lecturing (allow the parent to proceed at own pace)
8. Supply the parent with emotional support without fostering dependency
9. Promote the parent's self-respect and confidence by praising achievements with child

D. EVALUATION/OUTCOMES

1. Demonstrates a positive response to interventions
2. Gains weight steadily
3. Parents demonstrate ability to care for child

▼ SHAKEN BABY SYNDROME

Data Base

A. A form of child abuse caused by vigorously shaking while the child is held by the shoulders or upper extremities
B. Can cause fatal intracranial trauma without external signs of abuse
C. Clinical findings
   1. Failure to thrive
   2. Seizures; coma
   3. Respiratory irregularities; apnea
   4. Vomiting associated with drowsiness to lethargy

▼ SUDDEN INFANT DEATH SYNDROME (SIDS)

Data Base

A. The third leading cause of death in infants between 1 month and 1 year of age; incidence of 0.6 in every 1000 live births
B. Peak age of occurrence: healthy infants 2 to 4 months of age—95% occur by 6 months
C. Prevention: infants should be placed on their backs or sides on a firm surface for sleep
D. Higher incidence in:
   1. Infants sleeping on abdomen or on softer bedding, pillows, comforters, quilts, and sheepskin
   2. Males
   3. Low birth weight: newborns with low Apgar scores
   4. Infants with CNS disturbances
   5. Infants with respiratory disorders such as bronchopulmonary dysplasia
   6. Maternal factors such as youth, smoking during pregnancy, substance abuse
E. Lower incidence in breastfed infants
F. May be a greater incidence in siblings of children with SIDS
G. Pulmonary edema and intrathoracic hemorrhages found on autopsy
H. Clinical findings
   1. Sudden, unexplained death of an infant under 1 year of age
   2. Frothy, blood-tinged fluid fills mouth and nose
I. Therapeutic interventions
   1. Avoid implying wrongdoing, abuse, or neglect
   2. Support parents
   3. Be nonjudmental about parents' attempts at resuscitation

Nursing Care of Families of Children with Sudden Infant Death Syndrome

A. ASSESSMENT

1. Parental knowledge of SIDS
2. Parental support system

B. ANALYSIS/NURSING DIAGNOSES

1. Readiness for enhanced family coping related to successfully coping with loss
2. Compromised family coping related to situational crisis
3. Interrupted family processes related to disruption of lifestyle
4. Dysfunctional grieving related to loss of child
5. Impaired parenting of other children related to grief

C. PLANNING/IMPLEMENTATION

1. Know signs of SIDS to distinguish it from child neglect or abuse; do or say nothing that instills guilt in the parents

2. Reassure the parents that they could not have prevented the death or predicted its occurrence
3. Reinforce that an autopsy should be done on every child to confirm diagnosis
4. Visit the parents at home to discuss the cause of death and help them with their guilt and grief
5. Refer the parents to a national SIDS parent group

D. EVALUATION/OUTCOMES
1. Family exhibits positive coping behavior
2. Family uses support services
3. Family exhibits appropriate bereavement behavior
4. Parents maintain supportive relationship with other children

▼ APNEA OF INFANCY (AOI)

Data Base
A. Apnea of 15 seconds or less is normal at any age
B. Pathologic apnea lasts at least 20 seconds
C. May be symptomatic of sepsis, seizures, upper airway abnormalities, gastroesophageal reflux, hypoglycemia, or impaired regulation of sleep or feeding
D. No cause identified in 50% of cases
E. Less than 7% of SIDS cases
F. Clinical findings
   1. Usually presents as an apparent life-threatening event
   2. Is associated with cyanosis, marked pallor, hypotonia, or bradycardia
G. Therapeutic interventions
   1. Continuous home monitoring of cardiorespiratory rhythm
   2. Use of respiratory stimulant medication such as theophylline
   3. Treatment discontinued when child has gone 2 to 3 months without a significant number of alarms or with apneic episodes that did not require intervention

Nursing Care of Children with Apnea
A. ASSESSMENT
1. Parental fears and concerns
2. Knowledge about cardiopulmonary resuscitation (CPR) and home monitoring
3. Description of apparent life-threatening event

B. ANALYSIS/NURSING DIAGNOSES
1. Ineffective breathing pattern related to periods of apnea
2. Caregiver role strain related to constant monitoring
3. Interrupted family processes related to constant monitoring

4. Fear related to possible loss of child

C. PLANNING/IMPLEMENTATION
1. Monitor type and quality of apneic episodes
2. Teach parents about home monitoring and how to stimulate/resuscitate infant
3. Assist parents to identify support system

D. EVALUATION/OUTCOMES
1. Maintains respiratory functioning
2. Parents demonstrate proper use of equipment for home monitoring
3. Parents demonstrate CPR
4. Parents verbalize fears
5. Parents identify support system

▼ DIARRHEA

Data Base
A. Frequent, watery stools caused by increased peristalsis resulting from a variety of causes, local or systemic
B. Classification
   1. Acute: sudden change in frequency and consistency of stools; leading cause of illness in children younger than 5 years
   2. Chronic: persists longer than 2 weeks; often caused by chronic conditions such as malabsorption syndromes, inflammatory bowel disease, food allergy, lactose intolerance, or chronic nonspecific diarrhea
C. Clinical findings
   1. Frequent, watery stools
   2. If fluid loss is severe
      a. Weight loss greater than 10% (moderate dehydration)
      b. Diminished skin turgor and dry mucous membranes
      c. Depressed fontanels and sunken eyeballs
      d. Decreased urine output, increased specific gravity, and increased hematocrit
      e. Irritability, stupor, and seizures from loss of intracellular water and decreased plasma volume
      f. Metabolic acidosis, which decreases available bicarbonate
D. Therapeutic interventions
   1. In severe diarrhea correct fluid and electrolyte imbalance
   2. Identify the causative agent and institute proper therapy (antibiotics are used if a bacterial agent is present)

Nursing Care of Children with Diarrhea
A. ASSESSMENT
1. Assess diarrhea: number, volume, characteristics

2. State of hydration
3. Possible source of infection

B. **ANALYSIS/NURSING DIAGNOSES**
1. Risk for infection related to presence of infectious organisms
2. Imbalanced nutrition: less than body requirements related to increased peristalsis with decreased absorption of nutrients
3. Impaired skin integrity related to frequent loose stools
4. Deficient fluid volume related to fluid losses in stools

C. **PLANNING/IMPLEMENTATION**
1. Isolate the infant until stool culture results are reported as negative
2. Explain to the parents why antibiotics and an increase in food are ineffective in treating viral diarrhea
3. Teach parents progressive increase in diet; alterations in diet may control mild diarrhea
   a. Clear fluids to decrease inflammation of the intestinal mucosa
   b. If tolerated, use half-strength formula
   c. Regular diet of bland foods

D. **EVALUATION/OUTCOMES**
1. Consumes sufficient calories and fluids
2. Maintains skin integrity
3. Child and family do not transmit infection to others

▼ VOMITING

Data Base

A. Common symptom in childhood, usually minor and of short duration
B. Associated hazard: aspiration with risk of asphyxiation, atelectasis, or pneumonia
C. Forcible ejection of stomach contents: usually associated with nausea
D. Causes
1. Most commonly caused by infection
2. Response to allergen, drug ingestion
3. Recurrent or prolonged vomiting may be caused by increased intracranial pressure
E. Clinical findings
1. One or more episodes of regurgitation or emesis
2. If vomiting is severe
   a. Dehydration
   b. Tetany and convulsions in severe alkalosis resulting from hypokalemia and hypocalcemia
   c. Metabolic alkalosis from loss of hydrogen ions
F. Therapeutic intervention: correction of underlying disorder

Nursing Care of Children with Vomiting

A. **ASSESSMENT**
1. Amount and character of vomitus
2. Circumstances preceding vomiting
3. Child's behavior

B. **ANALYSIS/NURSING DIAGNOSES**
1. Imbalanced nutrition: less than body requirements related to vomiting
2. Deficient fluid volume related to losses with vomiting

C. **PLANNING/IMPLEMENTATION**
1. Maintain in side-lying position with body inclined at 30 degrees at all times
2. Do not disturb infant after feeding
3. If associated with gastroesophageal reflux or cardiac sphincter problems: thicken the consistency of foods and provide small volume feedings every 2 to 3 hours

D. **EVALUATION/OUTCOMES**
1. Demonstrates evidence of rehydration
2. Consumes adequate nutrients for growth and development

▼ COLIC

Data Base

A. Paroxsymal abdominal pain or cramping
B. More common in infants of less than 3 months
C. May be caused by cow's milk sensitivity, but often no cause is found
D. May be associated with excessive swallowing of air, size of nipple opening or shape of nipple, too rapid feeding or overfeeding, tenseness or anxiety in the caregiver, maternal diet
E. Clinical findings
1. Pulling up of arms and legs
2. Red-faced crying over long periods of time
3. Presence of excessive gas
F. Therapeutic intervention: correction of the underlying cause when identified

Nursing Care of Children with Colic

A. **ASSESSMENT**
1. Characteristics of the cry (duration and intensity)
2. Diet of breastfeeding mother
3. When the attacks occur in relationship to feeding
4. Activity of caregiver around time of attack
5. Mother's habits, such as smoking
6. Measures to relieve crying and their effectiveness

B. **ANALYSIS/NURSING DIAGNOSES**
1. Compromised family coping related to alterations in family lifestyle and relationships
2. Acute pain related to abdominal cramping
3. Disturbed sleep patterns related to pain; interrupted sleep from infant crying

C. **PLANNING/IMPLEMENTATION**
1. Watch the parent feed the infant before attempting to counsel
2. Provide smaller, frequent feedings
3. Teach parents to bubble infant frequently and to position on side after feeding
4. Encourage the caregiver to take time away from the infant
5. Reassure parents that the condition is not life-threatening, the infant will gain weight, and the condition will eventually subside

D. **EVALUATION/OUTCOMES**
1. Decreased pain episodes
2. Parents and child are rested and ready to deal with activities of daily living
3. Parents demonstrate proper feeding practices
4. Family can discuss the impact of infant's colic

▼ CONSTIPATION

Data Base
A. Hard, dry stools that are difficult to pass or are infrequent
B. Usually a result of diet, although may have a psychologic component
C. May be indicative of Hirschsprung's disease
D. Classification
1. Obstipation: long periods between defecation
2. Encopresis: constipation with fecal soiling
E. Clinical findings
1. "Stool withholding" behavior
2. Pain on defecation
F. Therapeutic interventions
1. Dietary: increased fiber and fluid
2. If mineral oil is used, it should not be given with foods, because it decreases the absorption of nutrients
3. Enemas should be avoided; bowel retraining should be instituted

Nursing Care of Children with Constipation
A. **ASSESSMENT**
1. History of bowel habits, diet
2. Stool characteristics, frequency
3. Parent/child knowledge of elimination
B. **ANALYSIS/NURSING DIAGNOSES**
1. Constipation related to inadequate fluid and fiber intake
2. Imbalanced nutrition: less than body requirements related to inadequate intake of fiber
3. Acute or chronic pain related to bowel distention; alteration in bowel motility
C. **PLANNING/IMPLEMENTATION**
1. Teach parents to provide foods with fiber and avoid those that bind

2. Teach parents to increase amount of fluid given to infant
3. Place infant in knee-chest position if distention or cramping is present
4. Cuddle infant to provide comfort as necessary
D. **EVALUATION/OUTCOMES**
1. Consumes appropriate amount of fiber and fluid
2. Remains free from pain when defecating

▼ RESPIRATORY TRACT INFECTIONS

Data Base
A. Frequent cause of morbidity
B. Young children have four to five infections per year
C. Children between 6 months and 3 years react more severely
D. Acute infection may be bacterial or viral
E. Respiratory syncytial virus (RSV) is the single most important respiratory pathogen for infants and young children; causes 50% of pediatric hospitalizations for bronchiolitis in children under one year of age
F. Classification: acute nasopharyngitis (common cold); pneumonia; bronchitis; tonsillitis; epiglottitis; croup; acute laryngotracheobronchitis
G. Clinical findings
1. Infection: elevated temperature; purulent discharge from nose, ears, lungs; enlarged cervical lymph nodes
2. Cough; wheeze
3. Cyanosis
H. Therapeutic interventions
1. Supportive therapy
2. Treat underlying cause if infectious

Nursing Care of Children with Respiratory Tract Infections
A. **ASSESSMENT**
1. Respirations: rate, depth, ease, and rhythm
2. Color: cyanosis
3. Adventitious breath sounds
4. Nasal discharge; presence of sputum
5. Cough; occurrence of laryngeal spasms
B. **ANALYSIS/NURSING DIAGNOSES**
1. Ineffective airway clearance related to mechanical obstruction; inflammation; increased secretions; pain when coughing
2. Ineffective breathing pattern related to inflammatory process; pain
3. Acute pain related to inflammatory process; excessive coughing
C. **PLANNING/IMPLEMENTATION**
1. Increase fluid intake to prevent dehydration from fever, perspiration, and to loosen thickened secretions

2. Increase humidity and environmental coolness
   a. Liquifies secretions
   b. Decreases febrile state and limits inflammation of the mucous membrane
   c. Causes vasoconstriction and bronchiolar dilation
3. Promote nasal and pulmonary drainage
   a. Clean the nares with a bulb syringe
   b. Suction the oronasal pharynx
   c. Perform postural drainage and chest physiotherapy
4. Decrease stimulation to promote rest
5. Administer oxygen
6. Never use tongue blade to visualize posterior pharynx in children with epiglottitis
7. Keep a tracheotomy set at the bedside; if a tracheostomy is necessary see Medical-Surgical Nursing for Tracheotomy Care

D. EVALUATION/OUTCOMES
1. Rests and sleeps with unlabored respirations
2. Maintains patent airway
3. Remains free of pain

▼ OTITIS MEDIA

Data Base

A. Acute infection of the middle ear; causative organism usually *Streptococcus pneumoniae* or *Haemophilus influenzae*
B. One of most common diseases of early childhood
C. Highest incidence between ages 6 months to 2 years
D. Classification
   1. Otitis media: inflammation of middle ear without reference to cause or pathogenesis
   2. Acute otitis media: rapid, short onset of signs and symptoms lasting about 3 weeks
   3. Otitis media with effusion: middle ear inflammation with fluid present
   4. Chronic otitis media with effusion: lasts more than 3 months
E. Clinical findings
   1. Acute otitis media
      a. Pain: infant frets and rubs ear or rolls head from side to side
      b. Drum bulging, red, may rupture; no light reflex
   2. Otitis media with effusion
      a. No pain or fever, but "fullness" in the ear
      b. Drum appears gray, bulging
      c. Possible loss of hearing from scarring of the drum
F. Therapeutic interventions
   1. Antibiotic therapy

2. Surgery including myringotomy or insertion of tympanotomy tubes

Nursing Care of Children with Otitis Media

A. ASSESSMENT
1. Pain
2. Signs and symptoms of infection
3. Allergies

B. ANALYSIS/NURSING DIAGNOSES
1. Risk for infection related to inadequate treatment; infectious organism
2. Acute pain related to pressure caused by inflammatory process

C. PLANNING/IMPLEMENTATION
1. Teach parents proper administration of antibiotics; stress importance of full course of therapy
2. Teach parent proper instillation of ear drops: in children under 3 years, pull the auricle down and back; for an older child, pull the auricle up and back
3. Minimize recurrence; eliminate environmental allergens and tobacco smoke; feed in upright position
4. Encourage medical follow-up to check for complications such as chronic hearing loss, mastoiditis, or possible meningitis

D. EVALUATION/OUTCOMES
1. Sleeps and rests without signs of discomfort
2. Remains free from infection
3. Parents verbalize techniques to minimize otitis media
4. Parents verbalize importance of antibiotic therapy

▼ MENINGITIS

Data Base

A. Most common CNS infection of infants and children
B. Inflammation of the meninges by microorganisms that travel via the cerebral spinal fluid
C. Classification: culture of cerebrospinal fluid used to identify organism
   1. Bacterial: caused by pus-forming bacteria, especially meningococcus, pneumococcus, and influenza bacillus
   2. Tuberculous: caused by tubercle bacillus
   3. Viral or aseptic: caused by a wide variety of viral agents
D. Clinical findings
   1. Opisthotonos: rigidity and hyperextension of the neck
   2. Irritability; high-pitched cry
   3. Signs of increased intracranial pressure; headache

4. Fever; nausea and vomiting
5. Meningococcal meningitis: petechiae and purpuric skin rash

E. Therapeutic intervention: massive doses of intravenous antibiotics

Nursing Care of Children with Meningitis

A. **ASSESSMENT**
1. Fever
2. Headache, irritability; vomiting
3. Seizures; nuchal rigidity

B. **ANALYSIS/NURSING DIAGNOSES**
1. Interrupted family processes related to having a child with a serious illness
2. Risk for infection related to presence of infective organisms
3. Risk for injury related to disease process

C. **PLANNING/IMPLEMENTATION**
1. Provide for rest; decrease environmental stimuli (control light and noise)
2. Position on the side with head gently supported in extension
3. Institute droplet precautions for at least 48 hours
4. Maintain fluid balance because of meningeal edema: intake and output; monitor intravenous fluids, daily weights; correct deficits
5. Administer antibiotic therapy as prescribed
6. Provide emotional support for parents, because onset of illness is sudden
7. Monitor for complications such as septic shock and circulatory collapse

D. **EVALUATION/OUTCOMES**
1. Demonstrates a positive response to interventions
2. Parents verbalize fears regarding child's prognosis

▼ FEBRILE SEIZURES

Data Base

A. Caused by elevation of temperature
B. Usually occur in children between 6 months and 3 years of age
C. Affects 3% to 5% of children in this age group
D. Classification
1. Simple seizure: brief; generalized
2. Complex seizure: prolonged; may have focal features

E. Clinical findings
1. Associated with disease outside the CNS
2. Fever usually exceeds 102° F (38.8° C); seizures occur on rise
3. 30% to 40% of children have a recurrence

F. Therapeutic interventions

1. Control seizure with medication
2. Reduce temperature
3. Treat underlying cause

Nursing Care of Children with Febrile Seizures

A. **ASSESSMENT**
1. Description of seizure
2. History of present illness

B. **ANALYSIS/NURSING DIAGNOSES**
1. Ineffective airway clearance related to decreased level of consciousness
2. Risk for aspiration related to seizures
3. Risk for injury related to environmental hazards
4. Hyperthermia related to altered hypothalamic regulating center

C. **PLANNING/IMPLEMENTATION**
1. Reduce fever with antipyretic drugs; monitor tympanic or axillary temperature
2. General seizure precautions
   a. Protect the child from injury; do not restrain; pad crib rails; do not use tongue blade
   b. Place in side-lying position to prevent aspiration
   c. Observe and record the time of seizure, duration, and body parts involved
   d. Suction the nasopharynx and administer oxygen after seizure as required
   e. Observe the degree of consciousness and behavior after the seizure
   f. Provide rest after the seizure
3. Teach parents to give antipyretics at first sign of increased temperature
4. For further discussion of seizures see Epilepsy (Seizure Disorders) in Medical-Surgical Nursing

D. **EVALUATION/OUTCOMES**
1. Maintains patent airway
2. Remains free from injury during and after seizure

▼ ATOPIC DERMATITIS (ECZEMA)

Data Base

A. Atopic manifestation of a specific allergen that may have an emotional component
B. Most common during first 2 years of life
C. Involves periods of remissions and exacerbations
D. Majority of children with infantile form have a family history of allergies
E. Classification
1. Infantile: begins between 2 and 6 months of age; spontaneous remission by 3 years
2. Childhood: occurs at 2 to 3 years of age; 90% manifest the disease by 5 years

3. Preadolescent and adolescent: begins at about 12 years and continues into adulthood
F. Clinical findings
   1. Erythema and edema from dilation of capillaries
   2. Papules, vesicles, and crusts
   3. Seen mostly on cheeks, scalp, neck, and flexor surfaces of arms and legs
   4. Itching that may precipitate infection from scratching
G. Therapeutic interventions
   1. Relieve pruritus
   2. Hydrate skin
   3. Reduce inflammation
   4. Prevent or control secondary infection

Nursing Care of Children with Atopic Dermatitis

A. **ASSESSMENT**
   1. Family history of allergies
   2. Environmental or dietary factors associated with previous exacerbations
   3. Skin lesions: distribution, type, presence of secondary infection
   4. Parent/child attitude toward lesions
B. **ANALYSIS/NURSING DIAGNOSES**
   1. Ineffective family therapeutic regimen management related to complex medical regimen
   2. Risk for infection related to skin impairment
   3. Impaired skin integrity related to eczematous lesions
   4. Disturbed sleep pattern related to physical discomfort; schedule of therapies
C. **PLANNING/IMPLEMENTATION**
   1. Support the parents—this long-term problem is often discouraging because the infant is difficult to comfort
   2. Restrain hands to keep the infant from scratching when unsupervised, but provide supervised, unrestrained play periods
   3. Pick up frequently because the infant is irritable, fretful, and anorectic
   4. Keep skin hydrated
   5. Provide the parent with a list of foods permitted or omitted on an elimination or restricted diet
   6. Instruct the parent how to apply topical ointments prescribed
D. **EVALUATION/OUTCOMES**
   1. Remains free from injury and infection in affected area
   2. Child and parents rest/sleep adequate amounts for age
   3. Parents demonstrate ability to follow medical regimen

▼ HUMAN IMMUNODEFICIENCY VIRUS (HIV) AND ACQUIRED IMMUNODEFICIENCY SYNDROME (AIDS)

Data Base
A. Infection with human immunodeficiency virus (HIV)
B. Viral infection occurs either:
   1. Vertically from an HIV-infected mother to child (breastfeeding has been identified as a source of the virus)
   2. Horizontally by sexual contact or parenteral exposure to blood
C. Immunosuppression results from decreased number of CD4 T cells as well as functional defects in B cells
D. Three populations of pediatric clients
   1. Children exposed during the perinatal period
   2. Children who have received blood products prior to 1987
   3. Adolescents who are infected after engaging in high-risk behaviors
E. Clinical findings
   1. Failure to thrive
   2. Hepatosplenomegaly
   3. Diffuse lymphadenopathy
   4. Chronic or recurrent diarrhea
   5. Oral candidiasis
   6. Parotitis
   7. *Pneumocystis carinii* pneumonia
   8. Neurologic involvement
F. Therapeutic interventions
   1. Use of medication to suppress viral replication; zidovudine (AZT, Retrovir), didanosine (ddl, Videx)
   2. Routine injections of gamma globulin
   3. Immunizations
      a. HIV asymptomatic: DTP is given; inactivated polio virus (Salk vaccine) is used rather than the oral polio virus (Sabin vaccine); measles, mumps, and rubella (MMR) vaccine is given; child monitored to observe results; varicella vaccine is avoided
      b. HIV symptomatic: immunizations are not usually given
   4. Prevention and management of secondary infections
   5. Treatment of pain
   6. Nutritional support

Nursing Care of Children with AIDS
A. **ASSESSMENT**
   1. Family support; who is able to care for child
   2. History to determine source of infection
   3. Health status

B. ANALYSIS/NURSING DIAGNOSES
1. Disturbed body image related to having a serious illness
2. Interrupted family processes related to having a child with a life-threatening disease
3. Anticipatory grieving related to having a child with a potentially fatal illness
4. Ineffective protection related to impaired immune response
5. Risk for caregiver role strain related to significant home care needs

C. PLANNING/IMPLEMENTATION
1. Prevent transmission of virus
   a. Standard and transmission-based precautions
   b. Education of child and parent about modes of transmission
2. Provide emotional support to child and family
3. Monitor child for signs and symptoms of sepsis and other complications

D. EVALUATION/OUTCOMES
1. Does not transmit the HIV virus
2. Remains free of opportunistic infections and other complications
3. Child and family maintain positive interpersonal relationships
4. Family members demonstrate appropriate care of child
5. Family members demonstrate appropriate bereavement behavior

▼ EMOTIONAL DISORDERS

For common emotional disorders of infancy see Disorders Usually First Evident in Infancy, Childhood, or Adolescence in Mental Health Nursing

THE TODDLER

GROWTH AND DEVELOPMENT
Developmental Timetable
15 months
A. Motor
1. Walks well alone by 14 months with a wide-based gait; creeps up stairs
2. Builds tower of two blocks; enjoys throwing objects and picking them up
3. Drinks from a cup and can use a spoon
B. Vocalization and socialization
1. Can use four to six words, including name
2. Has learned: "no," which may be said while doing a requested demand

18 months
A. Physical
1. Growth has decreased and appetite lessened—

"physiologic anorexia"
2. Anterior fontanel is usually closed
3. Abdomen protrudes, larger than chest circumference
B. Motor
1. Runs clumsily; climbs stairs or up on furniture
2. Imitates strokes in drawing
3. Drinks well from a cup; manages a spoon well
4. Builds tower of three to four cubes
C. Vocalization and socialization
1. Says 10 or more words
2. Has new awareness of strangers
3. Begins to have temper tantrums
4. Very ritualistic, has favorite toy or blanket, thumb-sucking may be at peak

2 years
A. Physical
1. Weight—about 11 to 12 kg (26 to 28 lb)
2. Height—about 80 to 82 cm (32 to 33 inches)
3. Teeth—16 temporary; begin visits to dentist
B. Motor
1. Gross motor skills quite refined
2. Can walk up and down stairs, both feet on one step at a time, holding onto rail
3. Builds tower of six to seven cubes or will make cubes into a train
C. Sensory
1. Accommodation well developed
2. Visual acuity 20/40
D. Vocalization and socialization
1. Vocabulary of about 300 words; uses short, two- to three-word phrases, also pronouns
2. Obeys simple commands; shows signs of increasing autonomy and individuality; makes simple choices when possible
3. Still very ritualistic, especially at bedtime
4. Can help undress self and pull on simple clothes
5. Does not share possessions, everything is "mine"

30 months
A. Physical
1. Full set of 20 temporary teeth
2. Decreased need for naps
B. Motor
1. Walks on tiptoe; stands on one foot momentarily
2. Builds tower of eight blocks
3. Copies horizontal or vertical line
4. May attend to own toilet needs
C. Vocalization and socialization
1. Beginning to see self as a separate individual from reflected appraisal of significant others
2. Still sees other children as objects
3. Increasingly independent, ritualistic, and negativistic

Major Learning Events

A. Toilet training: most important task of the toddler
   1. Physical maturation must be reached before training is possible; approach and attitude of parents play a vital role
      a. Sphincter control adequate when the child can walk
      b. Able to retain urine for at least 2 hours
      c. Usual age for bowel training: 24 to 30 months
      d. Daytime bowel and bladder control: during second year
      e. Night control: by 3 to 4 years of age
   2. Psychologic readiness
      a. Aware of the act of elimination
      b. Able to inform the parent of the need to urinate or defecate
      c. Desire to please the parent
   3. Process of training
      a. Usually begins with bowel, then bladder
      b. Accidents and regressions frequently occur
   4. Parental response
      a. Choose a specific word for the act
      b. Have a specific time and place
      c. Do not punish for accidents
B. Need for independence without overprotection; the parents should:
   1. Be consistent; set realistic limits
   2. Reinforce desired behavior
   3. Be constructive, geared to teach self-control
   4. Punish immediately after a wrongdoing; punish appropriately

Play During Toddlerhood (Parallel Play)

A. The child plays alongside other children but not with them
B. Mostly free and spontaneous, no rules or regulations
C. Attention span is still very short, and change of toys occurs at frequent intervals
D. Safety is important; there is danger of:
   1. Breaking a toy through exploration and ingesting small pieces
   2. Ingesting lead from lead-based paint on toys
   3. Being burned by potentially flammable toys
E. Imitation and make-believe play begins by end of the second year
F. Suggested toys
   1. Play furniture, dishes, cooking utensils, telephone
   2. Puzzles with a few large pieces
   3. Pedal-propelled toys, such as tricycle; straddle toys such as rocking horse
   4. Clay, sandbox toys, crayons, finger paints
   5. Pounding toys; blocks; push-pull toys

HEALTH PROMOTION FOR TODDLERS

Childhood Nutrition

A. Nutritional objectives
   1. Provide adequate nutrient intake to meet continuing growth and development needs
   2. Provide a basis for support of psychosocial development in relation to food patterns, eating behavior, and attitudes
   3. Provide sufficient calories for increasing physical activities and energy needs
B. Diet: calorie and nutrient requirements increase with age
   1. Increased variety in types and textures of foods
   2. Increased involvement in the feeding process, stimulation of curiosity about food environment, language learning
   3. Consideration for the child's appetite, choices, motor skills
C. Possible nutritional problem areas
   1. Anemia: increase foods containing iron (e.g., enriched cereals, meat, egg, green vegetables)
   2. Obesity or underweight: increase or decrease calories; maintain core foods
   3. Low intake of calcium, iron, vitamins A and C; usually caused by dietary fads
   4. Often omitting breakfast
   5. Influence of commercialism on selection of foods and emphasis on fast foods, "empty-calorie" snacks, and high-carbohydrate convenience foods

Injury Prevention

A. Leading cause of death in children between 1 and 4 years of age
B. Children under 5 years of age account for over half of all accidental deaths during childhood
C. More than half of accidental child deaths are related to automobiles and fire
D. Accidents can be viewed in terms of the child's growth and development, especially curiosity about the environment
   1. Motor vehicle
      a. Walking or running, especially chasing after objects thrown into the street
      b. Inability to determine speed, lack of experience to foresee danger
      c. Child often unseen because of small size; can be run over by a car backing out of the driveway, or when playing in leaves or snow
      d. Failure to restrain in a car (sitting in a person's lap, improper use of seat belts rather than appropriate car restraint)
   2. Burns
      a. Investigating: pulls a pot off the stove; plays with matches; inserts an object into wall socket

b. Climbing: reaches the stove, oven, ironing board and iron, cigarettes on the table
3. Poisons
  a. Learning new tastes and textures, puts everything into mouth
  b. Developing fine motor skills: able to open bottles, cabinets, jars
  c. Climbing to previously unreachable shelves and cabinets
4. Drowning
  a. Child and parents do not recognize the danger of water
  b. Child is unaware of inability to breathe under water
5. Aspirating small objects and putting foreign bodies in ear or nose
  a. Puts everything in mouth
  b. Very interested in body and newly found openings
6. Fractures
  a. Climbing, running, and jumping
  b. Still developing sense of balance
E. Prevention, through parent education and child protection, is the goal

HEALTH PROBLEMS MOST COMMON IN TODDLERS
Hospitalization

A. Toddler experiences basic fear of loss of love, fear of unknown, fear of punishment
B. Immobilization and isolation represent additional crises to the toddler
C. Regression to earlier behaviors may occur
D. Stages of separation anxiety: the specific response of toddler
  1. Protest
    a. Prolonged loud crying, consoled by no one but the parent or usual caregiver
    b. Continually asks to go home
    c. Rejection of the nurse or any other stranger
  2. Despair
    a. Alteration in sleep pattern
    b. Decreased appetite and weight loss
    c. Diminished interest in environment and play
    d. Relative immobility and listlessness
    e. No facial expression or smile
    f. Unresponsive to stimuli
  3. Detachment or denial
    a. Cheerful, undiscriminating friendliness
    b. Lack of preference for parents

General Nursing Diagnoses for Toddlers with Health Problems

A. Anxiety related to strange environment; perception of impending event; separation; anticipated discomfort; knowledge deficit; discomfort; difficulty breathing
B. Readiness for enhanced family coping related to successful parenting
C. Compromised, family coping related to situational crisis
D. Ineffective coping related to situational crisis
E. Deficient diversional activity related to lack of sensory stimulation; frequent or prolonged hospitalization
F. Interrupted family processes related to situational crisis; knowledge deficit; temporary family disorganization; inadequate support systems
G. Fear related to separation from support systems; uncertain prognosis
H. Anticipatory grieving (parental) related to expected loss; gravity of child's physical status
I. Impaired home maintenance related to knowledge deficit; inadequate support system
J. Risk for injury related to use of specific therapies and appliances; incapacity for self-protection; immobility
K. Acute/chronic pain related to disease process; interventions
L. Parental role conflict related to illness of child; inability to care for child
M. Risk for impaired parenting related to separation; skill deficit; family stress
N. Risk for impaired parent/infant/child attachment related to inability of parents to meet child's needs; separation; illness of child
O. Feeding, bathing/hygiene, dressing/grooming, toileting self-care deficits related to developmental level
P. Disturbed sensory perception related to protected environment
Q. Risk for impaired skin integrity related to immature structure and function; immobility
R. Disturbed sleep pattern related to excessive crying; frequent assessment; therapies
S. Spiritual distress (parental) related to inadequate support systems; decisions regarding "right to life" conflicts

General Nursing Care of Toddlers with Health Problems

A. Prevent separation anxiety
  1. Encourage the parents to stay with the child in hospital or to visit frequently
  2. Provide a consistent caregiver
  3. Provide individual attention, physical touch, sensory stimulation, and affection
  4. Prepare the parents for the child's reaction to separation
  5. Involve the parents in the child's care as much as possible

6. If a parent is unable to visit, establish phone contact
7. Establish routine similar to the child's home routine
8. Provide the child with favorite items from home; e.g., a blanket, a toy, a bottle, or a pacifier
9. Maintain the child's familiarity with home by talking about the parents, having the child listen to a tape recording of family members' voices, and showing photographs of family members
10. When family members leave, stay with child for comfort and to reassure parents
11. Associate the parents' visits with familiar events, such as "Mommy is coming after lunch"
12. Encourage the parents to visit at frequent intervals for shorter times, rather than one long visit

B. Prepare parents and the child for hospitalization
1. Give primary consideration to maintaining the parent-child relationship by limiting separation
2. Based on assessment, establish routines and rituals that the child is accustomed to in the areas of toilet training; feeding; bathing; sleep patterns; recreational activities
3. Prepare the parent for regression of the child to previous modes of behavior and loss of newly learned skills
4. Avoid teaching the child new skills during hospitalization
5. Allow the child's release of tension, especially aggression, through play (banging a drum, knocking blocks over, scribbling on paper)
6. Recognize that only minimal advance preparation of the child for hospitalization is possible, because cognitive ability to grasp verbal explanation is limited

▼ BURNS

See Medical-Surgical Nursing for additional information

Data Base

A. Second and third most common cause of death by trauma in individuals less than 15 years of age for boys and girls, respectively
B. Causative agents: thermal (flame, hot water); chemical; electrical; radiation
C. Classification
1. Superficial (first degree): tissue damage minimal; pain predominant symptom
2. Partial thickness (second degree): involves epithelium and part of dermis; severity and rate of healing depend on the amount of damaged dermis; very painful

3. Full thickness (third degree): all layers of skin destroyed; systemic effects can be life-threatening; requires skin grafting
D. Clinical findings
1. Local response
a. Edema formation
b. Fluid loss from nonprotected skin
c. Circulatory stasis occurs; usually restored within 24 to 48 hours in partial-thickness burns
2. Systemic response
a. "Burn shock" causes a precipitous drop in cardiac output; returns to normal in 24 to 36 hours
b. Metabolic rate greatly increased
E. Therapeutic interventions
1. Stop the burning process
a. Remove from source of danger
b. Remove smoldering clothes
c. For superficial burns, immerse the affected area in cool water
2. Administer prompt first aid
a. Maintain a patent airway
b. For superficial burns, cleanse the area, apply sterile dressing soaked in sterile saline if possible
c. Do not apply creams, butter, or any household remedies
d. Do not give oral fluids for severe burns (more than 10% of body)
3. Transport the client to a proper health care facility
a. Children are hospitalized with burns of 5% to 12% of body surface or more
b. Child's large body surface in proportion to weight results in greater potential for fluid loss
c. Shock: primary cause of death in first 24 to 48 hours
d. Infection: primary cause of death after initial period
4. Treat fluid and electrolyte loss
a. Greatest in first 24 to 48 hours because of tissue damage
b. Immediate replacement of both fluids and electrolytes is essential
c. Determination of hematocrit, hemoglobin, and chemistries should be done daily to provide a guide for replacement

Nursing Care of Children with Burns
A. ASSESSMENT
1. Wound assessment/classification; presence and extent of pain
2. Vital signs; respiratory status
3. Fluid balance; nutritional needs

B. ANALYSIS/NURSING DIAGNOSES
1. Disturbed body image related to perception of appearance; impaired mobility
2. Interrupted family processes related to situational crisis (seriously injured child)
3. Risk for infection related to injured skin
4. Imbalanced nutrition: less than body requirements related to increased metabolic need
5. Acute pain related to skin trauma; therapies
6. Impaired physical mobility related to pain; impaired joint movement
7. Impaired skin integrity related to thermal injury

C. PLANNING/IMPLEMENTATION
1. Monitor fluids and electrolytes
   a. Administer prescribed fluids accurately, both time and volume
   b. Accurate measurement of intake and output is critical (daily weights, diaper count, and weight)
2. Maintain isolation precautions
   a. The child has feelings of guilt and punishment
   b. Children under 5 years of age rarely understand the reason for isolation
   c. Furthers separation between parents and the child
   d. Encourage the child to express feelings
3. Compensate for touch deprivation
   a. Touch, a child's main means of comfort and security, is now painful
   b. Pleasurable touch must be reestablished (apply lotion to unaffected areas)
   c. Maximize the use of other senses to promote security and comfort
4. Provide for adequate nutrition
   a. High in protein, vitamins, and calories
   b. The child is frequently anorectic because of discomfort, isolation, emotional depression
   c. Provide the child's food preferences when feasible; do not force eating or use it as a weapon; encourage parent participation
   d. Alter the diet as needs change, especially when high-calorie foods are no longer needed and can cause obesity
5. Prevent contractures
   a. Make moving a game; use play that uses the affected part, such as throwing a ball for arm movement
   b. Provide for functional body alignment; place the child so attention is focused on an object that will keep the body in specific position
   c. Do passive exercises during bath or whirlpool
   d. Give analgesics before exercise
6. Meet child's emotional needs
   a. Allow the child to play with gown, mask, gloves, and bandages so that they are less strange
   b. Prepare the child for baths and whirlpool treatments, which can be frightening and painful
   c. Allow child to reenact treatments and care on a doll to work through feelings
   d. Help child deal with changes in body
      (1) For the younger child, more of a concern to parents (whose reactions are communicated to the child)
      (2) For the older child, especially the adolescent, body appearance is of great concern
      (3) Emphasize what can be done to improve looks (plastic surgery, wigs, appropriate clothing, makeup)
7. Help limit pain
   a. Assess extent of pain by observing behavior of the young child, as well as verbal complaints
   b. Distinguish pain from fear of dark, being left alone, or being in strange surroundings
   c. Administer analgesics before procedures; often narcotics may be required; IV is the preferred route
8. Teach prevention of burn injuries
   a. Educate children regarding fire safety
      (1) Tell the child to leave the house as soon as smoke is smelled or flames are seen, without stopping to retrieve a pet or toy
      (2) Involve all members of the family in fire drills
      (3) Demonstrate and practice "stop, drop, and roll," rather than running, if clothes are on fire
   b. Educate parents especially in regard to the child's growth and development and specific dangers at each age level
   c. Help parents prevent fires in the home
      (1) Supervise children at all times; maintain escape route
      (2) Teach cautious use of heaters, barbecue, and fireplace; place shield in front of heating unit
      (3) Maintain integrity of the electrical system
      (4) Regulate water heater to safe level
      (5) Use and maintain smoke detectors

D. EVALUATION/OUTCOMES
1. Remains comfortable
2. Maintains fluid and nutritional balance
3. Heals with minimal scarring and free from infection
4. Regains flexibility and functional capacity of joints

5. Child and family members verbalize feelings and concerns about appearance

▼ POISONING

Data Base

A. Ingestion of a toxic substance or an excessive amount of a substance
B. More than 90% of poisonings occur in the home
C. Highest incidence occurs in children under 4
D. Improper storage is the major contributing factor to poisonings

General Nursing Care of Children with Poisoning

A. ASSESSMENT

1. Vital signs
2. Need for respiratory or cardiac support
3. See Clinical Findings under type of poisoning

B. ANALYSIS/NURSING DIAGNOSES

1. Risk for poisoning related to child's immature judgment; sources of toxic substances in the environment
2. Interrupted family processes related to sudden hospitalization and emergency aspects of illness
3. Fear related to sudden hospitalization and treatment (e.g., multiple injections for lead poisoning)

C. PLANNING/IMPLEMENTATION

1. Terminate the exposure
   a. Empty the mouth of pills, plant parts, or other material
   b. Thoroughly flush eyes with tap water if they were involved
   c. Flush skin and wash with soap and soft cloth
   d. Remove clothing, especially if pesticide, acid, alkali, or hydrocarbon involved
   e. Bring the victim into fresh air if an inhalation poisoning
2. Communicate that a poisoning has occurred
   a. Call the local poison control center, emergency facility, or physician for immediate advice regarding treatment
   b. Save all evidence of poison (e.g., container, vomitus, urine)
3. Do not induce vomiting
   a. If the person is comatose, in severe shock, or convulsing or has lost the gag reflex; these conditions can increase the risk of aspiration
   b. If the poison is a low-viscosity hydrocarbon; once aspirated, it can cause a severe chemical pneumonitis
   c. If the poison is a strong corrosive (acid or alkali), emesis of the corrosive redamages the mucosa of the esophagus and pharynx

4. Remove the poison
   a. Dilute with water
   b. Administer activated charcoal (1 g per kg) 30 to 60 minutes after inducing vomiting
   c. Prepare equipment for gastric lavage
5. Prevent aspiration if child is vomiting
   a. Keep the child's head lower than the chest
   b. When alert, place the head between the legs
   c. When unconscious, position on the side
6. Observe for latent symptoms and complications of poisoning
   a. Monitor vital signs
   b. Treat as appropriate (e.g., institute seizure precautions, keep warm and position correctly in case of shock, reduce temperature if hyperpyretic)
7. Support the child and parent
   a. Keep calm and quiet
   b. Do not admonish or accuse the child or parent of wrongdoing
8. Teach prevention of poisoning
   a. Assess possible contributing factors in the occurrence of an accident, such as discipline, parent-child relationship, developmental ability, environmental factors, and behavior problems
   b. Institute anticipatory guidance for possible future accidents based on the child's age and developmental level
   c. Refer to an appropriate agency for evaluation of the home environment and the need for safety measures
   d. Provide assistance with environmental manipulation when necessary
   e. Educate the parents regarding safe storage of all substances
   f. Teach children the hazards of ingesting non-food items without supervision
   g. Caution against keeping large amounts of drugs on hand, especially children's varieties
   h. Discourage transferring drugs to containers without safety caps
   i. Discuss problems of discipline and children's noncompliance

D. EVALUATION/OUTCOMES

1. Recuperates free from complications
2. Parents and child demonstrate knowledge concerning prevention of future poisoning

▼ ACETAMINOPHEN POISONING

Data Base

A. One of the most common drugs taken by children
   1. Toxic dose 150 mg/kg body weight

2. Therapeutic use of 150 mg/kg/day for several days has resulted in toxicity
B. Clinical findings: symptoms of overdose
   1. Nausea; vomiting; profuse diaphoresis; decreased urine output
   2. Pallor; weakness; slow, weak pulse
   3. Jaundice; pain in right upper quadrant; coagulation abnormality; liver failure
   4. Confusion; coma
C. Therapeutic interventions
   1. IV fluid
   2. Administration of antidote (acetylcysteine)

Specific Nursing Care of Children with Acetaminophen Poisoning

A. Identify ingested substance and amount
B. Monitor the electrocardiograph
C. Measure intake and output
D. Measure and record the vital signs frequently
E. Obtain blood for hepatic and renal function tests
F. Support the child and family

▼ SALICYLATE TOXICITY AND POISONING

Data Base

A. Toxic dose: 300 to 500 mg per kilogram of body weight or 7 adult aspirins (28 baby aspirin) for a 9 kg (20 lb) child
B. Clinical findings
   1. Mild salicylate toxicity (subjective symptoms are of little value in small children)
     a. Dehydration: diaphoresis; nausea; vomiting; oliguria
     b. Hyperpyrexia; hyperpnea
     c. Ringing in the ears; dizziness; disturbances of hearing and vision
     d. Delirium
   2. Salicylate poisoning
     a. Hyperventilation: confusion; coma
     b. Metabolic acidosis: anorexia; diaphoresis; increased temperature
     c. Bleeding, especially if chronic ingestion
C. Therapeutic interventions
   1. Gastric lavage, activated charcoal, saline cathartics
   2. IV fluids
   3. Vitamin K if bleeding
   4. Peritoneal dialysis in severe cases
   5. Hypothermia blanket when hyperthermia is present

Specific Nursing Care of Children with Salicylate Poisoning

A. Identify the salicylate overdose

B. Assess blood gases and serum electrolyte concentration frequently
C. Administer sodium bicarbonate, electrolytes, and vitamin K as indicated
D. Maintain on a hypothermia blanket if hyperthermia is present

▼ PETROLEUM DISTILLATE POISONING

Data Base

A. Distillates include kerosene, turpentine, gasoline, lighter fluid, furniture polish, metal polish, benzene, naphthalene, some insecticides, and cleaning fluid
B. Clinical findings
   1. Gagging; choking; and coughing
   2. Nausea; vomiting
   3. Weakness; alterations in sensorium, such as lethargy
   4. Respiratory symptoms of pulmonary involvement: tachypnea; cyanosis; substernal retractions; grunting
C. Therapeutic interventions
   1. Vomiting not induced: aspiration is a particular lar danger because of the risk of a chemical pneumonia
   2. Gastric lavage followed by water, milk, or mineral oil

Specific Nursing Care of Children with Petroleum Distillate Poisoning

A. Identify ingestion of distillates
B. Prevent further irritation
   1. Avoid causing emesis
   2. Implement gastric lavage only as ordered

▼ CORROSIVE CHEMICAL POISONING

Data Base

A. Corrosive chemicals include oven and drain cleaners, electric dishwasher granules, and strong detergents
B. Clinical findings
   1. Severe burning pain in the mouth, throat, and stomach
   2. White, swollen mucous membranes; edema of the lips, tongue, and pharynx (respiratory obstruction)
   3. Violent vomiting; hemoptysis; hematemesis
   4. Signs of shock
   5. Anxiety and agitation
C. Therapeutic intervention: never induce vomiting because regurgitation of the substance will further damage the mucous membranes

Specific Nursing Care of Children with Corrosive Chemical Poisoning

A. Identify ingestion
B. Maintain a patent airway
   1. Examine the pharynx for burns; monitor for respiratory difficulty
   2. Have emergency equipment available; provide an airway if necessary
   3. Administer steroids if prescribed
C. Prevent further irritation
   1. Avoid causing emesis
   2. Give nothing by mouth except as ordered and tolerated; dilute with water and/or give a weak vinegar solution to neutralize acid if ordered
D. Provide comfort and support to the child and family
   1. Administer analgesics as ordered
   2. Remain with the child
   3. Keep parents informed of the child's progress

▼ LEAD POISONING (PLUMBISM)

Data Base

A. A prevalent, significant, preventable health problem that causes neurologic and intellectual damage from even low levels of lead
B. Blood lead concentration should be less than 10 mg per 100 ml of blood
C. Associated with increased levels of lead in the environment and pica: most common source is lead-based paint; soil, dust, or drinking water with lead; parental occupations; hobbies involving lead
D. Clinical findings (chronic ingestion)
   1. Anemia; pallor; listlessness; fatigue
   2. Lead line on teeth and long bones; joint pains
   3. Protein in urine as a result of proximal tubular damage
   4. Behavioral changes: impulsiveness; irritability; hyperactivity; lethargy
   5. Headache; insomnia; brain damage; convulsions; death
E. Therapeutic interventions
   1. Objective: reduce concentration of lead in the blood and soft tissue by promoting its excretion and deposition in bones
      a. Calcium disodium edetate (Calcium Disodium Versenate, calcium EDTA)
         (1) Urine lead content monitored; peak excretion in 24 to 48 hours
         (2) Adverse effects; acute tubular necrosis, malaise, fatigue, numbness of extremities, GI disturbances, fever, pain in muscles and joints
      b. Dimercaprol (BAL)
         (1) Generally used in conjunction with calcium disodium edetate

         (2) Adverse effects: local pain at the site of injection; may cause persistent fever in children receiving therapy; rise in blood pressure accompanied by tachycardia after injection
      c. d-Penicillamine
         (1) Oral chelating agent: increases urinary excretion, but less effective than calcium EDTA
         (2) Adverse effects: transient decrease in white blood cells and platelets; rash; enuresis; abdominal pain
   2. Prevention of further ingestion

Specific Nursing Care of Children with Lead Poisoning

A. Determine environmental exposure
B. Screen children at risk by recognizing clinical findings, especially behavior changes
C. Plan preparation of the child and rotation of injection sites if therapeutic intervention includes IM chelating agents; warm moist applications may relieve discomfort of injections
D. Use therapeutic play including a syringe and doll to help child express feelings
E. Prevent future lead poisoning by parental and child education, appropriate environment, and supervision of child and siblings

▼ FRACTURES

See Medical-Surgical Nursing for additional information

Data Base

A. An interruption in the integrity of a bone
B. In children, bones are more easily injured; fractures can result without major injury to surrounding tissue
C. Healing occurs rapidly in children; rapidity of healing is inversely related to the age of the child
D. Classification
   1. Bend: bone is bent, not broken
   2. Buckle or torus fracture: bone is compressed; appears as a bulge
   3. Greenstick fractures: incomplete break and bending of a long bone, occurs in young children because the bones are soft and not fully mineralized
   4. Complete fractures: bone fragments are divided; may be connected by a periosteal hinge; types include transverse, oblique, spiral
E. Clinical findings
   1. Generalized swelling
   2. Pain or tenderness

3. Diminished function or use of part

F. Therapeutic interventions
   1. Splints; traction
   2. Casts: hard or soft to promote bone alignment and prevent further damage

Nursing Care of Children with Fractures

A. ASSESSMENT
   1. The five Ps associated with neurovascular assessment
      a. Pain and point of tenderness
      b. Pulse distal to fracture site
      c. Pallor
      d. Paresthesia; sensation distal to fracture site
      e. Paralysis; movement distal to fracture site
   2. Cause of injury

B. ANALYSIS/NURSING DIAGNOSES
   1. Fear related to discomfort; unfamiliar apparatus
   2. Risk for injury related to altered mobility; application of devices
   3. Acute pain related to physical injury
   4. Impaired physical mobility related to musculoskeletal impairment
   5. Deficient diversional activity related to limitations in play activities

C. PLANNING/IMPLEMENTATION
   1. Administer analgesics as ordered
   2. Monitor neurovascular status of distal extremity
   3. Provide activity to keep child occupied and entertained
   4. Maintain functional alignment
      a. Keep child positioned by using supportive devices
      b. Jacket restraint may be necessary to prevent twisting or turning

D. EVALUATION/OUTCOMES
   1. Maintains neurovascular status in affected extremity
   2. Experiences minimal discomfort
   3. Maintains skin integrity
   4. Regains tone and flexibility in muscles and joints respectively
   5. Plays and interacts with others

▼ ASPIRATION OF FOREIGN OBJECTS

Data Base

A. Obstruction of the airway by a foreign object; can occur anywhere from larynx to bronchi

B. Most common in children 1 to 3 years of age; leading cause of accidental death in children less than 1 year of age

C. Foods that cause asphyxiation include hot dogs, round candy, peanuts, grapes, and popcorn

D. Classification
   1. Partial obstruction has time interval (hours to days) without symptoms
   2. Complete obstruction is an emergency

E. Clinical findings
   1. Complete obstruction: substernal retractions; inability to cough or speak; increased pulse and respiratory rate; cyanosis
   2. Partial obstruction: persistent respiratory infection; hoarseness or garbled speech; wheeze; stridor

F. Therapeutic interventions
   1. Incomplete obstruction: no intervention; allow child to continue coughing until object is dislodged
   2. Complete obstruction: immediate first aid
      a. Try to pull the object out if possible without forcing it further down
      b. Turn the small child upside down (head lower than chest) and deliver up to five quick, sharp back blows with the heel of the hand; turn the child over and deliver up to five quick chest thrusts using the technique for CPR
      c. Abdominal thrust for children aged 1 year and older (Heimlich maneuver): grasp the victim from behind around the upper abdomen and squeeze, forcing the diaphragm up
   3. Medical removal by bronchoscopy
   4. Surgical relief by a tracheotomy below level of the object

Nursing Care of Children Who Aspirate Foreign Objects

A. ASSESSMENT
   1. Breathing pattern
   2. Absence of speech
   3. Color

B. ANALYSIS/NURSING DIAGNOSES
   1. Ineffective airway clearance related to obstruction
   2. Anxiety related to parents' perceived threat to life of child; child's inability to breathe
   3. Risk for suffocation related to lack of knowledge about risk factors

C. PLANNING/IMPLEMENTATION
   1. Keep small objects such as balloons, buttons, and batteries out of the child's reach; inspect larger toys for removable objects
   2. Avoid giving young children foods easily aspirated, such as nuts or hot dogs
   3. Teach the child: not to run or laugh with food or fluid in the mouth; to chew food well before swallowing

D. EVALUATION/OUTCOMES
   1. Regains a patent airway

2. Child and parents verbalize ways to prevent future airway obstruction

▼ CHILD MALTREATMENT (ABUSE)

Data Base

A. One of the most significant social problems affecting children
B. Intentional physical abuse or neglect, emotional abuse or neglect, and sexual abuse of children
C. Family characteristics
   1. Difficulty controlling aggressive impulses
   2. Use of violence to resolve conflict
   3. Unpredictable, unstable family environment
   4. Inability to deal with serial crises
   5. Low trust for outsiders and family members
   6. Isolation from community and social supports
D. Child characteristics
   1. Temperament
   2. Position in family
   3. Additional physical needs
   4. Activity level
   5. Degree of sensitivity to parental needs
E. Environmental characteristics
   1. Atmosphere of chronic stress
   2. Presence of alcohol or substance abuse
F. Classification
   1. Neglect: the most common form of maltreatment; includes emotional neglect, physical neglect, and emotional abuse
   2. Physical abuse: minor physical abuse responsible for more reported cases than major physical abuse, which results in increased mortality
   3. Sexual abuse: incest; molestation; exhibitionism; pedophilia; child pornography or prostitution
G. Clinical findings
   1. Physical evidence of abuse/previous injuries
   2. Conflicting stories about injury
   3. Inappropriate parental response
   4. Inappropriate response of child
H. Therapeutic interventions
   1. Treat injury
   2. Identify and protect child from further abuse

Nursing Care of Children Who are Maltreated

A. ASSESSMENT
   1. History of injury
   2. Physical status; evidence of past injuries
   3. Parent-child interaction
   4. Developmental level of child
B. ANALYSIS/NURSING DIAGNOSES
   1. Fear related to negative interpersonal interaction; repeated maltreatment

2. Powerlessness related to inability to protect self; lack of safe place to go
   3. Impaired parenting related to abusive or neglectful caregiver(s); situational characteristics
   4. Risk for trauma related to characteristics of child; caregiver(s)
C. PLANNING/IMPLEMENTATION
   1. Be alert for clues that indicate child neglect or abuse
      a. The child has many unexplained injuries, scars, bruises
      b. Parents offer inconsistent stories explaining child's injuries when questioned
      c. Emotional response of parents is inconsistent with the degree of the child's injury
      d. Parents may resist or fail to be present for questioning
      e. The child exhibits physical signs of neglect: malnourished, dehydrated, unkempt
      f. The child cringes when physically approached and appears unduly afraid
      g. The child responds in a manner that indicates avoiding punishment rather than gaining reward
      h. The child has excessive interest in sexual matters
      i. The child has a sexually transmitted disease
   2. Be aware of child abuse laws; most states mandate reporting
   3. Recognize that the main objective is to protect the child from further abuse
   4. Focus on helping parents with their own dependency needs; use group therapy; home visiting; foster grandparents
   5. Help parents learn to control frustration through other outlets
   6. Educate parents about the child's normal needs and development, new modes of discipline, and realistic expectations
   7. Use therapeutic play to help child express feelings
   8. Provide emotional support and therapy for the child because children frequently grow up to be abusing parents
D. EVALUATION/OUTCOMES
   1. Remains free from injury or neglect
   2. Parents demonstrate effective parenting activities

▼ MENTAL RETARDATION (COGNITIVE IMPAIRMENT)

Data Base

A. Causes
   1. Infection and intoxication: congenital rubella;

syphilis; maternal alcohol or drug consumption; chronic lead ingestion; kernicterus (high bilirubin level)
   2. Injury to the brain suffered during the prenatal, perinatal, or postnatal periods; intracranial hemorrhage; anoxia; physical injury
   3. Inadequate nutrition and metabolic or endocrine disorders such as PKU or hypothyroidism
   4. Unknown prenatal influences, including cerebral and cranial malformations such as microcephalus and hydrocephalus
   5. Gestational disorders including low birth weight, prematurity, or postmaturity
   6. Chromosomal abnormalities such as Down syndrome and fragile X syndrome
   7. Environmental influences including deprived environment associated with parents and siblings with mental retardation
B. Conditions that may lead to a false diagnosis of mental retardation
   1. Emotional disturbance (e.g., autism, maternal deprivation)
   2. Sensory problems (e.g., deafness, blindness)
   3. Cerebral dysfunctions (e.g., cerebral palsy, learning disorders, hyperkinesia, seizure disorders)
C. Classification
   1. Normal: 90 to 110 IQ
   2. Borderline: 71 to 89 IQ
   3. Mild: 50/55 to 70 IQ
      a. Educable: can achieve a mental age of 8 to 12 years
      b. Can learn to read, write, do arithmetic, achieve a vocational skill, and function in society
   4. Moderate: 35/40 to 50/55 IQ
      a. Trainable: can achieve a mental age of 3 to 7 years
      b. Can learn the activities of daily living, social skills; can be trained to work in a sheltered workshop
   5. Severe: below 20/25 to 35/40 IQ
      a. Barely trainable: can achieve a mental age of 0 to 2 years
      b. Totally dependent on others and in need of custodial care
   6. Profound: below 20/25 IQ
      a. May attain mental age of young infant
      b. Requires total care
D. Clinical findings
   1. Delayed milestones: infant fails to suck; head lag after 4 to 6 months of age; slow in learning self-help; slow to respond to new stimuli; slow or absent speech development
   2. Mental abilities are concrete; abstract ability is limited; may repeat words (echolalia)
   3. Lacks power of self-appraisal; does not learn from errors
   4. Cannot carry out complex instructions; learns rote responses and socially acceptable behavior
   5. Does not relate to peers; more secure with adults; comforted by physical touch
   6. Short attention span, but usually attracted to music
E. Therapeutic interventions
   1. Prevent causes that damage brain cells such as hypoxia, untreated PKU
   2. Identify condition early
   3. Minimize long-term consequences: treatment of associated problems; infant stimulation; parental education

Nursing Care of Children Who Are Cognitively Impaired

A. ASSESSMENT
   1. Developmental screening
   2. Associated illnesses/risk factors

B. ANALYSIS/NURSING DIAGNOSES
   1. Interrupted family processes related to having a child who is cognitively impaired
   2. Compromised family coping related to situational/developmental crisis
   3. Delayed growth and development related to impaired cognitive function

C. PLANNING/IMPLEMENTATION
   1. Consider the child's developmental, not chronologic, age
      a. Educate the parent regarding developmental age
      b. Near adolescence, sexual feelings accompany maturation and need to be explained according to the child's mental capacity
   2. Set realistic goals; teach by simple steps for habit formation rather than for understanding or transference of learning
      a. Break down the process of skills learning into simple steps that can be easily achieved; ensure each step is learned completely before teaching the child the next step
      b. Recognize that behavior modification is a very effective method of teaching these children; praise accomplishments to develop the child's self-esteem
      c. Keep discipline simple, geared toward learning acceptable behavior rather than developing judgment
      d. Recognize that routines are the foundation of the child's lifestyle; hospital routines should be based on the child's normal schedule

D. EVALUATION/OUTCOMES
   1. Performs activities of daily living at optimum level

2. Family members make realistic decisions based on their needs and capabilities

▼ CEREBRAL PALSY

Data Base

A. Nonspecific term for a neuromuscular disability or difficulty in controlling voluntary muscles (caused by damage to some portion of the brain, with associated sensory, intellectual, emotional, or seizure disorders)

B. Characteristics of cerebral palsy
   1. Affects young children, usually becoming evident before 3 years of age
   2. Nonprogressive, but persists throughout life
   3. Some motor dysfunction always present
   4. Mental deficiency may be present; language deficit may be present

C. Major causes
   1. Prenatal brain abnormalities
   2. Prematurity
   3. Anoxia of the brain caused by a variety of insults at or near the time of birth
   4. Trauma; cerebral vascular accident
   5. No identified cause in 24% of affected children

D. Classification (based on predominant clinical manifestations)
   1. Spastic type: hypertonicity with poor control of posture, balance, and coordinated movements; impairment of gross and fine motor skills
   2. Dyskinetic type: abnormal involuntary movement
      a. Athetosis; characterized by slow, worm-like, writhing movements
      b. Involvement of mouth and throat that results in drooling
   3. Ataxic type: wide-based gait; rapid repetitive movements performed inadequately
   4. Mixed type: combination of spasticity and athetosis

E. Clinical findings
   1. Difficulty in feeding, especially sucking and swallowing
   2. Delayed motor development; abnormal motor performance; asymmetry of motion or contour of body
   3. Delayed speech development
   4. Reflex abnormalities (e.g., hyperreflexia)
   5. Any of the muscular abnormalities listed under classification

F. Therapeutic interventions
   1. Multidisciplinary approach
   2. Mobility devices
   3. Surgery to correct spastic muscle imbalance
   4. Medications, such as skeletal muscle relaxants and anticonvulsants
   5. Physiotherapy, occupational and speech therapy

Nursing Care of Children with Cerebral Palsy

A. ASSESSMENT
   1. Presence of prenatal/perinatal risk factors
   2. Ineffective feeding
   3. Muscles for rigidity, tenseness, hypotonia
   4. Delayed developmental milestones

B. ANALYSIS/NURSING DIAGNOSES
   1. Disturbed body image related to physical disability; appearance
   2. Interrupted family processes related to the birth of a child with special needs
   3. Fatigue related to increased energy expenditure
   4. Risk for injury related to neuromuscular impairments; cognitive-perceptual impairments
   5. Impaired physical mobility related to neuromuscular impairment
   6. Feeding, bathing/ hygiene, dressing/grooming, toileting self-care deficits related to impaired neuromuscular development
   7. Impaired verbal communication related to neuromuscular impairment

C. PLANNING/IMPLEMENTATION
   1. Feeding
      a. Recognize drooling results from difficulty in swallowing
      b. Use a spoon and blunt fork, with plate attached to the table, for easier self-feeding
      c. Provide increased calories because of excessive energy expenditure, increased protein for muscle activity, and increased vitamins (especially B_6) for amino acid metabolism
   2. Relaxation: provide rest periods in an area with few stimuli; set limits and control activity level
   3. Safety
      a. Protect from accidents resulting from altered sensation, impaired balance, and lack of muscle control
      b. Provide helmet for protection against head injuries
      c. Evaluate need for restraint
   4. Play
      a. Keep safety as main objective; do not overstimulate
      b. Play should have educational value, appropriate to developmental level and ability
   5. Elimination
      a. Recognize difficulty in toilet training results from poor muscle control
      b. Provide special bowel and bladder training
   6. Speech

a. Recognize poor coordination of lips, tongue, cheeks, larynx, and poor control of diaphragm make formation of words difficult
b. Refer for speech therapy

7. Breathing
a. Recognize impaired control of the intercostal muscles and diaphragm makes the child prone to respiratory tract infection
b. Protect the child from exposure to infection as much as possible; be alert for symptoms of aspiration pneumonia

8. Dental problems
a. Recognize problems in muscular control affect development and alignment of teeth
b. Explain that frequent dental caries occur and that there is a great need for dental supervision and care
c. Teach the parent to brush the child's teeth if muscular dysfunction is present

9. Vision
a. Recognize that common ocular problems such as strabismus and refractive errors may be related to poor muscular control
b. Look for such disorders to prevent further problems such as amblyopia

10. Hearing
a. Recognize hearing problems may be present, depending on the area brain damage
b. Encourage parents to have child's hearing checked periodically

11. Mobility
a. Perform passive and encourage active range-of-motion exercises to prevent contractures
b. Encourage use of leg braces if prescribed to stretch heel cords
c. Encourage the use of assistive devices such as a wheeled walker to promote stability

D. EVALUATION/OUTCOMES
1. Remains safe from injury
2. Consumes adequate nutrients for growth
3. Communicates needs to caregivers
4. Performs self-care activities within capabilities
5. Exhibits behavior indicative of positive self-image
6. Family verbalizes effect of child's disability on family

▼ HEARING IMPAIRMENT

Data Base
A. Causes
1. Family history of childhood hearing impairment
2. Anatomic malformations, Down syndrome, cerebral palsy

3. Perinatal factors; low birth weight; severe perinatal asphyxia; infection (cytomegalovirus, rubella, herpes, syphilis, toxoplasmosis, bacterial meningitis)
4. Chronic ear infections
5. Ototoxic drugs such as gentamicin
6. Environmental: continuous exposure to noises made by equipment in a neonatal intensive care unit; loud noises such as gunfire or continuous exposure to less intense noises

B. Types of hearing loss
1. Conductive: loss results from interference of transmission of sound to middle ear
a. Interferes mainly with loudness of sound
b. Most frequent cause is recurrent otitis media
c. Most common of all types of hearing loss
2. Sensorineural: damage to inner ear structures of the auditory nerve
a. Distortion in clarity of words
b. Problem in discrimination of sounds
c. Common causes: kernicterus, ototoxic drugs, excessive noise exposure
3. Mixed conductive-sensorineural
4. Central auditory imperception
a. Not explained by other three causes
b. The child hears but does not understand

C. Classification
1. Hard of hearing (16-25 decibels): has difficulty hearing faint or distant speech, usually unaware of problem; may have some problems in school; no speech defects
2. Mild (26-40 decibels): can miss 25% to 40% of discussions; may have some speech difficulties
3. Moderate (41-55 decibels): understands face-to-face conversational speech at a distance of 3 to 5 feet. Limited vocabulary and imperfect speech production
4. Moderately severe (56-70 decibels—hard of hearing): unable to understand conversational speech unless loud; considerable difficulty with classroom discussion; requires speech training
5. Severe (71-90 decibels—deaf): may hear loud noises if nearby; may be able to identify loud environmental noises; requires speech training
6. Profound (>90 decibels—deaf): may hear only loud noises; requires extensive speech training

D. Clinical findings
1. Lack of the Moro reflex in response to a sharp clap; failure to respond to loud noise
2. Failure to locate a source of sound at 2 to 3 feet after 6 months of age
3. Absence of babble by 7 months of age
4. Inability to understand words or phrases by 12 months of age
5. Use of gestures rather than verbalization to establish wants

6. History of frequent respiratory tract infections and otitis media
E. Therapeutic interventions
 1. Conductive loss: tympanostomy tubes for chronic otitis media; hearing aids to amplify sounds
 2. Sensorineural: cochlear implants; hearing aids of less value
 3. Central auditory imperception: may not respond to any therapy

Nursing Care of Children with Impaired Hearing
A. ASSESSMENT
 1. History that places child at risk
 2. Response to auditory stimuli
 3. Failure to develop intelligible speech by 24 months
B. ANALYSIS/NURSING DIAGNOSES
 1. Interrupted family processes related to situational crisis; difficulty in communication
 2. Delayed growth and development related to impaired communication
 3. Risk for injury related to perceptual impairment
 4. Disturbed sensory perception (auditory) related to hearing impairment
 5. Impaired verbal communication related to loss of hearing before speech is established
C. PLANNING/IMPLEMENTATION
 1. Observe for manifestations beginning at birth
 2. Face the child to facilitate lip reading; have a good light on speaker's face
 3. Be level with the child's face and speak toward the unaffected ear; do not walk back and forth while talking
 4. Always enunciate and articulate carefully; do not talk too loudly, especially if the loss is sensorineural
 5. Use facial expressions, since verbal intonations are not communicated
 6. Encourage active play to express feelings and build self-confidence
D. EVALUATION/OUTCOMES
 1. Remains safe
 2. Uses a hearing aid
 3. Engages in activities appropriate to developmental level
 4. Child/family communicates effectively

▼ VISUAL IMPAIRMENT

Data Base
A. Definition: Visual impairment general term referring to visual loss that cannot be corrected with regular prescription glasses

1. School vision (partially sighted): visual acuity is between 20/70 and 20/200; able to participate in school with usual size print
2. Legal blindness: visual acuity between 20/200 or less or a visual field of 20 degrees or less in the better eye; child is eligible for special services
B. Strabismus: imbalance of the extraocular muscles causing a physiologic incoordination of the eye
 1. Amblyopia develops in the weak eye from disuse; must be corrected before 4 years of age to prevent blindness
 2. Treatment: patch the unaffected and exercise the weak eye to force the weak eye to fixate; surgery to lengthen or shorten the extraocular muscles
C. Causes other than strabismus
 1. Perinatal infections: herpes; rubella; gonococci
 2. Congenital cataracts
 3. Retinopathy of prematurity
 4. Postnatal infections: meningitis
 5. Postnatal: trauma; tumor; diabetes mellitus
D. Clinical findings
 1. Delayed motor development
 2. Rocking for sensory stimulation
 3. Squinting; rubbing eyes; sitting close to television; holding book close to face
 4. Clumsiness (e.g., bumping into objects)
E. Therapeutic interventions
 1. Surgical intervention for strabismus and cataracts
 2. Corrective lenses

Nursing Care of Children with Impaired Vision
A. ASSESSMENT
 1. Factors that indicate children at risk
 2. Behavior indicative of vision loss
 3. Visual acuity and signs of ocular disorders
B. ANALYSIS/NURSING DIAGNOSES
 1. Readiness for enhanced family coping related to situational/developmental crisis
 2. Delayed growth and development related to sensory/perceptual alterations (visual)
 3. Risk for injury related to perceptual impairment
C. PLANNING/IMPLEMENTATION
 1. Assess for early signs of visual problems
 2. Explain to and encourage parents to follow treatments for strabismus and other conditions
 3. Talk clearly; use noise so the child can locate your position
 4. Help the child learn through other senses, especially touch, with play activities
 5. Facilitate eating
  a. Arrange food on the plate at clock hours and teach the child its location
  b. Provide finger foods when possible

c. Provide a light spoon and deep bowl so the child can feel weight of food on spoon

D. EVALUATION/OUTCOMES

1. Remains free from injury
2. Engages in appropriate activities for level of development
3. Child and other family members demonstrate a positive relationship

▼ LYME DISEASE

See Medical-Surgical Nursing for Lyme Disease

▼ CELIAC DISEASE

Data Base

A. Known as gluten-sensitive enteropathy and celiac-sprue
B. Chronic intestinal malabsorption and inability to digest gluten, a protein found mostly in wheat, rye, oats, and barley
C. Identified several months after introduction of gluten-containing grain into the diet; usually between 1 and 5 years of age
D. Progression of illness
   1. Fat absorption affected in early stage of disease
   2. Protein, carbohydrate, mineral, and electrolyte absorption then affected
   3. Growth failure and muscle wasting finally occur
E. Clinical findings
   1. Progressive malnutrition: anorexia; muscle wasting; distended abdomen
   2. Secondary deficiencies: anemia and rickets
   3. Behavioral changes: irritability, fretfulness, apathy
   4. Watery, pale, foul-smelling stool
   5. Celiac crisis: severe episode of dehydration and acidosis from diarrhea
F. Therapeutic intervention: dietary
   1. Low in glutens; no wheat, rye, oats, or barley
   2. High in calories and protein
   3. Low fat
   4. Small, frequent feedings; adequate fluids
   5. Vitamin supplements, all in water-miscible form; supplemental iron

Nursing Care of Children with Celiac Disease

A. ASSESSMENT

1. Nutritional status
2. Parent/child knowledge of dietary regimen

B. ANALYSIS/NURSING DIAGNOSES

1. Risk for injury related to knowledge deficit about diet and food composition
2. Imbalanced nutrition: less than body requirements related to impaired intestinal absorption

C. PLANNING/IMPLEMENTATION

1. Teach parents and child about dietary restrictions
2. Explain need for frequent health supervision
3. Provide support to facilitate adherence to dietary regimen

D. EVALUATION/OUTCOMES

1. Parent/child verbalizes correct dietary information
2. Consumes adequate calories for growth and development

▼ CYSTIC FIBROSIS

Data Base

A. Autosomal recessive disorder affecting the exocrine glands
B. Most common serious pulmonary and genetic disease of children
C. Elevation in sweat electrolytes: sodium and chloride are three to five times higher than normal; chloride levels above 60 mEq/L are diagnostic
D. Increased viscosity of mucous gland secretions is responsible for clinical findings
   1. Pancreas: becomes fibrotic, with a decreased production of pancreatic enzymes (late complication is diabetes mellitus)
      a. Lipase: causes steatorrhea (fatty, foul, bulky stools)
      b. Trypsin: causes increased nitrogen in stool
      c. Amylase: inability to break down polysaccharides
   2. Rectal prolapse
   3. Respiratory system: increased viscous mucus in the trachea, bronchi, and bronchioles that interferes with expiration (emphysema) and increases the incidence of infection
   4. Liver: possible cirrhosis from biliary obstruction, malnutrition, or infection; portal hypertension leads to esophageal varices
   5. Sexual organs: infertility may occur
E. Clinical findings
   1. Early manifestations during infancy
      a. Meconium ileus at birth (about 15%)
      b. Failure to regain normal 10% weight loss at birth
      c. Presence of cough or wheezing during first 6 months of age
   2. Respiratory involvement evidenced by clubbing of fingers, barrel-shaped chest, cyanosis, distended neck veins
   3. Cardiac enlargement, particularly right ventricular hypertrophy (cor pulmonale)

F. Therapeutic interventions
1. Pulmonary problems: chest physiotherapy; bronchodilators; antibiotic therapy as indicated
2. Gastrointestinal problems: pancreatic enzyme supplements; balanced nutritional intake

Nursing Care of Children with Cystic Fibrosis (CF)

A. ASSESSMENT
1. Respiratory status
2. Gastrointestinal status
3. Failure to thrive

B. ANALYSIS/NURSING DIAGNOSES
1. Activity intolerance related to imbalance between oxygen supply and demand
2. Ineffective airway clearance related to secretion of thick, tenacious mucus
3. Risk for infection related to stasis of respiratory secretions
4. Interrupted family processes related to having a child with a chronic illness
5. Disturbed body image related to changes in body configuration as disease progresses
6. Imbalanced nutrition: less than body requirements related to impaired digestive process

C. PLANNING/IMPLEMENTATION
1. Prevent respiratory tract infections
   a. Postural drainage, percussion, and vibration between feedings
   b. Use of expectorants, antibiotics, aerosol therapy; avoid antitussives and antihistamines
2. Promote optimal nutrition
   a. Administer pancreatic enzymes with cold food in middle of meal
   b. Administer fat-soluble vitamins in water-miscible form
   c. Encourage high-protein diet of easily digested food, normal fat, high calories
3. Promote mobility and activity
   a. Encourage activity and regular exercise
   b. Help the child regulate activity to own tolerance
4. Promote a positive body image
   a. Help child deal with barrel-shaped chest, low weight, thin extremities, bluish coloring, smell of stools
   b. Encourage hygiene and select clothes that compensate for protuberant abdomen and emaciated extremities
5. Provide for emotional support and counseling for child and family
   a. Recognize that CF is a long-term problem that causes financial and emotional stresses
   b. Understand that this chronic illness can become a major controlling factor in the family

(1) The child begins to recognize that wheezing brings attention and uses this knowledge
(2) Parents can deal with such behavior by recognizing false attacks and using consistent discipline
c. Encourage the family to join the Cystic Fibrosis Foundation
d. Refer family for genetic counseling

D. EVALUATION/OUTCOMES
1. Engages in activity that has a balance between oxygen supply and demand
2. Maintains a patent airway
3. Consumes adequate calories for growth and development
4. Family members demonstrate ability to care for child

▼ IRON DEFICIENCY ANEMIA

Data Base

A. Most prevalent nutritional disorder among children in the United States; caused by lack of adequate sources of dietary iron
1. Infant usually has iron reserve for 6 months
2. Premature infant lacks reserve
3. Children receiving only milk have no source of iron (milk babies)
B. Insidious onset: usually diagnosed because of an infection or chronic GI problems
C. Causes
1. Decreased intake
2. Increased loss
D. Clinical findings
1. Pallor; weakness; tachycardia; dizziness
2. Slow motor development; poor muscle tone
3. Hemoglobin level below normal for age (general rule: below 11 g/dl)
E. Therapeutic interventions
1. Food sources rich in iron
   a. Iron-fortified formula
   b. Iron-fortified infant cereal
2. Iron replacement
   a. Oral iron sources
      (1) Ferrous sulfate—most absorbable form of iron
      (2) Adverse effects: nausea, vomiting; fatalities in children who ingest enteric-coated tablets, thinking they are candy
   b. Parenteral iron sources for children with iron malabsorption or chronic hemoglobinuria
      (1) Iron-dextran injection (Imferon)

(2) Adverse effects: tissue staining (use Z track for intramuscular injection), fever, lymphadenopathy, nausea, vomiting, arthralgia, urticaria, severe peripheral vascular failure, anaphylaxis, secondary hematochromatosis

Nursing Care of Children with Iron Deficiency Anemia

A. ASSESSMENT
1. Nutritional history and status
2. History of chronic infection
3. Family history of hematologic disorder
4. Eating habits: pica; ingestion of lead
5. Bowel habits; blood in stools

B. ANALYSIS/NURSING DIAGNOSES
1. Ineffective tissue perfusion (cardiovascular) related to decreased oxygen carrying capacity of the blood
2. Activity intolerance related to imbalance between oxygen supply and demand
3. Imbalanced nutrition: less than body requirements related to knowledge deficit of appropriate foods

C. PLANNING/IMPLEMENTATION
1. Prevent development of anemia
   a. Teach pregnant women the importance of their iron intake
   b. Encourage feeding of iron-fortified infant formula or breastfeeding
   c. Encourage feeding iron-fortified infant cereal
   d. Introduce foods high in iron
2. Provide for proper administration of supplemental iron
   a. Vitamin C aids absorption
   b. Folic acid acts as a coenzyme in the formation of heme; proteins are necessary for the synthesis of hemoglobin; ascorbic acid promotes the conversion of folic acid to folinic acid
   c. Oxalates, phosphate, and caffeine decrease absorption
   d. Provide a straw because some liquid preparations stain teeth
   e. Colors stools blackish-green; may cause gastric irritation or constipation

D. EVALUATION/OUTCOMES
1. Engages in appropriate activities without fatigue
2. Consumes adequate nutrients for correction of anemia
3. Parents can verbalize dietary requirements of child

▼ SICKLE CELL ANEMIA

Data Base
A. Autosomal disorder affecting hemoglobin
B. Defective hemoglobin causes red blood cells to become sickle shaped and clump together under reduced oxygen tension; initially fetal hemoglobin prevents sickling
C. Classification
   1. Sickle cell anemia: homozygous for sickle cell gene
   2. Sickle cell trait: heterozygous for sickle cell gene
D. Clinical findings
   1. Vaso-occlusive crisis (preferably called "painful episode"): most common and non–life threatening
      a. Results from sickled cells obstructing blood vessels, causing occlusion, ischemia, and potential necrosis
      b. Symptoms include fever, acute abdominal pain (visceral hypoxia), hand-foot syndrome, priapism, and arthralgia without an exacerbation of anemia
   2. Sequestration crisis
      a. Results from the spleen pooling large quantities of blood, which causes a precipitous drop in blood pressure and ultimately shock
      b. Acute episode occurs most commonly in children between 8 months and 5 years of age; can result in death from anemia and cardiovascular collapse
      c. Chronic manifestation is termed functional asplenia
   3. Aplastic crisis: diminished red blood cell production
      a. May be triggered by a viral or other infection
      b. Profound anemia results from rapid destruction of red blood cells combined with a decreased production
   4. Hyperhemolytic crisis: increased rate of red blood cell destruction
      a. Characterized by anemia, jaundice, and reticulocytosis
      b. Rare complication that frequently suggests a coexisting abnormality such as glucose-6-phosphate dehydrogenase deficiency
   5. Stroke: sudden and severe complication with no related illnesses
      a. Sickled cells block the major blood vessels in the brain
      b. Repeat strokes in 60% of children who have experienced previous one
   6. Chest syndrome: clinically similar to pneumonia
   7. Overwhelming infection: Streptococcus pneumonia; *Haemophilus influenzae* type B
E. Therapeutic interventions
   1. Prevention of sickling phenomenon
      a. Adequate oxygenation

b. Adequate hydration
c. Administration of hydroxyurea to increase fetal hemoglobin
d. Blood transfusions to decrease production of cells with sickle hemoglobin
2. Treatment of crisis
   a. Pain management; rest
   b. Hydration/electrolyte replacement
   c. Antibiotic therapy
   d. Blood products

Nursing Care of Children with Sickle Cell Anemia

A. ASSESSMENT
1. Vital signs; neurologic signs
2. Vision/hearing
3. Location and intensity of pain
4. Spleen size

B. ANALYSIS/NURSING DIAGNOSES
1. Disturbed body image related to impaired growth and maturation; chronic illness
2. Fear related to unfamiliar environment; separation from support system
3. Pain related to tissue ischemia
4. Ineffective tissue perfusion (cardiovascular) related to decreased oxygen tension
5. Interrupted family processes related to having a child with a chronic illness

C. PLANNING/IMPLEMENTATION
1. Avoid dehydration
   a. May cause rapid thrombus formation and crisis
   b. Daily fluid intake should be calculated according to body weight (130 to 200 ml per kilogram)
   c. During crisis, fluid needs to be increased, especially if the child is febrile
2. Prevent crisis
   a. Avoid infection, dehydration, and other conditions causing strain on body, which precipitates a crisis; prophylactic use of pneumococcal, meningococcal, and *Haemophilus* flu vaccines; hepatitis B for those children who did not receive it with routine immunizations
   b. Avoid hypoxia; treat respiratory tract infections immediately
3. During crisis provide for
   a. Adequate hydration (may need IV therapy)
   b. Proper positioning (head of bed elevated; joints supported); careful handling
   c. Exercise as tolerated (immobility promotes thrombus formation and respiratory problems)
   d. Adequate ventilation
   e. Control of pain; use comfort measures; administer ordered narcotics; schedule medication administration to prevent pain
   f. Blood transfusions for severe anemia
4. Provide for genetic counseling
   a. Disorder mostly of blacks; can be found in Mediterranean people
   b. Parents need to know the risk of having other children with trait or disease
   c. If both parents are carriers, each pregnancy has 25% chance of producing a child with the disease
   d. Screen young children for the disorder because clinical manifestations usually do not appear before 6 months of age
5. Support parents

D. EVALUATION/OUTCOMES
1. Reports minimal pain
2. Verbalizes feelings about disease process
3. Demonstrates behaviors reflective of a positive body image
4. Remains free from crisis

▼ β-THALASSEMIA (COOLEY'S ANEMIA)

Data Base
A. Autosomal disorder with varied expressivity
B. Basic defect seems to be a deficiency in the synthesis of β-chain polypeptides, which results in a decreased rate of production of the globin molecule
C. Classification
1. Thalassemia trait: heterozygous, mild anemia
2. Thalassemia intermedia: splenomegaly, severe anemia
3. Thalassemia major: severe anemia; incompatible with life without transfusions
D. Clinical findings
1. Severe anemia
2. Unexplained fever; headache
3. Anorexia; impaired feeding
4. Enlarged abdomen; splenomegaly; hepatomegaly
5. Impaired physical growth
6. Listlessness; exercise intolerance
E. Therapeutic interventions
1. Use of blood transfusions to maintain adequate hemoglobin levels
2. Iron-chelating agents such as deferoxamine (Desferal) are given to reduce iron storage; transfusions greatly increase the risk of hemosiderosis (excessive iron storage in various tissues of the body, especially the spleen, liver, lymph glands, heart, and pancreas), hemochromatosis (excessive iron storage with resultant cellular damage), HF, and pulmonary edema
3. Bone marrow transplantation

Nursing Care of Children with β-Thalassemia (Cooley's Anemia)

A. ASSESSMENT
1. Family history
2. Red blood cells for significant anemia

B. ANALYSIS/NURSING DIAGNOSES
1. Activity intolerance related to general weakness
2. Disturbed body image related to impaired growth and maturation; chronic illness
3. Interrupted family processes related to situational crisis (child with a disability/serious illness)
4. Fear related to unfamiliar environment; separation from support system
5. Anticipatory grieving related to perceived potential loss of child

C. PLANNING/IMPLEMENTATION
1. Be alert for signs and symptoms in older infants or young children of Mediterranean descent (Italian, Greek, Syrian)
2. Prevent infection: avoid contact with persons who have infections; administer prophylactic antibiotics
3. Prevent complications
   a. Monitor during transfusions
   b. Administer chelating agents and folic acid as ordered
   c. Teach to avoid activities that increase risk of fractures
   d. Observe for signs of cholecystitis in the adolescent
4. Assist the child in coping with the disorder and its effects
   a. Explore the child's feelings about being different from other children
   b. Emphasize the child's abilities and focus on realistic endeavors
   c. Encourage quiet activities, creative efforts, and "thinking" games
   d. Encourage interaction with peers; introduce the child to other children who have adjusted well to this or a similar disorder
   e. Help plan therapies and medical care so they do not interfere with the child's regular activities and social interaction
   f. Assist the child with vocational planning
5. Support parents
   a. Explore feelings regarding the hereditary nature of the disease
   b. Emphasize the need for the child to lead as normal a life as possible
   c. Help the family deal with the potentially fatal nature of the disease
6. Prevent the occurrence of β-thalassemia: refer for genetic counseling; reinforce and clarify counseling information

D. EVALUATION/OUTCOMES
1. Participates in appropriate activities for energy level
2. Verbalizes feelings about disease/hospitalization
3. Demonstrates behaviors reflective of a positive body image
4. Parents demonstrate ability to care for child
5. Parents verbalize feelings and concerns about seriousness of illness

▼ PINWORMS

Data Base

A. Most common intestinal parasite in United States
B. Children reinfest themselves by fingers-to-anus-to-mouth route; can also be infested by breathing airborne ova
C. Crowded conditions such as classrooms and day-care centers increase risk of transmission
D. Clinical findings
   1. Severe pruritus of the anal area; pinworm eggs isolated from the perianal area; cellophane-tape test done first thing in the morning before first bowel movement
   2. Irritability and insomnia
   3. Anorexia; weight loss
   4. Eosinophilia
   5. Signs of complications: vaginitis; appendicitis
E. Therapeutic interventions: Mebendazole (Vermox) is drug of choice
   1. Selectively and irreversibly inhibits uptake of glucose and other nutrients of pinworms
   2. Adverse effects: occasional, transient abdominal pain and diarrhea

Nursing Care of Children with Pinworms

A. ASSESSMENT
1. Perianal area for signs of inflammation
2. Cellophane-tape test in AM before a bowel movement

B. ANALYSIS/NURSING DIAGNOSES
1. Pain related to severe itching in the rectal area
2. Risk for impaired skin integrity related to irritation of the perianal area

C. PLANNING/IMPLEMENTATION
1. Prevent reinfestation
   a. Wash anal area thoroughly at least once a day
   b. Place a tight diaper or underpants on child; change child's clothes and bedding daily and wash in hot water
   c. Do not allow the child to scratch the anus; keep fingernails short; child may need to wear mittens
   d. Air out bedroom; dust and vacuum house thoroughly

2. Teach parents about administration of medication
   a. Increasing dose will not produce a quicker recovery
   b. Stools contain worms; may turn bright red from medication
   c. Additional series of medication may be used depending on medication; frequently 2 weeks after initial dose; all family members are usually treated
D. **EVALUATION/OUTCOMES**
   1. Maintains intact perianal skin
   2. Produces stool that is free of infestation

▼ EMOTIONAL DISORDERS

For common emotional disorders of the toddler see Disorders Usually First Evident in Infancy, Childhood, or Adolescence in Mental Health Nursing

THE PRESCHOOLER

GROWTH AND DEVELOPMENT
Developmental Timetable
3 years
A. Physical
   1. Usual weight gain 1.8 to 2.7 kg (4 to 6 lb)
   2. Usual height gain 7.5 cm (3 inches)
B. Motor
   1. Jumps off bottom step; walks upstairs alternating feet
   2. Rides a tricycle using pedals
   3. Constructs three-block bridge; builds tower of 9 or 10 cubes
   4. Can unbutton front or side button; uses a spoon
   5. Usually toilet trained at night
C. Sensory: visual acuity 20/30
D. Vocalization and socialization
   1. Vocabulary of about 900 words; uses three-to four-word sentences; uses plurals; may have normal hesitation in speech pattern
   2. Begins to understand ideas of sharing and taking turns
E. Mental abilities
   1. Beginning understanding of the past, present, future, or any aspect of time
   2. Stage of magical thinking
4 years
A. Physical
   1. Height and weight increases are similar to previous year
   2. Length at birth is doubled
B. Motor

1. Skips and hops on one foot; walks up and down stairs like an adult
2. Can button buttons and lace shoes
3. Throws ball overhand; uses scissors to cut outline
C. Vocalization and socialization
   1. Vocabulary of 1500 words or more
   2. May have an imaginary companion
   3. Tends to be selfish and impatient but takes pride in accomplishments; exaggerates, boasts, and tattles on others
D. Mental abilities
   1. Unable to conserve matter
   2. Can repeat four numbers and is learning number concept
   3. Knows which is the longer of two lines; has poor space perception
5 years
A. Physical: height and weight increases are similar to previous year
B. Motor
   1. Gross motor abilities well developed; can balance on one foot for about 10 seconds; can jump rope, skip, and roller skate
   2. Can draw a picture of a person; prints first name and other words as learned
   3. Dresses and washes self; may be able to tie shoelaces
C. Sensory
   1. Color recognition is well established
   2. Minimal potential for amblyopia to develop
D. Vocalization and socialization
   1. Vocabulary of about 2100 words; talks constantly; asks meaning of new words
   2. Generally cooperative and sympathetic toward others
   3. Basic personality structure is well established
E. Mental abilities (Piaget's phase of intuitive thought)
   1. Beginning understanding of time in terms of days as part of a week
   2. Beginning understanding of conversion of numbers
   3. Has not mastered the concept that parts equal a whole regardless of their appearance; difficulty with abstract thought

Play during Preschool Years (Cooperative Play)
A. Loosely organized group play where membership changes readily, as do rules
B. Through play, the child deals with reality, learns control of feelings, and expresses emotions more through action than through words
C. Play is still physically oriented but is also imitative and imaginary
D. Increasing sharing and cooperation among preschool children, especially 5-year-old children

E. Suggested toys
  1. Dress-up clothes; dolls; doll house; small trucks; animals; puppets; etc.
  2. Painting sets, coloring books, paste, and cutout sets
  3. Illustrated books; puzzles with large pieces and more shapes
  4. Tricycle; swing; slide; other playground equipment

HEALTH PROMOTION FOR PRESCHOOLERS

See Health Promotion for Toddlers

HEALTH PROBLEMS MOST COMMON IN PRESCHOOLERS
Hospitalization

A. Reaction of the child
  1. Fears about body image and bodily harm are now greater than fear of separation
  2. The fears include:
    a. Intrusive experiences: needles, thermometer, otoscope
    b. Punishment and rejection
    c. Pain
    d. Castration and mutilation
B. If possible, parents can be helped to prepare the child beforehand because increased cognitive and verbal ability makes explanations possible

General Nursing Diagnoses for Preschoolers with Health Problems

A. Anxiety related to strange environment; perception of impending event; anticipated discomfort; feelings of lack of control; knowledge deficit
B. Readiness for enhanced family coping related to adaptive tasks effectively addressed
C. Compromised, family coping: related to situational crises
D. Ineffective coping related to situational crises
E. Decisional conflict related to multiple alternatives
F. Deficient diversional activity related to lack of sensory stimulation; frequent or prolonged hospitalization
G. Interrupted family processes related to situational crisis; temporary family disorganization; inadequate support system
H. Fear related to separation from support systems; potential change in body
I. Anticipatory grieving (parental) related to gravity of child's physical status; potential death of child
J. Impaired home maintenance related to knowledge deficit; inadequate support systems
K. Risk for injury related to use of specific therapies and appliances; incapacity for self-protection; immobility

L. Acute/chronic pain related to disease process; interventions
M. Parental role conflict related to sick child; inability to care for child
N. Risk for impaired parenting related to separation; skill deficit; family stress
O. Feeding, bathing/hygiene, dressing/grooming, toileting self-care deficits related to fatigue; pain; developmental level; limitations of treatment modalities
P. Disturbed sensory perception related to protected environment
Q. Risk for impaired skin integrity related to immobility
R. Disturbed sleep pattern related to excessive crying; frequent assessment; therapies
S. Spiritual distress (parental) related to decisions regarding life or death conflicts; perceived threat to value system

General Nursing Care of Preschoolers with Health Problems

A. Begin preparing for elective hospitalization a few days before but not too early because of the child's poor concept of time
B. Clarify cause and effect because of the child's phenomenalistic thinking (in the child's mind, proximity of two events relates them to each other)
C. Explain routines of hospital admission but not all procedures at one time, because this would be overwhelming
D. Recognize play is an excellent medium for preparation (use dolls, puppets, make-believe equipment, dress-up doctor and nurse clothes)
E. Provide time for play as an outlet for fear, anger, and hostility, as well as a temporary escape from reality
F. Keep verbal explanation as simple as possible and always honest
G. Add details about procedures, drugs, surgery, and the like as the child's cognitive level and personal experiences increase
H. Encourage parents to visit as often as possible
I. Facilitate therapeutic play for emergent hospitalization
J. See Nursing Care under each disorder

▼ LEUKEMIA

Data Base

A. Malignant neoplasm of blood-forming organs; overproduction of immature, nonfunctioning leukocytes (blast-cell or stem-cell leukemia)
B. The most common type of childhood cancer; peak incidence between 2 and 6 years of age; more common in males than females after the age of 1; prognosis is improving

C. Classification
   1. Acute lymphoid; most common; 75% long-term disease-free survival
   2. Acute myelogenous or acute nonlymphoid: 40% survival rate
D. Clinical findings
   1. Anemia: pallor, weakness, irritability
   2. Infection: fever
   3. Tendency toward bleeding: petechiae and bleeding into joints
   4. Pain in joints caused by seepage of serous fluid
   5. Tendency toward easy fracture of bones
   6. Enlargement of spleen, liver, lymph glands
   7. Abdominal pain and anorexia resulting in weight loss
   8. Necrosis and bleeding of gums and other mucous membranes
   9. Later symptoms: CNS involvement and frank hemorrhage
E. Therapeutic interventions
   1. Induce remission by chemotherapy (see Related Pharmacology under Neoplastic Disorders in Medical Surgical Nursing)
      a. Prednisone: steroid
      b. Vincristine: plant alkaloid
      c. Methotrexate: folic acid antagonist
      d. L-Asparaginase: enzyme
      e. 6-Mercaptopurine: purine antagonist
      f. Cyclophosphamide: alkylating agent
      g. Doxorubicin hydrochloride: cytotoxic antibiotic
   2. CNS prophylactic therapy: irradiation and intrathecal methotrexate, because leukemic cells invade the brain, but most antileukemic drugs do not pass the blood-brain barrier
   3. Transfusions to replace and provide needed blood factors such as red blood cells, platelets, and white blood cells
   4. Bone marrow transplantation

Nursing Care of Children with Leukemia
A. **ASSESSMENT**
   1. Hematologic status: anemia; thrombocytopenia; neutropenia
   2. Activity level
   3. Complications of therapy/disease process
B. **ANALYSIS/NURSING DIAGNOSES**
   1. Activity intolerance related to decreased oxygen carrying capacity of blood; disease process
   2. Disturbed body image related to loss of hair; moon face; debilitation
   3. Interrupted family processes related to situational crisis (child with life-threatening disease)
   4. Fear related to diagnostic tests; procedures
   5. Anticipatory grieving related to perceived potential loss of child
   6. Risk for infection related to decreased immune response
   7. Risk for injury related to decreased strength and endurance; pain and discomfort; decreased platelets
   8. Imbalanced nutrition: less than body requirements related to loss of appetite; increase in metabolic rate
   9. Acute/chronic pain related to physiologic effect of neoplasia; treatment
   10. Impaired physical mobility related to decreased strength and endurance; pain and discomfort; neuromuscular impairment
   11. Risk for impaired skin integrity related to immobility; administration of antimetabolites; disease process
C. **PLANNING/IMPLEMENTATION**
   1. Encourage adjustment to chronic illness; stress need for maintaining regular lifestyle
   2. Deal with the child's idea of death; discussion should be appropriate to level of understanding
      a. Preschooler: concept that death is reversible; greatest fear is separation
      b. Child 6 to 9 years of age: concept that death is personified; a person actually comes and removes the child
      c. Child over 9 years of age: adult concept of death as irreversible and inevitable
   3. Support the child experiencing side effects of drugs
      a. Cytoxan: severe nausea, vomiting, cystitis, and alopecia
      b. Vincristine: constipation, alopecia, neurotoxicity
      c. Methotrexate: oral and rectal ulcers
      d. Corticosteroids: mood swings, fluid retention
   4. Teach prevention of infection: hand washing; avoid contact with people who have active infections; avoid crowded places
   5. Handle the child carefully because of pain and risk for hemorrhage; administer analgesics for pain
   6. Provide gentle oral hygiene; soft, bland foods; increased liquids
   7. Provide for frequent rest periods; quiet play
D. **EVALUATION/OUTCOMES**
   1. Participates in developmental, age-appropriate activities
   2. Remains comfortable
   3. Consumes adequate calories for growth
   4. Remains free from complications (infection, bleeding, anemia, impaired skin)
   5. Expresses feelings about altered body image
   6. Family and child discuss fears, concerns, and needs

▼ WILMS' TUMOR (NEPHROBLASTOMA)

Data Base

A. Most common malignant neoplasm of the kidney in children
B. Estimated frequency is 8.1 cases per million white children less than 15 years old
C. Peak age at diagnosis is 3 years of age; 80% are diagnosed by 5 years of age
D. May be associated with congenital anomalies: aniridia (congenital absence of iris); hemihypertrophy; hypospadias; cryptorchidism
E. Prognosis
   1. Stages I and II with localized tumor: 90% cure with multimodal therapy
   2. Factors that favorably affect the success of further therapy
     a. Initial treatment with only vincristine and dactinomycin
     b. Relapse to the lungs only
     c. Relapse to the abdomen only with no prior abdominal radiation
     d. Relapse more than 12 months after diagnosis
F. Clinical findings
   1. Swelling or nontender mass in abdomen; confined to one side of midline
   2. Weight loss; fever; fatigue; malaise
   3. Hematuria occurs in less than 25%
   4. Hypertension occasionally occurs
   5. Other symptoms associated with compression of neighboring organs or metastasis (e.g., lungs: cough, dyspnea, shortness of breath)
G. Therapeutic interventions
   1. Surgery: should be scheduled soon after confirmation of renal mass
     a. Tumor, kidney, and associated adrenal gland removed; precautions taken not to rupture the capsule of the tumor
     b. Contralateral kidney is inspected; when bilateral kidney involvement, partial nephrectomy is done on the less affected side
     c. Regional lymph nodes and organs inspected and biopsied; when indicated, they are removed
   2. Chemotherapy
     a. Indicated for all stages; continued for 6 to 15 months
     b. Drugs used include actinomycin D, vincristine, adriamycin
   3. Radiation therapy: indicated for children with large tumors, metastasis, residual disease after surgery, and unfavorable cell type

Nursing Care of Children with Wilms' Tumor

A. ASSESSMENT
   1. Manifestations of Wilms' tumor
     a. Abdomen for mass or swelling; firm, nontender; does not cross midline
     b. Red blood cells for anemia; weight loss
   2. Symptoms of compression
   3. Signs of metastasis: dyspnea; cough; shortness of breath

B. ANALYSIS/NURSING DIAGNOSES
   1. Anxiety related to the unknown; strange environment
   2. Interrupted family processes related to situational crisis (child with a serious illness)
   3. Risk for infection related to lowered body defenses; abdominal surgery
   4. Risk for injury related to presence of encapsulated tumor
   5. Imbalanced nutrition: less than body requirements related to loss of appetite
   6. See Nursing Care of Children with Leukemia

C. PLANNING/IMPLEMENTATION
   1. Preoperative
     a. Handle and bathe carefully to prevent trauma to the abdomen, which may result in rupture of the tumor capsule; place sign over bed: "Do not palpate abdomen"
     b. Monitor blood pressure and intake and output
     c. Prepare parents and child for large size of incision and drainage
     d. Begin teaching family about chemotherapy and radiation therapy
   2. Postoperative
     a. Monitor blood pressure and intake and output
     b. Encourage child to turn, cough, and deep breathe to prevent pulmonary complications
     c. Teach parents to identify untoward reactions from chemotherapy and radiation therapy
   3. See Nursing Care of Children with Leukemia

D. EVALUATION/OUTCOMES
   1. Remains free from complications (infection, rupture of encapsulated tumor)
   2. Maintains blood pressure within acceptable range
   3. Consumes adequate calories for growth
   4. Child and family members discuss feelings and concerns

▼ NEPHROTIC SYNDROME (MINIMAL CHANGE NEPHROTIC SYNDROME)

Data Base

A. Pathology: abnormal, increased permeability of the glomerular basement membrane to plasma albumin; cause unknown

B. Peak incidence: 2 to 7 years of age
C. Classification
 1. Minimal change nephrotic syndrome (80% incidence)
 2. Secondary nephrotic syndrome
 3. Congenital nephrotic syndrome (usually die by second year of life without kidney transplant)
D. Clinical findings
 1. Weight gain
 2. Puffiness of face
 3. Abdominal swelling (ascites)
 4. Generalized edema
 5. Irritability
 6. Easily fatigued
 7. Blood pressure normal or slightly decreased
 8. Decreased urinary volume, may be frothy
 9. Proteinuria
E. Therapeutic interventions
 1. Supportive therapy
 2. Sodium restricted diet
 3. Corticosteroid therapy; prednisone drug of choice
  a. Response to therapy usually within 7 to 21 days
  b. Lower dose or gradually discontinue when satisfactory response noted
 4. Immunosuppressant therapy for children who do not respond to steroids or those who have frequent relapses; cyclophosphamide (Cytoxan) is drug of choice

Nursing Care of Children with Nephrotic Syndrome

A. **ASSESSMENT**
 1. Vital signs particularly blood pressure
 2. Fluid balance: daily weight; edema; abdominal girth
 3. Urine studies: specific gravity; albumin
B. **ANALYSIS/NURSING DIAGNOSES**
 1. Ineffective breathing pattern related to pressure of ascites
 2. Disturbed body image related to change in appearance
 3. Interrupted family processes related to situational crisis (child with a serious illness)
 4. Risk for deficient fluid volume related to loss of protein; loss of fluid
 5. Risk for infection related to presence of infective organisms; lowered body defenses
 6. Imbalanced nutrition: less than body requirements related to loss of appetite; loss of protein
 7. Risk for impaired skin integrity related to edema
C. **PLANNING/IMPLEMENTATION**
 1. Prevent infection: both disease state and drug therapy increase susceptibility

  a. Protect the child from others who are ill
  b. Teach parents the signs of impending infection and encourage them to seek medical care
 2. Prevent malnutrition: caused by loss of protein and anorexia
  a. Provide regular diet; encourage selection of foods from high-protein choices
  b. Restrict fluids if ordered; teach child and parents about sodium-restricted diet
 3. Promote respirations: respiratory difficulty caused by ascites
  a. Place in a Fowler's position to decrease pressure against the diaphragm
  b. Monitor vital signs and respiratory status
 4. Promote comfort: discomfort caused by edema, pressure areas
  a. Provide some relief by positioning and giving skin care
  b. Support the genitalia if edematous
 5. Promote a positive body image: altered body image as a result of edema and steroids
  a. Recognize that this becomes a greater problem as the child gets older
  b. Emphasize clothes, hairdo, etc., that make the child attractive
  c. Stress that "diets" will not help weight loss
 6. Provide emotional support: irritability and depression commonly occur
  a. Help parents understand that mood swings are influenced by illness
  b. Encourage the child to participate in own care
  c. Encourage diversionary activities that provide satisfaction
D. **EVALUATION/OUTCOMES**
 1. Engages in activities appropriate to capabilities
 2. Maintains fluid balance
 3. Adheres to dietary regimen
 4. Remains free from infection
 5. Maintains skin integrity
 6. Child and family members discuss feelings and concerns

▼ URINARY TRACT INFECTION (UTI)

Data Base

A. Most common in females because of anatomy of the lower urinary tract: urethra is short and meatus is close to the anus
B. Peak incidence occurs at 2 to 6 years of age
C. Classification
 1. Bacteriuria: asymptomatic; symptomatic
 2. Recurrent UTI
 3. Persistent UTI

4. Febrile UTI
5. Cystitis
6. Urethritis
7. Pyelonephritis
8. Urosepsis
D. Clinical findings
1. In children under 2 years of age symptoms mimic gastrointestinal disorders
2. Enuresis; daytime incontinence
3. Dysuria
4. Urgency; frequency of urination
E. Therapeutic interventions
1. Antibiotics to eliminate infection
2. Identify and correct structural anomalies if present
3. Bland, high-protein, high-carbohydrate diet
4. Prevent recurrence; preserve renal function

Nursing Care of Children with Urinary Tract Infections

A. ASSESSMENT
1. Discomfort on urination
2. Pattern of urinary elimination
3. Urine sample

B. ANALYSIS/NURSING DIAGNOSES
l. Impaired urinary elimination related to microbiologic stress
2. Risk for injury related to kidney damage from chronic infection

C. PLANNING/IMPLEMENTATION
1. Encourage to void when necessary as opposed to holding urine in bladder
2. Increase fluids, particularly those that acidify urine
3. Encourage routine health care supervision

D. EVALUATION/OUTCOMES
1. Resolves infection
2. Receives follow-up health care supervision

▼ ASTHMA

Data Base

A. Chronic inflammatory disorder of airways characterized by increased responsiveness and inflammation of the airway, spasms of bronchi and bronchioles, edema of mucous membranes, increased secretions; respiratory acidosis results from buildup of carbon dioxide
B. Results from exposure to a substance that has been inhaled or ingested or that has contacted the skin; increased incidence in inner cities thought to be related to exposure to rodent feces
C. The incidence, severity, and mortality associated with asthma are increasing; it is the most common chronic disease of childhood; primary cause of school accidents; and a leading cause of pediatric hospitalizations
D. Classification
1. Mild intermittent: symptoms two or fewer times each week; brief exacerbations; nighttime symptoms two or fewer times each month
2. Mild persistent: symptoms more than two times per week but no more than one per day; Exacerbations affect activity; nighttime symptoms more than twice per month
3. Moderate persistent asthma: daily symptoms; daily use of inhaled short-acting beta agonists; frequent nighttime symptoms; limited physical activity
4. Severe persistent asthma; continual symptoms; frequent exacerbations; frequent nighttime symptoms; limited physical activity
E. Clinical findings
1. Wheezing, especially on expiration
2. Labored breathing; flaring nares
3. Cough; increased secretions
4. Distended neck veins
F. Therapeutic interventions
1. Theophylline derivatives: aminophylline; theophylline
   a. Action
      (1) Relax bronchial smooth muscle to decrease spasm; relax smooth muscle of the vasculature
      (2) Stimulate myocardium increasing cardiac output, which improves blood flow to kidneys
      (3) Act on renal tubules to increase excretion of sodium and chloride ions
   b. Adverse effects: oral forms cause gastric irritation; may cause hypotension
2. β-adrenergic agonists: epinephrine hydrochloride is drug of choice in respiratory emergency, such as status asthmaticus; albuterol (Proventil); metaproterenol (Alupent); terbutaline (Brethine)
   a. Action
      (1) Act on beta-adrenergic receptors in the bronchi to relax smooth muscle and increase respiratory volume
      (2) Inhalants cause vasoconstriction, which reduces congestion or edema
   b. Adverse effects: cardiac palpitation; overuse of inhalants may cause "congestive rebound"
3. Nonsteroidal antiinflammatory drug: cromolyn sodium (Intal)
   a. Action: prevents release of mediators of type I allergic reactions (histamine, slow-reacting substance of anaphylaxis) from sensitized mast cells; prophylactic use lessens bronchoconstriction

b. Adverse effects: similar to bronchodilator group; anxiety, nervousness, tremors, nausea, vomiting, headache, dizziness

4. Corticosteroids
   a. Action: antiinflammatory effect diminishes the inflammatory component of asthma and reduces airway obstruction; used for status asthmaticus; however, less often for long-term control because of adverse effects
   b. Adverse effects: immunosuppressive effect increases risk of infection

Nursing Care of Children with Asthma

A. ASSESSMENT
1. Respiratory status
2. History of current and previous attacks
3. Precipitating events/environmental factors
4. Knowledge of drug therapy

B. ANALYSIS/NURSING DIAGNOSES
1. Risk for suffocation related to bronchospasm; increased mucous secretions; edema
2. Ineffective breathing pattern related to bronchospasm; increased mucous secretions; edema
3. Activity intolerance related to imbalance between oxygen supply and demand
4. Disturbed sleep pattern related to difficulty breathing
5. Social isolation related to recurrent hospitalization; need to avoid environments that precipitate asthma attacks
6. Interrupted family processes related to situational crisis (acute, sudden illness of child); chronic illness

C. PLANNING/IMPLEMENTATION
1. Administer parenteral drugs slowly over a 4- to 5-minute period to avoid peripheral vasodilation (hypotension, facial flushing), cerebral vascular constriction (headache, dizziness), cardiac palpitation, and precordial pain; recognize that cumulation of drug can occur unless dosage is regulated
2. Teach parents how to give antispasmodic drugs and bronchodilators and why they must be given even if child does not have an attack
3. Teach parents chest physiotherapy, need for increased fluids, and the use of a cool mist humidifier to provide high humidity in the home
4. Improve ventilating capacity
   a. Position in a high-Fowler's, or the orthopneic position
   b. Teach breathing exercises and controlled breathing
5. Teach parents that a controlled environment can limit attacks
   a. Keep environment as allergen free as possible

b. Avoid exertion, exposure to cold air, cold fluids, and people with infections

D. EVALUATION/OUTCOMES
1. Breathes without dyspnea when at rest or engaging in activities
2. Manages respiratory secretions
3. Obtains sufficient sleep to feel rested
4. Maintains family and peer-group relationships
5. Child and family members cope with impact of chronic illness

▼ MUCOCUTANEOUS LYMPH NODE SYNDROME (KAWASAKI DISEASE)

Data Base

A. Acute febrile illness of unknown cause; principally involving the cardiovascular system, with extensive perivasculitis of arterioles, venules, capillaries, including the coronary arteries; panvasculitis and perivasculitis of the main coronary arteries may cause stenosis or obstruction with aneurysm formation, pericarditis, interstitial myocarditis and endocarditis, and phlebitis of the larger veins

B. Geographic and seasonal outbreaks

C. Clinical findings
1. Fever for 5 or more days; cervical lymphadenopathy
2. Bilateral congestion of the ocular conjunctiva without exudation
3. Changes of the mucous membranes of the oral cavity, such as erythema, dryness, and fissuring of lips, oropharyngeal reddening, or "strawberry tongue"
4. Changes in the extremities, such as peripheral edema, peripheral erythema and desquamation of the palms and soles, particularly periungual peeling; polymorphous rash, primarily of the trunk
5. Extreme irritability
6. Joint stiffness and pain

D. Therapeutic interventions
1. Primarily supportive and directed toward controlling fever, preventing dehydration, and minimizing possible cardiac complications; cardiac monitoring
2. Intravenous gamma globulin
3. Large doses of aspirin initially, then low-dose therapy

Nursing Care of Children with Kawasaki Disease

A. ASSESSMENT
1. Cardiac status; signs of heart failure
2. Fluid balance
3. Symptoms associated with syndrome

B. ANALYSIS/NURSING DIAGNOSES
1. Anxiety related to concern for child's prognosis
2. Pain related to disease process
3. Risk for impaired skin integrity related to edema; desquamation

C. PLANNING/IMPLEMENTATION
1. Administer aspirin to control fever; assess for early signs of toxicity
2. Monitor for signs of cardiac complications, especially dysrhythmias
3. Observe for allergic reaction to and side effects of IV gamma globulin
4. Administer analgesics for joint pain
5. Minimize skin discomfort: cool baths; non-scented lotions; soft, loose clothing
6. Provide emotional support to child and parents; child is often inconsolable

D. EVALUATION/OUTCOMES
1. Regains skin integrity
2. Remains free from complications (cardiac problems, ASA toxicity)
3. Remains comfortable
4. Child and parents discuss feelings

▼ TONSILLECTOMY AND ADENOIDECTOMY

Data Base
A. Not done routinely, because lymphoid tissue helps prevent invasion of organisms
B. Indications for surgical removal
   1. Recurrent tonsillitis or otitis media
   2. Enlargement that interferes with breathing or swallowing
C. Contraindications for removal
   1. Occasional infections that clear up rapidly
   2. Cleft palate, hemophilia, or debilitating disease such as leukemia
D. Clinical findings: postoperative
   1. Postsurgical hemorrhage: first 24 hours after surgery because of trauma; 5 to 10 days after surgery because of sloughing of tissue
   2. Signs of hemorrhage: frequent swallowing; bright-red blood in the vomitus; restlessness; increased pulse rate; pallor

Nursing Care of Children Having a Tonsillectomy and/or Adenoidectomy
A. ASSESSMENT
1. Presence of bleeding
2. Presence and extent of pain
3. Swallowing ability

B. ANALYSIS/NURSING DIAGNOSES
1. Ineffective airway clearance related to discomfort when swallowing and coughing; edema

2. Risk for deficient fluid volume related to vomiting; difficulty drinking fluids
3. Imbalanced nutrition: less than body requirements related to difficulty swallowing; nausea and vomiting
4. Acute pain related to surgical trauma

C. PLANNING/IMPLEMENTATION
1. Keep positioned on the side to allow secretions to drain from mouth
2. Give child cool liquids that are not red in color, thick, or mucus producing
3. Ask the child to talk; provide assurance that it is possible
4. Apply an ice collar to decrease edema
5. Administer analgesics as necessary for comfort; avoid salicylates

D. EVALUATION/OUTCOMES
1. Maintains patent airway
2. Manages respiratory secretions
3. Reports minimal pain
4. Maintains fluid and nutritional status

▼ EMOTIONAL DISORDERS

For common emotional disorders of the preschooler see Disorders Usually First Evident in Infancy, Childhood, or Adolescence in Mental Health Nursing

SCHOOL-AGED CHILDREN

GROWTH AND DEVELOPMENT
Developmental Timetable
A. Physical growth
   1. Permanent dentition, beginning with 6-year molars and central incisors at 7 or 8 years of age
   2. Tends to look lanky because bone development precedes muscular development
      a. 6 years: height and weight gain slower, 2 inches and 2 to 3 kg ($4\frac{1}{2}$ to $6\frac{1}{2}$ lb) a year
      b. 7 years: continues to grow, 5 cm (2 inches) and 2.5 kg ($5\frac{1}{2}$ lb) a year
      c. 8 to 9 years: continues to grow, 5 cm (2 inches) and 3 kg ($6\frac{1}{2}$ lb) a year
      d. 10 to 12 years: slow growth in height compared to rapid weight gain, 6.25 cm ($2\frac{1}{2}$ inches) and 4.5 kg (10 lb) a year; pubescent changes may begin to appear, especially in females
B. Motor
   1. Refinement of coordination, balance, and control occurs
   2. Motor development necessary for competitive activity becomes important

C. Sensory: visual acuity of 20/20
D. Mental abilities
   1. Readiness for learning, especially in perceptual organization: names months of year, knows right from left, can tell time, can follow several directions at once
   2. Acquires use of reason and understanding of rules; needs consistency
   3. Trial-and-error problem solving becomes more conceptual rather than action oriented
   4. Reasoning ability allows greater understanding and use of language
   5. Concrete operations (Piaget): knows that quantity remains the same even though appearance differs

Play During School-Aged Years

A. Play activities vary with age; number of play activities decreases, whereas the amount of time spent in one particular activity increases
B. Likes games with rules because of increased mental abilities
C. Likes games of athletic competition because of increased motor ability
D. Should learn how to work as well as play, with a beginning appreciation for economics and finances
E. In beginning of school years, boys and girls play together but gradually separate into sex-oriented type of activities
F. Suggested play for 6- to 9-year-olds
   1. More housekeeping toys that work; doll accessories; paper-doll sets; simple sewing machine; needlework; building toys
   2. Simple word and number games that require increased skills
   3. Physically active games such as hopscotch, jump rope, climbing trees, bicycle riding
   4. Collections and hobbies such as stamp collecting and building simple models
G. Suggested play for 9- to 12-year-olds
   1. Handicrafts of all kinds; model kits; pottery clay; hobbies; collections
   2. Archery; dart games; chess; jigsaw puzzles
   3. Science toys; magic sets

HEALTH PROBLEMS MOST COMMON IN SCHOOL-AGED CHILDREN
Hospitalization

A. Reactions of the school-aged child
   1. Usually handles separation well but prefers parents to be near
   2. Fears the unknown, especially when dependency or loss of control is expected; fears bodily harm, especially disfigurement
   3. Possesses realistic concept of death by 9 to 10 years of age
   4. Self-image about reaction to pain is important; may use avoidance to deal with physical discomfort
   5. Wants to know scientific rationale for treatments and procedures
B. If possible parents can be helped to prepare the child beforehand, since increased cognitive and verbal ability makes explanations possible

General Nursing Diagnoses for School-Aged Children with Health Problems

A. Anxiety related to strange environment; perception of impending event; anticipated discomfort; uncertain prognosis
B. Readiness for enhanced family coping related to successful parenting
C. Compromised family coping related to situational crises
D. Disabled family coping related to situational crises
E. Deficient diversional activity related to lack of sensory stimulation; frequent or prolonged hospitalization
F. Interrupted family processes related to situational crisis; temporary family disorganization; inadequate support system
G. Fear related to separation from support systems; potential change in body
H. Anticipatory grieving (parental) related to gravity of child's physical status; potential for death of child
I. Impaired home maintenance related to complexity of health care regimen
J. Risk for injury related to use of specific therapies and appliances; incapacity for self-protection; immobility
K. Acute/chronic pain related to disease process; interventions
L. Parental role conflict related to sick child; inability to care for child
M. Risk for impaired parenting related to separation; skill deficit
N. Feeding, bathing/hygiene, dressing/grooming, toileting self-care deficits related to fatigue; pain; developmental level; limitations of treatment modalities
O. Disturbed sensory perception related to protected environment
P. Risk for impaired skin integrity related to immobility
Q. Disturbed sleep pattern related to excessive crying; frequent assessment; therapies
R. Spiritual distress (parental) related to decisions regarding life or death conflicts

General Nursing Care of School-Aged Children with Health Problems

A. Begin preparing child for hospitalization before admission if possible

B. Provide explanations that are simple and honest and at the child's level of understanding; add details about procedures, drugs, surgery, and the like as the child's cognitive level and personal experiences increase
C. Involve child and parents in planning care
D. Provide time for play as an outlet for fear, anger, and hostility, as well as a temporary escape from reality
E. Encourage and allow child to express feelings, emotions, and fears; expect and accept regression
F. Provide for tutoring if absence from school is prolonged
G. Encourage visits from siblings and peers and the formation of new peer relationships
H. Recognize that although play is diversional, this age group enjoys games with challenge and skill
I. Allow dependency but foster independence as much as possible
J. See Nursing Care under each disorder

▼ DIABETES MELLITUS

Data Base

A. Peak incidence in the school-aged group
B. Differences in diabetes in children and adults
   1. Onset: rapid in children; insidious in adults
   2. Obesity: not a factor in type 1 diabetes; becoming an increasing factor in both children and adults with type 2 diabetes factor in adults
   3. Dietary treatment: rarely adequate for children; may be beneficial for some adults
   4. Oral hypoglycemics: contraindicated for children; may be used for some adults
   5. Insulin: almost universally necessary in children with type 1 diabetes; may be necessary for type 2
   6. Hypoglycemia and ketoacidosis: frequent in children; more uncommon in adults
   7. Degenerative vascular changes: develop after adolescence in children; may be present at the time of diagnosis in adults
C. Classification
   1. Type 1 diabetes: onset usually in childhood but can be anytime; both genetic and immunologic factors are associated with onset
   2. Type 2 diabetes: appears to involve resistance to insulin action and defective glucose-mediated insulin secretion
   3. Maturity-onset diabetes of the young (MODY)
   4. Secondary: caused by exogenous factors; usually reversible if primary disorder corrected
D. Clinical findings
   1. Onset is rapid and obvious
   2. Child usually thin, underweight
   3. Three Ps: polydipsia, polyphagia, polyuria
   4. Hyperglycemia: ketoacidosis or diabetic coma

    a. Causes
      (1) Decreased insulin
      (2) Emotional stress
      (3) Physical stress such as fever, infection
      (4) Increased food intake
    b. Symptoms
      (1) Onset: gradual (days)
      (2) Mood: lethargic
      (3) Mental status: dulled sensorium, confused
      (4) Subjective symptoms: thirst, weakness, nausea/vomiting, abdominal pain
      (5) Skin: flushed, signs of dehydration
      (6) Mucous membranes: dry and crusty
      (7) Respirations: deep and rapid (Kussmaul)
      (8) Pulse: less rapid and weak than baseline
      (9) Breath odor: fruity and acetone
     (10) Neurologic: diminished reflexes and paresthesia
     (11) Ominous signs: acidosis and coma
     (12) Blood glucose: high, 250 mg/dl or higher
     (13) Urine output: polyuria (early), oliguria (late), enuresis, and nocturia
     (14) Vision: diplopia
   6. Hypoglycemia: insulin-therapy related
    a. Causes
      (1) Overdose of insulin
      (2) Decreased food intake
      (3) Excessive physical exercise: increases muscle activity and movement of glucose into muscle cells
    b. Symptoms
      (1) Onset: rapid
      (2) Mood: labile, irritable, and nervous
      (3) Mental status: difficulty concentrating, speaking, and focusing
      (4) Subjective symptoms: shaky feeling, hunger, headache, and dizziness
      (5) Skin: pallor and sweating
      (6) Mucous membranes: normal
      (7) Respirations: shallow, normal
      (8) Pulse: tachycardia and palpitations
      (9) Breath odor: normal
     (10) Neurologic: tremors, hyperflexia, dilated pupils
     (11) Ominous signs: shock and coma
     (12) Blood glucose: below 60 mg/dl
     (13) Urine output: normal
     (14) Vision: diplopia
E. Therapeutic interventions
   1. Control calorie, carbohydrate, fat, and protein intake
   2. Insulin (see Related Pharmacology under the Endocrine System in Medical Surgical Nursing)
   3. Exercise
   4. Hyperglycemia: hospitalization with administration of fluids, electrolytes, and insulin

5. Hypoglycemia: immediate supply of readily available glucose followed by a complex carbohydrate and protein

Nursing Care of Children with Diabetes Mellitus

A. ASSESSMENT
1. Knowledge of disease management
2. Blood glucose monitoring
3. Signs of hypoglycemia/hyperglycemia
4. Early signs of complications

B. ANALYSIS/NURSING DIAGNOSES
1. Disturbed body image related to dependence on insulin
2. Risk for injury related to hypoglycemia; hyperglycemia
3. Imbalanced nutrition: less than body requirements related to altered ability/inability to use nutrients
4. Powerlessness related to diagnosis of chronic illness
5. Situational low self-esteem related to need to restrict diet; need for insulin injections; feeling of being different from peers
6. Risk for deficient fluid volume related to polyuria
7. Ineffective therapeutic regimen management related to complexity of regimen; lack of judgment because of developmental level; desire not to be different from peers; fear of giving self injections

C. PLANNING/IMPLEMENTATION
1. Explain the differences between Type I and Type II diabetes to parents
2. Teach factors that affect insulin requirements and signs of insulin overdose and diabetic coma
   a. Provide a written list explaining symptoms and appropriate interventions
   b. Emphasize that skim milk can be given if insulin reaction is suspected but that insulin should not be increased if diabetic ketoacidosis is developing; physician should be notified
   c. Explain orders for insulin coverage
3. Teach need for prevention of infection: skin care; frequent baths; properly fitting shoes; prompt treatment of any small cut; protection from undue exposure to illness
4. Encourage well-balanced diet, with fairly equal quantities of food eaten frequently and regularly; usually unrestricted within reason
5. Help plan exercise and adjust food and insulin to meet child's requirements
6. Teach child how to do blood glucose testing to increase independence
7. Teach child how to administer insulin (by injection or pump)
   a. The child should be taught as early as motor and mental abilities allow, usually by 7 to 9 years of age
   b. Explanations should be simple; diagrams for administration sites should be used
   c. Periodic observation by an adult to ensure proper technique
8. Allow child to make choices when possible for sense of control
9. Encourage continued health care supervision

D. EVALUATION/OUTCOMES
1. Maintains blood glucose levels within acceptable range
2. Consumes adequate calories for growth and development
3. Remains free from complications (insulin coma; ketoacidosis)
4. Demonstrates behaviors reflective of a positive self-image
5. Child and parents demonstrate the ability to follow health care regimen

▼ HEMOPHILIA

Data Base
A. Defect in clotting mechanism of blood
B. Genetic disorder; X-linked recessive transmission
C. Usually occurs in males; females are carriers but do not have the disease
D. Classification
   1. Factor VIII deficiency (classic hemophilia): hemophilia A
   2. Factor IX deficiency (Christmas disease): hemophilia B
E. Clinical findings
   1. Prolonged bleeding anywhere from or within the body
   2. Bleeding into the joints (hemarthrosis), resulting in pain, deformity, and impaired growth
   3. Intracranial hemorrhage
   4. Severity of bleeding
      a. Mild: factor VIII activity of 5% to 50%; bleeding with severe trauma or surgery
      b. Moderate: factor VIII activity of 1% to 5%; bleeding with trauma
      c. Severe: factor VIII activity of 1%; spontaneous bleeding without trauma
F. Therapeutic interventions
   1. Control of bleeding
   2. Prevention of bleeding with use of factor replacement
      a. Drugs that replace deficient coagulation factors
         (1) Factor VIII concentrate from recombinant DNA

(2) Factor IX concentrate from recombinant DNA; complex contains factors II, VII, IX, X (concentrated)

b. Adjunctive measures

(1) DDAVP (l-deamino-8-D-arginine vaso-pressin) treatment of choice in mild hemophilia and von Willebrand disease; vigorous treatment to prevent joint bleeding is done if child responds to this drug therapy

(2) NSAIDs such as ibuprofen are effective in relieving pain caused by synovitis; they must be used with caution because of potential effect on platelet function

(3) Corticosteroids used for hematuria, acute hemarthrosis, and chronic synovitis

(4) Amicar (aminocaproic acid) oral administration or local application prevents clot destruction; use limited to mouth or trauma surgery

(5) Regular program of exercise and physical therapy to strengthen muscles around joints and minimize bleeding

Nursing Care of Children with Hemophilia

A. ASSESSMENT

1. Parent/child knowledge of disease process and injury prevention
2. Location and extent of bleeding
3. Mobility of joints

B. ANALYSIS/NURSING DIAGNOSES

1. Acute pain related to bleeding into joints/tissues
2. Disturbed body image related to perception of self as different; inability to participate in selected activities
3. Interrupted family processes related to situational crisis; chronic illness
4. Risk for infection related to frequent transfusions
5. Risk for injury (hemorrhage) related to deficient blood clotting
6. Impaired physical mobility related to effects of hemorrhages into joints and other tissues

C. PLANNING/IMPLEMENTATION

1. Instruct the child and parents about the treatment of bleeding, especially of joints
   a. Rest the area
   b. Application of cool/ice compresses
   c. Compression of the area
   d. Elevation of the body part
2. Provide for appropriate activity that lessens the chance of trauma, which is often difficult because boys are so physically active
3. Select safe toys and inform parents to safe-proof house to minimize injuries; secure throw rugs
4. Avoid use of aspirin or ibuprofen

5. Control joint pain so the child uses extremities to prevent muscle atrophy
6. Provide counseling, because disease is genetic
7. Encourage parents to avoid overprotection or overpermissiveness

D. EVALUATION/OUTCOMES

1. Reports minimal pain
2. Remains free from injury (hemorrhage)
3. Maintains range of motion of joints
4. Participates in desired activities
5. Child and parents discuss feelings and concerns

▼ RHEUMATIC FEVER (RF)

Data Base

A. Inflammatory disease affecting heart, joints, central nervous system, and subcutaneous tissue; most significant sequela is rheumatic heart disease with damage and scarring of the mitral valve

B. Strong relationship between upper respiratory tract infection with group A streptococci and RF

C. Clinical findings
   1. Heart: mitral and aortic stenosis may occur
   2. Joints: edema, inflammations, and effusion, especially in knees, elbows, hips, shoulders, and wrists
   3. Skin: erythematous macules with a clear center and wavy demarcated border usually on trunk and proximal extremities
   4. Neurologic: chorea
   5. Low-grade fever, epistaxis, abdominal pain, arthralgia, weakness, fatigue, pallor, anorexia, and weight loss

D. Therapeutic interventions
   1. Antibiotic therapy to eradicate organism and prevent recurrence; prophylactic therapy before dental work or invasive procedures for life
   2. Prevention of permanent cardiac damage
   3. Palliation of other symptoms
   4. Prevention of recurrences

Nursing Care of Children with Rheumatic Fever

A. ASSESSMENT

1. Presence of symptoms
2. Activity level
3. Compliance with drug regimen

B. ANALYSIS/NURSING DIAGNOSES

1. Decreased cardiac output related to disease process
2. Fatigue related to decreased metabolic energy production
3. Risk for injury related to autoimmune response
4. Imbalanced nutrition: less than body requirements related to anorexia; fatigue

5. Acute pain related to inflammation of joints
6. Impaired physical mobility related to joint pain

C. PLANNING/IMPLEMENTATION
1. Encourage bed rest to reduce workload of the heart; gradually increase activities over a period of weeks to months
2. Handle painful joints carefully; maintain functional alignment to prevent deformities
3. Monitor need for pain medication and administer when necessary
4. Provide small, frequent, meals; encourage intake of nutritious fluids
5. Prevent invalidism by emphasizing abilities rather than limitations; stimulate the development of quiet hobbies and collections
6. Maintain child's status in home and school by keeping communication channels open; encourage child to do schoolwork and keep up with class

D. EVALUATION/OUTCOMES
1. Maintains cardiac output within acceptable limits
2. Consumes adequate calories for growth
3. Reports minimal pain
4. Maintains mobility of joints
5. Participates in activities with sufficient energy

▼ JUVENILE RHEUMATOID ARTHRITIS

Data Base
A. Inflammatory disease of unknown cause; slight tendency to run in families
B. Two peak ages of onset: 1 to 3 and 8 to 10 years of age; females affected somewhat more frequently than males
C. Classification
1. Systemic onset
2. Monoarticular or pauciarticular: involves a few joints; usually fewer than five
3. Polyarticular: simultaneous involvement of five or more joints
D. Clinical findings
1. Joint enlargement; spindle-fingers with thick proximal joint and slender tip; chronic stiffness, pain, and limited motion, especially in morning on awakening
2. Low-grade fever; tachycardia; fatigue; weakness; weight loss
3. Erythematous rash on the trunk and extremities
4. Enlargement of the spleen, liver, and lymph nodes
E. Therapeutic interventions
1. Physical therapy
2. Nonsteroidal antiinflammatory drugs (NSAIDS) are first drugs used; therapy initiated with ibuprofen, naproxen, or tolmetin sodium because of reduced side effects
3. Cytotoxic drugs used for children with severe arthritis in whom NSAIDs have failed; low-dose methotrexate is an established therapy
4. Slow-acting antirheumatic drugs (SAARDs) require months to be effective and work in combination with NSAIDs; drugs are hydroxychloroquine, sulfasalazine, gold, and D-penicillamine
5. Corticosteroids are used for incapacitating arthritis
6. Immunologic modulators aimed at altering the immune response

Nursing Care of Children with Juvenile Rheumatoid Arthritis
A. ASSESSMENT
1. Status of involved joints
2. Physical restrictions
3. Location and extent of pain
4. Child's response to disease process

B. ANALYSIS/NURSING DIAGNOSES
1. Disturbed body image related to perception of self as different; inability to participate in selected activities
2. Interrupted family processes related to having a child with a chronic illness
3. Chronic pain related to joint inflammation
4. Impaired physical mobility related to discomfort
5. Feeding, bathing/hygiene, dressing/grooming, toileting self-care deficits related to pain; musculoskeletal impairment

C. PLANNING/IMPLEMENTATION
1. Emphasize that medication must be taken regularly, even in periods of remission, to decrease inflammation and pain
2. Promote functional alignment; provide passive range of motion; encourage non–weight-bearing exercises such as swimming
3. Encourage a warm bath in the morning to decrease stiffness and increase mobility
4. Encourage parents to accept the child's illness but to limit the use of the disease to foster dependency or control relationships
5. Encourage verbalization of feelings; emphasize abilities rather than limitations

D. EVALUATION/OUTCOMES
1. Reports minimal pain
2. Maintains mobility of joints
3. Participates in activities with minimal discomfort and sufficient energy
4. Participates in self-care to fullest extent of abilities
5. Child and family maintain health care regimen

▼ SKIN INFECTIONS

Nursing Care of Children with Skin Infections

A. ASSESSMENT
1. Type of skin lesion
2. Location and extent of discomfort or itching
3. Knowledge of cause, prevention and treatment

B. ANALYSIS/NURSING DIAGNOSES
1. Disturbed body image related to perceived appearance
2. Acute risk for infection related to breaks in skin and transmission to others
3. Pain related to skin lesions
4. Impaired skin integrity related to disease process; results of scratching
5. Social isolation related to self-concept disturbance

C. PLANNING/IMPLEMENTATION
1. Prevent secondary infection: keep nails short to prevent injury from scratching; administer medications to limit pruritus
2. Encourage daily bathing with tepid water; dry thoroughly; expose area to light and air
3. Encourage completion of the full regimen of antimicrobial medication
4. Prevent spread of infection to other members of the family: prevent direct contact between children; keep oozing lesions covered; prevent athlete's foot by not walking barefooted, drying feet carefully, wearing lightweight shoes to decrease heat, disinfecting shoes and socks
5. Teach proper hygiene: hair care; frequent bathing; clean clothes; avoidance of strong alkalis such as bleach when washing clothes
6. Encourage screening in schools to identify the source of infection

D. EVALUATION/OUTCOMES
1. Confines skin lesions to primary site and infection to self
2. Remains free from secondary infection
3. Remains free from discomfort
4. Child and parents verbalize how to prevent future infection

▼ PEDICULOSIS (LICE)

Data Base

A. Highly infectious infestation of head, body, or pubic hair; nits (grayish-white, oval eggs) attach to hair
B. Severe itching may lead to secondary infection
C. Therapeutic intervention:
   a. Special shampoo; use of fine-toothed comb to remove nits
   b. All bed linens and clothes must be washed in hot water and detergent

▼ SCABIES

Data Base

A. Produced by itch mite; female burrows under skin to lay eggs (usually in folds)
B. Intensely pruritic; scratching can lead to secondary infection with the development of papules and vesicles
C. Therapeutic intervention: all members of the family must be treated, because it is highly contagious; wash with sulfur or other special soap; wear clean clothes

▼ RINGWORM (FUNGAL DISEASE)

Data Base

A. Scalp (tinea capitis)
   1. Reddened, oval or round areas of alopecia
   2. Head should be covered to prevent spread of infection
B. Feet (athlete's foot, tinea pedis)
   1. Scaly fissures between toes, vesicles on sides of feet, pruritus
   2. Particularly common in summer; contracted in swimming areas and gymnasium locker rooms
C. Therapeutic intervention
   1. Griseofulvin, micronized (Fulvicin-U/F, Grifulvin V, Grisactin); topical or oral
   2. Terbinafine (Lamisil); topical cream

▼ INTERTRIGO

Data Base

A. Excoriation of any adjacent body surfaces
B. Caused by moisture and chafing

▼ IMPETIGO

Data Base

A. Bacterial infection of skin by streptococci or staphylococci
B. Highly contagious; other areas of body frequently become infected
C. Therapeutic intervention: antibiotics systemically and locally; isolate child; keep from scratching other areas of the body

▼ REYE SYNDROME

Data Base

A. Acute toxic encephalopathy associated with characteristic organ involvement

B. Usually follows viral illness, influenza, or varicella; associated with aspirin administration
C. Use of aspirin and NSAIDs, such as ibuprofen, are not recommended for children with varicella or influenza
D. Classification
1. Stage I: Vomiting; lethargy; drowsiness; liver dysfunction
2. Stage II: Disorientation; delirium; combativeness; hyperventilation; hyperactive reflexes; liver dysfunction
3. Stage III: Obtundity; coma; hyperventilation; decorticate rigidity
4. Stage IV: Deepening coma; decerebrate rigidity; loss of oculocephalic reflexes; large, fixed pupils; loss of doll's eye reflex; loss of corneal reflexes
5. Stage V: Seizures; loss of deep tendon reflexes; flaccidity; respiratory arrest; high serum ammonia levels
E. Clinical findings
1. Prodromal symptoms: malaise; cough; rhinorrhea; sore throat; fever; vomiting
2. Worsening cerebral signs as seen in the clinical stages
F. Therapeutic interventions
1. Early diagnosis with aggressive therapy
2. Treatment: determined by the clinical stage of the disease
a. Stage I: primarily supportive and directed toward restoring blood sugar levels, controlling cerebral edema, correcting acid-base imbalances, and eliminating factors known to increase intracranial pressure
b. Stages II through V: require invasive support, intracranial pressure monitoring, and tracheal intubation with controlled ventilation; a radical approach is curarization and sedation

Nursing Care of Children with Reye Syndrome

A. ASSESSMENT
1. Vital signs and neurologic status
2. Fluid balance
3. Level of consciousness
4. Signs of impaired coagulation (related to hepatic dysfunction)

B. ANALYSIS/NURSING DIAGNOSES
1. Risk for aspiration related to vomiting; decreased level of consciousness
2. Ineffective breathing pattern related to increased intracranial pressure
3. Interrupted family processes related to situational crisis (acute illness of child)
4. Fear (parental) related to possible death of child
5. Risk for deficient fluid volume related to intractable vomiting

6. Risk for injury related to disorientation; delirium; impaired coagulation

C. PLANNING/IMPLEMENTATION
1. Maintain a patent airway
2. Monitor vital signs; neurologic status; hemodynamic monitoring
3. Monitor fluid balance
4. Assist with numerous invasive procedures
5. Keep parents informed of child's progress; include parents in child's care whenever possible; provide emotional support
6. Foster dissemination of information concerning the role of aspirin in relation to viral disease and the development of Reye syndrome

D. EVALUATION/OUTCOMES
1. Maintains a patent airway and appropriate breathing pattern
2. Remains free from injury
3. Maintains fluid balance
4. Parents can verbalize questions and concerns about child's status

▼ LEGG-CALVÉ-PERTHES DISEASE (COXA PLANA)

Data Base

A. A disturbance of circulation to the femoral capital epiphysis producing an ischemic aseptic necrosis of the femoral head, epiphysis, and acetabulum; cause unknown
B. Occurs between 3 to 12 years of age; most common in males 4 to 8 years of age; more common in whites than in blacks (10:1)
C. In 10% to 15% of incidences, both hips are involved; most children have skeletal ages below chronologic age
D. Stages: Stage I—avascular; Stage II—fragmentation or revascularization; Stage III—reparative; Stage IV—regenerative
E. Clinical findings
1. Insidious onset
2. Persistent pain in the affected hip(s)
3. Limitation of movement in the affected hip(s); limp
F. Therapeutic interventions
1. Aim is to keep the head of the femur in the acetabulum and maintain a full range of motion
2. Conservative therapy must be continued for 2 to 4 years, whereas surgical correction returns the child to normal activities in 3 to 4 months
3. Use of non–weight-bearing devices such as an abduction brace, leg casts, or a leather harness sling that prevents weight bearing on the affected limb

4. Use of abduction-ambulation braces or casts after a period of bed rest and traction
5. Surgical reconstructive and containment procedures

Nursing Care of Children with Legg-Calvé-Perthes Disease

A. **ASSESSMENT**
  1. Extent of pain
  2. Extent of joint dysfunction
B. **ANALYSIS/NURSING DIAGNOSES**
  1. Disturbed body image related to perception of self as different; use of appliance; inability to participate in selected activities
  2. Risk for injury related to musculoskeletal impairment; use of appliance
  3. Impaired physical mobility related to pain
  4. Chronic pain associated with condition
C. **PLANNING/IMPLEMENTATION**
  1. Educate the child and parents regarding correct use of appliances
  2. Instruct the child and parents regarding what constitutes non–weight-bearing (e.g., no standing or kneeling on the affected leg)
  3. Assist the child and family in selecting activities according to the child's age, interests, and physical limitations (e.g., quiet games; hobbies; collections; model building; crafts; indoor gardening)
  4. Encourage peer interaction; help the child determine alternatives to weight-bearing activity (e.g., scorekeeping, sideline "coach")
  5. Help the child devise explanations for appliances
D. **EVALUATION/OUTCOMES**
  1. Reports minimal pain
  2. Remains free from injury
  3. Participate in activities with immobilizing device
  4. Discusses feelings and concerns

▼ EMOTIONAL DISORDERS

For common emotional disorders of the school-aged child see Disorders Usually First Evident in Infancy, Childhood, or Adolescence in Mental Health Nursing

THE ADOLESCENT

GROWTH AND DEVELOPMENT
Developmental Timetable

A. Physical growth: includes the physical changes associated with puberty such as secondary sexual characteristics

B. Pubertal growth spurt
  1. Females between 10 and 14
    a. Weight gain 7 to 25 kg {15 to 55 Ib), mean 17.5 kg (38 Ib)
    b. Approximately 95% of mature height achieved by the onset of menarche or skeletal age of 13 years; height gain 5 to 25 cm (2 to 10 inches), mean 20.5 cm ($8^{1}/_{4}$ inches)
  2. Males between 12 and 16 years
    a. Weight gain 7 to 30 kg (15 to 65 Ib), mean 23.7 kg (52 lb)
    b. Approximately 95% of mature height achieved by skeletal age of 15 years; height gain 10 to 30 cm (4 to 12 inches), mean 27.5 cm (11 inches)
C. Mental abilities
  1. Abstract thinking
    a. New level of social communication and understanding: can comprehend satire and double meanings; can say one thing and mean another
    b. Can conceptualize thought; more interested in exploring ideas than facts
    c. Can appreciate scientific thinking, problem solve, and theoretically explore alternatives
  2. Perception
    a. Can appreciate nonrepresentational art
    b. Can understand that the whole is more than the sum of its parts
  3. Learning
    a. Much longer span of attention
    b. Learns through inference, intuition, and surmise, rather than repetition and imitation
    c. Enjoys regressing in terms of language development by using jargon to suit changing moods
D. Social patterns
  1. Peer-group identity
    a. One of the strongest motivating forces of behavior
    b. Extremely important to be part of the group and like everyone else in every way
    c. Clique formation; usually based on common denominators such as race, social class, ethnic group, or special interests
  2. Interpersonal relationships
    a. Major goal is learning to form a close intimate relationship with the opposite sex
    b. Adolescents may develop crushes and worship many idols
    c. Time of sexual exploration and questioning of one's sexual role
  3. Independence
    a. By 15 or 16 years of age, adolescents feel they should be treated as adults

b. Ambivalence: adolescent wants freedom but is not happy about corresponding responsibilities and frequently yearns for more carefree days of childhood

c. Parental ambivalence and discipline problems are common as parents try to allow for increasing independence but continue to offer constructive guidance and enforce discipline

HEALTH PROMOTION DURING ADOLESCENCE
Adolescent Nutrition

A. Nutritional objectives
   1. Provide optimum nutritional support for demands of rapid growth and high energy expenditure
   2. Support development of appropriate eating habits through variety of foods, regular pattern, good quality snacks (high in protein; low in refined carbohydrate, primarily sugar)
B. Nutrient needs increased in all respects, so adequate intake of all nutrients should form basis of diet
C. Nutritional problems
   1. Low intake of calcium, vitamin A and C, and iron in females
   2. Anemia
   3. Obesity or underweight
D. Possible causes of nutritional deficiencies
   a. Psychologic factors: food aversions, emotional problems
   b. Fear of overweight: crash diets, mainly in girls; cultural pressure
   c. Fad diets: caused by misinformation; need for effective counseling
   d. Poor choice of snack foods: usually high in sugar and fat
   e. Irregular eating pattern
   f. Pregnancy that requires a higher intake of protein and calories
E. Nutrition education may be made through association with teenagers' concerns about physical appearance, figure control, complexion, physical fitness, athletic ability

Injury Prevention

A. Appropriate education regarding sexual maturity, reproduction, and sexual behavior
B. Driver education
C. Education regarding use and abuse of drugs, especially alcohol
D. Education about health hazards associated with smoking

Areas Needing Health Guidance During Adolescence

A. Accidents: leading cause of death, with motor vehicle accidents causing the most fatalities
B. Homicide and suicide: next two causes of death among adolescents
C. Alcoholism; drug abuse
D. Sexually transmitted diseases; pregnancy
E. Anorexia nervosa and bulimia nervosa; obesity
F. Delinquency
G. Acne
H. Orthopedic problems
I. Cancer

HEALTH PROBLEMS MOST COMMON IN ADOLESCENTS
Hospitalization

A. Reaction of the adolescent
   1. Increased need for privacy, sense of control, and independence
   2. Increased concern for mutilation, disfigurement, and loss of function; needs to be like peers; body image important
   3. Concerned about separation from peers and possible loss of status in group
B. Parents and health team members can help prepare the adolescent for hospitalization by providing full explanations and answering questions completely and honestly

General Nursing Diagnoses for Adolescents with Health Problems

A. Anxiety related to perception of impending event; separation from family/peer group; anticipated discomfort; prognosis; knowledge deficit
B. Disturbed body image related to change in body characteristics; perceived developmental imperfections
C. Compromised family coping related to situational crisis
D. Ineffective coping related to situational crisis
E. Deficient diversional activity related to frequent or prolonged hospitalization; separation from peer group
F. Interrupted family processes related to situational crisis; temporary family disorganization
G. Anticipatory grieving related to potential for death
H. Impaired home maintenance related to knowledge deficit; multiple therapies
I. Risk for injury related to use of specific therapies or appliances; incapacity for self-protection
J. Acute/chronic pain related to disease process; interventions
K. Parental role conflict related to ill child; inability to care for child

L. Impaired parenting related to separation; skill deficit
M. Risk for impaired skin integrity related to radio-therapy; use of an appliance
N. Spiritual distress related to decisions regarding life or death conflicts
O. Disturbed sensory perception (auditory) related to loud music and noises

General Nursing Care of Adolescents with Health Problems

A. Recognize that problems of adolescence are magnified by an illness during this period of development
B. Involve the adolescent in planning care
C. Be as open as possible concerning feelings, care, and prognosis; answer questions honestly and directly
D. Foster independence as much as possible
E. Provide for contact with peers
F. Encourage compliance with health program
G. Arrange for continuity in schoolwork
H. Encourage involvement of positive support systems
I. Accept the adolescent's self-appraisal but point out reality
J. Encourage use of clothing or makeup to minimize perceived shortcomings

▼ SCOLIOSIS

Data Base

A. Lateral curvature of spine usually associated with a rotary deformity that eventually causes cosmetic and physiologic alterations in the spine, chest, and pelvis
B. No apparent cause in most cases (termed idiopathic); possible genetic etiology
C. Most common spinal deformity; more frequent in adolescent girls during growth spurt
D. Classification
   1. Nonstructural scoliosis: curve is flexible and corrects by bending
   2. Structural scoliosis: curve fails to straighten on side-bending characterized by changes in the spine and its supporting structures
E. Clinical findings
   1. Curve in the vertebral spinous process alignment
   2. Prominence of one hip
   3. Prominence of one scapula; difference in shoulder or scapular height
   4. Deformity of the rib cage; breasts appear unequal in size
   5. Other clues: clothes do not fit right; skirt hems are uneven
F. Therapeutic interventions
   1. Screening for scoliosis; diagnosis confirmed by x-ray examination
   2. Exercise can be used in nonstructural scoliosis

   3. Mild to moderate curvature
      a. Boston brace
      b. Brace worn 23 hours a day; gradually weaned over a 1- to 2-year period; then worn only at night until the spine is mature
      c. Electrical stimulation to the convex side of the curvature may prevent progression of the scoliosis
   4. More severe curves usually require surgery: techniques consist of spinal realignment and straightening by way of external or internal fixation and instrumentation combined with bony fusion (arthrodesis) of the realigned spine (Harrington rods); L-rod segmental instrumentation
   5. Most severe scoliotic curvatures require traction devices and exercises for a time before spinal fusion to provide partial correction and more flexibility

Nursing Care of Adolescents with Scoliosis

A. ASSESSMENT
   1. Symmetry of the shoulders and hips while the child stands erect clothed only in underpants (and bra if older girl); observation occurs from behind
   2. Symmetry or prominence of the ribs while the child bends forward so the back is parallel with the floor; observation occurs from the side
B. ANALYSIS/NURSING DIAGNOSES
   1. Disturbed body image related to perceived alteration in body structure; altered appearance when using supportive device
   2. Delayed growth and development related to disease process
   3. Risk for injury related to use of supportive devices
   4. Impaired physical mobility related to use of supportive devices
   5. Risk for impaired skin integrity related to presence of brace; use of electrical stimulation
   6. Acute pain related to therapies
C. PLANNING/IMPLEMENTATION
   1. Maintain spinal alignment
   2. Examine skin surfaces in contact with the brace or electrical stimulator for signs of irritation; implement corrective action to treat or prevent skin breakdown
   3. Reinforce instructions about plan of care, use of appliance, activities permitted or restricted, adolescent's and parents' responsibilities in therapy
   4. Help in selection of the appropriate wearing apparel to wear over the brace to minimize altered appearance and footwear to maintain proper balance
   5. Prepare for surgery if required

D. **EVALUATION/OUTCOMES**
 1. Demonstrates proper use of brace
 2. Reports minimal pain
 3. Maintains skin integrity
 4. Verbalizes feelings and concerns
 5. Engages in activities appropriate to limitations and developmental level

▼ BONE TUMORS

Data Base
A. Neoplastic disease that can arise from any tissues involved in bone growth
B. Less than 1% of all malignant neoplasms; more common in children than adults; peak ages 15 to 19 years
C. Classification
 1. Osteogenic sarcoma
  a. Most frequent bone tumor in children
  b. Primary tumor site: metaphysis (wider part of the shaft) of a long bone, especially the femur
  c. Arises from osteoid tissue
 2. Ewing's sarcoma
  a. Most frequent sites: shaft of the long and trunk bones, especially the femur, tibia, fibula, humerus, ulna, vertebra, scapula, ribs, pelvic bones, and skull
  b. Arises from medullary tissue (marrow)
D. Clinical findings
 1. Symptoms
  a. Localized pain in the affected site
  b. Limp; voluntary curtailment of activity
  c. Inability to hold heavy objects
  d. Weight loss; frequent infections
 2. Diagnosis
  a. X-ray examination; computerized tomography (bone); bone scan
  b. Bone marrow aspiration
  c. Surgical biopsy (Ewing's sarcoma)
E. Therapetic interventions
 1. Osteogenic sarcoma: amputation of the affected bone followed by high-dose methotrexate with citrovorum factor rescue or preoperative and postoperative use of chemotherapy with en bloc resection of the primary tumor followed by a prosthetic replacement; approximately 65% to 75% can expect long-term survival
 2. Ewing's sarcoma: intensive irradiation of the involved bone and chemotherapy; prognosis is best when no metastasis is present at diagnosis

Nursing Care of Adolescents with Bone Tumors
A. **ASSESSMENT**
 1. Location and extent of pain
 2. Functional status of involved area
 3. Inflammation at site; lymph node involvement
 4. Systemic involvement
B. **ANALYSIS/NURSING DIAGNOSES**
 1. Anxiety related to diagnosis; treatment; prognosis
 2. Disturbed body image related to altered physical appearance after amputation; chemotherapy
 3. Ineffective coping related to therapeutic interventions
 4. Decisional conflict related to variety of treatment modalities
 5. Interrupted family processes related to child with a life-threatening illness
 6. Fear related to therapeutic interventions; potential for death
 7. Anticipatory grieving (adolescent) related to possible loss of limb
 8. Anticipatory grieving (parental) related to potential loss of child
 9. Acute pain related to disease process; therapeutic interventions
 10. Impaired physical mobility related to amputated extremity
 11. Social isolation related to hospitalization; changes in appearance
C. **PLANNING/IMPLEMENTATION**
 1. Care for the child having surgery
  a. Employ straightforward honesty; avoid disguising the diagnosis with terms such as "infection"
  b. Answer questions regarding information presented by the surgeon and clarify any misconceptions; avoid overwhelming the child or parents with too much information
  c. Emphasize lack of alternatives if amputation is planned
  d. Assist the child in becoming adept at using the prosthesis
  e. Help the child select clothing to camouflage the prosthesis
 2. Care for the child having radiotherapy (Ewing's sarcoma)
  a. Explain the procedure; explain the side effects
  b. Suggest and/or implement measures to reduce the physical effects of radiotherapy: select loose-fitting cotton clothing over the irradiated areas to decrease additional irritation; protect the area from sunlight and sudden changes in temperature; avoid use of ice packs, heating pads
  c. Help child cope with the side effects of radiotherapy
 3. Care for the child receiving chemotherapy
  a. Explain the procedure stressing the importance of therapy

b. Explain the probable side effects of antimetabolites (e.g., nausea, hair loss, stomatitis)

c. Help the child cope with the side effects of chemotherapy; discuss supportive therapies (e.g., antiemetics, nutrition)

d. Encourage hygiene, grooming, and items to enhance appearance such as a wig

4. Provide emotional support to child and family members

a. Clarify misconceptions and provide technical information as needed

b. Allow the time and opportunity to go through the grief process

c. Allow for expression of feelings regarding losses and the undesirable effects of therapy

d. Allow dependence but encourage independence

e. Impress on child and family the need for continuing regular activities, interactions, and behaviors

D. EVALUATION/OUTCOMES

1. Reports minimal pain

2. Child and parents express feelings and concerns

3. Child and parents demonstrate positive coping skills

4. Child and parents verbalize understanding of therapies and side effects

5. Child and parents adjust to alterations in child's appearance

6. Resumes peer relationships and activities commensurate with abilities

▼ EMOTIONAL DISORDERS

For common emotional disorders of the adolescent see Disorders First Evident in Infancy, Childhood, or Adolescence in Mental Health Nursing

▼ OTHER HEALTH PROBLEMS

Many problems of adolescence are similar to those of adults; see specific areas in Childbearing and Women's Health Nursing and Medical-Surgical Nursing for further discussion

PEDIATRIC NURSING
REVIEW QUESTIONS

Emotional Needs Related to Health Problems

1. The response that would be unusual in infants subjected to prolonged hospitalization would be:
   1. Lack or slowness of weight gain
   2. Limited emotional response to stimuli
   3. Excessive crying and clinging when approached
   4. Looking at ceiling lights rather than at persons caring for them

2. Before administering a tube feeding to an infant, the nurse should:
   1. Irrigate the tube with water
   2. Slowly instill 10 ml of formula
   3. Provide the baby with a pacifier
   4. Place in the Trendelenburg position

3. The nurse, realizing that the mother of a 2-month-old boy with colic needs help coping, suggests that she:
   1. Give her son a warm bath to calm him down
   2. Arrange for some time away from her son each day to rest
   3. Provide her son with warm sweetened tea when he begins to cry
   4. Sit comfortably in a quiet, darkened room to hold her son when he cries

4. Before surgery to relieve an intestinal obstruction, a 3-month-old is kept NPO and has a nasogastric tube in place. To calm the infant, as well as meet developmental needs best, the nurse should:
   1. Allow the infant to suck on a pacifier
   2. Allow the infant to hold onto a favorite toy
   3. Hang a brightly colored mobile in the infant's crib
   4. Place the infant on the abdomen and permit crawling

5. Attendance of parents during painful procedures on their toddlers should be:
   1. Based on individual assessment of the parents
   2. Based on the type of procedure to be performed
   3. Discouraged for the benefit of the parents and the child
   4. Encouraged and permitted if the child desires their presence

6. At 2 years of age, a child is readmitted to the hospital for additional surgery. The most important factor in preparing the child for this experience is:
   1. The child's previous hospital visits
   2. Assurance of affection and security
   3. Gratification of all the child's wishes
   4. Never leaving the child with strangers

7. The mother of a 2-year-old tells the nurse she is having difficulty disciplining her child. The nurse's response most appropriate to this comment would be;
   1. "This is a difficult age that your child is going through right now."
   2. "I'm not sure what you mean by difficulty. Tell me more about this."
   3. "I can understand what you mean; that's why it's called the terrible twos."
   4. "You know you have to be consistent with toddlers when you are disciplining them."

8. On the third day of hospitalization a 2-year-old who had been inconsolably crying and screaming begins to regress and is now lying quietly in the crib with a blanket. The nurse recognizes that the child is in the stage of:
   1. Denial
   2. Despair
   3. Mistrust
   4. Rejection

9. During the second week of hospitalization, a 2-year-old girl smiles easily, goes to all the nurses happily, and does not express a great deal of interest in her mother when she visits. The mother tells the nurse she is pleased about the adjustment but somewhat concerned about her child's reactions to her. Before responding to the mother, the nurse should understand that the behavior probably means that the child:
   1. Is repressing her feelings for her mother
   2. Has established a routine and feels safe
   3. Has given up fighting and accepts the separation
   4. Feels better physically so her behavior has improved

10. As a child with nephrosis gets older and has repeated attacks, it is most important for the nurse to help the child develop:
    1. A positive body image
    2. The ability to test urine
    3. Fine muscle coordination
    4. Acceptance of possible sterility

11. A 4-year-old male, being admitted for surgery, arrives on the ambulatory surgical unit crying and pulling at his hospital gown while clutching a teddy bear. The nurse's best response would be:
    1. "Oh come on now, stop crying! Nobody will hurt you."
    2. "Hello, my name is Ken. Let's go see where your room is."
    3. "Hi, there. I know you feel scared. Is this your special teddy bear?"
    4. "Hello young man. Let me show you to your room. Then we can play."

12. As a preschooler, the 4-year-old's response to hospitalization is influenced by:
    1. Fear of separation
    2. Fear of bodily harm
    3. Belief in death's finality
    4. Belief in the supernatural

13. When the nurse brings a dinner tray to a 4-year-old girl with pneumonia, the child says, "I'm too sick to feed myself." The nurse should respond:
    1. "Let it go until you feel better."
    2. "Try to eat as much as you can."
    3. "Wait 5 minutes and I will help you."
    4. "Be a big girl and don't act like a baby."

14. A 6-year-old, admitted to the hospital 2 days ago, tells the nurse, "I'm too sick to feed myself." The nurse recognizes that this statement is most likely indicative of:
    1. Immaturity
    2. Loneliness
    3. Regression
    4. Temper tantrum

15. A hospitalized 5-year-old is apathetic about eating. Nursing care directed toward supporting the child's nutrition should include:
    1. Asking the parents to visit at mealtime
    2. Giving only the foods the child likes best
    3. Providing diversional activity at mealtime
    4. Eliminating all between-meal nourishment

16. A 6-year-old girl begins thumb-sucking after surgery. This was not the child's behavior preoperatively. The nurse should:
    1. Accept the thumb-sucking
    2. Distract her by playing checkers
    3. Report this behavior to the physician
    4. Tell her thumb-sucking causes buckteeth

17. A 15-year-old male comes with his mother to the diabetic outpatient clinic. He has type 1 diabetes. The adolescent sits back in his chair with his arms folded and a frown on his face. He displays an "I don't care" attitude toward his diabetes and argues with his mother in front of the nurse. The approach that would be best for the nurse to use in dealing with this adolescent and his mother is to:
    1. Encourage them to work out their differences together and return to the room afterward
    2. Ask the mother to wait in the waiting room while her son meets with the physicians and other staff
    3. Encourage the adolescent to take more responsibility for treatment of his diabetes because he is almost an adult
    4. Speak separately with the adolescent and the mother, encouraging each of them to ventilate and recognize their anger

18. A 14-year-old is severely hurt while on a skateboard and develops contractures in all the limbs. The adolescent refuses to move, so the nurse should encourage movement by:
    1. Allowing friends to visit every day
    2. Explaining that some pain is inevitable
    3. Setting strict limits to increase the adolescent's security
    4. Permitting the adolescent to make decisions regarding care

19. To give the most support to the parents of an infant with an obvious physical defect, the nurse should:
    1. Discourage them from talking about the baby
    2. Encourage them to express their worries and fears
    3. Tell them not to worry because the defect can be repaired
    4. Show them postoperative photographs of babies who had similar defects

Drug-Related Responses

20. A child who is known to have the human immun-odeficiency virus (HIV) is admitted with the diagnosis of *Pneumocystis carinii* pneumonia. The physician orders trimethoxazole sulfamethoxazole (Bactrim) and pentamidine. When administering Bactrim to a child with AIDS the nurse should monitor for the most common side effect of:
    1. Jaundice
    2. Headache
    3. Toxic nephrosis
    4. Hypersensitivity reactions

21. An 8-year-old with juvenile rheumatoid arthritis is receiving salicylate therapy. During the salicylate therapy the nurse should observe the child for:
    1. Nausea, dizziness, edema, headache
    2. Gastric distress, nausea, vomiting, tinnitus
    3. Constipation, deafness, nausea, headache
    4. Diarrhea, gastric distress, edema of the face

22. The nurse should be aware that sodium salicylate is classified as an:
    1. Analgesic and sedative
    2. Antipyretic and hypnotic
    3. Antibiotic and antipyretic
    4. Analgesic and antipyretic

23. An 18-month-old, hospitalized with a severe asthma attack is given prednisone, 15 mg po bid. The nurse should:
    1. Prevent exposing the child to infection
    2. Check the child's eosinophil count daily
    3. Have the child rest as much as possible
    4. Keep the child NPO except for medications

24. Following orthopedic surgery, codeine sulfate is given for pain to an adolescent. About 8 hours later, the adolescent complains of itching. A drug that can he ordered to relieve this symptom is:
    1. Nitrofurazone (Furacin)
    2. Hyaluronidase (Wydase)
    3. Acetylsalicylic acid (Ecotrin)
    4. Chlorpheniramine (Chlor-Trimeton)

25. An 11-year-old with juvenile rheumatoid arthritis will be on continued aspirin medication at home. Before discharge the nurse should teach the child and the parents to closely monitor for the toxic effects of this drug, including:
    1. Tinnitus
    2. Diarrhea
    3. Jaundice
    4. Hypothermia

26. A 7-year-old female develops a urinary tract infection. The physician orders a sulfonamide preparation. A major nursing responsibility when administering this drug is to:
    1. Weigh the child daily
    2. Give milk with the medication
    3. Monitor the temperature frequently
    4. Administer the drug at the prescribed times

27. A child with acute leukemia is started on chemotherapy, including prednisone. A side effect of prednisone that may be exhibited is:
    1. Alopecia
    2. Anorexia
    3. Weight loss
    4. Mood changes

28. Methotrexate is prescribed as part of a child's cancer therapy. The nurse is aware this chemotherapeutic agent accomplishes its action by:
    1. Intervening in mitosis, thus inhibiting the growth of the malignant cells
    2. Acting as an antibiotic to control the spread of infected white blood cells
    3. Depressing bone marrow function, thus decreasing white blood cell production
    4. Competing for essential structural components, thus inhibiting white blood cell production

29. An adolescent client is started on a chemotherapeutic drug regimen for cancer that includes prednisone, vincristine, and L-asparaginase. The side effect of these drugs that requires early preparation of this client is:
    1. Alopecia
    2. Constipation
    3. Retarded growth in height
    4. Generalized short-term paralysis

30. The primary reason for using prednisone in the treatment of acute leukemia in children is that it is able to:
    1. Decrease inflammation
    2. Reduce irradiation edema
    3. Suppress mitosis in lymphocytes
    4. Increase appetite and sense of well-being

31. A combination of drugs, which includes vincristine (Oncovin) and prednisone, is prescribed for a child with leukemia. Because of the toxicity of vincristine the nurse should expect:
    1. Anemia and fever
    2. Irreversible alopecia
    3. Neurologic symptoms
    4. Gastrointestinal symptoms

32. A young child with acute nonlymphoid leukemia is started on induction chemotherapy. Nursing interventions that would be appropriate to avoid the complications associated with neutropenia include:
    1. Encouraging a well-balanced diet, including iron-rich foods, and helping the child avoid overexertion
    2. Placing the child in a private room, restricting ill visitors, and using strict handwashing techniques
    3. Avoiding rectal temperatures, avoiding injections, and applying direct pressure for 5 to 10 minutes after venipuncture
    4. Offering a moist, bland, soft diet, using toothettes rather than a toothbrush, and providing frequent saline mouthwashes

33. A client and her 6-year-old come to the clinic because they both have severe upper respiratory tract infections. The physician plans to prescribe tetracycline (Achromycin). The nurse reminds the physician that the child is 6 years old and that the client is in her eighteenth week of pregnancy. These data are important because the drug may cause:
    1. Changes in the bone structure of young children and pregnant women
    2. Persistent vomiting when given to small children and pregnant women
    3. Tooth enamel defects in children under 8 years of age and in the maturing fetus
    4 Lower red blood cell production at times in their development when anemia is a common problem

34. A 4-year-old has a seizure disorder and has been taking phenytoin (Dilantin) for 3 years. An important nursing measure for the child would be to:
    1. Offer the urinal frequently
    2. Check for pupillary reaction
    3. Observe for flushing of the face
    4. Administer scrupulous oral hygiene

35. An 8-year-old is receiving tetracycline (Achromycin). The fever is down and secretions have lessened, but the child is eating poorly, is withdrawn, lethargic, and irritable, and sobs readily. The nurse should promptly discuss the problem with the physician because:
    1. The child needs a higher food intake to fight the infection
    2. Anemia is a frequent occurrence after infection and treatment with antibiotics

    3. Concurrent bladder infection may be present as an extension of the gram-negative infection
    4. Generalized physical symptoms and behavior problems may precede drug-induced liver damage

36. Based on developmental norms for a 5-year-old, the nurse should withhold a scheduled dose of digoxin (Lanoxin) elixir and notify the physician when the child's apical pulse rate first drops below:
    1. 60 beats per minute
    2. 80 beats per minute
    3. 90 beats per minute
    4. 100 beats per minute

37. After administration of mebendazole (Vermox) to a 4-year-old for pinworms, the nurse should observe the child for:
    1. Constipation
    2. Hypertension
    3. Intestinal bleeding
    4. Worms in the stool

38. Following a tonsillectomy, a 20 kg 8-year-old is complaining of pain in the throat. The pain medication that would be best for the child at this time would be
    1. Aspirin, 300 mg
    2. Tylenol, 300 mg
    3. Demerol, 50 mg
    4. Phenobarbital, 15 mg

39. A toddler is admitted to the hospital in the terminal stage of leukemia with episodes of severe bone pain. The nurse should plan to administer:
    1. Analgesics when pain is severe
    2. IM analgesics as often as possible
    3. Oral analgesics between IM analgesics
    4. Analgesics before pain becomes severe

40. A child with a high blood level of lead is started on a regimen of chelation therapy that consists of calcium disodium edetate (EDTA) and dimercaprol (BAL) q4h for 5 days. The nurse understands that this combination of drugs:
    1. Removes lead from the bone marrow more efficiently
    2. Eliminates lead from the body more rapidly through the urine
    3. Has fewer side effects and removes lead from the brain more effectively
    4. Removes lead from the blood more rapidly and increases deposition in the bones

41. Calcium EDTA is to be used intravenously as the chelating agent for a preschooler with plumbism (lead poisoning). During the preschooler's hospital stay, it is most important for the nurse to recognize that this drug therapy requires that the staff:
    1. Test the child's stool for occult blood (Hematest)
    2. Assess the child's diet because no "junk food" is allowed
    3. Monitor the child for adequate hydration and urine output
    4. Administer the child's medication only at night to reduce the associated pain

42. If an adolescent with diabetes takes Humulin N insulin at 7:30 AM, the time of day that an insulin reaction is likely to occur would be:
    1. 8:30 AM
    2. 2:30 PM
    3. 7:30 PM
    4. 1:30 AM

Growth and Development

43. The major depriving factor in long-term hospitalization of which the nurse should be aware is usually the:
    1. Lack of play objects
    2. Lack of multisensory inputs
    3. Care provided only by a mother substitute
    4. Absence of interaction with a mother figure

44. To meet a major developmental need of a newborn in the immediate postoperative period the nurse should:
    1. Give the infant a pacifier
    2. Put a mobile over the infant's crib
    3. Provide the infant with a soft cuddly toy
    4. Warm the infant's formula before feeding

45. When reviewing the data recorded on a newborn's chart, the information that would indicate to the nurse that this baby requires special attention would be:
    1. Birth weight of 3500 g
    2. The Apgar score at birth was 3
    3. The infant has a positive Babinski reflex
    4. 20 ml of milky-colored fluid aspirated from stomach

46. The nurse is aware that children born with a missing chromosome are most likely to have:
    1. Cretinism
    2. Phenylketonuria
    3. Down syndrome
    4. Turner's syndrome

47. Play during infancy is:
    1. Initiated by the child
    2. A way of teaching how to share
    3. More important than in later years
    4. Mostly used for physical development

48. A characteristic of infants and young children who have experienced maternal deprivation is:
    1. Extreme activity
    2. Proneness to illness
    3. Responsiveness to stimuli
    4. Tendency toward overeating

49. When a mother with a 3-month-old infant comes to the well-baby clinic, the nurse should include in the accident prevention teaching plan the need to:
    1. Remove all tiny objects from the floor
    2. Cover electric outlets with safety plugs
    3. Keep crib rails up to the highest position
    4. Remove poisonous substances from low areas

50. When teaching a mother how to prevent accidents while caring for her 6-month-old, the nurse should emphasize that at this age child can usually:
    1. Sit up
    2. Roll over
    3. Crawl lengthy distances
    4. Stand while holding onto furniture

51. The mother of a 7-month-old infant who is to be catheterized to obtain a sterile urine specimen expresses fear that this procedure may traumatize the child psychologically. The nurse reassures the mother that:
    1. Her fear is justified and the nurse will obtain a "clean catch" specimen
    2. She has every right to refuse the catheterization; her concerns are realistic
    3. Her concern is appropriate but the need for a sterile specimen is a higher priority
    4. The procedure, though slightly uncomfortable, should not have any damaging effect

52. In terms of preventive teaching for the parents of a 1-year-old, the nurse would speak to them about:
    1. Accidents
    2. Toilet training
    3. Adequate nutrition
    4. Sexual development

53. A nurse who works in the parent-child center of a large city hospital is responsible for assessment of both child and parent, discharge teaching, and the orientation of new nurses to the various pediatric units. The nurse shares with the parents of one of the children that it is most challenging to perform a physical examination on a child who is:
    1. In the early school years
    2. From 1 to 4 years of age
    3. In the first 6 months of life
    4. Between 6 and 12 months old

54. The primary task to be accomplished between 12 and 15 months of age is to learn to:
    1. Walk erect
    2. Climb stairs
    3. Use a spoon
    4. Say simple words

55. A 15 month old is playing in the playpen. The nurse evaluates the child's ability to perform physical tasks is at the age-related norm when the child is able to:
    1. Build a tower of six blocks
    2. Walk across the playpen with ease
    3. Throw all the toys out of the playpen
    4. Stand in the playpen holding onto the sides

56. A father brings his 18-month-old son to the clinic. He asks the nurse why his son is so difficult to please, has temper tantrums, and annoys him by throwing food from the table. The nurse should explain that:
    1. Toddlers need to be disciplined at this stage to prevent the development of antisocial behaviors
    2. The child is learning to assert independence, and his behavior is considered normal for his age
    3. This is the usual way that a toddler expresses his needs during the initiative stage of development
    4. It is best to leave the child alone in his crib after calmly telling him why his behavior is unacceptable

57. A mother tells the nurse that each morning she offers her 24-month-old son juice and he always shakes his head and says, "No." She asks the nurse what to do, because she knows the child needs fluids. The nurse suggests that the mother:
    1. Distract him with some food
    2. Be firm and hand him the glass
    3. Let him see that he is making her angry
    4. Offer him a choice of two things to drink

58. A 2-year-old boy, admitted to the hospital for further surgical repair of a clubfoot, is standing in his crib crying. The child refuses to be comforted and calls for his mother. As the nurse approaches the crib to provide morning care the child screams louder. The nurse, recognizing that this behavior is typical of the stage of protest, decides to:
    1. Pick him up and carry him around the room
    2. Fill the basin with water and proceed to bathe him
    3. Sit by his crib and bathe him later when his anxiety decreases
    4. Skip the bath because a child this upset does not really need a bath

59. When successfully learning autonomy and independence, the toddler would be learning:
    1. Superego control
    2. Trust and security
    3. Roles within society
    4. To accept external limits

60. The nurse observes a 2-year-old at play and notes that this age toddler:
    1. Builds houses with blocks
    2. Is extremely possessive of toys
    3. Attempts to stay within the lines when coloring
    4. Amuses self with a picture book for 15 minutes

61. A mother asks when to take her 2-year-old to the dentist. For dental prophylaxis, the nurse encourages her to take the child:
    1. Before starting school
    2. Between 2 and 3 years of age
    3. When the child begins to lose deciduous teeth
    4. The next time another family member goes to the dentist

62. The nurse explains to the mother of a 2-year-old girl that the child's negativism is normal for her age and that it is helping her meet her need for:
    1. Trust
    2. Attention
    3. Discipline
    4. Independence

63. When ordering a regular diet for a young toddler the nurse should choose foods such as:
    1. SpaghettiOs and raisins
    2. Corn dog and french fries
    3. Hamburger with bun and grapes
    4. Hot dog with bun and potato chips

64. During a nap, a 3-year-old hospitalized boy wets the bed. The best approach by the nurse would be to:
1. Tell him to help with remaking the bed
2. Change his clothes and make no issue of it
3. Change his bed, putting a rubber sheet on it
4. Explain that big boys should try to call the nurse

65. When evaluating a 3-year-old's developmental progress, the nurse should recognize that development is delayed when the child is unable to:
1. Copy a square
2. Hop on one foot
3. Catch a ball reliably
4. Use a spoon effectively

66. The nurse understands that a good snack for a 2-year-old with a diagnosis of acute asthma would be:
1. Grapes
2. Apple slices
3. A glass of milk
4. A glass of cola

67. To teach the correct way to administer eardrops to a small child, the nurse should instruct the parent to position the child on the side and instill the drops while pulling the auricle:
1. Forward
2. Up and back
3. Straight back
4. Down and back

68. When observing a toddler playing with other children in the playroom, the nurse would expect the toddler to engage in:
1. Parallel play
2. Solitary play
3. Competitive play
4. Tumbling-type play

69. The nurse is aware that an appropriate toy for a young toddler during hospitalization would be a:
1. Mobile
2. Tricycle
3. Ten-piece puzzle
4. Carton of Play-Doh

70. The nurse teaches a toddler with cystic fibrosis how to use an inhaler. To evaluate the toddler's understanding the nurse should ask the toddler:
1. To show the nurse how to use the inhaler
2. If there are any questions about using the inhaler

3. To tell the nurse about all the things that have been learned
4. If the toddler can explain how the inhaler will be used at home

71. Preschool children role play. This is an important part of socialization because it:
1. Encourages expression
2. Helps children think about careers
3. Teaches children about stereotypes
4. Provides guidelines for adult behavior

72. The nurse observes that a 4 year old is having difficulty relating with the other children in the playroom. The nurse understands that it is normal for this age child to:
1. Engage in parallel or solitary play
2. Be almost totally dependent on parents
3. Exaggerate and boast to impress others
4. Have fierce temper tantrums and negativism

73. When providing nursing care to a preschooler the nurse should remember that the child's fear is of:
1. Pain
2. Death
3. Isolation
4. Intrusive procedures

74. A mother tells the nurse that the pediatrician has expressed concern that her 4-year-old child exhibits developmental delays. The mother expresses readiness to place her child in a preschool program for retarded children. The nurse should:
1. Praise the mother for her acceptance and encourage her plan
2. Advise the mother to have the pediatrician help choose an appropriate program
3. Ask the mother for more specific information related to the developmental delays
4. Tell the mother that this is probably a premature action because developmental delays often disappear

75. The nurse should attempt to involve a preschooler in therapeutic play to give the child the opportunity to:
1. Meet other children on the unit
2. Work out ways of coping with fears
3. Learn to accept the hospital situation
4. Forget the reality of the situation for a while

76. The nurse plans to talk to a mother about toilet training a toddler, knowing that the most important factor in the process of toilet training is the:
    1. Child's desire to be dry
    2. Ability of the child to sit still
    3. Parent's willingness to work at it
    4. Approach and attitude of the parent

77. A mother asks the nurse what to do when her toddler has temper tantrums. The nurse suggests that the mother allow the child another way of expressing anger such as by the use of a:
    1. Ball and bat
    2. Punching bag
    3. Pounding board
    4. Wad of clay or Play-Doh

78. When a young toddler's mother is getting ready to take the toddler home after a prolonged hospitalization, she asks the nurse what type of behavior she should expect to be displayed. The nurse informs the mother that the toddler will probably be:
    1. Hostile toward her
    2. Making excessive demands on both parents
    3. Cheerful but have a shallow attachment to all adults
    4. Apathetic and withdrawn from all emotional ties to her

79. The average 5 year old is incapable of:
    1. Tying shoelaces
    2. Abstract thought
    3. Making decisions
    4. Hand-eye coordination

80. A 6-year-old child is admitted to the hospital with a diagnosis of acute leukemia. When planning play activities for this six-year-old child the nurse should include:
    1. Action toys such as a hula hoop
    2. Stuffed animals, large puzzles, and large blocks
    3. Table games, checkers, simple card games, and crayons
    4. A record player, portable radio, and children's magazines

81. The nurse should encourage two 6-year-old boys in the playroom to play with:
    1. Clay
    2. Checkers
    3. A board game
    4. A building set

82. A 9 year old who is in bed convalescing becomes very bored and irritable. The nurse plans activities that a school-age child would like and suggests the child:
    1. Play chess
    2. Start a collection
    3. Do arithmetic puzzles
    4. Watch game shows on TV

83. Postoperatively, to help relieve the anxiety of a young school-aged child, the nurse should:
    1. Allow the child time to talk about feelings
    2. Tell a story about a child with similar surgery
    3. Ask the mother to room with the child for a few days
    4. Provide the child with bandages, tape, scissors, and a doll

84. An 11-year-old male has gained weight. His mother is concerned that her son, who loves sports, may become obese. The nurse:
    1. Advises an increase in activity
    2. Urges a decreased caloric intake
    3. Explains this is normal for a preadolescent
    4. Discusses the relationship of genetics and weight gain

85. Therapeutic communication with an adolescent is best accomplished by:
    1. Using teen language
    2. Relating on a peer level
    3. Dealing in concrete terms
    4. Establishing a relationship over time

86. The nurse is aware that a characteristic that often affects an adolescent's approach to illness and treatment is that adolescents are:
    1. Accurately in touch with their feelings
    2. Striving for industry as a developmental task
    3. Concerned more with the present than with the future
    4. Using thinking that is both concrete and reality oriented

Respiratory

87. The nurse teaching a mothers' class tells them that the best way to position their infants during the first couple of weeks of life is to lay them on their:
    1. Stomachs with their heads flat
    2. Backs or sides with their heads flat
    3. Right side with their heads slightly elevated
    4. Stomachs with their heads slightly elevated

88. A newborn of a few hours appears to be less cyanotic when crying. The nurse recognizes that this may be related to:
    1. Sternal retractions of respiratory distress syndrome
    2. Twitching of the body resulting from neurologic damage
    3. Asymmetry of chest expansion associated with atelectasis
    4. Alterations in heart rate associated with an atrioventricular septal defect

89. A 17-year-old female, smelling of alcohol, arrives in the emergency clinic with her 3-month-old son who she states stopped breathing for "a while." The baby continues to have difficulty breathing. The assessment data obtained on this baby that should alert the nurse to suspect shaken baby syndrome (SBS) would be:
    1. The baby was born at 28 weeks' gestation
    2. Lack of stridor and adventitious breath sounds
    3. Previous episodes of apnea lasting 10 to 15 seconds
    4. Retractions and use of accessory respiratory muscles

90. A mother talks to the nurse about her sick infant, and she is disturbed because she did not realize the baby was ill. A major indication of illness in an infant is:
    1. Profuse perspiration
    2. Longer periods of sleep
    3. Grunting and rapid respirations
    4. Desire for increased fluids during the feedings

91. One of the primary nursing diagnoses for an older child with chronic bronchitis is "ineffective airway clearance related to retained secretions." Plans to decrease retained secretions should include:
    1. Administering oxygen as ordered
    2. Placing the client in a high-Fowler's position
    3. Gargling periodically with warm normal saline
    4. Increasing fluid intake to at least 2000 ml/day

92. A newborn is admitted to the intensive care nursery with the diagnosis of choanal atresia. The nurse is aware that choanal atresia is an anomaly located in the:
    1. Anal area
    2. Nasopharynx
    3. Intestinal tract
    4. Pharynx and larynx

93. While feeding a newborn with the diagnosis of choanal atresia, the nurse notices that the newborn:
    1. Chokes on the feeding
    2. Lacks a swallowing reflex
    3. Does not appear to be hungry
    4. Takes only about half of the feeding

94. An infant is in pediatric intensive care after open-heart surgery for the repair of a ventricular septal defect. A nursing priority should be to:
    1. Monitor the infant's urinary output
    2. Ascertain the infant's pulmonary status
    3. Determine the status of the operative site
    4. Check the patency of the intravenous catheter

95. The earliest clinical sign in idiopathic respiratory distress syndrome in a young infant is usually:
    1. Grunting
    2. Cyanosis
    3. Rapid respiration
    4. Sternal and subcostal retractions

96. The most critical factor in the immediate care of an infant after repair of a cleft lip would be the:
    1. Prevention of vomiting
    2. Maintenance of a patent airway
    3. Administration of parenteral fluids
    4. Administration of drugs to reduce oral secretions

97. A toddler is admitted to the hospital because of sudden hoarseness and continuous, somewhat unintelligible speech. When talking with the mother, the nurse will be particularly concerned about:
    1. Retropharyngeal abscess
    2. Acute respiratory tract infection
    3. Undetected laryngeal abnormality
    4. Respiratory tract obstruction caused by a foreign body

98. When preparing for the admission of a child with acute laryngitis (croup), the nurse on the pediatric unit should first:
    1. Arrange for a quiet, cool room
    2. Pad the side rails of the croup tent
    3. Set up a cot so that a parent can stay
    4. Obtain a tracheostomy set for the bedside

99. When caring for a child with croup, the priority nursing action should be to:
    1. Initiate measures to reduce fever
    2. Constantly assess respiratory status
    3. Provide support to reduce apprehension
    4. Ensure delivery of 40% humidified oxygen

100. A 2-year-old is admitted to the pediatric unit with a diagnosis of acute asthma. A blood sample is obtained to measure the child's arterial blood gases. The nurse should expect:
    1. An elevated pH
    2. A raised oxygen level
    3. A decreased bicarbonate level
    4. An increased carbon dioxide level

101. When planning discharge teaching for the parents of a child with asthma, the nurse should include telling the parents to increase the child's fluid intake and to have the child:
    1. Avoid foods high in fat
    2. Increase the usual calorie intake
    3. Avoid exertion and exposure to cold
    4. Stay in the house for at least 2 weeks

102. When preparing a child with asthma for discharge, the nurse must emphasize to the family that:
    1. A cold dry environment is best for the child
    2. Limits should not be placed on child's behavior
    3. When the child is asymptomatic, the disease is gone
    4. Medications must be continued even if the child is asymptomatic

103. A 7-year-old is admitted for surgery. Preoperatively it is essential that the nurse:
    1. Observe the child's ASO titer
    2. Provide the child with a favorite toy
    3. Check for loose teeth and report the findings to the physician
    4. Encourage a parent to stay until the child goes to the operating room

104. The nurse is aware that the primary pathology that produces the clinical manifestations of cystic fibrosis is:
    1. Hyperactivity of the eccrine (sweat) glands
    2. Hypoactivity of the autonomic nervous system
    3. Mechanical obstruction of mucus-secreting glands
    4. Atrophic changes in the mucosal lining of the intestines

105. Although there is no history of cystic fibrosis in a 5-year-old's family, the nurse is aware that cystic fibrosis is inherited through chromosomes that are:
    1. X-linked
    2. Mutant in nature
    3. Autosomal dominant
    4. Autosomal recessive

106. The primary purpose of chest physiotherapy (CPT) for the child with cystic fibrosis is to:
    1. Mobilize secretions
    2. Prevent barrel chest
    3. Dilate the bronchioles
    4. Provide humidification

107. The problem of cystic fibrosis is sometimes first noted by the nurse in the newborn nursery because of the infant's:
    1. Excessive crying
    2. Sternal retractions
    3. Increased heart rate
    4. Abdominal distention

108. The nurse, when planning care, recalls that chest percussion and postural drainage for a toddler with cystic fibrosis are best done:
    1. After suctioning
    2. Before aerosol therapy
    3. One hour before meals
    4. Immediately after meals

109. When caring for the child with cystic fibrosis the nurse should:
    1. Prevent coughing
    2. Perform postural drainage
    3. Encourage active exercise
    4. Provide small, frequent feedings

110. A child with cystic fibrosis is predisposed to bronchitis mainly because of:
    1. Neuromuscular irritability that causes spasm and constriction of the bronchi
    2. Increased salt content in saliva that can irritate and necrose mucous membranes in nasopharynx
    3. The associated heart defects of cystic fibrosis that cause congestive heart failure and respiratory depression
    4. Tenacious secretions that obstruct the bronchioles and respiratory tract and provide a favorable medium for growth of bacteria

111. The nurse provides clapping, percussion, and postural drainage every 4 hours for a 3-month-old infant with cystic fibrosis. The nurse is aware that the best time for scheduling this chest physiotherapy is:
    1. After every feeding
    2. Before every feeding
    3. During every feeding
    4. Midway between feedings

112. A father of three young children is diagnosed as having tuberculosis. Members of this family who have a positive reaction to the tuberculin test are candidates for treatment with:
    1. BCG vaccine
    2. INH and PAS
    3. Old tuberculin
    4. Purified protein derivative of tuberculin

113. If a person has been exposed to tuberculosis but shows no signs or symptoms except a positive tuberculin test, prophylactic drug therapy is usually continued after the last exposure for a period of:
    1. 3 weeks
    2. 4 months
    3. 9 months
    4. 2 years

114. Children in the family of a person who has tuberculosis who have been exposed to but show no evidence of the disease:
    1. Can be considered to be immune
    2. Should be given antitubercular drugs
    3. Are usually given massive doses of penicillin
    4. Are given X-ray examinations every 6 months

115. Selection of drugs of choice for the treatment of pneumonia depends primarily on:
    1. Tolerance of the client
    2. Selectivity of the organism
    3. Sensitivity of the organism
    4. Preference of the physician

116. Nursing care most likely to be effective in alleviating the fretfulness of a 5-year-old girl hospitalized with pneumonia would be:
    1. Reading a story to her
    2. Giving her a jigsaw puzzle
    3. Letting her play with a doll
    4. Putting her in a room by herself

117. A 6-year-old child is admitted to the hospital with pneumonia. An immediate priority in this child's nursing care would be:
    1. Rest
    2. Exercise
    3. Nutrition
    4. Elimination

118. It is expected that after a thoracotomy lung expansion will recur within:
    1. 1 hour
    2. 4 hours
    3. 12 to 48 hours
    4. 48 to 72 hours

119. Following a tonsillectomy, the nurse suspects hemorrhage postoperatively when the child:
    1. Snores noisily
    2. Becomes pale
    3. Complains of thirst
    4. Swallows frequently

120. A 17-year-old high school student with a history of asthma is brought to the emergency department. The nurse recognizes that the adolescent is experiencing an acute asthma exacerbation when assessment reveals:
    1. Lethargy, hypotension, and fever
    2. Confusion, tachypnea, and crackles
    3. Tachycardia, anxiety, and wheezing
    4. Hypertension, bradycardia, and tremor

Reproductive and Genitourinary

121. After circumcision of a 6-month-old infant, the most essential nursing action during the initial postoperative period is to assess the infant for:
    1. Infection
    2. Hemorrhage
    3. Shrill, piercing cry
    4. Decreased urinary output

122. The nurse is aware that an additional defect associated with exstrophy of the bladder is:
    1. Absence of one kidney
    2. Congenital heart disease
    3. Pubic bone malformation
    4. Tracheoesophageal fistula

123. A child born with exstrophy of the bladder is admitted to the hospital for urinary diversion surgery wherein the ureters are transplanted to a resected section of the colon with one end attached to the abdominal wall as an ileostomy. The nurse is aware that this procedure is called:
    1. A cystostomy
    2. An ileal conduit
    3. An ureterosigmoidostomy
    4. A cutaneous ureterostomy

124. The best choice for between-meal nourishment for a preschool-age child with a urinary infection would be:
    1. Skim milk
    2. Fresh fruit
    3. Hard candy
    4. Creamed soup

125. The nurse snould observe a child with acute glomerulonephritis primarily for:
    1. Polyuria, high fever
    2. Oliguria, hypotension
    3. Dehydration, hematuria
    4. Hypertension, circumocular edema

126. A child is admitted with the diagnosis of glomerulonephritis. When performing a physical assessment, the nurse should expect to find:
    1. Anorexia, hematuria, proteinuria (1+), and decreased blood pressure
    2. Normal blood pressure, anorexia, proteinuria (1+), and glycosuria (3+)
    3. Lowered blood pressure, periorbital edema, proteinuria (1+), and decreased specific gravity (1.001)
    4. Moderately elevated blood pressure, periorbital edema, proteinuria (4+), and increased specific gravity (1.030)

127. When planning nursing care for a 5-year-old with acute glomerulonephritis, the nurse realizes that the child needs help in understanding the necessary restrictions, one of which is:
    1. Daily doses of IM penicillin
    2. A bland diet high in protein
    3. Bed rest for at least 4 weeks
    4. Isolation from other children with infections

128. The parents of a child with acute glomerulonephritis are very concerned about activity restrictions after discharge. The nurse bases the answer to them on the fact that after the urinary findings are nearly normal:
    1. Activity must be limited for 1 month
    2. The child must not play active games
    3. The child must remain in bed for 2 weeks
    4. Activity does not affect the course of the disease

129. The mother of a child with glomerulonephritis asks why the child is being weighed every morning. The nurse's best response would be:
    1. "It is the best way to measure your child's fluid balance."
    2. "When weight loss stops it indicates the disease process is over."
    3. "It gives the doctors a good idea of how much protein is being lost."
    4. "The dietitian plans the daily caloric intake according to the daily weight change."

130. The most important nursing intervention for a 3-year-old child with a diagnosis of nephrosis is:
    1. Encouraging fluids
    2. Regulating the diet
    3. Preventing infection
    4. Maintaining bed rest

131. During a clinic visit a child with nephrotic syndrome who has a muddy, pale appearance, complains of not wanting to eat and feeling tired. The nurse suspects that the child is:
    1. In impending renal failure
    2. Being too active in school
    3. Developing a viral infection
    4. Not taking the ordered medication

132. The nurse explains to a parent group that the most important complication of mumps in postpubertal males is:
    1. Sterility
    2. Hypopituitarism
    3. Decrease in libido
    4. A decrease in androgens

133. One of the earliest signs of sexual maturity in young girls that occurs about the age of 12 years is:
    1. Attention to grooming
    2. Interest in the opposite sex
    3. An increase in the size of the breasts
    4. The appearance of axillary and pubic hair

134. A physician orders the following for a young child with the diagnosis of Wilms' tumor. The nurse should question the physician regarding orders related to preparation for:
    1. An IVP
    2. A renal biopsy
    3. A nephrectomy
    4. An abdominal CT scan

Neuromuscular

135. The finding a nurse would consider most unusual in a full-term infant would be the presence of:
    1. Plantar creases covering the entire sole
    2. Ears contain cartilage with the pinna firm
    3. Square window sign (wrist forms a 90° angle)
    4. Testes both descended with rugae covering scrotum

136. When performing a physical assessment of a newborn with Down syndrome, the nurse should carefully evaluate the infant's:
    1. Heart sounds
    2. Anterior fontanel
    3. Pupillary reaction
    4. Lower extremities

137. A viral disease caused by one of the smallest human viruses that infect the motor cells of the anterior horn of the spinal cord is:
   1. Rubella
   2. Rubeola
   3. Chickenpox
   4. Poliomyelitis

138. When picked up by the mother or the nurse, an 8-month-old infant screams and seems to be in pain. The nurse notes the behavior and talks to the mother about:
   1. Accidents and injuries and the importance of their prevention
   2. Any other behavior of the infant that may have been noticed by the mother
   3. The food and specific vitamins that should be given to infants, including vitamins C and D
   4. Limiting the play time and activities that this infant has with other children in the family

139. A mother expresses concerns about her 9-month-old's development, noting that her infant no longer has the same strong grasp that was present shortly after birth, nor does the infant have a similar response to noise. The nurse should explain that:
   1. It would be advisable to have a neurologic examination
   2. Failure of these responses may be related to mental retardation
   3. These responses are usually replaced by voluntary activity at 5 to 6 months of age
   4. The infant needs additional sensory stimulation to aid in the return of these responses

140. Studies of young children institutionalized for some time indicate that they show signs of retarded development. Least affected by this type retardation is the child's:
   1. Sense of hearing
   2. Ability to understand
   3. Ability for self-expression
   4. Neuromuscular development

141. A 10-month-old is brought to the emergency room for a head injury after falling down the stairs. An immediate CT scan is ordered. In preparing a 10-month-old for a CT scan the nurse should:
   1. Shave the infant's head
   2. Administer the prescribed sedative
   3. Start the prescribed intravenous infusion
   4. Give the infant an explanation of the procedure

142. A female toddler has a tonic-clonic seizure because of a high fever. During the tonic-clonic stage of the seizure the nurses's priority should be to:
   1. Turn her on her side
   2. Protect her from injury
   3. Call for additional help
   4. Establish a patent airway

143. When explaining the occurrence of febrile convulsions to a parents' class, the nurse should include that they are common in children and:
   1. May occur in minor illnesses
   2. The cause is usually readily identified
   3. Usually occur after the first year of life
   4. Occur more frequently in females than males

144. A mother indicates her 3-year-old has had a fever for several days and is now vomiting. While instituting nursing measures to reduce the child's fever, the nurse recognizes that it is important to:
   1. Encourage oral fluids
   2. Measure output every hour
   3. Limit exposure to prevent shivering
   4. Monitor vital signs every 10 minutes

145. A 2-year-old has been admitted to rule out a seizure disorder. The nurse would establish the highest priority nursing diagnosis as:
   1. Disturbed body image related to hospitalization
   2. Disturbed sensory perception related to seizures
   3. Feeding self-care deficit related to developmental stage
   4. Risk for injury related to abnormal neuro-electrical activity

146. One morning, the nurse notes that a 3-year-old child in a crib has a clamped jaw and is having a tonic-clonic seizure. The priority nursing responsibility at this time is to:
   1. Start oxygen at 10 L
   2. Insert a plastic airway
   3. Restrain the child to prevent injury to soft tissue
   4. Protect the child from harm from the environment

147. If a child develops cyanosis early during a tonic-clonic seizure, it is most appropriate for the nurse to:
   1. Insert an airway
   2. Administer oxygen
   3. Use a padded tongue blade
   4. Observe without intervening

148. A child sitting on a chair in a playroom begins a tonic-clonic seizure with a clenched jaw. The nurse's best initial action would be to:
    1. Phone for assistance
    2. Attempt to open the jaw
    3. Lower the child to the floor
    4. Place a large pillow under the head

149. The nurse assesses a 6-year-old child transported to the emergency department following a closed head injury. The sign/symptom that indicates an increase in intracranial pressure would be:
    1. Bradycardia
    2. Hyperalertness
    3. A bulging fontanel
    4. A decreased systolic blood pressure

150. An infant is diagnosed as having communicating hydrocephalus. When helping the parents understand the physician's explanation of the baby's problem, the nurse should state:
    1. "Too much cerebrospinal fluid is produced within the ventricles of the brain."
    2. "The cerebrospinal fluid is prevented from proper absorption by a blockage in the ventricles of the brain."
    3. "The part of the brain surface that normally absorbs cerebrospinal fluid after its production is not functioning adequately."
    4. "There is a flow of cerebrospinal fluid between the brain cells and the ventricles, which do not empty properly into the spinal cord."

151. Hydrocephalus, if untreated, can cause mental retardation because:
    1. CSF dilutes blood supply, causing cells to atrophy
    2. Hypertonic CSF disturbs normal plasma concentration, depriving nerve cells of vital nutrients
    3. Increasing head size necessitates more oxygen and nutrients than normal blood flow can supply
    4. Gradually increasing size of the ventricles presses the brain against the bony cranium; anoxia and decreased blood supply result

152. Nursing care of a baby with increased intracranial pressure should include:
    1. Weighing the infant daily before feeding
    2. Elevating the infant's head higher than the hips
    3. Checking the infant's reflexes every 15 minutes
    4. Stimulating the infant frequently to monitor consciousness

153. The parents of an infant who has just had a ventriculoperitoneal shunt inserted for hydrocephalus are concerned about the prognosis. The nurse should explain that:

1. The prognosis is excellent and the valve is permanent
2. The shunt may need to be revised as the child grows older
3. If any brain damage has occurred, it is reversible during the first year of life
4. Hydrocephalus usually is self-limiting by 2 years of age and then the shunt is removed

154. An infant who was born with a meningomyelocele develops hydrocephalus. After discussion with the physician, the parents carefully consider options and decide in favor of having a shunt inserted. On return from the operating room, the infant has a ventriculoperitoneal (VP) shunt in place. Nursing care for the infant during the first 24 hours would involve:
    1. Sedating the infant frequently for pain
    2. Placing the infant in a high-Fowler's position
    3. Positioning the infant on the side that has the shunt
    4. Monitoring the infant for increasing intracranial pressure

155. The discharge of an infant with a surgically repaired spina bifida is anticipated at about 2 weeks of age. In preparation for home care related to the infant's diagnosis, the nurse should plan to include:
    1. Discussing the need to limit the infant's fluid intake to formula only
    2. Demonstrating restrictive positions to prevent the infant from turning
    3. Explaining the need to provide the infant with a quiet environment to limit external stimuli
    4. Teaching the parents how to do passive range-of-motion exercises to the infant's lower extremities

156. A 4-year-old has a revision of a ventriculoperitoneal shunt. A sign of an infected shunt that the nurse should assess for would be:
    1. Lethargy
    2. Headache
    3. Stiff neck
    4. Decreased pulse

157. The nurse should be aware that an assessment in an infant that would indicate a possible increase in intracranial pressure after the revision of a ventriculoperitoneal shunt would be:
    1. Hypoactive reflexes
    2. An increased pulse rate
    3. Tense anterior fontanel
    4. A decreased blood pressure

158. When caring for an infant with a meningomyelocele before surgical correction, a primary nursing goal would be to:
1. Prevent infection
2. Prevent trauma to the sac
3. Observe for increasing paralysis
4. Observe for bowel and bladder control

159. A newborn who has a meningomyelocele is admitted to the high-risk nursery. The newborn's Apgar scores were 9/10. During the first 24 hours it would be most appropriate for the nurse to:
1. Wash the genital area with Betadine
2. Perform neuro checks above the site of the lesion
3. Apply disposable diapers to monitor intake and output
4. Place the infant prone in a slight Trendelenburg position

160. After closure of a newborn's meningomyelocele, it is essential that the nursing care include:
1. Strict limitation of leg movement
2. Decrease of environmental stimuli
3. Measurement of head circumference daily
4. Observation of serous drainage from the nares

161. During discharge planning, the parents of an infant who had closure of a neural tube defect express concern about skin care and ask what they can do to avoid problems. The nurse plans to reinforce that:
1. Powder can be used with each diaper change to keep their infant dry
2. Their infant needs thorough cleaning and more frequent diaper changes to protect the skin
3. Their infant doesn't need anything more than routine cleansing and routine diaper changes
4. Vitamin A and D ointment should be used with each change to protect their infant's skin

162. At the age of 7 years, a child with cerebral palsy is admitted to the hospital for a tendon-lengthening procedure. While in bed after the surgery, the child must wear braces and shoes for at least 8 hours a day. This is to:
1. Encourage ambulation as soon as possible
2. Continue the child's acceptance of physical restraints
3. Maintain hip and knee alignment and help prevent footdrop
4. Stretch the child's ligaments and strengthen muscle tone

163. A child with diminished sensation in the legs because of cerebral palsy should be taught special safety precautions, including:
1. Testing the temperature of water in any water-related activity
2. Setting the clock two times during the night to change position
3. Tightening straps and buckles more than usual on braces when ambulating
4. Looking down at the lower extremities when crutch walking to determine proper positioning of the legs

164. When planning long-term care for a child with cerebral palsy, it is important for the nurse to recognize that the:
1. Illness is not progressively degenerative
2. Child probably has some degree of mental retardation
3. Effects of cerebral palsy are unstable and unpredictable
4. Child should have genetic counseling before planning a family

165. A child with cerebral palsy is to be taught the four-point alternate crutch gait. The nurse is aware that this gait was probably chosen because:
1. There are always two points of support on the floor
2. It provides for equal but partial weight bearing on each limb
3. The child has no power or step ability in the lower extremities
4. The child has more power in upper extremities than in lower extremities

166. The exact sociocultural reason for lead poisoning in children is:
1. Considered to be an environment with lead available for oral exploration
2. Attributed to an indigent and passive mother who fails to supervise children
3. Clearly understood to be caused by the child's ingestion of nonfood substances
4. Unknown, but groups at high risk include children with pica and those exposed to environmental hazards

167. Although lead poisoning affects various organ systems, its irreversible side effects are exerted mainly on the:
1. Urinary system
2. Skeletal system
3. Hematologic system
4. Central nervous system

168. For a child with the diagnosis of lead poisoning, the nursing diagnosis with the highest priority would be:
    1. Constipation related to the ingestion of lead
    2. Risk for injury related to the ingestion of lead
    3. Delayed growth and development related to inadequate parenting
    4. Imbalanced nutrition, less than body requirements, related to decreased iron intake

169. If a child cannot be given oral chelating agents, parenteral medication must be used. To effectively prepare a child to cope with this painful treatment, the nurse should give priority to:
    1. Rotating the injection sites and adding procaine to the chelating agents to lessen the discomfort
    2. Role playing with puppets dressed as physicians and nurses to minimize the child's fear of unfamiliar adults
    3. Allowing the child to play with a syringe and a doll before the therapy is initiated and after receiving each injection
    4. Carefully explaining the rationale for the injections so that the child does not view them as a punishment for bad behavior

170. Nursing care for an adolescent admitted with tetanus following a puncture wound should be primarily directed toward:
    1. Decreasing external stimuli
    2. Maintaining body alignment
    3. Encouraging high intake of fluid
    4. Carefully monitoring urinary output

171. The nurse should maintain isolation of a child with a diagnosis of bacterial meningitis:
    1. For 12 hours after admission
    2. Until the cultures are negative
    3. Until antibiotic therapy is completed
    4. For 48 hours after antibiotic therapy begins

172. Three days after admission, a 2-year-old with the diagnosis of meningitis appears clinically improved. A spinal tap is done to assess the child's response to therapy. The nurse correctly interprets that the child's condition is improving when the report of the spinal fluid indicates:
    1. Decreased protein
    2. Decreased glucose
    3. Increased cell count
    4. Increased specific gravity

173. When caring for a child with meningococcal meningitis, the nurse should observe for the:
    1. Identifying purpuric skin rash
    2. Low-grade nature of the fever
    3. Presence of severe glossitis
    4. Continual tremors of the extremities

174. To identify possible increasing intracranial pressure, the nurse should monitor a 2-year-old with the diagnosis of meningitis for:
    1. Restlessness, anorexia, rapid respirations
    2. Vomiting, seizures, complaints of head pain
    3. Anorexia, irritability, subnormal temperature
    4. Bulging fontanels, decreased blood pressure, elevated temperature

175. The most serious complication of meningitis in young children is:
    1. Epilepsy
    2. Blindness
    3. Peripheral circulatory collapse
    4. Communicating hydrocephalus

176. If monocular strabismus in children is not corrected early enough:
    1. Dyslexia will develop
    2. Peripheral vision will disappear
    3. Amblyopia develops in the weak eye
    4. Vision in both eyes will be diminished

177. After many episodes of otitis media a child is to have tubes implanted surgically in the ears. Discharge planning should include teaching the parents to:
    1. Apply Vaseline to the ear canal daily
    2. Use cotton swabs to clean the inner ears
    3. Keep the child out of day care for 1 week
    4. Have the child use ear plugs when bathing

178. An adolescent has arrived at the clinic complaining of buzzing in the ears. The nurse's assessment should be centered on information related to:
    1. Emotional upsets
    2. Music preferences
    3. Childhood ear infections
    4. Familial history of deafness

179. After surgery for the repair of a ruptured appendix, a 12-year-old was provided with morphine sulfate for pain control via a patient-controlled analgesia infusion. A bolus of morphine can be delivered every 6 minutes. The mother will be staying with the child for the immediate postoperative period. The nurse recognizes that the instructions about the PCA were understood when the mother states:
    1. "My son needs to push the PCA button when he determines that he needs pain medication."
    2. "When my son is sleeping I will wake him up on a regular basis to remind him to press the PCA button."
    3. "I will press the button every 6 minutes so that my son receives adequate pain control while he is sleeping."
    4. "Because my son is not allowed anything by mouth if the PCA is not effective, he will have to tolerate the pain."

180. During a well-child visit parents tell the nurse that their 5-year-old daughter has an attitude problem and does not listen to them when they speak to her. After an auditory screening, the nurse determines that the child has a mild hearing loss. The nurse is aware that a mild hearing loss:
    1. Will not require immediate follow-up
    2. Will progress to a severe hearing deficit
    3. May not interfere with progress in school
    4. May require hearing aids and speech therapy

Skeletal

181. A 3-month-old infant with a severe developmental dysplasia of the hip has a spica cast applied from below the axilla to below the knee. To prevent a serious complication that often occurs in infants in a spica cast, the nurse teaches the infant's parents to:
    1. Feed the infant a low-calorie diet
    2. Change the infant's diapers frequently
    3. Limit the infant's movement to prevent cast damage
    4. Seek immediate medical care if the infant develops a cough

182. When elevating the head of an infant in a spica cast, the nurse should be aware that it is important to:
    1. Limit this position to 1 hour at a maximum
    2. Use folded diapers around the edge of the cast
    3. Place at least two pillows under the shoulders
    4. Raise the entire mattress or bed at the head of the bed

183. Developmental dysplasia of the hip is often discovered by the nurse in the newborn nursery when the infant's assessment reveals:
    1. A depressed dance reflex
    2. Asymmetry of the gluteal folds
    3. Limitation in adduction of the leg
    4. Shortening of the leg on the unaffected side

184. A week-old infant has been in the pediatric unit for clubfoot casting for 18 hours when the nurse notes that the respiratory rate is below 30. No other changes are noted, and because the infant is apparently well, no record or report is made. Several hours later the infant experiences severe respiratory distress and emergency care is necessary. Legal responsibility in this instance would have to take into consideration that:
    1. Most infants experience slow respirations with skeletal deformities or discomfort
    2. A reading outside normal parameters is significant and should have been reported
    3. Respirations in young infants are often irregular and a drop is rarely important
    4. The respiratory tract is underdeveloped in young infants and the respiratory rate is not significant

185. A 7-year-old has recently been diagnosed with rheumatoid arthritis. The parents are concerned about the lifelong effects of the disease. Their daughter is already having difficulty going to school in the morning. The parents are investigating other therapies to use with the medications. The nurse should recommend a referral for:
    1. Physical therapy
    2. Special education
    3. Nutritional therapy
    4. Herbal supplements

186. To prevent loss of joint function in a child with juvenile rheumatoid arthritis, the nurse should teach the parents to avoid letting the child:
    1. Ride a bicycle
    2. Walk to school
    3. Do frequent isometric exercises
    4. Watch TV for prolonged periods

187. Range-of-motion exercises are prescribed for a child with rheumatoid arthritis. The nurse knows that the exercises have been effective when the:
    1. Child continues to experience pain
    2. Child's pedal pulses are diminished
    3. Subcutaneous nodules at the joints recede
    4. Affected knees can be flexed and extended

188. A 9-year-old has a fractured tibia and a full leg cast has been applied. The nurse should immediately notify the physician if assessment demonstrates:
    1. A pedal pulse of 90
    2. An increased urinary output
    3. An inability to move the toes
    4. A plaster cast that is still damp after 4 hours

189. A child has a plaster cast applied for a fractured ankle. To hasten drying of the cast the nurse should include in the care plan:
    1. Using a blow dryer
    2. Exposing the casted extremity
    3. Covering the cast with a light sheet
    4. Opening the window slightly to circulate air

190. A male adolescent sustains a sport-related fracture of the femur and an open reduction and internal fixation with a rod insertion is performed. After the surgery the adolescent is very upset. One potential explanation for the client's being upset is he:
    1. Will be unable to participate in sports for several years
    2. Will have to use a wheel chair to be able to get around
    3. Perceives the rod as an unacceptable intrusion on his body
    4. May have to continue taking pain medication until the bone heals

191. The nurse notes that the weights of a child in traction are touching the floor. The nurse should immediately:
    1. Raise the foot of the bed
    2. Lengthen the traction rope
    3. Notify the doctor to reapply the traction
    4. Move the child up toward the head of the bed

192. Following orthopedic surgery, a 15-year-old complains of pain and is given 15 mg of codeine sulfate as ordered q 3 hours prn. Two hours after being given this medication the adolescent complains of severe pain. The nurse should;
    1. Report that the adolescent has an apparent idiosyncrasy to codeine
    2. Tell the adolescent that additional medication cannot be given for 1 more hour
    3. Request that the physician evaluate the adolescent's need for additional medication
    4. Administer another dose of codeine within 30 minutes, because it is a relatively safe drug

193. A 12-year-old is diagnosed as having idiopathic scoliosis. Because proper exercise and avoidance of fatigue are essential components of care, the nurse is aware that the most therapeutic sport for this child would be:
    1. Golf
    2. Bowling
    3. Swimming
    4. Badminton

194. To assist curvature correction in scoliosis, the preadolescent is fitted with a brace. The nurse explains to the child and parents that the length of time the brace must be worn varies, but it is usually worn until:
    1. The iliac crests are at equal levels
    2. Pain on prolonged standing diminishes
    3. The curvature of the spine is completely straightened
    4. Cessation of bone growth occurs at the time of physical maturity

195. The nurse is aware that steroids, usually effective in adult clients with rheumatoid arthritis, will not be administered as a first choice drug to a preadolescent because of their adverse effects on:
    1. Growth
    2. Sexuality
    3. Emotions
    4. Body image

Endocrine

196. When planning a teaching program for a child who is newly diagnosed as having diabetes mellitus, the nurse should be especially concerned that:
    1. The child is taught to self-administer injections
    2. The parents receive instruction about blood glucose monitoring
    3. The child's activity be limited and the parents understand the need for this
    4. The parents and child be helped to understand their feelings about diabetes

197. An evening snack is planned for a child receiving Humulin N insulin. The nurse understands that this will provide:
    1. Added calories to help the child gain weight
    2. Encouragement for the child to stay on a diet
    3. High-carbohydrate nourishment for immediate utilization
    4. Nourishment with a latent effect to counteract late insulin activity

198. When reviewing the pathophysiology of diabetes mellitus with an 8-year-old, newly diagnosed child, the nurse's plan should take into consideration that:
    1. The child is in the abstract level of cognition
    2. Peer influence will decrease in importance to the child
    3. The child will respond favorably to opportunities to participate in self-care
    4. The child's current developmental task involves achieving a sense of identity

199. An 11-year-old child, newly diagnosed with diabetes mellitus, receives Humulin N insulin and Humulin R insulin at 7 AM. The nurse is aware that the child's response before lunch at noon will be controlled by:
    1. The increasing effects of the Humulin N insulin
    2. The Humulin N insulin rather than the Humulin R insulin
    3. Equal effects of the Humulin R and the Humulin N insulin
    4. Increasing effects of the Humulin R and the Humulin N insulin

200. When teaching an insulin-dependent adolescent client about dietary management, the nurse should instruct the client to:
    1. Eat all meals at home
    2. Weigh all food on a gram scale
    3. Always carry a concentrated form of glucose
    4. Have the parent prepare food separately from the rest of the family

201. At 7 AM, the nurse received the information that a diabetic child's 6 AM fasting blood glucose is 180 mg/dl. At this time the nurse should:
    1. Encourage the child to get up and exercise
    2. Ask the child to obtain an immediate glucometer reading
    3. Give the child a complex carbohydrate such as milk or cheese
    4. Have the child administer the prescribed dose of regular insulin

202. The nurse tells a male adolescent with type 1 diabetes that if he begins to experience an insulin reaction while at a basketball game, he should:
    1. Call his parents immediately
    2. Buy a Coke and hamburger to eat
    3. Administer regular insulin as soon as possible
    4. Rest in a quiet place until his symptoms subside

203. One nutritional principle to be followed in clients with type 1 diabetes is to provide for compensatory changes. The nurse reviews with a client how compensation for increased physical activity can be achieved and instructs the client to:
    1. Take the oral hypoglycemic medication on days of heavy exercise
    2. Increase dietary intake when there is a plan to exercise more than usual
    3. Lower the insulin dose in the morning when extra exercise is anticipated
    4. Eat more rapidly absorbed simple sugars to compensate for extra exercise

204. A 3-month-old infant has been diagnosed as having congenital hypothyroidism. If care is not instituted until after early infancy, the child will probably have:
    1. Myxedema
    2. Thyrotoxicosis
    3. Some mental retardation
    4. Abnormal deep tendon reflexes

205. A 10-year-old is diagnosed with lymphocytic thyroiditis. The nurse should explain to the parents and child that this condition is:
    1. Chronic
    2. Inherited
    3. Difficult to treat
    4. Probably temporary

206. A 14-year-old who has been on prolonged steroid therapy develops a cushingoid appearance. A nursing assessment of this child would probably reveal:
    1. Increased linear growth
    2. Loss of hair, including body hair
    3. Hypotension and hyponatremia
    4. Thin extremities with truncal obesity

Integumentary

207. When teaching parents at the school about communicable diseases, the nurse reminds them that these diseases are serious, and that encephalitis can be a complication of:
    1. Pertussis
    2. Chickenpox
    3. Poliomyelitis
    4. Scarlet fever

208. A mother asks the nurse how to tell the difference between measles (rubeola) and German measles (rubella). The nurse tells the mother that with rubeola the child has:
    1. A high fever and Koplik's spots
    2. A rash on the trunk with pruritus
    3. Nausea, vomiting, and abdominal cramps
    4. Symptoms similar to a cold, followed by a rash

209. Chickenpox can sometimes be fatal to children who are receiving:
    1. Insulin
    2. Steroids
    3. Antibiotics
    4. Anticonvulsants

210. A viral infection characterized by a red, blotchy rash and Koplik's spots in the mouth is:
    1. Mumps
    2. Rubella
    3. Rubeola
    4. Chickenpox

211. A viral disease that begins with respiratory inflammation and skin rash and may result in grave complications is:
    1. Rubella
    2. Rubeola
    3. Yellow fever
    4. Chickenpox

212. Under certain circumstances the virus that causes chickenpox can also cause:
    1. Athlete's foot
    2. Herpes zoster
    3. German measles
    4. Infectious hepatitis

213. A skin infection that can be a sequela of a staphylococcal infection or glomerulonephritis is:
    1. Scabies
    2. Impetigo
    3. Intertrigo
    4. Herpes simplex

214. An infection caused by the yeast *Candida albicans*, often occurring in infants and debilitated individuals, is:
    1. Thrush
    2. Dysentery
    3. Malta fever
    4. Typhoid fever

215. A 3-year-old is admitted with partial- and full-thickness burns over 30% of the body. Nursing observations in the first 48 hours of hospitalization are directed primarily toward preventing:
    1. Shock
    2. Pneumonia
    3. Contractures
    4. Hypertension

216. A 6-year-old has received partial-thickness burns of the face and chest in a house fire. For the first 24 hours after hospitalization, the nurse should primarily observe this child for:
    1. Wound sepsis
    2. Separation anxiety
    3. Pulmonary distress
    4. Fluid and electrolyte imbalance

217. A child was bitten on the hand by a dog who had recently received a rabies shot. The nursing priority for this child would be directed toward ensuring that the:
    1. Suture line remains red and dry
    2. Child does not develop a fear of dogs
    3. Rabies antibodies develop within 48 hours
    4. Mobility of the hand returns to a preinjury state in 1 week

218. A 15-year-old male is admitted with partial- and full-thickness burns of the arms and upper torso. The nurse plans for the administration of pain medication intravenously rather than intramuscularly because this method of administration:
    1. Decreases the risk of tissue irritation
    2. Reduces severe pain more effectively
    3. Bypasses impaired peripheral circulation
    4. Provides for more prolonged relief of pain

219. A 15-year-old camper contacts the camp nurse because of an itchy, erythematous area on the abdomen and abdominal pain. The nurse completes an assessment and suspects:
    1. IV drug use
    2. A spider bite
    3. Sickle cell crisis
    4. Diabetic ketoacidosis

Gastrointestinal

220. During a home visit, the mother asks the nurse how often she should burp her infant during bottlefeeding. Recognizing that the baby has a strong sucking reflex and no physical problems, the nurse could best respond:
1. "Burp the baby five to six times during each feeding for the first month."
2. "You should burp your baby at the end of the feeding only. Babies can become confused at having their feeding stopped."
3. "Burp your baby periodically; usually in the middle and at the end of a feeding. If the baby has been crying, you can burp before starting."
4. "With new infants we recommend burping every 5 to 10 minutes. That gets your baby used to a routine and lets you see how much formula is taken."

221. A mother brings her week-old infant to the clinic because the infant continually regurgitates. Chalasia is suspected. The nurse instructs the mother to:
1. Keep the infant prone following feedings
2. Prevent the infant from crying for prolonged periods
3. Administer a minimum of 8 oz of formula at each feeding
4. Keep the infant in a semisitting position, particularly after feedings

222. A mother asks the nurse how she should introduce pureed foods to her 9-month-old infant. The nurse's best response would be:
1. "Mix the pureed food in with the formula twice a day."
2. "Introduce one food at a time, usually at intervals of 4 to 7 days."
3. "Give the pureed foods by spoon after the infant has had formula."
4. "Keep the formula intake fairly constant regardless of the solid food intake."

223. The sequence for introducing other foods into a baby's diet after the introduction of cereals is:
1. Meats, fruits, vegetables, table foods
2. Vegetables, table foods, meats, fruits
3. Table foods, fruits, vegetables, meats
4. Fruits, vegetables, meats, table foods

224. The major influence on eating habits of the early school-aged child is the:
1. Availability of food selections
2. Smell and appearance of food
3. Example of parents at mealtime
4. Food preferences of the peer group

225. A mother brings her 9-month-old son to the pediatric clinic and asks about the introduction of new foods. The nurse suggests:
1. "Offer a new food every day until he likes one."
2. "Offer a new food after he has had his regular feeding."
3. "Offer a new food after he has had some milk when he is still hungry."
4. "Mix the pureed food with the formula and give through the bottle to help him learn new tastes."

226. An 8-month-old infant has a gastrostomy tube and is given 240 ml of tube feeding q4h. One of the primary nursing responsibilities is to:
1. Open the tube 1 hour before feeding
2. Position on the right side after feeding
3. Give 10 ml of normal saline before and after feeding
4. Elevate the tube 30 cm (12 inches) above the mattress

227. A nurse can assist in confirming a suspected diagnosis of intestinal infestation with pinworms in a 6-year-old child by:
1. Asking the mother to collect stools for 3 consecutive days for culture
2. Instructing the mother to do an anal Scotch-tape test early in the morning
3. Having the mother bring in the child's stools for visual examination for 3 days
4. Assisting the mother to schedule a hypersensitivity test of the child's blood serum

228. Nursing care for an infant after the surgical repair of a cleft lip should include:
1. Keeping the baby NPO
2. Keeping the infant from crying
3. Placing the infant in a semisitting position
4. Spoonfeeding for the first 2 days after surgery

229. A cleft lip predisposes an infant to infections primarily because of:
1. Poor nutrition from disturbed feeding
2. Poor circulation to the defective area
3. Waste products that accumulate along the defect
4. Mouth breathing, which dries the oropharyngeal mucous membranes

230. At 2 years of age, a child born with a cleft lip and palate is readmitted for palate surgery. A toothbrush would not be used immediately after palate surgery because the:
    1. Suture line might be injured
    2. Child would probably have no teeth
    3. Toothbrush might be frightening to the child
    4. Child would not be accustomed to a brush at home

231. In a baby born with a unilateral cleft lip and palate, feeding will probably be:
    1. Limited to IV fluids
    2. With a soft, large-holed nipple
    3. Too difficult because of breathing problems
    4. With a rubber-tipped syringe or medicine dropper

232. A toddler has swallowed a liquid drain cleaner containing lye. The immediate intervention is to administer:
    1. Syrup of ipecac
    2. Two ounces of milk
    3. Dilute vinegar solution
    4. Sodium bicarbonate and water

233. An infant is diagnosed as having pyloric stenosis. When palpating this infant's abdomen, the nurse would expect to find:
    1. An impacted and distended colon
    2. Marked tenderness around the umbilicus
    3. An olive-sized mass in the right upper quadrant
    4. Rhythmic peristaltic waves in the lower abdomen

234. Vomiting caused by pyloric stenosis is usually not bile stained because:
    1. The bile duct is also obstructed
    2. The obstruction is above the opening of the common bile duct
    3. The sphincter of the bile duct is connected to the hypertrophied pyloric muscle
    4. The obstruction of the cardiac sphincter prevents bile from entering the esophagus

235. The nurse should carefully observe the infant with a tentative diagnosis of pyloric stenosis for:
    1. Quality of cry
    2. Quality of stool
    3. Signs of dehydration
    4. Coughing and gagging after feeding

236. Surgery to correct a pyloric stenosis is performed on a 2-week-old and the infant's condition is stable. The nurse caring for the infant notices that the postoperative orders are similar to those for other infants having undergone such surgery and include:
    1. Thickened formula 24 hours after surgery
    2. Withholding all feedings for the first 24 hours
    3. Regular formula feeding 24 hours after surgery
    4. Additional glucose feedings as desired after the first 24 hours

237. Corrective surgery for pyloric stenosis is completed and the infant is returned in stable condition to the pediatric unit with an intravenous infusion and a nasogastric tube in place. The priority nursing action should be to:
    1. Apply adequate restraints
    2. Administer a mild sedative
    3. Connect the IV to an infusion pump
    4. Attach the nasogastric tube to wall suction

238. An infant has corrective surgery for pyloric stenosis. To reduce vomiting, the nurse should teach the mother that immediately after feeding the infant she should:
    1. Rock the baby for 20 minutes
    2. Place the baby in an infant seat
    3. Place the baby flat on the right side
    4. Keep the baby awake with sensory stimulation

239. Exposure to hepatitis B may occur in hospitals because of:
    1. Careless handling of feces by staff
    2. Increasing use of ventilating systems
    3. Needle sticks and mucous membrane exposure
    4. Early diagnosis and improved treatment of hepatitis A

240. One symptom common in children with celiac disease is stools that are:
    1. Small, pale, mucoid
    2. Large, frothy, dark green
    3. Large, pale, foul smelling
    4. Moderate, green, foul smelling

241. In cystic fibrosis, frequent stools and tenacious mucus often produce:
    1. Anal fissures
    2. Intussusception
    3. Meconium ileus
    4. Rectal prolapse

242. Children with cystic fibrosis are usually small and underdeveloped for their age primarily because they:
    1. Ingest little food because of an extremely poor appetite
    2. Secrete less than normal amounts of pituitary growth hormone
    3. Develop muscular and bony atrophy from lack of motor activity
    4. Are unable to absorb nutrients because of a lack of pancreatic enzymes

243. The foul-smelling, frothy characteristic stool in cystic fibrosis results from the presence of large amounts of:
    1. Undigested fat
    2. Sodium and chloride
    3. Semidigested carbohydrates
    4. Lipase, trypsin, and amylase

244. Medications that will probably be used in the therapeutic regimen for a child with cystic fibrosis include:
    1. A steroid and an antimetabolite
    2. Pancreatic enzymes and antibiotics
    3. Aerosol mists, decongestants, and fat-soluble vitamins
    4. Antibiotics, a multivitamin preparation, and cough drops

245. The most effective time for the nurse to perform a cellophane-tape test for pinworms is:
    1. Just following a BM
    2. Immediately after meals
    3. At bedtime before bathing
    4. Early morning before arising

246. Pinworms cause a number of symptoms besides anal itching. A complication of pinworm infestation, although rare, that the nurse should observe for is:
    1. Hepatitis
    2. Stomatitis
    3. Appendicitis
    4. Pneumonitis

247. A clinic nurse explains to the mother of a child with a pinworm infestation how pinworms are transmitted. The nurse can best evaluate the effectiveness of the teaching when the mother states:
    1. "I'll have to be sure that the cat stays off my children's bed."
    2. "I'll have to reinforce my child's handwashing techniques before eating or handling food."
    3. "I'll be sure to disinfect the toilet seat after every bowel movement for the next several days."

    4. "My child contracted this infestation from the dirty school toilets, and I'll report that to the school nurse."

248. Mebendazole (Vermox) 100 mg bid 3 days is ordered for a child with pinworms. It is advisable that this drug also be administered to:
    1. The child's younger brother who is 1 year old
    2. All members of the child's family who test positive
    3. All people using the same toilet facilities as the child
    4. The child's mother, father, and siblings even though they are symptom free

249. Dietary treatment of children with PKU includes a:
    1. Protein-free diet
    2. Low-phenylalanine diet
    3. Phenylalanine-free diet
    4. Dietary supplement of phenylalanine

250. When teaching the parents of an infant diagnosed with PKU, the nurse should plan to include the fact that:
    1. Mental retardation occurs if PKU is untreated
    2. Treatment for PKU includes lifelong medications
    3. PKU is transmitted by an autosomal dominant gene
    4. The infant is tested for PKU immediately after delivery

251. A test that is done on all neonates to detect PKU is:
    1. Phenistix test
    2. Guthrie blood test
    3. Ferric chloride urine test
    4. Clinitest serum phosphopyruvic acid

252. In terms of dietary counseling, the parents of a newborn with PKU need help and support in adhering to specific regimens. A frequent question asked by parents is, "How long will my child have to be on this diet?" An appropriate response by the nurse would be:
    1. "No one knows, but why don't you discuss it with your doctor?"
    2. "Usually, if the child does well for 1 year, regular foods can gradually be introduced."
    3. "Unfortunately, this is a lifelong problem and dietary management must always be maintained."
    4. "As of now, research shows that a child needs to be on this diet at least until adolescence and possibly longer."

253. The nurse plans to discuss childhood nutrition with parents of children with Down syndrome in an attempt to minimize a common nutritional problem encountered in children with Down syndrome, namely:
1. Rickets
2. Anemia
3. Obesity
4. Rumination

254. In a 3-month-old infant with bile-stained vomitus and abdominal distention, the nurse should observe for:
1. Bounding pulse and hypotonicity
2. High-pitched cry and weak thready pulse
3. Paroxysmal pain and grunting respirations
4. Constant severe pain and absence of stools

255. The behavior of an infant with colic is usually suggestive of:
1. An allergic response to certain proteins in milk
2. Inadequate peristalsis resulting in constipation
3. Paroxysmal abdominal pain caused by excessive gas
4. A protective mechanism designed to rid the GI tract of foreign proteins

256. Twenty-four hours after birth a newborn has not passed meconium and Hirschsprung's disease is suspected. To help relieve the obstruction and confirm the diagnosis the physician will probably order:
1. Multiple saline enemas
2. Surgical intervention
3. Insertion of a rectal tube prn
4. Placement of a nasogastric tube

257. The mother of a 20-month-old female has questions about her daughter's bowel training. The nurse advises the mother that training will be more successful if she:
1. Starts while her daughter is still on formula
2. Sits her daughter on the toilet every 2 hours
3. Begins by placing her daughter on a potty chair
4. Begins the bowel training when her daughter is about 24 months old

Fluid and Electrolytes

258. A three-year-old preschooler has been hospitalized with nephrotic syndrome. The best way to detect fluid retention would be to:
1. Have the child urinate in a bedpan
2. Measure the child's abdominal girth daily
3. Weigh the child at the same time every day
4. Test the child's urine for hematuria and proteinuria

259. The maintenance of fluid and electrolyte balance is more critical in children than in adults because:
1. Cellular metabolism is less stable than in adults
2. The proportion of water in the body is less than in adults
3. Renal function is immature in children below 4 years of age
4. The extracellular fluid requirement per unit of body weight is greater than in adults

260. The physician orders a tap-water enema for a 6-month-old infant. The nurse considers that a tap-water enema could:
1. Result in loss of necessary nutrients
2. Cause a fluid and electrolyte imbalance
3. Increase the infant's fear of intrusive procedures
4. Result in shock from a sudden drop in temperature

261. The physician orders an isotonic enema for a 2-year-old child with constipation. The nurse is aware that the maximum amount of fluid to be given a small child without a physician's specific order is:
1. 100 to 150 ml
2. 155 to 250 ml
3. 255 to 360 ml
4. 365 to 500 ml

262. An infant is receiving parenteral therapy. The IV orders are 400 ml of D5/0.45NS to run in 8 hours. A minidropper with a drop factor of 50 gtt per milliliter is used. The nurse should set the rate to deliver:
1. 38 drops per minute
2. 42 drops per minute
3. 46 drops per minute
4. 50 drops per minute

263. A 5 month old develops severe diarrhea and is given IV fluids. The rate of flow must be observed often by the nurse to:
1. Avoid IV infiltration
2. Replace all fluids lost
3. Prevent increased output
4. Prevent cardiac overload

264. An essential nursing action when caring for the small child with severe diarrhea is to:
1. Encourage fluids
2. Take daily weights
3. Replace lost calories
4. Keep body temperature below 100° F

265. A child has been admitted for surgery to correct a congenital megacolon. Enemas are ordered preoperatively to cleanse the bowel. The nurse should use:
1. Tap water
2. Soap suds
3. Isotonic saline
4. Hypertonic phosphate

266. Of primary importance when the nurse plans for the discharge of a child following a sickle cell crisis (pain episode) is the child's need for:
1. A high caloric diet
2. Rigorous exercise and play
3. At least 14 hours of sleep per day
4. Ingestion of large quantities of liquids

267. When vomiting is uncontrolled in an infant, the nurse should observe for signs of:
1. Tetany
2. Acidosis
3. Alkalosis
4. Hyperactivity

268. When administering IV fluids to a dehydrated infant, the most critical factor confronting the nurse is the:
1. Assurance of sterility
2. Calculation of the total necessary intake
3. Maintenance of the prescribed rate of flow
4. Maintenance of the fluid at body temperature

269. An infant is receiving 500 ml of IV fluid per 24 hours. Using an IV set with a drop rate of 60 drops/ml, the nurse should plan to regulate the IV at:
1. 8 drops per minute
2. 13 drops per minute
3. 21 drops per minute
4. 24 drops per minute

270. The acid-base imbalance resulting from a severe asthma attack is:
1. Metabolic alkalosis caused by excessive production of acid metabolites
2. Respiratory alkalosis caused by the accelerated respirations and loss of carbon dioxide
3. Respiratory acidosis caused by the impaired respirations and increased formation of carbonic acid
4. Metabolic acidosis caused by the kidneys' inability to help compensate for the increased carbonic acid formed

271. The nurse is aware that infants are at greater risk for a fluid volume deficit and hyperosmolar imbalance primarily because:
1. They have a decreased glomerular filtration rate
2. Body fluid loss is proportionately greater per kilogram of weight
3. A generalized response to insensible fluid loss has not yet developed
4. They have increased metabolic processes and increased water production

Cardiovascular

272. The nurse doing a newborn assessment counts the infant's cord vessels. In a normal infant there are:
1. Two vessels: one vein and one artery
2. Three vessels: two veins and one artery
3. Three vessels: one vein and two arteries
4. Four vessels: two veins and two arteries

273. A disorder, following a *streptococcal* infection, characterized by swollen joints, fever, and the possibility of endocarditis and death is:
1. Tetanus
2. Measles
3. Rheumatic fever
4. Whooping cough

274. A 5-month-old is brought to the pediatric clinic for a monthly checkup. The nurse is aware that the assessment finding that would need the most immediate follow-up would be:
1. Strabismus
2. Tachycardia
3. Mild hypotonia
4. Inability to sit with support

275. Among the last signs of heart failure in the infant and child is:
1. Orthopnea
2. Tachypnea
3. Tachycardia
4. Peripheral edema

276. A common finding in most children with cardiac anomalies is:
1. Mental retardation
2. Delayed physical growth
3. Cyanosis and clubbing of fingertips
4. A family history of cardiac anomalies

277. A 2-year-old has a congenital right-to-left shunt defect of the heart. The nurse would expect to observe:
    1. Orthopnea
    2. An elevated hematocrit
    3. Absence of pedal pulses
    4. Edema in the extremities

278. Children with cardiac problems who are awaiting corrective surgery are placed on long-term antibiotic prophylaxis to prevent:
    1. Myocarditis
    2. Pericarditis
    3. Upper respiratory infections
    4. Subacute bacterial endocarditis

279. Anticipating that a 4-year-old, scheduled for open-heart surgery, will have chest tubes postoperatively, the nurse plans to explain to the mother that if they are present they are used to:
    1. Increase tidal volumes
    2. Allow drainage of air and fluid
    3. Regulate pressure of chest wall
    4. Promote positive intraplural pressure

280. After discussion with the pediatric cardiologist, the parents of an infant ask the nurse to explain once again what patent ductus arteriosus is. The nurse tells them that it is:
    1. A narrowing of the pulmonary artery
    2. An enlarged aorta and pulmonary artery
    3. A connection between the pulmonary artery and the aorta
    4. An abnormal opening between the right and left ventricles

281. The nurse, caring for a child with a left-to-right shunt of the heart, should be aware that the major common symptom of this type congenital disorder is:
    1. Polycythemia
    2. Severe retarded growth
    3. Clubbing of fingers and toes
    4. The presence of an audible heart murmur

282. A young child has coarctation of the aorta. When taking the child's vital signs, the nurse can expect to observe:
    1. Notching of the clavicle
    2. Bounding femoral pulses
    3. Weak, thready radial pulses
    4. Higher BP in upper extremities

283. A 1-year-old child is admitted with a suspected diagnosis of tetralogy of Fallot. The parents report that their child had difficulty feeding as a newborn. The nurse should be aware that:
    1. Feeding problems are fairly common in newborns
    2. Poor sucking is usually insignificant in the absence of cyanosis
    3. Poor sucking and swallowing may be early indications of a heart defect
    4. Many babies retain mucus that may interfere with feeding for several days

284. A 3 year old is scheduled for a cardiac catheterization. Nursing care after this procedure should include:
    1. Encouraging early ambulation
    2. Monitoring the site for bleeding
    3. Restricting fluids until blood pressure is stabilized
    4. Comparing blood pressure in the affected and unaffected extremities

285. Down syndrome is suspected in a newborn. When doing a physical assessment of this infant, the nurse should carefully evaluate the infant's:
    1. Heart sounds
    2. Anterior fontanel
    3. Lower extremities
    4. Pupillary changes

286. The cardiac defects associated with tetralogy of Fallot include:
    1. Right ventricular hypertrophy, atrial and ventricular defects, and mitral valve stenosis
    2. Origin of the aorta from the right ventricle and of the pulmonary artery from the left ventricle
    3. Right ventricular hypertrophy, ventricular septal defect, stenosis of pulmonary artery, and overriding aorta
    4. Abnormal connection between the pulmonary artery and the aorta, right ventricular hypertrophy, and atrial septal defects

287. The laboratory analysis for a 5 year old admitted for repair of tetralogy of Fallot indicates a high red blood cell count. The nurse recognizes that this polycythemia can best be understood as a compensatory mechanism for:
    1. Low BP
    2. Cardiomegaly
    3. Low iron level
    4. Tissue oxygen need

288. The nurse is aware that a common adaptation of children with tetralogy of Fallot is:
    1. Clubbing of fingers
    2. Slow, irregular respirations
    3. Subcutaneous hemorrhages
    4. Decreased red blood cell counts

289. A child undergoes heart surgery to repair the defects associated with tetralogy of Fallot. Postoperatively it is essential that the nurse prevent:
    1. Crying
    2. Coughing
    3. Constipation
    4. Unnecessary movement

290. An infant who has had cardiac surgery for a congenital defect is to be discharged. The nurse's teaching to the parents regarding the infant's prescribed prophylactic antibiotic therapy should stress the importance of:
    1. Keeping the medicine in the refrigerator after it has been opened
    2. Making sure the infant receives the antibiotic prophylactically as prescribed
    3. Shaking the bottle of medicine thoroughly before administering it to the infant
    4. Waiting 2 hours after the last feeding before administering the antibiotic to the infant

291. The nurse understands that gavage feeding is often indicated for weak infants following repair of a congenital heart defect because:
    1. Vomiting is prevented
    2. The feeding can be given quickly, so handling is minimized
    3. The amount of food given can be more accurately regulated
    4. It conserves the infant's strength and does not depend on the swallowing reflex

292. When observing a newborn with Down syndrome, the nurse should be aware that a common defect associated with this condition is:
    1. Deafness
    2. Hydrocephaly
    3. Muscular hypertonicity
    4. Congenital heart defect

Blood and Immunity

293. Immunity by antibody formation during the course of a disease is:
    1. Active natural immunity
    2. Active artificial immunity
    3. Passive natural immunity
    4. Passive artificial immunity

294. Occasionally infants are born without an immune system. They can live normally with no apparent problems during their first months after birth because:
    1. Exposure to pathogens during this time can be limited
    2. Limited antibodies are produced by the infant's colonic bacteria
    3. Antibodies are passively received from the mother through the placenta and breast milk
    4. Limited antibodies are produced by the fetal thymus during the eighth and ninth months of gestation

295. When evaluating the laboratory reports for a 1-year-old child, the nurse recalls that the normal hematocrit range for a child of this age would be:
    1. 19% to 32%
    2. 29% to 41%
    3. 37% to 47%
    4. 42% to 69%

296. The nurse explains to a mother whose child has just received a tetanus toxoid injection that the toxoid confers:
    1. Lifelong passive immunity
    2. Long-lasting active immunity
    3. Lifelong active natural immunity
    4. Temporary passive natural immunity

297. Using live virus vaccines against measles is contraindicated in children receiving corticosteroid, antineoplastic, or irradiation therapy because these children may:
    1. Have had the disease or have been immunized previously
    2. Be unlikely to need this protection during their shortened life span
    3. Be susceptible to infection because of their depressed immune response
    4. Have an allergy to rabbit serum, which is used as a basis for these vaccines

298. The mother of a child who has received all of the primary immunizations asks the nurse which ones the child should receive before starting kindergarten. The nurse suggests the child receive the following boosters:
    1. DTaP and lVP
    2. IVP and Hep-B
    3. Measles and rubella
    4. DTaP and tuberculin test

299. When reviewing the immunization schedule for an 11 month old, the nurse would expect that the infant had been previously immunized against:
    1. Pertussis, tetanus, polio, and measles
    2. Polio, pertussis, tetanus, and diphtheria
    3. Measles, mumps, rubella, and tuberculosis
    4. Measles, rubella, polio, tuberculosis, and pertussis

300. A mother asks the nurse how the DTaP injection works. The nurse, in formulating a response, recalls that in active immunity:
    1. Lipid agents are formed by the body against antigens
    2. Protein antigens are formed in the blood to fight invading antibodies
    3. Protein substances are formed by the body to destroy or neutralize antigens
    4. Blood antigens are aided by phagocytes in defending the body against pathogens

301. To ensure immunity, children who are 5 years old and entering school, must have received at least:
    1. One dose of diphtheria toxoid; one dose each of poliomyelitis vaccine, live measles, live rubella, and mumps vaccines
    2. Two doses of diphtheria toxoid and poliomyelitis vaccine; one dose each of live measles, live rubella, and mumps vaccine
    3. Three doses of diphtheria toxoid and poliomyelitis vaccine; one dose each of live measles, live rubella, and mumps vaccines
    4. Five doses of diphtheria toxoid; four doses of poliomyelitis vaccine; one dose each of live measles, live rubella, and mumps vaccines

302. A child is to receive a blood transfusion. If an allergic reaction to the blood occurs, the nurse's first intervention should be to:
    1. Call the physician
    2. Slow the flow rate
    3. Stop the blood immediately
    4. Relieve the symptoms with an ordered antihistamine

303. Nutritional anemia a problem encountered in children and adults, involves several different nutrients. The nutrients include proteins, iron, vitamin B_{12}, and:
    1. Calcium
    2. Thiamine
    3. Folic acid
    4. Carbohydrates

304. The nurse's background knowledge of the basic nutrients that act as partners in building red blood cells will form the basis of a teaching plan for a child with nutritional anemia. These nutrient partners of iron are:
    1. Calcium and vitamins
    2. Vitamin D and riboflavin
    3. Proteins and ascorbic acid
    4. Carbohydrates and thiamine

305. A pale, lethargic 1 year old, who weighs 12.6 kg (28 pounds), has an enlarged heart and a hemoglobin level of 8 g. The mother tells the nurse that her infant spits out food fed with a spoon so she provides a quart of milk per day from a bottle. The nurse suggests that the mother:
    1. Immediately begin the weaning process
    2. Take the infant to the metabolic clinic for a checkup
    3. Give the infant finger foods such as raisins and chopped meat
    4. Put a large hole in the nipple and put baby food in with the milk

306. During a period of heavy play activity, a first grader with a known history of anemia complains of feeling woozy. The school nurse's best initial response would be to:
    1. Check the child's pulse and blood pressure
    2. Have the child sit until the dizziness subsides
    3. Use spirits of ammonia to prevent the child from fainting
    4. Assist the child to the nurse's room and place the child in a supine position

307. A child with β thalassemia is admitted to the ambulatory care unit for a transfusion. When developing the nursing care plan, the discharge instructions should include teaching the parents to:
    1. Encourage fluids
    2. Restrict activity
    3. Prevent infection
    4. Provide small, frequent meals

308. Infants with sickle cell anemia may not be diagnosed as having this disorder because of:
    1. The absence of any respiratory disorders
    2. General good health and an excellent growth curve
    3. The presence of fetal hemoglobin during the first 6 months of life
    4. Compensation of increased hematocrit and hemoglobin if well fed

309. To prevent thrombus formation in capillaries, as well as other problems from stasis and clotting of blood in the sickling process, the nurse should:
1. Administer oxygen
2. See that the client maintains bed rest
3. Increase fluids by mouth and use a humidifier
4. Administer ordered heparin or other anti-coagulants

310. The outpatient clinic nurse is caring for a 7-year-old child with sickle cell anemia. The child has a history of having a splenectomy at age four. At this time the nurse's priority of care would be:
1. Assessing for jaundice
2. Monitoring serial hematocrit readings
3. Frequent assessments of the abdomen
4. Keeping the child away from infectious contacts

311. An adolescent in sickle cell crisis (pain episode) is complaining of right-knee pain. The best nursing intervention would be to:
1. Decrease IV fluids
2. Wrap the right knee in a cold pack
3. Apply a warm soak to the right knee
4. Give morphine sulfate 0.5 mg as ordered

312. The nurse teaching the inservice group emphasizes that the common nursing care that helps prevent both sickle cell crisis and celiac crisis is:
1. Limitation of activity
2. Protection from infection
3. High-iron, low-fat, high-protein diet
4. Careful observation of all vital signs

313. A 6-year-old child with sickle cell disease is admitted with a vaso-occlusive crisis. Priority nursing concerns would be:
1. Nutrition and hydration
2. Nutrition and antibiotics
3. Hydration and pain management
4. Pain management and antibiotics

314. To control bleeding in a child with hemophilia A, the nurse would expect to give:
1. Albumin
2. Fresh frozen plasma
3. Factor VIII concentrate
4. Factor II, VII, IX, X complex

315. When discussing hemophilia with the parents of a child recently diagnosed with this disorder, the nurse should explain that:
1. Hemophilia is an autosomal dominant disorder in which the woman carries the trait
2. Hemophilia follows regular laws of Mendelian inherited disorders such as sickle cell anemia
3. This disorder can be carried by either male or female but occurs in the sex opposite that of the carrier
4. Hemophilia is an X-linked disorder in which the mother is usually the carrier of the illness but is not affected by it

316. The mother of a toddler with hemophilia has just told the nurse, "Every time my son bumps his head I'll give him two children's aspirin. Is that right?" The nurse's best response would be:
1. "That is exactly right; use aspirin or acetaminophen."
2. "Are you concerned about giving drugs to your child?"
3. "No. Give him acetaminophen every day to prevent bleeding."
4. "Aspirin will only cause more bleeding. Give him acetaminophen instead."

317. The parents of a 10-year-old boy with hemophilia are very worried about their other children, two girls and another boy, and want to know what the chances are concerning their having the disorder or being a carrier. An appropriate answer to this question would be that:
1. All the girls will be normal and the other son a carrier
2. All the girls will be carriers and one half the boys will be affected
3. Each son has a 50% chance of being either affected or a carrier, and the girls will all be carriers
4. Each son has a 50% chance of being affected and each daughter a 50% chance of being a carrier

318. When examining the laboratory reports of a newly diagnosed child with acute lymphoid leukemia, the nurse notes that the child is neutropenic. This alteration is a result of:
1. Overwhelming infection
2. Increased internal bleeding
3. Increased immature cell growth
4. Decreased intake of iron-rich nutrients

319. With the diagnosis of acute lymphoid leukemia (ALL) the nurse should consider it unusual to observe:
1. Marked fatigue, pallor
2. Multiple bruises, petechiae
3. Enlarged lymph nodes, spleen, and liver
4. Marked jaundice and generalized edema

320. In addition to the symptoms of pallor, loss of appetite, listlessness, and tiredness, the nurse would expect an infant with acute nonlymphoid leukemia to demonstrate:
    1. Oliguria
    2. Few stem cells
    3. Difficulty swallowing
    4. Depressed bone marrow

321. When preparing an infant who is immunosuppressed following chemotherapy for discharge, the nurse explains to the parents that the measles, mumps, and rubella (MMR) immunization must:
    1. Be discussed with the pediatrician on the next visit
    2. Not be given until the infant is at least 2 years of age
    3. Not be given as long as the infant is receiving chemotherapy
    4. Be given to protect the infant from getting any of these diseases

322. A 4 year old, newly diagnosed with leukemia, is placed on bed rest. While assisting with morning care, the nurse notes bloody expectorant after the child has brushed the teeth. The nurse should first:
    1. Secure a smaller toothbrush for the child's use
    2. Tell the child to be more careful when brushing the teeth
    3. Record and report the incident without alarming the child

4. Rinse the child's mouth with half-strength hydrogen peroxide

323. A child receiving chemotherapy for the treatment of cancer is at risk for mouth lesions from the chemotherapy. The nurse teaching the child and the mother should stress the importance of:
    1. Brushing with a soft toothbrush
    2. Frequent rinsing with undiluted mouthwash
    3. Brushing three times a day with a toothbrush
    4. Frequent mouth rinsing with hydrogen peroxide

324. A child with the diagnosis of acute lymphoid leukemia (ALL) is scheduled to receive cranial radiation. The teaching plan should reflect the fact that this is done to:
    1. Improve the quality of life
    2. Reduce the risk of systemic infection
    3. Avoid metastasis to the lymphatic system
    4. Prevent central nervous system involvement

325. When providing physical hygiene and comfort for a child with leukemia who is receiving cancer chemotherapy, the nurse should avoid the use of:
    1 Straws
    2 Mouthwash
    3 Any powder
    4 A firm toothbrush

PEDIATRIC NURSING
ANSWERS AND RATIONALES

Emotional Needs Related to Health Problems

1. **3** Excessive crying and clinging are the usual responses of an infant who expects to be comforted, not one who has experienced prolonged separation from a parent because of illness. (1; CJ; AS; PS; EH)
   1 Prolonged hospitalization and separation from parenting can cause delayed growth or even death in infants.
   2 Withdrawing active attention is the infant's way to "turn off" and may be learned from multiple failures in interactions with stimuli.
   4 Inattentiveness to focus may be learned from failure to gain response from humans in previous experiences.

2. **3** A pacifier should be given during the feeding to help the infant associate sucking with feeding and the sense of fullness. (2; CJ; IM; PS; EH)
   1 This would cause complications if the tube is not in the stomach.
   2 This would be done after placement and a residual are ascertained.
   4 Upright positioning is essential to prevent regurgitation or reflux and subsequent aspiration.

3. **2** Peak crying times are early evening and night, which exhaust the mother. She needs time away from the baby to rest and should be encouraged to or make some arrangements for time alone. (1; MR; IM; ED; EH)
   1 Providing warmth through a hot-water bottle or heating pad over the abdomen may be helpful for some children but not for others.
   3 Many treatments, including this one, may not be effective; children do outgrow colic, so parents need support to help them manage until that time.
   4 Treatment is usually based on relieving abdominal cramping by stimulating peristalsis; quiet environments may help prevent, not treat, the problem.

4. **1** Sucking is a primary need of infancy. It decreases anxiety and does not interfere with gastric decompression. (2; CJ; IM; PS; EH)
   2 This would be more helpful if the client were a toddler.
   3 This will probably not help to calm the infant.
   4 This will probably increase the pain from abdominal distention; 3-month-olds are not developmentally ready to crawl.

5. **1** If able to handle personal anxiety and give comfort to the child, parents can be a real help to the staff as well as the child. If the parents are extremely anxious, their anxiety can be transmitted, making the child even more anxious. (2; MR; AS; PS; EH)
   2 It is how the parents cope with the situation, rather than the situation itself, that helps determine how helpful their presence may be.
   3 Parents can be helpful to the child and the staff; they often want to participate in the child's care.
   4 Toddlers are cognitively unable to make decisions of this nature.

6. **2** The 2-year-old is still attached to and dependent on the parents. Fear of separation is a great stress. (2; CJ; PL; PS; EH)
   1 Most likely these will not be remembered accurately.
   3 This is neither possible nor desirable.
   4 This is not possible in a health care setting.

7. **2** The nurse needs to obtain clarification as to what the mother is concerned about in regard to the child's behavior (2; CJ; IM; ED; EH)
   1 Although this may be true, it cuts off communication; further cornmunication should be encouraged.
   3 Inappropriate response; the nurse is making a statement without really knowing what the mother means.
   4 This response assumes the mother has been inconsistent; the nurse needs more information.

8. **2** The second stage of separation anxiety is despair, in which the child is depressed, lonely and disinterested in the surroundings. (2; CJ; EV; PS; EH)

1 The third stage of separation, denial or detachment, is a more advanced stage than that demonstrated in the situation.

3 The nurse must recognize that the child is suffering from separation anxiety, which does not include a stage of mistrust.

4 The nurse must recognize that the child is suffering from separation anxiety, which does not include a stage of rejection.

9. **1** Detachment is the result of trying to escape the emotional pain of desiring the mother by repressing feelings for her. (3; CJ; EV; PS; EH)

2 This interpretation is not appropriate to the situation cited.

3 This conclusion cannot be drawn from the situation cited.

4 This response lacks insight.

10. **1** Children with nephrosis have a characteristic pale, overweight appearance from the malnutrition and edema. They may become very sensitive about these changes as they grow older. (2; CJ; IM; PS; EH)

2 Although this may be indicated, body-image problems pose a much greater threat.

3 Engaging in usual childhood activities between attacks should promote normal development of fine muscle coordination.

4 Sterility is not associated with nephrosis.

11. **3** This focuses on the child's feelings and a familiar object of security. (3; CJ; IM; PS; EH)

1 Trying to control the child is inappropriate and will only increase anxiety; the child will experience pain as part of the treatment, so the statement is untruthful.

2 Diverting the child will not alleviate fear and anxiety.

4 Same as answer 2.

12. **2** Fear of mutilation is typical of the older preschooler. (2; CJ; AN; PS; EH)

1 Toddlers and younger preschoolers fear separation from parents.

3 Preschoolers do not view death as final.

4 Preschoolers do not associate death with a supernatural being as does the school-age child.

13. **3** A few minutes will be enough time for the child to begin self-feeding. The nurse should provide both physical and emotional support, because the child's request for help indicates the need for dependence during a period of stress. (1; CJ; IM; PS; EH)

1 It may be awhile until the child feels better; in the meantime, adequate nourishment to provide for healing is needed.

2 This does not provide the child the help that may be needed.

4 A nurse should never make a statement like this; it can cause stress, feelings of guilt, and embarrassment to a sick child.

14. **3** Regression is the retreat to a past level of behavior as a way of minimizing stress or controlling anxiety. Increased dependence, such as being fed by another person, is a form of regression. (1; CJ; AN; PS; EH)

1 The child's statement does not reflect immaturity.

2 Although loneliness may be a factor, it is not the key one in the child's statement.

4 The child's statement can hardly be construed as a temper tantrum.

15. **1** Dinner is frequently a family activity. Having the parents visit during meals may provide the child with additional emotional, social, and physical support, resulting in an improved nutritional intake. (1; MR; PL; TC; EH)

2 If given full rein, a young child will not select the most nutritional foods.

3 This will further inhibit the child's nutritional intake.

4 This may not influence the child's overall intake.

16. **1** Regression is normal in times of stress. It is a transient need that should be accepted, because it helps reduce anxiety. (1; CJ; IM; PS; EH)

2 Distraction works only as long as it is employed.

3 This behavior is unrelated to medical progress.

4 Cause (thumb sucking) and future effect (buckteeth) will not be meaningful to a 6-year-old.

17. **4** Anger interferes with communication; recognition and ventilation of anger help to resolve it and can help increase productive communication. (3; CJ; PL; PS; EH)
   1 They are too angry with each other to work this out alone; they may express anger to each other, which most likely will escalate the conflict in their relationship.
   2 The mother should be involved with the therapy and therefore must be present when treatment is discussed.
   3 Anger is interfering with the acceptance of responsibility and must be dealt with first.

18. **4** Decision making fosters and supports independence, a developmental need of the adolescent. It also increases a sense of self-worth and control (2; MR; IM; PS; EH)
   1 This does not ensure movement but social interaction.
   2 Although this may be true, it is not motivating.
   3 Limit setting meets the security needs of young children.

19. **2** This helps and encourages parents to put their fears and feelings into words. Once these sentiments are expressed, they can at least be examined and addressed. (2; CJ; IM; PS; EH)
   1 This would not assist the parents in coping with the problem. Neither would it demonstrate the supportive and empathetic roles of the nurse.
   3 This response lacks insight. Parents will worry about their infant anyway.
   4 This may or may not be helpful.

Drug-Related Responses

20. **4** Hypersensitivity reactions such as skin rash, erythema, fever, and pruritus occur with much greater frequency in clients with AIDS. (2; CJ; EV; PA; DR).
   1 Hepatic side effects, such as jaundice, may occur but are not common.
   2 CNS side effects, such as headache, are rare adverse reactions.
   3 This is a rare side effect.

21. **2** Salicylates in large doses cause irritation of the gastric mucosa (gastric distress, nausea, vomiting) and also affect the CNS (tinnitus, dizziness, disturbance in hearing and vision). (1; CJ; EV; TC; DR)
   1 Although nausea, dizziness, and severe headache may be associated with salicylate ingestion, edema is not.
   3 Constipation is not a problem.
   4 Edema is not a problem.

22. **4** Salicylates act as analgesics by protecting peripheral pain receptors from bradykinin, a component in the inflammatory process. Salicylates act as antipyretics by affecting the heat-regulating center in the hypothalamus and increasing the elimination of heat through peripheral blood vessel dilation and evaporation of increased perspiration. (1; CJ; AN; TC; DR)
   1 Salicylates have no capacity to act as a sedative and calm individuals.
   2 Salicylates have no capacity to act as a hypnotic and induce sleep.
   3 Salicylates have no capacity to destroy or control a microorganism's effect.

23. **1** Prednisone reduces the individual's resistance to certain infectious processes. Also prednisone is an antiinflammatory drug that masks infection. (2; CJ; IM; TG: PR).
   2 Eosinophil counts are often consistently elevated in children with asthma.
   3 The child will limit own activity based upon the respiratory status.
   4 The child will need adequate hydration to assist with loosening and removing mucus.

24. **4** Chlorpheniramine (Chlor-Trimeton) is an antihistamine that prevents histamine from reaching its site of action by competing for the receptors. (2; CJ; lM; TC; DR)
   1 Nitrofurazone is a bactericidal agent used especially with burns.
   2 Hyaluronidase is a mucolytic enzyme that promotes diffusion and absorption of injected fluids, exudates, and transudates.
   3 This is a salicylate.

25. **1** Too much aspirin is toxic to the eighth cranial nerve; the ensuing ear involvement causes tinnitus (ringing) and vertigo. (1; CJ; EV; PA; DR)
   2 This can occur but is not a sign of toxicity.
   3 Aspirin does not cause hepatotoxicity.
   4 Same as answer 2.

26. **4** To maintain the desired blood level, the drug must be given in the exact amount at the times directed. If the blood level of the drug falls, the organisms have an opportunity to build up resistance to the drug. (2; LE; PL; TC; DR)
 1 Weighing a client is important with drugs that affect fluid balance.
 2 Giving medication with milk or meals is important with drugs that cause GI distress.
 3 Monitoring temperature would be important with antipyretic drugs.

27. **4** Euphoria and mood swings may result from steroid therapy. (2; CJ; EV; TC; DR)
 1 Alopecia does not result from steroid therapy.
 2 An increased appetite, not anorexia, results from steroid therapy.
 3 Weight gain, not weight loss, results from steroid therapy.

28. **1** Generally, antineoplastic drugs act by interfering with, or inhibiting, synthesis of DNA in malignant cells. (3; CJ; AN; PA; DR)
 2 Malignant cells are not infected, in the normal sense of the term; therefore this drug does not act in this manner.
 3 Bone marrow depression is a side effect of this drug, not a desired action.
 4 This is the activity of the malignant cells themselves.

29. **1** A side effect of vincristine is alopecia. To adolescents, who are very concerned with identity, this represents a tremendous threat to their self-image. (1; CJ; PL; ED; DR)
 2 Constipation, although very serious, does not require early preparation.
 3 This will not be immediately obvious.
 4 Although neurological side effects are serious, the adolescent need not be prepared for this early.

30. **1** Prednisone is a synthetic glucocorticoid that has an active antiinflammatory effect by stabilizing lysosomal membranes and thus inhibiting proteolytic enzyme release. (2; CJ; AN; PA; DR)
 2 There is no indication the child is receiving radiation.
 3 Prednisone does not affect mitosis, but inhibits proteolytic enzyme release.
 4 Although prednisone increases the appetite and creates a sense of well-being, these are not the reasons it is administered.

31. **3** Vincristine is highly neurotoxic, causing paresthesias, muscle weakness, ptosis, diplopia, paralytic ileus, vocal cord paralysis, and loss of deep tendon reflexes. (3; CJ; EV; TC; DR)
 1 Hematologic effects are rare with vincristine.
 2 Alopecia is reversible with cessation of the drug.
 4 The most severe problems associated with vincristine are neurologic and neuromuscular.

32. **2** Children with leukemia most often die of infection; a lowered neutrophil count results after induction with myelosuppressant therapy (2; MR; PL; TC; DR)
 1 These measures are not appropriate to prevent infection; appropriate for treating the anemia.
 3 These measures are not appropriate to prevent infection; more appropriate for preventing hemorrhage.
 4 These measures are not appropriate to prevent infection; used to treat stomatitis.

33. **3** The tetracyclines are not recommended during periods of tooth development (children under 8 years of age or in pregnant women during the latter half of pregnancy) because they may permanently discolor teeth yellow, gray, or brown. (2; CJ; EV; TC; DR)
 1 Tetracycline does not interfere with bone structure of school-age children or pregnant women.
 2 This is not an expected complication of tetracycline.
 4 Anemia is not a common condition for 6-year-olds.

34. **4** A common side effect of long-term phenytoin (Dilantin) therapy is hyperplasia of the gingiva. (3; CJ; IM; TC; DR)
 1 Dilantin does not affect urinary output.
 2 Dilantin does not influence pupillary response.
 3 Dilantin does not cause flushing.

35. **4** Tetracycline is potentially hepatotoxic because it is metabolized in the liver. Signs of hepatotoxicity are lethargy, anorexia, behavioral changes, jaundice, and fatty necrosis. (3; LE; EV; TC; DR)
 1 The decreasing fever and secretions indicate that the infectious process is under control.
 2 Anemia may cause fatigue but is not associated with withdrawal and irritability.
 3 Common symptoms of bladder infection include burning upon urination, frequency or hesitancy, abdominal pain, and low-grade fever.

36. **2** The purpose of digoxin (Lanoxin) is to slow and strengthen the apical rate. The normal apical rate for a child of 5 years is 90 to 110 beats per minute. If the apical rate is slow (10 to 20 beats below normal), administration of the drug could lower the apical rate to an unsafe level. (1; LE; EV; TC; DR)
    1 This rate is well below that which necessitates withholding Lanoxin for children; it is the correct rate for withholding Lanoxin in adults.
    3 This is within the normal range of the heart rate of 5-year-olds and does not necessitate withholding Lanoxin.
    4 Same as answer 3.

37. **4** This is the expected response because medication causes, death of the worms. (2; CJ; EV; TC; DR)
    1 Transient diarrhea, not constipation could occur.
    2 Hypertension does not occur as a result of this medication.
    3 Neither the drug nor the worms cause intestinal bleeding.

38. **2** Acetaminophen relieves pain and does not cause bleeding tendencies, as does aspirin. The correct dose for this age is 300 mg. (3; CJ; EV; TC; DR)
    1 Aspirin affects platelet function.
    3 Demerol may be given, although a narcotic is not usually necessary for children after tonsillectomy; however, 50 mg would be the normal dose for an adult.
    4 Phenobarbitol will not relieve the pain; it will only sedate the client.

39. **4** For maximum benefit, the drug should be given before the pain becomes severe; scheduled medication times can be individualized for the client. (2; CJ; PL; PA; DR)
    1 The medication is not as effective when pain is severe.
    2 If oral analgesics are effective, they are preferable to giving the child an injection.
    3 If appropriate and the child is able to swallow, oral medications are preferable to intramuscular medications.

40. **3** Fewer side effects are desirable. Better elimination of the lead prevents further irreversible damage. (2; CJ; AN; TC; DR)
    1 The combination is preferred because it removes lead more effectively from the brain rather than from bone marrow.

2 There is no marked difference in the rate of urinary elimination when these agents are used together.
4 Each drug is able to accomplish this, but singly given each can cause more side effects.

41. **3** Urinary output must be sufficient to carry away lead and the metabolized chelating agent; in addition, EDTA can damage kidney tissue. (3; CJ; EV; PA; DR)
    1 Calcium EDTA is not irritating to intestinal mucosa because it is excreted by the kidneys.
    2 A regular diet with some "junk food" is permitted.
    4 Calcium EDTA does not cause pain when given intravenously.

42. **2** The peak action of Humulin N insulin is 6 to 8 hours. (1; CJ; EV; PA; DR)
    1 This is the peak time for regular insulin, not Humulin N insulin.
    3 The peak action of Humulin N insulin is 6 to 8 hours; this is too late.
    4 Same as answer 3.

Growth and Development

43. **4** The child experiencing long-term hospitalization is forced to relate to a variety of significant adults instead of to a single figure providing mothering. The lack of continuity creates anxiety. (1; CJ; AN; PS; GD)
    1 Even with sufficient play objects, the child will still suffer from the lack of a mother figure.
    2 Even with sufficient sensory stimulation, the young child will still suffer from the lack of a mother figure.
    3 Although mother surrogates are helpful, they do not replace the mother figure.

44. **1** Sucking meets oral needs, which are primary during infancy. (3; CJ; IM; PS; GD)
    2 An infant of a few days is probably too young to focus well on a mobile; in addition, the infant will be placed in a side-lying position postoperatively and thus would not be able to focus on the mobile.
    3 Two-day-old infants are not yet developmentally capable of enjoying a soft, cuddly toy.
    4 This is not a developmental need.

45. **2** An Apgar score of 3 indicates neonatal distress and should signal the nurse that the infant requires close supervision and support. (2; CJ; EV; TC; GD)
 1 Average birth weight is about 3200 g.
 3 A positive Babinski is normal through the age of 2 years.
 4 Infants often swallow in utero.

46. **4** Turner's syndrome results from a missing X chromosome; these females have an XO configuration rather than XX. (2; CJ; AS; FA; GD)
 1 This occurs when there is a thyroid deficiency.
 2 This will result from an autosomal recessive single gene disorder.
 3 This will result from an extra chromosome 21.

47. **4** Play during infancy (solitary) promotes physical development. For example, mobiles strengthen eye movement, large beads promote fine finger movement, and soft toys encourage tactile sense. (1; CJ; AN; ED; GD)
 1 Play during infancy is usually initiated by the parent.
 2 Children do not begin to share until the preschool years.
 3 Play is important throughout childhood.

48. **2** Infants who have experienced maternal deprivation usually exhibit failure to thrive (i.e., weight below third percentile, developmental retardation, clinical signs of deprivation, and malnutrition). These physical and emotional factors predispose the infant to a variety of illnesses. (2; CJ; AS; PS; GD)
 1 Infants who have experienced maternal deprivation are usually quiet and nonresponsive.
 3 Responsiveness to stimuli is limited or nonexistent.
 4 Weight below the third percentile is characteristic.

49. **3** By 4 months of age infants are able to turn over and can easily fall from an inadequately guarded height. (1; CJ; lM; TC; GD)
 1 Although infants are capable of putting small things in their mouth, they are not yet able to crawl and would probably not be placed on the floor.
 2 At 4 months of age infants are not yet able to explore the environment to the point that electric outlets pose a problem.

 4 Infants are still too small and have not yet developed motor capabilities to get into containers of poison.

50. **2** Muscular coordination and perception are developed enough at 6 months so the infant can roll over. If unaware of this ability of the infant, the mother could leave the child unattended for a moment to reach for something and the child could roll off the crib. (2; CJ; IM; ED; GD)
 1 Sitting up unsupported is accomplished by most children at 7 to 8 months.
 3 Crawling takes place at about 9 months of age.
 4 Standing by holding onto furniture is accomplished by most children between 8 and 10 months.

51. **4** The 7-month-old is used to having the perineal area exposed and cared for and is not in a developmental stage where fears related to sexuality are present. (2; CJ; IM; ED; GD)
 1 A "clean catch" at this age is often contaminated; the physician ordered a catheterization.
 2 The mother does have the right to refuse but concerns are not realistic for this age infant.
 3 The mother's concern is not appropriate for the developmental age of the infant.

52. **1** Because of the infant's increasing mobility, high level of oral activity, and relative lack of fear or appreciation for danger, accidents are the primary cause of death in children above 1 year of age. (3; CJ; IM; ED; GD)
 2 This is too early for discussions about toilet training.
 3 This is best discussed with the mother prenatally or soon after delivery.
 4 This is too early for discussions of psychosexual development.

53. **2** The child from 1 to 4 years of age is learning to use the body and manipulate and experiment with all aspects of the environment; these abilities challenge the examiner and may require many modifications when doing a physical examination. (2; CJ; AS; ED; GD)
 1 The school-age child is able to cooperate and understand during the examination; however, modesty should be respected.
 3 The infant often enjoys having clothing removed and is easily distracted with sounds and smiles.
 4 From 6 to 12 months of age it is usually easier for the examination to be done with the infant held on the parent's lap to limit stranger anxiety.

54. **1** Walking is the primary developmental task of this age group. The other choices are not applicable to this age group. (2; CJ; AN; ED; GD)
    2 A child learns to climb stairs at around 18 months of age.
    3 The ability to use a spoon is not developed until 18 months.
    4 Learning to walk takes precedence over learning to talk; speaking is not a primary task at this age.

55. **2** At 15 months, strength and balance have improved, and the toddler can stand and walk alone. (2; CJ; EV; ED; GD)
    1 This is not usually true until the child is 2 years old.
    3 Infants are very capable of throwing toys.
    4 Infants 9 to 12 months of age can stand with support.

56. **2** The psychosocial need during the early toddler age is the development of autonomy. The toddler objects strongly to discipline. (2; CJ; AN; ED; GD)
    1 This is untrue; excessive discipline leads to feelings of shame and self-doubt, the major crisis at this stage of development.
    3 The sense of initiative is attained during the preschool age, not during the toddler age.
    4 It is frightening for a child to be left alone; it leaves the child with feelings of rejection, isolation, and insecurity.

57. **4** Children who are expressing negativism need to have a feeling of control. One way of achieving this within reasonable limits is for the parent or caregiver to provide a choice of two items, rather than force one on the child. (1; CJ; IM; ED; GD)
    1 This will not achieve the goal of giving fluids.
    2 This will probably not be successful with a toddler; it will probably end in disaster.
    3 This will complicate the situation and further inhibit the child's willingness to take fluids.

58. **3** The nurse recognizes the child's protest over the mother's absence and tries to comfort by staying near until the child feels more relaxed. The bathing can be postponed until the child has had time to test out the environment and is less anxious. (2; CJ; IM; ED; GD)
    1 This may frighten the child more.
    2 This action does not attempt to relieve the child's anxiety and will probably cause it to increase.

    4 This is probably true, although the nurse has not attempted to reduce anxiety.

59. **4** Appropriate limit setting and discipline are necessary for children to develop self-control while learning the boundaries of their abilities. (2; CJ; AN; ED; GD)
    1 Superego control begins in the preschooler.
    2 Trust and security are tasks that the infant learns.
    3 Roles within society are learned by the school-aged child.

60. **2** Common developmental norms of the toddler, who is struggling for independence, are inability to share easily, egotism, egocentrism, and possessiveness. (2; CJ; AS; PS; GD)
    1 This task is too advanced for toddlers and more accurate for preschoolers.
    3 This is true of 4-year-olds.
    4 One characteristic of toddlers is their short attention span; 15 minutes is too much to expect.

61. **2** The child should be taken to the dentist between 2 and 3 years of age, when most of the 20 deciduous teeth have erupted. (1; MR; IM; ED; GD)
    1 This is too late.
    3 Same as answer 1.
    4 This is too indefinite.

62. **4** The toddler is in Erikson's stage of acquiring a sense of autonomy. The negativism is the result of the child's need to express her will and test out her environment. (1, CJ; IM; ED; GD)
    1 This is the developmental task achieved in infancy.
    2 Although this is a factor, toddlers assert themselves in an attempt to attain more autonomy.
    3 Children do not assert themselves to obtain discipline.

63. **1** These are foods that a toddler likes and can handle; they provide good nutrition. (2; CJ; IM; ED; GD)
    2 These foods are not very nutritious, and the child may choke on corn dogs.
    3 Grapes are dangerous because toddlers may choke on the skins.
    4 The skin of a hot dog may cause choking and potato chips are not very nutritious.

PEDIATRIC **ANSWERS**

64. **2** Bed-wetting accidents are not uncommon in this age group, especially during hospitalization when regression may occur. Therefore the best approach is to ignore the event. (2; CJ; IM; PS; GD)
   1 The child may interpret this as punishment. Punishment for regressive behavior is inappropriate.
   3 Because skin breakdown is a concern, rubber sheets are contraindicated; they would hold moisture close to the skin.
   4 This may tend to make the child feel guilty for the behavior.

65. **4** This is a task expected of the 3-year-old. (1; CJ; AS; ED; GD)
   1 This is a task expected of the 4- or 5-year-old.
   2 This is a task expected of the 4-year-old.
   3 Same as answer 2.

66. **2** Of these foods and fluids an apple provides the best nutrition for a toddler and does not produce mucus. (3; CJ; PL; ED; GD)
   1 Unsafe; a toddler could choke on the skins of the grapes.
   3 Contraindicated; theories suggest that milk may produce mucus and may further compromise breathing.
   4 Cola is lacking in nutritional value and could be too much of a stimulant.

67. **4** In small children the eustachian tube is shorter, wider, and straighter. Pulling the auricle down and back facilitates passage of fluid to the drum. (2; CJ; IM; ED; GD)
   1 Pulling the auricle down and back, not forward, helps straighten the canal.
   2 Pulling the auricle up and back is used for older children and adults.
   3 Pulling the auricle down and back helps straighten the canal for passage of the drops.

68. **1** The toddler is still dependent on the mother, is narcissistic, and still plays alone, but is aware of others playing nearby (1; CJ; AS; ED; GD)
   2 Solitary play or onlookers' play is characteristic of the 1- to 2-year-old.
   3 Competitive play would be seen in school-aged children.
   4 Tumbling-type play is not a commonly accepted term used to refer to how play incorporates other children.

69. **4** Play-Doh is age appropriate; manipulating, rolling, and pounding it may help work out anger at being hospitalized (2; CJ; PL; ED; GD)
   1 An infant would enjoy a mobile.
   2 This is too advanced for a 2-year-old child.
   3 This could be too complicated for toddler to do.

70. **1** The nurse can best evaluate teaching by asking the learner for a demonstration; a child can show what has been learned more readily by behavior than by words. (2; CJ; EV; ED; GD)
   2 The child may be too young to know if there are any questions.
   3 This would be difficult for even 5-year-olds; their vocabularies are still growing.
   4 A demonstration rather than an explanation can be evaluated more readily.

71. **1** Role playing encourages expression of through behavior, since children's ability to verbalize feelings is limited. (2; CJ; AN; PS; GD)
   2 The preschooler is too young to think about careers.
   3 This may occur, but it is not a purpose of role playing.
   4 Although preschoolers try to imitate adults, providing guidelines for adult behavior is premature.

72. **3** Four year olds boast, exaggerate, and are impatient, noisy, and selfish. (3; CJ; EV; PS; GD)
   1 Four year olds engage in more advanced cooperative play.
   2 This is highly unusual for 4 year olds as they are striving toward more initiative and less dependence.
   4 The tendency toward tantrums and negativism should have waned by 4 years of age.

73. **4** Fear of mutilation and intrusive procedures is most common at this age because of fantasies and active imagination. These children also connect illness with being bad and view intrusion as punishment. (3; CJ; IM; PS; GD)
   1 A child this age usually has little previous contact with pain and therefore little experience upon which to base fear.
   2 Death is seen as reversible and not final.
   3 Fear of isolation from peers is a problem for school-aged children and adolescents.

74. **3** More information is needed; developmental delay suggests some milestone for age is not being met at the average time; it is not synonymous with retardation. (2; CJ; AS; ED; GD)
    1 This would be inappropriate as more information must be obtained.
    2 Although the physician may help, it is not yet known if such a program is needed.
    4 The nurse does not know this without more information.

75. **2** Because their verbal ability is limited, children act out their feelings via play. (1; CJ; IM; PS; GD)
    1 Therapeutic play does not necessarily involve other children.
    3 Acceptance of the hospital situation is not as important as dealing with feelings.
    4 The child needs to cope with feelings rather than forget them.

76. **4** The parents attitude, approach, and understanding of the child's physical and psychologic readiness are essential to letting the child proceed at his or her own pace with appropriate interventions by the parent. (2; MR; PL; ED; GD)
    1 This will not be the major motivation for toilet training.
    2 Although this will definitely be a factor, it is not a major one.
    3 This, of course, is a factor; but the major factor is the child, who is strongly influenced by the parents' attitudes and approach.

77. **3** A pounding board is a safe toy for toddlers, because it is fairly large, easy to manipulate, and sturdy. A pounding board provides a way for anger to be sublimated. (2; CJ; IM; PS; GD)
    1 The child's motor and hand-eye coordination is too immature for using these.
    2 This would be appropriate for an older child with more mature motor coordination to compensate for a moving object.
    4 This is not as safe because toddlers may eat clay.

78. **4** Until trust has been reestablished, the child will be unable to develop an emotional tie to the mother. (2; CJ; IM; PS; GD)
    1 At this stage of separation anxiety, the child would be too detached to be hostile.
    2 In extreme cases of separation, the child will be withdrawn from the parents.
    3 The child will be despairing and withdrawn.

79. **2** Piaget stresses that age 7 is the turning point in mental development. New forms of organization appear at this age that mark the beginning of logic, symbolism, and abstract thought. (1; CJ; AN; ED; GD)
    1 A 5 year old is capable of tying laces.
    3 A toddler is capable of making simple decisions.
    4 An infant is capable of hand-eye coordination.

80. **3** School-aged children enjoy competition, have manipulative skills, and are creative. (2; CJ; IM; ED; GD)
    1 This activity is inappropriate during an acute illness because it requires too much energy.
    2 These toys are appropriate for the toddler who is developing fine motor skills.
    4 Magazines would interest an older child.

81. **4** Six year olds are aware of their hands as tools and enjoy building simple structures. (2; CJ; IM; ED; GD)
    1 This is more appropriate for preschoolers.
    2 This is more useful for an older school-age child, with a longer attention span and a better ability to follow instructions.
    3 Same as answer 2.

82. **2** School-aged children have an interest in hobbies or collections of various kinds as a means of gathering information and knowledge about the world in which they live. (2; CJ; PL; ED; GD)
    1 This is too advanced for the average 9 year old.
    3 This would not interest a 9 year old.
    4 These would probably not interest a 9 year old.

83. **4** Because young children have difficulty verbalizing their fears or anxiety, play is a therapeutic way for these feelings to be expressed. The school-age child also likes to role play. (2; CJ; IM; PS; GD)
    1 A child this age is unable to express feelings entirely through words.
    2 Young school-aged children are still somewhat egocentric and therefore interested in their own experiences and sensations.
    3 This may be helpful for a toddler or preschooler.

PEDIATRIC   ANSWERS

84. **3** Normally there may be a weight gain caused by the influence of hormones before the growth spurt. Also, 10- to 12-year-old children can eat an adult-size meal without the increased metabolic needs of adolescence. (2; CJ; IM; ED; GD)

   1 Before advising increased activity, the nurse would need to assess the client's present activity level.

   2 This weight gain is normal and adequate calorie intake is needed for the growth spurt occurring in adolescence.

   4 Family eating patterns appear to have more effect on weight than do genetics.

85. **4** Several meetings with an adolescent provide an opportunity to develop trust and establish a relationship. (3; CJ; IM; PS; GD)

   1 This is not necessary and may not help in establishing a relationship.

   2 This is not realistic because the nurse is not the teenager's peer.

   3 It is not necessary to deal in concrete terms, because the average adolescent is above this level.

86. **3** The future seems far away, and immediate gratification takes priority. (2; CJ; AN; ED; GD)

   1 Adolescents are often confused about their feelings.

   2 This is the developmental task of children 6 to 12 years; identity is the developmental task of the adolescent.

   4 School-age children (7 to 11 years) use concrete operational reasoning; adolescents are learning to think abstractly and use formal operational reasoning.

Respiratory

87. **2** These positions have lowest risk for SIDS. (1; CJ; IM; ED; RE)

   1 This position has been associated with the incidence of SIDS and should be avoided.

   3 More than one position should be used.

   4 Same as answer 1.

88. **3** Crying increases the amount of air being brought into the lungs. The flow of air coming into the lungs creates an increase in positive pressure, which helps expand the alveoli and improve gas exchange, thereby decreasing cyanosis. In atelectasis some of the alveoli do not expand; as evidenced by a lack of chest expansion on the affected side. (3; CJ; EV; PA; RE)

   1 The signs of respiratory distress syndrome are much more severe than transient cyanosis.

   2 Decreasing cyanosis with crying is not indicative of neurologic damage.

4 The heart rate will not provide information about atrioventricular septal defects.

89. **2** In an emergency, respiratory distress or apnea without stridor or adventitious sounds is the most commonly seen symptom with shaken baby syndrome (SBS); this indicates a central cause of the distress; in addition, the youth of the mother and the influence of alcohol are stressors increasing the risk of SBS. (3; CJ; AS; PA; RE)

   1 The present age of this infant is beyond the time at which respiratory distress because of immaturity would occur.

   3 Short periods of apnea of less than 15 seconds can be normal at any age.

   4 These are indicative of laryngotracheobronchitis, which is common in children under 5 years of age.

90. **3** Grunting and rapid respirations are signs of respiratory distress in an infant. Grunting is a compensatory mechanism whereby an infant attempts to keep air in the alveoli to increase arterial oxygenation; increased respirations increase oxygen and carbon dioxide exchange. (2; CJ; AS; TC; RE)

   1 Sweating in infants is usually scanty because of immature functioning of the exocrine glands; profuse sweating is rarely seen in the sick infant.

   2 This is not necessarily a sign of illness.

   4 This is not necessarily indicative of illness.

91. **4** Increased fluids help to liquefy respiratory secretions, which promotes expectoration. (2; CJ; PL; PA; RE)

   1 Oxygen may be drying, which would thicken secretions.

   2 This position promotes retention of secretions; supine, prone, and Trendelenburg positions promote removal of secretions via gravity.

   3 Retained secretions are in the bronchi and trachea; gargling occurs in the oropharynx.

92. **2** Choanal atresia is a lack of an opening between one or both of the nasal passages and the nasopharynx. (3; CJ; AN; PA; RE)

   1 Rectal atresia involves the rectum's ending in a pouch and the normal anal canal's opening into the other (nonconnected) end of the rectum.

   3 Atresias associated with the GI tract include esophageal and intestinal atresia involving the ileum, jejunum, or colon.

   4 An atresia involving the pharynx and larynx is not commonly seen.

93. **1** There is little or no opening between the nasal passages and the nasopharynx; therefore the infant can breathe only through the mouth. When feeding, the infant cannot breathe without aspirating some of the fluid; this causes choking. (2; CJ; EV; TC; RE)
 2 The swallowing reflex is normal.
 3 Because it is difficult if not impossible to eat, the infant will be very hungry.
 4 If choanal atresia is unilateral, there may be no symptoms and infant will eat normally; if bilateral, sucking will be almost impossible.

94. **2** A patent airway and adequate pulmonary ventilation are always priorities after surgery. (1; CJ; AS; PA; RE)
 1 It is too soon for output to be a priority; however, it certainly must be assessed later.
 3 This is important, but adequate ventilation is the priority.
 4 The IV lines would be checked once the airway, breathing, and circulation are determined to be functioning well.

95. **4** Immaturity of the diaphragm and the intercostal and abdominal musculature in young infants inhibits adequate ventilation, which causes lung expansion to be inadequate; consequently the infant must use tremendous effort. (3; CJ; AS; TC; RE)
 1 Grunting more commonly occurs when the baby is chilled or cold.
 2 Cyanosis is a later manifestation; it is more common with congenital heart defects.
 3 Rapid respirations are normally present in young infants.

96. **2** These children frequently have difficulty in handling secretions as well as breathing after surgery. Nursing measures, such as using the partial side-lying position or gently aspirating secretions from the mouth or nasopharynx, may be necessary to prevent aspiration and respiratory complications. (1; CJ; IM; TC; RE)
 1 Although this is important, maintaining a patent airway is essential.
 3 Fluids are usually administered carefully by mouth.
 4 This is not necessary.

97. **4** Respiratory tract obstructions usually occur in the larynx, trachea, or major bronchi (usually right). Hoarseness may indicate vocal cord injury. Unintelligible speech may indicate an interference in the flow of air out of the respiratory tract and/or obstruction or injury to the larynx. (2; CJ; AS; TC; RE)
 1 A retropharyngeal abscess would not produce the clinical signs listed.
 2 Acute respiratory infection usually has a gradual onset.
 3 In view of the sudden onset of clinical signs and the age of the child, this is unlikely.

98. **4** A patent airway is the first priority, and necessary equipment must be immediately available. (2; CJ; PL; PA; RE)
 1 Although this would be helpful, it is not the priority.
 2 Convulsions are not necessarily associated with croup; respiratory promotion is the priority.
 3 Although appropriate, this is not the priority.

99. **2** Laryngeal spasms can occur abruptly; patency of airway is determined by constant assessment for signs of respiratory distress. (2; CJ; AS; PA; RE)
 1 This is important, but maintenance of respiration has priority.
 3 Same as answer 1.
 4 Same as answer 1.

100. **4** Gas exchange is limited because of narrowing and swelling of the bronchi; the Pco_2 rises. (2; CJ; AS; PA; RE)
 1 The pH would decrease; the child is in respiratory acidosis, not alkalosis.
 2 The O_2 level would be decreased, not increased.
 3 This would be increased to compensate for acidosis.

101. **3** Cold can precipitate bronchospasm, and increased exercise depletes oxygen. (2; CJ; PL; ED; RE)
 1 Treatment of asthma does not involve a low-fat diet.
 2 Although increased calories may be needed to support the child during a coexisting bacterial infection in the acute stage, by discharge a return to usual habits is indicated.
 4 Asthma is a chronic condition. Return to usual activities after the acute stage is essential for normal growth and development.

102. **4** The bronchodilator and antispasmodic medications must be continued to prevent attacks; it is the medications that are keeping the child asymptomatic. (3; MR; PL; TC; RE)
    1 This is untrue; some environmental moisture is necessary for these children; cold environments should be avoided.
    2 Consistent limits should be placed on the child's behavior regardless of the disease; a chronic illness does not remove the need for limit setting.
    3 The child's symptoms are being controlled by medications that are necessary to keep the child asymptomatic.

103. **3** School-aged children lose their primary teeth, which could be aspirated during surgery. The anesthesiologist must take special precautions to maintain client safety. (1; LE; IM; TC; RE)
    1 There is no reason to obtain an antistreptolysin O (ASO) titer on the client.
    2 This is a comforting gesture but is not essential.
    4 This is important but not essential and not always possible.

104. **3** Mucous secretions are increased in viscosity and precipitate or coagulate to form concentrations in glands and ducts which in turn cause obstructions. (3; CJ; AN; PA; RE)
    1 The eccrine (sweat) glands are not hyperactive, but there is an increased concentration of sweat electrolytes, namely sodium and chloride.
    2 The autonomic nervous system does not play a role in the pathology of cystic fibrosis.
    4 There is no alteration in the mucosal lining of the intestines; decreased amounts or absence of pancreatic enzymes causes impairment in the digestion and absorption of nutrients.

105. **4** Both parents are carriers; however, the gene for cystic fibrosis is recessive and the parents do not have the disease. (3; CJ; AN; ED; RE)
    1 The gene for cystic fibrosis is not located on the X or Y chromosome.
    2 Untrue; the gene for cystic fibrosis is recessive.
    3 The gene for cystic fibrosis is handed down as a recessive gene.

106. **1** Cupping and clapping over the chest (CPT) helps to break up mucus and mobilize secretions. (1; CJ; AN; PA; RE)
    2 Chest physiotherapy will not alter the physical changes that have occurred as a result of the disease process.
    3 Medications are required to dilate the bronchioles.

4 Chest physiotherapy does not humidify the bronchial tree.

107. **4** The first usual indication of cystic fibrosis is meconium ileus. The small intestine is blocked with a thick, tenacious, mucilaginous meconium, usually near the ileocecal valve. This causes intestinal obstruction with abdominal distention, vomiting, and fluid and electrolyte imbalance. (2; CJ; AS; PA; RE)
    1 This does not have special significance in cystic fibrosis.
    2 This is not an early sign of cystic fibrosis.
    3 Same as answer 1.

108. **3** This regimen will give the child an opportunity to rest before eating. (2; CJ; PL; TC; RE)
    1 The child should be encouraged to cough; if it is not effective, suctioning can be done after chest percussion and postural drainage.
    2 Chest percussion and drainage should be done after aerosol therapy.
    4 This action could cause the child to vomit.

109. **2** In cystic fibrosis the mucous glands secrete thick mucoid secretions that accumulate, reducing ciliary action and mucus flow. Expectoration is greatly hindered. Postural drainage promotes the removal of mucopurulent secretions by means of gravity. (2; CJ; IM; PA; RE)
    1 Coughing should be encouraged.
    3 The nurse should encourage activities appropriate for the child's physical capacity; this will include helping the child conserve energy during acute phases of illness.
    4 This is not necessary with cystic fibrosis.

110. **4** Cystic fibrosis is characterized by an overproduction of viscid mucus by exocrine glands in the lungs. The mucus traps bacteria and foreign debris that adhere to the lining and cannot be expelled by the cilia, thus obstructing the airway and favoring growth of organisms and infection. (1; CJ; AN; PA; RE)
    1 Neuromuscular irritability of the bronchi does not occur in cystic fibrosis.
    2 Although there is increased sodium and chloride in the saliva, it does not irritate or necrose mucous membranes.
    3 Cardiac defects are not associated with cystic fibrosis.

111. **4** Chest physiotherapy is done midway between feedings to lessen vomiting and increase drainage for suctioning. (2; CJ; IM; TC; RE)
 1 Doing chest physiotherapy at this time may cause the infant to vomit the feeding.
 2 Doing chest physiotherapy at this time will tire the infant and possibly lead to an impaired nutritional intake.
 3 This is inadvisable; the infant may vomit and nutritional intake will be impaired.

112. **2** These drugs are tuberculostatic and are prophylactic against tuberculosis. (3; CJ; PL; PA; RE)
 1 Bacille Calmette-Guérin (BCG) vaccine is the only successful vaccine for tuberculosis to date, but greater protection is afforded by daily prophylactic administration of INH.
 3 Old tuberculin is one type of skin test used to detect tuberculosis.
 4 Purified protein derivative (PPD) is a widely used skin test for detecting tuberculosis.

113. **3** Tubercle bacilli multiply in caseous lesions, which have a poor vascular supply. These areas receive lower levels of the drugs and as a result therapy must be prolonged. (2; CJ; PL; TC; RE)
 1 The length of therapy is insufficient to eradicate the bacilli.
 2 Because lower levels of drug reach caseous lesions, longer treatment periods are needed.
 4 Treatment for infected persons is usually less than a year.

114. **2** Family members who have been exposed are at high risk and should receive prophylactic therapy. (2; CJ; PL; TC; RE)
 1 This is an assumption, symptoms generally do not contribute significantly to a diagnosis of tuberculosis.
 3 Tubercle bacilli are not responsive to penicillin treatment.
 4 Too frequent; in addition prophylactic therapy should be started.

115. **3** When the causative organism is isolated, it is tested for antimicrobial susceptibility (sensitivity) to various antimicrobial agents. When an organism is sensitive to a medication, the medication is capable of destroying the organism. (2; CJ; AS; TC; RE)

 1 Although this is considered, the selection of drugs is based primarily on the ability of the drug to destroy the specific organism.
 2 This is an inappropriate answer.
 4 Although the physician's preference is considered, the selection of drugs is based primarily on the ability of the drug to destroy the specific organism.

116. **1** Nonstrenuous, diversional activities involving interpersonal relationships with another person provide better support and resting conditions than does more active play. (1; CJ; PL; PA; RE)
 2 A jigsaw puzzle is too complicated for a 5-year-old and does not provide the human contact needed.
 3 Although a doll is appropriate for a 5-year-old, it does not provide the human contact needed.
 4 This will probably increase the child's fretfulness and does not provide the human contact needed.

117. **1** Rest reduces the need for oxygen and minimizes metabolic needs during the acute, febrile stage of the disease. (1; CJ; AN; TC; RE)
 2 The child with pneumonia is usually confined to bed and needs to reduce activity to conserve oxygen.
 3 This is not a priority, and the child will be anorectic during the febrile phase.
 4 Elimination is not usually a problem except as a result of immobility.

118. **3** Following a thoracotomy, negative intrathoracic pressure is reestablished and the alveoli reexpand within 12 to 48 hours. (2; CJ; EV; PA; RE)
 1 This time is inadequate for reexpansion to occur.
 2 This time is inadequate for expecting reexpansion.
 4 In most instances, reexpansion will occur sooner than 48 hours; 72 hours is too prolonged.

119. **4** The seeping of blood from the operative site increases secretions, which the child adapts to by swallowing frequently. (2; CJ; EV; TC; RE)
 1 Snoring can be expected in a child who is postoperative from a tonsillectomy.
 2 This may be a later sign of hemorrhage. Frequent swallowing would be an initial sign.
 3 The child has been NPO for an extended time and is not able to ingest fluids easily because of a sore throat; the child will probably be thirsty.

120. **3** Bronchial constriction with mucus production will decrease arterial oxygenation producing an increase in heart rate and wheezing on auscultation; anxiety is characteristic of hypoxia. (1; CJ; AS; PA; RE)
1 These are characteristic of sepsis.
2 Confusion and tachypnea are seen with hypoxia, but crackles are not expected with asthma.
4 Hypertension may be seen in acute asthma, but the heart rate would be expected to increase; tremor is not specific to asthma.

Reproductive and Genitourinary

121. **2** This is an extremely vascular area and the infant must be closely observed for bleeding. (1; CJ; IM; TC; RG)
1 It is too soon to observe for signs of infection.
3 Generally the infant is not too uncomfortable after circumcision; this may, with other signs, be indicative of central nervous system difficulty.
4 If gauze is not wrapped too tightly around the penis, this should be no problem.

122. **3** Incomplete formation of the pubic bone is associated with exstrophy of the bladder. (2; CJ; AS; PA; RG)
1 This defect is not associated with exstrophy of the bladder.
2 Same as answer 1.
4 Same as answer 1.

123. **2** This is the transplantation of the ureters to a section of the colon with one end attached to the abdominal wall as an ileostomy. (2; CJ; AN; TC; RG)
1 This is an opening into the bladder through the abdominal wall that allows urine to flow out.
3 This is when the ureter is transplanted into the colon with urine excreted through the rectum.
4 This is when the ureter is transplanted through the abdomen and attached to the skin.

124. **1** A bland, high-protein, high-carbohydrate snack provides adequate nutrition in the face of infection and fever. (1; CJ; PL; PA; RG)
2 This does not provide the protein needed for the healing process.
3 These are empty calories.
4 This is too heavy for a between-meal snack and contains fats, which are not helpful in the healing process.

125. **4** The decreased filtration of plasma in the glomeruli results in an excess accumulation of water and sodium, producing edema that is first evident around the eyes. Hypertension is thought to be due to hypervolemia, although its exact cause is unclear. (2; CJ; AS; TC; RG)
1 Oliguria, not polyuria, is a sign of glomerulonephritis.
2 The client is usually hypertensive, not hypotensive.
3 Although hematuria is found, dehydration is not

126. **4** The glomerular filtration rate is reduced, resulting in sodium retention, protein loss, and fluid accumulation producing these symptoms. (2; CJ; AS; PA; RG)
1 None of these symptoms support the diagnosis of glomerulonephritis.
2 Not all of these symptoms support the diagnosis of glomerulonephritis.
3 Same as answer 2.

127. **4** During the acute stage, anorexia and the loss of protein lower the child's resistance to infection. (2; MR; PL; TC; RG)
1 Antibiotics are not necessary for all children with acute glomerulonephritis, only those with persistent streptococcal infections.
2 A bland diet is not necessary, and high protein should be avoided.
3 Bed rest is necessary only during the most acute stage; 4 weeks is too long.

128. **4** When urinary findings are normal, such as no evidence of hematuria or proteinuria, the child may resume preillness activities. (2; CJ; EV; TC; RG)
1 This restriction is unnecessary.
2 Same as answer 1.
3 Bed rest is unnecessary at this stage.

129. **1** Daily changes in weight are good indicators of fluid changes; loss or gain of muscle and fat do not usually cause apparent daily fluctuations in weight. (2; CJ; IM; ED; RG)
2 When weight gain, not loss, stops, the disease is being controlled.
3 Protein molecules do not weigh enough to be reflected in the child's weight on a daily basis.
4 It is not beneficial to plan the child's daily caloric intake on weight loss or gain.

130. 3 Infection is a constant threat because of a poor general state of nutrition, a tendency toward skin breakdown in edematous areas, corticosteroid therapy, and lowered immunoglobulin levels. (3; CJ; IM; TC; RG)

1 Fluid monitoring, not encouraging, is important in determining whether restriction is indicated.

2 The nurse should encourage intake of foods with high nutritional value and restrict salt during massive edema; the priority is preventing infection.

4 Bed rest may be used for severe stages, but generally ambulation is encouraged.

131. 1 Anemia accounts for the pallor; poor appetite and decreased energy are associated with the accumulation of toxic waste. (2; CJ; AN; PA; RG)

2 Once remission has occurred, usual activities can be resumed with discretion.

3 An elevated temperature probably would be present but an infection would not cause a muddy pallor.

4 Discontinuing the corticosteroids and diuretics that are usually prescribed would probably result in recurrence of edema in steroid-dependent children.

132. 1 Mumps can cause orchitis (inflammation of the testes) in males and oophoritis (inflammation of the ovaries) in females. Although rare, both can render the postpubescent child sterile. (2; CJ; IM; TC; RG)

2 This symptom is not associated with mumps.

3 Same as answer 2.

4 Same as answer 2.

133. 4 The hypothalamic-pituitary-gonadal-adrenal mechanism is responsible for the physiologic and structural changes that occur at puberty. In girls the adrenal glands secrete androgens that are responsible for the appearance of axillary and pubic hair, generally between 11 and 14 years of age. Menarche usually occurs 2 years after initial pubescent changes. (2; CJ; AS; PA; RG)

1 This is not an indicator of sexual maturity.

2 This is not a reliable indicator of sexual maturity.

3 This is not an appropriate indicator of sexual maturity in females.

134. 2 Renal biopsy is an invasive procedure. In early stages, Wilms' tumor is encapsulated. Any disruption of the tumor capsule would allow metastasis. (3; MR; EV; TC; RG)

1 IVP is helpful in making a diagnosis.

3 Surgical removal of the involved kidney is the preferred treatment.

4 Abdominal CT scan is helpful in making a diagnosis.

Neuromuscular

135. 3 The angle the wrist forms with the arm decreases as gestation increases; the angle is zero at term. (3; CJ; AS; ED; NM)

1 Sole creases develop progressively, covering the entire foot at term.

2 In immature infants the ears contain little cartilage and are very springy when folded; at term the ears contain cartilage and the pinna is firm.

4 In immature infants the testes are undescended; rugae develop, progressively covering the scrotum.

136. 1 Cardiac anomalies often accompany other genetic problems such as Down syndrome; 30% to 40% of these infants have congenital heart defects. (3; CJ; AS; PA; NM)

2 No need for special evaluation; routine assessment would be sufficient.

3 Same as answer 2.

4 Same as answer 2.

137. 4 The virus for polio damages the anterior horn cells of the spinal cord with a typical irregular and asymmetric pattern. The cervical and lumbar regions contain more anterior horn cells, and therefore the extremities are more frequently affected than the trunk. (2; CJ; AN; PA; NM)

1 The virus for rubella does not affect the motor cells of the anterior horn of the spinal cord.

2 The virus for rubeola does not affect the motor cells of the anterior horn of the spinal cord.

3 The virus for chickenpox does not affect the motor cells of the anterior horn of the spinal cord.

138. 2 When taking a health history, any areas of concern should be explored fully before a nursing diagnosis is made. (1; CJ; AS; PS; NM)

1 The nurse needs to gather more data to be able to determine the basis for the problem.

3 Data are inadequate to focus immediately on nutrition.

4 More data are needed before recommendations can be made

139. **3** Touching the palms of the hands causes flexion of the fingers (grasp reflex); this usually lessens after 3 months of age. An unexpected loud noise causes abduction of the extremities and then flexion of the elbows (startle reflex); this usually disappears by 4 months of age. Persistence of primitive reflexes usually is indicative of a cerebral insult. (2; CJ; IM; ED; NM)
  1 These changes are consistent with normal growth and development.
  2 The data do not support making this comment and would cause needless concern.
  4 Sensory stimulation at this age is directed toward experiences to add new motor, language, and social skills.

140. **1** Hearing is a sense that is not greatly influenced by emotional response in the young child. (2; CJ; AN; PA; NM)
  2 The emotional trauma of institutionalization will influence the child's cognitive development.
  3 The trauma of institutionalization may also result in speech and other expressive delays.
  4 Institutionalized children often manifest delays in neuromuscular development.

141. **2** A 10-month-old is unable to comply with directions to remain still and may be extremely frightened by the equipment used. (3; CJ; IM; TC; NM)
  1 This is not necessary; head must remain still but need not be shaved.
  3 This is not necessary unless a contrast medium is being used.
  4 The child is too young to understand details.

142. **2** This, together with observation and recording of seizure activity, is the primary nursing care for a client with a tonic-clonic seizure. (1; CJ; PL; TC; NM)
  1 This would aid with establishing an airway after the seizure but is an unsafe action during a seizure.
  3 The primary responsibility is to remain with the client to observe seizure activity and protect the client from injury.
  4 This is done after the tonic-clonic stage; the mouth should not be pried open to insert an airway during a seizure because injury may occur.

143. **1** Febrile convulsions are not necessarily associated with major neurologic problems but often accompany fever. Such convulsions may be partially accounted for by the overall brain immaturity in children. (2; CJ; PL; ED; NM)
  2 The cause of febrile convulsions is still uncertain.
  3 Febrile convulsions are more common in the infant and young toddler.
  4 Boys are affected about twice as often as girls.

144. **3** Shivering increases the metabolic rate, which intensifies the body's need for oxygen and raises the body temperature. (3; CJ; PL; TC; NM)
  1 Encouraging fluids is contraindicated because the child is vomiting.
  2 Although monitoring output will provide information about the client's level of hydration, it is more important to take affirmative action toward preventing increases in fever.
  4 Monitoring vital signs is not as important as taking affirmative action to prevent increases in fever.

145. **4** A child who has a seizure may be injured unless precautions are taken. (2; CJ; AN; PA; NM)
  1 A 2-year-old has not developed a concept of body image; there is a fear of pain.
  2 The priority is to prevent injury to the child during a seizure.
  3 Preventing injury is the priority and the nurse could provide age-appropriate feeding.

146. **4** Because the child is in a crib, the nurse should remain, observe, and protect the child from injury to the head or extremities during the seizure activity. (1; CJ; IM; TC; NM)
  1 Useless until the seizure is over; child is apneic during seizure.
  2 Contraindicated; attempts at inserting a plastic airway are futile; this could damage the child's teeth and jaws.
  3 Never restrain an individual during a seizure; fractured bones or torn muscles and ligaments can result.

147. **4** Cyanosis is expected because the child will not breathe until the tonic-clonic phase of the convulsion is over. Observation and prevention of injury are the priorities at this time. (2; CJ; IM; TC; NM)
  1 Insertion of a foreign body into the mouth during the tonic-clonic phase of a convulsion may cause injury.
  2 This is useless until the child breathes.
  3 Same as answer 1.

148. **3** This limits the danger of falling and striking the head. (2; CJ; IM; TC; NM)
  1 Never leave a client having a seizure unattended.
  2 Attempting to open the jaw may result in injury.
  4 This may cause airway occlusion by forcing the chin onto the neck.

149. **1** Bradycardia is a classic sign of increased intracranial pressure. (3; CJ; AS; PA; NM)
  2 With increased intracranial pressure there would be decreased alertness or loss of consciousness.
  3 The fontanels are closed in a 6-year-old.
  4 Systolic blood pressure increases with increased intracranial pressure

150. **3** This is what occurs in communicating hydrocephalus. (3; CJ; IM; ED; NM)
  1 This is often caused by a choroid plexus tumor and does not interfere with the flow of cerebrospinal fluid through the ventricles.
  2 This reflects the pathophysiologic process of noncommunicating hydrocephalus.
  4 This is an inaccurate answer; brain cells and the spinal cord are not involved.

151. **4** Cellular destruction occurs as the brain is pressed against the unyielding skull. This occludes blood vessels and deprives the cells of oxygen. (1; CJ; AN; PA; NM)
  1 The increased CSF does not dilute the blood supply; pressure on vessels diminishes the blood supply, causing atrophy and death of cells.
  2 Hydrocephalus results when CSF is produced in too great quantities or is not adequately circulated or absorbed; there is no change in the concentration of CSF or plasma.
  3 Oxygen deprivation occurs when blood vessels are occluded secondary to the pressure in the skull caused by hydrocephalus.

152. **2** Elevation of the head helps decrease intracranial pressure by gravity. (3; CJ; IM; TC; NM)
  1 This is done routinely for all neonates; it is not specific for this problem.
  3 This may be disturbing to the infant and impair the ability to rest.
  4 Frequent stimulation may cause further irritability to an already traumatized CNS.

153. **2** Shunts need to be revised; as the child grows, the length of tubing needs to be changed. The shunts are also prone to malfunction and may need revision. (1; CJ; IM; ED; NM)
  1 Although treatment of hydrocephalus by shunt replacement is quite successful, there is danger of malfunction and infection of the shunt.
  3 Damage to brain cells is irreversible.
  4 Hydrocephalus necessitates treatment for the life of the child.

154. **4** The shunt may obstruct and lead to increased cerebrospinal fluid (CSF) in the head; accumulated fluid raises the intracranial pressure, which leads to brainstem hypoxia. (3; CJ; EV; PA; NM)
  1 Sedation is contraindicated to allow determination of the level of consciousness (LOC).
  2 Positioning the infant flat helps prevent complications resulting from too rapid reduction of intracranial fluid.
  3 The infant is positioned off the shunt to prevent pressure on the valve and incisional area.

155. **4** The affected limbs should be exercised to promote circulation and prevent atrophy. (2; MR; PL; PA; NM)
  1 Fluids should be encouraged to provide adequate kidney function and prevent constipation.
  2 Normal development should be encouraged; the child's motion should not be restricted.
  3 Child needs stimulation to develop mentally and socially.

156. **3** An infectious process causes meningitis that results in a stiff neck. (3; CJ; EV; TC; NM)
  1 Irritability rather than lethargy would result; lethargy is more often associated with increased intracranial pressure.
  2 Headache is associated with increased intracranial pressure.
  4 The pulse would be increased with an infection; a decreased pulse is associated with increased intracranial pressure.

157. **3** The anterior fontanel would be widened and tense because of the increased volume of cerebral spinal fluid. (3; CJ; EV; TC; NM)
1 The reflexes would be increased with increased intracranial pressure.
2 The pulse rate would be decreased with increased intracranial pressure.
4 The blood pressure would be increased with increased intracranial pressure.

158. **2** The meningomyelocele sac is thinly covered and fragile; trauma to the sac can damage functioning neural tissue; an intact sac reduces a potential portal of entry for microorganisms. (2; CJ; AN; TC; NM)
1 Although this is always an important nursing measure, care of the sac is even more important because an intact sac reduces a portal of entry for microorganisms.
3 Although observation of paralysis is an important nursing measure, care of the meningomyelocele sac is of primary importance.
4 A meningomyelocele will influence the client's ability to control these functions, but control is not developed until the toddler and preschool years.

159. **4** This would be the best position for preventing pressure on the sac. (3; CJ; IM; TC; NM)
1 Betadine is not used.
2 Assessment of the area below the defect is essential to determine motor and sensory function.
3 Diapers should not be applied because they might irritate or contaminate the sac.

160. **3** The surgical closure of the sac decreases absorptive surface and eliminates a route by which the spinal fluid drains. Skull bones are soft and will expand as fluid increases, causing hydrocephalus. (2; CJ; EV; TC; NM)
1 Most infants with meningomyelocele are partially or completely paralyzed in the lower extremities; careful range-of-motion exercises are one of the important parts of nursing care for these infants.
2 There is no reason to decrease environmental stimuli for infants with hydrocephalus unless they also have seizures.
4 This is not expected because damage to the meninges of the brain is not a factor in the surgical treatment of meningomyelocele.

161. **2** These children often have frequent dribbling of urine; they need frequent skin care and diaper changes to prevent skin breakdown. (3; CJ; PL; TC; NM)
1 This is not sufficient to replace frequent cleansing and diaper changes.
3 Untrue; constant dribbling of urine and seepage of feces cause skin breakdown unless areas are cleansed frequently.
4 Insufficient; the need is for frequent diaper changes.

162. **3** Braces are used to enable the spastic child to control motions. They also prevent deformities from poor alignment. (1; MR; AN; PA; NM)
1 Early ambulation is promoted by maintaining muscle strength and tone.
2 Because the child is at the age when self-reliance is important (Erikson's stage of industry versus inferiority) and depends on the braces for self-care, it is unlikely that they would be rejected.
4 Exercises are used to stretch ligaments and improve muscle strength and tone.

163. **1** Clients whose thermoreceptive senses are impaired are unable to detect changes or degrees of temperature. They must be taught to test the temperature in any water-related activity to prevent scalding and burning. (1; MR; IM; ED; NM)
2 The child with cerebral palsy normally has uncontrolled movement of voluntary muscles and does not need to be awakened at night to prevent skin breakdown.
3 Overtightening straps and buckles may lead to circulatory impairment and/or skin breakdown.
4 This is dangerous because this action alters the center of gravity; with practice the child will be able to place the legs in the appropriate position for walking without looking down.

164. **1** The damage is fixed. It does not progressively increase. (3; CJ; AN; PA; NM)
2 Although mental retardation may be present in some children with cerebral palsy, it cannot be assumed that all children with this disorder are mentally retarded.
3 Cerebral palsy is a nonprogressive chronic condition.
4 The etiology of cerebral palsy is related to anoxia in the prenatal, perinatal, or postnatal periods and is not genetic.

165. **2** The four-point alternate crutch gait is a simple, slow, but stable gait, because there are always three points of support on the floor with equal but partial weight bearing on each limb. (2; CJ; AN; TC; NM)
 1 The four-point gait provides for three points of support.
 3 The child has uncoordinated movement in the lower extremities because of the cerebral palsy.
 4 A four-point gait divides weight bearing equally among the limbs.

166. **4** The exact reason is unknown, but three factors appear to influence it: a child prone to pica, lead in the environment, and a high-fat diet. (3; CJ; AS; PA; NM)
 1 The environment is only one of the three etiologic factors.
 2 The role of the mother is not an identified factor.
 3 A child prone to pica is only one of the three etiologic factors.

167. **4** Damaged nerve cells do not regenerate. Once mental retardation has occurred, it is not reversible. (2; CJ; AN; PA; NM)
 1 Damage to kidneys is reversible with treatment.
 2 Skeletal changes are not significant and are reversible as lead leaves the body.
 3 Effects of lead in bone marrow are reversible when lead is mobilized for excretion in urine or deposition in bone by chelation therapy.

168. **2** Irreversible neurologic and intellectual damage are the most serious consequences of lead intoxication because of cortical atrophy and lead encephalopathy; protecting the child from injury is the priority. (1; CJ; AN; TC; NM)
 1 Although constipation can occur, it is not the priority.
 3 Although this could be true, there is not enough information to conclude that altered parenting is the etiology of this nursing diagnosis.
 4 Anemia occurs because lead is toxic to the biosynthesis of heme, not because of an inadequate intake of iron.

169. **3** The child should be given an outlet for tension, and syringe play is the most appropriate. (2; CJ; PL; PS; NM)
 1 This may ease discomfort, but an outlet for feelings should be provided.
 2 Fear is not directed at unfamiliar adults but at the painful treatments.

 4 This is part of the preparation, but is not the most important; the child must be allowed to express feelings.

170. **1** The slightest stimulation sets off a wave of very severe and very painful muscle spasms involving the whole body. Nerve impulses cross the myoneural junction and stimulate muscle contraction due to the presence of exotoxins produced by *Clostridium tetani*. (3; MR; PL; TC; NM)
 2 Body alignment is not an important consideration in tetanus.
 3 Oral intake of fluids may not be possible because of excessive secretions and laryngospasm.
 4 Monitoring output is not a major nursing concern with tetanus.

171. **4** Most children are no longer contagious after 24 to 48 hours when receiving IV antibiotics. (3; MR; IM; PA; NM)
 1 This time period would be inadequate even if antibiotics were started immediately.
 2 This would be an excessive time period.
 3 Same as answer 2.

172. **1** Decreased protein in spinal fluid indicates lessening of infection; meninges are becoming less inflamed. (3; CJ; EV; PA; NM)
 2 Glucose levels would be normal.
 3 Cell count would be decreased.
 4 Specific gravity would be decreased.

173. **1** Meningococcal meningitis is identified by its epidemic nature and purpuric skin rash. (3; CJ; AS; TC; NM)
 2 The fever of meningitis is usually high.
 3 This is not characteristic of meningococcal meningitis.
 4 Same as answer 3.

174. **2** Because cranial sutures are closed by this age, increased pressure could cause headache; irritation of cerebral tissue would cause seizures and pressure on vital centers would cause, vomiting. (3; CJ; AS; TC; NM)
 1 Pressure on the respiratory center results in a decreased respiratory rate.
 3 The inflammatory process of meningitis would elevate the temperature; the other two symptoms are possible.
 4 Blood pressure would be elevated in the toddler with closed fontanels because of increased intracranial pressure.

175. **3** Peripheral circulatory collapse (Waterhouse-Friderichsen syndrome) is a serious complication of meningococcal meningitis caused by bilateral adrenal hemorrhage. The resultant acute adrenocortical insufficiency causes profound shock, petechiae and ecchymotic lesions, vomiting, prostration, and hypotension. (2; CJ; AN; TC; NM)
1 Although this may occur, it is controllable and not as serious as peripheral circulatory collapse.
2 Although this may occur, it is not as serious a complication as peripheral circulatory collapse.
4 Although this may occur, it is rare and not as serious as peripheral circulatory collapse.

176. **3** Amblyopia is reduced visual acuity that may occur when an eye weakened by strabismus is not forced to function. (3; CJ; AN; TC; NM)
1 The lack of binocularity could result in impaired depth and spatial perceptions, not dyslexia.
2 Depth and spatial perceptions are impaired when vision in one eye is severely impaired.
4 Only vision in the affected eye will be diminished.

177. **4** Water in the ears after a myringotomy may be a source of infection. (2; MR; PL; ED; NM)
1 This will clog the ear canal and serves no purpose.
2 These may be used occasionally in the outer ear but should not be inserted into the inner ear.
3 No reason child cannot be around other children because there is no infectious process.

178. **2** Tinnitus in adolescents is largely related to hearing loud music, especially via headphones. (2; CJ; AS; PA; NM)
1 Ear noises are a real, not imagined, phenomenon.
3 Long-resolved ear infections usually have no sequelae, such as buzzing in the ears.
4 Familial deafness is more related to the deafness of aging.

179. **1** Morphine, an analgesic, relieves pain; when control of pain is given to the client, anxiety and pain are usually less, resulting in a decreased need for narcotics. (1; MR; EV; ED; NM)
2 If the adolescent is sleeping then the pain is under control; waking the client would interfere with his rest.

3 If the adolescent is sleeping then the pain is under control; also, this would result in an unnecessary and excessive amount of narcotic to be administered.
4 If the therapeutic regimen is ineffective the practitioner should be notified so that the regimen can be adjusted or changed.

180. **4** This degree of hearing loss causes the child to miss approximately 25% to 40% of conversations; this loss may result in speech deficits if not corrected; hearing aids usually can help improve functioning. (2; MR; PL; TC; NM)
1 The significance of the hearing loss requires further analysis and intervention.
2 There is no evidence that this hearing loss is progressive.
3 The child is missing approximately 25% to 40% of conversations, which would interfere with the educational process unless corrected.

Skeletal

181. **4** Hypostatic pneumonia can develop from decreased activity. Also the cast prevents full chest expansion. (1; MR; IM; ED; SK)
1 This is not necessary or desirable.
2 Soiling of the cast with excreta, although problematic, is not a serious complication.
3 Cast damage, although problematic, is not a serious complication.

182. **4** Pillows under the head or shoulders of a child in a spica cast will thrust the chest forward against the cast, causing discomfort and respiratory distress. Therefore, when elevation of the head is desired, the entire mattress or bed should be raised at the head of the bed. (2; CJ; IM; TC; SK)
1 There is no reason to place a time limit on this position.
2 This will not help in any way.
3 This will thrust the chest forward against the cast, causing discomfort and respiratory distress.

183. **2** Gluteal folds should be symmetric, as should all planes and folds of the body. An abnormality of the hips will cause asymmetry and/or a shorter leg on the affected side. (1; CJ; AS; PA; SK)
1 The dance reflex is not affected.
3 In developmental dysplasia of the hip there is usually a limited abduction of the leg at the hip.
4 The affected side is shorter.

184. **2** A respiratory rate below 30 in the young infant is not within the normal range; normal is 30 to 60 breaths per minute; a drop below 30 per minute is a significant change and should have been reported. (2; LE; EV; TC; SK)

1 This is untrue; more likely respirations will accelerate when discomfort is increased.

3 Any significant change should be reported immediately.

4 The respiratory tract is fully developed, and respiratory rate is a cardinal sign of the infant's well-being.

185. **1** A physical therapist can prescribe an exercise protocol to keep the joints as mobile as possible; a routine can be developed to help the child alleviate morning stiffness. (2; MR; IM; TC; NM)

2 Although this might be necessary in the future, there is no evidence that it is needed at this time.

3 Although nutrition is an appropriate part of therapy, it is the physical therapy program that can most directly influence movement.

4 Over-the-counter medications should not be used without the supervision of the practitioner.

186. **4** Prolonged sitting or lying in one position can lead to stiffness and flexion contractures and should be avoided. (2; MR; PL; ED; SK)

1 This helps maintain joint mobility.

2 This promotes normal functional movement.

3 This helps maintain muscle tone.

187. **4** The exercises are done to preserve joint function. (2; CJ; EV; PA; SK)

1 Exercises do not necessarily relieve pain.

2 Circulation is not affected by the arthritic process.

3 Exercising does not affect the subcutaneous nodules.

188. **3** A cast is not flexible and can inhibit circulation. Cold toes, loss of sensation in toes, pain, and inability to move toes should be reported to the physician immediately. (3; CJ; EV; TC; SK)

1 The normal pulse for a 9-year-old ranges from 70 to 110.

2 This may be related to increased fluid intake.

4 It takes 24 to 48 hours for a plaster cast to dry.

189. **2** This is the safest way to dry the cast evenly. (2; CJ; PL; TC; SK)

1 Besides the danger of burning the client, the cast may dry on the outside and remain damp within.

3 This would impede the circulation of air and delay drying.

4 May create a draft and be uncomfortable for the client.

190. **3** Adolescents are concerned about body image and fitting in with a peer group; the stabilizing rod may be viewed as an insult to the intactness of his body. (1; CJ; EV; ED; NM)

1 After open reduction and internal fixation with a rod insertion, clients generally may return to activities after 4 months.

2 Weight bearing can be prevented with crutches, which provide greater mobility than a wheelchair.

4 This is unnecessary; the need for pain medication will decrease as the trauma from the injury and surgery subsides.

191. **4** This is an independent nursing intervention that will produce sufficient countertraction and will keep the weights off the floor. (2; CJ; IM; TC; SK)

1 This decreases countertraction and is contraindicated.

2 This is contraindicated because it will not raise the weights off the floor.

3 There is no need to notify physician for reapplication of the traction.

192. **3** The nurse made the assessment that the medication was ineffective in relieving the child's pain for the duration ordered. This information should be communicated to the physician for evaluation. (1; MR; IM; TC; SK)

1 There are no data to support this. The amount of medication was probably inadequate for the client's pain tolerance level.

2 The nurse should not ignore the client's need for pain relief.

4 The physician's order is for administration only every 3 hours. Legally it can be given only within these guidelines.

193. **3** The hyperextension required in swimming aids in strengthening back muscles and increases deeper respirations, both of which are necessary before surgery and/or wearing a brace or cast. (l; CJ; IM; TC; SK)

1 This will not be especially therapeutic for a child with this condition.

2 Same as answer 1.

4 Same as answer 1.

PEDIATRIC   ANSWERS

194. 4 Continuing growth causes changes in muscle, bone structure, and position. Adolescents have a rapid growth spurt. The brace is worn for 6 months after physical maturity, which is proved by x-ray examination to show cessation of bone growth. (2; MR; IM; ED; SK)

1 This is not an appropriate criterion for removal of the brace.
2 Pain is not usually a symptom of scoliosis.
3 The brace is used to halt the progression of the curvature, not correct it.

195. 1 Preadolescence is a critical period of growth, and steroids could lead to growth retardation. (3; CJ; AN; ED; NM)

2 The effect of steroids on sexuality is unclear.
3 The effect of steroids on emotions is unclear and can vary with each individual; mood changes, however, have been documented.
4 Poor body image is a result of many variables, not just medications.

Endocrine

196. 4 Helping families understand their feelings about diabetes is essential in assisting them to develop positive attitudes for optimal control of the disease and promotion of a normal life for the child. (1; MR; PL; PS; EN)

1 This is important; however, if feelings are not dealt with first, compliance with insulin injections is less likely.
2 Instruction in specific psychomotor tasks should be preceded by an assessment of the family's acceptance of the diagnosis and knowledge about the disease.
3 The client should participate in activities normal for the age group. Adequate exercise is an important part of the treatment regimen for diabetes.

197. 4 A bedtime snack is needed for the evening. Humulin N insulin lasts for 24 to 28 hours. Protein and carbohydrate ingestion before sleep prevents hypoglycemia during the night, when the action of Humulin N insulin will still be high. (1; MR; PL; PA; EN)

1 There are no data to indicate such a need; a bedtime snack is routinely provided to help cover intermediate-acting insulin during sleep.
2 The snack is important for diet/insulin balance during the night, not encouragement.
3 The snack must contain mainly protein-rich foods to help cover the intermediate-acting insulin during sleep.

198. 3 An 8-year-old is in the stage of industry and strives to complete assigned tasks. (2; CJ; PL; ED; EN)

1 This is true of an older age group (adolescent).
2 Peer influences increase rather than decrease as a child grows.
4 This is true in the period of adolescence.

199. 1 Peak action of Humulin R insulin is 2 to 4 hours; peak action of Humulin N insulin is 6 to 8 hours. (2; CJ; AN; PA; EN)

2 Humulin R insulin duration is 6 to 8 hours.
3 Humulin R insulin onset is 30 minutes to 1 hour; Humulin N insulin onset is 1 to 2 hours.
4 The opposite is true; peak action of Humulin R insulin is 2 to 4 hours; peak action of Humulin N insulin is 6 to 8 hours.

200. 3 An insulin-dependent diabetic client must carry a source of concentrated glucose (glucose tablets, Insta-glucose, sugar-containing candy such as Life Savers) as a rapid source of carbohydrate in the event of signs of hypoglycemia; this should be followed by complex carbohydrate and a protein. (1; MR; IM; ED; EN)

1 This is an unrealistic and unnatural pattern for an adolescent.
2 This is an unnecessary and a time-consuming procedure.
4 The client should be made to feel a part of the family; the diabetic diet will have foods that will be nutritious for the entire family.

201. 4 A blood sugar of 180 mg/dl is above the normal range, and regular insulin, which is fast acting, is needed. (2; MR; IM; TC; EN)

1 Exercise will not correct the problem; regular insulin is needed.
2 This action will not correct the problem: the blood glucose is already known.
3 Food intake would increase the blood sugar at this time.

202. 2 The client needs immediate and easily absorbable sugar, such as cola, and long-lasting complex carbohydrates and protein, which are supplied by the bun and hamburger. (2; MR; IM; ED; EN)

1 This can be done after the client ingests some sugar; otherwise, the client's hypoglycemia can become severe.
3 Extra insulin will further aggravate the problem.
4 Same as answer 1.

203. **2** By increasing the diet, that is, increasing the client's carbohydrate intake, a hypoglycemic reaction caused by exercise is less likely to occur. (2; MR; IM; ED; EN)
    1 An oral hypoglycemic is an inappropriate treatment for dependent diabetes mellitus.
    3 This is not an appropriate reason for altering the insulin dosage.
    4 This type of intake is less effective than other nutrients absorbed more slowly, which provide a more consistent blood glucose level.

204. **3** Congenital hypothyroidism is the result of insufficient secretion by the thyroid gland because of an embryonic defect. The decreased thyroid hormone has been affecting the infant since before birth during cerebral development, so it is likely that mental development will be retarded. Treatment before 3 months will prevent further damage. (2; CJ; AS; TC; EN)
    1 Congenital hypothyroidism does not become myxedema.
    2 This is a term for hyperthyroidism.
    4 Treatment corrects abnormal responses.

205. **4** The goiter associated with this disease (Hashimoto's disease) is usually transient and regresses spontaneously in a year or two; the client is usually euthyroid but may be slightly hypo- or hyperthyroid. (2; CJ; lM; ED; EN)
    1 This is not a chronic disease.
    2 There seems to be a strong genetic predisposition, but no mode of inheritance has been identified.
    3 This is not an untreatable or fatal disorder; it can be controlled with a medical regimen.

206. **4** There are both an increased appetite with increased deposition of fat in the stomach and trunk and muscle wasting, which causes thin extremities. (2; CJ; AS; PA; EN)
    1 Increased excretion of calcium causes a retarded linear growth with a short stature.
    2 Because of the excess production of androgens, virilization and hirsutism occur.
    3 Increased salt and water retention cause hypernatremia and hypertension.

Integumentary

207. **2** Chickenpox is caused by a virus and may be followed by encephalitis; it is characterized by skin lesions. (3; CJ; IM; ED; IT)
    1 Pertussis is caused by a bacterium and does not result in encephalitis.
    3 Although polio is caused by a virus, it does not result in encephalitis.

    4 Scarlet fever is caused by a bacterium and does not result in encephalitis.

208. **1** Rubeola signs and symptoms include a high fever, photophobia, Koplik's spots (white patches on mucous membranes of the oral cavity), and a rash. Rubella usually does not cause a high fever, runs a 3- to 6-day course, and never causes Koplik's spots. (3; CJ; AS; ED; IT)
    2 The rash spreads over most of the body.
    3 These symptoms are not associated with rubeola.
    4 Some symptoms may be similar to those of a severe cold, but are associated with high fever.

209. **2** Steroids have an antiinflammatory effect. It is believed that resistance to certain viral diseases, including chickenpox, is greatly decreased when the child is taking steroids regularly. (2; CJ; EV; TC; IT)
    1 There is no known correlation between chickenpox and insulin.
    3 Because chickenpox is viral, antibiotics would have no effect.
    4 There is no known correlation between chickenpox and anticonvulsants.

210. **3** Rubeola, or measles, is generally a viral-induced childhood disease, diagnosed on or about the second day by the presence of Koplik's spots on the oral mucosa. (1; CJ; AS; TC; IT)
    1 Neither a rash nor Koplik's spots occur with mumps.
    2 Rubella is manifested by a rash, but not by Koplik's spots.
    4 Chickenpox is manifested by a maculopapular rash; no Koplik's spots are present.

211. **2** Rubeola, or measles, produces coldlike respiratory symptoms and, after 3 or 4 days, a dark-red macular or maculopapular skin rash. Complications include convulsions in young children and secondary infection with hemolytic streptococci, pneumococci, or staphylococci. Such infection can result in otitis media and pneumonia, which are especially dangerous in children under 2 years of age. (3; CJ; AN; PA; IT)
    1 This is the most benign communicable disease; complications are rare.
    3 Yellow fever does not have respiratory complications.
    4 Chickenpox does not usually include respiratory inflammation, although pneumonia may occur as a complication.

PEDIATRIC ANSWERS

212. **2** Invasion of the posterior (dorsal) root ganglia by the same virus that causes chickenpox can result in herpes zoster, or shingles. This may be caused by reactivation of a previous chickenpox virus that has lain dormant in the body or by fresh contact with an individual who has chickenpox. (1; CJ; AS; PA; IT)

   1 Athlete's foot is caused by a fungus.
   3 German measles is caused by a virus, but not the herpesvirus.
   4 Hepatitis type A is caused by a virus, but not the herpesvirus.

213. **2** Impetigo is a bacterial infection of the skin caused by streptococci or staphylococci. Group A hemolytic streptococci can cause rheumatic fever and glomerulonephritis. (2; CJ; AN; PA; IT)

   1 This infectious condition of the skin is a result of infestation by mites; it is not associated with rheumatic fever or glomerulonephritis.
   3 Intertrigo is a superficial dermatitis in the folds of the skin; it is not associated with rheumatic fever or glomerulonephritis.
   4 This is a viral condition; not associated with rheumatic fever or glomerulonephritis.

214. **1** Thrush, also called moniliasis, usually affects the mucous membranes of the oral cavity, causing painful white patches. Individuals with immunologic deficiencies or those receiving prolonged antibiotic therapy are particularly susceptible to this organism. (2; CJ; AN; TC; IT)

   2 This is usually caused by an amoeba or a bacterium; it is not common in infants.
   3 This is not caused by yeast and is not common in the U.S. or in infants.
   4 This is not caused by yeast, nor does it occur often in infants.

215. **1** The immediate postburn period is marked by dramatic alterations in circulation because of large fluid losses through the denuded skin, vasodilation, and edema formation, affecting the contractility of the heart muscle. The precipitous drop in cardiac output causes shock. (2; CJ; AN; PA; IT)

   2 Pneumonia would be a later complication associated with immobility.
   3 Contractures are a later complication associated with scarring and aggravated by improper positioning and splinting.
   4 Hypotension, not hypertension, occurs with hypovolemic shock.

216. **3** Inhalation burns are usually present with facial burns, regardless of the depth; the immediate threat to life is asphyxia from irritation and edema of the respiratory passages and lungs. (2; CJ; AS; TC; IT)

   1 Although wound sepsis is a possible complication, it would not be evident until the third to fifth day.
   2 This child is too old for separation anxiety; however, complications related to stress can occur later.
   4 Fluid losses can be extremely high but reach their maximum about the fourth day; the initial priority is the airway.

217. **4** Injury to delicate hand structures requires nursing care to promote proper healing and functional mobility. (3; CJ; PL; PA; IT)

   1 A red suture line usually indicates infection.
   2 Psychologic effects of this incident usually develop after the injury heals.
   3 The child has not been exposed to rabies because the dog was immunized.

218. **3** Damage to tissues interferes with stability of peripheral circulation, precluding the use of intramuscular medications. (2; MR; PL; TC; IT)

   1 This is not a consideration in this situation.
   2 Mode of administration does not alter effectiveness of drug.
   4 Same as answer 2.

219. **2** Insect trauma is probably the cause of this adolescent's discomfort; it is associated with a small puncture wound, localized erythema, and abdominal pain. (1; CJ; AN; PA; IT)

   1 IV drug users have track marks, but do not generally complain of itching and abdominal pain.
   3 These symptoms are not a common presentation of sickle cell crisis.
   4 These symptoms are not a common presentation of diabetic ketoacidosis.

Gastrointestinal

220. **3** This is usually sufficient if no problems exist with sucking or palate; too frequent burping is confusing. (1; MR; IM; ED; GI)

   1 Excessive burping may confuse a new infant.
   2 Sucking too long without burping may result in regurgitation because of swallowed air.
   4 Same as answer 1.

221. **4** Chalasia is an incompetent cardiac sphincter, which allows a reflux of gastric contents into the esophagus and eventual regurgitation. Placing the infant in an upright position keeps the gastric contents in the stomach by gravity as well as limits the pressure against the cardiac sphincter. (2; MR; lM; ED; GI)
   1 This will promote regurgitation.
   2 This will probably have little effect on chalasia.
   3 This will promote vomiting because it is too much formula for a week-old infant.

222. **2** The introduction of one new food at a time permits the identification of any food allergies that might be present; multiple new foods make the identification of the causative foods more difficult. (2; MR; IM; TC; GI)
   1 This can create feeding problems; if the infant does not like a food taste it may be associated with the formula.
   3 Although this could be done, solid foods should be given when the infant is hungry to encourage intake.
   4 Formula intake should be decreased as solid food intake increases or the infant will be receiving excessive calories.

223. **4** Vegetables and fruits are introduced before meats because of the generous supply of vitamins and minerals; meats are high in saturated fats. Table foods are introduced once the infant can chew or bite (2; CJ; IM; ED; GI)
   1 This is an inappropriate sequence.
   2 Same as answer 1.
   3 Same as answer 1.

224. **3** The early school-aged child has become a cooperative member of the family and will mimic parents' attitudes and food habits readily. (2; MR; AN; ED; GI)
   1 This does not have a major influence on later eating habits.
   2 This certainly has some influence, though not major, on later eating habits.
   4 The peer group does not become highly influential until later school age and during adolescence.

225. **3** Offering a new food after giving some formula associates this activity with eating and takes advantage of the child's unsatisfied hunger. (2; MR; IM; ED; GI)
   1 New foods should be initiated one at a time and continued for 4 to 5 days to assess for an allergic reaction.

   2 Offering food after the regular feeding decreases the chance of success, because the infant's hunger is already satisfied.
   4 Solid food should be introduced by spoon to acquaint the child with new tastes and textures as well as the use of the spoon.

226. **2** Positioning on the right side after feeding facilitates digestion because the pyloric sphincter is on this side and gravity aids in emptying the stomach. (3; CJ; IM; PA; GI)
   1 Feeding may proceed immediately after opening the tube.
   3 Unsafe; placement of the tube and residual should be ascertained before administering any fluid.
   4 The usual height for elevation of the gastrostomy tube when feeding an infant is 6 to 8 inches above the child's stomach.

227. **2** Pinworms emerge nocturnally to lay eggs in the perianal area; eggs are caught on transparent tape in the morning before toileting. (1; MR: IM; TC; GI)
   1 A culture will not reveal the presence of parasites.
   3 Ova cannot be seen with the naked eye; the parasite is rarely observed in the stool.
   4 There is no such test to diagnose pinworms.

228. **2** Crying should be prevented because it places tension on the suture line. Frequently an appliance called a Logan bow is taped to the cheeks to relax the operative site, which helps prevent trauma. (2; MR; lM; TC; GI)
   1 This is not necessary or desirable.
   3 The infant may also be positioned on the side and on the back with surveillance.
   4 The feeding method of choice is by a rubber-tipped syringe or dropper.

229. **4** Infants with a cleft lip breathe through their mouths, bypassing the natural humidification provided by the nose. As a result, the mucous membranes become dry and cracked and are easily infected. (2; CJ; AN; PA; GI)
   1 Feeding can be adequate with special equipment and a slow approach.
   2 Circulation to the area is unimpaired.
   3 The area may be kept clean by washing with water after a feeding.

230. **1** A priority during the immediate postoperative period is protecting the operative site. (1; CJ; AN; TC; GI)
     2 Normal 2-year-olds have about 16 teeth; although tooth development may not be normal in these children, they usually have them.
     3 A toothbrush should be a familiar sight to a 2-year-old, not a frightening one.
     4 Same as answer 3.

231. **4** Because the infant with a cleft lip and palate is unable to form the vacuum needed for sucking, a rubber-tipped syringe or dropper is used. This allows formula to flow along the sides and back of the mouth, minimizing the danger of aspiration. (1; CJ; AN; TC; GI)
     1 Feeding can be accomplished with special equipment; IV fluids do not supply ample calories.
     2 A soft cross-cut nipple may be used with some infants, but rapid flow can cause aspiration.
     3 Feeding can be accomplished with the child in an upright position to facilitate swallowing and prevent choking; impaired sucking prevents breastfeeding in most situations.

232. **3** Lye, a basic solution, is neutralized by administration of a weak acid such as vinegar. (3; CJ; IM; TC; GI)
     1 This induces vomiting and would cause further burning of tissue when the lye was vomited back through the esophagus.
     2 Milk is useful to soothe irritated mucous membranes but will not inactivate the poison.
     4 Bicarbonate is used to neutralize acids.

233. **3** A characteristic description of what is found in children with pyloric stenosis. (2; CJ; AS; PA; GI)
     1 Obstruction is above colon area; there will be little or no fecal contents present.
     2 The baby does not have any significant tenderness in the abdomen.
     4 It is more likely that there will be an absence of peristalsis in the lower colon.

234. **2** The common bile duct enters the duodenum. The pyloric sphincter is located between the end of the stomach and the beginning of the duodenum; therefore, when it is hypertrophied, the tight sphincter prevents any mixing of formula with bile. (2; CJ; AS; PA; GI)

1 Pyloric stenosis involves hypertrophy and hyperplasia of the muscle of the pyloric sphincter, causing a severe narrowing between the stomach and the duodenal canal.
     3 The bile duct enters the duodenum at a site different from the pyloric sphincter and is uninvolved in pyloric stenosis.
     4 The area obstructed in pyloric stenosis is the pyloric sphincter, between the stomach and duodenum.

235. **3** Hypertrophy of the pyloric sphincter, at the distal end of the stomach, causes partial and then complete obstruction. Nonprojectile vomiting progresses to projectile vomiting, which rapidly leads to dehydration. (3; CJ; AS; TC; GI)
     1 The infant's cry is not affected by pyloric stenosis; there does not appear to be pain associated with this condition, except for the pain of hunger.
     2 The quality of the stool is not usually affected by pyloric stenosis.
     4 This can be expected with a tracheoesophageal fistula, but not with pyloric stenosis.

236. **3** Initial feedings of glucose in water or electrolyte solutions are given 4 to 6 hours after surgery. When clear fluids are retained, usually within 24 hours, formula feedings are begun. (3; CJ; PL; TC; GI)
     1 Regular formula should be started 24 hours after surgery in an attempt to gradually return the infant to a full feeding schedule.
     2 This is not necessary.
     4 Same as answer 2.

237. **1** Protecting the IV and nasogastric tube from becoming dislodged is a priority. (2; CJ; IM; TC; GI)
     2 This is not the priority action.
     3 Not a priority; visual monitoring of rate can be done at this time.
     4 Although this would eventually be done, it is not the priority at this time.

238. **2** An elevated position allows gravity to aid in preventing vomiting. (2; MR; IM; TC; GI)
     1 Movement increases the chance of vomiting.
     3 This would not prevent reflux and could result in aspiration.
     4 Activity increases the chance of vomiting.

239. 3 Hepatitis B virus is in the blood during the late incubation and acute stages of the disease. It may also persist in the carrier state for years. It is transmitted when the blood of an infected individual comes in contact with the blood or mucous membranes of another individual. Posttransfusion hepatitis has been reduced now that the surface antigen of hepatitis B (HBS Ag) and the antibody to hepatitis B core antigen tests are performed on blood donors and on the blood of carriers of type B virus. (1; CJ; PL; TC; GI)

    1 Hepatitis A is transferred principally through oral-fecal routes.

    2 Ventilating systems do not transmit this virus.

    4 This is unrelated to hepatitis B.

240. 3 This is because of the fact that celiac clients have a gluten-induced enteropathy and are unable to absorb fats from the intestinal tract. (2; CJ; AS; TC; GI)

    1 Stools are large and fatty or frothy, not mucoid.

    2 Although stools are large and frothy, they lack color because of incomplete absorption.

    4 Stools are foul smelling, in large quantities, and without color because of incomplete absorption.

241. 4 Rectal prolapse is a common GI complication and results from wasting of perirectal supporting tissues, secondary to malnutrition. (3; CJ; AN; PA; GI)

    1 Anal fissures may or may not occur with cystic fibrosis.

    2 Intussusception is not associated with cystic fibrosis.

    3 Meconium ileus, associated with cystic fibrosis in newborns, prevents passage of meconium; not caused by frequent stools.

242. 4 Production of tenacious mucus in the pancreatic ducts prevents the flow of digestive enzymes into the intestines. Thus fats, proteins, and (to a lesser extent) carbohydrates cannot be digested and absorbed. (2; CJ; EV; PA; GI)

    1 Anorexia is not a usual problem found with cystic fibrosis.

    2 Cystic fibrosis does not influence the secretion of growth hormone.

    3 These are not problems associated with cystic fibrosis.

243. 1 Because of a lack of the pancreatic enzyme lipase, fats remain unabsorbed and are excreted in excessive amounts in the stool. (1; CJ; AN; PA; GI)

    2 This does not cause the foul smell of stools.

    3 Same as answer 2.

    4 These are the pancreatic enzymes, whose passage into the intestine is prevented by blocked pancreatic ducts.

244. 2 Pancreatic enzymes are given as replacement because of the lack of their production by the pancreas. Antibiotics are prescribed to control respiratory tract infection. (1; CJ; PL; TC; GI)

    1 These are not indicated in the treatment of cystic fibrosis.

    3 Mists and expectorants may be used but are not as vital as pancreatic enzymes and antibiotics; fat-soluble vitamins must be given in water-miscible preparations; decongestants provide little relief.

    4 These may be used but are not specific for cystic fibrosis.

245. 4 The adult pinworm lives in the rectum or colon and emerges onto the perirectal skin during the hours of sleep, depositing its eggs during this time. (2; CJ; lM; TC; GI)

    1 Pinworms attach to the bowel wall and do not emerge from the rectum at this time.

    2 Same as answer 1.

    3 Same as answer 1.

246. 3 The worm attaches itself to the bowel wall in the cecum and appendix and can damagg the mucosa, causing appendicitis. (3; CJ; AS; TC; GI)

    1 The pinworm does not migrate to the liver.

    2 Although pinworms (and their ova) are ingested by mouth, they do not attach there; inflammation of the mouth is not a complication of pinworm.

    4 The pinworm does not migrate to the respiratory system.

247. 2 This infestation is transferred by the oral-anal route, and effective handwashing is the best method to prevent transmission. (2; MR; EV; ED; GI)

    1 Cats do not transmit this disease.

    3 This is not the usual mode of transmission; the oral-anal cycle must be completed.

    4 This is not the usual mode of transmission; the oral-anal cycle must be completed.

PEDIATRIC **ANSWERS**

248. **4** All household members should be treated at the same time unless they are younger than 2 years or pregnant. (3; CJ; PL; TC; GI)
    1 This drug is not recommended for children under the age of 2.
    2 Positive testing is not a criterion for administration to family members.
    3 This is not a significant criterion for administration of medication because eggs are airborne.

249. **2** Because phenylalanine is an essential amino acid, it must be provided in quantities sufficient for promoting growth while maintaining safe blood levels. (3; CJ; PL; TC; GI)
    1 All proteins do not contain phenylalanine.
    3 Phenylalanine is an essential amino acid and cannot be totally removed from the diet.
    4 In PKU phenylalanine accumulates in the blood, causing irreversible CNS damage; additional phenylalanine must be avoided.

250. **1** In PKU the absence of the hepatic enzyme phenylalanine hydroxylase prevents normal metabolism (hydroxylation to tyrosine) of the amino acid phenylalanine. The increased fluid levels of phenylalanine in the body and the alternate metabolic by-products (phenylketones) are associated with severe mental retardation (exact mechanism not known). (2; MR; PL; ED; GI)
    2 Medications are not part of therapy.
    3 PKU is transmitted by an autosomal recessive gene.
    4 Testing for PKU cannot be done until after several days of milk ingestion.

251. **2** The Guthrie blood test reliably detects abnormal phenylalanine levels as early as 4 days of age, provided the infant has been fed a milk diet. (1; CJ; AS; TC; GI)
    1 This is used for screening large groups of infants but cannot be used until after 6 weeks of age.
    3 This is not used because it takes too long for the phenylpyruvic acid to appear in the urine. By this time (10 to 14 days), brain damage may have occurred.
    4 This is an inappropriate test for PKU.

252. **4** Maintaining low phenylalanine levels is recommended until brain growth is almost completed, usually by adolescence. (2; MR; IM; ED; GI)
    1 This is untrue and is not helpful to the parents.
    2 Dietary management is necessary until the child is an adolescent or older.
    3 Same as answer 2.

253. **3** Obesity is a very common nutritional problem in children with Down syndrome; it is thought to be related to excessive caloric intake and impaired growth. (2; MR; PL; TC; GI)
    1 This is a nutritional disorder related to vitamin D deficiency; it is not especially encountered in these children.
    2 This is the most common nutritional problem in children (iron deficiency); it is not especially encountered in these children.
    4 This is a psychiatric eating disorder of infancy characterized by repeated regurgitation without gastrointestinal illness; it is not usually encountered in these children.

254. **3** Paroxysmal pain is related to peristaltic action associated with intestinal obstruction. Abdominal distention pushes up the diaphragm, causing respiratory distress characterized by grunting respirations. (3; CJ; AS; PA; GI)
    1 These symptoms do not usually accompany intestinal obstruction.
    2 These symptoms are not characteristic of intestinal obstruction.
    4 The pain of intestinal obstruction is paroxysmal.

255. **3** The traditional efforts to explain and treat colic center on control of gas in the intestinal tract that is causing the paroxysmal pain. (1; CJ; EV; PA; GI)
    1 Excessive intake of carbohydrates may cause flatus, but diet changes rarely prevent colic attacks.
    2 Colic is thought to be caused by excessive fermentation and gas production.
    4 The exact cause of colic is not known.

256. **1** This is the most effective method of relieving obstruction and restoring bowel mobility and function. (2; CJ; PL; TC; GI)
    2 This would not be done with a newborn.
    3 A rectal tube does not relieve the obstruction, because it only releases gas pressure.
    4 A nasogastric tube will remove stomach contents; this will not relieve the obstruction or confirm the diagnosis.

257. 3 The use of a potty chair allows the child to display its content with pride; sitting on top of a toilet seat is frightening for many children. (3; MR; IM; ED; GI)

1 A diet of more solid food will make stools more bulky and easier to control.
2 Sitting on a toilet seat can be frightening for a toddler; timing of bowel training should coincide with the gastrocolic reflex
4 Bowel training should begin when the child shows readiness.

Fluid and Electrolytes

258. 3 Daily weights are an important direct way to assess fluid retention or loss. (1; CJ; AS; PA; FE)

1 This may not always happen and would not be accurate.
2 This is a measure for the degree of ascites; it would only measure fluid retention indirectly.
4 Assessment of urine for blood and protein gives information about the disease process, but not about the amount of fluid retention.

259. 4 The extracellular body fluid represents 45% at birth, 25% at 2 years of age, and 20% at maturity. Another measurement is percentage of total body weight, which is 80% at birth, 63% at 3, and approximately 60% at 12 years. (3; CJ; AN; PA; FE)

1 Cellular metabolism in children is not less stable than in adults.
2 The proportion of total body water in children (up to 2 years) is greater than in adults.
3 Renal function is immature during infancy only.

260. 2 Tap-water enemas are hypotonic and are contraindicated; they may cause increased absorption of fluid via the bowel and may upset the balance of fluid in the body. There also is interference with potassium ion balance; this electrolyte can be lost via the large intestine. (1; CJ; EV; TC; FE)

1 The enema would remove only waste products from the bowel.
3 Fear of intrusive procedures is typical of preschoolers.
4 The temperature of the water should be regulated so this does not occur.

261. 3 No more than 360 ml of solution should be administered to an infant or child unless ordered, because fluid and electrolyte balance in an infant or child is easily disturbed. (3; CJ; PL; PA; FE)

1 This quantity may be ordered for a small infant.
2 This quantity may be ordered for an older or larger infant.
4 This quantity is too large for small children.

262. 4 Total amount × Drop factor/Total time (in minutes)
$$\frac{400 \times 60}{8 \times 60} = \frac{24,000}{480} = 50 \text{ gtt}$$
(2; CJ; IM; PA; FE)

1 This is too slow to administer the fluid ordered.
2 Same as answer 1.
3 Same as answer 1.

263. 4 If the circulation is overloaded with too much fluid or the rate is too rapid, the stress on the heart becomes too great and cardiac embarrassment may occur. (2; LE; PL; TC; FE)

1 This is important, but an infiltrated IV is not as serious a complication.
2 Although fluid replacement is important, prevention of cardiac problems from fluid overload is critical.
3 Increased output is not the primary consideration.

264. 2 Weight is the best indicator of fluid loss if measured each day at the same time, on the same scale, and with the same amount of clothing. (2; CJ; EV; PA; FE)

1 In cases of severe diarrhea, an IV is usually employed until the diarrhea is controlled; oral fluids are gradually added as tolerated.
3 Because of the diarrhea, food will not be properly absorbed.
4 This temperature is not unusual in infants.

265. 3 Isotonic saline is compatible with body fluids. It is neither hypertonic nor hypotonic, so it does not cause a change in osmotic pressure and upset the balance of intracellular and extracellular fluid and electrolytes. (2; CJ; IM; TC; FE)

1 This hypotonic solution might cause fluid and electrolyte imbalance.
2 Soap-suds enemas are water with added soap products and are therefore usually hypotonic; this can cause fluid shifts and overloads.
4 This solution would cause excess fluid loss and therefore be dangerous.

266. **4** Dehydration promotes the sickling of erythrocytes. Increased fluid intake minimizes the chance that a sickle cell pain episode will occur. (3; MR; PL; ED; FE)

1 This is not necessary or helpful in sickle cell anemia.

2 Rigorous exercise will cause sickling because of decreased oxygen.

3 This is not necessary.

267. **3** In excessive vomiting there is an increased loss of hydrogen ions (hydrochloric acid), which leads to metabolic alkalosis, an excess of base bicarbonate. (2; CJ; AS; TC; FE)

1 Although some calcium is lost through vomiting, it is highly unusual that the infant would develop tetany.

2 This is caused by a retention of hydrogen ions and a loss of base bicarbonates. In vomiting, base bicarbonates are retained and hydrogen ions are lost.

4 Hyperactivity is not associated with vomiting.

268. **3** An infant's intravascular compartment is fairly limited and cannot accommodate large volumes of fluid administered in a short time. Equipment such as minidroppers, volume control chambers, and infusion pumps should be used, since they help control or limit the volume of fluid to be infused. (2; CJ; PL; TC; FE)

1 This is important for everyone receiving IV fluids.

2 This is the physician's role.

4 IV fluids can be administered at room temperature.

269. **3** $\dfrac{\text{Amount of fluid} \times \text{Drop factor}}{\text{Time (in minutes)}}$

$\dfrac{500 \times 60}{24 \times 60} = 21$ drops   (1; CJ; PL; PA; FE)

1 This would be too slow to infuse the desired amount.

2 Same as answer 1.

4 This would be too rapid; the fluid would run out before 24 hours had elapsed.

270. **3** The restricted ventilation accompanying an asthmatic attack limits the body's ability to blow off carbon dioxide. As carbon dioxide accumulates in the body fluids, it reacts with water to produce carbonic acid (H_2CO_3); the result is respiratory acidosis. (2; CJ; AN; PA; FE)

1 The problem basic to asthma is respiratory, not metabolic.

2 Respiratory alkalosis is caused by exhaling large amounts of carbon dioxide; asthma causes carbon dioxide retention.

4 Asthma is a respiratory problem, not a metabolic one; metabolic acidosis can result from a gain of nonvolatile acids or a loss of base bicarbonate.

271. **2** Infants are not protected from water loss because they ingest and excrete a relatively greater daily water volume than adults; therefore the proportion of total body water is higher. (2; CJ; AN; TC; FE)

1 Infants have a high glomerular filtration rate; a decreased rate is common in the older adult.

3 Infants and children have a rapid generalized response to insensible fluid loss.

4 This is true of the adolescent and is related to the major rapid changes that occur in the anatomic and physiologic growth process.

Cardiovascular

272. **3** There are three vessels; one vein carries oxygenated blood to the fetus, and two arteries return deoxygenated blood to the placenta. (1; CJ; EV; PA; CV)

1 The umbilical cord has three vessels; a cord with two vessels is frequently associated with congenital abnormalities.

2 This is the right number of vessels, but there are two arteries and one vein.

4 The umbilical cord has three vessels, not four.

273. **3** Rheumatic fever is an inflammatory disease involving the joints, heart, CNS, and subcutaneous tissue. It is believed to be an autoimmune process that causes connective tissue damage. (2; CJ; AS; PA; CV)

1 Tetanus is not caused by a streptococcal infection and does not include the symptoms listed.

2 Measles is caused by a virus and does not include the symptoms listed.

4 Whooping cough is not caused by a streptococcal infection and does not include the symptoms listed.

274. 2 Tachycardia in infants is often a symptom of a heart defect; this infant should be examined for the presence of a heart defect. (2; CJ; AN; PA; CV)

1 This is frequently seen in young children; it is related to immature muscle control and does not require intervention unless it persists into toddlerhood.

3 This does not warrant immediate attention, but the infant should be reevaluated at the next visit; the infant may just be tired.

4 This finding at this age does not need immediate attention; however, the child should be monitored for the attainment of this and other developmental milestones at future visits.

275. 4 In heart failure there is a decrease in the blood flow to the kidneys, causing sodium and water reabsorption resulting in peripheral edema. The peripheral edema indicates severe cardiac decompensation. (2; CJ; AS; PA; CV)

1 This may be an early attempt by the body to compensate for decreased cardiac output.

2 Same as answer 1.

3 Same as answer 1.

276. 2 Children with cardiac anomalies often use increased energy in activities of daily living; decreased oxygen and increased energy output in the developing child causes a slow growth rate. (2; CJ; AS; ED; CV)

1 Mental retardation is not a common finding in children with congenital heart disease.

3 Cyanosis and clubbing are not characteristic of most children with cardiac anomalies, only of those with more serious hypoxia.

4 Cardiac anomalies are more often a result of prenatal, rather than genetic, factors.

277. 2 Polycythemia, reflected in an elevated hematocrit level, is a direct attempt of the body to compensate for the decrease in oxygenation to all body cells caused by the mixture of oxygenated and unoxygenated circulating blood. (3; CJ; AS; PA; CV)

1 This is not characteristic of right-to-left shunt heart disease in children.

3 This is characteristic of coarctation of the aorta.

4 Edema is not a common finding in right-to-left shunt heart disease.

278. 4 Prophylaxis before the procedure can prevent this disease, which often occurs in clients with abnormal heart structures. (2; CJ; AN; TC; CV)

1 This is not generally associated with congenital heart defects in children.

2 Same as answer 1.

3 Avoidance of crowds, not antibiotics, is recommended to prevent upper respiratory infections.

279. 2 The intrapleural space must be drained of fluid and air to facilitate the reestablishment of negative pressure. (2; MR; AN; PA; CV)

1 The tidal volume increases as the lung reexpands, but it is not the reason for the insertion of chest tubes.

3 Closed chest drainage is related to intrapleural not chest wall pressure.

4 Intrapleural pressure should be negative, not positive; positive intrapleural pressure would promote collapse of the lung.

280. 3 In the fetus, oxygenated blood is shunted directly into the systemic circulation via the ductus arteriosus, a connection between the pulmonary artery and the aorta. Normally after birth the increased oxygen tension causes a functional closure of the ductus arteriosus. Occasionally, particularly in premature infants, this vessel remains open and is known as patent ductus arteriosus. (3; MR; IM; ED; CV)

1 This is known as pulmonic stenosis.

2 This is not the problem in patent ductus arteriosus.

4 Patent ductus arteriosus does not involve ventricular septal defects.

281. 4 In left-to-right shunt heart disease there are holes in the septum of the heart that cause a murmuring sound as the blood is pumped through. (3; CJ; AS; PA; CV)

1 This is not a common clinical finding in left-to-right shunt heart disease.

2 This is not a common finding in left-to-right shunt heart disease; tissue perfusion is usually adequate.

3 Clubbing is a finding in right-to-left shunt heart disease.

PEDIATRIC

ANSWERS

282. **4** Coarctation of the aorta is a narrowing, usually in the thoracic segment, causing decreased blood flow below the constriction and increased blood volume above it. (3; CJ; EV; PA; CV)
   1 This has nothing to do with coarctation of the aorta.
   2 In coarctation of the aorta, femoral pulses would be weak or absent, and blood pressure in the lower extremities would be decreased.
   3 In coarctation of the aorta, radial pulses would be full and bounding.

283. **3** Compromised heart functioning in the infant often results in cyanosis and fatigue while sucking and swallowing because of decreased cardiac output. (3; CJ; AN; PA; CV)
   1 Untrue; when a feeding problem persists in a newborn, it is generally an indication of some pathology.
   2 Poor sucking is never insignificant; it may be indicative of many problems, such as CNS involvement or immaturity.
   4 Generally most infants are free from mucus within 24 to 48 hours after birth.

284. **2** Hemorrhage is a major life-threatening complication, because arterial blood is under pressure and an artery has been entered (punctured) by a catheter. (2; LE; IM; TC; CV)
   1 The child is kept in bed for 6 to 8 hours after the procedure.
   3 Fluids may be given as soon as tolerated.
   4 Pulses, not blood pressure, must be checked for quality and symmetry.

285. **1** Children with Down syndrome have a high incidence of congenital heart defects, which alter normal heart sounds. (2; CJ; AS; PA; CV)
   2 This is comparable to the fontanel of a normal newborn.
   3 No differentiation exists from the extremities of a normal newborn.
   4 The infant with Down syndrome does not have any extraordinary pupillary changes.

286. **3** Tetralogy of Fallot classically consists of four defects. Three of them are anatomic: ventricular septal defect, pulmonic stenosis, and overriding aorta. The fourth defect, right ventricular hypertrophy, is secondary to increased resistance to blood flow in that ventricle. (2; CJ; AN; PA; CV)
   1 Right ventricular hypertrophy is correct, the other anomalies are not.

2 These are the characteristics of transposition of the great vessels.
   4 Same as answer 1.

287. **4** Decreased tissue oxygenation stimulates erythropoiesis, resulting in excessive production of red blood cells. (1; CJ; EV; PA; CV)
   1 This would not be a direct cause of polycythemia.
   2 Same as answer 1.
   3 This may or may not affect the production of red blood cells.

288. **1** Hypoxia leads to poor peripheral circulation; clubbing occurs as a result of tissue hypertrophy and additional capillary development in the fingers. (2; CJ; AS; PA; CV)
   2 The respirations are generally rapid to compensate for O_2 deprivation.
   3 This is not an adaptation that occurs in children with tetralogy of Fallot.
   4 These children have polycythemia.

289. **3** Forceful evacuation results in the child's taking a deep breath, holding it, and straining (Valsalva maneuver). This increased intrathoracic pressure puts excessive strain on the heart sutures. (2; CJ; PL; TC; CV)
   1 Crying is not a problem after cardiac surgery; it may, in fact, help prevent respiratory complications.
   2 Coughing and deep breathing are essential for the prevention of postoperative respiratory complicatipns.
   4 Activity is gradually increased postoperatively.

290. **2** This is a priority because inadequate antibiotic therapy may predispose the child to the development of endocarditis. (2; MR; IM; ED; CV)
   1 This is not a priority because instructions are usually printed on the label.
   3 Same as answer 1.
   4 Same as answer 1.

291. **4** Gavage feeding is preferred for weak infants, those with respiratory distress or poor sucking-swallowing coordination, and those who are easily fatigued because of physical stress such as surgery. (2; CJ; AN; TC; CV)
   1 This is not a reason for instituting gavage; however, vomiting may be lessened with gavage feeding because the amount and rapidity of feeding can be controlled.
   2 Feeding the infant quickly is not desirable; vomiting with aspiration may occur.
   3 The amount can be regulated with bottle-feeding as well.

292. **4** Babies with Down syndrome have a high incidence of congenital heart disease, especially atrial defects. (2; CJ; PL; PA; CV)
1 Deafness is not usually a problem in Down syndrome.
2 Infants with Down syndrome usually do not have a problem with hydrocephaly.
3 The muscles of infants with Down syndrome are usually hypotonic.

Blood and Immunity

293. **1** In active natural immunity, the infected person's immune system responds to the invading organism by producing antibodies specific for the invader. (3; CJ; AN; PA; BI)
2 Active artificial immunity is acquired by the injection of antigens, after which the individual develops antibodies.
3 Passive natural immunity is acquired by the fetus from the mother.
4 Passive artificial immunity is acquired through injection of antibodies.

294. **3** Antibodies received in utero through the placenta and in the newborn via mother's milk provide the baby with immunity against most viral, bacterial, and fungal infections during the first several weeks after birth. Then, as the titer of maternal antibodies drops and is not replaced by the child's own antibodies, prolonged and repeated infection occurs. (1; CJ; EV; PA; BI)
1 This is not enough to prevent infections in these children.
2 Bacteria do not produce antibodies.
4 This probably does not occur in children born without an immune system.

295. **2** This is the normal hematocrit range for a 1 year old. (3; CJ; EV; PA; BI)
1 This would be too low; it would only occur with a problem such as prolonged blood loss.
3 This is too high; this would be normal for an adult female.
4 This is too high; this would be normal for a newborn.

296. **2** Toxoids are modified toxins that stimulate the body to form antibodies that last up to 10 years against the specific disease. (2; MR; IM; ED; BI)
1 Passive immunity, even the natural type derived from the mother, does not last longer than the first year of life.
3 Only having the disease can provide lifelong natural immunity.
4 This is provided by tetanus immune globulin.

297. **3** Corticosteroids (e.g., cortisol) cause involution of lymphatic tissue and resultant depression of the immune response. Antineoplastic drugs or high-energy radiation preferentially destroy tissues with high mitotic rates, including lymphatic tissue and bone marrow, where antibody production and other immune responses take place. (1; CJ; EV; TC; BI)
1 This is an inappropriate answer; it is no more true for these children than for other children.
2 This is not a reason to withhold immunizations.
4 The measles vaccine does not contain rabbit serum.

298. **1** Adequate immunizations for normal preschool children include DTaP, IVP, and measles at 4 to 6 years (usually required by law). (3; MR; IM; PA; BI)
2 Hepatitis immunization is given in three doses between birth and 9 months with no booster.
3 Rubella vaccine is given between 12 and 15 months and may be repeated at this age, but DTaP and IVP should be given.
4 The tuberculin test is not an immunization.

299. **2** The recommended immunization schedule for infants is administration of the combined diphtheria, pertussis, and tetanus vaccine and the polio virus at ages 2, 4, and 6 months. (2; MR; EV; PA; BI)
1 Measles vaccine is not usually administered until the child is 12 months old.
3 Measles, mumps, and rubella vaccines are not given until 12 months; there is no tuberculosis vaccine.
4 Measles and rubella vaccines are not usually given until 12 months of age; there is no tuberculosis vaccine.

300. **3** The body's immune system constructs proteins called antibodies that possess a specificity toward another protein called the antigen. The antibody may neutralize or damage the antigen and thus render it harmless. (3; MR; IM; ED; BI)
1 Antibodies are protein substances.
2 Antibodies are produced to fight antigens.
4 Antigens are harmful to the body.

301. **4** This is the schedule for active immunization recommended by the American Academy of Pediatrics (2; LE; PL; TC; BI)
1 This regimen does not follow the schedule for active immunization.
2 Same as answer 1.
3 Same as answer 1.

302. 3 The child is having an allergic reaction, and flow of blood should be stopped immediately to prevent serious complications. (2; LE; IM; TC; BI)
1 Physician should be called after blood has been stopped.
2 Slowing the rate of infusion will not halt the allergic reaction to the blood.
4 This is dangerous as an initial action because the degree of allergic reaction cannot be determined at this time; blood must be stopped.

303. 3 Folic acid acts as a necessary coenzyme in the formation of heme, the iron-containing protein in hemoglobin. (3; CJ; AN; PA; BI)
1 Calcium is not involved in the production of red blood cells.
2 This is a coenzyme in carbohydrate metabolism.
4 The production of red blood cells does not involve carbohydrates.

304. 3 Proteins are essential for the synthesis of the blood proteins, albumin, fibrinogen, and hemoglobin. Ascorbic acid influences the removal of iron from ferritin (making more iron available for production of heme) and influences the conversion of folic acid to folinic acid. (2; CJ; PL; PA; BI)
1 These are not involved in building red blood cells.
2 Same as answer 1.
4 Same as answer 1.

305. 3 A diet of milk only is not sufficient to meet iron needs. Raisins and meat are high in iron, and finger foods are appropriate for toddlers. (2; MR; IM; ED; BI)
1 Weaning from the bottle is not the issue; supplementary iron intake is.
2 Although medical care and monitoring will be required, the metabolic clinic is not the appropriate referral.
4 This is not appropriate for a 1 year old, nor is it necessary or desirable.

306. 2 The child's immediate physical safety takes priority. The child must sit down to avoid falling. (2; MR; IM; TC; BI)
1 Immediate physical safety takes priority over further assessment.
3 The subjective symptom of dizziness alone does not warrant this; immediate physical safety takes priority.

4 Although gravity promotes cerebral blood flow in this position, immediate physical safety takes priority; walking at this time would be unsafe.

307. 3 Children with chronic illness should not be exposed to the additional stress of infection. (2; MR; PL; ED; BI)
1 A normal intake of fluid is recommended.
2 Activity is not restricted.
4 Regular meals with the family should be encouraged.

308. 3 High levels of fetal hemoglobin prevent sickling of red blood cells. The newborn has from 44% to 89% fetal hemoglobin, but this rapidly decreases during the first year. (3; CJ; AN; PA; BI)
1 Respiratory difficulties are not associated with sickle cell anemia except as a consequence of hypoxia during a crisis.
2 The diagnosis of sickle cell anemia is made on the basis of hematologic tests; general health and growth are not affected initially.
4 These will not affect the diagnosis of sickle cell anemia.

309. 3 Sickling is related to the concentration of hemoglobin within the cell. Because hypertonicity of the blood plasma increases the intracellular concentration of hemoglobin, dehydration promotes sickling. (3; CJ; IM; TC; BI)
1 This will not prevent thrombus formation.
2 The condition determines the activity level; although bed rest may be necessary during a pain episode, complete bed rest is rarely necessary.
4 Anticoagulants do not help prevent thrombus formation in sickle cell anemia.

310. 4 The spleen plays a role in immunity; without a spleen, a child is more prone to infection, which can precipitate crisis. (2; CJ; PL; PA; BI)
1 Jaundice, which may be chronic with sickle cell anemia or developing crisis, is not relevant to the child's compromised immune status because of the splenectomy.
2 Serial hematocrit readings would be necessary if the child were in crisis.
3 Abdominal assessments are important, but not required frequently in this situation.

311. **3** Warmth causes vasodilation, which will help lessen the pain of a vaso-occlusive crisis. (3; CJ; IM; PA; BI)
1 IV fluids, if ordered, should be increased to dilute the blood
2 Cold will cause more vasoconstriction and increase pain.
4 This is an inadequate dose for an adolescent.

312. **2** Both cause poor resistance to infection. With sickling it results from low oxygen levels, and with celiac disease it results from malnourishment and immunologic defects. (2; CJ; IM; ED; BI)
1 Activity does not need to be limited in celiac disease; strenuous activity should be limited in sickle cell anemia.
3 This specific diet is not particularly helpful for either sickle cell anemia or celiac disease.
4 Vital signs will not be abnormal except during a crisis in either condition.

313. **3** Hydration is necessary to promote and maintain hemodilution; pain in the area of involvement is a major problem in pain crises and demands priority care. (2; MR; PL; TC; BI)
1 Although hydration is a major concern, nutrition is not.
2 Neither of these factors are priority concerns in a pain episode.
4 Although antibiotics may be ordered to treat any preexisting infection that may have precipitated the crisis, it would be a medical, not a nursing, decision; pain management is a major nursing concern.

314. **3** Factor VIII is the missing plasma component necessary to control bleeding in hemophilia A. (2; CJ; PL; PA; BI)
1 Factor VIII, the missing component, would not be provided by this blood derivative.
2 Although fresh frozen plasma does contain factor VIII, it is an insufficient amount and a high volume is required.
4 Same as answer 1.

315. **4** Hemophilia is carried on the X chromosome but is recessive. Therefore the female is the carrier (an unaffected XO and an affected XH). If the male receives the affected XH (XHYO), the disease is manifest. (1; MR; IM; ED; BI)

1 Hemophilia is a sex-linked recessive disorder.
2 Hemophilia is carried by the female. Regular laws of Mendelian inheritance are not sex-specific.
3 Only females carry the trait; males are usually affected.

316. **4** Aspirin is an anticoagulant and would not be appropriate for a child with bleeding problems. (1; MR; IM; ED; BI)
1 This is unsafe; aspirin would cause bleeding.
2 This response does not respond to the mother's question; it could cause the mother to feel defensive.
3 Acetaminophen cannot prevent bleeding episodes.

317. **4** The mating of a carrier female (XOXH) and an unaffected male (XOYO) results in the following possible offspring: a carrier female (XOXH), an unaffected female (XOXO), an unaffected male (XOYO), or an affected male (XHYO). (2; MR; IM; ED; BI)
1 For each child there is a 50% chance of being normal.
2 For each child there is a 50% chance of being affected.
3 Males cannot carry the trait; females have a 50% chance of being carriers.

318. **3** The extensive growth of lymphoblasts suppresses the normal growth of red cells, white cells, and platelets. (2; CJ; AS; PA; BI)
1 Infection is a result of, not the cause of, leukopenia.
2 Internal bleeding does not cause neutropenia.
4 Iron-intake deficit will not result in neutropenia.

319. **4** Marked jaundice generally indicates liver damage or excessive hemolysis and is not a sign of leukemia unless hepatic damage from late effects of the disease or drugs has occurred. Edema is not a manifestation of the disease, because the pathophysiology does not involve transport of fluids. (1; CJ; AS; PA; BI)
1 Marked fatigue and pallor are the result of anemia associated with leukemia.
2 Multiple bruises and petechiae are the result of thrombocytopenia associated with leukemia.
3 Enlarged lymph nodes, spleen, and liver are the result of the infiltration of these organs with leukemic cells.

320. **4** Depressed bone marrow production of formed elements of blood leads to neutropenia and increased susceptibility to infection. (2; CJ; AS; PA; BI)

1 Urine output will be within normal limits; there is no kidney involvement at this stage of the disease.

2 There are more, not less, quantities of stem cells in the peripheral blood and bone marrow.

3 The swallowing reflex is not affected.

321. **3** MMR vaccine is composed of live viruses, and its administration could be life threatening for an immunosuppressed child. (3; MR; PL; TC; BI)

1 At discharge the parents need information about immunizations, because MMR vaccine is generally given at 15 months of age.

2 Inaccurate; this child will receive MMR vaccine when blood values return to normal regardless of age; normally it is given at 15 months.

4 Because the MMR vaccine is composed of live viruses, giving it can be as ife threatening as actually having the disease.

322. **3** Because of the increased capillary fragility and decreased platelet counts that accompany leukemia, even the slightest trauma can cause hemorrhage. Therefore the toothbrush can produce gingival hemorrhage, and the physician should be informed of this happening; this may also assist in defining the treatment plan. (2; CJ; IM; TC; BI)

1 It would be wiser to eliminate the use of a toothbrush and use a sponge-type applicator; therefore this is not necessary.

2 It cannot be assumed that a 4 year old would follow such direction.

4 This is inappropriate; if oral ulcers develop, washes with isotonic solution such as normal saline may be used.

323. **1** Soft toothbrushes should be used to reduce trauma to the oral mucosa. (1; MR; PL; ED; BI)

2 This may irritate the oral mucosa and should always be diluted, if used at all.

3 This will injure the oral mucosa.

4 This will irritate the mucosa and has an offensive taste.

324. **4** Radiation destroys leukemic cells in the brain because chemotherapeutic agents are poorly absorbed through the blood-brain barrier. (1; MR; AN; PA; BI)

1 This is not the primary reason for the treatment; it is a curative measure.

2 This is inaccurate; this is not the reason for cranial radiation.

3 This is inaccurate; ALL is an abnormality of the bone marrow and lymphatic system.

325. **4** Bristles may be irritating and cause hemorrhage of gums; soft brushes are used. (2; CJ; PL; TC; BI)

1 These can be used; the child may prefer to drink this way.

2 This can be used as long as it is diluted and does not irritate the mucous membrane.

3 This can be used, since it will not injure skin.

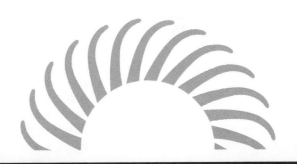

CHAPTER 6

Medical-Surgical Nursing

GROWTH AND DEVELOPMENT

▼ THE YOUNG ADULT (AGED 20 TO 45 YEARS)

Data Base
A. Physiologic development
1. Physical maturation occurs
2. Muscle strength and coordination peak
3. Biorhythms become established
4. Sexuality
   a. Established sex drive remains high for men
   b. Female sex drive reaches a peak during later phase of young adulthood
   c. Physiologically optimal period for child-bearing
5. Basal metabolic rate (BMR) decreases at rate of 2% to 4% per decade after 20 years of age
B. Psychosocial development
1. Mental abilities reflect formal operations (see Growth and Development of the Adolescent in Pediatric Nursing)
2. Resolving the developmental crisis of intimacy versus isolation
3. Establishing new family relationships and parenting patterns
4. Establishing the self in, and advancing in, a chosen occupation
C. Common health problems: accidents, AIDS, cancer involving the reproductive organs, hypertension, suicide, alcoholism, spousal abuse, fertility regulation, periodontal disease, unbalanced diet, and intimacy problems

General Nursing Care of Young Adults
A. **ASSESSMENT**
1. Obtain history of drug and alcohol use, sexual practices, and family relationships
2. Determine baseline height, weight, and dietary history
3. Measure vital signs to establish baseline
4. Question client about health practices related to cancer prevention and detection
B. **ANALYSIS/NURSING DIAGNOSES**
1. Risk for infection related to sexual activity
2. Risk for injury related to chemical impairment
3. Ineffective therapeutic regimen management related to feelings of invincibility
4. Impaired nutrition: risk for more than body requirements related to consumption of fast food and junk food
5. Ineffective sexuality patterns related to increased sex drives, sexual preference, and establishment of a family

C. **PLANNING/IMPLEMENTATION**
1. Encourage attendance at safety programs to promote accident prevention (e.g., defensive driving)
2. Increase public awareness of problems and availability of crisis counseling, support groups, and other community resources (e.g., hot lines, Alcoholics Anonymous, family planning clinics)
3. Teach safer sex practices
4. Promote awareness that optimal diet is essential to achieving and maintaining optimal health; encourage nutritional evaluation and consultation
5. Use exogenous supplemental vitamins with caution, especially vitamins A, D, and E; higher doses than necessary can cause health problems
6. Teach dietary guidelines following USDA recommendations
   a. Eat a variety of foods
   b. Maintain ideal weight
   c. Avoid too much fat, saturated fat, and cholesterol
   d. Eat a diet with adequate vegetables, fruit, and grain products; fruits are low in sodium
   e. Use salt in moderation
   f. Limit intake of alcoholic beverages to one drink for women and two drinks for men
   g. Maintain recommended daily caloric intake
7. Teach breast and testicular self-examination techniques and encourage regular medical checkups
D. **EVALUATION/OUTCOMES**
1. Establishes safe health care practices
2. Maintains ideal body weight
3. Maintains blood pressure within normal limits
4. Remains free from infection

▼ THE MIDDLE-AGED ADULT (AGED 45 TO 60 YEARS)

Data Base
A. Physiologic development
1. Greater diversity in physiologic conditioning resulting from established lifestyle
2. Early signs of aging (e.g., wrinkling, thinning hair, decreased muscle tone and nerve function)
3. Decreased BMR with subsequent weight gain unless caloric intake is reduced
4. Decreased production of sexual hormones
   a. Menopause (see Childbearing and Women's Health Nursing)
   b. Male climacteric; may pass unnoticed, especially in those with high self-esteem; symptoms may include diminished potency, less forceful ejaculation, thinning and graying hair, fatigue, and depression

B. Psychosocial development
   1. Cognitive abilities enhanced because of motivation and past experiences
   2. Resolving developmental crisis of generativity versus stagnation
   3. Adjusting to changes in family caused by aging parents and growing or returning children
   4. Maintaining satisfactory status of one's career
   5. Accepting physical changes associated with advancing age
   6. Developing social and civic activities that are personally satisfying
C. Health problems: cardiovascular disease, hypertension, alcoholism, sexual dysfunction, presbyopia, unbalanced or inadequate diet, and depression

General Nursing Care of Middle-Aged Adults

A. ASSESSMENT
1. Determine cardiovascular status: vital signs, peripheral pulses, peripheral edema, shortness of breath, and chest pain
2. Measure visual acuity
3. Obtain history of alcohol use, sexual patterns, and family relationships
4. Determine baseline height and weight and dietary history
5. Question client about leisure activities and retirement plans

B. ANALYSIS/NURSING DIAGNOSES
1. Risk for activity intolerance related to diminished physiologic conditioning
2. Risk for caregiver role strain related to aging parents
3. Impaired nutrition: risk for more than body requirements related to sedentary lifestyle and dietary indiscretions
4. Ineffective sexuality patterns related to decreased hormonal production

C. PLANNING/IMPLEMENTATION
1. Reinforce importance of regular exercise to prevent cardiovascular and neuromusculoskeletal disease
2. Stress dietary changes: reduction of calories, fats, and protein; increased calcium and fiber; encourage individuals to follow USDA recommendations
3. Emphasize need for regular medical evaluations as well as self-evaluations
4. Encourage attendance at self-help groups to stop substance dependency (e.g., smoking, alcohol, weight control)

D. EVALUATION/OUTCOMES
1. Maintains ideal body weight
2. Maintains blood pressure within normal limits
3. Establishes healthy dietary pattern
4. Participates in exercise regimen
5. Develops coping skills to manage stress

▼ THE YOUNG-OLDER ADULT (AGED 60 TO 75 YEARS)

Data Base
A. Physiologic development
   1. Slowing of reaction time
   2. Loss of sensory acuity
   3. Diminished muscle tone and strength
   4. Increased diversity in health status and function resulting from earlier lifestyle and development of chronic health problems
B. Psychosocial development
   1. Cognitive abilities may be affected by cardiovascular disease
   2. Adjusting to retirement: some individuals experience a loss of self-esteem, whereas others enjoy the freedom to explore other interests
   3. Coping with altered economic status; adjusting to fixed income
   4. Resolving death of parents and possibly spouse
   5. Accepting separation from their children and their families
C. Health problems: cardiovascular disease, cancer, presbyopia, accidents, respiratory disease, osteoporosis/osteoarthritis, hearing loss, especially for high-pitched sounds, unbalanced or inadequate diet, and depression

General Nursing Care of Young-Older Adults

A. ASSESSMENT
1. Determine cardiovascular status: vital signs, peripheral pulses, peripheral edema, shortness of breath, history of chest pain, and changes in sensation
2. Measure visual and auditory acuities
3. Obtain history relative to warning signs of cancer
4. Identify coping skills and support systems

B. ANALYSIS/NURSING DIAGNOSES
1. Risk for caregiver role strain related to illness of significant other
2. Ineffective coping related to chronic health problems and fear of disability
3. Impaired gas exchange related to respiratory and musculoskeletal changes
4. Risk for injury related to sensory perceptual alterations and weakness
5. Impaired nutrition: risk for less than body requirements related to anorexia and lack of interest in food preparation
6. Disturbed sensory perception (visual, auditory, and kinesthetic) related to changes associated with aging
7. Social isolation related to loss of hearing, changes in peer group, and death of spouse or friends

8. Ineffective tissue perfusion (cerebral, cardiopulmonary, and peripheral) related to cardiovascular changes

C. **PLANNING/IMPLEMENTATION**
1. Encourage individuals to maintain a schedule of regular medical, dental, and visual examinations to control or prevent health problems
2. Assess living conditions for possible hazards that could cause accidents
3. Refer widows and widowers to appropriate self-help groups as necessary
4. Encourage individuals to anticipate and plan for retirement and to develop new interests and support systems
5. Encourage nutritional assessment and consultation to prevent nutrient deficiencies and to provide for diet modifications with aging

D. **EVALUATION/OUTCOMES**
1. Participates in an exercise program
2. Verbalizes fears to health care providers
3. Remains free from injury
4. Maintains satisfying interpersonal relationships
5. Consumes nutritionally adequate diet

▼ THE MIDDLE-OLDER ADULT (AGED 75 TO 84 YEARS) AND OLD-OLDER ADULT (AGED 85+ YEARS)

Data Base

A. Physiologic development
1. Diminished sensation (visual and auditory) and diminished reaction time
2. Increased sensitivity to cold because of decreased subcutaneous tissue, decreased thyroid functioning, and impaired circulation
3. Decreased enzyme secretion in and motility of the gastrointestinal tract
4. Decreased glomerular filtration rate
5. Decreased cardiac output
6. Arteriosclerotic changes with diminished elasticity of blood vessels
7. Decreased lung capacity
8. Demineralization and other degenerative skeletal changes, particularly in weight-bearing bones
9. Muscle atrophy
B. Psychosocial development
1. Cognitive abilities not necessarily affected by age, but may be impaired as a result of disease, leading to diminished awareness
2. Resolving the developmental crisis of ego integrity versus despair
3. Adjusting to the death of important others
4. Adapting to decreased physical capacity and changes in body image

5. Adjusting to the economic burden of a fixed income
6. Recognizing the inevitability of death
7. Reminiscing increasingly about the past

C. Health problems, cardiovascular disease, cancer, accidents (e.g., falls, automobile accidents), respiratory disease, cerebral vascular insufficiency, malnutrition, and problems with perception (cataracts, glaucoma, hearing loss)

General Nursing Care of Middle-Older and Old-Older Adults

A. **ASSESSMENT**
1. Determine cardiovascular status: vital signs, peripheral pulses, peripheral edema, shortness of breath, history of chest pain, and changes in sensation
2. Identify neurologic deficits: level of consciousness, orientation, motor function, and sensory function
3. Determine respiratory function: respiratory rate, rhythm, and depth, use of accessory muscles, breath sounds, vital capacity, and arterial blood gases
4. Review nutritional status: dietary history, body height and weight, skin condition, and serum protein and albumin levels
5. Assess the individual's ability to cope

B. **ANALYSIS/NURSING DIAGNOSES**
1. Impaired gas exchange related to decreased vital capacity
2. Risk for injury related to neurologic deficits
3. Impaired nutrition: less than body requirements related to decreased appetite, decreased taste, poor-fitting dentures, and depression
4. Risk for peripheral neurovascular dysfunction related to age-related changes
5. Relocation stress syndrome related to inability to maintain own home
6. Self-care deficit related to altered motor/sensory function
7. Ineffective tissue perfusion related to cardiovascular changes

C. **PLANNING/IMPLEMENTATION**
1. Encourage individuals to maintain a schedule of regular medical supervision
2. Promote maximum degree of independence
3. Initiate appropriate referrals for individuals requiring assistance with activities of daily living
4. Open channels of communication for reality orientation, reminiscing, and emotional support; explain procedures and expectations; reinforce and repeat as necessary
5. Refer to social service and other resources that can provide economic assistance when necessary

6. Ensure that prosthetic devices (e.g., dentures, contact lenses, eye prosthetics, braces, limbs) fit comfortably and do not cause irritation; teach proper care of such devices

7. Encourage following the USDA recommendations

D. **EVALUATION/OUTCOMES**
1. Performs or assists with self-care activities
2. Remains free from injury
3. Uses community resources to maximize independence
4. Maintains nutritionally adequate diet
5. Maintains social relationships

PAIN

OVERVIEW

A. Definition: universally unpleasant emotional and sensory experience that occurs in response to tissue trauma; referred to as the *fifth vital sign;* subjective
B. Types
1. Acute pain: mild to severe pain lasting less than 6 months; usually associated with specific injury; involves sympathetic nervous system response
2. Chronic pain: mild to severe pain lasting longer than 6 months; associated with parasympathetic nervous system; client may not exhibit behaviors associated with acute pain; may lead to depression
C. Terminology
1. Pain threshold: minimum amount of stimulus required to cause sensation of pain
2. Pain tolerance: maximum pain a client is willing to endure
3. Referred pain: pain is experienced in an area different from the site of tissue trauma
4. Intractable pain: pain not relieved by conventional treatment
5. Neuropathic pain: pain caused by neurologic disturbance; may not be associated with tissue damage
6. Phantom pain: pain experienced in a missing body part
7. Radiating pain: pain experienced at the source and extending to other areas

REVIEW OF PHYSIOLOGY

A. Sensory neurons, nociceptors in the peripheral nervous system are stimulated by biochemical mediators (e.g., bradykinin, serotonin, histamine, potassium, and substance P) when there is mechanical, thermal, or chemical damage to tissue. (Viscera do not have special neurons for pain transmission; receptors respond to stretching, ischemia, and inflammation)
B. Pain impulses are transmitted to the spinal column
1. A delta fibers: myelinated, large-diameter neurons
2. C fibers: unmyelinated, narrow-diameter neurons
C. Impulse enters at the dorsal horn and ascends the spinothalamic tract to the thalamus
D. Impulse travels to the basal areas of the brain and to the somatic sensory cortex
E. Endogenous opioids, such as endorphin, are released and bind to receptors to modify pain transmission
F. Gate-control theory suggests that stimulation of the large-diameter fibers can block transmission of painful impulses through the dorsal horn.

 ## PHARMACOLOGIC CONTROL OF PAIN

Narcotic analgesics

A. Action
1. Bind to opiate receptors in central nervous system
2. Result in diminished transmission and perception of pain impulse
B. Examples: morphine sulfate, codeine, meperidine (Demerol), hydromorphine (Dilaudid), fentanyl (Sublimaze), propoxyphene (Darvon), lydrocodone (Vicodin)
C. Major side effects
1. Respiratory depression
2. Lethargy
3. Mental cloudiness
4. Nausea and vomiting
5. Hypotension
6. Constipation
7. Urinary retention
D. Nursing care
1. Monitor for side effects
2. Institute measures to support respiratory function, such as turning clients frequently, encouraging coughing and deep breathing
3. Ensure that a narcotic antagonist (nalmefene, naloxone HCl, or naltrexone) is available in case of overdose
4. Ensure medications are renewed at required intervals
5. Keep accurate count of narcotics
6. Use measures to promote elimination (e.g., fluids and roughage)
7. Maintain therapeutic levels of medication
8. Administer before pain becomes severe; medication less effective when pain is severe

Nonsteroidal Antiinflammatory Drugs (NSAIDs)

A. Action
1. Act on peripheral nerve endings and decrease inflammatory mediators by inhibiting prostaglandin synthesis
2. Have analgesic, antiinflammatory, and antipyretic effects
B. Examples: acetylsalicylic acid (aspirin), ibuprofen (Motrin, Advil), naproxen (Naprosyn)
C. Major side effects
1. Gastrointestinal (GI) ulceration and bleeding (most common)
2. Nausea and vomiting
3. Constipation or diarrhea
4. Bone marrow depression and impaired coagulation
5. Visual disturbances
6. Tinnitus
7. Confusion
8. Seizures
D. Nursing care
1. Administer with food or milk
2. Monitor for side effects
3. Monitor complete blood count (CBC)
4. Monitor liver function
5. Avoid use of alcohol or aspirin when taking other NSAIDs

Other Nonnarcotic Analgesics

A. Action
1. Analgesic effect may be caused by inhibition of CNS prostaglandin synthesis
2. No effect on peripheral prostaglandin synthesis; therefore, no antiinflammatory action
B. Example: acetaminophen (Tylenol)
C. Major side effects (few, if therapy is short-term)
1. Hemolytic anemia
2. Hepatotoxicity
3. Seizures
4. Coma and death
D. Nursing care
1. Do not crush extended relief products
2. Monitor CBC
3. Monitor liver function
4. Teach client to avoid alcohol and other over-the-counter products that contain acetaminophen

General Nursing Care of Clients in Pain

A. **ASSESSMENT**
1. Client's description of pain: location, intensity (using a numeric or picture scale), character, onset, duration, and aggravating and alleviating factors
2. Associated signs and symptoms: increased vital signs (may be decreased with visceral pain), nausea, vomiting, diarrhea, diaphoresis
3. Nonverbal cues: facial expression, body posture
4. Contributing factors: age (older adults may feel pain as normal or may fear addiction, so they may not complain), culture, past experience, anxiety, fear, uncertainty (lack of information), fatigue
5. Effect of pain on client's activities of daily living (ADL)

B. **ANALYSIS/NURSING DIAGNOSIS**
1. Acute or chronic pain related to tissue trauma
2. Ineffective coping related to intractable pain
3. Disturbed sleep pattern related to pain
4. Impaired physical mobility related to pain

C. **PLANNING/IMPLEMENTATION**
1. Continue to monitor and document client's pain and associated symptoms
2. Use nonpharmacologic techniques
   a. Massage and acupressure
   b. Teach relaxation techniques, guided imagery
   c. Use distraction
   d. Apply heat or cold
3. Administer prescribed analgesics
4. Teach client use of transcutaneous electric nerve stimulation (TENS) unit; electronic stimulation via surface electrodes to prevent complete depolarization or block transmission of pain impulses
5. Teach client use of patient-controlled analgesics (PCA) pump; infusion pump is programmed for dose and time interval, allowing client to control administration without overdose; may be intravenous, subcutaneous, or epidural
6. Provide preoperative and postoperative care for clients requiring surgical intervention
   a. Rhizotomy: posterior spinal nerve root is resected between the ganglion and the cord, resulting in permanent loss of sensation; the anterior root may be cut to alleviate painful muscle spasm
   b. Cordotomy: to alleviate intractable pain in the trunk or lower extremities; transmission of pain and temperature sensation is interrupted by creation of a lesion in ascending tracts, percutaneously using an electrode or surgically via laminectomy
   c. Sympathectomy: to control pain of vascular disturbances and phantom limb pain
   d. Dorsal column stimulator and peripheral nerve implant: direct attachment of electrode to sensory nerve; a transmitter attached to the electrode is carried by client so electric stimulation can be administered as needed
7. Provide information about other available pain management options (e.g., acupuncture, biofeedback)

D. **EVALUATION/OUTCOMES**
1. Reports a reduction in pain
2. Participates actively in ADLs

INFECTION

REVIEW OF PHYSIOLOGY

Immunity

A. Nonspecific immune response: that directed against all invading microbes
   1. Body surface barriers: intact skin and mucosa, cilia, and secretion of mucus
   2. Antimicrobial secretions: oil of skin, tears, gastric juice, and vaginal secretions
   3. Internal antimicrobial agents
      a. Interferon: substance produced within the cells in response to a viral attack
      b. Properdin: protein agent in blood that destroys certain gram-negative bacteria and viruses
      c. Lysozyme: destroys mainly gram-positive bacteria
   4. Phagocytes (microphages, macrophages): cells in the blood that ingest and destroy microbes; part of the reticuloendothelial system
   5. Inflammatory response
      a. First stage: release of histamine and chemical mediators (e.g., prostaglandin, bradykinin) leads to vascular dilatation and increased capillary permeability resulting in signs of inflammation: pain, heat, redness, edema, and loss of function
      b. Second stage: exudate production
      c. Third stage: reparative phase

B. Specific immune response: that directed against a specific pathogen (foreign protein) or its toxin; may be cell mediated or humoral
   1. Cell-mediated immunity
      a. Occurs within the cells of the immune system
      b. Involves T lymphocytes (T helper, T suppressor, T cytotoxic, lymphokines); each type plays a distinct role in the immune system
      c. Cluster designations: mature T cells carry markers on their surface that permit them to be classified structurally (e.g., CD_4 cells associated with AIDS)
      d. Function of cell-mediated immunity
         (1) Protect against most viral, fungal, protozoan, and slow-growing bacterial infections
         (2) Reject histioincompatible grafts
         (3) Cause skin hypersensitivity reactions (e.g., TB screening)
         (4) Survey for malignant cells
   2. Humoral immunity: concerned with immune responses outside of cell; involves B lymphocytes that differentiate into plasma cells and secrete antibodies
      a. Antigen: any substance, including allergens, that stimulates production of antibodies when introduced into the body; typically, antigens are foreign proteins, the most potent being microbial cells and their products
      b. Antibody: immune substance produced by plasma cells; antibodies are gamma globulin molecules; commonly referred to as immunoglobulin (Ig)
      c. Complement-fixation: group of blood serum proteins needed in certain antigen-antibody reactions; both the complement and the antibody must be present for a reaction to occur
      d. Types of immunoglobulins
         (1) Immunoglobulin M (IgM) antibodies: first antibodies to be detected after exposure to an antigen; protection from gram-negative bacteria
         (2) Immunoglobulin G (IgG) antibodies: make up more than 75% of the total immunoglobulins; highest increase in response to subsequent exposure to an antigen; only immunoglobulin that passes the placental barrier
         (3) Immunoglobulin A (IgA) antibodies: present in blood, mucus, and human milk secretions; play an important role against viral and respiratory pathogens
         (4) Immunoglobulin E (IgE) antibodies: responsible for hypersensitivity and allergic responses; cause mast cells to release histamine; protection from parasites
         (5) Immunoglobulin D (IgD) antibodies: help in differentiation of B lymphocytes

C. Types of immunity (Table 6-1)
   1. Active immunity: antibodies formed in the body
      a. Natural active immunity: antibodies formed by the individual during the course of the disease; may provide lifelong immunity (e.g., measles, chickenpox, yellow fever, smallpox)
      b. Artificial active immunity: use of a vaccine or toxoid to stimulate formation of homologous antibodies; revaccination (booster shot) is often needed to sustain antibody titer (anamnestic effect)
         (1) Killed vaccines: antigenic preparations containing killed microbes (e.g., pertussis vaccine, typhoid vaccine)
         (2) Live vaccines: antigenic preparations containing weakened (attenuated) microbes; typically such vaccines are more antigenic than killed preparations (e.g., oral [Sabin] poliomyelitis vaccine, measles vaccine)

TABLE 6-1	Adult immunization schedule	
Vaccine	**When to administer**	**Dose/route**
Influenza	One dose each fall	0.5 ml, IM
Tetanus-diphtheria	First dose	0.5 ml, IM
	Second dose 4 to 6 weeks later	
	Third dose 6 to 12 months after second dose	
	Booster shot every 10 years	
Polio	OPV: one dose	OPV: 0.5 ml on back of tongue
Pneumococcal disease	One dose anytime during the year	0.5 ml, IM or SC
Hepatitis A	First dose	1.0 ml, IM
	Second dose 6 to 12 months later	
Hepatitis B	First dose	1.0 ml, IM/deltoid
	Second dose 1 month later	
	Third dose 5 months after second dose	
Measles, mumps, and rubella	One dose	0.5 ml, SC/deltoid
Varicella	First dose	0.5 ml, SC/deltoid
	Second dose 1 to 2 months later	

(3) Toxoids: antigenic preparations composed of inactivated bacterial toxins (e.g., tetanus toxoids, diphtheria toxoids)
2. Passive immunity: antibodies acquired from an outside source
   a. Natural passive immunity: passage of preformed antibodies from the mother through the placenta or colostrum to the baby; during the first few weeks of life the newborn is immune to certain diseases to which the mother has active immunity
   b. Artificial passive immunity: injection of antisera derived from immunized animals or humans; provide immediate protection and also are of value in treatment (e.g., diphtheria antitoxin, tetanus antitoxin)

REVIEW OF MICROBIOLOGY

Pathology of Infection

A. Infection: invasion of the body by pathogenic microorganisms (pathogens) and the reaction of the tissues to their presence and to the toxins generated by them
   1. Pathogenicity: the ability of a microbe to cause disease
   2. Virulence: the degree of pathogenicity
B. Classifications
   1. Extent of involvement
      a. Local infection: limited to one locality of the body, such as a boil; may have systemic repercussions such as fever and malaise
      b. Focal infection: a local infection from which the organisms spread to other parts of body

(e.g., a tooth abscess that seeds organisms into the blood)
      c. Systemic infection: infectious agent is spread throughout the body (e.g., typhoid fever)
   2. Length of infectious process
      a. Acute infection: one that develops rapidly, usually resulting in a high fever and severe sickness; resolves in a short period of time
      b. Chronic infection: one that develops slowly, with mild but longer-lasting symptoms; sometimes an acute infection becomes chronic and vice versa
   3. Etiology of infectious process
      a. Primary infection: develops after initial exposure to antigen, unrelated to other health problems
      b. Secondary infection: develops when antigens take advantage of the weakened defenses resulting from a primary infection (e.g., staphylococcal pneumonia as a sequela of measles)
      c. Opportunistic infection: develops when host defenses are diminished because of disease process or therapeutic modalities (e.g., urinary tract infection following antibiotic therapy)
C. Chain of infection
   1. Infectious agent
   2. Reservoir: source of almost all pathogens is human or animal
      a. Persons exhibiting symptoms of disease
      b. Carriers: persons who harbor a pathogen in the absence of a discernible clinical disease

(1) Healthy carriers: those who have never had the disease in question

(2) Incubatory carriers: those in the incubation period of a disease

(3) Chronic carriers: those who have recovered from a disease but continue to harbor pathogens

3. Portals of exit: route by which microorganisms leave the body; blood, skin, and mucous membranes, and respiratory, genitourinary, and gastrointestinal tracts

4. Mode of transmission

a. Contact transmission

(1) Direct: contact between body surfaces

(2) Indirect: contact between susceptible host and a contaminated intermediate object

b. Droplet transmission: droplets from infected individual are propelled a short distance by coughing, sneezing, talking, or suctioning before settling to the floor

c. Airborne transmission: small droplet nuclei (≤5 microns) or dust particles that contain the pathogen remain suspended in the air for an extended period

d. Common vehicle transmission: microorganisms are transmitted by contaminated food, water, medication, equipment, or devices

e. Vector-borne transmission: microorganisms are transmitted by vectors such as mosquitoes, flies, ticks, and rats

5. Portals of entry: same as portals of exit

6. Susceptible host

a. Developmental level: extremes of age

b. Inadequate nutritional status

c. Coexisting disease

d. Decreased immune responses

Types of Pathogens

Bacteria

A. Unicellular microbes without chlorophyll

B. Capsule: a material secreted by the cell protecting it from phagocytosis and increasing its virulence (e.g., *Diplococcus pneumoniae*)

C. Spores: the inactive resistant structures into which bacterial protoplasm can transform under adverse conditions; under favorable conditions a spore germinates into an active cell (e.g., *Clostridium tetani*)

D. Examples of medically important bacteria

1. Eubacteriales: divided into five families based on shape, Gram stain, and endospore formation

a. Gram-positive cocci

(1) Diplococci: occurring predominantly in pairs (e.g., *Diplococcus pneumoniae*)

(2) Streptococci: occurring predominantly in chains (e.g., *Streptococcus pyogenes*)

(3) Staphylococci: occurring predominantly in grapelike bunches (e.g., *Staphylococcus aureus*)

b. Gram-negative cocci include *Neisseria gonorrhoeae* and *Neisseria meningitidis*

c. Gram-negative rods include enterobacteria such as *Escherichia*, *Salmonella*, and *Shigella* species

d. Gram-positive rods that do not produce endospores include *Corynebacterium diphtheriae*

e. Gram-positive rods producing endospores include *Bacillus anthracis*, *Clostridium botulinum*, and *Clostridium tetani*

2. Actinomycetales (actinomycetes): moldlike microbes with elongated cells, frequently filamentous (e.g., *Mycobacterium tuberculosis* and *Mycobacterium leprae*)

3. Spirochaetales (spirochetes): flexuous, spiral organisms (e.g., *Treponema pallidum*)

4. Mycoplasmatales (mycoplasmas): delicate, nonmotile microbes displaying a variety of sizes and shapes

Viruses

A. Obligate intracellular parasite; can replicate only within a cell of another organism; composed of either ribonucleic acid (RNA) or deoxyribonucleic acid (DNA), not both

B. Examples of medically important viruses

1. Human immunodeficiency virus: AIDS

2. Hepatitis B virus (HBV): hepatitis type B

3. Haemophilus influenza virus: influenza

4. Varicella zoster virus: chickenpox, herpes zoster, shingles

Fungi

A. A saprophytic organism that lives on organic material

B. Molds: fuzzy growths of interlacing filaments called hyphae; reproduce by spores

C. Yeasts: organisms that usually are single-celled and usually reproduce by budding

D. Examples of medically important fungi

1. *Candida albicans*, a yeast: monilias ("thrush")

2. *Histoplasmosis capsulatum*: histoplasmosis

3. *Trichophyton rubrum*: tinea pedis ("athlete's foot")

Control of Microorganisms

A. Medical asepsis

1. Standard precautions (e.g., handwashing, personal protective equipment)

2. Transmission-based precautions (e.g., airborne, droplet, and contact)

B. Surgical asepsis

C. Disinfection: removal or destruction of pathogens
D. Sterilization: removal or destruction of all microbes
E. Antiseptic: inhibits microbial growth
F. Heat sterilization
　1. Moist heat
　　a. Steam under pressure (autoclave)
　　b. Boiling objects in water; some spores resist boiling
　2. Dry heat
G. Radiation: all types of radiation injurious to microbes
　1. Gamma rays: used to sterilize food and drugs
　2. Ultraviolet light: used to inhibit the microbial population of air in operating rooms, nurseries, and laboratories

PHARMACOLOGIC CONTROL OF INFECTION

Definition of Terms
A. Bactericidal effect: destroys bacteria at low concentrations
B. Bacteriostatic effect: slows reproduction of bacteria
C. Superinfection (secondary infection): emergence of microorganism growth when natural protective flora is destroyed by antiinfective drug
D. Bacterial resistance: a natural or acquired characteristic of an organism preventing destruction by a drug to which it was previously susceptible

Antibiotics
A. Description
　1. Used to destroy bacteria or inhibit bacterial reproduction to control infection
　2. Available in oral, parenteral, and topical, including ophthalmic and ear drop preparations
B. Antibiotic sensitivity tests: identifies antibiotics that are effective against a particular organism
C. Examples
　1. Penicillins: interfere with bacterial cell wall synthesis; e.g., broad spectrum amoxicillin (Amoxil) and penicillin G potassium (Pentids)
　2. Cephalosporins: interfere with bacterial cell wall synthesis; e.g., broad spectrum cefazolin sodium (Ancef, Kefzol) and cephalexin monohydrate (Keflex)
　3. Erythromycins: inhibit mRNA synthesis of bacterial protein; e.g., clindamycin HCl (Cleocin), azithromycin (Zithromax), erythromycin (E-mycin)
　4. Tetracyclines: inhibit bacterial protein synthesis by blocking tRNA attachment to ribosomes; e.g., broad spectrum doxycycline (Vibramycin) and tetracycline (Achromycin, Sumycin)
　5. Aminoglycosides: disrupt bacterial protein synthesis by providing a substitute for essential nucleotide required by mRNA; e.g., broad

spectrum gentamicin sulfate (Garamycin), neomycin sulfate (Mycifradin), streptomycin sulfate
　6. Quinolones: interfere with DNA gyrase, an enzyme necessary for the synthesis of bacterial DNA (e.g., broad spectrum ciprofloxacin [Cipro] and levofloxacin [Levaquin])
　7. Polymyxin group: decreases bacterial cell membrane permeability; e.g., polymyxin B sulfate (Aerosporin)
　8. Vancomycin: inhibits bacterial cell wall synthesis (e.g., Lyphocin and Vancocin)
D. Major side effects
　1. Depressed appetite (altered taste sensitivity)
　2. Nausea, vomiting (normal flora imbalance)
　3. Diarrhea (normal flora imbalance)
　4. Suppressed absorption of a variety of nutrients including fat; protein; lactose; vitamins A, D, K, and B$_{12}$; and the minerals calcium, iron, and potassium (normal flora imbalance)
　5. Increased excretion of water-soluble vitamins and minerals (normal flora imbalance)
　6. Superinfection (normal flora imbalance)
　7. Allergic reactions, anaphylaxis (hypersensitivity)
　8. Nephrotoxicity (direct kidney toxic effect)
　9. Tetracyclines
　　a. Hepatotoxicity (direct liver toxic effect)
　　b. Phototoxicity (degradation to toxic products by ultraviolet rays)
　　c. Hyperuricemia (impaired kidney function)
　　d. Enamel hypoplasia, dental caries, and bone defects in children under 8 years of age (drug binds to calcium in tissue)
　10. Aminoglycosides
　　a. Ototoxicity (direct auditory [eighth cranial] nerve toxic effect)
　　b. Leukopenia (decreased WBC synthesis)
　　c. Thrombocytopenia (decreased platelet synthesis)
　　d. Headache, confusion (neurotoxicity)
　　e. Peripheral neuropathy (neurotoxicity)
　　f. Nephrotoxicity (direct kidney toxic effect)
　　g. Respiratory paralysis (neuromuscular blockade)
　11. Vancomycin
　　a. Ototoxicity (hearing loss)
　　b. Nephrotoxicity (kidney damage)
E. Nursing care
　1. Assess client for history of drug allergy
　2. Instruct client regarding:
　　a. How to take the drug (frequency, relation to meals)
　　b. Completing the prescribed course of therapy; prevent the emergence of resistant strains of microorganisms such as methicillin-resistant *Staphylococcus aureus* (MRSA)

c. Symptoms of allergic response

d. Side effects, including superinfection; suggest ingestion of yogurt or food supplements containing *Lactobacillus acidophilus* when dairy products cannot be tolerated; suggest nutritional consultation when drug therapy may have an impact on client's nutritional status

3. Shake liquid suspensions to mix thoroughly

4. Administer most preparations 1 hour before meals or 2 hours after meals for best absorption

5. Administer at equal intervals around the clock to maintain blood levels

6. Assess vital signs during course of therapy

7. Tetracyclines
   a. Avoid use during last half of pregnancy or by children younger than 8 years
   b. Assess for potentiation if client is receiving oral anticoagulants
   c. Teach client to avoid direct sunlight
   d. Advise client to avoid dairy products, antacids, or iron preparations, because they reduce effectiveness

8. Aminoglycosides: assess for potentiation if client is receiving neuromuscular blocking agents, a general anesthetic, or parenteral magnesium

9. Vancomycin: peak and trough blood levels need to be assessed because it has a narrow therapeutic range

Antivirals

A. Description
   1. Used to provide prophylaxis when exposure to viral infection has occurred; prevent entrance of the virus into host cells
   2. Available in oral, parenteral (IV), and topical, including ophthalmic, preparations

B. Examples: acyclovir sodium (Zovirax) amantadine HCl (Symmetrel), and vidarabine (Vira-A)

C. Major side effects
   1. Central nervous system (CNS) stimulation (direct CNS effect)
   2. Orthostatic hypotension (depressed cardiovascular system)
   3. Dizziness (hypotension)
   4. Constipation (decreased peristalsis)
   5. Nephrotoxicity (direct kidney toxic effect)
   6. Local irritation (direct local tissue effect)

D. Nursing care
   1. Assess vital signs during course of therapy
   2. Support natural defense mechanisms of client; encourage intake of foods rich in the immune-stimulating nutrients, such as vitamins A, C, and E, and the minerals selenium and zinc
   3. Encourage intake of high-fiber foods to reduce potential of constipation

4. Monitor disease symptoms and laboratory data
5. Evaluate client's response to medication

Sulfonamides

A. Description
   1. Antiinfective drugs used primarily to treat urinary tract infections substitute a false metabolite for paraaminobenzoic acid (PABA) that is required in the bacterial synthesis of folic acid
   2. Available in oral, parenteral (IM, IV), and topical, including ophthalmic, preparations

B. Examples: sulfisoxazole (Gantrisin) and combination products such as sulfamethoxazole and trimethoprim (Bactrim, Septra)

C. Major side effects
   1. Nausea, vomiting; decreased absorption of folacin (irritation of gastric mucosa)
   2. Skin rash (hypersensitivity)
   3. Malaise (decreased RBCs)
   4. Blood dyscrasias (decreased RBCs, WBCs, platelet synthesis)
   5. Crystalluria (drug precipitation in acidic urine)
   6. Stomatitis (GI irritation)
   7. Headache (CNS effect)
   8. Photosensitivity (hypersensitivity)
   9. Allergic response, anaphylaxis (hypersensitivity)

D. Nursing care
   1. Assess client for history of drug allergy
   2. Promote increased fluid intake
   3. Caution client to avoid direct exposure to sunlight
   4. Assess vital signs during course of therapy
   5. Maintain alkaline urine
   6. Administer at routine intervals around the clock to maintain blood levels; obtain blood specimens for peak and trough levels
   7. Monitor blood work during therapy; potential for megaloblastic anemia caused by folacin deficiency
   8. Assess for potentiation of oral anticoagulant and oral hypoglycemic effects
   9. Evaluate client's response to medication

Antifungals

A. Description
   1. Used to treat systemic and localized fungal infections; destroy fungal cells (fungicidal) or inhibit the reproduction of fungal cells (fungistatic)
   2. Available in oral, parenteral (IV), topical, vaginal, and intrathecal preparations

B. Examples
   1. Amphotericin B (Fungizone) and nystatin (Mycostatin, Nilstat): disrupts fungal cell membrane permeability
   2. Fluconazole (Diflucan): disrupts fungal cell membrane function

3. Griseofulvin (Grisactin): disrupts fungal nucleic acid synthesis
C. Major side effects
   1. Nausea, vomiting (irritation to gastric mucosa)
   2. Headache (neurotoxicity)
   3. Blood dyscrasias (effect on bone marrow)
   4. Paresthesia (neurotoxicity)
D. Nursing care
   1. Assess vital signs during course of therapy
   2. Review proper method of application with client
   3. Amphotericin B
      a. Use infusion control device for IV administration
      b. Protect solution from light during IV infusion
      c. Monitor blood work during therapy; potential hypokalemia as well as increased urinary excretion of magnesium
      d. Premedicate with antipyretics, corticosteroids, antihistamines, and antiemetics before IV administration
   4. Griseofulvin
      a. Assess for antagonism if client is taking oral anticoagulants
      b. Instruct client to avoid direct exposure to sunlight
   5. Evaluate client's response to medication

Antiparasitics
A. Description
   1. Used to treat parasitic diseases; interfere with parasite metabolism and reproduction; helminthic (pinworm and tapeworm) as well as protozoal (amebiasis and malaria) infestations respond well to these drugs
   2. Available in oral, parenteral (IM, SC, IV), vaginal, and rectal preparations
B. Examples
   1. Anthelmintics: mebendazole (Vermox) and pyrivinium pamoate (Povan)
   2. Amebicides: chloroquine HCl (Aralen) and metronidazole (Flagyl)
   3. Antimalarials: chloroquine HCl (Aralen), hydroxychloroquine sulfate (Plaquenil), and quinine sulfate (Quinamm)
C. Major side effects
   1. Anthelmintics
      a. Gastrointestinal irritation (direct tissue irritation)
      b. CNS disturbances (neurotoxicity)
      c. Skin rash (hypersensitivity)
   2. Amebicides
      a. Gastrointestinal irritation (direct tissue irritation)
      b. Blood dyscrasias (decreased RBCs, WBCs, platelet synthesis)
      c. Skin rash (hypersensitivity)

d. Headache (neurotoxicity)
e. Dizziness (CNS effect)
3. Antimalarials
   a. Nausea, vomiting (irritation to gastric mucosa)
   b. Blood dyscrasias (decreased RBCs, WBCs)
   c. Visual disturbances (impairment of accommodation; retinal and corneal changes)
D. Nursing care
   1. Administer drug with meals to decrease GI irritability
   2. Assess vital signs during course of therapy
   3. Monitor blood work during therapy
   4. Instruct client regarding proper hygiene to prevent spread of disease
   5. Use safety precautions (supervise ambulation) if CNS effects are manifested
   6. Antimalarials: encourage frequent visual examinations
   7. Evaluate client's response to medication

General Nursing Care of Clients at Risk for Infection
A. ASSESSMENT
   1. Obtain history to identify factors affecting chain of infection
   2. Obtain baseline vital signs
   3. Monitor baseline WBC
   4. Review results of culture and sensitivity tests
B. ANALYSIS/NURSING DIAGNOSES
   1. Deficient fluid volume related to insensible fluid losses associated with fever
   2. Hyperthermia related to infectious process
   3. Risk for infection related to impaired immune response
C. PLANNING/IMPLEMENTATION
   1. Decrease host susceptibility
      a. Maintain skin and mucous membranes as first line of defense
      b. Reinforce or maintain natural protective mechanisms such as coughing, pH of secretions, resident flora
      c. Maintain nutrition and encourage rest and sleep to promote tissue repair and production of lymphocytes and antibodies
      d. Educate client about immunizations
   2. Use principles of asepsis
      a. Medical asepsis: Limits the growth and spread of microorganisms by confining them to a specific area
      b. Surgical asepsis
         (1) Absence of all microorganisms and spores; prevents microorganisms from entering a specific area
         (2) Contamination occurs if a sterile article:
            (a) Touches an unsterile article

(b) Is placed outside a 1-inch inside border of a sterile field

(c) Is below waist level or above shoulder level

(d) Is beyond the field of vision

(e) Rests on a wet, permeable surface, which enables contamination by capillary action

(f) Is exposed to airborne microorganisms

3. Limit or eliminate the microbiologic agent
   a. Disinfection and sterilization
   b. Administration of antimicrobial agents
4. Prevent transmission
   a. Employ hand-washing techniques
      (1) Before client contact; after client contact; after contact with blood, body fluids, secretions, excretions, mucous membranes, or nonintact skin
      (2) Use friction, soap, and warm water to loosen and flush microorganisms
   b. Use standard precautions (Table 6-2); used for all clients regardless of diagnosis or presumed infectious status
   c. Use transmission-based precautions (Table 6-2); employed in addition to standard precautions; designed for clients documented or suspected to be infected with highly transmissible or epidemiologically important pathogens; precautions may be combined for diseases that have multiple routes of transmission
   d. Correctly dispose of contaminated material
      (1) Use impervious bags to dispose of contaminated material
      (2) Do not recap or break needles after administering injections; use rigid container for disposal
5. Monitor vital signs, particularly temperature; ensure consistency of measurement (Celsius or Fahrenheit); conversion from one temperature scale to another is accomplished by using the formula:

$$F = 9/5 \; C + 32$$

6. Employ measures to decrease body temperature as prescribed (tepid bath, antipyretics, hypothermia blanket); prevent shivering, which raises the BMR and thus temperature, pulse, and respirations
7. Ensure adequate fluid intake

D. EVALUATION/OUTCOMES
1. Complies with medical regimen
2. Establishes health practices that enhance immunity
3. Maintains body temperature within normal range
4. Maintains fluid balance

5. Becomes infection free
6. Remains free from infection

FLUID, ELECTROLYTE, AND ACID-BASE BALANCE

FLUID AND ELECTROLYTE BALANCE
Basic Concepts
A. Volume of blood plasma, interstitial fluid, and intracellular fluid, and the concentration of electrolytes in each, remain relatively constant (Table 6-3)
B. Intake must approximately equal output
C. The average adult contains about 40 L of water, comprising 60% of body weight; 25 L intracellular, 15 to 17 L extracellular; may be as high as 80% in infants and as low as 40% in the elderly
D. Extracellular fluid divided among:
   1. Interstitial compartment: 10 to 12 L
   2. Intravascular compartment: 3 L
   3. Small fluid compartments: 1 L (e.g., aqueous humor, serous and synovial fluid, lymphatic channels)
   4. Gastrointestinal tract: 1 L at any given time for all gastrointestinal organs
E. All body fluids are related and mix well with each other: plasma becomes interstitial fluid as it filters across the capillary wall; interstitial fluid can return to the capillary by osmosis or enter lymphatic channels, becoming lymph; interstitial fluid and intracellular fluid are in osmotic equilibrium across the cell membranes, regulated by the sodium ion (Na^+) concentration of interstitial fluid and the potassium ion (K^+) concentration of intracellular fluid

Water
A. Water is a combination of oxygen and hydrogen; most abundant compound; essential to life
B. Water enters the body through the digestive tract by liquids and food; it is also formed by the metabolism of foods
C. Water leaves the body via the kidneys, intestines, and lungs and skin (insensible losses); only the kidneys have a feedback mechanism

Solutions
A. Substances that dissolve in other substances form solutions
B. Substance dissolved is called the solute
C. Substance in which the solute is dissolved is called the solvent
D. Solutions can be administered intravenously; the potential energy of fluid in an IV bag is converted to kinetic energy when it flows through the tubing

TABLE 6-2   Precautions to prevent the spread of microorganisms

Category	Indications	Conditions	Room	Gown
STANDARD PRE-CAUTIONS	Used for all clients regardless of diagnosis when there is contact with: 1. Blood 2. Body fluid 3. Secretions 4. Excretions 5. Nonintact skin 6. Mucous membranes	Used for all clients, particularly those with acquired immunodeficiency syndrome (AIDS) and hepatitis type B	Private room indicated if personal hygiene is inadequate	Indicated if soiling with blood, body fluid, secretions, or excretions is likely (e.g., during client care activities that are associated with splashes of blood); should be impermeable to liquids
TRANSMISSION-BASED PRECAUTIONS*				
AIRBORNE PRE-CAUTIONS	Prevents transmission of droplet nuclei less than or equal to 5 microns or dust particles that contain the pathogen. These nuclei and particles remain suspended in the air for an extended period	Tuberculosis, varicella, rubeola	Negative-pressure isolation room with at least six air exchanges per hour. Door must be kept closed	See Standard Precautions
DROPLET PRE-CAUTIONS	Prevents transmission of particle droplets greater than 5 microns that are dispersed by coughing, sneezing, talking, or suctioning. These droplets travel up to 3 feet before settling to the floor or other surfaces	*Haemophilus influenzae* type B in children, meningococci meningitis, *Streptococcus pneumoniae* pneumonia, mycoplasmal pneumonia, streptococcal pharyngitis, scarlet fever, pertussis, rubella, mumps, diphtheria	Private room; clients infected with the same organism may share a room	See Standard Precautions
CONTACT PRE-CAUTIONS a. Direct b. Indirect	Prevents transmission of epidemiologically important microorganisms by direct contact with client's skin or indirect contact with contaminated items or surfaces	*Clostridium difficile* enteric infection, enterohemorrhagic *Escherichia coli*, shigella, hepatitis type A, herpes simplex virus, cellulitis, scabies	Private room; clients infected with the same organism may share a room	See Standard Precautions. Don gown when first entering room if contact with client or items in room is likely

*Used in addition to standard precautions for clients with documented or suspected infection with highly transmittable or epidemiologically important pathogens.

Gloves	Mask and Eye	Handwashing	Precautions
Required for touching blood, body fluids, secretions, excretions, contaminated items or surfaces, mucous membranes, and nonintact skin	Required if splashes of blood, body fluids, secretions, or excretions are likely	Required after touching blood, body fluids, secretions, excretions, or contaminated articles whether gloves were worn or not. Hands must be washed when gloves are removed, before contact with another client, and before touching a noncontaminated item or surface	Discard items contaminated with blood, body fluids, secretions, or excretions in a biohazard receptacle or handle equipment in a manner that will prevent transfer of microorganisms. Disinfect and sterilize reusable items. Dispose of used needles and other sharp devices in properly labeled, puncture-resistant container. Never recap used needles. Use ventilation devices instead of mouth-to-mouth resuscitation.
See Standard Precautions	See Standard Precautions. Use particular respirators such as HEPA mask (high efficiency particulate air filter respirator) when client has a known or suspected diagnosis of tuberculosis. People susceptible to varicella or rubeola should not enter the room	See Standard Precautions	See Standard Precautions. Confine client to room; transport only if absolutely essential; during transport have client wear a surgical mask to minimize droplet nuclei dispersal
See Standard Precautions	See Standard Precautions	See Standard Precautions	See Standard Precautions. See Airborne Precautions
See Standard Precautions. Apply gloves when entering room; change gloves after contact with substances such as feces or wound drainage that have high concentrations of microorganisms	See Standard Precautions	See Standard Precautions	See Standard Precautions. Confine client to room. Transport only if absolutely essential; during transport maintain precautions to limit transmission of microorganisms. If possible, equipment such as a stethoscope or sphygmomanometer should be used only for the infected client

TABLE 6-3   Average concentrations of major ions in extracellular and intracellular fluids (usually expressed in milliosmols per liter [mOsm/L] of H₂O)

Ion	Intracellular fluid	Extracellular fluid Plasma	Interstitial
Na⁺	10	144.0	137.0
K⁺	141	5.0	4.7
Cl⁻	4	107.0	112.7
HCO₃⁻	10	27.0	28.3
Ca⁺⁺	0	2.5	2.4
Mg⁺⁺	31	1.5	1.4
SO₄⁼	1	0.5	0.5
Phosphates (H₂PO₄⁻; HPO₄⁼)	11	2.0	2.0
Proteins	4	1.2	0.2

E. Types of solutions
1. Dilute: small amount of solute in a relatively large amount of solvent
2. Concentrated: large amount of solute in a relatively small amount of solvent
3. Percent solution: grams of solute per gram of solution
4. Molar solution (M): number of gram-molecular weights of solute per liter of solution
5. Isotonic solution: when the osmotic pressures of two liquids are equal, the flow of solvent is equalized and the two solutions are said to be isotonic to each other; physiologic saline (0.89% NaCl in distilled water) and 5% dextrose in water

Major Ions (Electrolytes)

A. When an atom loses or gains an electron it is no longer a neutral atom but a charged particle: an ion
B. A substance that, when dissolved in water, dissociates into an ion that is able to conduct an electric current
C. An ion that carries a positive charge is called a cation; an ion that carries a negative charge is called an anion
D. Cations (⁺)
1. Sodium (Na⁺)
   a. Most abundant cation in extracellular fluid
   b. Sodium pump in most body cells pumps sodium out of intracellular fluid
   c. Action potential of nervous and muscle fibers requires sodium; sodium is basic to communication between nerves and muscles
   d. Helps to regulate acid-base balance by exchanging hydrogen ions for sodium ions

in the kidney tubules; excess hydrogen ions (acid) are excreted
   e. Foods high in sodium include celery, processed foods, snack foods, condiments, smoked meats, and cheese
2. Potassium (K⁺)
   a. Most abundant cation of intracellular fluid
   b. Potassium pump brings potassium into cells
   c. Resting polarization and repolarization of nerve and muscle fibers depend on potassium
      (1) If potassium concentration of extracellular fluid rises above normal (hyperkalemia), the force of the contracting heart weakens; with extremely high concentrations the heart will not contract
      (2) If potassium concentration of extracellular fluid drops below normal (hypokalemia), the resting polarization in nerve and muscle fibers increases, resulting in weakness and eventual paralysis
   d. Foods high in potassium include bananas, avocados, oranges, dates, potatoes, and raisins
3. Calcium (Ca⁺⁺)
   a. Forms salts with phosphates, carbonate, and fluoride in bones and teeth to make them hard
   b. Required for correct functioning of nerves and muscles
      (1) If calcium concentration rises above normal levels (hypercalcemia), nervous system becomes depressed and sluggish
      (2) If calcium concentration falls below normal levels (hypocalcemia), nervous system becomes extremely excitable, resulting in cramps and tetany
   c. Calcium is required for blood clotting, acting as a cofactor in the formation of prothrombin activator and thrombin
   d. Foods high in calcium include milk, dairy products, canned fish with bones, whole grains, legumes, and leafy vegetables
4. Magnesium (Mg⁺⁺)
   a. Cofactor for many enzymes involved in energy metabolism
   b. Normal constituent of bone
   c. Foods high in magnesium include nuts, soy beans, cocoa, seafood, whole grains, dried beans, and peas
E. Anions (⁻)
1. Chloride (C⁻)
   a. Most abundant anion in extracellular fluid
   b. Helps balance sodium
   c. Major component of gastric secretions
   d. Dietary source of chloride is salt

2. Bicarbonate (HCO_3^-)
   a. Part of bicarbonate buffer system
   b. Reacts with a strong acid to form carbonic acid and a basic salt, thus limiting the drop in pH
3. Phosphate ($H_2PO_4^-$ and HPO_4^{--})
   a. Part of phosphate buffer system
   b. Functions in cellular energy metabolism: phosphate + ADP → ATP (the energy currency of the cell)
   c. Combines with calcium ions in bone, providing hardness
   d. Involved in structure of genetic material, DNA and RNA

Factors That Influence Fluid Balance

A. Regulation of fluid intake: thirst mechanism
   1. Dryness of the oral mucosa and dehydration of cells in the thirst center of the hypothalamus give rise to the thirst sensation
   2. Stretching of the stomach by fluid and moistening of the oral mucosa cancel the thirst sensation before the actual hydration of body fluids
B. Osmosis
   1. Osmosis is the movement of fluid across a semipermeable membrane from a lesser concentration to a greater concentration
   2. Pressure forcing the fluid across the membrane is called osmotic (oncotic) pressure
   3. Movement of fluid across the membrane continues until the concentrations of the solutions equalize
   4. Hypertonic solutions: when one solution has less osmotic pressure (is more concentrated) than another, it draws fluid from the other and is said to be hypertonic to it
   5. Hypotonic solutions: when one solution has more osmotic pressure (is more dilute) than another, it forces fluid into the other and is said to be hypotonic to it
C. Protein
   1. Protein molecules are very large and form colloid particles in solution
   2. Proteins are the tissue builders of the body; inadequate intake of protein will result in negative nitrogen balance.
   3. Albumin is most important in the development of the plasma colloid osmotic (oncotic) pressure, which helps control (through osmosis) the flow of water between the plasma and interstitial fluid; during a condition such as starvation, a fall in the albumin level of the blood results in a fall in the plasma colloid osmotic pressure, which leads to edema because less fluid is being drawn by osmosis into the capillaries from the interstitial spaces

D. Circulatory system
   1. Blood hydrostatic pressure: pressure within the intravascular compartment that moves fluid from the vessels to the interstitial compartment
   2. Blood osmotic (oncotic) pressure: pressure that returns fluid to the vessels from the interstitial compartment
   3. Increased fluid intake increases the blood volume, which results in an increase in cardiac output and blood pressure and therefore glomerular filtration (GF); the opposite is true with a decrease in fluid intake
   4. Increased GF results in an increase in urinary output and a decrease in blood volume; the opposite is true with a decrease in GF
E. Osmoreceptor system
   1. Cells in the hypothalamus synthesize antidiuretic hormone, which is then stored in the posterior pituitary before release into the circulation
   2. Osmoreceptors respond to dehydration by increasing the ADH released; this increases water reabsorption in the kidney tubules and decreases urinary output; the opposite occurs with overhydration

Factors That Influence Electrolyte Balance

A. Active transport: the use of energy to move ions across a semipermeable membrane against a concentration, chemical, or electrical gradient
B. Diffusion
   1. Diffusion: the process in which particles in a fluid move across a semipermeable membrane from an area of greater concentration to an area of lesser concentration
   2. Movement of particles across the membrane continues until the concentrations of the solutions equalize
C. Aldosterone feedback mechanism
   1. Adrenal cortex secretes the steroid hormone aldosterone when extracellular fluid sodium concentrations decrease or potassium concentrations increase
   2. Aldosterone stimulates kidney tubules to reabsorb sodium; potassium reabsorption decreases as sodium reabsorption increases; sodium is salvaged while potassium is excreted; occurs during stress such as surgery
   3. This mechanism helps preserve normal sodium and potassium concentrations in extracellular fluid
   4. Secondary effects of aldosterone
      a. Chloride conserved with sodium
      b. Water conserved because it is reabsorbed by osmosis as tubules reabsorb sodium

D. Parathyroid regulation of calcium
1. Parathyroid glands secrete parathormone when extracellular fluid calcium concentrations decrease
2. Parathormone stimulates the release of calcium from bone, calcium reabsorption in the small intestine (vitamin D required), and calcium reabsorption in kidney tubules
3. Increased extracellular fluid calcium concentrations result in decreased secretion of parathormone and gradual loss of excess calcium

ACID-BASE BALANCE
Basic Concepts
A. The pH denotes the power of strength of hydrogen (ions) in a solution
1. An acid solution has more H^+ than OH^-
2. A basic solution has more OH^- than H^+
B. When the body is in a state of acid-base balance it maintains a stable hydrogen ion concentration in the extracellular (intravascular and interstitial compartments) fluid in the narrow range of 7.35 to 7.45 (slightly alkaline); a pH of 7 or less or 7.8 or more can result in death
1. A state of uncompensated acidosis exists if blood pH decreases below 7.35
2. A state of uncompensated alkalosis exists if blood pH increases above 7.45
C. Certain body fluids have a pH different from the norm of 7.35 to 7.45; gastric juice has a pH of 1 or 2 caused by presence of hydrochloric acid; bile is alkaline; urine may be acidic or alkaline

Acids
A. Acid: a compound that yields hydrogen ions when dissociated in solution
B. Properties of an acid
1. Acts as an electrolyte in water
2. Reacts with bases to form water and a salt (neutralization)
3. In high concentration destroys body tissues (corrosive)
C. Common acids
1. Hydrochloric acid: secreted by the parietal cells of the stomach; transforms pepsinogen into pepsin, which is a protein-digesting enzyme of gastric juice
2. Carbonic acid
a. One form in which CO_2 is transported in the blood
b. Part of the bicarbonate buffer system, which is the most important buffer system regulating the pH of body fluids
3. Acetic acid: vinegar

4. Lactic acid: builds up in muscle tissue during exercise and is transported to the liver via the circulatory system, where it is completely oxidized into CO_2, water, and energy (as adenosine triphosphate [ATP])

Bases
A. Base: a compound that combines with an acid to form water and a salt (neutralization)
B. Properties of a base: acts as an electrolyte in water; destroys body tissues (corrosive) in high concentrations
C. Common bases
1. Magnesium hydroxide: water solution marketed under trade name Milk of Magnesia; antacid, mild laxative
2. Aluminum hydroxide: component of antacids
3. Ammonium hydroxide: household cleaner

Salts
A. Salt: the compound (besides water) formed when an acid is neutralized by a base
B. Properties of a salt: acts as an electrolyte in water; is crystalline in nature; "salty" taste
C. Common salts
1. Sodium chloride: salt of extracellular compartment
2. Potassium chloride: salt of intracellular spaces
3. Calcium phosphate: bone and tooth formation
4. Barium sulfate: when taken internally, outlines internal structures for x-ray studies
5. Silver nitrate: antiseptic
6. Ferrous sulfate: treatment of anemia
7. Sodium bicarbonate: antacid

Mechanisms That Maintain Acid-Base Balances
A. Buffer mechanism: first line of defense (takes seconds)
1. Combine with relatively strong acids or bases to convert them to weaker acids or bases to prevent marked changes in blood pH levels
2. Often referred to as a buffer pair because it consists of not one but two substances, a weak acid and its basic salt
3. Bicarbonate buffer system
a. The most important buffer in body fluids because its components, base bicarbonate (HCO_3) and carbonic acid (H_2CO_3), are actively and constantly regulated by the action of the respiratory and urinary systems
b. When the body is in a state of acid-base balance blood contains 27 mEq base bicarbonate per liter and 1.35 mEq carbonic acid per liter, the base bicarbonate/carbonic acid ratio:

$$\frac{27 \text{ mEq base bicarbonate } (HCO_3)}{1.35 \text{ mEq carbonic acid } (H_2CO_3)} = \frac{20}{1}$$

4. Phosphate buffer system; more important in intracellular fluids, where its concentration is considerably higher
5. Protein buffer system; hemoglobin, a protein buffer, promotes the movement of chloride across the RBC membrane in exchange for bicarbonate ions

B. Respiratory mechanism: second line of defense (takes minutes)
   1. Carbon dioxide is carried in the body in the forms of carbonic acid and bicarbonate
   2. Controls rate of carbon dioxide exhalation from lungs
      a. When there are increased amounts of CO_2 in the body the medulla is stimulated to increase the rate and depth of respirations
      b. When there are decreased amounts of CO_2 in the body the rate and depth of respirations decrease
   3. During body metabolism CO_2 is produced, which reacts with water to form carbonic acid, resulting in a decrease in pH (as acidity increases, pH decreases)
   4. In the lung carbonic acid breaks down into CO_2 and H_2O; increased exhalation of CO_2 results in an increase in pH (as acidity decreases, pH increases)

C. Renal mechanism: third line of defense (takes hours to days)
   1. The kidneys function to increase the blood's sodium bicarbonate content and decrease its carbonic acid content, thereby increasing the base bicarbonate/carbonic acid ratio and blood pH
   2. When there are high levels of hydrogen ions in the body the kidneys
      a. Secrete hydrogen ions and reabsorb sodium ions (Fig. 6-1)
      b. Form ammonia that combines with hydrogen ions to form ammonium ions (NH_4^+); ammonium ions are excreted in the urine in exchange for sodium ions, which are reabsorbed into the blood (Fig. 6-2)
   3. When there are low levels of hydrogen ions in the body the kidneys retain hydrogen ions to form bicarbonate

Acid-Base Imbalances

A. Respiratory acidosis
   1. Carbonic acid excess; increased retention of carbon dioxide; PCO_2 is greater than 45 mm Hg (hypercapnia)
   2. pH is below 7.35
   3. Common causes
      a. Inadequate ventilation: e.g., apnea, holding the breath
      b. Respiratory obstruction: mechanical (e.g., tumors) or functional (e.g., asthma)
      c. Impaired gas exchange in the alveoli: e.g., emphysema
      d. Neuromuscular impairment: e.g., spinal cord injury

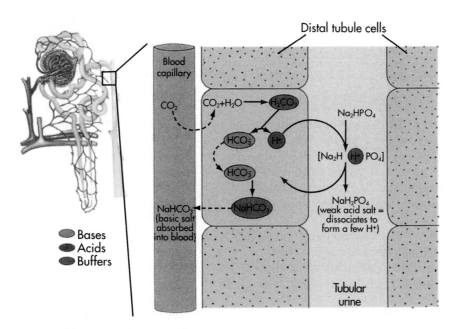

FIGURE 6-1 Acidification of urine and conservation of base by the distal renal tubular excretion of hydrogen ions (H^+) from the urine and the reabsorption of sodium ions (Na^+) into the blood in exchange for the H^+ excreted into it. (From Thibodeau GA, Patton KT: *Anatomy and physiology,* ed 4, St. Louis, 1999, Mosby.)

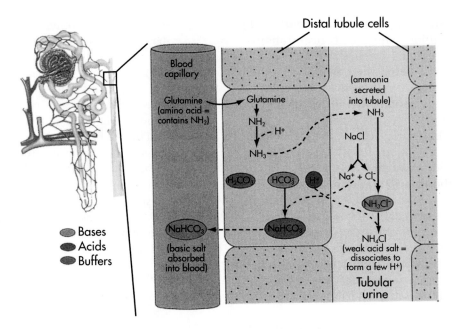

FIGURE 6-2 Acidification of urine by the tubular excretion of ammonia (NH_3). An acid (glutamine) leaves the blood, enters a tubule cell, and is deaminized to form ammonia. The ammonia is excreted into the urine, where it combines with hydrogen to form the ammonium ion (NH_4^+). In exchange for NH_4^+ the tubule cell reabsorbs Na^+. (From Thibodeau GA, Patton KT: *Anatomy and physiology*, ed 4, St. Louis, 1999, Mosby.)

4. Signs of respiratory acidosis: dyspnea, irritability, disorientation, tachycardia, cyanosis, and coma
5. Compensatory mechanisms
   a. The urinary system excretes increased hydrogen ions to compensate for the respiratory system's inability to blow off CO_2
   b. The urinary system retains sodium to facilitate the body's attempt to increase sodium bicarbonate
   c. The rate and depth of respirations increase; however, that is inefficient because the primary dysfunction involves the respiratory system
   d. With chronic hypoxia decreased oxygen levels become the stimulant to breathe; normally elevated carbon dioxide levels stimulate breathing
B. Metabolic acidosis:
   1. Base bicarbonate deficit; excess acid other than carbonic acid (a respiratory acid) accumulates beyond the body's ability to neutralize it; bicarbonate is below 22 mEq/L
   2. pH is below 7.35
   3. Common causes
      a. Cellular breakdown: e.g., starvation, terminal cancer
      b. Increased ketones: ketoacidosis, dieting

   c. Renal insufficiency: acute and chronic renal failure
   d. Direct loss of bicarbonate: loss of intestinal and pancreatic secretions via diarrhea
4. Signs of metabolic acidosis: weakness, headache, disorientation, deep rapid breathing (Kussmaul), fruity odor to the breath, nausea and vomiting, and coma
5. Compensatory mechanisms
   a. The respiratory system compensates by hyperventilation in an attempt to blow off CO_2 and raise the pH
   b. The urinary system excretes hydrogen ions to remove excess hydrogen ions and sodium is retained to help increase sodium bicarbonate
C. Respiratory alkalosis
   1. Carbonic acid deficit; hyperventilation blows off excessive CO_2; Pco_2 is less than 35 mm Hg
   2. pH is above 7.45
   3. Common causes
      a. Hyperventilation related to anxiety, panic, or hysteria
      b. Excessive mechanical ventilation
   4. Signs of respiratory alkalosis: deep, rapid breathing, lightheadedness, tingling and numbness, tinnitus, loss of concentration, and unconsciousness

5. Compensatory mechanisms: the urinary system may decrease the excretion of hydrogen ions to maintain the pH in the normal range
D. Metabolic alkalosis
   1. Base bicarbonate excess; bicarbonate is above 26 mEq/L
   2. pH is above 7.45
   3. Common causes
      a. Loss of gastric juices: e.g., vomiting, nasogastric decompression, lavage
      b. Excessive ingestion of alkaline drugs: e.g., sodium bicarbonate (baking soda)
      c. Potent diuretics may precipitate hypokalemia: in the presence of hypokalemia the kidneys conserve potassium and excrete hydrogen, intracellular potassium moves into the interstitial compartment, and hydrogen moves into cells; as a result of these processes the plasma hydrogen level is decreased and the base bicarbonate level is increased
   4. Signs of metabolic alkalosis: muscle hypertonicity (tetany), tingling, tremors, shallow and slow respirations, dizziness, confusion, and coma
   5. Compensatory mechanisms for metabolic alkalosis
      a. The respiratory system compensates by decreasing the rate and depth of breathing in an attempt to retain CO_2 and decrease the pH
      b. The urinary system excretes sodium bicarbonate

General Nursing Care of Clients with Fluid and Electrolyte Problems

A. **ASSESSMENT**
   1. Obtain history to identify etiology of fluid and electrolyte imbalances (Table 6-4)
   2. Monitor vital signs
   3. Evaluate skin turgor, hydration, and temperature
   4. Auscultate breath sounds
   5. Weigh client daily
   6. Monitor intake and output
   7. Evaluate changes in behavior, energy level, and level of consciousness
   8. Review laboratory tests: urinary specific gravity; serum pH and arterial blood gases; serum electrolytes; hematocrit; blood urea nitrogen; and creatinine clearance

B. **ANALYSIS/NURSING DIAGNOSES**
   1. Ineffective breathing pattern related to anxiety, impaired respiratory mechanics, and muscle weakness
   2. Decreased cardiac output related to cardiac dysrhythmias and electrolyte imbalances
   3. Deficient fluid volume related to diarrhea, loss of gastric contents, diaphoresis, and polyuria

4. Excess fluid volume related to anuria, decreased cardiac output, altered regulatory mechanisms and trapping of fluid in third space (extracellular fluid accumulates and is physiologically unavailable to the body)

C. **PLANNING/IMPLEMENTATION**
   1. Manage fluid and electrolyte intake
      a. Fluids may be encouraged to correct deficit (usually 3000 ml/day; may be restricted to prevent excess); 1 ounce is equal to 30 ml
      b. Nutritional intake can be increased or restricted to correct electrolyte disturbances (e.g., sodium, potassium, calcium)
   2. Administer intravenous therapy
      a. Fluids
         (1) Dextrose in water
            (a) Provides fluid and limited calories (1 L of 5% dextrose provides 170 calories)
            (b) Used to correct dehydration, ketosis, and hypernatremia
         (2) Dextrose in sodium chloride (NaCl): used to correct fluid loss from excessive perspiration or vomiting and to prevent alkalosis
         (3) NaCl: used to manage alkalosis, fluid loss, and adrenal cortical insufficiency
         (4) Ringer's solution
            (a) Contains sodium, chloride, potassium, and calcium
            (b) Used to correct dehydration from vomiting, diarrhea, or inadequate intake
         (5) Lactated Ringer's solution
            (a) Contains sodium, chloride, potassium, calcium, and lactate
            (b) Lactate is metabolized by liver and forms bicarbonate
            (c) Used to correct extracellular fluid shifts and moderate metabolic acidosis
         (6) Plasma expanders
            (a) Used to increase blood volume in trauma or burn victims
            (b) Examples: albumin, plasma, Plasmanate, dextran, and hetastarch
            (c) Need to be administered slowly
      b. Regulation of intravenous flow rates
         (1) Manual regulation of gravity flow with clamp

$$\text{Per minute drop rate} = \frac{\text{Milliliters to be infused} \times \text{drop factor (drops per 1 ml)}}{\text{Number of hours} \times 60 \text{ minutes}}$$

         (2) Use of infusion pump or controller

TABLE 6-4   Etiology, manifestations, and treatment of major fluid and electrolyte imbalances

Fluid/electrolyte imbalance	Etiology	Signs and symptoms	Treatment
Extracellular fluid deficit	Decreased fluid intake Prolonged fever Vomiting Excessive use of diuretics	Increased thirst Dry skin and mucous membranes Increased temperature Flushed skin Rapid, thready pulse Increased Hct, Na^+, and specific gravity	Administration of hypotonic or isotonic fluids
Extracellular fluid excess	Heart failure Liver disease Malnutrition (decreased plasma protein) Renal disease Excessive parenteral fluids	Weight gain Crackles Edema Ascites Confusion Weakness Decreased Hct	Administration of diuretics Fluid restriction
Hypokalemia	Diarrhea Vomiting Diabetic acidosis Diuretics Inadequate intake	Loss of muscle tone Cardiac dysrhythmias Abdominal distension Vomiting Decreased serum K^+	Parenteral/oral administration of potassium supplement Increased dietary intake of potassium
Hyperkalemia	Advanced kidney disease Severe burns or tissue trauma Excessive dosages of potassium	Cardiac irregularities Weakness Diarrhea Nausea Irritability Increased serum K^+	Administration of potassium-free fluids Dialysis Potassium-removing resin
Hyponatremia	Diuretics Electrolyte-free IV fluids Diarrhea GI suction Excessive perspiration followed by increased water intake	Abdominal cramps Convulsions Oliguria Decreased serum Na^+ and specific gravity	Administration of IV solutions containing NaCl Administration of NaCl tablets
Hypernatremia	Diabetes insipidus Excess NaCl IV fluid intake	Dry, sticky mucous membranes Oliguria Firm tissue turgor Dry tongue Increased serum Na^+ and specific gravity	Low Na^+ diet Increased Na^+-free fluid intake
Hypocalcemia	Removal of parathyroid glands Administration of electrolyte-free solutions	Tingling of extremities Tetany Cramps Convulsions	Oral/parenteral calcium replacement
Hypercalcemia	Hyperparathyroidism Prolonged immobility Excessive intake of Ca^+ or vitamin D	Flank pain (renal calculi) Deep bone pain Relaxed muscles	Correction of primary problem Increased fluid intake

(a) Drop control: usually drops per minute (follow manufacturer's instructions when setting desired rate of flow)

(b) Volume control: usually milliliters per hour (follow manufacturer's instructions when setting desired rate of flow)

c. Monitor client for complications

(1) Infiltration

(a) Catheter is displaced, allowing fluid to leak into tissues

(b) Insertion site is pale, cool, and edematous; flow rate decreases

(c) IV must be removed and restarted in a new site

(2) Phlebitis

(a) Vein is irritated by catheter or medications

(b) Insertion site is red, painful, and warm; flow rate is decreased

(c) IV must be removed and restarted in a new site; warm compresses are applied to inflammation

(3) Circulatory overload

(a) Flow rate exceeds cardiovascular system's capability to adjust to the increased fluid volume

(b) Client exhibits dyspnea, crackles, distended neck veins, and increased blood pressure

(c) Rate is decreased to keep the vein open; physician is notified and diuretics, if prescribed, are administered

(4) Infection

(a) Change of solution bag every 24 hours because risk of contamination is increased after this time

(b) Client exhibits signs of inflammation at insertion site, lymphatic streaking, and fever

3. Administer pharmacologic agents

a. Diuretics (e.g., thiazide, potassium-sparing, loop, or osmotic diuretics)

b. Electrolyte replacement (e.g., sodium chloride, potassium chloride, calcium gluconate)

c. Potassium-removing resin: sodium polystyrene sulfonate (Kayexalate)

4. Provide care (e.g., skin care, safe environment) based on specific clinical findings

D. EVALUATION/OUTCOMES

1. Maintains fluid balance

2. Maintains serum electrolyte levels within normal limits

3. Maintains vital signs within normal limits

PERIOPERATIVE CARE

 ## PHARMACOLOGY RELATED TO PERIOPERATIVE CARE

General Anesthetics

A. Description

1. Used in a "balanced" combination to produce varying levels of loss of consciousness, pain control, and/or skeletal muscle relaxation

2. Depress the CNS through a progressive sequence (4 stages)

3. Paralyzing agents: inhibit transmission of nerve impulses by binding with cholinergic receptor sites, antagonizing action of acetylcholine

4. Available in parenteral (IM, IV) and inhalation preparations; ultrashort-acting IV barbiturates are useful in the induction of anesthesia because they quickly penetrate the blood-brain barrier; IV and IM nonbarbiturates produce a special type of anesthesia in which the client appears to be awake but dissociated from the environment, resulting in amnesia for the surgical experience

B. Examples

1. Inhalation anesthetics: halothane (Fluothane); nitrous oxide

2. IV barbiturates: high lipoid affinity provides prompt effect on cerebral tissue

a. Methohexital sodium (Brevital)

b. Thiopental sodium (Pentothal)

3. IV and IM nonbarbiturates: induce a cataleptic state and produce amnesia for the procedure

a. Midazolam HCl (Versed)

b. Combination product: fentanyl (Sublimaze) and droperidol (Innovar)

4. Conscious sedation: uses IV or nasal routes of sedation to depress consciousness but maintains airway and ventilations (e.g., midazolam [Versed], ketamine [Ketalar], and fentanyl [Sublimaze])

5. Paralyzing agents

a. Pancuronium (Pavulon)

b. Succinylcholine chloride (Anectine)

C. Major side effects

1. Inhalation anesthetics

a. Excitement and restlessness (initial CNS stimulation)

b. Nausea and vomiting (stimulation of chemoreceptor trigger zone in medullary vomiting center)

c. Respiratory distress (depression of medullary respiratory center)

2. IV barbiturates

a. Respiratory depression (depression of medullary respiratory center)

b. Hypotension and tachycardia (depression of cardiovascular system)

c. Laryngospasm (depression of laryngeal reflex)

3. IV and IM nonbarbiturates

a. Respiratory failure (depression of medullary respiratory center)

b. Changes in blood pressure: hypertension; hypotension (alterations in cardiovascular system)

c. Rigidity (enhancement of muscle tone)

d. Psychic disturbances (emergence reaction-recovery period)

4. Paralyzing agents

a. Hypotension (increased vagal stimulation; increased release of histamine; ganglionic blockade)

b. Respiratory depression (neuromuscular blockade)

c. Dysrhythmias (increased vagal stimulation)

D. Nursing care

1. Assess for allergies and other medical problems that could alter the client's response to the anesthetic agents

2. Have O_2 and emergency resuscitative equipment available

3. Assess vital signs before, during, and after anesthetic administration

4. Maintain a calm environment during induction of anesthesia

5. Use safety precautions with flammable agents

6. Protect client during this period because of decreased sensory awareness

7. Judiciously administer narcotics (opioids) in the initial postanesthetic period

8. Provide care for the client receiving a paralyzing agent

a. Administer sedation; have O_2 and emergency resuscitative equipment available

b. Assess vital signs before, during, and after administration

c. Administer under direct medical supervision

Local Anesthetics

A. Description

1. Used to produce pain control without rendering the client unconscious; useful for obstetric, dental, and minor surgical procedures; block nerve impulse conduction in sensory, motor, and autonomic nerve cells by decreasing nerve membrane permeability to sodium ion influx

2. Available in topical, spinal, regional, and nerve block preparations; epinephrine may be added to enhance the duration of the local anesthetic effect

B. Examples

1. Topical: local infiltration of tissue (e.g., benzocaine; lidocaine HCl [Xylocaine], also used for nerve block; tetracaine HCl [Pontocaine], also used for spinal anesthesia and nerve block)

2. Spinal: injected into the spinal subarachnoid space (e.g., lidocaine HCl [Xylocaine]; procaine HCl [Novocain], also used for nerve block)

3. Epidural: injected into the epidural space of the spinal column (e.g., bupivacaine HCl [Marcaine]; lidocaine HCl [Xylocaine])

4. Nerve block: injected at perineural site distant from desired anesthesia site (e.g., bupivacaine HCl [Marcaine]; chloroprocaine HCl [Nesacaine]; mepivacaine HCl [Carbocaine])

C. Major side effects

1. Allergic reactions; anaphylaxis (hypersensitivity)

2. Respiratory arrest (depression of medullary respiratory center)

3. Dysrhythmias; cardiac arrest (depression of cardiovascular system)

4. Convulsions (depression of central nervous system)

5. Hypotension (depression of cardiovascular system)

D. Nursing care

1. Assess for allergies and other medical problems that could alter the client's response to the anesthetic agent

2. Have O_2 and emergency resuscitative equipment available

3. Assess vital signs before, during, and after anesthetic administration

4. Protect anesthetized body parts from mechanical and/or thermal injury

5. Maintain a calm environment while the client is anesthetized

6. Keep client flat for a specified period (usually 6 to 12 hours) after spinal anesthesia to prevent severe headache; avoid pillows; monitor for hypotension

7. Use safety precautions (side rails up) and maintain bed rest until sensation returns to lower extremities after spinal anesthesia

8. Maintain side-lying position to prevent aspiration after general anesthesia

9. Restrict oral intake after client has had general anesthesia until ability to swallow has returned

Sedatives/Hypnotics

A. Description

1. Used for clients experiencing anxiety-related situations and insomnia

2. Act by depressing the CNS; produce sedation in small doses and sleep in larger doses

3. Available in oral, parenteral (IV, IM), and rectal preparations
B. Examples
 1. Barbiturates: depress CNS starting with diencephalon; amobarbital (Amytal), pentobarbital sodium (Nembutal), secobarbital (Seconal)
 2. Nonbarbiturates: depress CNS and relax skeletal muscles; chloral hydrate (Noctec), temazepam (Restoril)
C. Major side effects
 1. Drowsiness (depression of CNS)
 2. Hypotension (depression of cardiovascular system)
 3. Dizziness (hypotension)
 4. Gastrointestinal irritation (local oral effect)
 5. Skin rash (hypersensitivity)
 6. Blood disorders (hematologic alterations)
 7. Drug dependence
 8. Barbiturates
  a. Hangover (persistence of low barbiturate concentration in body caused by decreased metabolism)
  b. Photosensitivity (hypersensitivity)
  c. Excitement in children and elderly (paradoxic reaction)
D. Nursing care
 1. Avoid administration with other CNS depressants
 2. Caution client to avoid engaging in hazardous activity; avoid concurrent use of alcohol
 3. Assess for signs of dependence
 4. Use safety precautions at night for hospitalized clients
 5. Implement supportive measures to promote sleep (back rub; warm milk)
 6. Instruct client to avoid placing medication within reach to prevent possible overdose while drowsy
 7. Monitor blood work during long-term therapy
 8. Administer controlled substances according to appropriate schedule restrictions

CLASSIFICATION OF SURGERY

A. Surgery may be classified as elective, diagnostic, urgent (emergency), ablative, palliative, or curative
B. Ambulatory surgery
 1. Hospital-based outpatient settings
  a. Diagnostic workup in hospital several days before surgery
  b. Direct admission to the ambulatory surgical unit
  c. Discharged from the postanesthesia or clinical unit the same day as the surgery is performed; if complications occur, the client is admitted to the hospital

 2. Private surgical offices
  a. Surgical procedures are performed in a private office, which has a surgical suite and surgical staff
  b. Preoperative workup is performed by hospital, physician, or clinic before surgery
C. Inpatient surgical care: client is admitted to the hospital setting for surgical care

General Nursing Care of Clients During the Preoperative and Intraoperative Periods

A. ASSESSMENT
 1. Obtain history of current health problems and factors that may influence recovery
 2. Perform physical assessment to identify potential health problems
 3. Determine client's understanding of disease and treatment plan
 4. Identify client's emotional state and coping skills
B. ANALYSIS/NURSING DIAGNOSES
 1. Fear related to surgical procedure
 2. Anxiety related to prognosis and lack of knowledge
 3. Disturbed sleep pattern related to anxiety
 4. Risk for injury related to perioperative positioning
 5. Risk for injury related to lowered level of consciousness
C. PLANNING/IMPLEMENTATION
 1. Explain all procedures to the client and give reasons for them
 2. Explain to the client what to expect in the operating room, postanesthesia unit, and/or intensive care units, including use of anticipated equipment
 3. Allow the client and family time to ask questions about procedures and surgery
 4. Determine the client's level of understanding of operative procedure to ascertain whether signature on permit represents informed consent
 5. Allow and encourage the client to ventilate feelings about diagnosis and surgery
 6. Provide a spiritual counselor if desired by the client or family
 7. Teach the client the activities that will be instituted after surgery related to ventilatory function: diaphragmatic breathing, coughing, incentive spirometry, splinting, and turning
 8. Teach the client physical exercises that will be used to promote circulation after surgery: leg exercises (dorsiflexion, plantar flexion, eversion, inversion), ambulation routines, isometric exercises
 9. Inform the client to expect some discomfort after surgery and teach importance of requesting medication for pain or using patient-controlled analgesia

10. Make certain that history, physical examination results, recent laboratory tests, and chest x-ray report are entered on the chart
11. Inform all members of the medical team of the client's allergies and other health problems and prominently mark the chart
12. Implement preoperative preparation orders: e.g., enemas (often until clear returns), douches, medications for bowel surgery
13. Inform the client not to take anything by mouth after midnight the night before surgery; remove fluid from the bedside unit
14. Provide care for the client on the day of surgery
    a. Before surgery check the client's vital signs and assess overall physical status; record and report any deviations to physician
    b. Before surgery assess the client's emotional status; notify the physician if the client expresses an impending sense of doom
    c. Complete the preoperative checklist: includes preoperative tests and identification and allergy bands
    d. Provide hygiene and have the client void
    e. Remove any prosthetics such as dentures, contact lenses, and wigs
    f. Apply antiembolic stockings as ordered
    g. Arrange for insertion of any tubes as ordered: nasogastric tube, indwelling urinary catheter, intravenous line
    h. Administer prescribed preoperative medications as ordered: e.g., antianxiety agents, sedatives, narcotic analgesics, anticholinergics
    i. Put side rails up after administering medications
15. Provide care for the client in the operative suite
    a. Assume role of client advocate during the intraoperative phase
    b. Complete preoperative checklist
    c. Perform skin preps as ordered: e.g., shaving, scrubs
    d. Transfer client to the operating room; a laminar airflow room is often used for orthopedic surgery
    e. Apply monitoring devices as needed
    f. Allay client's anxiety; ambulatory surgical clients remain aware during most of their stay in the operating room because local anesthetics are frequently used
    g. Anesthesia is introduced to produce four stages of anesthesia
       (1) Stage 1: Client becomes drowsy and loses consciousness
       (2) Stage 2: Stage of excitement; muscles are tense, breathing may be irregular
       (3) Stage 3: Depression of vital signs and reflexes; operation begins during this phase
       (4) Stage 4: Complete respiratory depression
    h. Position and drape client for surgery

D. **EVALUATION/OUTCOMES**
1. Verbalizes fears concerning operative process
2. Controls long-standing health problems
3. Demonstrates an understanding of preoperative teaching
4. Remains free from injury

General Nursing Care of Clients During The Postoperative Period

A. **ASSESSMENT**
1. Verify patency of airway
2. Establish baseline vital signs, breath sounds
3. Determine level of consciousness
4. Observe tubes for patency and placement and drainage for characteristics
5. Inspect dressing if present; observe for spitting up or vomiting of blood with oral or nasal surgery
6. Determine if client has sufficient urinary output
7. Assess for signs of normal wound healing after initial postoperative period

B. **ANALYSIS/NURSING DIAGNOSES**
1. Ineffective airway clearance related to prolonged sedation
2. Risk for aspiration related to reduced level of consciousness
3. Ineffective breathing pattern related to incisional pain
4. Constipation related to decreased peristalsis
5. Fear related to surgical procedure and prognosis
6. Risk for deficient fluid volume related to inadequate intake, wound drainage, and gastric decompression
7. Hyperthermia related to inflammatory process
8. Risk for infection related to surgical wound
9. Risk for injury related to anesthesia and sedation
10. Pain related to surgical incision
11. Disturbed sleep pattern related to anxiety and pain
12. Urinary retention related to effects of anesthesia

C. **PLANNING/IMPLEMENTATION**
1. Provide immediate care
   a. Respiratory needs: anesthesia depresses respiratory function
      (1) Maintain a patent airway by keeping the artificial airway in place until gag reflex returns; suction before removal to clear mucous plugs and secretions as needed

(2) Position client on one side with neck slightly extended to prevent aspiration and accumulation of mucous secretions

(3) Monitor the rate, rhythm, symmetry of chest movement, breath sounds, pulse oximeter, behavior, and color of mucous membranes

(4) Suction artificial airway and the oral cavity as needed to remove secretions

(5) Administer oxygen as ordered or needed

(6) Encourage coughing and deep breathing as soon as the client is able to cooperate

b. Circulatory needs: anesthesia and immobilization during surgery may result in circulatory compromise

(1) Monitor the heart rate and rhythm as well as the blood pressure at frequent intervals, approximately every 15 minutes

(2) Monitor peripheral circulation by noting the color, temperature, capillary refill, and presence of pulses to ensure tissue perfusion

(3) Monitor for hemorrhage by measuring blood pressure for hypotension and observing and measuring wound drainage; report signs of hemorrhage immediately

c. Neurologic needs: medications and anesthetic agents depress the central nervous system

(1) Monitor the client's level of consciousness

(2) Monitor pupillary blink and gag reflexes

(3) Monitor motor and sensory status of extremities

(4) Call client by name; reorient to time, place, and situation

(5) Answer questions as honestly and simply as possible; repeat as needed

d. Wound care

(1) Note the location of the wound and the color, odor, amount, and consistency of drainage

(2) Circle drainage on the dressing to allow for objective assessment

(3) Reinforce postoperative dressings because surgeons generally perform the first dressing change

e. Care of drains and tubes

(1) Maintain patency of tubing (e.g., gravity, negative pressure, instillation, or irrigation as indicated)

(2) Attach tubing to appropriate collection containers; maintain negative pressure in portable wound drainage systems (e.g., empty when half full and compress before closing port)

(3) Monitor output of drains for amount and color

f. Fluid and electrolyte needs

(1) Maintain intravenous therapy as ordered

(2) Record intake and output accurately

(3) Monitor for electrolyte imbalances

g. Comfort needs

(1) Assess the client's pain (e.g., location, intensity, duration, precipitating factors, and effectiveness of pain management)

(2) Medicate as ordered to reduce pain and increase postoperative compliance with breathing, coughing, and activity regimens

(3) Teach client how to use patient-controlled analgesia (PCA)

2. Provide care for the ambulatory surgical client

a. All care included under immediate postoperative care applies to the ambulatory surgical client

b. When the client is responsive, encourage sips of water and ambulate to chair

c. Provide a light meal when tolerated

d. When the client is stable, has retained foods, and has voided, reinforce postoperative teaching and discharge planning with client and family members; evaluate understanding of teaching

3. Provide care for the inpatient surgical client

a. Protect the client from injury

b. Turn frequently; encourage deep breathing and coughing and use of incentive spirometer to prevent the development of atelectasis or hypostatic pneumonia; assess for diminished breath sounds in lower lobes of lung

c. Perform or encourage range of motion and isometric exercises and early ambulation to prevent phlebitis, paralytic ileus, and circulatory stasis; notify physician if complications occur

d. Maintain patency of tubing (e.g., urinary catheter, gastric tube, T-tube, chest tubes, incisional drains) to promote drainage and maintain decompression to reduce pressure on suture line

e. Use aseptic technique when changing dressings or as necessary when irrigating tubing or emptying portable wound drainage systems to prevent infection

f. Monitor intake and output to prevent dehydration, electrolyte imbalance, and urinary suppression or retention; encourage client to void; provide privacy

g. Assess for urinary retention; client must void in 8 to 12 hours following surgery or a catheter is inserted

h. Observe for abdominal distention; ambulation, rectal tube (usually for 30 minutes), or Harris flush may be ordered

i. Administer medication for pain as ordered to prevent discomfort and restlessness

j. Regulate IV therapy to prevent overload or circulatory collapse

k. Encourage the client to support and splint the incisional site when coughing, moving, or turning to prevent tension on the suture line

l. Position the client as required by type of surgery to prevent misalignment and prevent accumulation of fluid or blockage of the drainage tubes

m. Provide emotional support; assist client to cope with changes in body image

4. Provide for nutritional needs

a. Maintain IV therapy to provide water and electrolytes

b. Monitor parenteral nutrition (total parenteral nutrition [TPN] and peripheral parenteral nutrition [PPN]); parenteral nutrition is of high nutrient density; solutions of amino acids, glucose, electrolytes, minerals, vitamins; fat emulsions (intralipids); TPN usually inserted into larger veins (inferior or superior vena cava) to avoid thrombosis in peripheral veins; used in clients with major tissue trauma, injury, or extensive surgery

c. Gradually increase oral intake as permitted

(1) Liquid diets

(a) Clear liquid: clear broth, bouillon, juices, plain gelatin, fruit-flavored water, ices, ginger ale, coffee, tea

(b) Full liquid: may add milk and items made with milk, such as cream soups, milk drinks, sherbet, ice cream, puddings, custard

(2) Soft diet: may add all soft, cooked foods, such as refined cereals; pasta; rice; white bread and crackers; eggs; cheese; meat; potatoes; cooked whole vegetables; cooked fruits; few soft ripe, plain fruits without membranes or skins; simple desserts

(3) Regular diet: full, well-balanced diet of all foods as desired and tolerated

d. Provide for special nutritional needs

(1) Protein: increased need caused by protein losses and the anabolism of recovery and tissue healing; approximate requirement for adult is 1.2 to 2 g/kg/day

(2) Calories: adequate amount to supply energy and spare protein for tissue building

(3) Vitamins and minerals: need for most will be increased following surgery and the nutrition program must be designed to ensure that individual requirements are met: zinc increases the strength of the healing wound (4 to 6 mg/day recommended); vitamin C required for collagen formation (500 to 1000 mg/day recommended)

D. EVALUATION/OUTCOMES

1. Avoids respiratory complications
2. Remains free of infection
3. Experiences relief of pain
4. Maintains fluid balance
5. Reestablishes urinary function
6. Reestablishes bowel function
7. Demonstrates ability to care for self
8. Copes with changes resulting from surgery

NEOPLASTIC DISORDERS

CLASSIFICATION OF NEOPLASMS

A. Benign neoplasia

1. Cells adhere to each other and the growth remains circumscribed
2. Generally not life threatening unless they occur in a restricted area (e.g., skull)
3. Classified according to the tissue involved, e.g., glandular tissue (adenoma), bone (osteoma), nerve cells (neuroma), fibrous tissue (fibroma)

B. Malignant neoplasia

1. Cells infiltrate surrounding tissue
2. Cells invade other tissues and produce secondary lesions
3. May spread (metastasize) by direct extension, lymphatic permeation and embolization, and diffusion of cancer cells by mechanical means
4. Tumors are classified according to the tissue involved, e.g., glandular epithelial tissue (adenocarcinoma), epithelial surface tissue (carcinoma), connective tissue (sarcoma), melanocytes (melanoma)
5. Tumors are often classified by a universal system of staging classification, the TNM system

a. T designates a primary tumor
b. N designates lymph node involvement
c. M designates metastasis
d. A 0 to 4 after any of the above letters designates degree of involvement
e. TIS designates carcinoma in situ or one that is noninfiltrating

RELATED PHARMACOLOGY

Basic Concepts

A. Used to destroy malignant cells by interfering with reproduction of the cancer cell
B. Act at specific points in the cycle of cell division (cell-cycle specific) or at any phase of the cycle of cell division (cell-cycle nonspecific)
C. Affect any rapidly dividing cell within the body, thus having the potential for toxicity development in healthy, functional tissue (bone marrow, hair follicles, GI mucosa); to reduce the possibility of toxicity, combination therapy is often used
D. Available in oral, parenteral (IM, SC, IV), intraarterial, intrathecal, and topical preparations

Antineoplastic Drugs

Alkalating agents

A. Cell-cycle nonspecific; attack the DNA of rapidly dividing cells
B. Examples:
   1. Nitrosourea: carmustine (BCNU)
   2. Nitrogen mustard: chlorambucil (Leukeran), cyclophosphamide (Cytoxan)
   3. Inorganic heavy metal: cisplatin (Platinol)

Anthracyclines

A. Cell-cycle nonspecific; interfere with DNA and RNA synthesis
B. Examples: doxorubicin (Doxil)

Vinca alkaloids

A. Cell-cycle specific; work during "M" phase; interfere with mitosis
B. Examples: vincristine (Oncovin), vinblastine (Velban)

Antibiotics

A. Cell-cycle specific; inhibit RNA and protein synthesis of rapidly dividing tissue
B. Examples: doxorubicin hydrochloride (Adriamycin), mithramycin (Mithracin)

Antimetabolites

A. Cell-cycle specific; inhibit protein synthesis in rapidly dividing cells during "S" phase
B. Examples: azathioprine (Imuran), fluorouracil (5-FU), hydroxyurea (Hydrea), methotrexate (Mexate)

Hormones

A. Tissue specific; inhibit RNA and protein synthesis in tissues that are dependent on the opposite (sex) hormone for development
B. Examples: androgens, estrogens (estramustine phosphate sodium [Emcyt]), progestins, steroids (prednisone [Meticorten]), and hormone antagonists such as mitotane (Lysodren), a cortisol antagonist, and tamoxifen citrate (Nolvadex), an estrogen antagonist

Immune agents

A. Involve introduction of noncancerous antigens or other agents into the body to stimulate production of lymphocytes and antibodies
B. Examples
   1. Bacillus Calmette-Guérin (BCG) vaccine: provides active immunity
   2. Interferon alfa-2a (Roferon-A), interferon alfa-2b (Intron A): suppresses cell proliferation
   3. Filgrastim (Neupogen): granulocyte colony-stimulating factor

Miscellaneous agents

A. Leucovorin calcium: a reduced form of folic acid; acts as an antidote to folic acid antagonists
B. Paclitaxel (Taxol): inhibits the reorganization of the microtubule network that is needed for interphase and mitotic cellular functions and causes abnormal bundles of microtubules during cell cycle and multiple esters of microtubules during mitosis

Common combinations of neoplastic agents

A. ABVD: doxorubicin hydrochloride (Adriamycin), bleomycin sulfate (Blenoxane), vinblastine sulfate (Velban), dacarbazine (DTIC-Dome)
B. CHOP: cyclophosphamide (Cytoxan), doxorubicin hydrochloride (Adriamycin), vincristine sulfate (Oncovin), prednisone
C. CMF (referred to as CMFP when prednisone is included): cyclophosphamide (Cytoxan), methotrexate (Mexate), fluorouracil (5-FU)
D. COPP (referred to as A-COPP when Adriamycin is included): cyclophosphamide (Cytoxan), vincristine sulfate (Oncovin), procarbazine hydrochloride (Matulane), prednisone
E. CVP: cyclophosphamide (Cytoxan), vincristine sulfate (Oncovin), prednisone
F. FAC: fluorouracil (5-FU), doxorubicin hydrochloride (Adriamycin), cyclophosphamide (Cytoxan)
G. MOPP: mechlorethamine hydrochloride (nitrogen mustard, Mustargen), vincristine sulfate (Oncovin), procarbazine hydrochloride (Matulane), prednisone
H. VAC: vincristine sulfate (Oncovin), dactinomycin (Actinomycin D), cyclophosphamide (Cytoxan)

Major side effects

A. Anorexia, nausea, vomiting, stomatitis (irritation of GI tract; quick uptake by rapidly dividing alimentary tract tissue)
B. Diarrhea (irritation of GI tract; quick uptake by rapidly dividing alimentary tract tissue)
C. Bone marrow depression (quick uptake by rapidly dividing myeloid tissue)
D. Blood dyscrasias (bone marrow depression)
E. Alopecia (rapid uptake by rapidly dividing hair follicle cells)
F. CNS disturbances (neurotoxicity)
G. Hepatic disturbances (hepatotoxicity)
H. Hyperuricemia (release of large quantities of breakdown products—uric acid)
I. Kidney failure (direct kidney toxic effect)
J. Doxorubicin: cardiac toxicity (direct toxic effect)
K. BCG: allergic reactions, anaphylaxis

RADIATION

Purpose

A. Diagnosis
B. Treatment: curative, palliative, adjuvant (used in conjunction with chemotherapy or surgery)

Examples

A. Alpha particle: fast-moving helium nucleus; slight penetration
B. Beta particle: fast-moving electron; moderate penetration
C. Gamma ray: similar to light ray; high penetration
D. Gold (^{198}Au): effective for ascites; pleural effusions
E. Sodium iodide (^{131}I): effective for thyroid gland
F. Sodium phosphate (^{32}P): effective for erythrocytes

Major Side Effects

A. Localized skin irritation
B. Vary based on site
   1. Gastrointestinal tract: nausea, vomiting, diarrhea
   2. Gonads: temporary or permanent sterility
   3. Bone marrow: leukopenia, thrombocytopenia, anemia
   4. Respiratory tract: pneumonitis
   5. Genitourinary tract: cystitis

Methods of Delivery

A. External beam radiotherapy or teletherapy delivers radiation to a tumor by means of an external machine (cobalt or linear accelerator) at a predetermined distance
B. Internal radiation therapy or brachytherapy delivers radiation by systemic, interstitial, or intracavity means
   1. Systemic (metabolized) involves administration by intravenous or oral routes
   2. Interstitial involves implantation of needles, wires, or seeds into the tissue
   3. Intracavity radiation involves placing an implant into a body cavity and may require a surgical procedure

BONE MARROW TRANSPLANTATION

Purpose

A. Treatment of hematologic cancer
B. Treatment of certain solid tumor recurrences that require ablative chemotherapy, which destroys bone marrow

Types

A. Autologous: bone marrow is removed from the client and reinfused after high-dose chemotherapy
B. Allogenic: bone marrow from a donor with compatible human leukocyte antigen (HLA); infused after the client's own bone marrow is destroyed by chemotherapy or radiation
C. Syngeneic: bone marrow is obtained from an identical twin
D. Peripheral stem cell transplantation: after stem cell production is stimulated by administration of growth factor, cells are collected by apheresis and reinfused after high-dose chemotherapy

Major Side Effects

A. Infection, fever, chill
B. Cutaneous reactions
C. Gastrointestinal: nausea, vomiting, diarrhea
D. Cardiovascular: hypotension, hypertension, tachycardia, chest pain, bleeding
E. Respiratory: shortness of breath, pneumonia

General Nursing Care of Clients with Neoplastic Disorders Receiving Either Chemotherapy or Radiation Therapy

A. **ASSESSMENT**
   1. Obtain a description of onset and progression of symptoms
   2. Perform physical assessment to determine general state of health and nutrition
   3. Determine client's understanding of disease and treatment plan
B. **ANALYSIS/NURSING DIAGNOSES**
   1. Decisional conflict (choice or continuation of treatment modality) related to values and beliefs
   2. Fatigue related to depletion of body reserve, therapy, and increased metabolic rate
   3. Fear related to dependency, intractable pain, and death
   4. Risk for infection related to altered immune response
   5. Imbalanced nutrition: less than body requirements related to disease process and therapeutic modalities
   6. Impaired oral mucous membrane related to disease process and therapeutic modalities
   7. Pain related to disease process and therapeutic modalities
   8. Powerlessness related to diagnosis and prognosis
   9. Impaired tissue integrity related to treatment modalities
C. **PLANNING/IMPLEMENTATION**
   1. Instruct client regarding special measures to limit infection; instruct client to report temperature higher than 100° F (37.7° C)
   2. Teach client special measures to limit injury (e.g., gentle oral hygiene, prevention of pathologic fractures)

3. Explain side effects that influence appearance and encourage positive adaptations (e.g., purchase of wigs, scarves, hats)
4. Implement measures to reduce or eliminate nausea such as antiemetics, hypnosis, relaxation modalities, small frequent feedings, adjustment of meal times in relation to therapy, avoidance of spicy foods
5. Monitor blood work during therapy
   a. White blood cells, red blood cells, platelets
   b. Tumor markers: alpha-fetoprotein—liver, testes; CA-125—gastrointestinal, ovaries; carcinoembryonic antigen (CEA)—breast, colon, lung; prostatic specific antigen (PSA)—prostate
6. Administer prescribed colony-stimulating factors to stimulate the production of white and red blood cells (e.g., erythropoietin, human granulocyte colony-stimulating factors)
7. Offer emotional support to client and family; answer questions and encourage verbalization of fears
8. Encourage conservation of client's decreasing energy
9. Encourage client to enroll in American Cancer Society's "Look Good, Feel Better" program
10. Support natural defense mechanisms of client; encourage intake of foods rich in the immune-stimulating nutrients, especially vitamins A, C, and E, and the mineral selenium, which is found in whole grains and seeds
11. Encourage optimal intake of high-nutrient–density foods; bland or mechanical soft diet may be indicated if stomatitis exists; routinely monitor weight
12. Encourage women of childbearing age to use birth control measures while receiving therapy because of mutagenic/teratogenic effects; avoid use of birth control pill
13. Counsel male clients regarding use of sperm bank if permanent infertility may result
14. Keep client well hydrated (3000 ml/24 hr); monitor intake and output
15. Assess client for pain; administer analgesics or antidepressant to control the pain; provide for client comfort
16. Encourage client to become involved in decision making; support client's decisions whenever possible, even if they differ from the nurse's philosophy
17. Specific care for clients receiving chemotherapy
   a. Monitor intravenous infusion site for infiltration to prevent local tissue necrosis
   b. Follow established protocols for handling chemotherapeutic agents and equipment to minimize exposure of the nurse

   c. Institute protective isolation if WBCs are low
   d. Wear double gloves when handling urine and other excretions
   e. Observe for signs of bleeding; avoid anticoagulants because of decreased platelets
   f. Avoid use of rectal thermometers, enemas, IM injections, and razor blades because of increased bleeding tendency
   g. Monitor renal function for nephrotoxicity
   h. Monitor vital signs; monitor for cardiac toxicity
   i. Encourage client to check with physician before consuming over-the-counter drugs, such as aspirin; avoid alcohol
18. Specific care for clients receiving external radiation
   a. Avoid washing off the port marks
   b. Assess skin for erythema, dryness, burning; avoid creams, soaps, powders, and deodorants in the area during the treatment periods
   c. Instruct client to wear loose-fitting cotton clothing; protect skin from sunlight
   d. Apply a nonadherent dressing to areas of skin breakdown
   e. Reassure others that the client will not be a source of radiation
19. Specific care for clients receiving internal radiation
   a. Avoid overexposure to the client and use the principles of time, distance, and shielding; supervise exposure of staff and visitors; use dosimeter badges to monitor exposure
   b. Postpone routine hygiene while implant is in place
   c. Prevent dislodgement of intracavity radiation implants; bed rest, urinary retention catheter, low-residue diet, antidiarrheal agents
   d. Ascertain if body excreta has to be placed in lead containers for disposal when systemic (metabolized) radiation is used
   e. Store radioactive material in lead containers to prevent contamination of the environment

D. EVALUATION/OUTCOMES
1. Remains free from infection
2. Verbalizes feelings about disease and treatment
3. Maintains skin integrity
4. Consumes nutritionally adequate diet
5. Verbalizes details concerning self-care related to treatment regimen

EMERGENCY SITUATIONS

FIRST AID

A. Maintain or establish the ABCs
   1. Airway

2. Breathing
3. Circulation

B. Provide for physical safety
  1. Remove client from immediate danger
  2. Control bleeding
  3. Avoid unnecessary movement of spinal column or extremities; use neck brace and back board
  4. Control pain
  5. Monitor level of consciousness

C. Establish priority for care
  1. Triage: system of client evaluation to establish priorities and assign appropriate treatment or personnel
  2. Determination of priority
    a. Emergency situations: greatest risk receives priority
    b. Major disasters: classification based on principles to benefit the largest number; those requiring highly specialized care may be given minimal or no care; those requiring minimal care to save their lives or to be available to help others should be treated first

D. Offer psychologic support
  1. Reduce panic to prevent its spread
  2. Establish and maintain open communication with the client and family to mediate feelings of loss of control
  3. Allow contact between the client and family as soon as feasible

Specific Emergencies

A. Near-drowning
  1. Assessment
    a. Possible airway obstruction from bronchospasm
    b. Adventitious or absent breath sounds
    c. Hypoxia, hypercarbia, and acidosis
    d. Possible pulmonary edema
      (1) Salt water: high osmotic pressure of aspirated water draws additional fluid into alveolar spaces from the vascular bed
      (2) Fresh water: removes surfactant, leading to alveolar collapse
  2. Treatment and nursing care
    a. Establish an airway and ventilate with 100% oxygen and positive pressure
    b. Correct the acidosis
    c. Insert a nasogastric tube and decompress the stomach to prevent aspiration of gastric contents
    d. Treat pulmonary edema and hypothermia if present

B. Heatstroke
  1. Assessment

    a. Risk factors: advanced age, strenuous exercise in heat, medications such as anticholinergics that interfere with perspiring
    b. Hot, dry, flushed skin progressing to pallor in late circulatory collapse
    c. Elevation of body temperature above 105° F (40.5° C)
    d. Complaints of dizziness, nausea, and headaches
    e. Convulsions
    f. Altered level of consciousness
  2. Treatment and nursing care
    a. Rapidly reduce temperature: hypothermia blanket, cool-water baths, and cool enemas
    b. Administer oxygen to meet increased metabolic demands
    c. Institute seizure precautions

C. Hypothermia
  1. Assessment
    a. Risk factors: exposure to cold; submersion in cold water; age (elderly and very young)
    b. Local (frostbite): pallor, paresthesia, pain to absence of sensation of involved body part
    c. Systemic: core temperature less than 94° F (34.4° C), weak and irregular pulse, decreased level of consciousness
  2. Treatment and nursing care
    a. Monitor core temperature
    b. Continually assess cardiac status, arterial blood gases, electrolytes, glucose, and blood urea nitrogen (BUN)
    c. Rewarm: to prevent cardiovascular collapse, core rewarming with heated oxygen and/or irrigations must precede surface rewarming
    d. Correct fluid and electrolyte imbalances

CIRCULATORY SYSTEM

REVIEW OF ANATOMY AND PHYSIOLOGY

Functions of the Circulatory System

A. Primary function: transportation of hormones, nutrients, wastes, respiratory gases, vitamins, minerals, enzymes, water, leukocytes, antibodies, and buffers
B. Secondary function: contributes directly or indirectly to all the body's metabolic functions

Structures of the Circulatory System
Blood

A. Blood components
  1. Serum: plasma with fewer or no coagulating proteins
  2. Plasma

a. Water: 3 L in average adult; constitutes 90% of plasma
b. Ions: see fluid and electrolytes
c. Albumin (major plasma protein)
 (1) Acts as a buffer
 (2) Maintains plasma colloid osmotic pressure
d. Glucose: prime oxidative metabolite
3. Formed elements
 a. Erythrocytes
  (1) Shape: pliable biconcave disc that maximizes surface area proportional to volume for ease of diffusion of gases
  (2) Number: males: 4.5 to $6.2 \times 10^6/mm^3$; females: 4.0 to $5.5 \times 10^6/mm^3$
  (3) Formation: erythropoiesis
   (a) Location: red marrow of vertebrae, sternum, ribs, iliac crests, clavicles, scapulae, and skull
   (b) Liver and kidneys secrete proteins that help form erythropoietin, which stimulates erythrocyte production
   (c) Maturation process: mature erythrocytes are mainly sacs of hemoglobin without a nucleus, mitochondria, ribosomes, endoplasmic reticula, or Golgi bodies; process requires folic acid and vitamin B_{12}; vitamin B_{12} plus intrinsic factor from the parietal cells of the stomach form hemopoietic factor, which stimulates erythrocyte formation (see Pernicious Anemia)
  (4) Principal component is hemoglobin
   (a) Functions to bind O_2 through iron in heme and CO_2 through globulin portion; can carry both simultaneously
   (b) Formed within the erythrocyte utilizing copper, cobalt, iron, nickel, and vitamin B_6
  (5) Erythrocytes live for about 120 days; old or deteriorated ones are removed by reticuloendothelial cells of the liver, spleen, and bone marrow; heme is converted to bilirubin, which is excreted from the liver as part of bile
 b. Leukocytes
  (1) Types
   (a) Granulocytes (polymorphonuclear): neutrophils, eosinophils, and basophils
   (b) Agranulocytes (mononuclear): monocytes that become macrophages in tissue spaces and lymphocytes

  (2) Functions
   (a) Phagocytosis of bacteria by neutrophils and macrophages; phagocytosis of antibody-antigen complexes by eosinophils
   (b) Antibody synthesis: B lymphocytes produce antibodies; they also become plasma cells, which produce most circulatory antibodies
   (c) Destruction of transplanted tissues and cancer cells by T lymphocytes, which form in lymphoid tissue and mature in the thymus
  (3) Leukocytes live for a few hours or days; some T lymphocytes live for many years and provide long-term immunity
 c. Platelets (thrombocytes)
  (1) Number: 150,000 to 500,000/mm^3
  (2) Function in blood coagulation
   (a) Adhere to each other and to damaged areas of circulatory system to limit or prevent blood loss
   (b) Release chemicals that constrict damaged blood vessels
  (3) Thrombocytopenia may cause bleeding tendencies
B. Physical properties of blood
 1. Volume: males: 5 to 6 L; female: 4.5 to 5.5 L
 2. Hematocrit is percent blood volume occupied by red cells: males: 45% to 52%; females: 37% to 48%
 3. Viscosity: about 5.5 times as viscous as pure water; the higher the RBCs the greater the viscosity
C. Blood groups
 1. There are 4 blood types: A, B, AB, and O; type indicates antigens on or in the red blood cell membrane (e.g., type A blood has A antigens and type O blood has no antigens)
 2. Blood can be either Rh positive or negative; blood does not usually contain anti-Rh antibodies. However, Rh-negative blood will contain anti-Rh antibodies if the individual has been transfused with Rh-positive blood or has carried an Rh-positive fetus without treatment; Rh-positive blood never contains anti-Rh antibodies
 3. Plasma: normally contains no antibodies against antigens present on its own red blood cells, but does contain antibodies against other A or B antigens not present on its red blood cells
 4. The potential danger in transfusing blood is that the donor's blood may be agglutinated (clumped) by the recipient's antibodies
D. Hemostasis: arrest of bleeding
 1. Vasoconstriction

2. Aggregation of platelets: adhere to damaged blood vessel walls forming plugs
3. Blood coagulation (clotting): blood becomes gel as soluble fibrinogen is converted to insoluble fibrin
   a. Extrinsic clotting mechanism: trigger for mechanism is blood contacting damaged tissue
   b. Intrinsic clotting mechanism: trigger for mechanism is release of chemicals (platelet factors such as thromboplastin) from platelets aggregated at the site of an injury
   c. Liver cells synthesize prothrombin, fibrinogen, and other clotting factors; adequate amounts of vitamin K must be present in blood for the liver to make normal amounts of prothrombin
   d. Normal blood prothrombin content: 10 to 15 mg/100 ml of plasma; calcium acts as a catalyst to convert prothrombin to thrombin
   e. Normal blood fibrinogen content: 350 mg/100 ml of plasma
   f. Fibrin is an insoluble protein formed from the soluble protein fibrinogen in the presence of thrombin; fibrin appears as a tangled mass of threads in which blood cells become enmeshed

Heart

A. Location: in mediastinum
B. Structure
   1. Pericardium (covering)
      a. Parietal layer: lines inner surface of fibrous pericardium
      b. Visceral layer (epicardium): adheres to outer surface of the heart; pericardial space, lying between the parietal and visceral layers, contains a few drops of lubricating pericardial fluid that reduces friction
   2. Heart wall: myocardium (cardiac muscle cells); endocardium (endothelial inner lining)
   3. Cavities: upper two called atria; lower two called ventricles
   4. Valves and openings
      a. Atrioventricular valves between atria and ventricles: tricuspid on right, mitral (bicuspid) on left; valves consist of three parts: flaps or cusps, chordae tendineae, papillary muscles
      b. Pulmonary semilunar valve between right ventricle and pulmonary arteries
      c. Aortic semilunar valve between left ventricle and the aorta
   5. Blood supply to myocardium (heart muscle)
      a. Left coronary artery branches to the left anterior decending artery, the circumflex artery, and the right coronary artery
      b. Right coronary artery branches mainly supply the right side of the heart but also carry some blood to the left ventricle
      c. Most abundant blood supply goes to the myocardium of the left ventricle
      d. Greatest flow of blood into myocardium occurs when the heart relaxes as a result of decreased arterial compression
      e. Relatively few anastomoses exist between the larger branches of the coronary arteries (poor collateral circulation); hence, if one of these vessels becomes occluded, little or no blood can reach the myocardial cells supplied by that vessel
   6. Nerve supply to heart
      a. Sympathetic fibers (in cardiac nerves) and parasympathetic fibers (in the vagus nerve) form the cardiac plexuses
      b. Fibers from the cardiac plexuses terminate mainly in the sinoatrial node
      c. Sympathetic impulses tend to accelerate and strengthen heartbeat
      d. Parasympathetic (vagal) impulses slow the heartbeat
   7. Conduction system of heart
      a. Sinoatrial (SA) node: located in the right atrial wall
      b. Atrioventricular (AV) node: located in the base of the right atrium
      c. AV bundle of His: originates in the AV node and extends by two branches down the two sides of the interventricular septum (right and left bundle branches); an error in conduction here is called a bundle branch block
      d. Purkinje fibers: extend from the AV bundles throughout the wall of the ventricles
      e. Normally a nerve impulse begins at the SA node and spreads through both atria to the AV node; after a short delay it is conducted by the bundle of His and the Purkinje fibers to the lateral walls of the ventricles
C. Physiology of heart
   1. Cardiac cycle: pumps varing amounts of blood through the vessels as the needs of cells change
      a. Consists of systole (contraction) and diastole (relaxation) of atria and ventricles; atria contract, and as they relax ventricles contract
      b. Time required: about 0.8 seconds for one cardiac cycle; 60 to 80 cycles or heartbeats per minute
   2. Auscultatory events (heart sounds): first sound (S_1), "lub," occurs at the beginning of ventricular systole because of the closing of the atrioventricular valves (tricuspid and mitral); second sound (S_2), "dub," occurs at the end of

ventricular systole as a result of the closing of the semilunar valves

Blood vessels

A. Kinds
1. Arteries: carry blood away from the heart (all arteries except pulmonary artery carry oxygenated blood); branch into smaller and smaller vessels called arterioles, which branch into microscopic capillaries
2. Veins: vessels that carry blood toward the heart (all veins except the pulmonary veins carry deoxygenated blood); branch into venules, which collect blood from capillaries; veins in the cranial cavity formed by the dura mater are called sinuses
3. Capillaries: carry blood from arterioles and unite to form small veins or venules, which, in turn, unite to form veins; exchange of substances between blood and interstitial fluid occurs in capillaries

B. Structure of blood vessels
1. Arteries: lining (tunica intima) of endothelium; middle coat (tunica media) of smooth muscle, elastic, and fibrous tissues, which permits constriction and dilation; outer coat (tunica adventitia or externa) of fibrous tissue; this firmness makes arteries stand open instead of collapsing when cut
2. Veins: same three coats, but thinner and fewer elastic fibers allowing veins to collapse when cut; semilunar valves present in most veins over 2 mm in diameter
3. Capillaries: only lining coat present (intima); wall only one cell thick

Physiology of Circulation

A. Definitions
1. Circulation: blood flow through circuit of vessels
2. Systemic circulation: blood flow from left ventricle into aorta, other arteries, arterioles, capillaries, venules, and veins to right atrium of heart
3. Pulmonary circulation: blood flow from right ventricle to pulmonary artery to lung arterioles, capillaries, and venules, to pulmonary veins, to left atrium
4. Hepatic portal circulation: blood flow from capillaries, venules, and veins of stomach, intestines, spleen, pancreas, and gallbladder into portal vein, liver sinusoids, to hepatic veins, to inferior vena cava
5. Cardiac output (CO): volume of blood pumped per minute by the ventricles; average for adult at rest is approximately 3 to 5 liters per minute
   a. Preload: extent to which left ventricle stretches at the height of diastole
   b. Afterload: force required to overcome arterial resistance and eject contents of the left ventricle during systole

B. Regulation of cardiac output
1. Starling's law of the heart: within physiologic limits, the heart, when stretched by an increased returning volume of blood, contracts more strongly and pumps out the extra returned blood; the heart pumps in proportion to peripheral demand, resistance, and blood viscosity
2. Venous return: sum of all volumes of blood flowing through all capillary beds of the body; initiates Starling's law of the heart
3. Nervous and hormonal influences on heart: physiologic limit on heart's ability to increase output as venous return increases; maximum at about 15 L/minute; sympathetic stimulation and epinephrine raise upper limit of cardiac output to 25 to 30 L/minute in normal individuals; parasympathetic stimulation decreases heart rate and stroke volume
4. Neural influence on veins: venous constriction caused by sympathetic stimulation milks blood toward heart

C. Principles of circulation
1. Blood circulates because a blood pressure gradient exists in the vessels; blood moves from regions where its pressure is greater to regions where the pressure is less
2. Normal range of systolic blood pressure is 100 to 139 mm Hg; difference between systolic and diastolic pressures is the pulse pressure, normally between 30 and 40 mm Hg
3. Blood pressure normally remains relatively constant over a wide range of activities as a result of:
   a. Neural regulation: maintains blood pressure; increase in arterial pressure stimulates baroreceptors in the aorta and carotid sinus, which leads to increased parasympathetic impulses to the heart via the vagus nerve, which slow the heart rate; a decrease in arterial pressure inhibits baroreceptors in the aorta and carotid sinus and thereby leads to decreased parasympathetic impulses and increased sympathetic impulses to the heart, which in turn cause an increased cardiac output
   b. Intrinsic circulatory regulation: maintains blood pressure; increased blood pressure raises the hydrostatic pressure of plasma, leading to increased filtration of plasma from the circulatory system to interstitial spaces; this results in reduced venous return, decreased cardiac output, and decreased blood pressure

c. Kidney regulation: provides long-term regulation of blood pressure; increased blood pressure drives more blood through the kidneys, increasing urine output, which decreases venous return, cardiac output, and blood pressure

4. Blood flow through the capillary bed: plasma filters through capillary wall and becomes interstitial fluid; fluid flows over cells in the capillary bed, and diffusion of nutrients and wastes occurs between fluid and cells

5. Regulation of blood flow in the circulatory system: rate of flow in liters per minute is directly proportional to blood pressure gradient and diameter of blood vessels; rate of flow is inversely proportional to blood vessel length and blood viscosity; peripheral resistance refers to the combined effects of blood vessel radius and length and blood viscosity

6. Under nonpathologic conditions, blood pressure remains relatively constant; because vessel length and blood viscosity are constant, the rate of flow depends almost entirely on blood vessel radius (constriction and dilation)
   a. Sympathetic discharge constricts muscular arteries and arterioles leading to the viscera, kidneys, and skin and dilates those leading to skeletal muscles; also constricts blood reservoirs such as the veins, and propels blood toward the heart
   b. Postural reflexes (baroreceptor system): arterioles are constricted when one suddenly stands after sitting or lying down; this raises blood pressure to ensure adequate perfusion of brain cells

D. Pulse
   1. Definition: alternate expansion and elastic recoil of blood vessel
   2. Cause: variations in pressure within vessel caused by each ventricular contraction; pulse can be felt wherever an artery lies near the surface and over a firm background such as bone, because of elasticity of arterial walls
   3. Pulse sites: *Apical*—5th to 6th intercostal space in left midclavicular line; *radial*—at wrist; *temporal*—in front of ear, or above and to outer side of eye; *carotid*—along anterior edge of sternocleidomastoid muscle, at level of lower margin of thyroid cartilage; *brachial*—at bend of the elbow, along the inner margin of the biceps muscle; *femoral*—in groin; *popliteal*—behind knee; *posterior tibial*—behind the medial malleolus; *dorsalis pedis*—on anterior surface of the foot, just below the bend of the ankle
   4. Venous pulse: in large veins only; produced by changes in venous pressure brought about by

alternate contraction and relaxation of the atria
   5. A pulse rate of less than 60 beats per minute is bradycardia; a pulse rate greater than 100 beats per minute is tachycardia

Lymphatic System
Lymph vessels
A. Structure: lymph capillaries similar to blood capillaries in structure; larger lymphatics similar to veins but are thinner walled, have more valves, and have lymph nodes in certain places along their course
B. Functions
   1. About 60% of fluid filtered out of blood capillaries returns to circulation via lymphatics rather than by osmosis into venous ends of capillaries; about 50% of total blood proteins leak out of capillaries per day and can only return to blood via lymphatics
   2. Lymph return is essential for homeostasis of blood proteins and blood volume
   3. Interference with the return of proteins to the blood results in edema, caused by the loss of protein and changes in colloid osmotic pressure

Lymph nodes
A. Usually occur in clusters:
   1. Submental and submaxillary groups in floor of mouth; drain lymph from nose, lips, and teeth
   2. Superficial cervical nodes in neck, along sternocleidomastoid muscle; drain lymph from head and neck
   3. Superficial cubital nodes at bend of elbow; drain lymph from hand and forearm
   4. Axillary nodes in armpit; drain lymph from arm and upper part of the chest wall, including the breast
   5. Inguinal nodes in groin; drain lymph from the leg and external genitals
B. Functions
   1. Help defend the body against injurious substances (notably, bacteria and tumor cells) by filtering them out of lymph and thereby preventing their entrance into bloodstream
   2. Lymphatic tissue of lymph nodes carries on the process of hemopoiesis; specifically, it forms T and B lymphocytes

Lymph
Fluid in lymphatics is derived from interstitial fluid that has entered the lymphatic capillaries
Spleen
A. Location: left hypochondrium, above and behind cardiac portion of the stomach
B. Structure: lymphatic tissues: size varies; contains numerous spaces filled with venous blood
C. Functions

1. Defense: phagocytosis of particles such as microbes, red blood cell fragments, and platelets by reticuloendothelial cells of spleen (reticuloendothelial system—phagocytic cells, located mainly in the liver, spleen, bone marrow, and lymph nodes; also, macrophages of connective tissue and microglia in the brain and cord); antibody formation by plasma cells of spleen
2. Hemopoiesis: lymphatic tissue of the spleen forms lymphocytes and possibly monocytes
3. Spleen serves as blood reservoir; sympathetic stimulation causes constriction of its capsule, squeezing out an estimated 200 ml of blood into general circulation within 1 minute

REVIEW OF MICROORGANISMS

A. *Streptococcus pyogenes:* gram-positive streptococcus; the most virulent strain (group A beta hemolytic) causes scarlet fever, septic sore throat, tonsillitis, cellulitis, puerperal fever, erysipelas, rheumatic fever, and glomerulonephritis
B. *Streptococcus viridans:* gram-positive streptococcus; distinguishable from *S. pyogenes* by its alpha hemolysis (rather than beta) of red blood cells; the most common cause of subacute bacterial endocarditis

 ## RELATED PHARMACOLOGY

Cardiac glycosides
A. Description
1. Produce a positive inotropic effect (increased force of contraction) by increasing permeability of cardiac muscle membranes to the calcium and sodium ions required for contraction of muscle fibrils
2. Improve the pumping ability of the heart, thus increasing cardiac output
3. Produce a negative chronotropic effect (decreased rate of contraction) by an action mediated through the vagus nerve, which slows firing of the SA node and impulse transmission at the AV node
4. Effective in treating congestive heart failure and atrial flutter and fibrillation
5. Available in oral and parenteral (IM, IV) preparations
6. Initially, loading dose is administered to digitalize the client; after the desired effect is achieved, the dosage is lowered to a maintenance level, which replaces the amount of drug metabolized and excreted each day
B. Examples: digitalis; digoxin (Lanoxin)
C. Major side effects: diarrhea (local effect), malabsorption of all nutrients (nausea, vomiting, diarrhea); bradycardia (increased vagal tone at AV node)

D. Toxicity: premature ventricular beats (increased spontaneous rate of ventricular depolarization); xanthopsia/yellow vision (effect on visual cones); muscle weakness (CNS effect, neurotoxicity, hypokalemia); blurred vision (CNS effect); anorexia, vomiting (local effect stimulates chemoreceptor zone in medulla)
E. Nursing care
1. Check apical pulse before administration: in adults if pulse is below 60 or over 120 withhold dose and notify physician
2. Administer oral preparations with meals to reduce GI irritation
3. Encourage intake of high nutrient density foods
4. Assess client for signs of impending toxicity (anorexia, nausea, vomiting, dysrhythmias, xanthopsia)
5. Monitor the client for hypokalemia, which potentiates the effects of digitalis; ECG will indicate depressed T waves with hypokalemia
6. Instruct the client to: count radial pulse and record before each administration; notify, physician of any side effects; report any changes in heart rate to physician (irregular heartbeats; increased or decreased rate)
7. Digoxin—monitor blood level during therapy (normal serum: 0.9 to 2.0 ng/ml)

Antidysrhythmics
A. Description
1. Treat abnormal variations in cardiac rate and rhythm; also prevent dysrhythmias
2. Available in oral and parenteral (IM, IV) preparations
B. Examples
1. Calcium ion antagonists control atrial dysrhythmias by decreasing cardiac automaticity and impulse conduction: diltiazem (Cardizem), nifedipine (Procardia), verapamil (Calan)
2. Beta-adrenergic blockers control supraventricular dysrhythmias by decreasing cardiac impulse conduction through a blocking action: propranolol (Inderal), metoprolol (Lopressor)
3. Disopyramide phosphate (Norpace): controls ventricular dysrhythmias by decreasing the rate of diastolic depolarization
4. Lidocaine HCl: controls ventricular irritability by shortening the refractory period and suppressing ectopic foci
5. Procainamide HCl (Pronestyl): controls ventricular and atrial dysrhythmias by prolonging the refractory period and slowing conduction of cardiac impulses
6. Quinidine preparations: control atrial dysrhythmias by prolonging the effective refractory period and slowing depolarization

7. Amiodarone (Cordarone): controls ventricular dysrhythmias by prolonging action potential and refractory period; slows the sinus rate

C. Major side effects: hypotension (decreased cardiac output caused by vasodilation); dizziness (hypotension); nausea, vomiting (irritation of gastric mucosa); heart block (direct cardiac toxic effect; cardiac depressant); anticholinergic effect (decreased parasympathetic stimulation); blood dyscrasias (decreased RBCs, WBCs, and platelet synthesis)

D. Toxicity: diarrhea (GI irritation), CNS disturbances (neurotoxicity), sensory disturbances (neurotoxicity)

E. Nursing care
1. Assess vital signs during course of therapy; monitor drug blood levels
2. Use cardiac monitoring during IV administration; ensure follow-up ECGs
3. Use infusion-control device for continuous IV administration
4. Administer oral preparations with meals to reduce GI irritation
5. Use safety precautions (supervise ambulation, side rails up) when CNS effects are manifested
6. Instruct client to: notify physician of any side effects; report any changes in heart rate or rhythm to physician (irregular beats, increased or decreased rate)

Cardiac stimulants
A. Description
1. Increase the heart rate
2. Act by either indirect or direct mechanisms affecting the autonomic nervous system
3. Available in parenteral (IM/IV), endotracheal, and intracardiac preparations

B. Examples
1. Atropine sulfate: suppresses parasympathetic nervous system control at SA and AV nodes, thus allowing heart rate to increase
2. Epinephrine HCl (Adrenalin): stimulates the rate and force of cardiac contraction via the sympathetic nervous system
3. Isoproterenol HCl (Isuprel): stimulates beta-adrenergic receptors of the sympathetic nervous system, thus increasing heart rate

C. Major side effects: tachycardia (sympathetic stimulation); headache (dilation of cerebral vessels); CNS stimulation (sympathetic stimulation); cardiac dysrhythmias (cardiovascular system stimulation); atropine: anticholinergic effects (dry mouth, blurred vision, urinary retention as a result of decreased parasympathetic stimulation)

D. Nursing care: assess vital signs during course of therapy; use cardiac monitoring during IV administration; ensure follow-up ECGs

Coronary vasodilators
A. Description
1. Decrease cardiac work and myocardial oxygen requirements by their vasodilatory action to decrease preload and afterload
2. Nitrates act directly at receptors in smooth muscles causing vasodilation, which decreases the preload, thus decreasing cardiac workload
3. Calcium ion antagonists inhibit the influx of the calcium ion across the cell membrane during depolarization of the cardiac and vascular smooth muscle
4. Effective in the treatment of angina pectoris
5. Available in oral, sublingual, buccal, and topical, including transdermal, preparations

B. Examples
1. Nitrates (sublingual): isosorbide dinitrate (Isordil, Sorbitrate); nitroglycerin
2. Nitrates (oral): isosorbide dinitrate (Isordil, Sorbitrate)
3. Nitrates (topical):
   a. Nitroglycerin ointment (Nitro-Bid; Nitrol)
   b. Nitroglycerin transdermal (Nitro-Dur; Transderm-Nitro)
4. Calcium ion antagonists (calcium channel blockers): amlodipine (Norvasc); nifedipine (Procardia); verapamil (Calan, Isoptin)

C. Major side effects: headache (dilation of cerebral vessels); flushing (peripheral vasodilation); orthostatic hypotension (loss of compensatory vasoconstriction with position change); tachycardia (reflex reaction to severe hypotension); dizziness (orthostatic hypotension)

D. Nursing care
1. Assess for hypotension before administering; if present, withhold drug
2. Encourage client to change positions slowly
3. Use safety precautions
4. Nitroglycerin: instruct client to: take sublingual preparations before angina-producing activities; note slight stinging, burning, tingling under the tongue that indicate potency of drug; avoid placing the drug in heat, light, moisture, or plastic; store in original amber glass container; obtain a new supply every 3 to 4 months; take sublingual preparations every 5 minutes, not to exceed 3 in 15 minutes for chest pain; if pain persists, get emergency care

Antihypertensives
A. Description
1. Promote dilation of peripheral blood vessels, thus decreasing blood pressure and afterload
2. Available in oral, parenteral (IM, IV), and transdermal preparations

B. Examples
1. Angiotensin-converting enzyme (ACE) inhibitors: captopril (Capoten); enalapril maleate (Vasotec)

2. Sympatholytics: clonidine (Catapres); guanethidine sulfate (Ismelin); methyldopa (Aldomet)
3. Direct smooth muscle relaxants: diazoxide (Hyperstat IV), promotes hyperglycemia; hydralazine HCl (Apresoline), increases excretion of vitamin B_6; nitroprusside sodium (Nipride), reduces serum B_{12} level; prazosin HCl (Minipress)
4. Beta-adrenergic blocker (sympatholytic): atenolol (Tenormin) metoprolol (Lopressor)
5. Alpha-adrenergic blocker (sympatholytic): phentolamine (Regitine)

C. Major side effects
1. Orthostatic hypotension (loss of compensatory vasoconstriction with position change)
2. Dizziness (orthostatic hypotension); drowsiness (cerebral hypoxia)
3. Cardiac rate alteration: bradycardia (sympatholytics) (decreased sympathetic stimulation to the heart); tachycardia (direct relaxers) (reflex reaction to severe hypotension)
4. Sexual disturbances (failure of erection or ejaculation caused by loss of vascular tone)
5. Blood dyscrasias (decreased RBCs, WBCs, platelet synthesis)

D. Nursing care
1. Assess vital signs, especially pulse and monitor blood pressure in standing and supine positions during therapy
2. Monitor urinary output during initial titration
3. Protect nitroprusside IV solution from light during administration
4. Instruct client to: follow a low-sodium diet; eat foods high in B-complex vitamins; change positions slowly; continue to take medication as prescribed because therapy is usually for life; report occurrence of any side effects to physician; avoid engaging in hazardous activities when initially placed on antihypertensive drug therapy

Diuretics

A. Description
1. Interfere with sodium reabsorption in the kidney
2. Increase urine output, which reduces hypervolemia; decreases preload and afterload
3. Available in oral and parenteral (IM, IV) preparations

B. Examples
1. Thiazides: chlorothiazide (Diuril); hydrochlorothiazide (HydroDIURIL); interfere with sodium ion transport at loop of Henle and inhibit carbonic anhydrase activity at distal tubule sites
2. Potassium-sparers: spironolactone (Aldactone); triamterine (Dyrenium); interfere with aldosterone-induced reabsorption of sodium

ions at distal nephron sites to increase sodium chloride excretion and decrease potassium ion loss
3. Loop diuretics: ethacrynic acid (Edecrin); furosemide (Lasix); interfere with active transport of sodium ions in loop of Henle and inhibit sodium chloride and water reabsorption at proximal tubule sites

C. Major side effects: GI irritation (local effect); hyponatremia (inhibition of sodium reabsorption at the kidney tubule); orthostatic hypotension (reduced blood volume); hyperuricemia (partial blockage of uric acid excretion); dehydration (excessive sodium and water loss)
1. All diuretics except potassium-sparers: hypokalemia (increased potassium excretion); increased urinary excretion of magnesium and zinc
2. Potassium-sparers: hyperkalemia (reabsorption of potassium at the kidney tubule); hypomagnesemia (increased excretion of magnesium at kidney tubule); increased urinary excretion of calcium
3. Furosemide (Lasix) competes with aspirin for renal excretion sites and can cause aspirin toxicity
4. Thiazides and loop diuretics: may cause hyperglycemia in clients with diabetes

D. Nursing care
1. Maintain intake and output; weigh daily (same time, scale, clothing); assess for signs of fluid-electrolyte imbalance
2. Administer the drug in the morning so that the maximal effect will occur during the waking hours
3. Assess vital signs, especially pulse and blood pressure; instruct client to change position slowly
4. Encourage intake of foods high in calcium, magnesium, zinc, and potassium (except for potassium-sparers)
5. Be alert for signs of hypokalemia except for potassium sparers (muscle weakness, cramps)

Peripheral vasoconstrictors

A. Description
1. Constrict peripheral blood vessels through alpha-adrenergic stimulation
2. Elevate blood pressure
3. Available in parenteral (IV) preparations

B. Examples: levarterenol bitartrate (Levophed); metaraminol bitartrate (Aramine); phenylephrine HCl (Neo-Synephrine); dopamine (Depostat); vasopressin

C. Major side effects: hypertension (compression of cerebral blood vessels); headache (increase in blood pressure); GI disturbance (autonomic dysfunction)

D. Nursing care
   1. Assess vital signs; monitor blood pressure frequently; titrate IV depending on blood pressure readings to prevent hypertension
   2. Assess for IV infiltration; may lead to tissue necrosis
   3. Encourage intake of high-fiber foods to reduce the potential of constipation

Anticoagulants
A. Description
   1. Prevent fibrin formation by interfering with the production of various clotting factors in the coagulation process
   2. Prevent clot formation and clot extension
   3. Available in oral and parenteral (SC, IV) preparations; may be given concurrently until oral medication reaches therapeutic level
B. Examples: parenteral—heparin sodium (Calciparine); enoxaparin (Lovenox); and oral—warfarin sodium (Coumadin)
C. Major side effects: fever, chills (hypersensitivity); skin rash (hypersensitivity); hemorrhage (interference with clotting mechanisms); diarrhea (GI irritation)
D. Nursing care
   1. Monitor blood work during course of therapy, especially coagulation studies; International Normative Ratio (INR), PT (for warfarin derivatives) and PTT (for heparin therapy), blood platelets; PT and PTT values would be 1.5 to 2 times normal values; INR values would be 2.0 to 3.5
   2. Assess client for signs of bleeding
   3. Have appropriate antidote available: vitamin K for warfarin; protamine sulfate for heparin
   4. Avoid administration of salicylates and IM injections during anticoagulant therapy
   5. Instruct client to: carry a medical alert card; immediately report any signs of bleeding to the physician; avoid any medications containing aspirin and the ingestion of alcohol; use an electric razor and soft toothbrush; follow schedule for coagulation studies
   6. Subcutaneous heparin is generally administered in the abdomen; the nurse does not aspirate or massage the area

Antianemics
A. Description
   1. Promote RBC production; effective in the treatment of iron-deficiency and nutritional anemias
   2. Include iron-containing compounds and vitamin replacements
   3. Available in oral and parenteral (IM, IV [SC for vitamin B_{12}]) preparations
B. Examples
   Iron compounds (oral): ferrous gluconate, ferrous sulfate; iron compounds (parenteral): iron

dextran (Imferon), iron sorbitex (Jectofer); vitamin replacements: cyanocobalamin—vitamin B_{12} (Redisol), folic acid—vitamin B_9 (Folvite)
C. Major side effects
   1. Iron replacements: nausea, vomiting (irritation of gastric mucosa); constipation (delayed passage of iron and stool); black stools (presence of unabsorbed iron in stool); stained teeth (liquid preparations that come into contact with enamel); tissue staining (injectable preparations that leak iron into tissue)
   2. Vitamin replacements: local irritation (local tissue effect); allergic reactions, anaphylaxis (hypersensitivity); diarrhea (GI irritation)
D. Nursing care
   1. Iron replacements
      a. Inform client about side effects of therapy
      b. Administer IM using Z-track method; administer liquid preparations, diluted with water or fruit juice, through a straw on an empty stomach if possible for optimum absorption; ascorbic acid (vitamin C) increases absorption; encourage oral hygiene
      c. Encourage intake of foods high in iron, vitamin B_{12}, and folic acid and intake of high-fiber foods to reduce the potential of constipation
      d. Deferoxamine mesylate (Desferal) is the antidote for iron toxicity
   2. Vitamin replacements
      a. Vitamin B_{12}: inform client that this drug cannot be administered orally; therapy is for life in pernicious anemia
      b. Folic acid: instruct client about dietary sources of folic acid (fresh fruits, vegetables, and meats)

Antilipidemics
A. Description
   1. Lower serum lipid levels by reducing cholesterol or triglyceride synthesis or both
   2. Available in oral preparations
B. Examples
   1. HMG-CoA reductase inhibitors: pravastatin (Pravachol), lovastatin (Mevacor), simvastatin (Zocor)
   2. Fibrates: gemfibrozil (Lopid), clofibrate (Atromids)
   3. Bile acid sequestrant: cholestyramine (Questran)
   4. Niacins
C. Major side effects
   1. Nausea, vomiting (irritation to gastric mucosa); diarrhea (GI irritation)
   2. Musculoskeletal disturbances (direct musculoskeletal tissue effect)
   3. Hepatic disturbances (hepatic toxicity)
   4. Skin rash (hypersensitivity)

5. Reduced absorption of fat and fat-soluble vitamins (A, D, E, K) as well as vitamin B_{12} and iron
6. Lovastatin and gemfibrozil: visual disturbances (ocular alterations)

D. Nursing care
   1. Encourage the following dietary program:
      a. Low cholesterol, low fat (especially saturated)
      b. Replace vegetable oils high in polyunsaturated fatty acid (PUFA) with those high in monounsaturated fatty acid (MUFA), such as olive, avocado
      c. Eat fish high in omega-3 fatty acids several times per week (salmon, tuna)
      d. Increase intake of high-fiber foods, such as fruits, vegetables, cereal grains, and legumes; soluble fiber is particularly effective in reducing blood lipids (oat bran, legumes)
   2. Administer "statins" at hour of sleep to enhance effectiveness; administer other medications with meals to reduce GI irritation
   3. Monitor serum cholesterol and triglyceride levels; hemoglobin and RBC levels; fat-soluble vitamin levels; and liver function tests
   4. Cholestyramine: mix with full glass of liquid
   5. Lovastatin and gemfibrozil: assess for visual disturbances with prolonged use

Thrombolytics

A. Description
   1. Convert plasminogen to plasmin, which initiates local fibrinolysis
   2. Dissolve occluding thrombi in the coronary arteries
   3. Administered intravenously or intraarterially (via cardiac catheterization)
   4. Initially, loading dose is administered
   5. Therapy must be instituted within 4 to 12 hours of the onset of the myocardial infarction

B. Examples: streptokinase (Streptase); tissue plasminogen activator (t-PA) (Activase)

C. Major side effects: bleeding (increased fibrinolytic activity especially GI if there is a history of peptic ulcer disease); allergic reactions (introduction of a foreign protein); low-grade fever (resulting from absorption of infarcted tissue)

D. Nursing care
   1. Observe for signs of bleeding; monitor partial thromboplastin time (PTT) and fibrinogen concentration; monitor vital signs and neurologic status
   2. Assess for signs of allergic reactions such as chills, urticaria, pruritus, rash, and malaise
   3. Keep aminocaproic acid (Amicar), a fibrinolysis inhibitor, available
   4. Maintain continuous IV infusion of heparin following thrombolytic therapy

RELATED PROCEDURES

Angiography

A. Definition: an x-ray examination using contrast dye to visualize patency of arteries

B. Nursing care
   1. Inform the client of risks (allergic reaction, embolus, cardiac dysrhythmia)
   2. Administer mild sedative as ordered before procedure
   3. Postprocedure care: check injection site for bleeding and inflammation; maintain pressure over site; assess circulatory status of extremities; enforce bed rest

Angioplasty

A. Definition
   1. Percutaneous transluminal coronary angioplasty (PTCA) is the introduction of a balloon-tipped catheter into the coronary artery to the stenosis to reduce or eliminate the occlusion; may be used with laser angioplasty that vaporizes the plaque
      a. Performed via coronary catheterization using fluoroscopy; heparin infusion is used to prevent thrombus formation
      b. Thrombolytic therapy may be combined with PTCA in some situations
      c. Intracoronary stents may be inserted to maintain patency; clients would require long-term anticoagulation therapy
      d. If lesions are calcified and cannot be removed by PTCA, an atherectomy to mechanically remove the plaque by shaving and retrieving it from the vessel's lumen can be done
      e. Complications include arterial spasm or perforation and thrombus formation; emergency open-heart surgery may be necessary
   2. Percutaneous transluminal angioplasty is used to dilate stenotic vessels by stretching the artery wall away from the plaque; used in aorta, iliac, femoral, popliteal, tibial, renal vessels and arteriovenous dialysis shunts; stent placement generally follows procedure

B. Nursing care: see care for Cardiac Catheterization; administer vasoactive drugs such as calcium channel blockers and nitroglycerin before, during, and after this procedure, as ordered; monitor client for angina, dysrhythmias, bleeding, and evidence of restenosis and reocclusion

Blood Transfusion

A. Purpose: restore blood volume after hemorrhage; maintain hemoglobin levels in severe anemias; replace specific blood components

B. Sources of blood for transfusions
   1. Homologous: random collection of blood by volunteer donors

2. Autologous: donation of a client's own blood before hospitalization; possible when donor's hemoglobin remains over 11 g/dl; donations can be saved for 5 weeks
3. Directed donation: donation of blood by a donor specifically for a client
4. Blood salvage: a method by which a client's blood is suctioned from a closed body cavity (operative site, trauma site, joint) and processed to be transfused; must be used within 6 hours of collection

C. Blood components
1. Whole blood: contains red blood cells and plasma
2. Red blood cells: contains red blood cells
3. Platelets
4. Fresh frozen plasma: contains plasma, antibodies, clotting factors
5. Cryoprecipitate: contains factor VIII, fibrinogen, and factor XIII
6. Albumin
7. Plasma protein factor

D. Nursing care
1. Obtain and document informed consent
2. Check that blood or blood components have been typed and cross-matched for compatibility; it is advisable for two nurses to verify the blood type, Rh factor, client identification and blood numbers, and expiration date
3. Blood must be hung within 30 minutes of arriving on the unit
4. Obtain baseline vital signs before administration
5. An IV with normal saline infusing through a large-bore angiocath and a blood administration set containing a filter are used to start the infusion; solutions containing glucose should not be used
6. Maintain standard precautions when handling blood or IV equipment; assure client that the risk for AIDS is minimal becaused blood is screened
7. Invert the container gently to suspend the red blood cells within the plasma
8. Administer at appropriate rate
   a. Platelets, plasma, and cryoprecipitate may be infused rapidly, assessing for signs of circulatory impairment
   b. Blood transfusions should be completed within 4 hours
9. Observe for signs of hemolytic reaction, which generally occur within the first 10 to 15 minutes: shivering; headache; lower back pain; increased pulse and respiratory rate; hemoglobinuria; oliguria; hypotension
10. Infuse with a controller, regulating rate by gravity; pressure in pumps may cause RBC hemolysis
11. Observe for signs of febrile reaction, which usually occur within 30 minutes: shaking; headache; elevated temperature; back pain; confusion; hematemesis
12. Observe for allergic reaction: hives; wheezing; pruritus; joint pain
13. If any reaction occurs: stop infusion immediately; notify the physician; maintain patency of the IV with normal saline; send blood to the laboratory; monitor vital signs and I and O frequently; send a urine specimen to the laboratory if a hemolytic reaction is suspected; evaluate hemoglobin and hematocrit

Bone Marrow Aspiration
A. Definition: puncture to collect tissue from the bone marrow of the sternum, vertebral body, iliac crest, or the tibia in infants; performed to study the cells involved in blood production
B. Nursing care: allay anxiety of the client; pain is brief, only during aspiration (conscious sedation may be used); position the client to expose site; apply pressure for several minutes or for 1 hour if biopsy is done

Cardiac Catheterization
A. Definition: introduction of a catheter into the heart via a peripheral vessel
1. Injection of contrast material for visualization of chambers, coronary circulation, and great vessels
2. Withdrawal of blood samples to evaluate cardiac function
3. Measurement of pressures within chambers and blood vessels (e.g., pulmonary wedge pressure)
B. Nursing care
1. Inform client of the procedure's purpose, its possible complications (e.g., hemorrhage, CVA), and the sensations it causes (e.g., urge to cough, nausea, heat); allow time for verbalization of fears
2. Identify allergies to iodine
3. Keep NPO for 8 to 12 hours before the procedure; administer sedatives as ordered before the procedure
4. After catheterization: monitor vital signs frequently; cardiac dysrhythmias are more common during the procedure but may occur afterward; assess the puncture site for bleeding (sandbags or ice packs may be ordered if the femoral artery is used); assess the involved extremity for signs of ischemia (e.g., absence of peripheral pulses, changes in sensation, color, and temperature); maintain bed rest for the prescribed number of hours; increase fluids to eliminate dye

Cardiac Monitoring

A. Definition
1. Electric observation of the conductivity patterns of the heart by the use of skin electrodes and a monitoring device; the heart's electric activity is conducted to the surface of the skin by the salty fluids bathing the cells and tissues
2. Used when danger of dysrhythmias is apparent (e.g., heart disease, surgery, invasive procedures)
3. Conduction from the SA node through the atria causes atrial contraction and gives rise to the P wave; conduction from the AV node down the bundle of His to Purkinje's fibers to the lateral walls of the ventricles and out the Purkinje's fibers causes ventricular contraction and gives rise to the QRS wave; ventricular repolarization is associated with the T wave
4. Holter monitor allows cardiac tracings to be recorded on an ambulatory basis to assess for dysrhythmias
B. Nursing care
1. Explain the procedure to client and attempt to allay anxiety
2. Prepare the skin on the chest for electrode attachment; cleanse area with alcohol to remove dirt and oils; shave area if necessary
3. Place electrodes on the skin and attach to the monitor cable as indicated: RA (attach to right upper chest); LA (attach to left upper chest); RA (attach to right lower chest [ground]); LA (attach to left lower chest)
4. Turn on the monitor scope and set the machine's sensitivity when a clear picture is obtained; observe the monitor for changes in rate and rhythm
5. Set the alarm and readout attachment (if available) so an electric printout will be made if there is a change in cardiac activity
6. Intervene immediately when life-threatening dysrhythmias occur; brain damage will occur if client is anoxic for more than 4 minutes
   a. Ventricular fibrillation: repetitive rapid stimulation from ectopic ventricular foci to which the ventricles are unable to respond; ventricular contraction is replaced by uncoordinated twitching; circulation ceases, and death ensues: defibrillate immediately; inject medications per protocol; institute CPR; document the dysrhythmia and notify the physician; prepare for possible automatic implantable defibrillator (AICD) insertion
   b. Ventricular tachycardia: series of 3 or more bizarre premature ventricular beats that occur in a regular rhythm; this electric activity results in decreased cardiac output and may rapidly convert to ventricular fibrillation: administer medications per protocol; administer cardioversion if medications fail; be prepared to administer defibrillation and cardiopulmonary resuscitation; document the dysrhythmia and notify the physician; prepare for possible automatic implantable defibrillator (AICD) insertion
   c. Premature ventricular beats: originate in the ventricles and occur before the next expected sinus beat; they can be life threatening when they occur close to the T wave because cardiac repolarization is interfered with and ventricular fibrillation may ensue: administer medications per protocol; document the dysrhythmia and notify the physician; long-term institution of oral antidysrhythmics may be indicated
   d. Third-degree atrioventricular block (complete heart block) occurs when there is no electric communication between the atria and ventricles and each beats independently; this activity will not provide long-term adequate circulation, and syncope, heart failure, or cardiac arrest may ensue: document the dysrhythmia and notify the physician; administer medications per protocol; prepare for pacemaker insertion (see procedure)
   e. Cardiac standstill (asystole) occurs when there is no cardiac activity (flat line on ECG tracing); this terminates in death unless intervention is begun immediately: institute cardiopulmonary resuscitation; document the dysrhythmia and notify the physician; cardiac stimulants may be given via IV or intracardiac route; pacemaker insertion may be indicated (see procedure)
   f. Atrial fibrillation: results from rapid firing of atrial ectopic foci, between 400 and 700/minute; ECG shows no p waves, rather irregular forms; pulse deficit is common; danger from blood pooling in quivering atria leading to emboli; heparin may reduce incidence of stroke until rhythm is controlled

Cardioversion

A. Definition: elective procedure during which current is administered to the myocardium in a synchronized fashion to depolarize all cells simultaneously, allowing SA node to resume pacemaker function; may be useful in treating tachydysrhythmias, atrial fibrillation, supraventricular tachycardia, and ventricular tachycardia
B. Nursing care
1. Obtain informed consent

2. Maintain NPO and ascertain patent IV line
3. Ensure that no one is touching the bed/client when shock is delivered
4. Monitor cardiac status for dysrhythmias for several hours after procedure

Basic Life Support (Cardiopulmonary Resuscitation, CPR)

A. Definition: institution of artificial ventilation and circulation with rescue breathing and external cardiac compression
B. Nursing care
   1. Assess level of consciousness: shake victim's shoulder and shout, "Are you OK?"; if no response, call for help or activate the EMS system
   2. Establish an airway: use head tilt or jaw thrust maneuver; determine if air is being exchanged by looking to see if the chest is moving, listening if air can be head escaping during exhalation, and feeling if air can be felt escaping during exhalation (<10 seconds)
   3. Initiate rescue breathing: maintain the head-tilt or jaw-thrust maneuver and pinch the victim's nostrils; give two slow breaths using pocket mask or bag-mask
   4. Assess circulation; palpate carotid pulse
   5. Deliver external cardiac compressions: ensure that the victim is on a firm surface and in the supine position; place heel of hand over lower half of body of sternum, interlock hands and compress the chest 3.8 to 5 cm ($1^1/_2$ to 2 inches for an adult)
   6. Maintain the ventilation/compression ratio: one or two rescuers—two breaths after every 15 compressions (rate of 100 per minute); reassess carotid pulse after first four cycles and then every few minutes
   7. Defibrillate using automated external defibrillator; part of BLS for health care providers
   8. Place client in recovery position if pulse and respirations resume; continue to monitor breathing regularly
   9. Terminate CPR as indicated: return of cardiac rhythm and spontaneous respirations; rescuer exhaustion; physician-ordered cessation

Cardiac Pacemaker Insertion

A. Definition: artificial pacemakers replace natural electric stimulation of the heart and are indicated in the treatment of:
   1. Third-degree atrioventricular block: impulses generated from the SA node of the heart do not reach the ventricles; the atria and ventricles beat independently of each other
   2. Second-degree atrioventricular block: intermittent failure of impulse to reach the ventricles

   3. Adams-Stokes syndrome: a sudden drop in ventricular rate that causes syncope and temporary loss of consciousness
B. Pacemakers: involve the insertion of an electrode catheter into the heart, which transmits the impulses generated by the pacing unit
   1. Demand pacemakers are most frequently used; the pacemaker will stimulate the ventricles to contract only if the client's ventricular rate falls below the rate set on the pacemaker
   2. May be temporary and worn externally or permanent and surgically placed under the skin
   3. May stimulate only right ventricle or right atrium and ventricle (physiologic pacing)
C. Nursing care
   1. Observe the cardiac monitor before, during, and after the procedure to verify pacemaker capture (QRS following pacemaker spike), and observe for dysrhythmias; note stimulation threshold; have emergency medications (e.g., lidocaine, atropine sulfate) available, as well as a defibrillator; ensure electrical equipment is grounded; monitor incision for hematoma and infection
   2. Teach the client how to take pulse, to keep a diary of pulse, and to notify the physician immediately if the rate falls below that set on the pacemaker and to remain under a physician's supervision because batteries must be replaced periodically; pacemaker function may be checked by special telephone devices
   3. Encourage the client to wear a bracelet or carry a medical alert card
   4. Teach client to avoid high magnetic fields such as airport security devices, high-tension wires, and magnetic resonance imaging (MRI); when in doubt consult physician

Nuclear Medicine Procedures

A. Multiple-gated angiographic radioisotope (MUGA) scan and equilibrium radionuclide angiography (ERNA)
   1. Involves intravenous injection of a radioisotope that has an affinity for red blood cells to study ventricular wall motion
   2. Volume of blood pumped during one ventricular contraction is compared with the total volume in the left ventricle, which yields an ejection fraction
   3. The ejection fraction gives important information on ventricular size and wall motion abnormalities
B. Myocardial perfusion imaging
   1. Intravenous injection of a radioisotope such as thallium or technetium-99m (TC-99m), which is taken up by the heart muscle

2. Damaged myocardial tissue takes up the isotope more slowly and retains it for a longer period
3. The isotope can be injected during and after exercise to determine myocardial perfusion

C. Positron-emission tomography (PET) scan
   1. A positron-emitting isotope is administered intravenously to study patency of vessels
   2. Provides detailed information about cardiac circulation
   3. Clients should be encouraged to drink fluids after the test to facilitate excretion of the isotope

D. Nursing care
   1. Review client's medications because some may affect results (e.g., beta blockers)
   2. Monitor client's vital signs before and after test
   3. Determine history of allergies and notify radiology before test
   4. Offer emotional support to client, who may be apprehensive about test and results; allay client's fears about the use of radioactive substances

Hemodynamic Monitoring with Pulmonary Artery Catheter

A. Definition: catheter used to measure pulmonary capillary wedge pressure, pulmonary artery pressure, and right atrial pressure (central venous pressure)
   1. The double-lumen catheter with a balloon tip is inserted into a vein and advanced through the superior vena cava into the right atrium and ventricle, and into the pulmonary artery; the catheter is guided further until, when the balloon is inflated, it is wedged in the distal arterial branch
   2. This catheter yields information on the client's circulatory status, left ventricular pumping action, and vascular tone

B. Nursing care
   1. Assist the physician in inserting the catheter using surgical aseptic technique
   2. Observe the insertion site for inflammation
   3. Observe the line for patency and air bubbles
   4. Take readings with client in supine position if possible with transducer at the level of the client's sternal notch
   5. Provide site care
   6. Notify the physician if the waveform changes or pressure readings are altered
   7. Ensure that balloon does not remain inflated after wedge pressure determination
   8. Normal readings
      a. Pulmonary capillary wedge pressure: 5 to 13 mm Hg
      b. Pulmonary artery pressure—systolic: 16 to 30 mm Hg; diastolic: 0 to 7 mm Hg
      c. Right atrial pressure: 2 to 6 mm Hg
      d. Cardiac output is determined by injecting iced or room-temperature saline through the proximal lumen of the pulmonary artery catheter; a thermistor unit can detect temperature changes in the right atrium that allow the computer to calculate cardiac output
   9. Keep emergency medications and a defibrillator available

MAJOR DISORDERS OF THE CIRCULATORY SYSTEM

▼ HYPERTENSION

Data Base
A. Etiology and pathophysiology
   1. Hypertension increases the risk of coronary artery disease, heart failure, myocardial infarction, cerebral vascular accidents (CVAs), and renal failure
   2. Risk factors
      a. Stress
      b. Obesity (apple-shaped form)
      c. Nutrition (high sodium, low calcium, magnesium, and potassium)
      d. Substance abuse (cigarettes, alcohol, cocaine)
      e. Family history
      f. Age
      g. Sedentary lifestyle
      h. Hyperlipidemia
   3. Often asymptomatic; diagnosis requires three assessments of elevated blood pressure on separate occasions
   4. Classification of blood pressure
      a. Optimal: systolic <129 mm Hg; diastolic <80 mm Hg
      b. Normal: systolic <130 mm Hg; diastolic <85 mm Hg
      c. High normal: systolic 130 to 139 mm Hg or diastolic 85 to 89 mm Hg
      d. Hypertension
         (1) Stage 1: systolic 140 to 159 mm Hg or diastolic 90 to 99 mm Hg
         (2) Stage 2: systolic 160 to 179 mm Hg or diastolic 100 to 109 mm Hg
         (3) Stage 3: systolic 180 mm Hg or diastolic 110 mm Hg
   5. Primary (essential) hypertension
      a. 90% to 95% of all cases of hypertension
      b. Etiology is complex; begins insidiously; changes in arteriolar bed cause increased resistance; increased blood volume may result from hormonal or renal dysfunction; arteriolar thickening causes increased peripheral vascular resistance; abnormal renin release constricts arterioles

6. Secondary hypertension
   a. Results from identifiable sources, including renovascular disease; primary hyperaldosteronism; Cushing's syndrome; diabetes mellitus; neurologic disorders; dysfunction of thyroid, pituitary, or parathyroid glands; coarctation of the aorta; and pregnancy
   b. The pathophysiology is related to the disease causing the rise in pressure

B. Clinical findings
   1. Subjective: headache (occipital area); lightheadedness; tinnitus; easy fatigue; visual disturbances; palpitations
   2. Objective: blood pressure greater than 140/90 mm Hg obtained on three separate occasions; retinal changes; renal pathology (e.g., azotemia); epistaxis; cardiac hypertrophy

C. Therapeutic interventions
   1. Treatment algorithm recommended by the Joint National Committee on Detection, Evaluation, and Treatment of High Blood Pressure
      a. Step 1: lifestyle modifications: sodium restriction (1 to 2 g daily); weight control or reduction; alcohol restriction; cessation of smoking; regular exercise program; stress management
      b. Steps 2 to 5: pharmacologies are added by steps if lifestyle modifications alone are ineffective
         (1) Step 2: diuretic, beta blocker, calcium antagonist, angiotensin-converting enzyme (ACE) inhibitor or a receptor blocker is prescribed based on client's other health problems
         (2) Step 3: if ineffective, the dosage of the drug is increased, a different drug is given, or a second drug of a different classification is added
         (3) Step 4: if still ineffective, a second drug is substituted or a third drug of a different classification is added
         (4) Step 5: if still ineffective, a third or fourth drug is added
   2. Relaxation modalities such as biofeedback and imagery

Nursing Care of Clients with Hypertension

A. ASSESSMENT
1. Vital signs with client in both upright and recumbent positions; use proper size cuff (its width should be 40% of the arm's circumference); avoid errors of parallax when reading sphygmomanometer
2. Baseline weight
3. Presence of risk factors and clinical findings

B. ANALYSIS/NURSING DIAGNOSES
1. Ineffective therapeutic regimen management related to side effects of treatment (e.g., impo-

tence) and lack of knowledge about treatment and disease process
2. Fear related to questionable prognosis and potential disability/death

C. PLANNING/IMPLEMENTATION
1. Monitor electrolytes, BUN, creatinine lipid profile, and urine for protein
2. Weigh client daily when there is a threat of heart failure
3. Teach client to monitor own BP; advise client to change position slowly and avoid hot showers to prevent orthostatic hypotension
4. Reassure and support any expression of emotions; encourage relaxation techniques
5. Reinforce that hypertension is not cured, but controlled
6. Educate the client and family regarding drugs, follow-up care, activity restrictions, and diet; note that many salt substitutes contain potassium chloride rather than sodium chloride and may be permitted by the physician if client has no renal impairment

D. EVALUATION/OUTCOMES
1. Maintains blood pressure at an acceptable level
2. Understands and adheres to therapeutic regimen
3. Verbalizes need for stress reduction

▼ CORONARY ARTERY DISEASE (CAD): ATHEROSCLEROSIS, ANGINA PECTORIS, MYOCARDIAL INFARCTION

Data Base
A. Etiology and pathophysiology
   1. Atherosclerosis: deposition of fatty plaques along inner wall of coronary arteries leads to smooth muscle cell proliferation, narrowing and possible obstruction; also affects peripheral and cerebral vessels
   2. Angina pectoris: episodic pain experienced when oxygen supplied by the blood cannot meet the metabolic demands of the muscle. In addition to atherosclerosis this temporary ischemia may be precipitated by coronary artery spasms, strenuous exercise, hyperthyroidism, exposure to cold and emotional stress; classified as unstable preinfarction, chronic stable, nocturnally resting (Prinzmetal)
   3. Myocardial infarction (MI): acute necrosis of the heart muscle caused by interruption of oxygen supply to the area (ischemia), resulting in altered function and reduced cardiac output

4. Risk factors
   a. Family history
   b. Increasing age
   c. Gender: males and females especially after menopause (estrogen seems to provide some degree of protection)
   d. Race: risk appears higher in African-Americans
   e. Cigarette smoking (contributes to vasoconstriction, platelet activation, arterial smooth muscle cell proliferation, and reduced oxygen availability)
   f. Hypertension
   g. Hyperlipidemia: increased cholesterol; increased low-density lipoprotein cholesterol (LDL); increased ratio of total cholesterol or LDL-C to HDL-C; decreased high-density lipoprotein cholesterol (HDL); HDL seems to protect against CAD; increased triglycerides
   h. Obesity (particularly abdominal obesity)
   i. Sedentary lifestyle (contributes to obesity and reduced HDL)
   j. Diabetes
   k. Stress (an innate competitive, aggressive type A personality seems less important than amount of stress and client's psychologic response)
B. Clinical findings
   1. Subjective: retrosternal chest pain; pain may radiate to arms, jaw, neck, shoulder or back; pain described as "pressure," "crushing," or "viselike"; pain of angina is associated with activity and generally subsides with rest; palpitations; apprehension, feeling of dread; dyspnea; nausea; asymptomatic with silent ischemia
   2. Objective
      a. ECG changes may reveal ischemia (inverted T wave, elevated ST segment) or evidence of MI (presence of Q wave); a Holter monitor may be used to detect changes associated with ADL
      b. Elevated serum enzymes and isoenzymes with MI
         (1) Cardiac troponin T (cTnT) levels increase within 3 to 6 hours and remain elevated for 14 to 21 days; very accurate for assessing cardiac disease
         (2) Cardiac troponin I (cTnI) levels rise 7 to 14 hours after an MI and remain elevated for 5 to 7 days; highly specific for myocardial damage
         (3) Creatinine kinase or creatinine phosphokinase (CK or CPK); elevated 3 to 6 hours after infarction, peaking at 24 hours, and returning to normal within 72 to 96 hours
         (4) CK isoenzymes or CPK isoenzymes (CK-MB or CPK-MB): elevated 4 to 6 hours after pain, peaking within 24 hours, and returning to normal within 72 hours; specific for myocardial damage
         (5) Lactic dehydrogenase (LDH): elevated on first day, reaching its peak on third to fourth day, and then gradually subsiding
         (6) LDH$_1$ and LDH$_2$: elevated in 4 hours and peaking 48 hours after infarction
         (7) LDH isoenzymes: following a myocardial infarction LDH$_1$ is greater than LDH$_2$
         (8) Aspartate aminotransferase (AST) (formerly SGOT): elevated on days 2 to 4
      c. Doppler flow studies
      d. Cardiac Nuclear Scanning (thallium, MUGA) or echocardiographic studies can help determine extent of vessels involved
      e. Sympathetic nervous system responses: pallor, rapid pulse, diaphoresis, vomiting
      f. Dysrhythmia, elevated temperature, sedimentation rate, and WBCs (MI)
C. Therapeutic interventions
   1. Prevention of MI
      a. Supervised exercise program to avoid ischemia but promote collateral circulation, increase HDL; weight control; smoking cessation; dietary restriction of cholesterol and total and saturated fat
      b. Pharmacologic management: nitrates, beta-blocking agents, calcium channel-blocking agents, antilipidemics, antiplatelet agents (ASA)
      c. Supplemental oxygen during anginal attack as needed
      d. Percutaneous transluminal coronary angioplasty (PTCA)
      e. Coronary artery bypass surgery if medical regimen not successful
      f. Intracoronary stent placement
      g. Transmyocardial revascularization: involves creating laser channels in the myocardium to promote vascular growth or angiogenesis
   2. Management of acute MI
      a. Improvement of perfusion
         (1) Administer ASA immediately, often enroute to hospital
         (2) Begin beta blockage and IV nitroglycerin
         (3) Thrombolytic therapy within 3 to 6 hours of MI with streptokinase, urokinase, t-PA, reteplase
         (4) Antidysrhythmics to maintain cardiac function

(5) Intraaortic balloon pump that inflates during diastole and deflates during systole to decrease cardiac workload by decreasing afterload

b. Promotion of comfort and rest

(1) Administer analgesics such as intravenous morphine sulfate

(2) Oxygen administration to alter tissue hypoxia

(3) Maintain bed rest to decrease oxygen tissue demands

(4) Diet therapy may be 2 g sodium diet or clear liquids, depending on presence of nausea

c. Monitoring client

(1) Pulse oximetry

(2) Cardiac monitoring

(3) Vital signs

(4) Swan-Ganz catheter

d. Assessment for complications of MI

(1) Shock

(2) Pulmonary edema

(3) Embolism

(4) Extension of MI

(5) Pericarditis

Nursing Care of Clients with Coronary Artery Disease

A. ASSESSMENT

1. History of chest, arm, shoulder, neck, jaw pain
2. Precipitating factors (e.g., exercise, cold)
3. Risk factors (nonmodifiable and modifiable)
4. Vital signs
5. Intake and output (fluid volume overload is dangerous if cardiac output is compromised)
6. Adventitious breath sounds and dependent edema with impending failure
7. Restlessness, dyspnea
8. Skin: diaphoresis; pallor; cyanosis
9. If MI is suspected, continuous ECG monitoring to detect: changes in rate, rhythm, and conduction of heartbeat; life-threatening dysrhythmias (ventricular fibrillation and ventricular standstill); dysrhythmias such as premature ventricular beats close to a T wave, ventricular tachycardia, and atrial fibrillation

B. ANALYSIS/NURSING DIAGNOSES

1. Activity intolerance related to pain
2. Decreased cardiac output related to myocardial ischemia
3. Ineffective sexuality pattern related to chest pain
4. Anxiety related to anticipated lifestyle changes

C. PLANNING/IMPLEMENTATION

1. Teach signs and management of cardiac ischemia (rest; nitrates; emergency care if ineffective)

2. Encourage prophylactic administration of nitrates
3. Reinforce need to avoid nonaerobic exertion (e.g., shoveling snow) and exposure to cold air
4. Support involvement in smoking cessation programs
5. Encourage the following dietary program

a. Low cholesterol, low fat (especially saturated)

b. Replace vegetable oils high in PUFA with those high in MUFA, such as olive and avocado

c. Eat fish high in omega-3 fatty acids several times per week (salmon, tuna)

d. Increase intake of high-fiber foods such as fruits, vegetables, cereal grains, and legumes; soluble fiber is particularly effective in reducing blood lipids (oat bran, legumes)

6. Educate client about medications
7. Provide emotional support regarding alteration in lifestyle
8. Care of client after acute MI

a. Document dysrhythmia and respond with medications per protocol, defibrillation, or CPR

b. Administer oxygen, analgesics, vasodilators, and other medications as ordered

c. Recognize risk of sensory overload: orient to unit and equipment; allow time to express feelings; encourage short visits by significant others

d. Use measures to prevent sequelae to diminished activity: thrombophlebitis, pneumonia

D. EVALUATION/OUTCOMES

1. Remains free of chest pain
2. Verbalizes a reduced level of anxiety
3. Adheres to prescribed regimen (dietary, pharmacologic, and exercise)
4. Maintains oxygen saturation at 92% on room air

▼ INFLAMMATORY DISEASES OF THE HEART: PERICARDITIS, MYOCARDITIS, INFECTIVE SUBACUTE BACTERIAL ENDOCARDITIS

Data Base

A. Etiology and pathophysiology

1. Pericarditis

a. Acute or chronic inflammation of the pericardium

b. May be idiopathic or result from: bacterial infection (streptococcal, staphylococcal, gonococcal, meningococcal organisms); viral infection (coxsackievirus, influenza); mycotic (fungal) infection; rickettsial and parasitic infestation; trauma; collagen disease; rheumatic fever; neoplastic disease secondary to lung and breast metastasis

 c. Sequelae: loss of periocardial elasticity or an accumulation of fluid within the sac; heart failure or cardiac tamponade

 2. Myocarditis

  a. Inflammation of the myocardium

  b. May result from: viral, bacterial, mycotic, parasitic, protozoal, or spirochetal infections or infestations; rheumatic fever; endocarditis; impaired immune system

  c. Sequelae: impaired contractility of the heart caused by the inflammatory process; myocardial ischemia and necrosis

 3. Infective subacute bacterial endocarditis

  a. Inflammation of the inner lining of the heart and valves

  b. May result from: *Streptococcus viridans,* bacterial, fungal, or rickettsial infections; rheumatic heart disease

  c. Sequelae: structural damage to the valves; pump failure; embolization

B. Clinical findings

 1. Subjective: precordial or substernal pain; dyspnea; chills; fatigue and malaise

 2. Objective: dysrhythmias; increased cardiac enzymes; fever; positive blood cultures; friction rubs evident on auscultation

C. Therapeutic interventions

 1. Oxygen therapy and bed rest

 2. Antibiotics to relieve underlying infection; corticosteroids; antidysrhythmics; and salicylates to suppress rheumatic activity

 3. Pericardectomy (surgical removal of scar tissue and the pericardium), if indicated

 4. Cardiac monitoring

Nursing Care of Clients with Inflammatory Disease of the Heart

A. ASSESSMENT

 1. Signs of shock, heart failure, and dysrhythmias

 2. Temperature to obtain baseline data

 3. Distention of neck veins

 4. Friction rub and murmur

 5. Overt and covert indicators of pain

B. ANALYSIS/NURSING DIAGNOSES

 1. Activity intolerance related to reduced cardiac reserve

 2. Ineffective tissue perfusion: cardiopulmonary/peripheral related to risk for development of emboli

 3. Acute or chronic pain related to biological injury, inflammation

C. PLANNING/IMPLEMENTATION

 1. Maintain a tranquil environment and help the client achieve maximum rest; medicate for discomfort as needed

 2. Explain posthospitalization therapy to improve compliance (lifelong doses of penicillin prophylactically when undergoing invasive procedures)

 3. Administer IV antibiotics as ordered

 4. Monitor temperature and blood cultures to evaluate antibiotic therapy

 5. If surgical intervention is undertaken, care for chest tubes and follow the postoperative chest surgery routine (see Cardiac Surgery)

D. EVALUATION/OUTCOMES

 1. Verbalizes pain is relieved

 2. Achieves afebrile state

 3. Maintains vital signs within normal limits

 4. Adheres to therapeutic regimen

▼ HEART FAILURE (HF)

Data Base

A. Etiology and pathophysiology

 1. Inability of the heart to meet the demands of the body

 2. Pump failure may be caused by cardiac abnormalities or conditions that place increased demands on the heart such as cardiac muscle disorders, valvular defects, hypertension, coronary atherosclerosis, hyperthyroidism, obesity, and circulatory overload

 3. When one side of the heart "fails," there is essentially a buildup of pressure in the vascular system feeding into that side; signs of right-ventricular failure will be evident in the systemic circulation, those of left-ventricular failure in the pulmonary system

B. Clinical findings

 1. Left-ventricular heart failure

  a. Subjective: dyspnea from fluid within the lungs; orthopnea; fatigue and restlessness; paroxysmal nocturnal dyspnea

  b. Objective: crackles; peripheral cyanosis; Cheyne-Stokes respirations; frothy, blood-tinged sputum; dry, nonproductive cough

 2. Right-ventricular failure

  a. Subjective: abdominal pain; fatigue; bloating; nausea

  b. Objective: Dependent, pitting edema that often subsides at night when legs are elevated; ankle edema is frequently the first sign of HF; ascites from increased pressure within the portal system; hepatomegaly; anorexia; respiratory distress; increased CVP; diminished urinary output

C. Therapeutic interventions

 1. Rest in Fowler's position to reduce cardiac workload

2. Morphine sulfate to reduce anxiety and dyspnea
3. Oxygen therapy; in acute ventricular failure endotracheal intubation and a ventilator
4. Decrease cardiac workload with diuretics, venous vasodilators, vein and arteriole dilators, ACE inhibitors, and beta-adrenergic antagonists
5. Increase pump performance with cardiac glycosides, inotropes
6. Potassium supplements to prevent digitalis toxicity and hypokalemia
7. Hemodynamic monitoring through a multilumen pulmonary artery catheter
8. Sodium-restricted diet to limit fluid retention and promote fluid-excretion
9. A paracentesis if ascites exists and is causing respiratory distress

Nursing Care of Clients with Heart Failure

A. ASSESSMENT
  1. Baseline vital signs
  2. Body weight; circumference of edematous extremities
  3. Baseline CVP and pulmonary wedge pressure, when indicated
  4. Electrolyte levels (sodium, chloride, potassium)
  5. Intake and output
B. ANALYSIS/NURSING DIAGNOSES
  1. Decreased cardiac output related to impaired cardiac function
  2. Excess fluid volume related to impaired excretion of sodium and water
  3. Impaired gas exchange related to excessive fluid in interstitial space
C. PLANNING/IMPLEMENTATION
  1. Maintain the client in high-Fowler's position
  2. Elevate extremities except when the client is in acute distress
  3. Frequently monitor vital signs
  4. Change position frequently
  5. Monitor intake and output and daily weight
  6. Restrict fluids as ordered
  7. Monitor invasive lines
  8. Refer to glycoside and diuretic medications for additional nursing actions
D. EVALUATION/OUTCOMES
  1. Maintains adequate tissue perfusion
  2. Reduces peripheral edema/ascites
  3. Verbalizes understanding of pharmacologic and diet therapy

▼ CARDIAC SURGERY

Data Base

A. May be used to:

1. Correct abnormalities; mitral stenosis or regurgitation; aortic stenosis or insufficiency; coronary occlusion; ventricular aneurysm
2. Replace failing heart (cardiac transplantation): terminal heart disease with life expectancy of less than 1 year; viral myocarditis; toxic injury to the myocardium; severe coronary artery disease

B. Types of procedures: open or closed heart surgery (when extracorporeal circulation or the heart-lung machine is used, it is called open heart surgery)
  1. Hypothermia may be used to decrease metabolic rate during cardiac surgery
  2. Percutaneous transluminal coronary angioplasty (PTCA) is indicated for individuals with single-vessel disease; procedure involves inserting a balloon-tipped catheter into the diseased vessel and inflating it to reduce stenosis
  3. Coronary artery bypass graft (CABG) surgery is done when severe arteriosclerotic disease causes angina pectoris; involves anastomosis of a graft or a segment of a vessel (often the internal mammary artery and the saphenous vein), bypassing the diseased portion of a coronary artery; one or more vessels may be bypassed
  4. Cardiac transplantation involves replacement of the client's diseased heart with one from a compatible donor
  5. Surgical removal (ablation) of foci and pathways of dysrhythmias; involves mapping cardiac electrophysiologic function to locate the source of the dysrhythmic foci; surgical resection of the focus is made through a sternotomy
  6. Surgical repair or replacement of valves

Nursing Care of Clients Following Cardiac Surgery

A. ASSESSMENT
  1. Hemodynamic monitoring
  2. Airway patency
  3. Tubes to ensure patency and to assess drainage
  4. Incision for signs of hemorrhage or infection
B. ANALYSIS/NURSING DIAGNOSES
  1. Decreased cardiac output related to ventricular ischemia, dysrhythmias, depressed cardiac function
  2. Fear related to surgical procedure and death
  3. Acute or chronic pain related to traumatic, extensive surgery
C. PLANNING/IMPLEMENTATION
  1. Monitor hemodynamic functioning
  2. Evaluate neurologic signs
  3. Monitor temperature closely because fever increases the workload of the heart

4. Maintain airway; the client will have an endotracheal tube in place postoperatively and require mechanical ventilation; suction as necessary
5. Monitor intake and output; weigh regularly
6. Assess pain (nature, site, duration, type) and provide relief
7. Monitor arterial blood gases
8. Maintain a Foley catheter in place; in addition to output, monitor specific gravity
9. Care for chest tubes: maintain patency of tubes; avoid kinked tubing; drainage should not be more than 200 ml/hour
10. Administer parenteral therapy, including electrolytes and blood
11. Provide relief of anxiety and fear by staying with the client and explaining procedures; encourage verbalization of feelings; provide emotional support
12. If saphenous vein has been used, assess the leg for signs of impaired circulation, edema, or infection
13. Monitor client for signs of complications
    a. Hemorrhage that can lead to hypovolemia: decreased blood pressure, increased pulse rate; restlessness, apprehension; lowered CVP; pallor
    b. Cardiac tamponade caused by collection of fluid or blood within pericardium: decreased arterial pressure; elevated CVP; rapid, thready pulse; diminished output
    c. Heart failure: dyspnea; elevated CVP; tachycardia; edema
    d. Myocardial infarction
    e. Renal failure
    f. Embolism
    g. Psychosis resulting from an inability to cope with anxiety associated with cardiac surgery

D. EVALUATION/OUTCOMES
1. Achieves adequate cardiac output
2. Maintains painless state
3. Performs self-care activities

▼ VASCULAR DISEASE: THROMBOPHLEBITIS, VARICOSE VEINS, AND PERIPHERAL VASCULAR DISEASE

Data Base
A. Etiology and pathophysiology
1. Thrombus: a clot composed of platelets, fibrin, clotting factors, and cellular debris attached to the interior wall of an artery or vein

2. Embolus: a clot or solid particle carried by the bloodstream, which may interfere with tissue perfusion in an artery or vein
3. Arterial disorders involve depriving oxygen to a body part or tissue. This is affected by blood pressure and presence of collateral circulation
   a. Reduced blood flow resulting from atherosclerosis, thrombus, or embolus
   b. Buerger's disease (thromboangiitis obliterans)
      (1) Peripheral circulation impaired by inflammatory occlusions of peripheral arteries; thromboses of arteries may occur
      (2) Incidence is highest in young adult males who smoke
   c. Raynaud's disease
      (1) Spasms of digital arteries thought to be caused by abnormal response of the sympathetic nervous system to cold or emotional stress, usually bilateral and primarily occurs in young females
      (2) Raynaud's phenomenon is episodic arterial spasm of the extremities secondary to another disease or abnormality
4. Venous disorders involve a problem with transportation of blood back to the heart from the capillary beds as a result of changes in smooth muscle around vessels
   a. Thrombophlebitis: inflammation of a vein associated with clot formation; risk factors include immobilization, venous stasis, vessel trauma, pregnancy, obesity, and pelvic surgery
   b. Varicose veins occur when veins in lower extremities become dilated, congested, tortuous as a result of weakness of valves or loss of elasticity of vessel walls; risk factors include family history, prolonged standing, pregnancy, leg trauma, thrombophlebitis
B. Clinical findings
1. Peripheral arterial disorders
   a. Subjective: paresthesia; aching to severe or burning pain
   b. Objective: pallor or cyanosis; gangrenous ulcers and diminished pulses in Buerger's disease
2. Varicose veins
   a. Subjective: heaviness and fatigue in legs with cramping that increases at night
   b. Objective: positive venogram; positive Trendelenburg test is diagnostic of varicose veins; brown skin discoloration; stasis ulcers
3. Thrombophlebitis
   a. Subjective: pain on dorsiflexion of affected extremity (Homans' sign); may be asymptomatic until embolus is released and occludes organ

    b. Objective: swollen limb with hard veins that are sensitive to pressure; redness and warmth of area along the vein; Doppler studies/flow studies of lower extremities indicate obstruction or decreased flow to the area suggest thrombus formation

C. Therapeutic intervention
1. Peripheral vascular disease
    a. Sympathectomy to sever the sympathetic ganglia supplying the area; there is local vasodilatation with improved circulation
    b. Femoropopliteal bypass grafting
    c. Amputation if vascular supply is severely impaired (see Neuromusculoskeletal System)
2. Varicose veins
    a. Sclerotherapy involves injection of a chemical irritant to the vein
    b. Surgical intervention involves ligation of the vein above the varicosity and removal of the involved vein; the great saphenous vein may be ligated near the femoral junction
    c. Postoperative early ambulation is essential to prevent formation of thrombi
3. Thrombophlebitis
    a. Prophylactic antiembolytic stockings and exercises to promote venous return
    b. Warm moist heat to promote vasodilation
    c. Elevation of extremity to reduce edema
    d. Anticoagulants to prevent recurrence of deep vein involvement
    e. Vasodilators to prevent vascular spasm
    f. Thrombolytic therapy to dissolve clot
    g. Transvenous filter or thrombectomy

Nursing Care of Clients with Vascular Disease

A. ASSESSMENT
1. Risk factors and subjective data
2. Affected extremity for pulses, color, temperature, and circumference
3. Mobility of involved extremity

B. ANALYSIS/NURSING DIAGNOSES
1. Ineffective tissue perfusion: peripheral related to venous stasis
2. Risk for impaired skin integrity related to altered peripheral tissue perfusion
3. Chronic pain related to vascular obstruction

C. PLANNING/IMPLEMENTATION
1. Observe frequently for signs of vascular impairment (e.g., pallor, cyanosis, coolness of involved extremities, and amplitude and symmetry of peripheral pulses)
2. Apply antiembolism stockings before ambulating and remove and replace as ordered; if thrombophlebitis is suspected maintain bed rest and notify physician
3. Instruct the client to avoid tight and constricting clothing that can affect peripheral vessels, cigarette smoking, massaging legs, maintaining one position for long periods; reduce weight when indicated
4. In arterial disease, keep extremities warm; instruct the client to wear gloves when exposed to cold and apply lubricants to keep skin supple
5. Observe for signs of pulmonary embolism (e.g., sudden pain, cyanosis, hemoptysis, shock)
6. Provide specific care if undergoing vascular surgery: monitor for hemorrhage; notify physician if bleeding is suspected; assess circulatory status of extremity; keep extremity elevated; allow out of bed as ordered; avoid prolonged hip flexion
7. Provide specific care for the client following a vein ligation: elevate the foot of the bed for the first 24 hours; observe for signs of hemorrhage; maintain compression dressings; assist with ambulation
8. Provide specific care for the client following endarterectomy and femoropopliteal bypass grafting
    a. Assess circulation of involved area by checking pulses, color, temperature, and neurologic function
    b. Observe blood pressure frequently because hypotension increases the possibility of thrombus formation
    c. Observe for signs of hemorrhage, pain, change in skin color, and alteration of vital signs
    d. Ambulate as ordered; sitting should be avoided in femoropopliteal bypass surgery
9. See care associated with amputation in Neuromusculoskeletal System

D. EVALUATION/OUTCOMES
1. Maintains tissue perfusion
2. Verbalizes reduction in pain

▼ ANEURYSMS

Data Base

A. Etiology and pathophysiology
1. Distention at the site of a weakness in the arterial wall
    a. Saccular aneurysm: pouchlike projection on one side of the artery
    b. Fusiform aneurysm: entire circumference of the artery wall is dilated
    c. Mycotic aneurysm: tiny weaknesses in arterial walls resulting from infection
    d. Dissecting aneurysm: tear in the inner lining of an arteriosclerotic aortic wall

causes blood to form a hematoma between layers of the artery compressing the lumen

2. Causes: congenital weakness; syphilis; trauma; atherosclerosis (most common cause of both thoracic and abdominal aortic aneurysms)
3. Represent surgical emergency if ruptured
4. Occur most frequently in middle-aged white males
5. Risk factors include history of hypertension, obesity, stress, hypercholesterolemia, cigarette smoking, familial tendency

B. Clinical findings
   1. Thoracic aortic aneurysm
      a. Subjective: may be asymptomatic; dyspnea; dysphagia; pain resulting from pressure against the nerves or vertebrae
      b. Objective: hoarseness, cough, and aphonia from impingement on laryngeal nerve; unequal pulses and arterial pressure in upper extremities; trachea may be displaced from midline because of adhesions between trachea and aneurysm
   2. Abdominal aortic aneurysm
      a. Subjective: may be asymptomatic; lower back or abdominal pain (severe if aneurysm is leaking); sensory changes in the lower extremities if aneurysm ruptures
      b. Objective: hypertension; pulsating abdominal mass; mottling of the lower extremities if aneurysm ruptures; increased abdominal girth if aneurysm ruptures
   3. Dissecting aortic aneurysm
      a. Subjective: restlessness; anxiety; severe pain
      b. Objective: diminished pulses; signs of shock

C. Therapeutic interventions
   1. Resection of the aneurysm and use of a Teflon or Dacron graft
   2. Surgical procedures involving the aorta would necessitate use of a heart-lung device (cardiopulmonary bypass)
   3. Medical treatment is aimed at decreasing cardiac output and blood pressure through the use of drugs

Nursing Care of Clients with Aneurysms

A. ASSESSMENT
1. History of risk factors
2. Pulsation in abdomen (palpate gently)
3. History of pain

B. ANALYSIS/NURSING DIAGNOSES
1. Health-seeking behaviors related to lack of knowledge concerning modifications necessary to reduce risk factors
2. Ineffectve tissue perfusion: peripheral related to impaired arterial circulation

3. Risk for deficient fluid volume: hemorrhage related to potential blood loss

C. PLANNING/IMPLEMENTATION
1. Perform neurovascular assessment of extremities
2. Monitor hemodynamic status
3. Record intake and output, because renal failure may occur after surgery
4. Administer narcotics as ordered to alleviate pain
5. Apply abdominal binders to provide support when the client is coughing, deep breathing, and ambulating
6. Prevent flexion of hip and knees to eliminate pressure on the arterial wall

D. EVALUATION/OUTCOMES
1. Maintains adequate peripheral circulation
2. Identifies ways to modify risk factors

▼ SHOCK

Data Base
A. Etiology and pathophysiology
   1. Hypovolemic: occurs when there is a loss of fluid resulting in inadequate tissue perfusion; caused by excessive bleeding, diarrhea, or vomiting; fluid loss from fistulas or burns
   2. Cardiogenic: occurs when pump failure causes inadequate tissue perfusion; caused by heart failure; myocardial infarction; cardiac tamponade
   3. Neurogenic: caused by rapid vasodilation and subsequent pooling of blood within the peripheral vessels; caused by spinal anesthesia; emotional stress; drugs that inhibit the sympathetic nervous system
   4. Anaphylactic: caused by an allergic reaction that causes a release of histamine and subsequent vasodilation
   5. Septic (similar to anaphylaxis) reaction to bacterial toxins (generally gram-negative infections), which results in the leakage of plasma into tissues

B. Clinical findings
   1. Subjective: apprehension; restlessness; paresis of extremities
   2. Objective: weak, rapid, thready pulse; diaphoresis; cold, clammy skin; pallor; decreased urine output; progressive loss of consciousness; decreased mean arterial pressure (normal 80 to 120 mm Hg)

C. Therapeutic interventions
   1. Aimed at correcting the underlying cause
   2. Fluid and blood replacement
   3. Oxygen therapy, ventilator
   4. Vasoconstricting drugs to increase blood pressure
   5. Cardiac and hemodynamic monitoring

6. Cardiotonics for cardiogenic shock
7. Adrenergic blockage: prevents effects of prolonged vasoconstriction; causes loss of fluid from vascular compartment
8. Antihistamines for anaphylactic shock
9. Antibiotics for septic shock based on blood cultures
10. Elevation of lower extremities to ensure circulation to vital organs
11. Intraaortic balloon pump may be used to aid the failing heart
12. MAST or pneumatic antishock garment causes resistance in the vessels and reduces vessel diameter in the legs and abdomen; used in trauma settings

Nursing Care of Clients in Shock

A. ASSESSMENT
1. History of causative and risk factors from client
2. Fluid intake and output over the previous 24 hours
3. Signs of covert bleeding: weak, thready pulse; hypotension; increased respirations; cold clammy skin
4. Mental status

B. ANALYSIS/NURSING DIAGNOSES
1. Ineffective tissue perfusion: cardiopulmonary, peripheral related to arterial/venous blood flow exchange problems
2. Risk for injury related to prolonged shock resulting in multiple organ failure
3. Deficient fluid volume related to loss of fluid

C. PLANNING/IMPLEMENTATION
1. Keep the client warm, place in supine position
2. Monitor hemodynamic status and vital signs
3. Monitor urine output and specific gravity
4. Allay client's anxiety
5. Administer intravenous fluids as ordered
6. Monitor oxygen saturation and provide oxygen therapy as indicated

D. EVALUATION/OUTCOMES
1. Reduces blood/fluid loss
2. Restores normal circulating volume
3. Maintains a urine output of 30 ml or more per hour
4. Remains oriented to time, place, and person
5. Maintains adequate cardiac output

▼ ANEMIAS AND BLOOD DISORDERS

Data Base
A. Etiology and pathophysiology
1. Iron deficiency anemia: most common cause is bleeding related to GI bleeding, menstruation, malignancy; other causes include inadequate dietary intake, malabsorption, and increased demand (e.g., pregnancy)
2. Folate deficiency: amount of folic acid absorbed or ingested is insufficient to synthesize DNA, RNA, and proteins; associated with alcoholism, malabsorption, pregnancy, lactation
3. Pernicious anemia: lack of intrinsic factor in the stomach prevents the absorption of B_{12}, which reduces the number of erythrocytes formed
4. Aplastic (hypoplastic) anemia: bone marrow is depressed or destroyed by a chemical or drug leading to leukopenia, thrombocytopenia, decreased erythrocytes, and decreased leukocytes (agranulocytosis)
5. Hemolytic anemia: excessive or premature destruction of red blood cells. There are many causes, which include sickle cell anemia, thalassemia, G-6-PD deficiency, antibody reactions, infection, and toxins
6. Polycythemia vera: a sustained increase in the number of erythrocytes, leukocytes, and platelets, with an increased viscosity of the blood.
7. Thrombocytopenia purpura: appears to result from the production of an antiplatelet antibody that coats the surface of platelets and facilitates their destruction by phagocytic leukocytes

B. Clinical findings
1. Subjective: fatigue, headache; paresthesias; dyspnea; sore mouth with pernicious anemia; gum bleeding and epistaxis with thrombocytopenic purpura
2. Objective
   a. Ankle edema
   b. Dry, pale mucous membranes
   c. Pallor (except polycythemia vera)
   d. Decreased hemoglobin, erythrocytes, ferritin, increased iron-binding capacity, megaloblastic condition of the blood with iron deficiency anemia
   e. Beefy red tongue, lack of intrinsic factor, positive Romberg test (loss of balance with eyes closed) with pernicous anemia
   f. Fever, bleeding from mucous membranes, decreased leukocytes, erythrocytes, and platelets with aplastic anemia
   g. Increased hemoglobin, purple-red complexion with polycythemia vera
   h. Low platelet count, ecchymotic areas, hemorrhagic petechiae with thrombocytopenic purpura

C. Therapeutic interventions
1. Improve diet: include ascorbic acid, which stimulates iron uptake
2. Vitamin supplements: iron, B_{12}, folic acid

3. Blood transfusions (except for polycythemia vera)
4. Corticosteroids and androgens to stimulate bone marrow function; bone marrow transplant; splenectomy when formed elements of the blood are destroyed (aplastic anemia); thrombocytopenic purpura
5. Phlebotomy, low iron diet, radioactive phosphorus, busulfan (Mylaran) (for polycythemia vera)
6. Removal of causative agent; splenectomy may be indicated for hemolytic anemias

Nursing Care of Clients with Anemias and Blood Disorders

A. **ASSESSMENT**
1. Obtain thorough history of dietary habits, symptoms, and causative agents
2. Observe status of skin, mucous membranes, and sclera
3. Obtain baseline vital signs

B. **ANALYSIS/NURSING DIAGNOSES**
1. Fatigue related to decreased oxygen supply to the body and increased cardiac workload
2. Ineffective protection related to impaired hemopoiesis (thrombocytopenic purpura)
3. Ineffective health maintenance related to knowledge deficit regarding nutritional and therapeutic regimen
4. Risk for infection related to altered immune response (aplastic anemia, leukopenia)

C. **PLANNING/IMPLEMENTATION**
1. Teach client about dietary modifications and medication administration
2. Explain the need for prevention of hemorrhage and phlebotomies (for polycythemia vera)
3. Provide postoperative care if splenectomy is performed

D. **EVALUATION/OUTCOMES**
1. States dietary sources of iron, folic acid, and vitamin B_{12}
2. Verbalizes understanding of long-term need for therapeutic supervision
3. Performs ADL
4. Remains afebrile and injury free

▼ DISSEMINATED INTRAVASCULAR COAGULATION (DIC)

Data Base
A. Etiology and pathophysiology
1. Body's response to overstimulation of clotting and anticlotting processes in response to injury or disease
2. Complicated by hemorrhage at various sites throughout the body

B. Clinical findings
1. Subjective: restlessness; anxiety
2. Objective
a. Laboratory tests indicate low fibrinogen and prolonged prothrombin and partial thromboplastin times, reduced platelets, elevated fibrin split products
b. Hemorrhage, both subcutaneous and internal

C. Therapeutic interventions
1. Relieve the underlying cause
2. Heparin to prevent the formation of thrombi
3. Transfusion of blood products
4. Antifibrinolytic therapy to prevent bleeding may be necessary

Nursing Care of Clients with Disseminated Intravascular Coagulation

A. **ASSESSMENT**
1. History of causative factors (generally septicemia, obstetric emergencies, and septic shock)
2. Subcutaneous hemorrhages

B. **ANALYSIS/NURSING DIAGNOSES**
1. Fear related to threat to well being/death
2. Ineffective tissue perfusion: peripheral related to hypovolemia and microemboli
3. Ineffective protection related to abnormal clotting mechanism

C. **PLANNING/IMPLEMENTATION**
1. Observe for bleeding
2. Minimize skin punctures
3. Prevent injury
4. Provide emotional support

D. **EVALUATION/OUTCOMES**
1. Maintains circulation to all tissues
2. Verbalizes a decrease in fears
3. Maintains adequate cardiac output

▼ LEUKEMIA

See Leukemia in Pediatric Nursing

Data Base
A. Etiology and pathophysiology
1. Incidence highest in children ages 2 to 6; declines until age 35, at which point there is a steady increase
2. Etiology unknown, although exposure to certain toxic substances such as radiation seems to increase the incidence
3. In general, an uncontrolled proliferation of white blood cells; classified according to the type of white blood cell affected
a. Acute lymphocytic leukemia (ALL): primarily occurs in children

b. Acute myelogenous leukemia (AML): occurs throughout life cycle; prognosis is poor with or without chemotherapy; leukocytes are immature and abnormal

c. Chronic myelogenous leukemia (CML): occurs after the second decade; prognosis is poor; results from abnormal production of granulocytic cells

d. Chronic lymphocytic leukemia (CLL): occurs most commonly in 50 to 70 year olds; life expectancy is 4 to 5 years; results from increased production of leukocytes and lymphocytes and proliferation of cells within the bone marrow, spleen, and liver

B. Clinical findings
1. Subjective: malaise; bone pain
2. Objective: anemia; thrombocytopenia; elevated leukocytes; decreased platelets; petechiae; gingival bleeding

C. Therapeutic interventions
1. Chemotherapy
2. Transfusions of whole blood or blood fractions
3. Analgesics
4. Bone marrow transplant
5. Radiation to areas of lymphocytic infiltration

Nursing Care of Clients with Leukemia

A. ASSESSMENT
1. History of infectious processes
2. Overt and covert bleeding
3. Baseline vital signs; observe for signs of anemia, thrombocytopenia, and neutropenia

B. ANALYSIS/NURSING DIAGNOSES
1. Acute or chronic pain related to leukocytic infiltration of systemic tissues
2. Fatigue related to anemia
3. Anticipatory grieving related to anticipated loss
4. Risk for infection related to ineffective immune system
5. Risk for injury related to thrombocytopenia

C. PLANNING/IMPLEMENTATION
1. Discuss the importance of follow-up care with the client and family
2. Provide emotional support for the client and family
3. Provide specific nursing care related to chemotherapeutic therapy, transfusion, or diagnostic tests
4. Provide a safe injury-free environment
5. Use appropriate infection control techniques
6. Pace care to avoid client fatigue and assist as necessary

D. EVALUATION/OUTCOMES
1. States signs of infection
2. Remains free from bleeding episodes
3. Verbalizes a decrease in fears
4. Plans strategies to avoid excessive energy expenditure
5. Remains free from infection

▼ HODGKIN'S DISEASE

Data Base
A. Etiology and pathophysiology
1. Cause unknown
2. Higher incidence in males and young adults
3. Proliferation of malignant cells (Reed-Sternberg cells) within lymph nodes
4. All tissues may eventually be involved, but chiefly lymph nodes, spleen, liver, tonsils, and bone marrow
5. Classification by staging and the presence or absence of systemic symptoms

B. Clinical findings
1. Subjective: pruritus; anorexia; dyspnea and dysphagia caused by pressure from enlarged nodes
2. Objective
a. Enlarged lymph nodes (generally cervical nodes are involved first)
b. Diagnosis confirmed by histologic examination of a lymph node
c. Progressive anemia
d. Elevated temperature
e. Enlarged spleen and liver may occur
f. Pressure from enlarged lymph nodes may cause symptoms of edema and obstructive jaundice
g. Thrombocytopenia if spleen and bone marrow involved

C. Therapeutic interventions
1. Radiotherapy
a. Vital organs must be shielded
b. Potential side effects: nausea; skin rashes; dry mouth; dysphagia; infections; pancytopenia
2. Chemotherapy: MOPP and ABVD protocols (see Related Pharmacology under Neoplastic Disorders)
3. Surgical intervention includes excision of masses to relieve pressure on other organs

Nursing Care of Clients with Hodgkin's Disease

A. ASSESSMENT
1. Lymph nodes to determine enlargement
2. Temperature for baseline data
3. Liver and spleen to determine enlargement

B. ANALYSIS/NURSING DIAGNOSES
1. Activity intolerance related to effects of disease and side effects of treatment
2. Risk for infection related to inadequate immune system
3. Anticipatory grieving related to anticipated loss

C. PLANNING/IMPLEMENTATION
1. Provide emotional support for the client and family

2. Protect from infection
3. Monitor temperature
4. Observe for signs of anemia; provide adequate rest
5. Examine sclera and skin for signs of jaundice
6. Encourage high nutrient density foods; observe for anorexia and nausea

D. EVALUATION/OUTCOMES
1. Remains afebrile
2. Conserves energy
3. Verbalizes feelings related to therapy and prognosis

▼ LYMPHOSARCOMA

See Hodgkin's Disease for Data Base and Nursing Care

RESPIRATORY SYSTEM

REVIEW OF ANATOMY AND PHYSIOLOGY

Functions of the Respiratory System

A. The upper portion of the respiratory system filters, moistens, and warms air during inspiration
B. The lower portion of the respiratory system enables the exchange of gases between blood and air to regulate serum Po_2, Pco_2, and pH

Structures of the Respiratory System

Nose
A. Structure
1. Anterior nares: exterior openings
2. Nasal cavities: lining is ciliated mucosa; divided by septum; turbinates (conchae) projected from lateral walls
3. Paranasal sinuses draining into the nose: frontal, maxillary, sphenoidal, ethmoidal
B. Functions
1. Passageway for incoming and outgoing air, filtering, warming, and moistening
2. Organ of smell: olfactory receptors located in the nasal mucosa
3. Aids in phonation

Pharynx
A. Structure: composed of muscle with mucous lining
1. Nasopharynx: behind the nose; opens into eustachian tubes; contains nasopharyngeal tonsils (adenoids)
2. Oropharynx: forms archway behind the mouth; contains palatine tonsils
3. Laryngopharynx: opens into esophagus and larynx
B. Functions: passageway to the respiratory and digestive tracts; aids in phonation; tonsils help destroy incoming bacteria

Larynx
A. Location: at upper end of the trachea, just below the pharynx
B. Structure
1. Formed by cartilage including the thyroid cartilage (Adam's apple); epiglottis (the lid cartilage); and cricoid (the signet ring cartilage)
2. Vocal cords
   a. False cords: folds of mucous lining
   b. True cords: fibroelastic bands stretched across the hollow interior of the larynx; the paired vocal cords (folds) and the posterior arytenoid cartilages make up the glottis
C. Functions: voice production: during expiration, air passing through the larynx causes the vocal cords to vibrate; short, tense cords produce a high pitch; long, relaxed cords, a low pitch; serves as part of the passageway for air and as the entrance to the lower respiratory tract

Trachea
A. Structure
1. Walls: smooth muscle; contain C-shaped rings of cartilage that keep the tube open at all times
2. Lining: ciliated mucosa
3. Extend from larynx to bronchi; 10 to 12 cm long
B. Function: furnishes open passageway for air going to and from lungs

Lungs
A. Structure
1. Divisions
   a. Root: consists of the primary bronchus and pulmonary artery and veins bound together by connective tissue
   b. Hilum: vertical slit on medial surface of the lung, through which root structures enter the lung
   c. Lobes: three in the right lung, two in the left
   d. Apex: pointed upper part of the lung
   e. Base: broad, inferior surface of the lung
2. Bronchial tree: consists of the following
   a. Bronchi: right and left, formed by branching of the trachea; right bronchus slightly larger and more vertical than left; each primary bronchus branches into segmental bronchi in each lung; primary and segmental bronchi all contain C-shaped cartilage
   b. Bronchioles: small branches off the secondary bronchi, distinguished by lack of C-shaped cartilage and a duct diameter of about 1 mm, which further branch into terminal bronchioles, respiratory bronchioles, and then alveolar ducts
   c. Alveoli: microscopic sacs composed of a single layer of extremely thin squamous epithelial cells enveloped by a network of lung capillaries

3. Covering of lung: visceral layer of pleura
B. Function
   1. Bronchi, bronchioles, alveolar ducts: passage to move air into and out of alveoli
   2. Alveoli: provide a surface area large enough and thin enough to allow rapid gas exchange
      a. Type I cells form walls
      b. Type II cells produce surfactant to prevent alveolar collapse

Physiology of Respiration

A. Mechanism of breathing
   1. Following phrenic nerve stimulation, the diaphragm and other respiratory muscles contract
   2. Thorax increases in size
   3. Intrathoracic and intrapulmonic pressures decrease
   4. Air rushes from positive pressure in the atmosphere to negative pressure in the alveoli
   5. Inspiration is completed
   6. Expiration reverses procedure of inspiration
B. Control of respiration
   1. Alveolar stretch receptors respond to inspiration by sending inhibitory impulses to inspiratory neurons in brainstem to prevent lung overdistention (Hering-Breuer reflex)
   2. Blood pH: decrease in pH stimulates respiration by direct stimulation of respiratory center (medulla)
   3. Blood Pco_2: increase in arterial Pco_2 results in decrease in pH and stimulation of respiration
   4. Blood Po_2: decrease in arterial Po_2 produces effects similar to decreased blood pH
C. Amount of air exchanged in breathing
   1. Directly related to gas pressure gradient between atmosphere and alveoli and inversely related to resistance that opposes air flow; pulmonary function can be evaluated with a spirometer
   2. Tidal volume: average amount expired after normal inspiration; approximately 500 ml
   3. Expiratory reserve volume (ERV): largest additional volume of air that can be forcibly expired after a normal inspiration and expiration; normal ERV 1000 to 1200 ml
   4. Inspiratory reserve volume (IRV): largest additional volume of air that can be forcibly inspired after a normal inspiration; normal IRV 3000 to 3300 ml
   5. Residual volume: air that cannot be forcibly expired from lungs; about 1200 ml
   6. Vital capacity: amount of air that can be forcibly expired after forcible inspiration; varies with size of thoracic cavity, which is determined by various factors (e.g., size of rib cage, posture, volume of blood and interstitial fluid in the lungs, size of the heart)

7. Forced expiratory volume (FEV): volume of air that can be forcibly exhaled within a specific time, usually 1 to 3 seconds
8. Positions such as orthopneic and Fowler's can lower abdominal organs and reduce pressure against diaphragm
D. Diffusion of gases between air and blood
   1. Occurs across alveolar-capillary membranes (i.e., in lungs between air in alveoli and venous blood in lung capillaries); adequate diffusion depends on a balanced ventilation-perfusion (V-Q) ratio
   2. Direction of diffusion
      a. Oxygen: net diffusion toward lower oxygen pressure gradient (i.e., from alveolar air to blood)
      b. Carbon dioxide: net diffusion toward lower carbon dioxide pressure gradient (i.e., from blood to alveolar air)
E. Blood transports oxygen as a solute (Po_2) and as oxyhemoglobin (oxygen saturation)
F. Blood transports carbon dioxide
   1. Primarily as a bicarbonate ion (HCO_3^-) formed by ionization of carbonic acid
   2. As a solute in plasma
   3. In combination with hemoglobin (carboxyhemoglobin)
G. Diffusion of gases between arterial blood and tissues occurs in tissue capillaries
   1. Oxygen: net diffusion of dissolved oxygen out of the blood into the tissues because of lower Po_2 there (perhaps 30 mm Hg, compared to arterial Po_2 of 100 mm Hg); diffusion of dissolved oxygen out of the blood lowers blood Po_2 from arterial to venous level (from 100 to 40 mm Hg); decreasing Po_2 as the blood moves through tissue capillaries causes oxygen to dissociate from hemoglobin, thereby releasing more oxygen for diffusion out of the blood to the tissue cells
   2. Carbon dioxide: net diffusion of carbon dioxide into the blood because of lower Pco_2 there (40 mm Hg compared with probably more than 50 mm Hg in tissues); diffusion of carbon dioxide into tissue capillaries increases blood Pco_2 from arterial to venous level (from 40 to 46 mm Hg); increasing Pco_2, similar to decreasing Po_2, tends to accelerate oxygen dissociation from hemoglobin
H. Normal breath sounds
   1. Bronchial sounds (over trachea, larynx): result of air passing through larger airways; sounds are loud, harsh, high pitched; expiration longer than inspiration
   2. Vesicular sounds (over entire lung field except large airways): result of air moving in and out

of alveoli; may reflect sound of air in larger passages that is transmitted through lung tissue; sounds are quiet, low pitched; inspiration longer than expiration

3. Bronchovesicular sounds (near main stem bronchi); result of air moving through smaller air passages; sounds are moderately pitched, breezy; inspiratory and expiratory phases equal

I. Adventitious breath sounds
   1. Fine crackles
      a. Result of sudden opening of small airways and alveoli that contain fluid
      b. Short, high-pitched bubbling sounds; sounds may be simulated by rubbing a few strands of hair between fingers next to the ear
      c. Most common during the height of inspiration
      d. Associated with conditions such as pneumonia and pulmonary edema
   2. Course crackles
      a. Rush of air passing through airway intermittently occluded by mucus
      b. Short, low-pitched bubbling sounds
      c. Most common on inspiration and at times expiration
      d. Associated with pneumonia and pulmonary edema
   3. Wheezes
      a. Result of air passing through narrowed small airways
      b. Sounds are high pitched and musical (sibilant wheezes), or low pitched and rumbling (sonorous wheezes or rhonchi)
      c. Most common on expiration
      d. Associated with conditions causing narrowing of airways, such as asthma, and with conditions that involve partial obstruction of airway by mucus, foreign body, or tumor
   4. Pleural friction rub
      a. Result of roughened pleural surfaces rubbing across each other
      b. Sounds are crackling, grating
      c. Most common during height of inspiration but can occur throughout the respiratory cycle
      d. Associated with conditions causing inflammation of the pleura

REVIEW OF MICROORGANISMS

A. Bacterial pathogens
   1. *Bordetella pertussis:* small, gram-negative coccobacillus; causes pertussis or whooping cough
   2. *Streptococcus pneumoniae:* gram-positive, encapsulated diplococcus; causes pneumococcal pneumonia (most commonly lobar) and often responsible for sinusitis, otitis media, and meningitis

   3. *Haemophilus influenzae:* small, gram-negative, highly pleomorphic bacillus; causes acute meningitis and upper respiratory tract infections
   4. *Klebsiella pneumoniae* (Friedlander's bacillus): gram-negative, encapsulated, nonspore-forming bacillus; causes pneumonia and urinary tract infections
   5. *Mycobacterium tuberculosis* (tubercle bacillus): acid-fast actinomycete causes tuberculosis
   6. *Pseudomonas aerucginosa:* gram-negative, non–spore-forming bacillus; important cause of hospital-acquired infections; respiratory equipment can be source; causes pneumonia, urinary tract infections, and the sepsis that complicates severe burns

B. Rickettsial pathogen: *Coxiella burnetii:* only Rickettsiae species not associated with a vector; causes Q fever, an infection clinically similar to primary atypical pneumonia

C. Viral pathogens
   1. DNA viruses: adenoviruses cause acute respiratory tract disease, adenitis, pharyngitis, and other respiratory tract infections, as well as conjunctivitis
   2. RNA viruses
      a. Coronaviruses: frequently associated with a mild upper respiratory tract infection
      b. Picornaviruses: cause poliomyelitis, coxsackie disease, common cold
      c. Retroviruses: invade T lymphocytes and are associated with malignancies, human immunodeficiency virus, and AIDS

D. Fungal pathogens:
   1. *Histoplasma capsulatum:* dimorphic fungus producing chlamydospores in infected tissue; causes histoplasmosis
   2. *Pneumocystis carinii:* a unicellular organism thought to be transmitted by air-borne droplets

 RELATED PHARMACOLOGY

Bronchodilators
A. Description
   1. Reverse bronchoconstriction, thus opening air passages in the lungs
   2. Act by stimulating beta-adrenergic sympathetic nervous system receptors, relaxing bronchial smooth muscle
   3. Available in oral, parenteral (IM, SC, IV), rectal, and inhalation preparations
B. Examples
   1. Adrenergics: act at beta-adrenergic receptors in bronchus to relax smooth muscle and increase respiratory volume: albuterol (Proventil); epinephrine HCl (Adrenalin; Sus-Phrine); metaproterenol sulfate (Alupent); salmeterol (Serevent)

2. Xanthines: act directly on bronchial smooth muscle, decreasing spasm and relaxing smooth muscle of the vasculature: aminophylline; theophylline (Elixophyllin; TheoDur)
3. Anticholinergics: inhibit action of acetylcholine at receptor sites on the bronchial smooth muscle: ipratropium (Atrovent)
4. Steroids: exert antiinflammatory effect on nasal passages: fluticasone (Flovent); beclomethasone
5. Leukotriene receptor antagonists: block action of leukotriene to reduce bronchoconstriction and inflammation associated with asthma; montelukast sodium (Singulair), zafirlukast (Accolate), zileuton (Zyflo)

C. Major side effects: dizziness (decrease in blood pressure); CNS stimulation (sympathetic stimulation); palpitations (beta-adrenergic stimulation); gastric irritation (local effect)

D. Nursing care
1. Avoid administration to clients with hypertension, hyperthyroidism, and cardiovascular dysfunction
2. Avoid concurrent administration of CNS stimulants (adrenergics) and bronchoconstricting agents (beta blockers)
3. Administer during waking hours
4. Assess vital signs, especially respirations
5. Assess intake and output
6. Administer with food

Mucolytic agents and expectorants

A. Description
1. Liquify secretions in the respiratory tract, promoting a productive cough
2. Mucolytics act directly to break up mucous plugs in tracheobronchial passages
3. Expectorants act indirectly to liquify mucus by increasing respiratory tract secretions via oral absorption
4. Mucolytic agents are available in inhalation preparations; expectorants are available in oral preparations

B. Examples: mucolytic: acetylcysteine (Mucomyst); expectorants: guaifenesin (Robitussin); potassium iodide (SSKI)

C. Major side effects: GI irritation (local effect); skin rash (hypersensitivity); oropharyngeal irritation and bronchospasm with mucolytics

D. Nursing care
1. Promote adequate fluid intake
2. Encourage coughing and deep breathing
3. Avoid administering fluids immediately after taking liquid expectorants
4. Assess respiratory status
5. Have suction apparatus available

Antitussives

A. Description
1. Suppress the cough reflex

2. Inhibit the cough reflex either by direct action on the medullary cough center or by indirect action peripherally on sensory nerve endings
3. Available in oral preparations

B. Examples: narcotic—codeine, hydrocodone bitartrate (Hycodan); nonnarcotic—dextromethorphan hydrobromide (Vicks 44), diphenhydramine HCl (Benadryl)

C. Major side effects: drowsiness (CNS depression); nausea (GI irritation); dry mouth (anticholinergic effect of antihistamine in combination products)

D. Nursing care
1. Provide adequate fluid intake
2. Avoid administering fluids immediately after liquid preparations
3. Encourage high-Fowler's position
4. Avoid use postoperatively and for clients with head injury
5. Administer narcotics cautiously: avoid giving with CNS depressants; caution client to avoid hazardous activity; assess for signs of dependence

Narcotic antagonist

A. Description
1. Displaces narcotics at respiratory receptor sites via competitive antagonism
2. Reverses respiratory depression caused by narcotic overdosage
3. Available in parenteral (IV, SC, IM) preparations

B. Example: naloxone HCl (Narcan)

C. Major side effects: CNS depression (acts on opioid receptors in CNS); nausea, vomiting

D. Nursing care
1. Assess vital signs, especially respirations
2. Have O_2 and emergency resuscitative equipment available

Antihistamines

A. Description
1. Block the action of histamine at receptor sites via competitive inhibition; also exert antiemetic, anticholinergic, and CNS depressant effects
2. Relieve symptoms of the common cold and allergies that are mediated by the chemical histamine
3. Available in oral and parenteral (IM, IV) preparations

B. Examples: brompheniramine maleate (Dimetane); diphenhydramine HCl (Benadryl); promethazine HCl (Phenergan); combination products: Drixoral; Triaminic

C. Major side effects
1. Drowsiness and dizziness (CNS depression); GI irritation (local effect); dry mouth (anticholinergic effect of decreased salivation); excitement (paradoxic effect)

D. Nursing care

1. Avoid administration with CNS depressants
2. Caution client to avoid engaging in hazardous activities
3. Administer with food or milk to avoid GI irritation
4. Offer gum or hard candy to promote salivation

Antituberculars

A. Description
   1. Used to treat tuberculosis; administered in combination (first-line and second-line drugs) over a prolonged time period to reduce the possibility of mycobacterial drug resistance
   2. Available in oral and parenteral (IM) preparations
B. Examples
   1. First-line drugs
      a. Ethambutol (Myambutol): interferes with mycobacterial RNA synthesis
      b. Isoniazid (INK, Nydrazid); interferes with mycobacterial cell wall synthesis
      c. Paraaminosalicylic acid preparations (PAS): interfere with mycobacterial folic acid synthesis
      d. Rifampin (Rifadin): interferes with mycobacterial RNA synthesis
      e. Streptomycin sulfate: inhibits mycobacterial protein synthesis
   2. Second-line drugs inhibit mycobacterial cell metabolism: e.g., capreomycin (Capastat), and cycloserine (Seromycin)
C. Major side effects
   1. GI irritation (direct tissue irritation)
   2. Suppressed absorption of fat and B complex vitamins, especially folic acid and B_{12}; depletion of vitamin B_6 by isoniazid
   3. Dizziness (CNS effect)
   4. CNS disturbances (direct CNS toxic effect)
   5. Liver disturbances (direct liver toxic effect)
   6. Blood dyscrasias (decreased RBCs, WBCs, platelet synthesis)
   7. Streptomycin: ototoxicity (direct auditory [eighth cranial] nerve toxic effect)
   8. Ethambutol: visual disturbances (direct optic [second cranial] nerve toxic effect)
   9. Rifampin: red discoloration of all body fluids
D. Nursing care
   1. Support natural defense mechanisms of client; encourage intake of foods rich in immune-stimulating nutrients such as vitamins A, C, and E, and the minerals selenium and zinc
   2. Obtain sputum specimens for acid-fast bacillus
   3. Monitor blood work during therapy
   4. Instruct the client to take the drugs regularly as prescribed; reinforce need for medical supervision
   5. Offer client emotional support during therapy

6. Use safety precautions (supervise ambulation) if CNS effects are manifested
7. Instruct client regarding nutritional side effects and encourage foods rich in B complex vitamins
8. Encourage client to avoid use of alcohol during therapy
9. Ethambutol: encourage frequent visual examinations
10. Rifampin: instruct client that body fluids may appear orange-red
11. Streptomycin: encourage frequent auditory examinations
12. Evaluate client's response to medication

RELATED PROCEDURES

Abdominal Thrust (Heimlich Maneuver)

A. Definition: short, abrupt pressure against the abdomen, two fingerbreadths above the umbilicus, to raise intrathoracic pressure, which will dislodge an obstruction such as a bolus of food or a foreign body
B. Symptoms of obstruction
   1. Partial: noisy respiration, dyspnea, lightheadedness, dizziness, flushing of face, bulging of eyes, repeated coughing
   2. Total: cessation of breathing, inability to speak or cough, extension of head, facial cyanosis, bulging of eyes, panic, unconsciousness
C. Nursing care
   1. Assess client no longer than 3 to 5 seconds
      a. Ask if client is choking
      b. Determine if victim can speak or cough
      c. Observe for universal choking sign (thumb and forefinger encircling throat under chin)
      d. Assess respirations: observe for rise and fall of chest; listen for escape of air from nose and mouth on expiration; feel for flow of air from nose and mouth on expiration
   2. Initiate intervention in the presence of a partial obstruction
      a. Allow the individual's expulsive cough to dislodge the obstruction
      b. Assess for signs of total obstruction
      c. Remove foreign bodies coughed up into the mouth
   3. Initiate intervention in the presence of a total obstruction
      a. Open the individual's mouth and remove the obstruction if possible
      b. Standing behind the conscious victim, encircle the waist and thrust upward and inward against the diaphragm with intertwined clenched fists

c. If victim becomes unconscious, activate EMS system; straddling the hips of the unconscious supine victim, place the heel of one hand on the other and thrust upward and inward against the diaphragm; activate emergency medical service (EMS) system
d. Repeat abdominal thrust several times (may require 6 to 10 thrusts) until foreign body is dislodged or until help arrives
e. Determine patency of airway; remove foreign objects from mouth; attempt rescue breathing
f. Continue pattern of abdominal thrusts if breathing is not reestablished.
g. If an airway cannot be established, an emergency cricothyrotomy may be necessary
h. Assess for signs of injury to liver or spleen; there is a higher risk when abdominal thrusts are performed with the victim in recumbent position

Bronchoscopy

A. Definition
1. Visualization of the tracheobronchial tree via a scope advanced through the mouth or nose into the bronchi
2. Performed to remove foreign body, to remove secretions, or to obtain specimens of tissue or mucus for further study
B. Nursing care
1. Obtain an informed consent
2. Keep NPO for 6 to 8 hours before procedure
3. Administer ordered preprocedure medications to produce sedation and decrease anxiety
4. Inform client to expect some soreness, dysphagia, and hemoptysis after the procedure
5. Advise client to avoid coughing or clearing throat
6. Observe for signs of hemorrhage and/or respiratory distress; keep head of bed elevated
7. Monitor vital signs until stable
8. Do not allow fluids until the gag reflex returns

Chest Physiotherapy

A. Definition: Activities that assist the client to mobilize respiratory secretions that could lead to atelectasis and/or pneumonia
B. Types of interventions
1. Incentive spirometer: mechanical device used to promote maximum inspiration and loosening of secretions; measures air inspired, providing visual feedback to client
2. Percussion (clapping): use of cupped hands to repeatedly strike chest wall over congested areas; action causes loosening of secretions
3. Vibration: palmar surface of hands are placed on chest over congested area and vibrated as client exhales; used with percussion to loosen secretions
4. Postural drainage: positioning client to permit gravity drainage of congested lung segments
C. Nursing care
1. Assess baseline breath sounds and ability of client to tolerate procedure
2. Administer prescribed bronchodilators, mucolytics, analgesics
3. Position client
a. Fowler's position for incentive spirometery and to drain upper lung segments
b. Sidelying and prone position with head lower than affected segment
4. Teach use of incentive spirometer
a. After exhaling, form seal around mouthpiece with lips
b. Take slow deep breath and hold inspiration for a few seconds before exhaling
c. Repeat 10 × per hour or as ordered
5. Perform percussion and vibration for several minutes over affected areas being managed with postural drainage
6. Encourage coughing and expectoration of secretions; provide tissues and appropriate receptacle
7. Allow rest periods as needed
8. Evaluate color, amount of secretion, quality of breath sounds after procedure
9. Encourage a 2- to 3-liter fluid intake daily to liquify secretions

Chest Tubes

A. Definition
1. Use of tubes and suction to return negative pressure to the intrapleural space, expanding lungs
2. To drain air from the intrapleural space, the chest tube is placed in the second or third intercostal space; to drain blood or fluid, the catheter would be placed at a lower site, usually the eighth or ninth intercostal space
B. Commercial drainage systems: (e.g., PleurEvac)
1. Calibrated collection chamber for drainage
2. Water seal chamber: prevents atmospheric air from entering pleural space; fluid level will normally fluctuate with respirations until lung is fully expanded; continuous bubbling may indicate an air leak.
3. Suction control chamber: controls amount of suction, usually 10 to 20 cm H_2O, if gravity drainage is insufficient; bubbling indicates that suction level is maintained; some systems use "dry" suction
C. Nursing care
1. Ensure that the tubing is not kinked; tape all connections to prevent separation

2. Milking and "stripping" chest tubes is not a safe practice because it increases negative intrapleural pressure and does not significantly affect tube patency
3. Maintain the drainage system below the level of the chest
4. Turn the client frequently, making sure the chest tubes are not compressed
5. Report drainage on dressing immediately; this is not a normal occurrence
6. Observe for fluctuation of fluid in water-seal chamber (tidaling); the level will rise on inhalation and fall on exhalation; if there are no fluctuations, either the lung has expanded fully or the chest tube is clogged; length of time for lung expansion depends on etiology
7. Palpate the area around the chest tube insertion site for subcutaneous emphysema or crepitus, which indicates that air is leaking into the subcutaneous tissue
8. Situate the drainage system to avoid breakage
9. Place two clamps at the bedside for use when changing systems or if a leak is suspected; clamps are used judiciously and only in emergency situations because they can cause tension pneumonthorax
10. Encourage movement, coughing, and deep breathing every 2 hours, splinting the area as needed; assess breath sounds
11. Assess for tracheal deviation, a sign of tension pneumothorax
12. Verify that chest x-rays have been done before chest tubes are removed
13. Instruct the client to exhale or strain (Valsalva's maneuver) as the tube is withdrawn by the physician; apply a gauze dressing immediately and firmly secure with tape to make an airtight dressing

Mechanical Ventilation

A. Definition: use of a mechanical device to instill a mixture of air and oxygen into the lungs using positive pressure; a device such as an Ambu-Bag can be used temporarily during a respiratory arrest
B. Types of ventilators
 1. Pressure cycled: delivers a volume of gas with positive press during inspiration
 2. Volume cycled: delivers a preset tidal volume of inspired gas regardless of pressure
 3. Time cycled: deliver volume of gas for a predetermined inspiratory time
C. Modes of ventilation
 1. Controlled mandatory ventilation (CMV): the client receives a specified volume and rate with no triggering of the machine by the client; the nurse may have to administer drugs such as pancuronium bromide (Pavulon) or morphine to decrease the client's own respiratory response
 2. Assist control ventilation (ACV): the client triggers the machine so that the rate may vary; however, if client has apnea, the machine will initiate respirations at a preset tidal volume
 3. Intermittent mandatory ventilation (IMV): the client receives a predetermined tidal volume and number of breaths per minute; the client controls respirations between mechanical ventilations; rate can be gradually reduced as a client is weaned from the ventilator; rarely used today
 4. Synchronized intermittent mandatory ventilation (SIMV): same as IMV but the ventilator breaths are synchronized with the client's own breaths; often used for weaning
 5. Pressure support ventilation (PSV): the client initiates all breaths, which are then supplemented by positive pressure, improving the tidal volume and reducing respiratory efforts; may be used alone or with IMV/SIMV
 6. Positive end expiratory pressure (PEEP): maintains positive pressure at the end of expiration to keep alveoli open, increasing the functional residual capacity (FRC)
 7. Continuous positive airway pressure (CPAP): similar to PEEP but exerts positive pressure throughout the respiratory cycle; the client must be breathing spontaneously; may be used without intubation or mechanical ventilation
D. Nursing care
 1. Maintain ventilator settings and notify the respiratory department and the physician if distress occurs
 2. Maintain a sealed system between the ventilator and the client so that volume to be delivered is kept constant and air is not lost around the tubing; this is accomplished by inflating the cuff of the endotracheal tube or tracheostomy tube to the minimum occlusive volume
 3. Perform suction as necessary; humidified oxygen helps to liquify secretions that must be removed
 4. Assess for signs of respiratory insufficiency, such as breath sounds, tachypnea, cyanosis, and changes in sensorium
 5. Check pulse oximetry and blood gases as ordered to determine effectiveness of ventilation
 6. Establish a means of communication because client will be unable to speak while on a ventilator

Oxygen Therapy

A. Definition: administration of supplemental oxygen to prevent or treat tissue hypoxia

B. Methods: depend on client's condition
   1. Nasal cannula: 1 to 6 liters per minute (24% to 43%), least restrictive
   2. Simple mask: 5 to 8 LPM (40% to 60%)
   3. Partial rebreathing mask: 8 to 11 LPM (50% to 90%)
   4. Nonrebreather mask: 12 to 15 LPM (90% to 100%)
   5. Venturi mask: delivers precise percentage of oxygen inspired
C. Nursing care
   1. Monitor for signs of hypoxia: agitatation, confusion, lethargy, pallor, diaphoresis, tachycardia, cyanosis (late)
   2. Monitor arterial oxygen saturation as ordered with pulse oximeter
      a. Attach sensor, usually to finger or ear lobe; avoid extremity with impediment to blood flow
      b. Check preset alarm for O_2 saturation (SaO_2); if less than 85%, adjustment is needed
   3. Maintain safety precaution (oxygen supports combustion): place "oxygen in use" sign on door; remind client and visitors not to smoke or use faulty electric devices; be aware of fire extinguishers and oxygen turn-off valve
   4. Verify client does not have COPD before administering high concentration of O_2 to prevent CO_2 narcosis
   5. Provide for humidification of oxygen flow rates greater than 4 LPM to prevent drying of secretions
   6. Specific care related to method
      a. Cannula—nares' care with water soluble lubricant
      b. Rebreather masks—ensure that bag does not deflate completely
      c. Venturi mask—set LPM to deliver specified FIO_2; use appropriate adapter to mix room air with oxygen; ensure ports are not obstructed

Suctioning of Airway

A. Definition
   1. Mechanical aspiration of mucous secretions from the tracheobronchial tree by application of negative pressure
   2. Used to maintain a patent airway, obtain a sputum specimen, or stimulate coughing
   3. May be nasotracheal, oropharyngeal, or through an endotracheal or tracheostomy tube
B. Nursing care
   1. Place client in semi-Fowler's position
   2. Assess proper functioning of equipment before and after using
   3. Hyperoxygenate by increasing flow rate; encourage deep breathing

   4. Lubricate the suction catheter with sterile saline or water or water-soluble gel
   5. Insert the catheter: if tracheal suction is being used, insert to the end of the tube (approximately 4 inches); if nasotracheal suction is being used, insert until the cough reflex is induced or resistance is met; when resistance is met withdraw catheter 2 cm before initiating suction
   6. Apply no suction while the catheter is being inserted
   7. Rotate and withdraw the catheter while suction is applied; do not exceed 10 to 15 seconds
   8. Clear the catheter with sterile solution and encourage the client to breathe deeply

Thoracentesis

A. Definition
   1. Removal of fluid or air from pleural space; this is done for diagnostic purposes or to alleviate respiratory distress
   2. No more than 1000 ml of fluid should be removed at a time; fluid withdrawn should be sent to the laboratory for culture and sensitivity, analysis of glucose, protein, and pH
   3. Complications include pneumothorax from trauma to the lung and pulmonary edema resulting from sudden fluid shifts
B. Nursing care
   1. Obtain an informed consent
   2. Ensure that chest x-ray examination is done before and after the procedure
   3. Assist and support the client in the sitting position
   4. Inform the client not to cough during the procedure to prevent trauma to lungs
   5. Assess pulse and respirations before, during, and after the procedure
   6. Note and record the amount, color, and clarity of the fluid withdrawn
   7. Place client on opposite side for 1 hour to promote lung expansion
   8. Observe the client for coughing, bloody sputum, and rapid pulse rate and report their occurrence immediately
   9. Monitor for subcutaneous emphysema (crepitus)

Tracheostomy Care

A. Definition: removal of dried secretions from the cannula to maintain a patent airway, prevent infection, and prevent irritation
B. Nursing care
   1. Provide tracheostomy care at least every 8 hours
   2. Suction to remove secretions from the lumen of the tube (see procedure for suctioning of airways)

3. If an inner cannula is present
   a. Remove disposable inner cannula and replace with new one
   b. Care for nondisposable inner cannula using surgical aspetic technique; remove and place in peroxide; remove secretions within the cannula with a sterile brush; rinse with normal saline; drain excess saline before reinserting the tube, which is then locked in place
4. Clean around the stoma with saline, using sterile technique; apply antiseptic ointment if ordered
5. Change the tracheostomy tape, being careful not to dislodge the cannula; tie with a double knot
6. Place a tracheostomy dressing or fenestrated 4 × 4 inch (unfilled) dressing below the stoma to absorb expelled secretions
7. Humidify inhaled air if ordered because air is bypassing normal humidification process in the nasopharynx

MAJOR DISORDERS OF THE RESPIRATORY SYSTEM

▼ PULMONARY EMBOLISM AND INFARCTION

Data Base
A. Etiology and pathophysiology
   1. Emboli develop from thrombi in peripheral circulation; associated with venous stasis resulting from immobility, coagulopathy, vascular disease, surgery, aging, oral contraceptives, obesity, and constrictive clothing
   2. When an embolus lodges in the pulmonary artery causing hemorrhage and necrosis of lung tissue it is called a pulmonary infarction
B. Clinical findings
   1. Subjective: severe dyspnea that occurs suddenly; anxiety; restlessness; sharp pleuritic pain
   2. Objective: increased temperature, pulse, and respirations; violent coughing with hemoptysis; diaphoresis; V/Q (ventilation-perfusion) lung scan CTs of the chest and pulmonary angiography are diagnostic measures
C. Therapeutic interventions
   1. Anticoagulation with heparin IV until therapeutic PTT is attained; sodium warfarin is used for maintenance therapy
   2. Thrombolytic therapy
   3. Angiography; if the condition is severe, an embolectomy may be indicated

4. Vena caval interruption; a filter may be implanted in the inferior vena cava preventing the passage of large thrombi (Greenfield or umbrella filters)

Nursing Care of Clients with Pulmonary Embolism and Infarction
A. **ASSESSMENT**
   1. Data related to causative factors, especially surgery of the pelvic floor or lower extremities
   2. Presence of clinical findings
B. **ANALYSIS/NURSING DIAGNOSES**
   1. Impaired gas exchange related to inadequate ventilation/perfusion imbalance
   2. Anxiety related to acute hypoxemia
C. **PLANNING/IMPLEMENTATION**
   1. Place in the high-Fowler's position and administer oxygen
   2. Monitor for hypoxemia and right heart failure
   3. Administer thrombolytics/anticoagulants as ordered; monitor for bleeding
   4. Administer analgesics to reduce pain and decrease anxiety
   5. Maintain calm environment to decrease fear
   6. Educate client regarding anticogulants and prevention of thrombophlebitis
D. **EVALUATION/OUTCOMES**
   1. Maintains normal breathing patterns
   2. Exchanges adequate gases to maintain tissue perfusion
   3. Verbalizes feelings of control over situation

▼ PULMONARY EDEMA

Data Base
A. Etiology and pathophysiology
   1. An acute emergency condition characterized by a rapid accumulation of fluid in interstitial spaces surrounding the alveoli resulting from increased pressure within the pulmonary system
   2. Possible causes include myocardial infarction, valvular disease, or hypertension leading to left-ventricular failure; circulatory overload, aspiration of gastric contents, drowning, or severe CNS damage
B. Clinical findings
   1. Subjective: history of premonitory symptoms such as shortness of breath, paroxysmal nocturnal dyspnea, wheezing, and orthopnea; acute anxiety, apprehension, restlessness
   2. Objective: rapid, thready pulse and rapid respirations; pink, frothy sputum; wheezing; crackles; pallor or cyanosis; low Po_2; elevated pulmonary capillary wedge pressure and central venous pressure

C. Therapeutic interventions
1. Oxygen in high concentrations or by CPAP as necessary
2. Fowler's position
3. Reduce preload with diuretics, nitrates for vasodilation and possible phlebotomy
4. Reduce afterload with antihypertensive drugs such as nitroprusside
5. Support cardiac function with inotropic drugs such as dobutamine
6. Hemodynamic monitoring and possible intraaortic balloon pump

Nursing Care of Clients with Pulmonary Edema

A. ASSESSMENT
1. Presence of clinical findings
2. Signs of hypoxemia
3. Precipitating factors

B. ANALYSIS/NURSING DIAGNOSES
1. Impaired gas exchange related to fluid overload
2. Activity intolerance related to impaired oxygenation
3. Anxiety related to shortness of breath

C. PLANNING/IMPLEMENTATION
1. Support client in the orthopneic, high-Fowler's or semi-Fowler's position with legs dependent
2. Observe and record vital signs and monitor cardiac activity and intake and output
3. Provide a reassuring environment to allay anxiety; administer morphine sulfate to relieve anxiety
4. Suction as needed to maintain a patent airway
5. Administer and monitor effects of medications to reduce preload and afterload
6. Educate client regarding pharmacology and prevention of heart failure

D. EVALUATION/OUTCOMES
1. Demonstrates activity tolerance within level of cardiac function
2. Maintains adequate gas exchange
3. Verbalizes decreased anxiety

▼ PNEUMONIA

Data Base

A. Etiology and pathophysiology
1. Inflammatory disease of the lung; may cause a collection of pus (empyema) or fluid (pleural effusion) within the pleural space; atelectasis
2. May be caused by an infectious agent (bacterial, viral, or fungal) but may also be caused by inhalation of chemicals and aspiration of gastric contents.
   a. Community-acquired pneumonia (CAP) is most commonly caused by *Streptococcus pneumoniae* (pneumococcal), *Haemophilus influenzae*, *Legionella pneumophila*, *Mycoplasma pneumoniae*; *Chlamydia* species (*Chlamydia pneumoniae*; more common *psittaci*); viruses
   b. Hospital-acquired pneumonia (HAP) is most commonly caused by *Staphylococcus aureus*, *Pseudomonas aeruginosa*, *Klebsiella pneumoniae* *Serratia marcescens*
   c. Aspiration pneumonia occurs when the normal flora of the upper respiratory tract, gastric contents, or chemicals are aspirated into the lung
   d. Pneumonia in the immunocompromised host include pneumonias that are generally uncommon in clients with healthy immune responses; examples include *Pneumocystic carinii* pneumonia and other fungal pneumonias (e.g., aspergillosis), and mycobacterium tuberculosis
3. Risk factors include age, COPD, alcoholism, smoking, neutropenia, ineffective cough, immobility, HIV infection
4. Pneumonia is commonly spread by respiratory droplets

B. Clinical findings
1. Subjective: lassitude; dyspnea; chest pain that increases on inspiration
2. Objective
   a. Elevated temperature, increased WBC
   b. Chest x-ray examination shows pulmonary infiltration
   c. Cough with sputum production
      (1) Pneumococcal: purulent, rusty sputum
      (2) Staphylococcal: yellow, blood-streaked sputum
      (3) *Klebsiella* species: red, gelatinous sputum
      (4) Mycoplasmal: nonproductive that advances to mucoid sputum

C. Therapeutic interventions
1. Culture and sensitivity tests will be done on blood and sputum to determine appropriate antibiotic
2. Antiviral therapy: *Aspergillus* infection is treated with amphotericin B, azole agents, such as intraconazole, or the newest antifungal agents echinocandins (e.g., caspofungin)
3. Respiratory support
4. Nutritional supplementation and fluid and electrolyte replacement
5. Bronchodilators
6. Chest physiotherapy and suctioning as needed

Nursing Care of Clients with Pneumonia

A. ASSESSMENT
1. Vital signs, breathing patterns
2. Color, amount, and consistency of sputum
3. Adventitious sounds on auscultation of lung

4. Mental status changes

B. ANALYSIS/NURSING DIAGNOSES
1. Ineffective airway clearance related to excessive secretions
2. Activity intolerance related to decreased oxygenation

C. PLANNING/IMPLEMENTATION
1. Encourage coughing and deep breathing after chest physiotherapy, splinting the chest as necessary
2. Collect sputum specimen for culture and sensitivity tests in sterile container; notify the physician if organism is resistant to the antibiotic being given
3. Increase fluid intake to 3 liters daily
4. Maintain semi-Fowler's position
5. Monitor for signs of respiratory distress, such as labored respirations, cool clammy skin, cyanosis and change in mental status
6. Plan rest periods
7. Instruct client to cover nose and mouth when coughing
8. Administer antibiotics as ordered
9. Teach preventive measures including: role of nutrition and fluids; avoiding respiratory irritants (e.g., aerosols); vaccination against *Streptococcus pneumoniae* and influenza; balance of activity and rest; cessation of smoking; oral hygiene

D. EVALUATION/OUTCOMES
1. Maintains patent airway
2. Performs activities of daily living (ADL) without assistance
3. Abstains from smoking

▼ PULMONARY TUBERCULOSIS

Data Base

A. Etiology and pathophysiology
1. Infection of lungs caused by *Mycobacterium tuberculosis,* an acid-fast bacterium, commonly transmitted by inhalation of droplets
2. Causes tubercles, fibrosis, and calcification within the lungs
3. Predisposing factors include debilitating diseases such as alcoholism, diabetes mellitus, cardiovascular disease, HIV infection, and cirrhosis, as well as poor nutrition and crowded living conditions
4. The emergence of drug-resistant tuberculosis has complicated management of the disease
5. Chronic, progressive, and reinfection phase is most frequently encountered in adults and involves progression or reactivation of primary lesions after months or years of latency.
6. Swallowing infected sputum may lead to laryngeal, oropharyngeal, and intestinal tuberculosis

B. Clinical findings
1. Subjective: malaise; pleuritic pain; easy fatigability
2. Objective
   a. Fever, night sweats, weight loss; cough that progressively becomes worse; hemoptysis
   b. Chest x-ray examination may reveal presence of active or calcified lesions, pleural effusion
   c. Analysis of sputum and gastric contents reveals presence of acid-fast bacilli
   d. Intradermal tuberculin testing: Mantoux, with purified protein derivative (PPD)
      (1) Determines antibody response to the tubercle bacillus, an induration of 10 mm or greater present 48 to 72 hours later indicates a positive finding; an induration of 5 mm may also be significant, particularly for an immunocompromised client
      (2) Indicates prior exposure to bacillus, which may or may not indicate active disease state (a sudden change from negative to positive requires follow-up testing)
      (3) Immunocompromised clients may not have a positive reaction despite being infected with *M. tuberculosis*
      (4) Clients who have received bacilli Calmette-Guerin (BCG) vaccine will also have a positive (significant) reaction

C. Therapeutic interventions
1. Program of two or more antituberculin drugs such as isoniazid INH, streptomycin, pyrazinamide, rifampin, ethambutol, and rifapentine (Priftin)
   a. Length of time the drug must be taken varies based on response
   b. When compliance is an issue, mandated directly observed therapy (DOT) ensures treatment is ongoing
2. Bed rest until symptoms abate or therapeutic regimen is established
3. Surgical resection of the involved lobe is necessary if symptoms such as hemorrhage develop or chemotherapy is unsatisfactory
4. Isoniazid preventive therapy (IPT) for 6 to 12 months to immediate contacts (all cases and follow-up of contacts must be reported to public health agency)
5. High-carbohydrate, high-protein, high-vitamin diet with supplemental vitamin B_6 to counter INH side effects

Nursing Care of Clients with Pulmonary Tuberculosis

A. ASSESSMENT

1. Detailed history related to exposure, travel, or BCG inoculation
2. Fatigue, anorexia, low-grade fever, and night sweats
3. Sputum for color, amount, and consistency

B. ANALYSIS/NURSING DIAGNOSES

1. Activity intolerance related to impaired oxygenation
2. Imbalanced nutrition: less than body requirements related to anorexia
3. Noncompliance related to long-term nature of treatment

C. PLANNING/IMPLEMENTATION

1. Teach client to provide for scheduled rest periods
2. Teach which foods to include in the diet and which are nutritious between-meal supplements
3. Help client plan a realistic schedule for taking the large number of necessary medications
4. Teach the importance of continued follow-up and adherence, without variation, to the drug program that has been established; monitor compliance
5. Instruct client to be alert to the early symptoms of adverse drug reactions (e.g., optic and peripheral neuritis, 8th cranial nerve damage, nephrotoxicity, hepatitis, dermatitis) and to contact the physician immediately if any occur
6. Teach the proper techniques to prevent spread of infection: frequent hand washing; cover the mouth when coughing; use and disposal of tissues; cleansing of eating utensils and disposal of food wastes; standard precautions and airborne precautions with high efficiency particulate air (HEPA) filter
7. Instruct client to be alert to the early symptoms of hemorrhage, such as hemoptysis, and to contact the physician immediately if any occur
8. Encourage coughing and deep breathing
9. Encourage client to express feelings about disease and the many ramifications (stigma, isolation, fear) it creates

D. EVALUATION/OUTCOMES

1. Performs ADL without shortness of breath
2. Maintains adequate body weight
3. Complies with treatment regimen

▼ OBSTRUCTIVE AIRWAY DISEASES

Data Base

A. Etiology and pathophysiology

1. Asthma: reversible bronchospasms and increased secretions that last from 1 to several hours; obstruction of the bronchioles characterized by attacks that occur suddenly and last from 30 to 60 minutes; an asthmatic attack that is difficult to control is referred to as status asthmaticus (asthma is no longer grouped together with other diseases that comprise the broad classification of COPD but is left here for review of common clinical findings and care)
2. Chronic obstructive pulmonary disease (COPD)
   a. Chronic bronchitis: inflammation of the bronchial walls with hypertrophy of the mucous goblet cells; characterized by a chronic cough
   b. Emphysema: characterized by distended, inelastic, or destroyed alveoli with bronchiolar obstruction and collapse; these alterations greatly impair the diffusion of gases through the alveolar capillary membrane
3. Clients with COPD become accustomed to an elevated residual carbon dioxide level and do not respond to high CO_2 concentrations as the normal respiratory stimulant; they respond instead to a drop in oxygen concentration in the blood
4. May precipitate pulmonary hypertension, cor pulmonale, and right ventricular heart failure

B. Clinical findings

1. Subjective: fatigue and weakness; dyspnea; headache; impaired sensorium
2. Objective
   a. Orthopnea, expiratory wheezing, stertorous breathing sounds, cough
   b. Barrel chest, cyanosis, clubbing of fingers, use of accessory muscles; pursed lip breathing
   c. Increased P_{CO_2} and decreased P_{O_2} of arterial blood gases; polycythemia
   d. Distended neck veins, peripheral edema (with right heart failure)

C. Therapeutic interventions

1. Steroids to prevent and reduce inflammation
2. Antibiotics to prevent/treat infection
3. Bronchodilators to reduce muscular spasm
4. Mucolytics and expectorants to liquify secretions and to facilitate their removal
5. Leukotriene receptor antagonist to prevent edema, bronchoconstriction, and mucus production associated with asthma
6. Oxygen at 1 to 3 L even it hypoxia is severe
7. Respiratory therapy program to include nebulizer therapy, postural drainage, and exercise
8. High-protein soft diet in small, frequent feedings is most easily tolerated

9. Phlebotomy to reduce blood volume if hematocrit is more than 60%; also reduces cardiac workload

Nursing Care of Clients with Obstructive Airway Disease

A. ASSESSMENT
1. History of increased symptoms: during early morning, in cold weather, when sleeping, and when smoking
2. Breathing patterns: abdominal, paradoxical, pursed lip, asynchronous; breath sounds
3. Frequency of respiratory infections
4. Evidence of chronic and acute hypoxia
5. Nutritional status

B. ANALYSIS/NURSING DIAGNOSES
1. Ineffective airway clearance related to bronchospasm and secretions
2. Powerlessness related to loss of self-care capability
3. Anxiety related to oxygen deprivation

C. PLANNING/IMPLEMENTATION
1. Advise the elimination of smoking and other external irritants, such as dust, as much as possible
2. Supervise client's respiratory exercises, such as pursed-lip or diaphragmatic breathing
3. Teach proper use of inhalers and other special equipment (e.g., spacer)
4. Carefully observe for symptoms of hypoxia and carbon dioxide intoxication (CO_2 narcosis) if oxygen is being administered
5. Teach client to adjust activities to avoid overexertion
6. Teach client to avoid people with respiratory infections
7. Teach the client to avoid the use of sedatives or hypnotics, which could compromise respirations
8. Teach client to maintain the highest resistance possible by getting adequate rest, eating nutritious food, dressing properly for weather conditions, maintaining fluid intake, receiving vaccinations against *S. pneumoniae* and influenza
9. Teach client to be alert to early symptoms of infection, hypoxia, hypercapnea, or adverse response to medications
10. Encourage client to continue with close medical supervision; monitor compliance
11. Encourage client to express feelings about disease and therapy
12. Accept feelings about lifelong restrictions in activity
13. Encourage client and family to take an active role in planning therapy

D. EVALUATION/OUTCOMES
1. Demonstrates pursed-lip breathing and diaphragmatic breathing
2. Describes and complies with treatment regimen
3. States methods for reducing/controlling feelings of anxiety/fear

▼ PNEUMOTHORAX/CHEST INJURY

Data Base
A. Etiology and pathophysiology
1. Collapse of a lung resulting from disruption of the negative pressure that normally exists within the intrapleural space caused by the presence of air in the pleural cavity; may be associated with fractured ribs
2. Reduces the surface area for gaseous exchange and leads to hypoxia and retention of carbon dioxide (hypercarbia)
3. Types
   a. Spontaneous or closed: thought to occur when a weakened area of the lung (bleb) ruptures; air then moves from the lung to the intrapleural space causing collapse; highest incidence is in men 20 to 40 years of age
   b. Open: laceration (e.g., a stab wound) through the chest wall into the intrapleural space
   c. Hemothorax: collection of blood within the pleural cavity
   d. Hydrothorax: accumulation of fluid in the pleural cavity
   e. Tension: buildup of pressure as air accumulates within the pleural space; the pressure increase is likely to induce a mediastinal shift; may occur from milking or stripping of chest tubes, which is unsafe practice
4. Mediastinal shift may occur toward the uninvolved side as a result of increased pressure within the pleural space; this involves the trachea, esophagus, heart, and great vessels
5. Flail chest: instability of chest wall related to fractures of the ribs or detached sternum; caused by crushing chest injuries
B. Clinical findings
1. Subjective: chest pain, usually described as sharp and increasing on exertion; dyspnea; drowsiness
2. Objective
   a. Tachycardia; hypotension; rapid, shallow respirations (nonsymmetric)
   b. Flail chest: loose chest segment moves inward during inspiration and outward during expiration (paradoxical respiration)
   c. Breath sounds on the affected side will be diminished or absent
   d. Chest x-ray examination will reveal extent of the pneumothorax

C. Therapeutic interventions
1. Bed rest initially
2. Analgesics and antibiotics
3. Negative pressure is returned to the intrapleural space by the insertion of chest tubes attached to underwater drainage
4. Restoration of blood volume loss as a result of trauma
5. Volume controlled ventilation

Nursing Care of Clients with Pneumothorax

A. ASSESSMENT
1. Auscultation of lung fields for diminished or absent breath sounds
2. Chest percussion for hyperresonance
3. Chest motion during inhalation for inequality
4. Paradoxical chest movement
5. Skin for changes in color

B. ANALYSIS/NURSING DIAGNOSES
1. Ineffective breathing pattern related to rib cage trauma
2. Ineffective airway clearance related to pain
3. Impaired gas exchange related to inadequate lung expansion

C. PLANNING/IMPLEMENTATION
1. Maintain constant supervision until stable
2. Maintain patency of chest tubes (see procedure for chest tubes)
3. Place in high-Fowler's position
4. Offer fluids frequently
5. Monitor vital signs, particularly respirations

D. EVALUATION/OUTCOMES
1. Maintains adequate gas exchange
2. Verifies reduction or absence of chest pain

▼ MALIGNANT LUNG TUMORS

Data Base
A. Etiology and pathophysiology
1. Carcinoma of the lungs may be primary or metastatic
2. Smoking is the most significant risk factor
3. Leading type of cancer that causes death
4. Incidence highest in men over the age of 40
5. Symptoms may occur after metastasis to other organs such as the ribs, liver, adrenal glands, mediastinal organs, kidneys, and brain
6. Classification and incidence of lung cancers: adenocarcinoma 35% to 40%; epidermoid (squamous cell) 30% to 35%; small cell (oat cell carcinoma) 20% to 25%; large cell (undifferentiated) 15% to 20%
B. Clinical findings
1. Subjective: dyspnea; chills; fatigue; chest pain
2. Objective: persistent cough; change in voice

quality: hemoptysis; unilateral wheeze; weight loss; clubbing of fingers; chest x-ray reveals pleural effusion and "coin" lesions; cytologic test of sputum positive
C. Therapeutic interventions
1. Surgical
a. Lobectomy: removal of one lobe of the lung when the lesion is limited to one area
b. Resection: removal of a small confined lesion; may also be done for biopsy
c. Pneumonectomy: removal of an entire lung
d. Exploratory thoracotomy: opening of the thoracic cavity to determine extent and further therapy
e. Thoracoplasty: removal of ribs to reduce the size of the pleural cavity; may be done to prevent complications after resection of lung
f. Laser surgery: removal of tumor via endoscope inserted between the ribs
g. Thoracentesis (see procedure)
2. Radiation therapy may be used as an adjunct therapy or to alleviate symptoms of pain, dyspnea, and hemoptysis
3. Chemotherapy (e.g., cydophosphamide, methotrexate, vincristine)

Nursing Care of Clients with Malignant Lung Tumors

A. ASSESSMENT
1. Sputum quantity and characteristics
2. Lung auscultation for absent breath sounds
3. Chest percussion for dullness over tumors
4. Respirations for shallowness, stridor, and use of accessory muscles
5. Persistent cough

B. ANALYSIS/NURSING DIAGNOSES
1. Impaired gas exchange related to decreased lung capacity
2. Ineffective airway clearance related to increased secretions and tumor obstruction
3. Pain related to direct pressure on tissues and tissue erosion

C. PLANNING/IMPLEMENTATION
1. Monitor temperature and vital signs
2. Encourage coughing and deep breathing
3. Change client's position frequently; semi-Fowler's or high-Fowler's promotes greater lung expansion
4. After pneumonectomy, position on operative side to promote lung expansion; assess position of trachea for mediastinal shift
5. Provide specific care based on therapy being used: care of client with chest tubes; radiation therapy; chemotherapy
6. Provide high-protein, high-calorie diet and supplements

7. Use interventions to manage pain: analgesics, distraction, relaxation, imagery

D. EVALUATION/OUTCOMES
1. Verbalizes a reduction of pain
2. Maintains patent airway
3. States understanding of treatment
4. Breathes with minimal effort

▼ CANCER OF THE LARYNX

Data Base

A. Etiology and pathophysiology
1. Most tumors of the larynx (vocal cords, epiglottis, and laryngeal cartilages) are squamous cell carcinoma
2. Cigarette smoking, air pollution, chronic respiratory infections, and heavy alcohol consumption appear to be related to increased incidence
3. More common in men 50 to 70 years of age

B. Clinical findings
1. Subjective: sore throat; dyspnea; dysphagia; weakness
2. Objective: increasing hoarseness; weight loss; enlarged cervical lymph nodes; foul breath

C. Therapeutic interventions
1. Radiation therapy
2. Chemotherapy is not curative but is used preoperatively to decrease tumor size; postoperatively, chemotherapy is used to decrease metastasis
3. Surgical intervention
   a. Thyrotomy: removal of tumor from the larynx via an incision through the thyroid cartilage
   b. Total laryngectomy: removal of total larynx with construction of a permanent tracheal stoma
   c. Radical neck dissection (used when the tumor has metastasized into surrounding tissue and lymph nodes): removal of larynx, surrounding tissue and muscle, lymph nodes, and glands with a permanent tracheal stoma; chest tubes may be needed if thoracic duct leakage occurs; TPN if needed
   d. Laser: to eradicate small tumors, vocal cord tumors, or in conjunction with chemotherapy

Nursing Care of Clients with a Total Laryngectomy

A. ASSESSMENT
1. Voice for hoarseness
2. Oropharyngeal inspection for masses
3. Neck palpation for masses and nodal enlargement

B. ANALYSIS/NURSING DIAGNOSES
1. Ineffective airway clearance related to impaired airway from tumor invasion
2. Risk for aspiration related to alteration of protective reflexes
3. Disturbed body image related to tumor and treatment modalities

C. PLANNING/IMPLEMENTATION
1. Provide time to discuss the diagnosis and the ramifications of surgery
2. Assist and encourage the client to express feelings
3. Answer questions as thoroughly and honestly as possible
4. Arrange for individuals with laryngectomies to visit and discuss the rehabilitative process
5. Instruct as to the method of communication that will be used after surgery (e.g., slate board and chalk, pencil and paper, sign language, electronic voice)
6. Observe for obstruction of airway by mucous plugs, edema, or blood (e.g., air hunger, dyspnea, cyanosis, gurgling); keep head elevated
7. Observe for signs of hemorrhage (e.g., increased pulse rate, drop in blood pressure, cold clammy skin, appearance of blood on dressing)
8. Provide, at the bedside, suction apparatus and catheters (additional laryngectomy tube and a surgical instrument set with additional hemostats should be immediately available in case tube becomes dislodged or blocked)
9. Suction the laryngectomy tube as necessary (see procedure for suctioning of airway)
10. Provide humidity to compensate for loss of normal humidification of air in the nasopharynx; later the stoma may be covered with a moistened, unfilled gauze pad
11. Expect and accept a period of mourning, but prevent withdrawal from reality by: involving in laryngectomy care; keeping channels of communication open; supporting strengths; encouraging a return to activities of daily living (ADL); allowing time to write responses or use gestures
12. Encourage the client to become involved in speech therapy and realistically support efforts and gains
13. Teach skills necessary to handle altered body functioning: tracheobronchial suctioning; changing, cleaning, and securing the laryngectomy tube; care of skin around the opening; providing humidified air for inspiration to prevent drying of secretions (can be achieved by use of moist dressing or cloth bib)

14. Teach the client to avoid activities that may permit water or irritating substances to enter the trachea; avoid showers (unless wearing a protective cover), swimming, dust, hair spray, and other volatile substances
15. Teach the client to avoid wearing clothes with constricting collars or necklines
16. Teach the client that certain other activities will be impossible (e.g., sipping through a straw, whistling, blowing the nose)

D. EVALUATION/OUTCOMES
1. States a reduction in feelings of fear
2. Maintains patent airway
3. States acceptance of body image

▼ ADULT RESPIRATORY DISTRESS SYNDROME (ARDS)

Data Base

A. Etiology and pathophysiology
1. Respiratory failure as a complication of trauma, aspiration, prolonged mechanical ventilation, severe infection, open-heart surgery, fat emboli, shock
2. Involves:
   a. Pulmonary capillary damage with loss of fluid and interstitial edema
   b. Impaired alveolar gas exchange and tissue hypoxia resulting from pulmonary edema
   c. Alteration in surfactant production; collapse of alveoli
   d. Atelectasis resulting in labored and inefficient respiration
B. Clinical findings
1. Subjective: restlessness; anxiety; dyspnea
2. Objective: tachycardia; grunting respirations; intercostal retractions; cyanosis; Pco_2 initially decreased and later increased and decreased Po_2 arterial blood gases; chest x-ray examination reveals pulmonary edema
C. Therapeutic interventions
1. Relieve the underlying cause
2. Mechanical ventilation with positive end expiratory pressure (PEEP): this setting on a mechanical ventilator maintains positive pressure within the lungs at the end of expiration, which increases the residual capacity, reducing hypoxia
3. Corticosteroids may be used
4. Nitric oxide (NO) prevents calcium influx into cells and causes vasodilation; inhaled it dilates capillary beds of lungs, which reduces pressure in pulmonary arteries
5. Alpha-antitrypsin, a scavenger of oxygen-free radicals is used to inhibit substances released by endotoxins

Nursing Care of Clients with Adult Respiratory Distress Syndrome

A. ASSESSMENT
1. Vital signs especially characteristics of respirations
2. Pain that increases on inspiration
3. Chest percussion for hyperresonance

B. ANALYSIS/NURSING DIAGNOSES
1. Impaired gas exchange related to unequal ventilation/perfusion
2. Anxiety related to fear of death

C. PLANNING/IMPLEMENTATION
1. Allow frequent rest periods between therapeutic interventions
2. Provide tranquil, supportive environment; sedation is contraindicated because of its depressant effect on respirations
3. Observe behavioral changes and vital signs because confusion and hypertension may indicate cerebral hypoxia
4. Auscultate breath sounds to observe for signs of pneumothorax when the client is on PEEP (lung tissue that is frail may not withstand increased intrathoracic pressure, and pneumothorax occurs)
5. Monitor arterial blood gases, as ordered; use a heparinized syringe
6. Maintain a patent airway
7. Care for the client on mechanical ventilation (see procedure for mechanical ventilation)
8. Measure central venous and pulmonary artery pressures
9. Place in prone position to improve oxygenation by altering distribution of perfusion
10. Inotropic pharmaceuticals may improve cardiac output

D. EVALUATION/OUTCOMES
1. Maintains adequate gas exchange
2. Communicates reduction in anxiety
3. Performs activities without respiratory distress or fatigue

▼ CARBON MONOXIDE POISONING

Data Base

A. Etiology and pathophysiology: carbon monoxide combines with hemoglobin more readily than does oxygen, resulting in tissue anoxia; caused by inadequately vented combustion devices
B. Clinical findings
1. Subjective: headache; faintness; vertigo; tinnitus
2. Objective: color normal, cyanotic, or flushed, but usually cherry pink; paralysis; loss of consciousness; ECG changes

C. Therapeutic interventions
   1. Mechanical ventilation with 100% oxygen until carboxyhemoglobin is reduced to less than 5% and respirations are normal
   2. Hyperbaric pressure chamber to increase oxygen concentration and accelerate formation of carbon dioxide, which can be exhaled

Nursing Care of Clients with Carbon Monoxide Poisoning

A. **ASSESSMENT**
   1. History to determine extent of exposure
   2. Color of skin
   3. Level of consciousness
B. **ANALYSIS/NURSING DIAGNOSES**
   1. Impaired gas exchange related to chemical imbalance
   2. Disturbed thought processes related to hypoxia
C. **PLANNING/IMPLEMENTATION**
   1. Remove the individual from the immediate area of poisoning
   2. Evaluate for cardiopulmonary function
   3. Institute cardiopulmonary resuscitation if necessary and maintain until additional help arrives
   4. Administer oxygen as prescribed
   5. Maintain respirations with assistance if needed
   6. Maintain body temperature
   7. Monitor vital signs, with special concern for respirations
D. **EVALUATION/OUTCOMES**
   1. Maintains adequate oxygen levels
   2. Remains conscious and alert

GASTROINTESTINAL SYSTEM

REVIEW OF ANATOMY AND PHYSIOLOGY

Functions of the Gastrointestinal System

Digestion
A. All changes that food undergoes in the alimentary canal so that it can be absorbed and metabolized
B. Types
   1. Mechanical digestion: all movements of the alimentary tract that:
      a. Change physical state of foods
      b. Propel food along the alimentary tract
         (1) Deglutition: swallowing
         (2) Peristalsis: wavelike movements that squeeze food downward in the tract
         (3) Sequential contractions: movements that mix intestinal contents with digestive juices
   2. Chemical digestion: series of hydrolytic processes dependent on specific enzymes; an addi-

tional substance may be necessary to act as a catalyst to facilitate the process

Absorption
A. Passage of substances through the intestinal mucosa into the blood or lymph
B. Accomplished mainly through the movement of molecules against a concentration gradient because of energy (ATP) expenditure (active transport) by the intestinal cells; makes it possible for both water and solutes to move through the intestinal mucosa in a direction opposite that expected in osmosis and diffusion
C. Majority occurs in the small intestine; most water is absorbed from large intestine

Metabolism
A. Definition: sum of all the chemical reactions in the body
B. Anabolism: synthesis of various compounds from simpler compounds
C. Catabolism: metabolic process in which complex substances are broken down into simple compounds; energy is liberated for use in work, energy storage, and heat production
D. Metabolism of carbohydrates
   1. Glucose transport through cell membranes and phosphorylation
      a. Insulin promotes this transport through cell membranes
      b. Glucose phosphorylation: conversion of glucose to glucose-6-phosphate; insulin increases the activity of glucokinase and promotes glucose phosphorylation, which is essential prior to both glycogenesis and glucose catabolism
   2. Glycogenesis: conversion of glucose to glycogen for storage; occurs mainly in the liver and muscle cells
   3. Glycogenolysis
      a. In muscle cells glycogen is changed back to glucose-6-phosphate, which is catabolized in the muscle cells
      b. In liver cells glycogen is changed back to glucose; glucagon and epinephrine accelerate liver glycogenolysis
   4. Glucose catabolism
      a. Glycolysis: anabolic reaction that breaks one glucose molecule down into two pyruvic acid molecules, with conversion of about 5% of energy stored in glucose to heat and ATP molecules
      b. Krebs' citric acid cycle with the electron transport chain: an aerobic chemical reaction in which two pyruvic acid molecules are broken down to six carbon dioxide and six water molecules, with the release of some energy as heat and some stored as ATP; the

aerobic reactions release about 95% of the energy stored in glucose, whereas the anaerobic reactions release only about 5%; the aerobic reactions occur in the mitochondria of cells

5. Gluconeogenesis: chemical reaction that converts protein or fat compounds into glucose: occurs in liver cells

6. Principles of carbohydrate metabolism
   a. Principle of preferred energy fuel: most cells first catabolize glucose, sparing fats and proteins; when the glucose supply becomes inadequate, most cells next catabolize fats; nerve cells require glucose, thus causing proteins to be sacrificed to provide the amino acids needed to produce more glucose (gluconeogenesis); also small amounts of glucose can be made from the glycerol portion of fats
   b. Principle of glycogenesis: glucose in excess of about 120 to 140 mg per 100 ml of blood brought to liver cells undergoes glycogenesis and is stored as glycogen
   c. Principle of glycogenolysis: when blood glucose decreases below the midpoint of normal, liver glycogenolysis accelerates and tends to raise the blood glucose concentration back toward the midpoint of normal
   d. Principle of gluconeogenesis: when blood glucose decreases below normal or when the amount of glucose entering the cells is inadequate, liver gluconeogenesis accelerates and raises blood glucose levels
   e. Principle of glucose storage as fat; when the blood insulin content is adequate, glucose in excess of the amount used for catabolism and glycogenesis is converted to fat

Structures of the Gastrointestinal System
Mouth (buccal cavity)
A. Lips and cheeks
B. Hard palate; soft palate
C. Gums (gingivae); teeth
D. Tongue
   1. Papillae: rough elevations on surface
   2. Taste buds: receptors of cranial nerves VII (facial) and IX (glossopharyngeal); located in papillae
E. Tonsils: lymphatic tissue that produces lymphocytes; defense against infection
F. Parotid glands
   1. Parotid, submandibular, and sublingual
   2. Produce saliva, a mixture of water, mucin, salts, and the enzyme, salivary amylase (ptyalin)

Esophagus
A. Posterior to the trachea; anterior to the vertebral column
B. Extends from the pharynx through an opening in the diaphragm (hiatus) to the stomach
C. Collapsible muscular tube; about 25 cm (10 inches) long
D. Secretes mucus; facilitates movement of food

Stomach
A. Size varies in different persons and according to degree of distention
B. Elongated pouch, with greater curve forming the lower left border
C. In epigastric and left hypochondriac portions of the abdominal cavity
D. Divisions
   1. Fundus: the uppermost portion; the bulge adjacent to and extending above the esophageal opening
   2. Body: central portion
   3. Pylorus: constricted lower portion
E. Sphincters
   1. Cardiac: at opening of the esophagus into the stomach
   2. Pyloric: at opening of the pylorus into the duodenum
F. Secretes gastric juice
   1. Stomach wall cells secrete gastrin that stimulates the flow of gastric juices
   2. Chief cells secrete pepsin
   3. Parietal cells secrete hydrochloric acid and intrinsic factor
   4. Goblet cells secrete mucin
G. Functions: food storage and liquefaction (chyme)

Small intestine
A. Size: approximately 2.5 cm (1 inch) in diameter; 6.1 m (29 feet) in length when relaxed
B. Divisions
   1. Duodenum: joins pylorus of the stomach; C shaped
   2. Jejunum: middle section
   3. Ileum: lower section; no clear boundary between jejunum and ileum
C. Functions: digestion and absorption; enzymes include sucrase, lactase, and maltase; cholecystokinin stimulates release of bile from the gallbladder
D. Process: mixing movements; peristalsis; secretion of water, ions, mucus; receives secretions from the liver, gallbladder, and pancreas

Large intestine
A. Size: approximately 6.3 cm (2.5 inches) in diameter; 1.5 m (5 to 6 feet) long when relaxed
B. Divisions
   1. Cecum: first 2 to 3 inches
   2. Colon: consists of ascending, transverse, descending, and sigmoid colon
   3. Rectum: last 7 to 8 inches
   4. Anus: terminal opening of the alimentary canal

C. Functions: water and sodium ion absorption; temporary storage of fecal matter; defecation

D. Process: weak mixing movements, mass movements, and peristalsis

Vermiform appendix

A. Blind-end tube off the cecum just beyond the ileocecal valve

B. Function: part of the immune system

Liver

A. Occupies most of the right hypochondrium and part of the epigastrium

B. Divided into thousands of lobules

C. Ducts
  1. Hepatic duct: from liver
  2. Cystic duct: from gallbladder
  3. Common bile duct: formed by the union of the hepatic and cystic ducts; drains bile into the duodenum at the sphincter of Oddi

D. Functions: plays a role in the metabolism of proteins, carbohydrates, and fats
  1. Carbohydrate metabolism: converts glucose to glycogen by glycogenesis, glycogen to glucose by glycogenolysis, and forms glucose from proteins and fats by gluconeogenesis
  2. Fat metabolism
    a. Ketogenesis: fatty acids are broken down into molecules of acetyl CoA (beta oxygenation), which then form ketone bodies (acetoacetic acid, acetone, beta-hydroxybutyric acid)
    b. Fat storage
    c. Synthesis of triglycerides, phospholipids, cholesterol, and B complex factor choline
  3. Protein metabolism
    a. Anabolism: synthesis of various blood proteins (e.g., prothrombin, fibrinogen, albumins, alpha and beta globulins, and clotting factors V, VII, IX, and X)
    b. Deamination: chemical reaction by which amino group is split off from amino acid to form ammonia and a keto acid
    c. Urea formation: converts most of ammonia formed by deamination to urea
  4. Secretes bile, a substance important for emulsifying fats prior to digestion and as a vehicle for excretion of cholesterol and bile pigments
  5. Detoxifies various substances (e.g., drugs, hormones)
  6. Vitamin metabolism: stores vitamins A, D, K, and B_{12}

Gallbladder

A. Lies on the undersurface of the liver

B. Sac made of smooth muscle, lined with mucosa arranged in rugae

C. Functions: concentrates and stores bile

Pancreas

A. Structure

  1. Fish-shaped, with body, head, and tail; extends from the duodenal curve to the spleen
  2. Both a duct and a ductless gland
    a. Pancreatic cells: secrete pancreatic juice via a duct to the duodenum; enzymes include trypsin, lipase, and amylase; stimulated by the duodenal hormones secretin and pancreozymin and parasympathetic impulses
    b. Islets of Langerhans: clusters of cells not connected with pancreatic ducts; composed of alpha and beta cells

B. Functions
  1. Pancreatic juice composed of enzymes that help digest carbohydrates, proteins, and fats
  2. Islet cells constitute the endocrine gland
    a. Alpha cells secrete the hormone glucagon, which accelerates liver glycogenolysis and initiates gluconogenesis; tends to increase blood glucose level
    b. Beta cells secrete insulin, which exerts a profound influence on the metabolism of carbohydrates, proteins, and fats
      (1) Accelerates the active transport of glucose, along with potassium and phosphate ions, through cell membranes; decreases blood glucose and increases glucose utilization by the cells for either catabolism or anabolism
      (2) Stimulates the production of liver cell glucokinase; promotes liver glycogenesis which lowers blood glucose
      (3) Inhibits liver cell phosphatase and therefore inhibits liver glycogenolysis
      (4) Accelerates the rate of amino acid transfer into cells promoting anabolism of proteins within the cells
      (5) Accelerates the rate of fatty acid transfer into cells, promotes fat anabolism (lipogenesis); inhibits fat catabolism

REVIEW OF PHYSICAL PRINCIPLES
Law of Motion

The greater the force of contraction of the intestinal wall and the more frequent the contractions, the more rapid the propulsion of food and fecal matter through the digestive tract

Light

A. Refraction: Total internal reflection in fiberoptics permits viewing of interior walls of stomach (gastroscopy) and intestines (sigmoidoscopy)

B. X-rays: GI series and barium enemas allow visualization of the soft tissues of the upper and lower gastrointestinal tract; the barium salts coat the inner walls of the tract and absorb the x-rays, outlining organ surfaces

REVIEW OF CHEMICAL PRINCIPLES
Oxidation and Reduction

A. Uniting oxygen with a substance results in oxidation
B. Uniting hydrogen with a substance results in reduction
C. Oxidation of nutrients such as glucose results in the formation of high-energy ATP molecules and heat
D. Some forms of life (anaerobes) can use substances other than oxygen for cellular oxidation (e.g., *Clostridium perfringens* found in gangrenous tissue)

Types of Compounds
Organic acids

A. Lactic acid: end product of anaerobic muscle metabolism
B. Citric acid: one intermediate in the Krebs' citric acid cycle

Amino acids

A. Able to act as an acid and as a base (amphoteric character)
B. Essential amino acids cannot be synthesized well enough in the body to maintain health and growth and must be supplied in the food

Carbohydrates

A. Include simple sugars, starches, celluloses, gums, and resins; contain carbon, hydrogen, and oxygen
B. Classification
   1. Monosaccharide: a simple sugar (e.g., glucose, fructose)
   2. Disaccharide (e.g., sucrose, lactose, maltose)
   3. Polysaccharide (e.g., starch, glycogen)

Lipids

A. Fatty acids are important constituents of all lipids except sterols
   1. Usually straight-chain carboxylic acids; 3 fatty acids and 1 glycerol molecule form a triglyceride
   2. Saturated fatty acids: have no double bonds between their carbon atoms; solid at room temperature; mainly animal fats
   3. Unsaturated fatty acids; have one or more double bonds between their carbon atoms; liquid at room temperature
   4. Essential fatty acids: cannot be synthesized by the body; must be taken in by diet
B. Cholesterol: a sterol found in human and animal tissue; important component of membranes; found in blood 150 to 200 mg/ml; high cholesterol associated with increased intake of saturated fats and arterial atherosclerosis

Proteins

A. Simple proteins
   1. Albumins: necessary for plasma colloid osmotic pressure (oncotic pressure), which helps control (through osmosis) the flow of water between the plasma and interstitial fluid; with starvation, a decreased serum albumin causes a fall in the plasma colloid osmotic pressure; this results in edema as less fluid is drawn by osmosis into the capillaries from the interstitial spaces
   2. Globulins: necessary to form antibodies (e.g., gamma serum globulin)
B. Compound proteins
   1. Lipoproteins: simple proteins combined with lipid substances
      a. Low-density lipoprotein cholesterol (beta lipoproteins)
         (1) LDL: Low-density lipoproteins that are chief carriers of cholesterol and are low in triglycerides
         (2) Contribute to atherosclerotic plaque formation
      b. High-density lipoprotein cholesterol (HDL) (alpha lipoproteins)
         (1) Consist of 50% protein and 20% cholesterol
         (2) Inversely associated with coronary artery disease
   2. Nucleoproteins: proteins complexed with nucleic acids; chromosomes are sometimes referred to as nucleoprotein structures
      a. Ribonucleic acid (RNA) and deoxyribonucleic acid (DNA) are nucleic acids
      b. RNA and DNA store and transmit genetic information from one generation to another
   3. Metalloproteins: proteins containing metal ions (e.g., ferritin, the iron transport compound of plasma)

REVIEW OF MICROORGANISMS

A. Bacterial pathogens
   1. Brucella: small, gram-negative bacilli cause brucellosis, an infection that can be acquired by drinking infected milk
   2. *Escherichia coli:* small, gram-negative bacillus that is part of the normal flora of the large intestine; certain strains cause urinary tract infections and diarrhea
   3. *Clostridium difficile:* anaerobic, spore-forming bacterial pathogen; produces toxins that affect bowel mucosa; major cause of nosocomial diarrhea
   4. Shigella: gram-negative bacilli, similar to salmonella; *Shigella dysenteriae* causes bacillary dysentery or shigellosis
B. Protozoal pathogens
   1. *Balantidium coli:* ciliated protozoan; causes enteritis
   2. *Entamoeba histolytica:* an amoeba; causes amoebiasis (amoebic dysentery)

3. *Giardia lamblia:* flagellated protozoan; causes enteritis
C. Parasitic pathogens
1. Nematodes (roundworms): include *Necator americanus* (hookworm), *Ascaris lumbricoides, Enterobius vermicularis* (pinworm), *Trichuris trichiura* (whipworm), all of which may be found in the intestine
2. Cestodes (tapeworm): may be found in adult form in the intestine; the larval stage (hydatid) of some forms may develop and form cysts in the liver, lungs, and kidneys
3. Trematodes (flukes): may be found in the lungs, liver, and abdominal cavity

 RELATED PHARMACOLOGY

Antiemetics
A. Description
1. Diminish the sensitivity of the chemoreceptor trigger zone (CTZ) to irritants or decrease labyrinthine excitability
2. Alleviate nausea and vomiting
3. Prevent and control emesis and motion sickness
4. Available in oral, parenteral (IM, IV), rectal, and transdermal preparations
B. Examples
1. Centrally acting agents: ondansetron HCl (Zofran); prochlorperazine (Compazine); trimethobenzamide HCl (Tigan)
2. Agents for motion sickness control: dimenhydrinate (Dramamine); meclizine HCl (Antivert, Bonine); promethazine HCl (Phenergan)
3. Agents that promote gastric emptying: metoclopramide (Reglan)
C. Major side effects: drowsiness (CNS depression); hypotension (vasodilation via central mechanism); dry mouth (decreased salivation from anticholinergic effect); blurred vision (pupillary dilation from anticholinergic effect); incoordination (an extrapyramidal symptom due to dopamine antagonism)
D. Nursing care
1. Observe occurrence and characteristics of vomitus
2. Eliminate noxious substances from the diet and environment
3. Provide oral hygiene
4. Caution client to avoid engaging in hazardous activities
5. Offer sugar-free chewing gum or hard candy to promote salivation
6. Instruct client to change positions slowly

Anorexiants
A. Description
1. Suppress the desire for food at the hypothalamic appetite centers; generally produce CNS stimulation
2. Available in oral preparations
B. Examples: amphetamine sulfate (Benzedrine); dextroamphetamine sulfate (Dexedrine)
C. Major side effects: nausea, vomiting (irritation of gastric mucosa); constipation (delayed passage of stool in GI tract); tachycardia (sympathetic stimulation); CNS stimulation (sympathetic activation)
D. Nursing care
1. Educate client regarding:
a. Drug misuse (controlled substances)
b. Concurrent exercise and diet therapy
c. Need for medical supervision during therapy
d. Possibility of affecting ability to engage in hazardous activities
2. Monitor weight

Antacids
A. Description
1. Provide a protective coating on the stomach lining and lower the gastric acid level; allows more rapid movement of stomach contents into the duodenum
2. Neutralize gastric acid; effective in the treatment of ulcers
3. Available in oral preparations
B. Examples: aluminum hydroxide gel (Amphojel); aluminum and magnesium hydroxides (Maalox); sodium bicarbonate: systemic antacid; may cause alkalosis
C. Major side effects
1. Constipation (aluminum compounds) (aluminum delays passage of stool in GI tract)
2. Diarrhea (magnesium compounds) (magnesium stimulates peristalsis in GI tract)
3. Alkalosis (systemic antacids) (absorption of alkaline compound into the circulation)
4. Reduced absorption of calcium and iron (increase in gastric pH)
D. Nursing care
1. Instruct the client regarding:
a. Prevention of overuse of antacids, which can result in rebound hyperacidity
b. Need for continued supervision
c. Dietary restrictions related to gastric distress
d. Foods high in calcium and iron
2. Caution client on a sodium-restricted diet that many antacids contain sodium
3. Shake oral suspensions well before administration
4. Administer with small amount of water of ensure passage to stomach

Anticholinergics
A. Description
1. Inhibit smooth muscle contraction in the GI tract

2. Alleviate pain associated with peptic ulcer
3. Available in oral and parenteral (IM, IV) preparations

B. Examples: atropine sulfate; dicyclomine HCl (Bentyl); glycopyrrolate (Robinul); propantheline bromide (Pro-Banthine)

C. Major side effects (all related to decreased parasympathetic stimulation)
   1. Abdominal distention and constipation (decreased peristalsis)
   2. Dry mouth (decreased salivation)
   3. Urinary retention (decreased parasympathetic stimulation)
   4. CNS disturbances (direct CNS toxic effect)

D. Nursing care
   1. Provide dietary counseling with emphasis on bland foods
   2. Provide oral hygiene

Antisecretory agents

A. Description
   1. Inhibit gastric acid secretion
   2. Act at the H_2 receptors of the stomach parietal cells to limit gastric secretion (H_2 antagonists)
   3. Inhibit hydrogen/potassium ATPase enzyme system to block acid production (proton pump inhibitors)
   4. Available in oral and parenteral (IM, IV) preparations

B. Examples
   1. H_2 antagonists: famotidine (Pepcid); ranitidine (Zantac)
   2. Proton pump inhibitors: omeprazole (Prilosec); lansoprazole (Prevacid)

C. Major side effects
   1. CNS disturbances (decreased metabolism of drug because of liver or kidney impairment)
   2. Blood dyscrasias (decreased RBCs, WBCs, platelet synthesis)
   3. Skin rash (hypersensitivity)

D. Nursing care
   1. Do not administer at same time as antacids; allow 1 to 2 hours between drugs
   2. Administer oral preparations with meals
   3. Assess for potentiation of oral anticoagulant effect
   4. Instruct client to follow prescription exactly
   5. Administration should not exceed 8 weeks without medical supervision

Antidiarrheals

A. Description
   1. Promote the formation of formed stools
   2. Alleviate diarrhea
   3. Available in oral and parenteral (IM) preparations.

B. Examples

1. Fluid adsorbents: decrease the fluid content of stool: bismuth subcarbonate; kaolin and pectin (Kaopectate)
2. Enteric bacteria replacements: enhance production of lactic acid from carbohydrates in intestinal lumen; acidity suppresses pathogenic bacterial overgrowth: *Lactobacillus acidophilus* (Bacid); *Lactobacillus bulgaricus* (Lactinex)
3. Motility suppressants: decrease GI tract motility so that more water will be absorbed from the large intestine: diphenoxylate HCl (Lomotil); loperamide HCl (Imodium)

C. Major side effects
   1. Fluid adsorbents: GI disturbances (local effect); CNS disturbances (direct CNS toxic effect)
   2. Enteric bacteria replacements: excessive flatulence (increased microbial gas production); abdominal cramps (increased microbial gas production)
   3. Motility suppressants: urinary retention (decreased parasympathetic stimulation); tachycardia (vagolytic effect on cardiac conduction); dry mouth (decreased salivation from anticholinergic effect); sedation (CNS depression); paralytic ileus (decreased peristalsis); respiratory depression (depression of medullary respiratory center)

D. Nursing care
   1. Monitor bowel movements for color, characteristics, and frequency
   2. Assess for fluid/electrolyte imbalance
   3. Assess and eliminate cause of diarrhea
   4. Motility suppressants
      a. Warn client of interference with ability to perform hazardous activities and risk of physical dependence with long-term use
      b. Offer sugar-free chewing gum and hard candy to promote salivation

Cathartics/laxatives

A. Description
   1. Alleviate or prevent constipation and promote evacuation of stool
   2. Available in oral and rectal preparations

B. Examples
   1. Intestinal lubricants: decrease dehydration of feces; lubricate intestinal tract: mineral oil; olive oil
   2. Fecal softners: lower surface tension of feces, allowing water and fats to penetrate; docusate calcium (Surfak); docusate sodium (Colace)
   3. Bulk-forming laxatives: increase bulk in intestinal lumen, which stimulates propulsive movements by pressure on mucosal lining: methylcellulose (Cellothyl); psyllium hydrophilic mucilloid (Metamucil)

4. Colon irritants: stimulate peristalsis by reflexive response to irritation of intestinal lumen; bisacodyl (Dulcolax); senna (Senokot)
5. Saline cathartics: increase osmotic pressure within intestine, drawing fluid from blood and bowel wall, thus increasing bulk and stimulating peristalsis: effervescent sodium phosphate (Fleet Phospho-Soda); magnesium citrate solution; Milk of Magnesia
C. Major side effects
1. Laxative dependence with long-term use (loss of normal defecation mechanism)
2. GI disturbances (local effect)
3. Intestinal lubricants: inhibit absorption of fat-soluble vitamins A, D, E, K; can cause anal leaking of oil (accumulation of lubricant near rectal sphincter)
4. Saline cathartics: dehydration (fluid volume depletion resulting from hypertonic state in GI tract); hypernatremia (increased sodium absorption into circulation; shift of fluid from vasculature to intestinal lumen)
D. Nursing care
1. Instruct the client regarding: overuse of cathartics and intestinal lubricants; increasing intake of fluids and dietary fiber; increasing activity level; compliance with bowel-retraining program
2. Monitor bowel movements for consistency and frequency of stool
3. Intestinal lubricants: use peripad to protect clothing
4. Bulk-forming laxatives: mix thoroughly in 8 oz of fluid and follow with another 8 oz of fluid to prevent obstruction
5. Administer at bedtime to promote defecation in the morning

Intestinal antibiotics
See Aminoglycosides in Pharmacologic Control of Infection

Pancreatic enzymes
A. Description
1. Replace natural endogenous pancreatic enzymes (protease, lipase, amylase); promote the digestion of proteins, fats, and carbohydrates
2. Available in oral preparations
B. Examples: pancreatin (Viokase); pancrelipase (Cotazym)
C. Major side effects: nausea and diarrhea (GI irritation)
D. Nursing care
1. Administer with meals or snacks
2. Avoid crushing preparations that are enteric coated
3. Provide a balanced diet to prevent indigestion

RELATED PROCEDURES
Colostomy Irrigation and Care
A. Definition
1. Instillation of fluid into the lower colon via a stoma on the abdominal wall to stimulate peristalsis and facilitate the expulsion of feces
2. Cleansing the colostomy stoma and collection of feces (stool consistency will depend on location of the ostomy: a colostomy of the sigmoid colon will tend to produce formed stools; a transverse or ascending colostomy will produce less formed stools)
B. Nursing care
1. Irrigate the stoma at the same time each day to approximate normal bowel habits
2. Insert a well-lubricated catheter tip into the stoma approximately 7 to 10 cm in the direction of the remaining bowel (anatomy of ascending, transverse, and descending colon should be considered)
3. Hold the irrigating container 12 to 18 inches above the colostomy; irrigating solution should be 105° F (40.5° C)
4. Stop the flow of fluid temporarily if cramping occurs
5. Provide privacy while waiting for fecal returns or permit the client to ambulate with the collection bag in place to further stimulate peristalsis
6. Cleanse the stoma; apply a protective skin barrier
7. Apply a colostomy bag or gauze dressing (if the colostomy is well regulated)
8. Teach the client to control odor when necessary by placing commercially available deodorizer in the colostomy bag

Endoscopy
A. Definition: visualization of the esophagus, stomach, biliary and pancreatic ducts, colon, or rectum using a hollow tube with a lighted end: gastroscopy—stomach; esophagoscopy—esophagus; colonoscopy—large colon; proctoscopy—rectum; endoscopic retrograde cholangiopancreatography (ERCP)—common bile and pancreatic ducts
B. Nursing care
1. Obtain an informed consent for the procedure
2. If rectal examination is indicated, administer cleansing enemas before the test
3. Restrict diet (NPO) before procedure
4. Following the procedure, observe for bleeding, changes in vital signs, or nausea
5. If the throat is anesthetized (as for a gastroscopy or esophagoscopy), check for the return of gag reflex before offering oral fluids
6. Assess for bleeding or signs of pancreatitis

Enemas

A. Definitions
1. Tap-water enema: introduction of water into the colon to stimulate evacuation
2. Soapsuds enema: introduction of soapy water into the colon to stimulate peristalsis by bowel irritation; contraindicated as a preparation for an endoscopic procedure because it may alter the appearance of the mucosa
3. Hypertonic enema: commercially prepared small-volume enema that works on the principle of osmosis
4. Harris flush or drip: repeated alternate introduction of water into the colon and drainage of that water from the colon through the same tubing to facilitate exit of flatus
5. Installation: introduction of a liquid (usually mineral oil) into the colon to facilitate fecal activity through lubricating effect

B. Nursing care
1. Provide privacy, place client in left side-lying position
2. Obtain the correct solution
3. Lubricate the tip of a rectal catheter with water-soluble jelly
4. Insert the catheter 4 to 6 inches into the rectum
5. Allow the solution to enter slowly; keep it no more than 12 to 18 inches (30.5 to 45.7 cm) above the rectum; temporarily interrupt flow if cramping occurs
6. Allow ample time for the client to expel the enema
7. Observe and record the amount and consistency of returns

Gastrointestinal Series

A. Definition: introduction of barium, an opaque medium, into the upper GI tract via the mouth (upper GI series) or the lower GI tract via the rectum for the purpose of x-ray visualization for pathologic changes

B. Nursing care
1. Prepare the client for the procedure by:
   a. Maintaining the client NPO for 8 to 10 hours before the test
   b. Administering cathartics and/or enemas as ordered to evacuate the bowel
2. Inspect stool after the procedure for the presence of barium
3. Administer enemas and/or cathartics as ordered if the stool does not return to normal
4. Encourage fluid intake

Gavage (Tube Feeding)

A. Definitions
1. Nasogastric: placement of a tube through the nose into the stomach (has the highest risk of aspiration of all types of feeding tubes)
2. Intestinal: placement of a tube through the nose into the small intestine
3. Surgically placed feeding tubes
   a. Cervical esophagostomy: tube is sutured directly into the esophagus for clients who have had head and neck surgery
   b. Gastrostomy: tube is placed directly into stomach through the abdominal wall and sutured in place; used for clients who require tube feeding on a long-term basis
   c. Jejunostomy: tube is inserted directly into the jejunum for clients with pathologic conditions of the upper GI tract
4. Percutaneous endoscopic gastrostomy (PEG) and low profile gastrostomy device (G-Button)
   a. Stomach is punctured during endoscopy procedure
   b. Associated with reduced risks but accidental removal may occur; low risk with button
   c. Dressing should be changed daily

B. Nursing care
1. Verify placement of tube before feeding
   a. Inject a small amount of air into the tube and, with a stethoscope placed over the epigastric area, listen for the passage of air into the stomach
   b. Aspirate for presence of stomach contents; reinstill to avoid electrolyte imbalance
   c. Test aspirate for acid pH
   d. Small-bore tube placement must be verified by x-ray examination
2. Aspirate contents of stomach before feeding to determine residual; reinstill to avoid electrolyte imbalance; withhold feeding if residual is greater than 160 ml or the amount specified by the agency's protocol
3. Intermittent feeding
   a. Position the client so that the head is elevated during the feeding
   b. Verify placement of tube
   c. Introduce 30 ml of water to verify the patency of the tube; the tube should not be allowed to empty during feeding
   d. Slowly administer the feeding at room or body temperature; observe and question the client to determine tolerance
   e. Administer 30 ml of water to clear the tube at the completion of the feeding
   f. Clamp the tubing and clean the equipment
   g. Place client in sitting position for 1 hour after feeding; place infant in right side-lying position
4. Continuous feeding
   a. Place prescribed feeding in gavage bag and

prime tubing to prevent excess air from entering stomach

b. Set rate of flow; rate of flow can be manually regulated by setting drops per minute or mechanically regulated by using an electric pump

c. Position the client to keep the head elevated throughout the feeding

d. Verify placement of tube when adding additional fluid to a continuous feeding

e. Flush tube intermittently with water to prevent occlusion of tube with feeding, change tubing per protocol

f. Monitor for gastric distention and aspiration; because smaller amounts of feeding are generally administered within a given period, gastric distention and subsequent aspiration are less frequent

g. Discard unused fluid that has been in gavage administration bag at room temperature for longer than 4 hours

5. Care common for all clients receiving tube feedings

a. Monitor for abdominal distention; changes in bowel sounds

b. Discontinue feeding if nausea and/or vomiting occur

c. Provide oral hygiene

d. When appropriate, encourage the client to chew foods that will stimulate gastric secretions while providing psychologic comfort; chewed food may or may not be swallowed

e. Provide special skin care; if the client has a gastrostomy tube sutured in place, the skin may become irritated from gastrointestinal enzymes; if the client has a nasogastric tube, the skin may become excoriated at point of entry because of irritation

Parenteral Replacement Therapy

A. Definitions

1. Peripheral parenteral nutrition (PPN)

a. Administration of isotonic lipid and amino acid solutions through a peripheral vein

b. Amino acid content should not exceed 4%; dextrose content should not be greater than 10%; helps maintain a positive nitrogen balance

c. Therapy usually limited to 2 weeks

2. Total parenteral nutrition (TPN)

a. Administration of carbohydrates, amino acids, vitamins, and minerals via a central vein

b. High osmolality solutions (25% dextrose) are administered in conjunction with 5% to 10% amino acids, electrolytes, minerals, and

vitamins; helps maintain a positive nitrogen balance

c. Long-term home nutritional therapy may be delivered by atrial catheters (Hickman/ Broviac or Groshong) that are surgically inserted

3. Intralipid therapy

a. Infusion of 10% to 20% fat emulsion that provides essential fatty acids

b. Provides increased caloric intake to maintain positive nitrogen balance

4. Total nutrient admixture (TNA or "3 in 1")

a. Combination of dextrose, amino acids, and lipids in one container; vitamins and minerals may be added

b. Administered through a central line over 24 hours

B. Nursing care

1. Infuse fluid through a large vein such as the subclavian because of the high osmolarity of the solution

2. Ensure proper placement of the tube by chest x-ray examination after insertion; accidental pneumothorax can occur during insertion

3. Precisely regulate the fluid infusion rate; an intravenous pump should be used

a. Rapid infusion may result in movement of the fluid into the intravascular compartment; dehydration, circulatory overload, and hyperglycemia can occur

b. Slow infusion may result in hypoglycemia because the body adapts to the high osmolarity of this fluid by secreting more insulin; for this reason, therapy is never terminated abruptly but is gradually discontinued

4. Use aseptic technique when handling the infusion or changing the dressing

5. Use a filter for TPN; filters cannot be used for lipids

6. Use surgically aseptic technique when changing tubing

7. Record daily weights and monitor urinary sugar and acetone or blood glucose levels frequently

8. Check laboratory reports daily, especially glucose, creatine, BUN, and electrolytes; serum lipids and liver function studies if lipids are administered

9. Monitor temperature every four hours because infection is the most common complication of TPN; if the client has a temperature elevation, order cultures of blood, urine, and sputum to rule out other sources of infection

Paracentesis

A. Definition: removal of fluid from the peritoneum to reduce intraabdominal tension or obtain fluid for culture

B. Nursing care
1. Obtain informed consent
2. Have client void before procedure
3. Position upright at edge of bed
4. Assess vital signs following procedure; assess for signs of hypovolemia, including pallor, oliguria, dyspnea, and tachycardia

MAJOR DISORDERS OF THE GASTROINTESTINAL SYSTEM

▼ FRACTURE OF THE JAW

Data Base
A. Etiology and pathophysiology
   1. Generally the result of trauma such as motor vehicle accidents or physical combat
   2. Blowout fractures of the orbit may accompany fractured jaw; these are stabilized surgically with wires, plates, and screws
B. Clinical findings
   1. Subjective: history of trauma to the face; pain in the face and jaw; double vision
   2. Objective: bloody discharge from the mouth; swelling of face on the affected side; difficulty opening or closing the mouth; malocculusion
C. Therapeutic interventions
   1. Separated fragments of the broken bone are reunited and immobilized by wires and rubber bands; usually placed without surgical incision
   2. Open reduction of the jaw is indicated for severely fractured or displaced bones; interosseous wiring is done

Nursing Care of Clients with Fracture of the Jaw
A. ASSESSMENT
1. Respiratory status for presence of distress
2. Presence of nausea and potential for vomiting
3. Structures of the face and neck for signs of edema
4. Assessment of drainage from nose or ears for prescence of CSF; CSF dries in concentric rings

B. ANALYSIS/NURSING DIAGNOSES
1. Risk for aspiration related to presence of oral wires
2. Imbalanced nutrition: less than body requirements related to inability to consume regular diet

C. PLANNING/IMPLEMENTATION
1. Postoperatively control vomiting and reduce the chance of aspiration pneumonia by positioning client on abdomen or side
2. Keep wire cutters at the bedside to release the wires and rubber bands if emesis occurs and aspiration cannot be prevented by suctioning

3. Initially establish an alternate means of communication
4. Explain diet to the client and family; no solid foods are permitted; encourage high-protein liquids or blenderized soft foods
5. Stress the importance of regular oral hygiene and institute it early in the postoperative period

D. EVALUATION/OUTCOMES
1. Adheres to nutritionally balanced safe diet
2. Demonstrates oral hygiene techniques
3. Describes technique for releasing wires and rubber bands if emesis occurs

▼ CANCER OF THE ORAL CAVITY

Data Base
A. Etiology and pathophysiology
   1. Primarily in clients who smoke and drink alcohol in large quantities
   2. Cancer of the lip easily diagnosed; prognosis is good; incidence highest in pipe smokers
   3. Cancer of the tongue usually occurs with cancer of the floor of the mouth; metastasis to the neck is common
   4. Cancer of the submaxillary glands; highly malignant and grows rapidly
B. Clinical findings
   1. Subjective: pain (not an early symptom); alterations of taste
   2. Objective: leukoplakia (white patches on mucosa), which is considered precancerous; ulcerated, bleeding areas in the involved structure
C. Therapeutic interventions
   1. Reconstructive surgery if indicated
   2. Radiation or implantation of radioactive material may arrest growth of tumor
   3. Total parenteral nutrition, enteral tube feedings

Nursing Care of Clients with Cancer of the Oral Cavity
A. ASSESSMENT
1. History of hemoptysis and pain
2. Baseline nutritional data including weight, dietary intake, and ability to chew
3. Characteristics of lesions in oral cavity

B. ANALYSIS/NURSING DIAGNOSES
1. Ineffective airway clearance related to tissue trauma from iatrogenic stresses
2. Impaired oral mucous membranes related to oral lesions
3. Imbalanced nutrition: less than body requirements related to decreased taste, dysphagia, and pain

C. PLANNING/IMPLEMENTATION

1. Maintain a patient airway; keep a tracheostomy set at the bedside
2. Maintain fluid, electrolyte, and nutritional balance; administer TPN, enteral tube feedings as ordered
3. If radiation therapy is indicated, relieve dryness of the mouth by frequent saline mouthwashes and ample fluids
4. Consider time and distance in relation to the radioactive implants when giving nursing care

D. EVALUATION/OUTCOMES

1. Maintains airway patency
2. Maintains nutritional status

▼ GASTROESOPHAGEAL REFLUX DISEASE (GERD)

Data Base

A. Etiology and pathophysiology
  1. Backflow of gastric contents into the esophagus, gradually breaking down esophageal mucosa
  2. Etiology includes inadequate lower esophageal sphincter (LES) tone, corrosive effects of gastric acid on the esophagus, and delayed esophageal and gastric emptying; may be associated with hiatal hernia, obesity, pregnancy, and caffeine, chocolate, and high-fat food ingestion
  3. May lead to Barrett's esophagus, a pathologic condition that can lead to esophageal cancer
B. Clinical findings
  1. Subjective: heartburn, water brash, dysphagia, burning pain after meals
  2. Objective: eructation, regurgitation, hoarseness, chronic cough, wheezing, recurrent pneumonia if severe; esophageal pH monitoring provides evidence of acid reflux; endoscopy reveals evidence of tissue damage
C. Therapeutic interventions
  1. Medical management with histamine receptor agonists, antacids, proton pump inhibitors, cholinergics
  2. Small, frequent feedings; avoiding spices, fats, and alcohol; or eating before lying down to diminish reflux
  3. Weight reduction if indicated
  4. Surgical intervention if medical management is unsuccessful
    a. Nissen fundoplication: suturing to tighten the fundus around the esophagus
    b. Hill procedure: narrows esophageal opening

Nursing Care of Clients with Gastroesophageal Reflux Disease

A. ASSESSMENT

1. History of heartburn, regurgitation, dysphagia
2. Establishment of baseline weight to determine need for weight loss
3. Dietary and medication history to determine contributing factors

B. ANALYSIS/NURSING DIAGNOSES

1. Acute pain related to tissue trauma resulting from reflux
2. Imbalanced nutrition: more than body requirements related to excess intake

C. PLANNING/IMPLEMENTATION

1. Teach client dietary guidelines
  a. Eat small, frequent meals to avoid gastric distention
  b. Limit fatty foods, which delay gastric emptying
  c. Avoid foods that decrease lower esophageal sphincter (LES) pressure, such as alcohol, caffeine, and chocolate
  d. Avoid eating or drinking 2 to 3 hours before bedtime
2. Teach client to maintain desirable body weight and avoid tight-fitting clothing and activities that increase intraabdominal pressure
3. Support smoking cessation efforts
4. Elevate the head of the bed on blocks and advise client to avoid exercise or lying down after meals

D. EVALUATION/OUTCOMES

1. Reports incidence of heartburn is greatly reduced
2. Maintains desirable body weight

▼ CANCER OF THE ESOPHAGUS

Data Base

A. Etiology and pathophysiology
  1. Occurs predominantly in persons with a history of alcohol abuse, ingestion of hot, spicy foods, smoking, or GERD
  2. Tumor may develop anywhere in the esophagus, but most commonly in the middle and lower third
B. Clinical findings
  1. Subjective: dysphagia; substernal burning pain, particularly after hot fluids
  2. Objective: regurgitation; esophagogastroduodenoscopy (EGD) with biopsy and brushings reveals malignant cells
C. Therapeutic interventions
  1. Surgical removal of the esophagus is the treatment of choice
    a. Esophagogastrostomy: resection of a portion of the esophagus; a portion of the bowel may be grafted between the esophagus and stomach, or the stomach may be brought up to the proximal end of the esophagus

b. Esophagectomy: removal of part or all of the esophagus, which is replaced by a Dacron graft

c. Gastrostomy: opening directly into the stomach in which a feeding tube is usually inserted to bypass the esophagus

2. Radiation and/or chemotherapy may be used before or instead of surgery as a palliative measure

3. Total parenteral nutrition, enteral tube feedings

4. Photodynamic therapy is used for palliative treatment; Photofrin is injected and several days later, a fiberoptic probe in the esophagus activates the absorbed drug in cancer cells, shrinking them

Nursing Care of Clients with Cancer of the Esophagus

A. ASSESSMENT
1. History of nutritional status and weight loss
2. Presence of pain and dysphagia
3. History of foul breath, eructation, nausea, and vomiting

B. ANALYSIS/NURSING DIAGNOSES
1. Ineffective airway clearance related to tumor
2. Imbalanced nutrition: less than body requirements related to dysphagia

C. PLANNING/IMPLEMENTATION
1. Observe for respiratory distress caused by pressure of tumor on the trachea; place in a semi-Fowler's or high-Fowler's position to facilitate respirations
2. Monitor vital signs, especially respirations
3. Provide oral care because dysphagia may result in increased accumulation of salvia in mouth
4. Maintain nutritional status by providing TPN, tube feedings, high-protein liquids, and vitamin and mineral replacements as ordered

D. EVALUATION/OUTCOMES
1. Maintains airway
2. Maintains nutritional status

▼ HIATAL HERNIA

Data Base
A. Etiology and pathophysiology
1. Portion of the stomach protruding through a hiatus (opening) in the diaphragm into the thoracic cavity
2. May result from a congenital weakness of the diaphragm or from injury, pregnancy, or obesity
3. Function of the cardiac sphincter is lost, gastric juices enter the esophagus causing inflammation
B. Clinical findings

1. Subjective: substernal burning pain or fullness after eating; dyspepsia in the recumbent position; nocturnal dyspnea
2. Objective: barium swallow, upper GI series, and endoscopy show protrusion of the stomach through the diaphragm; regurgitation

C. Therapeutic interventions
1. Small, frequent, bland feedings
2. Pharmacologic therapy and dietary management
3. Surgical repair (done infrequently)

Nursing Care of Clients with Hiatal Hernia
See Nursing Care of Clients with Gastroesophageal Reflux Disease

▼ PEPTIC ULCER DISEASE (PUD)

Data Base
A. Etiology and pathophysiology
1. Ulcerations of the gastrointestinal mucosa and underlying tissues caused by gastric secretions that have a low pH (acid)
2. Causes include conditions that increase the secretion of hydrochloric acid by the gastric mucosa or that decrease that tissue's resistance to the acid
   a. Infection of the gastric and/or duodenal mucosa by *Campylobacter pylori* or *Helicobacter pylori*
   b. Zollinger-Ellison syndrome: tumors secreting gastrin, which will stimulate the production of excessive hydrochloric acid
   c. Certain drugs such as aspirin, steroids, and indomethacin will decrease tissue resistance
   d. Smoking
3. Peptic ulcers may be present in the esophagus, stomach, or duodenum (the most common site)
4. Complications include pyloric or duodenal obstruction, hemorrhage, and perforation
B. Clinical findings
1. Subjective: gnawing or burning epigastric pain that occurs 1 to 2 hours after eating (gastric) or 2 to 4 hours after eating (duodenal); nausea; heartburn (pyrosis); relieved by food or antacids (duodenal)
2. Objective
   a. History of gastritis
   b. If bleeding occurs: signs of anemia; passage of tarry stools (melena); vomitus that is coffee ground to port-wine color
   c. Presence of *Helicobacter pylori* serum antibodies via urea breath test or via biopsy during esophagogastroduodenoscopy
C. Therapeutic interventions

1. Bland foods, and restriction of irritating substances such as nicotine, caffeine, alcohol, spices, and gas-producing foods
2. Antibiotic therapy if microorganism is identified; tetracycline, metronidazole, and bismuth
3. Histamine H_2 receptor antagonists or proton pump inhibitors to limit gastric acid secretion; antacids to reduce acidity
4. Sedatives, tranquilizers, anticholinergics, and analgesics for pain and restlessness
5. Antiemetics for nausea and vomiting
6. Type and cross-match so blood will be available if gastric hemorrhage occurs
7. A nasogastric tube for decompression, instillation of vasoconstrictors, and/or saline lavages when hemorrhage occurs
8. Surgical intervention
   a. Esophagogastroduodenoscopy to treat area with electrocoagulation or heater proble therapy
   b. Vagotomy: cutting the vagus nerve, which innervates the stomach, to decrease the secretion of hydrochloric acid
   c. Billroth I: removal of the lower portion of the stomach and attachment of the remaining portion to the duodenum
   d. Billroth II: removal of the antrum and distal portion of the stomach and subsequent anastomosis of remaining section to the jejunum
   e. Antrectomy: removal of the antral portion of the stomach
   f. Gastrectomy: removal of 60% to 80% of the stomach
   g. Common complications of partial or total gastric resection
      (1) Dumping syndrome: involves the rapid passage of food from the stomach to the jejunum; the food, being hypertonic (especially if high in carbohydrates), will draw fluid from the circulating blood into the jejunum causing diaphoresis, faintness, and palpitations
      (2) Hemorrhage
      (3) Pneumonia
      (4) Pernicious anemia

Nursing Care of Clients with Peptic Ulcer Disease

A. ASSESSMENT
1. Characteristics of pain and relationship to types of food ingested and time food is consumed
2. Abdomen for epigastric tenderness, guarding, and bowel sounds
3. History of dietary patterns, foods ingested, and alcohol consumption

B. ANALYSIS/NURSING DIAGNOSES
1. Pain related to gastric secretion
2. Deficient fluid volume related to hemorrhage or dumping syndrome

C. PLANNING/IMPLEMENTATION
1. Allow ample time for the client to express feelings and concerns
2. Administer and assess effects of sedatives, antacids, anticholinergics, H_2 receptor antagonists, antibiotics, and dietary modifications
3. Encourage hydration to reduce anticholinergic side effects and dilute the hydrochloric acid in the stomach
4. Instruct client to:
   a. Eat small to medium-sized meals because this helps prevent gastric distention; encourage between meal snacks to achieve adequate calories when necessary
   b. Avoid foods that increase gastric acid secretion or irritate gastric mucosa, such as alcohol, caffeine-containing foods and beverages, decaffeinated coffee, red or black pepper; replace with decaffeinated soft drinks and teas; use seasonings like thyme, basil, sage, etc. to replace pepper
   c. Avoid foods that cause distress; varies for individuals but common offenders are the gas producers (legumes, carbonated beverages, the cruciferous vegetables)
   d. Eat meals in pleasant, relaxing surroundings to reduce acid secretion
   e. Administer calcium and iron supplements as ordered if client's medication increases gastric pH
5. Refrain from administering drugs such as salicylates, NSAIDS, steroids, and ACTH
6. Observe for complications such as gastric hemorrhage, perforation, and drug toxicity
7. Provide postoperative care after gastric resection
   a. Monitor vital signs; assess the dressing for drainage
   b. Maintain a patent nasogastric tube to suction to prevent stress on the suture line
   c. Observe the color and amount of nasogastric drainage; excessive bleeding or the presence of bright red blood after 12 hours should be reported immediately
   d. Have the client cough, deep breathe, and change position frequently to prevent the occurrence of pulmonary complications
   e. Monitor intake and output
   f. Apply antiembolism stockings; have the client ambulate early to prevent vascular complications
   g. To prevent dumping syndrome, instruct the client to:

(1) Eat smaller meals at more frequent intervals
(2) Avoid high-carbohydrate intake and concentrated sweets
(3) Consume liquids only between meals
(4) Lie down or rest after eating

D. **EVALUATION/OUTCOMES**
1. States pain is reduced or relieved
2. Identifies signs of complications and the need for immediate medical care
3. Follows a nutritionally sound diet

▼ CANCER OF THE STOMACH

Data Base
A. Etiology and pathophysiology
1. Risk factors include *H. pylori* in the stomach; ingestion of smoked meats, salted fish, and nitrates
2. Often not diagnosed until metastasis occurs; the stomach is able to accommodate to the growth of a tumor, and pain occurs late in the disease
3. May metastasize by direct extension, lymphatics, or blood to the esophagus, spleen, pancreas, liver, or bone
4. Heredity apparently a factor in the development of carcinoma of the stomach, as is the presence of precursors such as ulcerative disease and pernicious anemia
5. Incidence higher in men more than 40 years of age; Japan has a 4 times greater rate of cancer of the stomach than does the United States

B. Clinical findings
1. Subjective: anorexia (lack of interest in food); nausea; belching (eructation); heartburn
2. Objective: weight loss; stools positive for occult blood; anemia; achlorhydria (absence of hydrochloric acid); pale skin and acanthosis nigricans (a hyperpigmented, velvety thickening of the skin in the neck, axilla, and groin)

C. Therapeutic interventions
1. Surgical resection
2. Radiation
3. Chemotherapy
4. Combination of radiation and chemotherapy after surgery

Nursing Care of Clients with Cancer of the Stomach

A. **ASSESSMENT**
1. History of causative factors, presence of pain, and weight loss
2. Axillary lymph nodes and left supraclavicular nodes for hardness indicative of metastasis
3. Skin for color and presence of lesions associated with cancer of the GI tract

B. **ANALYSIS/NURSING DIAGNOSES**
1. Pain related to pathologic processes
2. Imbalanced nutrition: less than body requirements related to anorexia, increased metabolic rate, and interruption in digestion
3. Hopelessness related to diagnosis of cancer

C. **PLANNING/IMPLEMENTATION**
1. Offer the client opportunity to verbalize fears (e.g., cancer, death, family problems, self-image)
2. Provide care after a gastric resection (see Peptic Ulcer for nursing care); in addition, if a total gastrectomy is performed, the chest cavity is usually entered, so the client will have chest tubes (see Chest Tube Procedure for nursing care)
3. Modify diet to include smaller, more frequent meals (see Peptic Ulcer for more dietary information)
4. If total gastrectomy has been performed, the client will have a vitamin B_{12} deficiency (see Pernicious Anemia)
5. Client may require gavage feedings (see procedure for gavage)

D. **EVALUATION/OUTCOMES**
1. States relief from discomfort and pain
2. Maintains adequate nutritional status
3. Verbalizes feelings

▼ CHOLELITHIASIS/CHOLECYSTITIS

Data Base
A. Etiology and pathophysiology
1. Inflammation of the gallbladder; usually caused by the presence of stones (cholelithiasis), which are composed of cholesterol, bile pigments, and calcium; may be related to hepatic helicobacter bacteria
2. Diseased gallbladder is unable to contract in response to fatty foods entering the duodenum because of obstruction by calculi or edema
3. When the common bile duct is completely obstructed, the bile is unable to pass into the duodenum and is absorbed into the blood
4. Incidence is highest in obese women in the fourth decade

B. Clinical findings
1. Subjective: indigestion after eating fatty or fried foods; pain, usually in the right upper quadrant of the abdomen, which may radiate to the back; nausea

2. Objective
a. Vomiting; elevated temperature and WBC; jaundice may be present
b. Diagnostic tests
(1) Serum bilirubin and alkaline phosphatase are elevated
(2) Ultrasonography determines the presence of gallstones
(3) Endoscopic retrograde cholangiopancreatography (ERCP) reveals presence of gallstones

C. Therapeutic interventions
1. Medical management
a. Nasogastric suctioning to reduce nausea and eliminate vomiting
b. Narcotics to decrease pain
c. Antispasmodics and anticholinergics to reduce spasms and contractions of the gallbladder
d. Antibiotic therapy if infection is suspected
e. When clients are poor surgical risks or radiolucent cholesterol stones are small, oral chenodiol (Chenix) or ursodiol (Actigall) for 6 to 12 months to dissolve the stones
f. Dissolution of stones by infusing a solvent such as methyl tertiary turbutyl ether (MTBE) into the gallbladder through ERCP
g. Endoscopic papillotomy via ERCP to retrieve stones in the common bile duct
h. Lithotripsy: fragmentation of stones by ultrasonic soundwaves enable their passage without surgical intervention
i. Low-fat diet to avoid stimulating the gallbladder, which constricts to excrete bile with subsequent pain; calories principally from carbohydrate foods in acute phases; if weight loss is indicated, calories may be reduced to 1000 to 1200; postoperatively clients may take fat-restricted diets initially but progress to regular diets
2. Surgical intervention
a. Cholecystotomy: incision into the gallbladder for the purpose of drainage
b. Abdominal cholecystectomy: removal of the gallbladder through an abdominal incision
c. Laparoscopic cholecystectomy: removal of the gallbladder through an endoscope inserted through the abdominal wall; also called endoscopic laser cholecystectomy (not used if infection is present)
d. Choledochotomy: incision into the common bile duct for removal of stones

Nursing Care of Clients with Cholelithiasis/Cholecystitis

A. ASSESSMENT
1. Characteristics of pain

2. Presence of pain in relation to ingestion of foods high in fat
3. Abdomen for rebound tenderness that increases on inspiration (peritoneal inflammation)
4. Stools for color (clay colored) and fat (steatorrhea); urine for color (dark)

B. ANALYSIS/NURSING DIAGNOSES
1. Imbalanced nutrition: less than body requirements related to inability to digest or absorb fats
2. Pain related to spasms of the gallbladder or surgery

C. PLANNING/IMPLEMENTATION
1. Teach dietary modification to achieve a low-fat intake because reduced bile flow will reduce fat absorption; supplementation with water-miscible forms of vitamins A and E may be prescribed
2. Relieve pain both preoperatively and postoperatively
3. Observe for signs of bleeding (vitamin K is fat soluble and is not absorbed in the absence of bile); administer vitamin K preparations as ordered
4. Provide care following a cholecystectomy
a. Monitor nasogastric tube attached to suction to prevent distention
(1) Maintain patency of the tube
(2) Assess and measure drainage
b. Provide fluids and electrolytes via intravenous route
(1) Monitor intake and output
(2) Check IV site for redness, swelling, heat, or pain
c. Keep the client in a low-Fowler's position
d. Have the client cough and deep breathe; splint the incision (incision is high and midline, making coughing extremely uncomfortable)
e. Provide care for the client with a T-tube (if the common bile duct has been explored, a T-tube is inserted to maintain patency)
(1) Secure the drainage bag; avoid kinking of the tube
(2) Measure drainage at least every shift; drainage during the first day may reach 500 to 1000 ml and then gradually decline
(3) Apply ordered protective ointments around tube to prevent excoriation
(4) When the tube is removed, usually in 7 days, observe stool for normal brown color, which indicates bile is again entering the duodenum

D. EVALUATION/OUTCOMES
1. Verbalizes a decrease in pain
2. Maintains nutritional status

▼ ACUTE PANCREATITIS

Data Base

A. Etiology and pathophysiology
1. Inflammation of pancreas caused by autodigestion by pancreatic enzymes, primarily trypsin
2. May result from gallstones, alcoholism, carcinoma, acute trauma to the pancreas or abdomen, or hyperlipidemia
3. Inflammation with or without edema of pancreatic tissues, suppuration, abscess formation, hemorrhage, necrosis, or duct obstruction

B. Clinical findings
1. Subjective
   a. Abrupt onset of aching, burning, stabbing, or pressing central epigastric pain that may radiate to shoulder, chest, and back
   b. Abdominal tenderness
   c. Nausea
   d. Pruritus associated with jaundice
2. Objective
   a. Elevated temperature
   b. Shallow respirations
   c. Vomiting, weight loss
   d. Change in character of stools
   e. Shock, tachycardia, hypotension
   f. Jaundice
   g. Grossly elevated serum amylase and lipase
   h. Decreased serum calcium
   i. Boardlike abdomen with peritonitis
   j. Abnormal pancreatic findings on CT scan
3. Severity of symptoms depends on the cause of the problem, the amount of fibrous replacement of normal duct tissue, the degree of autodigestion of the organ, the type of associated biliary disease if present, and the amount of interference in blood supply to the pancreas
4. Symptoms may be exaggerated by the development of complications such as pseudocysts, abscesses, and pancreatic fistulas

C. Therapeutic interventions
1. Neutralize gastric secretions
2. Narcotics to control pain; morphine is contraindicated because it causes spasms of the sphincter of Oddi; although this thinking is under investigation
3. Bed rest to decrease metabolic demands and promote healing
4. Nothing by mouth and nasogastric decompression to control nausea, reduce stimulation of the pancreas to secrete enzymes, and remove gastric hydrochloric acid
5. Anticholinergics to suppress vagal stimulation and decrease gastric motility and duodenal spasm
6. Antibiotics to prevent secondary infections and abscess formation
7. Diet regulated according to the client's condition: nothing by mouth; parenteral administration of fluids and electrolytes, total or peripheral parenteral nutrition; diet low in fats and proteins, with restriction of stimulants such as caffeine and alcohol; pancreatic rest until largely free of pain and bowel sounds return
8. Pancreatic enzymes and bile salts if necessary
9. Surgical intervention if the client fails to respond to medical management, exhibits persistent jaundice, develops a pseudocyst or bleeds; type of surgery is determined by the cause (e.g., biliary tract surgery, removal of gallstones, drainage of cysts, temporary stent placement

Nursing Care of Clients with Acute Pancreatitis

A. **ASSESSMENT**
1. History of causative factors, pain, and recent weight loss
2. Presence of jaundice
3. Abdomen for rigidity and guarding

B. **ANALYSIS/NURSING DIAGNOSES**
1. Pain related to inflammation of the pancreas
2. Ineffective breathing pattern related to pain and pulmonary infiltrates
3. Imbalanced nutrition: less than body requirements related to lack of pancreatic enzymes to digest food
4. Deficient fluid volume related to fluid shift into the peritoneal cavity

C. **PLANNING/IMPLEMENTATION**
1. Provide care for a client with a nasogastric tube
   a. Observe for electrolyte imbalances (manifested by symptoms such as tetany, irritability, jerking, muscular twitching, mental changes, and psychotic behavior)
   b. Observe for signs of adynamic ileus (e.g., nausea and vomiting, abdominal distention)
2. Be alert for hyperglycemic states
3. Monitor vital signs
4. Administer prescribed analgesics
5. Maintain NPO during the acute stage of illness; monitor intake and output
6. Use the semi-Fowler's position and encourage deep breathing and coughing to promote deeper respiration and prevent respiratory problems
7. Closely monitor parenteral therapy until oral feedings can be tolerated
8. Teach dietary modifications as required by the client's condition, usually starting with small feedings of low-fat, non–gas-producing liquids and progressing to a more liberalized diet that is low in fat but high in protein and carbohydrates; if fat malabsorption is severe, vitamins A and E may be necessary; daily supplements of calcium and zinc may also be needed; if

insulin secretion is impaired, an American Diabetes Association (ADA) diet is indicated
9. Teach the client and family the importance of dietary discretion, especially the avoidance of alcohol, coffee, spicy foods, and heavy meals
10. Teach importance of taking medication containing pancreatic enzymes (amylase, lipase, trypsin, etc.) with each meal to improve digestion of food if the disease becomes chronic

D. EVALUATION/OUTCOMES
1. Reports decrease in pain
2. Maintains nutritional status
3. Demonstrates adequate depth of respirations
4. Maintains fluid and electrolyte balance

▼ CANCER OF THE PANCREAS

Data Base

A. Etiology and pathophysiology
1. Malignant growth from the epithelium of the ductal system, producing cells that block the ducts of the pancreas
2. Fibrosis, pancreatitis, and obstruction of the pancreas
3. Lesion tends to metastasize by direct extension to the duodenal wall, splenic flexure of the colon, posterior stomach wall, and common bile duct
4. Heredity, environmental toxins, alcohol, a high-fat diet, and smoking are associated with increased incidence
5. History of chronic pancreatitis, diabetes mellitus, and alcoholism is common
6. More common in middle-aged men than women

B. Clinical findings
1. Subjective: anxiety; depression; anorexia; nausea; dull, achy pain progressing to severe pain; pruritus associated with jaundice
2. Objective
   a. Jaundice; weight loss; diarrhea and steatorrhea; clay-colored stools; dark urine; ascites
   b. Decreased serum amylase and lipase levels because of decreased secretion of enzymes
   c. Increased serum bilirubin and alkaline phosphatase levels when biliary ducts are obstructed

C. Therapeutic interventions
1. Preparation for surgical intervention: red blood cell and blood volume replacement; medications to correct coagulation problems and nutritional deficiencies
2. Chemotherapy with gemcitabine (Gemzar) is useful in inhibiting movement of cells from G_1 to S phase of cell cycle
3. Chemotherapy and radiation when surgery is not possible or desired to provide comfort, or in conjunction with surgery to limit metastasis
4. Medications to control diabetes if present
5. Drug therapy such as pancreatic enzymes, bile salts, and vitamin K to correct deficiencies
6. Analgesics and tranquilizers for pain
7. Surgery (the treatment of choice, although the postsurgical prognosis is grim): Whipple's procedure (removal of the head of the pancreas, the duodenum, a portion of the stomach, and the common bile duct) or a cholecystojejunostomy (creation of an opening between the gallbladder and jejunum)

Nursing Care of Clients with Cancer of the Pancreas

A. ASSESSMENT
1. Presence of jaundice
2. Stool for clay-color
3. Urine for dark-amber color and frothy appearance
4. Abdomen for enlargement of liver and gallbladder
5. Characteristics of pain
6. History of anorexia, nausea, and weight loss
7. Abdominal dullness on percussion indicating early ascites

B. ANALYSIS/NURSING DIAGNOSES
1. Imbalanced nutrition: less than body requirements related to increased metabolic rate, lack of pancreatic enzymes to digest food, and reduced food intake
2. Pain related to pathologic process
3. Deficient fluid volume related to fluid shifts into peritoneal cavity
4. Hopelessness related to diagnosis and prognosis

C. PLANNING/IMPLEMENTATION
1. Provide emotional support for the client and family, and set realistic goals when planning care
2. Administer analgesics as ordered and as soon as needed to promote rest and comfort
3. Use soapless bathing and antipruritic agents to relieve pruritus
4. Observe for complications such as peritonitis, gastrointestinal obstruction, jaundice, hyperglycemia, and hypotension
5. Observe the stools for undigested fat
6. Frequently monitor the vital signs, observing for wound hemorrhage caused by coagulation deficiency
7. Administer vitamin K parenterally as ordered
8. Monitor for respiratory tract infection caused by limited chest expansion because of pain and the site of the incision; encourage coughing, turning, and deep breathing

9. Monitor intake and output; measure abdominal girth
10. Observe for chemotherapeutic and radiation side effects (e.g., skin irritation, anorexia, nausea, vomiting)
11. Maintain skin markings for radiation therapy
12. Support natural defense mechanisms of the client by encouraging frequent and supplemental feedings of high nutrient density foods as tolerated; stress the immune-stimulating nutrients, especially vitamins A, C, and E, and the mineral selenium
13. Control nausea and vomiting before feedings, if possible
14. Administer vitamin supplements, bile salts, and pancreatic enzymes, as ordered
15. Provide oral hygiene and maintain a pleasant environment, especially at mealtime

D. EVALUATION/OUTCOMES
1. States that pain is controlled
2. Maintains nutritional status
3. Maintains fluid and electrolyte balance
4. Discusses feelings and concerns

▼ HEPATITIS

Data Base

A. Etiology and pathology
1. Hepatitis is an acute or chronic inflammation of the liver caused by bacterial or viral infection, parasitic infestation (usually by contaminated water or food), or chemical agents
2. Hepatic involvement may impair clotting mechanisms
3. Hepatitis A (formerly known as infectious hepatitis)
   a. Caused by hepatitis A virus (HAV)
   b. Transmitted via fecal-oral route, contamination associated with flood waters or contaminated food (e.g., shellfish)
   c. Excreted in large quantities in feces 2 weeks before and 1 week after the onset of symptoms
   d. Incubation period is 15 to 50 days
   e. Confers immunity on individual
   f. Carrier state is possible
   g. Serum studies
      (1) Anti-HAV: antibody usually apparent once symptoms appear and lasts up to 12 months
      (2) IgM anti-HAV: antibody indicates recent infection
4. Hepatitis B (formerly known as serum hepatitis)
   a. Caused by hepatitis B virus (HBV)
   b. Transmitted by:

(1) Contaminated blood products or articles (e.g., toothbrush, razor, needle)
(2) Other body secretions (e.g., saliva, semen, urine)
(3) Introduction of infectious material into eye, oral cavity, lacerations, or vagina
(4) Shared contaminated needles
   c. Incubation period is 28 to 160 days
   d. Serum studies
      (1) HBsAg—hepatitis B surface antigen: indicates infectious state
      (2) Anti-HBs: antibody to surface antigen indicates immune response
      (3) HBeAg—hepatitis B e antigen: indicates highly infectious state and possible progression to chronic hepatitis
      (4) Anti-HBe
      (5) HBcAg: coreantigen of hepatitis B; found in liver cells
      (6) Anti HBc: antibody most sensitive indicator of prior HBV infection
5. Hepatitis C
   a. Caused by hepatitis C virus (HCV)
   b. Transmitted through blood and blood products
   c. Incubation period is 15 to 160 days following exposure (average 50)
   d. Serum studies
      (1) Hepatitis C virus antibodies
      (2) Hepatitis C virus RNA
   e. Chronic carrier state possible; associated with hepatic cancer
6. Hepatitis D
   a. Caused by hepatitis D virus (HDV)
   b. Transmitted through blood and blood products and close personal contact
   c. Incubation period is unknown
   d. Chronic carrier state possible
   e. Serum studies
      (1) HDAg—hepatitis D antigen: can be detected early
      (2) Anti-HDV antibody: indicates past or present infection
7. Hepatitis E
   a. Caused by hepatitis E virus (HEV)
   b. Transmitted through fecal-oral route
   c. Incubation period is 15 to 65 days
   d. Onset of symptoms is similar to other types of hepatitis; symptoms are severe in pregnant women
8. Hepatitis G
   a. Caused by hepatitis G virus (HGV)
   b. Transmitted percutaneously through blood, needles, body fluids
   c. Incubation period unknown
   d. It is a blood-borne RNA virus frequently found in clients with HIV

9. Nonviral, toxic, or drug-induced hepatitis: may be caused by drug therapy or other chemicals (e.g., carbon tetrachloride, chloroform, gold compounds, INH, halothene, acetaminophen)
10. Phases of disease: prodromal (preicteric), icteric, and recovery
11. Progression to cirrhosis, hepatic coma, and death may occur

B. Clinical findings
   1. Prodromal (preicteric) phase: malaise, anorexia, nausea, vomiting, and weight loss; symptoms of upper respiratory tract infection; intolerance for cigarette smoke
   2. Icteric phase: jaundice, bile-colored urine that foams when shaken; acholic (clay-colored) stools
   3. Recovery phase: easy fatigability

C. Therapeutic interventions
   1. Rest
   2. Diet therapy
      a. High protein to heal liver tissue; total should approximate 75 to 100 g daily alcohol should be avoided
      b. High carbohydrate to meet energy needs and restore glycogen reserves; total should be 300 to 400 g
      c. Low fat
      d. High calorie to meet increased energy needs for disease process, tissue regeneration, and to spare protein for healing; total should be 2500 to 3000 calories daily
      e. Vitamins A and E when steatorrhea is present; mineral supplements of calcium and zinc
   3. Bile and sequestrants such as cholestryamine (Questran) to reduce pruritus
   4. Avoidance of hepatotoxic drugs such as acetaminophen, aspirin, chlorpromazine, and sedatives
   5. Antiviral agents such as interferon

Nursing Care of Clients with Hepatitis

A. ASSESSMENT
   1. History of exposure to virus
   2. History of exposure to environmental factors over previous 6 months
   3. Right upper quadrant for liver tenderness, firmness
   4. Presence of jaundice in skin, sclera, and mucous membranes
   5. Temperature to determine presence of fever (associated with type A) or low-grade fever (associated with types B and C); fatigue
   6. Presence of bleeding tendencies

B. ANALYSIS/NURSING DIAGNOSES
   1. Imbalanced nutrition: less than body requirements related to anorexia

2. Risk for injury related to altered clotting mechanisms
3. Fatigue related to pathologic processes

C. PLANNING/IMPLEMENTATION
   1. Encourage rest and quiet activities; protect from injury to prevent bleeding
   2. Attempt to stimulate the appetite
      a. Provide oral hygiene
      b. Select foods based on the client's preferences
      c. Provide a pleasant, unhurried atmosphere
      d. Provide small, frequent feedings that are usually tolerated better than large meals
   3. Use standard precautions to prevent the spread to others; for hepatitis A or E, use contact precautions when exposed to client's feces
   4. Teach prevention
      a. Thorough hand washing
      b. Contact precautions when exposure to feces, blood, or body secretions
      c. Careful handling of needles (dispose of needles without recapping to prevent self-injury and contamination, dispose of needles in hard-sided container)
      d. Administration of immune serum globulin (ISG) after exposure to HAV and hepatitis B immune serum globulin after exposure to HBV to provide passive immunity
      e. Vaccinations against HAV (Havrix, Vaqta) and against HBV (Recumbivax HB)
      f. When client has hepatitis that can be transmitted sexually, encourage the use of condoms

D. EVALUATION/OUTCOMES
   1. States a decrease in fatigue
   2. Adheres to prescribed diet
   3. Remains free from injury
   4. Follows appropriate precautions to prevent transmission

▼ HEPATIC CIRRHOSIS

Data Base

A. Etiology and pathophysiology
   1. Irreversible fibrosis and degeneration of the liver
   2. Types of cirrhosis
      a. Alcoholic (Laënnec's) cirrhosis: related to alcohol abuse
      b. Postnecrotic or macronodular: most common form worldwide; related to viral hepatitis B and C and industrial chemical exposure
      c. Biliary: related to biliary stasis in hepatic ducts; may be an autoimmune response
      d. Cardiac: results from long-term right-sided heart failure; least common form

3. Pressure rises in the portal system (which drains blood from the digestive organs), causing stasis and backup in digestive organs and lower extremities (portal hypertension)
4. There is a buildup of protein metabolic wastes and increased ammonia levels
5. As liver failure progresses, there is increased secretion of aldosterone, decreased absorption and utilization of the fat-soluble vitamins (A, D, E, K), and ineffective detoxification of protein wastes
6. Gastrointestinal bleeding results from esophageal varices
7. Hepatic coma (hepatic encephalopathy) may result from high blood ammonia levels when the liver is unable to convert the ammonia to urea

B. Clinical findings
   1. Subjective: anorexia; nausea; weakness; fatigue; abdominal discomfort; pruritus
   2. Objective
      a. Weight loss; ascites; esophageal varices resulting from portal hypertension; hemorrhoids; edema of extremities; hematemesis; hemorrhage resulting from decreased formation of prothrombin; jaundice; delirium caused by rising blood ammonia levels
      b. Elevated liver enzymes (aspartate aminotransferase [AST], alanine aminotransferase [ALT], alkaline phosphatase [ALP], gamma-glutamyl transferase [GGT])
      c. Decreased serum albumin; elevated serum bilirubin; prolonged prothrombin time

C. Therapeutic interventions
   1. Rest
   2. Restriction of alcohol intake
   3. Vitamin therapy: especially the fat soluble vitamins A, D, E, and K and vitamin B (thiamine chloride and nicotinic acid); zinc and calcium supplements
   4. Diuretics to control ascites and edema
   5. Neomycin and lactulose may be prescribed for elevated blood ammonia levels
   6. Paracentesis if respiratory distress occurs as a result of ascites
   7. Surgical intervention to decrease portal hypertension: a portal caval shunt, in which the circulation from the portal vein bypasses the liver and enters the vena cava; a peritoneovenous shunt (LeVeen or Denver) to move fluid from abdominal cavity to superior vena cava
   8. Balloon tamponade with Blakemore-Sengstaken tube for bleeding esophageal varices to apply direct pressure to the varices; vasopressin may be administered IV to control GI bleeding; sclerotherapy to varices via endoscopy

9. Dietary modification
   a. Cirrhosis
      (1) Protein as tolerated (80 to 100 g); with increasing liver damage, protein metabolism is hindered
      (2) High carbohydrate, moderate fat; provides for energy; vitamin, mineral, and electrolyte supplements
      (3) Low sodium (500 to 1000 mg daily); helps control increasing ascites
      (4) Soft foods if esophageal varices are present; prevents danger of rupture and bleeding
      (5) Supplementation with B vitamins and fat-soluble vitamins A, D, E, and K
      (6) Alcohol contraindicated to avoid irritation and malnutrition
   b. Hepatic coma
      (1) Protein: is reduced to 15 to 30 g when blood ammonia level rises to above 200 µg/dl
      (2) High calorie (1500 to 2000 g) to prevent catabolism and liberation of nitrogen
      (3) Fluid carefully controlled according to output and presence of ascites and edema

Nursing Care of Clients with Hepatic Cirrhosis

A. ASSESSMENT
   1. History of anorexia, dyspepsia, and weight loss
   2. Abdomen for pain and liver tenderness; dullness when percussing enlarged liver
   3. Abdominal girth measurements for baseline data relative to ascites
   4. Skin for presence of jaundice, dryness, petechiae, ecchymoses, spider angiomas, and palmar erythema
   5. Signs of hepatic coma such as confusion, flapping of extremities

B. ANALYSIS/NURSING DIAGNOSES
   1. Excess fluid volume related to edema and fluid shifts
   2. Disturbed thought processes related to elevated ammonia level
   3. Imbalanced nutrition: less than body requirements related to pathologic processes
   4. Risk for injury related to altered coagulation and altered sensorium

C. PLANNING/IMPLEMENTATION
   1. Observe for bleeding
   2. Provide special skin care and keep nails trimmed because pruritus is associated with jaundice
   3. Maintain the client in a semi-Fowler's position to prevent ascites from causing dyspnea
   4. Monitor intake and output, abdominal girth, and daily weight to assess fluid balance
   5. Assist with paracentesis

a. Have client void before procedure
b. Assist to a sitting or high-Fowler's position
c. Observe for shock
d. Maintain pressure to dressing over needle insertion site
6. Provide care when a Blakemore-Sengstaken tube is in place
  a. Maintain traction once the tube is passed and the gastric balloon is inflated to ensure proper placement
  b. Maintain the esophageal balloon at inflated level (30 to 35 mm Hg)
  c. Deflate the balloon for a few minutes at specific intervals if ordered to prevent necrosis
  d. Irrigate with saline if ordered
  e. Maintain a patent airway; orally as necessary because the client is unable to swallow saliva
7. Repeat instructions; ability of client to understand and remember is often impaired because of hepatic encephalopathy; include family in instructions
8. Monitor for signs of impending hepatic coma

D. EVALUATION/OUTCOMES
1. Complies with dietary regimen
2. Maintains fluid balance
3. Remains free from injury

▼ CANCER OF THE LIVER

Data Base
A. Etiology and pathophysiology
1. May be primary or metastatic carcinoma; primary carcinoma of the liver is rare
2. Contributing factors include hepatitis B and C, cirrhosis, and anabolic steroid use
3. Poor prognosis
B. Clinical findings
1. Subjective: anorexia; ache in epigastric area
2. Objective: weight loss; bleeding; anemia; jaundice; ascites; increased serum bilirubin; increased alkaline phosphatase
C. Therapeutic interventions
1. Generally palliative
2. Hepatic lobectomy if the tumor is confined
3. Percutaneous infusions with cytotoxic agents
4. External radiation therapy

Nursing Care of Clients with Cancer of the Liver
A. ASSESSMENT
1. Weight
2. Skin for jaundice, bleeding, and pallor
3. Presence of dullness when percussing over liver; ascites

4. Detailed history including exposure to any known causative agents
B. ANALYSIS/NURSING DIAGNOSES
1. Excess fluid volume related to edema and fluid shifts
2. Hopelessness related to prognosis
3. Risk for injury related to altered coagulation
C. PLANNING/IMPLEMENTATION
1. Provide for comfort
2. Be available to both the client and family members to discuss their feelings
3. Maintain fluid and electrolyte balance; monitor intake and output
4. Observe for signs of bleeding, hypoglycemia, and other metabolic dysfunctions resulting from impaired liver function
5. Have client cough, deep breathe, and change position frequently to prevent pulmonary and circulatory complications
6. Because the thoracic cavity may be entered during hepatic surgery, be aware of the care of a client with chest tubes
D. EVALUATION/OUTCOMES
1. Verbalizes feelings about diagnosis and prognosis
2. Maintains fluid balance
3. States relief from discomfort

▼ APPENDICITIS

Data Base
A. Etiology and pathophysiology
1. Compromised circulation and inflammation of the vermiform appendix; inflammation may be followed by edema, necrosis, and rupture
2. Causes include obstruction by a fecalith, foreign body, or kinking
B. Clinical findings
1. Subjective: anorexia; nausea; right lower quadrant pain (McBurney's point); rebound tenderness
2. Objective: vomiting; fever; leukocytosis; abdominal distention and paralytic ileus if appendix has ruptured
C. Therapeutic interventions
1. Surgical removal of the appendix without delay to decrease the chance of rupture and the risk of peritonitis
2. Prophylactic use of antibiotics
3. Fluid and electrolyte maintenance
4. Analgesics for pain

Nursing Care of Clients with Appendicitis
A. ASSESSMENT
1. History of characteristics of pain and presence of nausea and vomiting

2. Presence of anorexia or the urge to pass flatus
3. Presence of rebound tenderness when palpating abdomen
4. Presence of tenderness/rigidity when palpating McBurney's point
5. Temperature for baseline data
6. Presence and extent of bowel sounds

B. ANALYSIS/NURSING DIAGNOSES
1. Pain related to inflammatory process
2. Risk for infection related to rupture of appendix

C. PLANNING/IMPLEMENTATION
1. Provide emotional support because this condition is unanticipated and the individual needs to ventilate any fear of surgery
2. Monitor fluid and electrolyte balance
3. Assess the client for signs of infection; maintain a semi-Fowler's position to help localize infection if the appendix ruptures
4. Assess the client's return of bowel function (bowel sounds, flatus, bowel movement); encourage ambulation

D. EVALUATION/OUTCOMES
1. States pain is alleviated
2. Remains free from infection

▼ INFLAMMATORY BOWEL DISEASE REGIONAL ENTERITIS (CROHN'S DISEASE)

Data Base
A. Etiology and pathophysiology
1. There are various theories involving genetic predisposition, autoimmune reaction, or environmental causes
2. Cobblestone ulcerations along the mucosal wall of the terminal ileum, cecum, and ascending colon form scar tissue that inhibits food and water absorption
3. Ulceration of the intestinal submucosa accompanied by congestion, thickening of the small bowel, and fissure formations; fistulas and abcesses may form
4. Enlargement of regional lymph nodes
B. Clinical findings
1. Subjective: nausea; severe abdominal pain, cramping, and spasms; exacerbations related to emotional upsets or dietary indiscretions with milk, milk products, and fried foods
2. Objective
   a. Weight loss; fever; elevated WBC; diarrhea with mucus, electrolyte disturbances; presence of blood and fat in feces
   b. Fecal fat test determines fat content, an abnormal amount of which is significant in malabsorptive disorders or hypermotility

c. Erythema nodosum, conjunctivitis, and arthritis
d. D-xylose tolerance test determines absorptive ability of upper intestinal tract
e. CT scan shows bowel wall thickening and fistulas
C. Therapeutic interventions
1. Nothing by mouth and TPN when inflammatory episodes are severe
2. Clear fluid diet progressing to bland, low-residue, low-fat, but increased calories, carbohydrates, proteins, and vitamins, especially K and B_{12} (when a large portion of the ileum is involved)
3. Pharmacologic management: antidiarrheals such as loperamide (Imodium, Kaopectate II, Pepto-Bismol); antispasmotics such as propantheline bromide (Pro-Banthine); immunosuppressives such as infliximab (Remicade); anticholinergics; antiinfectives such as metronidazole (Flagyl) and ciprofloxacin (Cipro); and antiinflammatory therapy with steroids
4. Surgery when complications such as fistulas or intestinal obstruction occurs; anastomosis or temporary or permanent ostomy

Nursing Care of Clients with Crohn's Disease
A. ASSESSMENT
1. Weight, temperature, and intake and output
2. Feces for color, consistency, and steatorrhea
3. Tenderness and guarding of abdomen, especially right lower quadrant
4. Presence and extent of bowel sounds

B. ANALYSIS/NURSING DIAGNOSES
1. Imbalanced nutrition: less than body requirements related to hypermotility and malabsorption
2. Pain related to abdominal cramping
3. Diarrhea related to hypermotility
4. Deficient fluid volume related to diarrhea

C. PLANNING/IMPLEMENTATION
1. Encourage verbalization of feelings; encourage client and family to participate in the Crohn's and Colitis Foundation of America
2. Instruct client regarding dietary restrictions and modifications (see Ulcerative Colitis)
3. Observe for signs of fluid and electrolyte imbalances; monitor intake and output
4. Observe for signs of complications such as elevated temperature, increasing nausea and vomiting, abdominal rigidity
5. Assist with total parenteral nutrition (TPN) if ordered (see procedure)
6. Teach the client:
   a. To avoid taking laxatives and salicylates that irritate the intestinal mucosa
   b. How to take antidiarrheals and mucilloid drugs effectively

c. Skin care if the perineal area is irritated

d. The importance of seeking help early when exacerbations occur

D. EVALUATION/OUTCOMES

1. Reports a reduction in pain
2. Has a decrease in the number of bowel movements
3. Maintains nutritional status
4. Maintains fluid and electrolyte balance

▼ INFLAMMATORY BOWEL DISEASE ULCERATIVE COLITIS

Data Base

A. Etiology and pathophysiology

1. May be caused by emotional stress, an autoimmune response, or a genetic predisposition, or bacterial infection before onset
2. Edema of mucous membrane of colon leads to bleeding and shallow ulcerations
3. Abscess formation occurs, the bowel wall shortens, and becomes thin and fragile
4. Associated with increased risk of colon cancer

B. Clinical findings

1. Subjective: weakness; debilitation; anorexia; nausea
2. Objective: dehydration with tenting of skin; passage of bloody, purulent, mucoid, watery stools; anemia; hypocalcemia; low-grade fever

C. Therapeutic interventions

1. Dietary management
   a. During acute episode, low-residue diet progressing to a regular diet; raw bran may be effective in controlling bouts of diarrhea and constipation
   b. Unrestricted fluid intake if tolerated; high-protein, high-calorie diet; avoidance of food allergens, especially milk
2. Pharmacologic management: antiemetics, anticholinergics, corticosteroids, antibiotics, sedatives, analgesics, tranquilizers, and antidiarrheals
3. Replacement of fluids and electrolytes that are lost because of diarrhea; TPN may be instituted
4. Surgical intervention: indicated when medical management is unsuccessful
   a. Segmental or partial colectomy with anastomosis
   b. Total colectomy with ileostomy
   c. Total colectomy with continent ileostomy (Kock's pouch)
   d. Total colectomy with ileoanal anastomosis (creation of an ileal pouch that maintains anal sphincter function)

Nursing Care of Clients with Ulcerative Colitis

A. ASSESSMENT

1. Localized areas of tenderness found over diseased bowel on palpation
2. History of patterns and characteristics of bowel elimination
3. Feces for color, consistency, and characteristics
4. Temperature and weight for baseline data
5. Presence and extent of bowel sounds

B. ANALYSIS/NURSING DIAGNOSES

1. Diarrhea related to hypermotility
2. Imbalanced nutrition: less than body requirements related to hypermotility and malabsorption
3. Deficient fluid volume related to diarrhea

C. PLANNING/IMPLEMENTATION

1. Instruct client to adhere to the following dietary program
   a. Eat small, frequent feedings of high-protein, high-calorie foods; low fat helps decrease steatorrhea; if steatorrhea is present, vitamins A and E may be required as supplements
   b. Avoid irritating foods and spices
   c. Replace iron, calcium, and zinc losses with supplements; if there is ileal involvement, intramuscular injections of vitamin B_{12} may be prescribed monthly to reduce anemia
   d. Avoid all food allergens, especially milk; milk may be reintroduced when client is relatively asymptomatic; however, lactose intolerance is common and dairy restrictions may be permanent; lactase enzymes are available that can be added to milk products to hydrolyze lactose
2. Involve client in dietary selection; recognize preferences as much as possible
3. Initiate administration and recording of fluid, electrolyte, or blood replacements
4. Provide gentle, thorough perineal care as required
5. Observe for complications such as rectal hemorrhage, fever, dehydration
6. Allow the client and family time to verbalize feelings and participate in care; encourage participation in the Crohn's and Colitis Foundation of America
7. Postoperative care
   a. Maintain nasogastric suction during the immediate postoperative period
   b. Monitor fecal drainage and fluid balance
   c. Assess for signs of peritonitis
   d. Teach client ileostomy care
      (1) Ileostomy: skin care, continuous use of appliance because the stoma drains continuously
      (2) Continent ileostomy (Kock's pouch): pouch will stretch over time to hold over 500 ml; must be catheterized to

drain effluent every 4 to 6 hours; external appliance unnecessary; a small dressing covers the stoma
- e. Teach dietary guidelines
  - (1) Initial low-residue diet to promote healing
  - (2) Avoidance of kernels or seeds that can cause obstruction
  - (3) Increased fluid intake to compensate for losses
- f. Provide emotional support; involve enterostomal therapy nurse and local ostomy organizations
8. Anticipate that stress can precipitate peristalsis

D. EVALUATION/OUTCOMES
1. Maintains or regains weight
2. Adheres to dietary regimen
3. Establishes an acceptable pattern of soft, formed bowel movements
4. Client or family member demonstrates ability to perform ostomy care

▼ INTESTINAL OBSTRUCTION

Data Base
A. Etiology and pathophysiology
1. Interference with normal peristaltic movement of intestinal contents because of neurologic or mechanical impairments
2. Causes
   a. Carcinoma of the bowel
   b. Hernias
   c. Fecal impaction
   d. Adhesions (scar tissue that forms abnormal connections after surgery or inflammation)
   e. Intussusception (telescoping of the bowel on itself)
   f. Volvulus (twisting of the intestines)
   g. Paralytic ileus (interference with neural innervation of the intestines resulting in a decrease in or absence of peristalsis; may be caused by surgical manipulation, electrolyte imbalance, or infection)
   h. Mesenteric infarction (occlusion of arterial blood supply to bowel, which stops bowel function)
B. Clinical findings
1. Subjective: colicky abdominal pain; constipation that may be accompanied by urge to defecate without results and seepage of fecal liquid
2. Objective: abdominal distention; vomiting that may contain fecal matter; decreased or absent bowel sounds; signs of dehydration and electrolyte imbalance; obstipation; flat plate of the abdomen shows the bowel distended with air

C. Therapeutic interventions
1. Restriction of oral intake; administration of parenteral fluid and electrolytes
2. Surgical intervention: correction of cause (e.g., hernias, adhesions); colostomy, cecostomy, or ileostomy
3. Decompression of GI tract by means of a nasogastric or intestinal tube

Nursing Care of Clients with Intestinal Obstruction
A. ASSESSMENT
1. Detailed history to determine risk and causative factors
2. Abdomen for peristaltic waves, distention
3. Presence and characteristics of bowel sounds
4. Patterns and characteristics of bowel elimination

B. ANALYSIS/NURSING DIAGNOSES
1. Constipation related to mechanical or functional obstruction
2. Deficient fluid volume related to fluid shift into intestinal lumen and GI decompression

C. PLANNING/IMPLEMENTATION
1. Assess for dehydration and electrolyte imbalance; monitor intake and output
2. Auscultate for bowel sounds; note the passage of flatus
3. Administer oral hygiene frequently
4. Provide special care for the client with an intestinal tube
   a. Once the tube reaches the stomach, position the client on the right side to facilitate passage of tube through the pylorus; then in a semi-Fowler's position to continue the gradual advance into the intestines
   b. Coil and loosely attach extra tubing to the client's gown to avoid tension against peristaltic action
   c. Instill or irrigate as ordered to maintain patency
   d. Assess placement of the tube; record the level of advancement; advance as ordered
   e. When the tube is discontinued, remove gradually because it is being pulled against peristalsis

D. EVALUATION/OUTCOMES
1. Establishes a regular pattern of bowel elimination
2. Maintains fluid and electrolyte balance

▼ DIVERTICULAR DISEASE

Data Base
A. Etiology and pathophysiology

1. Diverticulosis: multiple pouchlike herniations of intestinal mucosa, as a result of weakness and increased intraabdominal pressure; may be asymptomatic
2. Diverticulitis: inflammation caused by food or feces trapped in a diverticulum; may lead to bleeding, perforation, peritonitis, and bowel obstruction
3. Most commonly occurs in the sigmoid colon, but could occur anywhere along the GI tract
4. Incidence increases with age; inadequate dietary fiber, history of constipation with straining at stool, and genetic predisposition are risk factors
B. Clinical findings
   1. Subjective: cramping, colicky pain in left lower quadrant; nausea; malaise
   2. Objective
      a. Altered bowel elimination: diarrhea or constipation; frank blood in stool; abdominal distention; fever; leukocytosis
      b. Diagnostic tests: CT scan, abdominal x-ray, and colonoscopy provide direct evidence of the disease
C. Therapeutic interventions
   1. Prevention through high-fiber diet
   2. Nothing by mouth or clear liquids during acute diverticulitis
   3. Pharmacologic management: analgesics (morphine sulfate is avoided because it can increase intracolonic pressure), antibiotics, antispasmodics, and bulk-forming laxatives and stool softeners
   4. Fluid and electrolyte replacement
   5. Surgery: hemicolectomy, temporary loop colostomy, and removal of involved bowel

Nursing Care of Clients with Diverticular Disease

A. ASSESSMENT
1. History of constipation and/or diarrhea with progression of symptoms
2. Stool for consistency and presence of blood
3. Abdomen for distention
4. Presence and extent of bowel sounds

B. ANALYSIS/NURSING DIAGNOSES
1. Constipation related to narrowed, inflamed intestine
2. Pain related to inflammation
3. Risk for deficient fluid volume related to gastric decompression

C. PLANNING/IMPLEMENTATION
1. Teach importance of high-fiber and high-fluid intake to prevent diverticulitis
2. Prevention of constipation with dietary bran and bulk laxatives

3. Maintain NPO and gastric decompression if ordered during acute episode
4. Monitor for signs of peritonitis: pain, hypotension, abdominal rigidity, abdominal distention, and leukocytosis
5. Administer fluid and electrolyte replacement
6. Teach client the importance of completing antibiotic regimen
7. Provide care related to bowel surgery (see Nursing Care of Clients with Cancer of the Small Intestine, Colon, and Rectum)

D. EVALUATION/OUTCOMES
1. Exhibits normal pattern of soft, formed bowel movements
2. Increases intake of high-fiber foods
3. Reports relief from pain
4. Maintains fluid and electrolyte balance

▼ CANCER OF THE SMALL INTESTINE, COLON, OR RECTUM

Data Base
A. Etiology and pathophysiology
   1. Tumor causes narrowing of lumen of bowel, ulcerations, necrosis, or perforation
   2. Predisposing factors include familial polyps, chronic ulcerative colitis, and bowel stasis, ingestion of food additives, and a high-fat, low-fiber diet
   3. Cancer of the colon is more common in males, and incidence increases after 50 years of age
   4. Cancer of the small intestine is rare; adenocarcinoma of the large intestine is relatively common
B. Clinical findings
   1. Subjective: abdominal discomfort or pain; weakness and fatigue
   2. Objective
      a. Alterations in usual bowel function (constipation or diarrhea or alternating constipation and diarrhea); pencil- or ribbon-shaped stool
      b. Abdominal distention
      c. Weight loss
      d. Frank or occult blood in stool; secondary anemia
      e. Digital examination detects any palpable masses
      f. Proctosigmoidoscopy visualizes the bowel directly and determines the presence of abnormalities; permits biopsy
      g. Cytologic examination of tissue from GI tract detects malignant cells
      h. Elevated alkaline phosphatase and aspartate aminotransferase (AST) levels detect metastasis to the liver

i. Elevated serum carcinoembryonic antigen (CEA) may indicate carcinoma of the colon

C. Therapeutic interventions

1. Surgical intervention to remove the mass and restore bowel function (e.g., hemicolectomy, abdominal perineal resection)
2. Radiation in nonsurgical situations may be used to limit symptoms; may be used preoperatively to reduce size of tumor or postoperatively to limit metastases
3. Chemotherapy to reduce the lesion and limit metastases
4. Preparation for surgery
   a. Antibiotics (e.g., neomycin or sulfonamides) to reduce bacteria in the bowel
   b. Type and cross-match of blood for transfusions to correct anemia
   c. Vitamin supplements to improve the nutritional status
   d. Gastric or intestinal decompression
   e. Bowel preparation

Nursing Care of Clients with Cancer of Small Intestine, Colon, or Rectum

A. **ASSESSMENT**

1. Detailed history of symptoms and risk factors
2. Stool for frequency, color, consistency, and shape
3. Weight for baseline data
4. Areas of abdominal discomfort on palpation
5. Presence and extent of bowel sounds

B. **ANALYSIS/NURSING DIAGNOSES**

1. Pain related to trauma of surgery and pathologic processes
2. Anxiety related to treatments and prognosis
3. Disturbed body image related to alteration in GI structure and function
4. Deficient fluid volume related to losses through ostomy
5. Imbalanced nutrition: less than body requirements related to malabsorption
6. Risk for impaired skin integrity related to fecal irritation

C. **PLANNING/IMPLEMENTATION**

1. Observe vital signs, increasing abdominal pain, nausea, and vomiting to detect early signs of complications
2. Monitor patency of gastric or intestinal tube; instill or irrigate with normal saline as ordered; note the amount and character of drainage
3. Implement mechanical cleansing and intestinal antisepsis preoperatively
4. Administer chemotherapeutic drugs if ordered; observe for significant side effects such as stomatitis, dehydration, nausea and vomiting, diarrhea, leukopenia
5. Administer electrolyte and parenteral fluid replacement as ordered in situations of bleeding, vomiting, and/or obstruction
6. Administer progressive diet as ordered; assess tolerance; teach dietary modifications to client and family, including nongas-forming foods, avoidance of stimulants, adequate fluid intake; diet should be as close to the client's normal as possible
7. Teach the importance of diet in supporting the body's natural defenses; emphasize high nutrient density foods from the fruit, vegetable, cereal grain, and legume groups with some lean meat, fish, and poultry; encourage client to eat as great a variety of foods as can be tolerated; vitamin and mineral supplements can be encouraged, especially the immune-stimulating factors
8. Assess the client's reaction to the colostomy, recognizing that it will depend on how the client sees it affecting lifestyle, physical and emotional status, social and cultural background, and place and role in the family; client may demonstrate the stages of grieving
9. Provide colostomy care (see procedure); encourage involvement in colostomy care as soon as physical and emotional status permits
10. Recognize that the client with a cecostomy or colostomy is especially sensitive to gestures, odors, and facial expressions
11. Teach the client and family care of the colostomy, measures to facilitate acceptance and adjustment, resumption of activities including sexual, and the need for regular medical supervision
12. Teach the client that colostomy drainage begins in 3 to 4 days and can be controlled by following a regular irrigation schedule and dietary modifications; adequate uninterrupted time for procedure is necessary
13. Arrange for follow-up care with community agencies as required (e.g., public health, home care programs, Cancer Society, ostomy resource person)

D. **EVALUATION/OUTCOMES**

1. Maintains adequate fluid and electrolyte balance
2. Resumes a regular pattern of bowel elimination
3. Client or family member demonstrates ability to perform ostomy care
4. Discusses feelings concerning diagnosis, prognosis, and ostomy
5. Maintains nutritional status

▼ PERITONITIS

Data Base

A. Etiology and pathophysiology
   1. Inflammation of the peritoneum (most commonly caused by *E. coli*)
   2. Generally caused by infection from perforation of GI tract or chemical stress
B. Clinical findings
   1. Subjective: abdominal pain, rebound tenderness; malaise; nausea
   2. Objective: abdominal muscle rigidity; vomiting; elevated temperature, WBCs, and neutrophil count
C. Therapeutic interventions
   1. Bed rest in a semi-Fowler's position to localize drainage to the dependent portion of the abdominal cavity
   2. Nasogastric decompression until the client passes flatus
   3. Fluids and electrolytes replaced parenterally; TPN
   4. Antibiotic therapy
   5. Surgery to correct the cause of peritonitis (e.g., appendectomy, incision and drainage of abscesses, closure of a perforation)

Nursing Care of Clients with Peritonitis

A. **ASSESSMENT**
   1. Temperature for baseline data
   2. Guarded movements and/or self-splinting
   3. Reduction or absence of bowel sounds
   4. Presence and characteristics of abdominal pain
B. **ANALYSIS/NURSING DIAGNOSES**
   1. Pain related to inflamed peritoneal membrane
   2. Deficient fluid volume related to gastric decompression and fluid shifts
C. **PLANNING/IMPLEMENTATION**
   1. Maintain the semi-Fowler's position
   2. Assess pain and vital signs, especially temperature
   3. Monitor IV therapy and GI decompression, monitor intake and output
   4. Auscultate for bowel sounds; note the passage of flatus
   5. Administer IV antibiotics
D. **EVALUATION/OUTCOMES**
   1. Reports absence of pain
   2. Maintains fluid and electrolyte balance
   3. Reestablishes regular pattern of bowel elimination

▼ HEMORRHOIDS

Data Base

A. Etiology and pathophysiology
   1. Varicosities of the rectum that can be internal or external
   2. Precipitated by constipation, prolonged sitting or standing, straining at defecation, and pregnancy
B. Clinical findings
   1. Subjective: anal pain; pruritus
   2. Objective: protrusion of varicosities around the anus; rectal bleeding and mucus discharge
C. Therapeutic interventions
   1. High-fiber diet (especially pectin-containing fruits and vegetables) to prevent constipation
   2. Low-roughage diet (elimination of raw fruits and vegetables) during acute exacerbations
   3. Laxatives and stool softeners to regulate bowel
   4. Analgesic suppositories and ointments; sitz baths or ice compresses for discomfort
   5. Internal hemorrhoids ligated with rubber bands; as necrosis occurs, tissue sloughs off
   6. Surgical intervention: generally in an ambulatory setting
      a. Ligation
      b. Cryosurgery
      c. Laser
      d. Sclerotherapy
      e. Hemorrhoidectomy

Nursing Care of Clients with Hemorrhoids

A. **ASSESSMENT**
   1. History of causative factors
   2. Presence and characteristics of pain
   3. Presence of hemorrhoids in perianal area
B. **ANALYSIS/NURSING DIAGNOSES**
   1. Constipation related to fear of pain on defecation
   2. Pain related to inflammation
C. **PLANNING/IMPLEMENTATION**
   1. Help relieve pain by sitz baths, ice compresses, local analgesics
   2. Provide privacy and sufficient time for defecation, especially after meals
   3. Encourage generous daily intake of high-fiber foods; promote intake of at least 8 glasses of fluid per day
   4. Discourage routine use of laxatives, which results in dependency; bulking agents such as Metamucil may be prescribed
   5. Provide care for the client having a hemorrhoidectomy
      a. Administer cleansing enemas preoperatively
      b. Observe for rectal hemorrhage and urinary retention postoperatively; explain that some bleeding with a bowel movement is expected
      c. Administer a retention enema on the second or third postoperative day if ordered to stimulate defecation and soften the stool

D. EVALUATION/OUTCOMES
1. Reports increased comfort, particularly on defecation
2. Complies with treatment regimen
3. Establishes a pattern of regular bowel movements

▼ HERNIAS

Data Base
A. Etiology and pathophysiology
1. Protrusion of an organ or structure through a weakening in the abdominal wall; may result from a congenital or acquired defect
2. If the protruding structure can be manipulated back in place, the hernia is said to be reducible; if it cannot, it is considered incarcerated
3. Strangulation occurs when blood supply to the tissues within the hernia is disrupted; this is an emergency situation, since gangrene occurs
4. Hernias are named by location: incisional, umbilical, femoral, inguinal
B. Clinical findings
1. Subjective: history of appearance of swelling after lifting, coughing, or exercise; pain caused by irritation or strangulation; nausea can accompany strangulation
2. Objective: swelling (lump) in the groin or umbilicus, or near an old surgical incision that may subside when the client is in a recumbent position; vomiting and abdominal distention when strangulation occurs
C. Therapeutic interventions
1. Manual reduction by gently pushing the mass back into the abdominal cavity
2. When the client is a poor surgical risk, a truss (pad worn next to skin held in place under pressure by a belt) may be ordered
3. Herniorrhaphy: repair of the defect in the abdominal musculature or fascia
4. Hernioplasty: insertion of wire, mesh, or plastic to strengthen abdominal wall

Nursing Care of Clients with Hernias
A. ASSESSMENT
1. History of potential causative factors
2. Presence or absence of bowel sounds on auscultation
3. Abdomen with client in standing and lying positions to determine if hernia reduces with positional change
B. ANALYSIS/NURSING DIAGNOSES
1. Pain related to pathologic processes
2. Risk for injury related to strangulation

C. PLANNING/IMPLEMENTATION
1. Avoid abdominal palpation if hernia is strangulated
2. Provide care following surgery
a. Instruct client to avoid coughing if possible; use deep breathing and incentive spirometry to prevent respiratory complications; encourage self-splinting
b. Administer mild cathartics as ordered to prevent straining and increased intraabdominal pressure
c. Apply an ice bag and scrotal support if the scrotum is edematous postoperatively to reduce the edema and pain
d. Administer medication for pain as ordered
e. Instruct the client to avoid lifting or strenuous exercise on discharge until permitted by the surgeon
D. EVALUATION/OUTCOMES
1. Reports decreased pain
2. Restates discharge instructions

▼ EATING DISORDERS

For anorexia nervosa and bulimia nervosa see Eating Disorders in Psychiatric/Mental Health Nursing. Although obesity is usually not related to a severe emotional disturbance, see Fundamental Principles When Caring for Clients with Eating Disorders.

ENDOCRINE SYSTEM

REVIEW OF ANATOMY AND PHYSIOLOGY
Function of the Endocrine System
Endocrine glands continuously secrete products called hormones, which are chemical messengers that deliver stimulatory or inhibitory signals to target cells as a result of a feedback mechanism.

Structures of the Endocrine System
Thyroid gland
A. Overlies thyroid cartilage below the larynx
B. Thyroid hormones: accelerate cellular reactions in most body cells
1. Thyroxine: stimulates metabolic rate; essential for normal physical and mental development
2. Triiodothyronine: inhibits anterior pituitary secretion of thyroid stimulating hormone
3. Calcitonin (thyrocalcitonin): decreases loss of calcium from bone; promotes hypocalcemia; action opposite that of parathormone

Parathyroid glands

A. Small glands (2 to 12) embedded in the posterior part of the thyroid
B. Parathyroid hormone (parathormone)
  1. Increases blood calcium concentration
     a. Breakdown of bone with release of calcium into blood (requires the active form of vitamin D)
     b. Calcium absorption from intestine into blood
     c. Kidney tubule reabsorption of calcium
  2. Decreases blood phosphate concentration by slowing its reabsorption from the kidneys, thereby decreasing calcium loss in urine

Testes and ovaries

See Structures of the Male Reproductive System under Urinary/Reproductive Systems in this chapter and Structures of the Female Reproductive System under Women's Health in Childbearing and Women's Health Nursing

Adrenal glands

A. Two closely associated structures, adrenal medulla and adrenal cortex, positioned at each kidney's superior border
B. Adrenal hormones
  1. Adrenal medulla: produces two catecholamines, epinephrine and norepinephrine
     a. Stimulate liver and skeletal muscle to break down glycogen
     b. Increase oxygen use and carbon dioxide production
     c. Increase blood concentration of free fatty acids through stimulation of lipolysis in adipose tissue
     d. Cause constriction of nearly all blood vessels of body, thereby greatly increasing total peripheral resistance and arterial pressure
     e. Increase heart rate and force of contraction and thereby raise cardiac output
     f. Inhibit contractions of gastrointestinal and uterine smooth muscle
     g. Epinephrine significantly dilates bronchial smooth muscle
  2. Adrenal cortex: secretes the mineralocorticoid aldosterone and the glucocorticoids cortisol and corticosterone
     a. Aldosterone
        (1) Markedly accelerates sodium and water reabsorption by kidney tubules
        (2) Markedly accelerates potassium excretion by kidney tubules
        (3) Aldosterone secretion increases as sodium ions decrease or potassium ions increase
     b. Cortisol and corticosterone
        (1) Accelerate mobilization and catabolism of tissue protein and fats
        (2) Accelerate liver gluconeogenesis (formation of glucose from mobilized proteins, a hyperglycemic effect)
        (3) Decrease antibody formation (immunosuppressive, antiallergic effect)
        (4) Slow the proliferation of fibroblasts characteristic of inflammation (antiinflammatory effect)
        (5) Decrease ACTH secretion
        (6) Mildly accelerate sodium and water reabsorption and potassium excretion by kidney tubules

Pancreas

A. Retroperitoneal in abdominal cavity
B. Pancreatic hormones: regulate glucose homeostasis through the action of insulin and glucagon
  1. Insulin: secreted by beta cells of islets of Langerhans
     a. Promotes the cellular uptake of glucose
     b. Stimulates intracellualr macromolecular synthesis, such as glycogen synthesis (glyconeogenesis), fat synthesis (lipogenesis), and protein synthesis
     c. Stimulates cellular uptake of sodium and potassium (latter is significant in the treatment of diabetic coma with insulin)
  2. Glucagon: secreted by alpha cells of islets of Langerhans
     a. Induces liver glycogenolysis; antagonizes the glycogen synthesis stimulated by insulin
     b. Inhibits hepatic protein synthesis; this makes amino acids available for gluconeogenesis and also increases urea production
     c. Stimulates hepatic ketogenesis and release of glycerol and fatty acids from adipose tissue

Thymus gland

A. Located at root of neck and anterior thorax
B. Thymic hormone (thymosin)
  1. Regulates immunologic processes
  2. Just after birth produces T lymphocytes that migrate to the lymph nodes and spleen to provide cell-mediated immunity
  3. Synthesizes hormones that regulate the rate of development of lymphoid cells, particularly T cells

Pineal gland

A. Located in midbrain attached to third ventricle
B. Pineal hormone (melatonin)
  1. May regulate diurnal fluctuations of hypothalamic-hypophyseal hormones
  2. Inhibits numerous endocrine functions, particularly gonadotropic hormones

Pituitary gland

A. Located in cranial cavity in sella turcica of sphenoid bone; near optic chiasm

B. Composed of an anterior lobe (adenohypophysis) and a posterior lobe (neurohypophysis)

C. Pituitary hormones

  1. Hormones secreted by the anterior lobe

    a. Growth hormone (GH)

      (1) Promotes protein anabolism

      (2) Promotes fat mobilization and catabolism

      (3) Slows carbohydrate metabolism

    b. Thyroid-stimulating hormone (TSH): stimulates synthesis and secretion of thyroid hormones

    c. Adrenocorticotropic hormone (ACTH)

      (1) Stimulates growth of adrenal cortex

      (2) Stimulates the secretion of glucocorticoids; slightly stimulates mineralocorticoid secretion

    d. Follicle-stimulating hormone (FSH)

      (1) Stimulates primary graafian follicle to grow and develop

      (2) Stimulates follicle cells to secrete estrogen

      (3) Stimulates development of seminiferous tubules and spermatogenesis

    e. Luteinizing hormone (LH)

      (1) Stimulates maturation of follicle and ovum; required for ovulation

      (2) Forms corpus luteum in ruptured follicle following ovulation; stimulates corpus luteum to secrete progesterone

      (3) In males, LH is called interstitial-cell–stimulating hormone (ICSH); stimulates testes to secrete testosterone

    f. Prolactin

      (1) Promotes breast development during pregnancy

      (2) Initiates milk production after delivery

      (3) Stimulates progesterone secretion by corpus luteum

  2. Hormones secreted by the posterior lobe

    a. Antidiuretic hormone (ADH); vasopressin

      (1) Increases water reabsorption by distal and collecting tubules of kidneys

      (2) Stimulates vasoconstriction, raising blood pressure

    b. Oxytocin

      (1) Stimulates contractions by pregnant uterus

      (2) Stimulates milk ejection from alveoli of lactating breasts into ducts

    c. Melanocyte-stimulating hormoen (MSH): stimulates synthesis and dispersion of melanin in skin, causing darkening

 RELATED PHARMACOLOGY

Antidiabetic agents

A. Description

  1. Used to treat diabetes mellitus

  2. Classified into two types: insulin for parenteral use and oral antidiabetics

  3. Insulin

    a. Acts to facilitate the transport of glucose across the cell membrane and to promote glycogenesis

    b. Available in three forms: human, beef, and pork; human and purified pork insulins are less antigenic; administered parenterally; brands or forms should not be substituted without medical supervision

    c. Available in rapid-acting, intermediate-acting, and long-acting forms; rapid-acting and intermediate-acting forms are available in mixed preparations (e.g., Humulin 70/30, which contains 70% NPH and 30% regular insulin)

  4. Oral antidiabetics

    a. Require some functioning beta cells

    b. Lower serum glucose in a variety of ways depending on the drug

B. Examples

  1. Insulin

    a. Rapid-acting: lispro (Humalog); onset: 10 to 15 minutes; peak: 1 hour; duration: 3 hours

    b. Short-acting: regular (Humulin R, Novolin R); onset: $1/2$ to 1 hour; peak: 2 to 3 hours; duration: 4 to 6 hours

    c. Intermediate-acting: NPH (Humulin N) and Lente; onset: 3 to 4 hours; peak: 4 to 12 hours; duration: 16 to 20 hours

    d. Long-acting

      (1) Ultralente: onset: 6 to 8 hours; peak: 12 to 16 hours; duration: 20 to 30 hours

      (2) Glargine (Lantus): slow, prolonged absorption leads to a relatively constant concentration over 24 hours without peaks

    e. Combination: NPH and regular (Humulin 70/30 or 50/50; Novolin 70/30)

  2. Oral antidiabetics

    a. Sulfonylureas: stimulate beta cells to produce insulin

      (1) First-generation sulfonylureas are rarely used: tolbutamide (Orinase), chlorpropramide (Diabinese), tolazamide (Tolinase), acetohyxamide (Dymelor)

      (2) Second-generation sulfonylureas: glipizide (Glucotrol), glyburide (Micronase), glimepiride (Amaryl)

    b. Biguanides: reduce the rate of endogenous glucose production by liver; increase the use of glucose by muscle and fat cells; metformin (Glucophage)

  c. Thiazolidinediones: improve insulin sensitivity, thus improving peripheral glucose uptake; rosiglitazone (Avandia), pioglitazone (Actos)

  d. Meglitinides: stimulate quick release of insulin by beta cells; repaglinide (Prandin), nateglinide (Starlix)

  e. Alpha-glucosidase inhibitors: block digestion of complex carbohydrates and slow absorption of glucose; acarbose (Precose), miglitol (Glyset)

  f. Combination: glyburide and metformin (Glucovance)

C. Major side effects

  1. Insulin: irritability, tremor (hypoglycemia); headache; confusion, convulsion (hypoglycemia); tachycardia (hypoglycemia); moist skin (hypoglycemia); hunger (hypoglycemia)

  2. Oral antidiabetics: hypoglycemia; skin rash, allergic reactions, pruritus (hypersensitivity); jaundice (hepatic alterations); thrombocytopenia and lactic acidosis (Glucophage); bloating, gas pains and diarrhea (Precose, Glyset); hepatotoxicity (Avandia)

D. Nursing care

  1. Assess clients for signs of hypoglycemia

  2. Instruct client to:

    a. Use proper medication administration procedure

    b. Comply with dietary program, including snacks

    c. Avoid alcohol, especially when taking Glucophage

    d. Perform self-monitoring of blood glucose (SMBG)

    e. Carry medical alert card

    f. Be prepared for hypoglycemic incidents; administer rapid-acting glucose (e.g., glucose solution or tablets) followed by complex carbohydrate and protein (e.g., cheese and crackers) to stabilize blood glucose

    g. Comply with regular laboratory test such as blood glucose, glycosylated hemoglobin (glycohemoglobin, Hgb A_{1c}), liver enzymes

  3. Administer insulin

    a. Administer all forms of insulin subcutaneously

    b. Use only regular insulin for IV administration

    c. If premixed insulin is not prescribed and two forms are to be mixed, draw up regular insulin first

    d. Rotate sites within same anatomic area; abdomen is preferred site because absorption is not influenced by exercise

    e. Dosage adjustment will be necessary for NPO status and when ill

  4. Offer emotional support to client; therapy is lifelong

  5. Withhold metformin before diagnostic studies requiring iodinated contrast media

Thyroid enhancers

A. Description

  1. Regulate the metabolic rate of body cells; aid in growth and development of bones and teeth; and affect protein, fat, and carbohydrate metabolism

  2. Replace thyroid hormone in clients experiencing a reduction in or absence of thyroid gland function

  3. Available in oral and parenteral (IV) preparations

B. Examples: levothyroxine sodium (Synthroid) is drug of choice; liothyronine sodium (Cytomel); thyroid (Thyrar)

C. Major side effects: increased metabolism (increased serum T_3, T_4); hyperactivity (increased metabolic rate); cardiac stimulation (increased cardiac metabolism)

D. Nursing care

  1. Instruct client to:

    a. Report the occurrence of any side effects to the physician immediately

    b. Take medication as scheduled at the same time daily; do not stop abruptly

    c. Take radial pulse; notify physician if greater than 100 beats/minute

    d. Carry medical alert card

    e. Keep all scheduled appointments with physician; medical supervision is necessary

  2. Assess client for potentiation of anticoagulant effect

  3. Offer emotional support to client; therapy usually is lifelong

  4. Assess client for signs of hyperthyroidism

Thyroid inhibitors

A. Description

  1. Interfere with the synthesis and release of thyroid hormone; inhibit oxidation of iodides to prevent their combination with tyrosine in formation of thyroxine

  2. Treat hyperthyroidism

  3. Available in oral and parenteral (IV) preparations

B. Examples: iodine (potassium iodide); methimazole (Tapazole); propylthiouracil (PTU)

C. Major side effects: agranulocytosis (decreased WBCs); skin disturbances (hypersensitivity); nausea, vomiting (irritation of gastric mucosa); decreased metabolism (decreased production of serum T_3, T_4); iodine: bitter taste, stains teeth (local oral effect on mucosa and teeth)

D. Nursing care
1. Instruct client to:
a. Report the occurrence of any side effects to physician, especially sore throat, jaundice, and fever
b. Avoid crowded places and potentially infectious situations
2. Administer liquid iodine preparations diluted in beverage of choice; use a straw
3. Assess client for signs of hypothyroidism

Adrenocorticoids
A. Description
1. Interfere with the release of factors important in producing the normal inflammatory and immune responses
2. Remove fluid accumulation from brain thereby decreasing cerebral edema
3. Increase glucose and fat formation and promote protein breakdown
4. Used for hormonal replacement therapy
5. Available in oral, parenteral (IM, IV), inhalation, intraarticular, and topical, including ophthalmic, preparations
B. Examples
1. Glucocorticoids
a. Long-acting: dexamethasone (Decadron)
b. Intermediate-acting: methylprednisolone (Medrol, Solu-Medrol)
c. Short-acting: hydrocortisone (Solu-Cortef)
2. Mineralocorticoids: fludrocortisone (Florinef)
C. Major side effects
1. Cushing-like symptoms (increased glucocorticoid activity)
2. Hypertension (promotion of sodium and water retention)
3. Hyperglycemia (increased carbohydrate catabolism; gluconeogenesis)
4. Mood changes (CNS effect)
5. GI irritation and ulcer formation (local GI effect)
6. Cataracts (hyperglycemia)
7. Hypokalemia (promotion of potassium excretion)
8. Decreased wound healing
9. Osteoporosis
D. Nursing care
1. Administer oral preparations with food, milk, or antacid
2. Monitor client's weight, blood pressure, and serum electrolytes during therapy
3. Avoid placing client in potentially infectious situations
4. Assess for GI bleeding; monitor blood glucose in people with diabetes
5. In addition to carrying a medical alert card, instruct client to:

a. Avoid exposure to infections; notify physician if fever or sore throat occurs; avoid immunizations during therapy
b. Avoid using salt; encourage foods high in potassium
c. Avoid missing, changing, or withdrawing drug suddenly
6. Withdraw drug therapy gradually to permit adrenal recovery

Antidiuretic hormone
A. Description
1. Promotes water reabsorption by the distal renal tubules and causes vasoconstriction and increased muscle tone of the bladder, GI tract, uterus, and blood vessels
2. Treatment for diabetes insipidus
3. Available in parenteral (IM, SC) or nasal preparation
B. Examples
Lypressin (Diapid) for intranasal administration; vasopressin (Pitressin)
C. Major side effects
1. Increased intestinal activity (direct peristaltic stimulant)
2. Hyponatremia (promotion of water reabsorption)
3. Pallor (hemodilution)
4. Water intoxication (promotion of water reabsorption
5. Cardiac disturbances (fluid/electrolyte imbalance)
6. Nasal irritation (lypressin has local effect on nasal mucosa)
D. Nursing care
1. Assess client for signs of water intoxication during therapy, monitor intake and output
2. Assess vital signs, especially blood pressure
3. If drug is administered to improve bladder or bowel tone, assess for continence or passage of flatus

MAJOR DISORDERS OF THE ENDOCRINE SYSTEM

▼ HYPERPITUITARISM

Data Base
A. Etiology and pathophysiology
1. May result from overactivity of gland or from an adenoma
2. Characterized by an excessive concentration of pituitary hormones (GH, ACTH, PRL) in the blood, overactivity, and changes in the anterior lobe of the pituitary gland
3. Two classifications of GH overproduction
a. Giantism: generalized increase in size, especially in children; involves the long bones

b. Acromegaly: occurs after epiphyseal closing, with subsequent enlargement of cartilage, bone, and soft tissues of body

4. ACTH overproduction leads to Cushing's disease

B. Clinical findings

1. Subjective: headaches; depression; weakness
2. Objective
   a. Increased soft tissue and bone thickness
   b. Facial features become coarse and heavy, with enlargement of lower jaw, lips, and tongue
   c. Enlarged hands and feet
   d. Increased growth hormone (GH), corticotrophic hormone (ACTH), or prolactin (PRL)
   e. X-ray examination of long bones, skull (sella turcica area), and jaw demonstrates change in structure
   f. Amenorrhea
   g. Signs of increased intracranial pressure such as vomiting, papilledema, focal neurologic deficits
   h. Diabetes and hyperthyroidism may also occur

C. Therapeutic interventions

1. Medications
   a. Somatostatin analog octreotide (Sandostatin)
   b. Dopamine agonist bromocriptine (Parlodel)
   c. Medications to relieve symptoms of other endocrine imbalances resulting from pituitary hyperfunctioning
2. Surgical intervention (hypophysectomy) or irradiation of the pituitary

Nursing Care of Clients with Hyperpituitarism

A. ASSESSMENT

1. Changes in energy level, sexual function and menstrual patterns
2. Face, hands, and feet for thickening, enlargement; and changes in the size of hat, gloves, rings, or shoes
3. Presence of dysphagia or voice changes
4. Presence of hypogonadism as a result of hyperprolactimia
5. Reaction to changes in physical appearance and sexual function

B. ANALYSIS/NURSING DIAGNOSES

1. Disturbed body image related to altered appearance
2. Disturbed sensory perception related to neurologic deficits
3. Sexual dysfunction related to hormonal imbalance

C. PLANNING/IMPLEMENTATION

1. Help the client accept the altered body image that is irreversible

2. Assist family to understand what the client is experiencing
3. Help the client recognize that medical supervision will be required for life
4. Help the client understand the basis for the change in sexual functioning
5. Assist the client in expressing feelings
6. Care for the client following a hypophysectomy
   a. Encourage following an established medical regimen
   b. Protect from stress situations
   c. Protect from infection
   d. Follow and maintain an established schedule for hormone replacement
7. Care for the client undergoing intracranial surgery
   a. Perform neurologic assessments
   b. Measure specific gravity of urine, monitor intake and output, and check daily weight to identify complication of diabetes insipidus
   c. Check clear nasal drainage for glucose to determine presence of CSF
   d. Encourage deep breathing, but not coughing
   e. Institute measures to prevent constipation because straining increases intracranial pressure

D. EVALUATION/OUTCOMES

1. Verbalizes an improved body image
2. Reports satisfying sexual relationship
3. Continues medical supervision

▼ HYPOPITUITARISM

Data Base

A. Etiology and pathophysiology

1. Deficiency of one or more anterior pituitary hormones
2. Total absence of pituitary hormones referred to as panhypopituitarism (Simmonds' disease)
3. Occurs when there is destruction of the anterior lobe of the gland by trauma, tumor, or hemorrhage
4. Clinical findings vary with target organs affected

B. Clinical findings

1. Subjective: lethargy; loss of strength and libido; decreased tolerance for cold
2. Objective
   a. Decreased temperature
   b. Postural hypotension
   c. Hypoglycemia
   d. Decreased levels of GH, ACTH, TSH, FSH, and LH
   e. Sterility; loss of secondary sexual characteristics

f. Visual disturbances if tumor impinges on optic nerve

C. Therapeutic interventions: replace hormones; intervene surgically if tumor is present

Nursing Care of Clients with Hypopituitarism

A. ASSESSMENT
1. Baseline vital signs
2. Sexual patterns: loss of libido; painful intercourse; inability to maintain an erection
3. Past and present menstrual patterns
4. Visual acuity
5. Loss of secondary sexual characteristics
6. Activity tolerance

B. ANALYSIS/NURSING DIAGNOSES
1. Activity intolerance related to decreased serum glucose
2. Disturbed body image related to loss of secondary sexual characteristics
3. Sexual dysfunction related to loss of libido

C. PLANNING/IMPLEMENTATION
1. Monitor effects of hormone replacement
2. Discuss the importance of adhering to medical regimen on a long-term basis
3. Allow the client ample time to verbalize feelings regarding the long-term nature of the disease and impact on daily life
4. Provide adequate rest periods

D. EVALUATION/OUTCOMES
1. Complies with medical regimen
2. Expresses positive feelings of body image
3. Establishes satisfying sexual relationship

▼ DIABETES INSIPIDUS

Data Base

A. Etiology and pathophysiology
1. A deficient production or secretion of the antidiuretic hormone (ADH) by the posterior pituitary gland decreasing reabsorption of water in nephron tubules; may be familial, idiopathic, secondary to trauma, surgery, tumors, infections, or autoimmune disorders
2. Neurogenic diabetes insipidus, a renal tubular defect resulting in decreased water absorption, may be familial or result from renal disorders, primary aldosteronism, or excessive water intake (primary polydipsia); results in impaired renal concentrating ability

B. Clinical findings
1. Subjective: polydipsia; craving for cold water
2. Objective
   a. Polyuria (5 to 25 L/24 hr)
   b. Dilute urine; specific gravity 1.001 to 1.005; osmolality 50 to 200 mOsm/kg

c. Increased serum sodium and plasma osmolality
d. Signs of dehydration (poor skin turgor, dry mucous membranes, elevated temperature)

C. Therapeutic interventions
1. Antidiuretic hormone replacement: vasopressin (Pitressin), lypressin (Diapid), desmopressin (DDAVP), vasopressin tannate (Pitressin Tannate)
2. Treatment of underlying cause
3. Hypophysectomy

Nursing Care of Clients with Diabetes Insipidus

A. ASSESSMENT
1. Intake and output, weight, and specific gravity of urine to establish baseline data
2. Results of serum electrolyte evaluation
3. Dryness of skin and mucous membranes

B. ANALYSIS/NURSING DIAGNOSES
1. Deficient fluid volume related to polyuria
2. Ineffective therapeutic regimen management related to chronicity of problem

C. PLANNING/IMPLEMENTATION
1. Monitor fluid and electrolyte status: intake and output, daily weight, skin turgor, electrolyte levels
2. Replace fluid by mouth or parenterally
3. Monitor response to ADH replacement
4. Teach client on long-term vasopressin therapy the need for daily weight records, recognition of polyuria, and wearing a medical alert bracelet; overdosage may cause syndrome of inappropriate antidiuretic hormone (SIADH), leading to water retention and hyponatremia
5. Advise client to avoid alcohol because it suppresses ADH secretion

D. EVALUATION/OUTCOMES
1. Maintains fluid balance
2. States signs of overmedication and undermedication with ADH replacement

▼ SYNDROME OF INAPPROPRIATE ANTIDIURETIC HORMONE SECRETION

Data Base

A. Etiology and pathophysiology
1. Excessive ADH secretion leads to fluid retention and dilutional hyponatremia
2. May be caused by head trauma, tumors, or infection; malignant tumor cells may produce ADH

B. Clinical findings
1. Subjective: anorexia; nausea; fatigue; headache
2. Objective

a. Reduced urine output
b. Decreased deep tendon reflexes
c. Change in mental status, seizures, coma
d. Signs of fluid retention such as weight gain, crackles, jugular vein distention
e. Decreased serum sodium and osmolality
C. Therapeutic interventions: fluid restriction; hypertonic parenteral fluids

Nursing Care of Clients with Syndrome of Inappropriate Antidiuretic Hormone Secretion

A. ASSESSMENT
1. History of malignancy, infection, or increased intracranial pressure
2. Intake and output, daily weight, vital signs
3. Serum and urine for sodium and osmolality
4. Neurologic evaluations

B. ANALYSIS/NURSING DIAGNOSES
1. Excess fluid volume related to fluid retention
2. Risk for injury related to altered neurologic function

C. PLANNING/IMPLEMENTATION
1. Monitor fluid and electrolyte status
2. Restrict fluid intake; administer hypertonic intravenous solutions as ordered
3. Institute seizure precautions
4. Provide supportive measures for related disorders

D. EVALUATION/OUTCOMES
1. Maintains fluid balance
2. Remains seizure free

▼ HYPERTHYROIDISM (GRAVES' DISEASE, THYROTOXICOSIS)

Data Base
A. Etiology and pathophysiology
1. Excessive concentration of thyroid hormones in the blood as a result of thyroid disease or increased TSH; leads to a hypermetabolic state
2. Etiology of Graves' disease is mediated by immunoglobulin G (IgG) antibody that activates TSH receptors on the surface of thyroid cells
3. Etiology of Graves' disease is believed to be involved with an autoimmune process of impaired regulation; associated with to other autoimmune disorders
4. The gland may also enlarge (goiter) as a result of decreased iodine intake; no increase in secretion of thyroid is present
B. Clinical findings
1. Subjective: polyphagia; emotional lability; apprehension; heat intolerance
2. Objective
   a. Weight loss; loose stools; tremors, hyperactive reflexes; diaphoresis; insomnia; exoph-

thalmos, corneal ulceration; increased systolic blood pressure, temperature, pulse, and respiration
b. Decreased TSH levels if thyroid disorder; increased TSH levels if secondary to a pituitary disorder
c. Graves' disease generally involves hyperthyroidism, goiter, and exophthalmos
d. Increased triiodothyronine (T_3), thyroxine (T_4), protein-bound iodine (PBI), long-acting thyroid simulator (LATS), and radioactive iodine uptake
e. Thyrotoxic crisis (thyroid storm): a state of hypermetabolism that may lead to heart failure; usually precipitated by a period of severe physiologic or psychologic stress, thyroid surgery, or radioactive iodine therapy
C. Therapeutic interventions
1. Antithyroid medications such as prophylthiouracil (PTU) and methimazole (Tapazole) to block the synthesis of thyroid hormone
2. Antithyroid medications such as iodine (potassium iodide, SSKI) to reduce the vascularity of the thyroid gland
3. Radioactive iodine ^{131}I to destroy thyroid gland cells, thereby decreasing the production of thyroid hormone (atomic cocktail)
4. Medications to relieve the symptoms related to the increased metabolic rate such as adrenergic blocking agents
5. Well-balanced, high-calorie diet with vitamin and mineral supplements
6. Surgical intervention involves a subtotal or total thyroidectomy

Nursing Care of Clients with Hyperthyroidism

A. ASSESSMENT
1. History of weight loss, diarrhea, insomnia, emotional lability, palpitations, and heat intolerance
2. Eyes for exophthalmos, tearing, and sensitivity to light
3. Neck palpation for enlarged thyroid gland
4. Weight and vital signs to establish baseline

B. ANALYSIS/NURSING DIAGNOSES
1. Ineffective coping related to emotional lability
2. Imbalanced nutrition: less than body requirements related to increased metabolic needs

C. PLANNING/IMPLEMENTATION
1. Use measures such as decreased stimulation, medications, and back rub to establish a climate for uninterrupted rest
2. Protect the client from stress-producing situations
3. Keep the room cool

4. Provide diet high in calories, proteins, and carbohydrates with supplemental feedings between meals and at bedtime; vitamin and mineral supplements should be given as prescribed

5. Understand that the client is upset by lability of mood and exaggerated response to environmental stimuli; take time to explain disease processes involved

6. Provide eye drops or patches as needed

7. Care for the client before a thyroidectomy
   a. Administer prescribed antithyroid medications to achieve euthyroid state
   b. Teach deep breathing exercises and use of hands to support neck and to avoid strain on suture line

8. Care for the client following a thyroidectomy
   a. Observe for signs of respiratory distress and laryngeal stridor caused by tracheal edema (keep tracheotomy set available)
   b. Provide humidity with cold steam nebulizer to keep secretions moist when at home
   c. Keep the bed in a semi-Fowler's position
   d. Observe dressings at the operative site and back of the neck and shoulders for signs of hemorrhage
   e. Observe for signs of thyroid storm such as high fever, tachycardia, irritability, delirium, coma; may result from manipulation of the gland during surgery, which releases thyroid hormone into bloodstream
   f. Notify the physician immediately if signs of thyroid storm occur; administer propanolol (Inderal), iodides, propylthiouracil, and steroids as ordered
   g. Observe for signs of tetany such as numbness or twitching of extremities, spasm of the glottis; hypocalcemia can occur after accidental trauma or removal of the parathyroid glands; if tetany occurs, give calcium gluconate or calcium chloride (IV) as prescribed
   h. Assess for hoareness; may result from endotracheal intubation or laryngeal nerve damage

9. Provide teaching regarding radioactive iodine therapy
   a. Following therapy client returns to the community
   b. Hospitalization in isolation may be required for several days if larger doses are used
   c. Symptoms of hyperthyroidism may take 3 to 4 weeks to subside

10. Teach client signs and symptoms of:
    a. Hypothyroidism as a result of treatment
    b. Hyperthyroidism as a result of thyroid storm or overmedication with thyroid hormone-replacement therapy

11. Teach the importance of taking antithyroid medications regularly and to observe for adverse effects

D. EVALUATION/OUTCOMES
   1. Maintains ideal body weight
   2. Establishes regular routine of activity and rest

▼ HYPOTHYROIDISM

Data Base

A. Etiology and pathophysiology
   1. Congenital thyroid defects
   2. Defective hormone synthesis
   3. Prenatal and postnatal iodine deficiency
   4. Therapy for hyperthyroidism: thyroid medication, thyroid surgery, radioactive iodine
   5. Autoimmune diseases such as Hashimoto's disease and sarcoidosis
   6. Classified according to the time of life in which it occurs
      a. Cretinism: hypothyroidism found at birth
      b. Lymphocytic thyroiditis most frequently appears after 6 years of age and peaks during adolescence; generally self-limiting
      c. Hypothyroidism without myxedema: mild degree of thyroid failure in older children and adults
      d. Hypothyroidism with myxedema: severe degree of thyroid failure in older individuals
   7. Decreased levels of thyroid hormones (T_3 and T_4) slows the basal metabolic rate (BMR); the decreased BMR affects lipid metabolism, increases cholesterol and triglyceride levels, and affects RBC production leading to anemia and folate deficiency
   8. Myxedema coma is the most severe degree of hypothyroidism, representing a potentially fatal endocrine emergency; precipitated by a severe physiologic stress, myxedema coma involves hypothermia, bradycardia, hypoventilation, and progressive loss of consciousness

B. Clinical findings
   1. Subjective: dull mental processes; apathy; lethargy; loss of libido; intolerance to cold; anorexia
   2. Objective
      a. Lack of facial expression; increase in weight; constipation; subnormal temperature and pulse; dry, brittle hair and nails; pale, dry, coarse skin; enlarged tongue; drooling; hoarseness; thinning of lateral eyebrows; scalp, axilla, and pubic hair loss; diminished hearing; anemia; periorbital edema
      b. Decreased basal metabolic rate (BMR)

c. Decreased thyroxine (T_4), triiodothyronine (T_3), and radioactive iodine uptake; delayed or poor response to TSH stimulation test in secondary hypothyroidism, increased TSH in primary hypothyroidism

C. Therapeutic interventions: administer thyroid hormones; maintain vital functions

Nursing Care of Clients with Hypothyroidism

A. ASSESSMENT

1. History that may have contributed to condition
2. Activity tolerance, bowel elimination, sleeping patterns, sexual function, and intolerance to cold
3. Skin and hair for characteristic changes
4. Weight and vital signs to establish baseline
5. Signs of anemia, atherosclerosis, or arthritis

B. ANALYSIS/NURSING DIAGNOSES

1. Activity intolerance related to decreased metabolic rate
2. Constipation related to decreased gastrointestinal activity

C. PLANNING/IMPLEMENTATION

1. Have patience with a lethargic client; activity tolerance and mental functioning will improve with therapy
2. Teach the client and family to be alert for signs of complications
   a. Angina pectoris: chest pain, indigestion
   b. Cardiac failure: dyspnea, palpitations
   c. Myxedema coma: weakness, syncope, slow pulse rate, subnormal temperature, slow respirations, lethargy
3. Teach the client to seek medical supervision regularly and when signs of illness develop
4. Explain the importance of continued hormone replacement throughout life
5. Review the signs of hypothyroidism and hyperthyroidism to help client recognize signs of undermedication or overmedication
6. Explain that incresed sensitivity to narcotic analgesics and tranquilizers necessitates dosage adjustment; OTC drugs should be avoided unless approved by physician
7. Help the client and family recognize that client's inability to adapt to cold temperature requires additional protection and modification of outdoor activity in cold weather
8. Teach the client to avoid constipation by the use of adequate hydration and roughage in the diet
9. Apply moisturizers to skin
10. Teach the need to restrict calories, cholesterol, and fat in the diet

D. EVALUATION/OUTCOMES

1. Completes activities of daily living (ADL) without fatigue
2. Complies with dietary, exercise, and medication regimen
3. Establishes regular pattern of bowel elimination

▼ HYPERPARATHYROIDISM

Data Base

A. Etiology and pathophysiology
   1. Hyperfunction of the parathyroid glands; usually caused by adenoma; hypertrophy and hyperplasia of the glands may also be responsible
   2. As a result the absorption of calcium and excretion of phosphorus by the kidneys is increased
   3. If dietary intake is not enough to meet calcium levels demanded by high levels of parathormone, demineralization of the bone occurs

B. Clinical findings
   1. Subjective: apathy, fatigue; muscular weakness; anorexia; nausea; emotional irritability; deep bone pain (if demineralization occurs); backache
   2. Objective
      a. Bone cysts, pathologic fractures
      b. Renal calculi composed of calcium; pyelonephritis; renal damage; polyuria
      c. Vomiting; constipation
      d. Elevated serum calcium and parathormone
      e. Decreased serum phosphorus
      f. Cardiac dysrhythmias

C. Therapeutic interventions
   1. Surgical excision of a parathyroid tumor
   2. Calcium intake restricted
   3. Administration of furosemide (Lasix) to increase renal excretion of calcium
   4. Administration of gallium nitrate, calcitonin, or plicamycin with glucocorticoid to lower calcium level

Nursing Care of Clients with Hyperparathyroidism

A. ASSESSMENT

1. Presence of GI disturbance or bone pain
2. History of renal calculi or fractures
3. Signs of renal calculi such as hematuria or flank pain
4. Use of thiazide diuretics or vitamin D, which can increase serum calcium
5. Serum calcium and phosphorus levels
6. Baseline vital signs, particularly heart rate and rhythm

B. ANALYSIS/NURSING DIAGNOSES

1. Risk for injury related to bone demineralization
2. Impaired urinary elimination related to obstruction by calculi

C. **PLANNING/IMPLEMENTATION**
1. Strain the urine, observing for calculi
2. Encourage fluid intake
3. Assist the client with ambulation, which helps prevent demineralization; instruct client to avoid high-impact activities
4. Monitor intake and output
5. Encourage foods with fiber to limit constipation
6. Instruct the client to limit intake of foods high in calcium, especially milk products
7. Provide cardiac monitoring if hypercalcemia is severe
8. If surgery is performed, provide postoperative care the same as for clients undergoing thyroidectomy (see Hyperthyroidism)

D. **EVALUTION/OUTCOMES**
1. Maintains skeletal intergrity
2. Remains free of urinary complications

▼ HYPOPARATHYROIDISM

Data Base

A. Etiology and pathophysiology
1. Parathyroid glands may not secrete a sufficient amount of parathormone after thyroid surgery, parathyroid surgery, or radiation therapy of the neck; idiopathic hypoparathyroidism rare
2. As levels of parathormone drop, the serum calcium also drops, causing signs of tetany; a concomitant rise in serum phosphate occurs

B. Clinical findings
1. Subjective: photophobia; muscle cramps; irritability; dyspnea; tingling of extremities
2. Objective
   a. Trousseau's sign (carpopedal spasm)
   b. Chvostek's sign (contraction of the facial muscle in response to tapping near the angle of the jaw)
   c. Decreased serum calcium and parathormone; elevated serum phosphate
   d. Stridor, wheezing from laryngeal spasm; tremors; convulsions
   e. X-ray examination reveals increased bone density
   f. Cardiac dysrhythmias; alkalosis; cataracts if the disease is chronic

C. Therapeutic interventions
1. Calcium chloride or calcium gluconate given IV for emergency treatment of overt tetany
2. Calcium salts administered orally (calcium carbonate, calcium gluconate)
3. Vitamin D (dihydrotachysterol, ergocalciferol) to increase absorption of calcium from the GI tract
4. Parathormone injections

5. High-calcium, low-phosphate diet
6. Aluminum hydroxide to decrease absorption of phosphorus from the GI tract

Nursing Care of Clients with Hypoparathyroidism

A. **ASSESSMENT**
1. History of muscle spasms, numbness or tingling of extremities, visual disturbances, or convulsions
2. Presence of neuromuscular irritability
3. Status of respiratory functioning
4. Heart rate and rhythm
5. Serum calcium and phosphate levels

B. **ANALYSIS/NURSING DIAGNOSES**
1. Ineffective airway clearance related to laryngeal spasm
2. Risk for injury related to neuromuscular irritability

C. **PLANNING/IMPLEMENTATION**
1. Observe for respiratory distress and have emergency equipment available for tracheostomy and mechanical ventilation
2. Maintain seizure precautions
3. Reduce environmental stimuli
4. Provide drug and dietary instruction including elimination of milk, cheese, and egg yolks because of high phosphorus content
5. Teach symptoms of hypocalcemia and hypercalcemia; instruct client to contact physician immediately if either should occur

D. **EVALUATION/OUTCOMES**
1. Remains free from neuromuscular irritability
2. Maintains respiratory functioning within normal limits

▼ DIABETES MELLITUS

Data Base

A. Etiology and pathophysiology
1. Hyperglycemia occurs when there is insufficient secretion of insulin, cells become insulin resistant, and/or hepatic glucose production is increased
2. Body attempts to rid itself of excess glucose by excreting some via kidneys; an osmotic force is created within the kidneys because of this glucose excretion and body fluid is lost
3. If the body is unable to use carbohydrates for cellular function fat is oxidized as a compensatory mechanism; oxidation of fats gives off ketone bodies
4. Risk factors
   a. Type 1: genetic predisposition; environmental factors such as toxins or viruses, age <30 years

b. Type 2: family history, obesity, usually age ≥45 years, history of gestational diabetes, increasing incidence in childhood and adolescence

5. Classification
   a. Type 1: formerly known as insulin-dependent diabetes mellitus (IDDM); destruction of beta cells leads to an inability to produce insulin; requires exogenous insulin
   b. Type 2: formerly known as non–insulin-dependent diabetes mellitus (NIDDM); has a gradual onset and the pancreas produces some insulin so that ketoacidosis is not likely; may be controlled with adherence to a diet and exercise program that promotes maintenance of a desirable weight; accounts for 90% of diabetes
   c. Gestational: detected during 24 to 28 weeks' gestation; glucose levels are generally normal 6 weeks postpartum; more likely to develop type 2 diabetes 5 to 10 years after delivery; neonate exhibits macrosomia, hypoglycemia, hypocalcemia, and hyperbilirubinemia
   d. Diabetes mellitus associated with other conditions or syndromes (formerly known as secondary diabetes); associated with conditions such as Cushing's disease, pancreatic disease, and glucocorticoid medication
   e. Impaired glucose tolerance; high glucose levels but not sufficiently high to be diagnostic for diabetes

6. Acute increases in serum glucose levels: diabetic ketoacidosis (DKA) and hyperglycemic hyperosmolar nonketotic syndrome (HHKS)
   a. Causes: insufficient insulin, major stresses (e.g., infection, surgery, trauma, pregnancy, emotional turmoil, nausea and vomiting), or drugs (steroids)
   b. Pathophysiology
      (1) DKA is associated with type 1; with inadequate insulin to support basal needs, proteins and fats are used; ketones are excreted via urine and breathing; dehydration and electrolyte imbalances occur
      (2) HHKS is associated with type 2; hyperglycemia increases intravascular osmotic pressure, leading to polyuria and cellular dehydration

7. Acute decrease in serum glucose: insulin shock or reaction
   a. Causes: excess insulin or oral antidiabetic medications; too little food or too much exercise when receiving antidiabetic medications
   b. Pathophysiology: excessive insulin lowers serum glucose as glucose is carried into cells; decreased food intake in relation to prescribed antidiabetic medications results in hypoglycemia; excessive exercise uses glucose for metabolism decreasing serum glucose

8. Long-term complications of diabetes include microangiopathy (retinopathy, nephropathy), macroangiopathy (peripheral vascular diseases, arterioatherosclerosis, coronary artery disease, cerebral vascular disease), neuropathy, skin problems (cellulitis, fungal infections, boils), periodontal disease

B. Clinical findings
   1. Subjective: polydipsia; polyphagia; fatigue; blurred vision (retinopathy; osmotic changes); peripheral neuropathy
   2. Objective
      a. Polyuria; weight loss; glycosuria; peripheral vascular changes; ulcers; gangrene
      b. Hyperglycemia: detected by fasting blood sugar, glucose tolerance test, 2-hour postprandial glucose, and glycosylated hemoglobin or hemoglobin A_{1c} (provides measure of average glucose level over preceding 2 to 3 months)
   3. DKA and HHKS
      a. Hyperglycemia, glycosuria, polyuria
      b. Dehydration: flushed, hot, dry skin, decreased skin turgor (tenting), hypotension, tachycardia, thirst, headache, confusion, drowsiness
      c. Metabolic acidosis (DKA only): Kussmaul respirations as body attempts to blow off carbon dioxide; ketonuria, sweet breath odor, anorexia, nausea, vomiting, decreased serum pH, decreased P_{CO_2}
   4. Hypoglycemia (insulin shock or reaction)
      a. Occurs as a result of sympathetic nervous stimulation or reduced cerebral glucose supply
      b. CNS effects: mental confusion, blurred vision, diplopia, slurred speech, fatigue, seizures
      c. SNS (adrenergic) effects: nervousness, weakness, pallor, diaphoresis, tremor, tachycardia, hunger

C. Therapeutic interventions
   1. Lifestyle changes
      a. Weight control: obesity leads to insulin resistance; this can be reversed by weight loss
      b. Exercise: increases insulin sensitivity but must be regular; brisk walking, swimming, and bicycling are recommended
      c. Diet: current recommendations include:
         (1) Caloric control to maintain ideal body weight
         (2) 50% to 60% of caloric intake should be from carbohydrates with emphasis on complex carbohydrates, high-fiber foods

rich in water-soluble fiber (oat bran, peas, all forms of beans, pectin-rich fruits and vegetables); foods with a high glycemic index should be avoided; glycemic index refers to effect of particular foods on blood glucose

(3) Protein: intake should be consistent with the U.S. Dietary Guidelines, usually between 60 and 85 g; should be 12% to 20% of daily calories

(4) Fat intake not to exceed 30% of daily calories (70 to 90 g/day); keep saturated fat intake low; emphasize mono- and polyunsaturated fats

(5) Dietary ratio: carbohydrate to protein to fat usually about 5:1:2

(6) Distribute food fairly evenly throughout the day in three or four meals, with snacks added between and at bedtime as needed in accordance with total food allowance and therapy (insulin or oral hypoglycemics)

(7) Basic tools for planning diet: Diabetes Food Guide Pyramid, food composition tables showing nutrient content and glycemic index of foods

d. Self-monitoring of blood glucose (SMBG)

2. Insulin administration

a. Adjusted after considering the client's physical and emotional stresses; a specific type of insulin and schedule is prescribed

b. Somogyi effect: insulin-induced hypoglycemia rebounds to hyperglycemia

(1) Epinephrine and glucagon are released in response to hypoglycemia

(2) These reactions cause mobilization of the liver's stored glucose and iatrogenically induce hyperglycemia

(3) Somogyi phenomenon is treated by gradually lowering insulin dosage while monitoring blood glucose, particularly during the night (when hypoglycemia is most likely to occur)

(4) Must be differentiated from the dawn phenomenon, early morning hyperglycemia attributed to increased secretion of growth hormone; this requires delaying administration of PM insulin or increased dosage

c. Insulin pump

(1) External battery-operated device that delivers insulin through a needle inserted into subcutaneous tissue

(2) Small (basal) doses of regular insulin are programmed into computer to be delivered every few minutes; bolus doses (extra preset amounts) are delivered before meals

(3) Improves glucose control for clients with wide variations in insulin need as a result of irregular schedules, pregnancy, or growth requirements

(4) A prescribed amount of insulin for 24 hours plus priming is drawn into syringe

(5) The administration set is primed and needle inserted aseptically, usually into subcutaneous tissue of abdomen

3. Oral antidiabetics for certain clients with type 2 diabetes who cannot be managed with lifestyle changes alone; must have some functioning beta cells in the islets of Langerhans

4. Other therapies include pancreatic islet cell grafts, pancreas transplants, implantable insulin pumps that continually monitor blood glucose and release insulin accordingly, cyclosporin therapy to prevent beta-cell destruction in type 1 diabetes

5. Management of DKA and HHKS

a. IV to provide fluid replacement and direct access to the circulatory system, and a Foley catheter to monitor urine output

b. Rapid-acting insulin based on serum glucose levels

c. Replacement of lost electrolytes, particularly sodium and potassium, using blood studies to determine dosage; when insulin is administered potassium reenters the cell resulting in hypokalemia

d. Cardiac monitoring if circulatory collapse is imminent or dysrhythmias associated with electrolyte imbalance occur

e. Treat acidosis according to cause

6. Management of hypoglycemia (insulin shock or reaction)

a. 10 to 15 g of simple sugar (e.g., glucose tablets, 4 to 6 ounces of juice or soda, hard candy) followed by complex carbohydrate and protein (e.g., cheese and crackers)

b. Establish an intravenous line for circulatory access

c. Administration of 50% dextrose solution

d. If unconscious, glucagon injection to stimulate glycogenolysis

Nursing Care of Clients with Diabetes Mellitus

A. ASSESSMENT

1. Familial history of diabetes mellitus

2. Cardinal signs of polyuria, polydipsia, and polyphagia

3. History of fatigue, visual changes, impaired wound healing, urinary tract infections, fungal infections, and altered sensation

4. Blood glucose levels, hemoglobin A_{1c}
5. Visual acuity and retinal changes
6. Vital signs and weight for baseline data
7. Urine for acetone, microalbumin
8. Renal function
9. Dietary and exercise patterns

B. ANALYSIS/NURSING DIAGNOSES
1. Ineffective therapeutic regimen management related to complexity of therapies and chronicity of the illness
2. Imbalanced nutrition: less than body requirements related to impaired carbohydrate, fat, and protein metabolism

C. PLANNING/IMPLEMENTATION
1. Assist the client and family to understand the disease process
2. Encourage the client to express feelings about illness and the necessary changes in lifestyle and self-image
3. Help the client with the administration of medication until self-administration is both physically and psychologically possible
4. Assist the client in recognizing the need for activities and diet that promote and maintain normal body weight
5. Monitor serum glucose with routine finger sticks
6. Test urine for ketones when glucose is high; obtain double voided specimen or specimen from port of retention catheter if in place
7. Teach client and family to:
   a. Use blood-glucose–monitoring system to test blood glucose
   b. Test urine for ketones when blood glucose is high
   c. Avoid infection
   d. Care for the legs, feet, and toenails properly; inspect, bathe, dry; lubricate feet except between toes; avoid exposure of feet to heat sources; wear shoes to protect feet
   e. Administer insulin by using sterile technique, rotating injection sites within an anatomic location, measuring dosage, noting types, strengths of insulin, and peak action periods; using insulin pump, need to carry carbohydrate source
   f. Use Diabetes Food Guide Pyramid and food tables when planning dietary intake
   g. Avoid tight shoes and smoking, which will constrict circulation
   h. Recognize signs of impending hypoglycemia (insulin shock, reaction)
   i. Recognize signs of impending hyperglycemia (DKA, HHKS)
8. Encourage the client to continue medical supervision and follow-up care, including visits to an eye care specialist and podiatrist

9. Encourage follow-up nutritional counseling

D. EVALUATION/OUTCOMES
1. Complies with medical regimen of diet, exercise, and medications
2. Maintains blood glucose and hemoglobin A_{1c} levels within an acceptable range

▼ PRIMARY ALDOSTERONISM (CONN'S SYNDROME)

Data Base
A. Etiology and pathophysiology
1. Aldosterone, a mineralocorticoid secreted in response to the renin-angiotensin system and ACTH, causes the kidneys to retain sodium and excrete potassium and hydrogen
2. Usually caused by an adenoma of the adrenal cortex, but may also be caused by hyperplasia or carcinoma
B. Clinical findings
1. Subjective: muscle weakness and cramping; polydipsia, polyuria; paresthesia
2. Objective: hypertension; hypokalemia, hypernatremia; alkalosis; elevated urinary aldosterone levels; renal damage: proteinuria, decreased urine specific gravity
C. Therapeutic interventions
1. Surgical removal of the tumor
2. Temporary management with spironolactone
3. Occasionally a bilateral adrenalectomy involving lifelong corticosteroid therapy is necessary

Nursing Care of Clients with Primary Aldosteronism
A. ASSESSMENT
1. Vital signs
2. Electrolyte levels
3. Intake and output, urine specific gravity
4. Motor and sensory functions for alterations
5. Cardiac dysrhythmias as a result of hypokalemia

B. ANALYSIS/NURSING DIAGNOSES
1. Fatigue related to muscle weakness
2. Deficient fluid volume related to polyuria
3. Excess fluid volume related to excess sodium retention

C. PLANNING/IMPLEMENTATION
1. Regulate fluid intake
2. Encourage continued medical supervision
3. Care for the client after a bilateral adrenalectomy
   a. Monitor vital signs, hemodynamic state, and blood glucose level
   b. Administer steroids with milk or antacid
   c. Protect the client from infection and stressful situations

d. Explain drug and side effects to client
e. Instruct the client to carry medical alert identification card
4. Provide dietary instruction; encourage intake of foods high in potassium and avoidance of foods that contain sodium

D. EVALUATION/OUTCOMES
1. Maintains blood pressure at an acceptable level
2. Selects foods low in sodium and high in potassium
3. Performs routine ADL without fatigue

▼ CUSHING'S SYNDROME

Data Base

A. Etiology and pathophysiology
1. Results from excess secretion of adrenocortical hormones
2. Caused by hyperplasia or by a tumor of the adrenal cortex; however, the primary lesion may occur in the pituitary gland, causing excess production of ACTH
3. Administration of excess glucocorticoids or ACTH will also cause Cushing's syndrome

B. Clinical findings
1. Subjective: weakness; decreased libido; mood swings; steroid psychosis
2. Objective
   a. Obese trunk, thin arms and legs; moon face; buffalo hump; acne; hirsutism; ecchymotic areas; purple striae on breast and abdomen; amenorrhea; increased susceptibility to infections
   b. Hypertension
   c. Hyperglycemia; hypokalemia; elevated plasma cortisol level
   d. Elevated 17-hydroxycorticosteroids and 17-ketosteroids in urine
   e. Osteoporosis; fractures; kyphosis
   f. Protein wasting, which causes muscle wasting and weakness
   g. Sodium and water retention with edema and hypertension

C. Therapeutic interventions
1. Reduce dosage of externally administered corticoids
2. If lesion on pituitary is causing hypersecretion of ACTH, a hypophysectomy or irradiation of the pituitary may be done
3. Surgical excision of adrenal tumors (adrenalectomy)
4. Adrenal enzyme inhibitors
5. Potassium supplements
6. High-protein diet with sodium restriction

Nursing Care of Clients with Cushing's Syndrome

A. ASSESSMENT
1. Baseline vital signs, weight, blood glucose and electrolytes
2. Urine specimens for diagnostic purposes
3. Physical appearance
4. Changes in coping and sexuality from history

B. ANALYSIS/NURSING DIAGNOSES
1. Disturbed body image related to altered appearance
2. Excess fluid volume related to sodium excess
3. Risk for infection related to altered immune response

C. PLANNING/IMPLEMENTATION
1. Monitor vital signs, daily weight, intake and output, blood glucose, and electrolytes
2. Protect the client from exposure to infections
3. Encourage ventilation of feelings by the client and spouse because changes in body image and sex drive can alter spousal support
4. Attempt to minimize stress in the environment by measures such as limiting visitors and explaining procedures carefully
5. Instruct client regarding diet and supplementation; encourage diet rich in nutrient-dense foods such as fruits, vegetables, whole grains, and legumes to improve and maintain nutritional status and prevent any possible drug-induced nutrient deficiencies
6. Care for the client following a bilateral adrenalectomy (see Primary Aldosteronism)
7. Care for the client following a hypophysectomy (see Hyperpituitarism)

D. EVALUATION/OUTCOMES
1. Maintains fluid balance
2. Remains free of infection
3. Discusses feelings regarding physical changes

▼ ADDISON'S DISEASE (PRIMARY ADRENAL INSUFFICIENCY)

Data Base

A. Etiology and pathophysiology
1. Hyposecretion of adrenocortical hormones
2. Generally caused by autoimmune destruction of the cortex or by idiopathic atrophy; may be seen in clients with AIDS and tuberculosis
3. Addisonian crisis (acute adrenal insufficiency) can be precipitated by stresses such as pregnancy, surgery, infection, dehydration, emotional turmoil; fatal if not treated
4. Risk factors include endocrine disorders, sudden cessation of glucocorticoids, adrenalectomy, tuberculosis

B. Clinical findings
1. Subjective: weakness, fatigue; anorexia, nausea
2. Objective
   a. Increased bronze pigmentation of skin
   b. Vomiting; diarrhea
   c. Hypotension
   d. Decreased serum cortisol, 17-ketosteroids, and 17-hydroxysteroids; increased plasma ACTH; hyponatremia; hypoglycemia; hyperkalemia
C. Therapeutic interventions
1. Replacement of hormones: glucocorticoids to correct metabolic imbalance and mineralocorticoids to correct electrolyte imbalance and hypotension
2. Correction of fluid, electrolyte, and glucose imbalances
3. High-carbohydrate, high-protein diet
4. Prevention of osteoporosis, which may develop with the use of steroid therapy that break down protein matrix in the bones

Nursing Care of Clients with Addison's Disease
A. ASSESSMENT
1. Baseline vital signs, weight, electrolytes, and serum glucose
2. 24-hour urine specimens for diagnostic purposes (17-hydroxycorticosteroids and 17-ketosteroids)
3. Appearance of skin
4. Changes in energy or activity from history

B. ANALYSIS/NURSING DIAGNOSES
1. Deficient fluid volume related to excess sodium loss
2. Decreased cardiac output related to electrolyte imbalances

C. PLANNING/IMPLEMENTATION
1. Monitor vital signs four times a day; be alert for elevation in temperature (infection, dehydration), alterations in pulse rate and rhythm (hyperkalemia), and alterations in blood pressure
2. Observe for signs of sodium and potassium imbalance
3. Monitor intake and output and weigh daily
4. Administer steroids as ordered; give with milk or an antacid to limit ulcerogenic factor of the drug
5. Put the client in a private room to prevent contact with clients having infectious diseases
6. Limit the number of visitors
7. Advise the client to avoid physical and emotional stress
8. Teach client need for lifelong hormone replacement with increased dosage during stress
9. Review signs of adrenal hypofunction or hyperfunction so client can recognize need for adjustment of steroid dose
10. Instruct client to wear medical alert band
11. Encourage diet consistent with the U.S. Dietary Goals with emphasis on diet high in nutrient-dense foods and adequate sodium
12. Administer antiemetics to prevent fluid and electrolyte loss by vomiting

D. EVALUATION/OUTCOMES
1. Maintains fluid balance
2. Maintains electrolyte balance

▼ PHEOCHROMOCYTOMA

Data Base
A. Etiology and pathophysiology
1. Catecholamine-secreting tumor of the adrenal medulla; usually benign
2. Causes increased secretion of epinephrine and norepinephrine (catecholamines)
3. Familial tendency; peak incidence 25 to 50 years
B. Clinical findings
1. Subjective: headache; visual disturbances; palpitations; anxiety; psychoneurosis
2. Objective
   a. Hypertension, postural hypotension; tachycardia; diaphoresis; tremors; hyperglycemia; CVA or blindness may occur
   b. Increased plasma and urinary catecholamines and vanillylmandelic acid (VMA), a product of catecholamine breakdown
C. Therapeutic interventions
1. Surgical removal of the tumor
2. Antihypertensive and antidysrhythmic drugs such as nitroprusside (Nipride), propranolol (Inderal), phentolamine (Regitine)

Nursing Care of Clients with Pheochromocytoma
A. ASSESSMENT
1. Blood pressures with client in upright and horizontal positions
2. Symptoms associated with hypertension
3. 24-hour urine specimens for VMA and catecholamine studies; instruct client to avoid coffee, chocolate, beer, wine, citrus fruit, bananas, and vanilla before the test for VMA

B. ANALYSIS/NURSING DIAGNOSES
1. Disturbed sensory perception related to sustained elevated blood pressure
2. Ineffective tissue perfusion related to sustained elevated blood pressure

C. PLANNING/IMPLEMENTATION
1. Administer parenteral fluids and blood as ordered before and after surgery to maintain blood volume

2. Decrease environmental stimulation
3. If bilateral adrenalectomy is performed, instruct the client regarding maintenance doses of steroids (see Care for the Client Following a Bilateral Adrenalectomy under Primary Aldosteronism)
4. Emphasize the importance of continued medical supervision and screening for other family members

D. EVALUATION/OUTCOMES
1. Maintains blood pressure at an acceptable level
2. Remains free of complications of hypertension

INTEGUMENTARY SYSTEM

REVIEW OF ANATOMY AND PHYSIOLOGY

Functions of the Integumentary System

A. Prevents loss of body fluids
B. Protects deeper tissues from pathogenic organisms, noxious chemicals, and short-wavelength ultraviolet radiation
C. Helps regulate body temperature
D. Provides location for sensory reception of touch, pressure, temperature, pain, wetness, tickle, etc.
E. Assists in vitamin D synthesis
F. Plays excretory role

Structures of the Integumentary System

A. Epidermis
1. Contains no blood or lymphatic vessels; nourished by diffusion from underlying dermal papillae
2. Melanocytes of the lower epidermis produce melanin, which colors skin
3. Exceptional epidermal regions
    a. Conjunctiva: epidermis so thin it is transparent
    b. Lips: epidermis very thin and highly vascular
B. Dermis
1. Vascular fabric of collagen and elastic fibers woven for strength and flexibility
2. Contains abundant touch receptors
3. Provides fingerprint pattern as unique arrangement of ridges projected to epidermal surface
4. Skin stretched beyond certain limits (e.g., during pregnancy) may rupture dermal collagen and elastic fibers; consequent scar tissue repair produces striae gravidarum
C. Glands
1. Eccrine: sweat glands opening in pores that secrete clear fluid
2. Apocrine: scent glands found in the axillary, mammary, and genital areas
3. Ceruminous: wax glands in external auditory canal
4. Sebaceous: small, saclike glands lacking innervation, usually forming close to hairs and opening into upper portion of hair follicle
5. Mammary: milk-secreting, alveolar glands developing to full extent only during pregnancy
D. Hair
1. About the same number of follicles in males and females; hormones stimulate differential growth
2. Arrector pili (smooth muscle) attached at one end to connective sheath in middle of the hair follicle and at other end to the dermal papillary region of the dermis; on contraction produces "goose-bumps"

Tissue Repair

A. Inflammation
1. Vascular changes: initially there is vasoconstriction; vessel walls lined with leukocytes (margination); then vasodilation and increased vessel permeability (effects of histamine from mast cells, kinins, and prostaglandins); lymphatics become plugged with fibrin to wall off damaged area
2. Leukocytes leave the vessels (diapedesis) and phagocytize foreign substances
3. Chronic inflammation: macrophages predominate and fibroblasts deposit collagen around each group of macrophages and foreign substances; stage of granuloma formation
B. Fibroplasia
1. Epithelization: epithelial cells of the epidermis begin to cover tissue defect
2. Deep in the wound, fibroblasts synthesize collagen and ground substance; process begins about fourth or fifth day and continues for 2 to 4 weeks
3. Capillaries regenerate and tissue becomes red
4. Fibrin plugs are lysed
C. Scar maturation
1. Collagen fibers rearranged into a stronger, more organized pattern
2. Scar remodels, gradually softens, and fades; if collagen synthesis exceeds breakdown, a hypertrophic scar or keloid forms
3. Contraction of wound margins begins about 5 days after injury; fibroblasts migrate into the wound and assist in closing the defect; may result in contractures that can be debilitating

REVIEW OF PHYSICAL PRINCIPLES: HEAT

A. Conduction: transfer of heat from one object to another by direct contact

B. Evaporation: sweat evaporating cools the body surface and acts to drain heat from the body interior

C. Radiation: transfer of heat from one object to another without actual contact

D. Convection: transfer of heat away from the body by air movement

 RELATED PHARMACOLOGY

Pediculicides/scabicides

A. Description
1. Act at the parasite's nerve cell membrane to produce death of the organism
2. Destroy parasitic arthropods
3. Available in topical preparations

B. Examples: lindane (Kwell); malathion (Prioderm lotion)

C. Major side effects: skin irritation (hypersensitivity); contact dermatitis (local irritation)

D. Nursing care
1. Inspect skin, particularly the scalp, for scabies and pediculosis before and after treatment; assess for skin irritation
2. Use gown, gloves, and cap to prevent spread of parasitic arthropods
3. Keep linen of an infected client separate to prevent reinfection of client or family
4. Avoid drug contact with the eyes and mucous membranes

Antiinfectives

A. Description
1. Have bactericidal effect on the bacterial cell wall or alter cellular function
2. Available in topical preparations

B. Examples: mafenide acetate (Sulfamylon); silver nitrate 0.5% solution; silver sulfadiazine (Silvadene)

C. Major side effects
1. Silver sulfadiazine: skin irritation; hemolysis in clients with G-6-PD deficiency
2. Mafenide acetate: metabolic acidosis; burning sensation when first applied
3. Silver nitrate: electrolyte imbalance; brownish black discoloration of skin

D. Nursing care
1. Adhere to strict surgical asepsis, cleanse and debride before application
2. Apply prescribed medications
   a. Silver sulfadiazine: apply to a thickness of $^{1}/_{16}$ inch; monitor G-6-PD level before treatment
   b. Mafenide acetate: assess client for signs of acidosis during course of therapy
   c. Silver nitrate: apply dressings soaked in silver nitrate; avoid contact with drug; assess for signs of electrolyte imbalance during course of therapy

Antipruritics

A. Description
1. Inhibit sensory nerve impulse conduction at the local site and exert a local anesthetic effect
2. Relieve itching and promote comfort
3. Available in topical preparations

B. Examples: benzocaine (Anbesol, Solarcaine), tetracaine HCl (Pontocaine)

C. Major side effects: skin irritation (hypersensitivity); contact dermatitis (local irritation)

D. Nursing care
1. Assess the lesion, including location, size, irritation
2. Discourage client from scratching; keep nails well trimmed
3. Advise medical follow-up because these medications provide only temporary relief of symptoms

Antiinflammatory agents

A. Description
1. Reduce signs of inflammation
2. Produce vasoconstriction, which decreases swelling and pruritus
3. Available in topical preparations

B. Examples: dexamethasone (Decaderm; Hexadrol); hydrocortisone (Acticort), triamcinolone (Aristocort, Kenalog, Trimalone)

C. Major side effects: skin irritation (hypersensitivity); contact dermatitis (local irritation); skin atrophy; adrenal insufficiency if absorbed systemically (suppression of hypothalamic-pituitary-adrenal axis)

D. Nursing care
1. Assess lesions for color, location, and size
2. Protect skin from scratching or rubbing
3. Avoid contact with eyes
4. Cleanse skin before application
5. Assess client for signs of sensitivity
6. Avoid occlusive dressings unless directed otherwise

Dermal agents

A. Description
1. Inhibit keratinization and sebaceous gland function to improve cystic acne and reduce sebum excretion
2. Available preparation: oral

B. Examples: isotretinoin (Accutane), vitamin A acid (Retin-A)

C. Major side effects: visual disturbances: corneal opacities, decreased night vision (vitamin A toxicity—effect on visual rods); papilledema, headache (pseudotumor cerebri); hepatic dysfunction (hepatotoxicity); cheilitis (vitamin A toxicity); pruritus, skin fragility (dryness); hypertriglyceridemia (increased plasma triglycerides)

D. Nursing care
1. Assess visual and hepatic status before administration

2. Monitor blood lipids before and during therapy
3. Instruct client to:
   a. Avoid pregnancy during and for 1 month after therapy; use contraception if sexually active to avoid pregnancy
   b. Avoid vitamin A supplements
   c. Side effects are reversible when therapy is discontinued

MAJOR DISORDERS OF THE INTEGUMENTARY SYSTEM

Skin Lesions

Primary lesions

A. Macule: flat circumscribed area from 1 to several centimeters in size, without elevation (freckle, flat pigmented moles, Rocky Mountain spotted fever)
B. Papule: raised circumscribed area less than 1 cm in size (acne)
C. Nodule: raised solid mass that extends into the dermis and is 1 to 2 cm in size (pigmented nevi)
D. Tumor: solid raised mass that extends into the dermis and is over 2 cm in size (dermatofibroma)
E. Wheal: flattened collection of fluid 1 mm to several centimeters in size (mosquito bites)
F. Vesicle: raised collection of fluid less than 1 cm in size (chickenpox, herpes simplex)
G. Bulla: fluid-filled vesicle over 1 cm in size (second-degree burn, pemphigus)
H. Pustule: vesicle or bulla filled with pus, over 1 cm in size (acne vulgaris)
I. Cyst: mass of fluid-filled tissue that extends to the subcutaneous tissues or dermis, over 1 cm in size (epidermoid cyst)
J. Plaque: bright red, well-demarcated lesion covered with silvery scales (psoriasis)

Secondary lesions

A. Fissure: a linear crack in the skin (athlete's foot)
B. Erosion: nonbleeding loss of superficial dermis (chickenpox rupture)
C. Ulcer: deep loss of skin surface that may bleed (stasis ulcer)
D. Crust: dried residue from blood or pus (impetigo)
E. Scale: flake of exfoliated epidermis (dandruff)

▼ PRESSURE ULCERS (DECUBITUS ULCERS)

Data Base

A. Etiology and pathophysiology
   1. Caused by interruption of circulation when pressure on the skin exceeds capillary pressure of 32 mm Hg

   2. Pressure compresses capillaries and microthrombi form to occlude blood flow; tissue becomes damaged as a result
   3. Most ulcers commonly occur over bony prominences: sacrum, greater trochanter, heels, scapulae, elbows, malleoli, occiput, ears, and ischial tuberosities
   4. Contributing factors
      a. Immobility—results in prolonged pressure
      b. Aging—decreased epidermal thickness, elasticity, and secretion by sebaceous glands
      c. Moisture—causes skin maceration
      d. Inadequate nutrition—loss of subcutaneous tissue reduces padding; inadequate protein intake leads to negative nitrogen balance
      e. Pyrexia—causes increased cellular demand for oxygen
      f. Inadequate tissue oxygenation—edema, anemia and circulatory disturbances result in less oxygen delivered to tissues
      g. Incontinence—substances in urine and feces irritate the skin
      h. Dryness—skin less supple
      i. Shearing force or friction—exerts excessive tension on skin
      j. Cognitive impairments—client not aware of discomfort and does not take protective precautions
      k. Equipment—causes pressure, tension, or shearing forces on skin
   5. Staging determined by:
      a. Depth of tissue damage
         (1) Stage I: nonblanchable area of erythema; skin is intact
         (2) Stage II: partial thickness ulceration of epidermis and/or dermis; presents as an abrasion, blister, or shallow crater
         (3) Stage III: full-thickness ulceration involving the epidermis and dermis, as well as subcutaneous tissue; presents as a deep crater with or without undermining
         (4) Stage IV: extensive tissue damage involving full-thickness skin loss, as well as damage to muscle, bone, and/or supporting structures
      b. Color of wound
         (1) Black: necrotic
         (2) Yellow: exudate and yellow fibrous debris
         (3) Red: pink to red granulation
B. Clinical findings
   1. Subjective: pain; loss of sensation if sensory nerve damage is present
   2. Objective: erythema; tissue damage (see staging of pressure ulcers); exudate; pyrexia and leukocytosis if systemic infection is present

C. Therapeutic interventions
1. Elimination of pressure on the ulcer through positioning and supportive devices (e.g., air-fluidized beds, low-air-loss beds, or kinetic beds)
2. Administration of protein supplements or TPN to prevent negative nitrogen balance if client has serum albumin <3.5 g, is anorexic, or is <80% of ideal body weight
3. Administration of vitamin and mineral supplements to promote wound healing, particularly vitamin C and zinc
4. Debridement of necrotic tissue, which interferes with healing and promotes bacterial growth: mechanical irrigation; chemical debridement with enzyme preparations; surgical debridement; wet to damp dressings
5. Dressings to promote wound healing
   a. Moist gauze: maintains wound humidity that promotes epithelial cell growth
   b. Polyurethane film: provides barrier to bacteria and external fluid, promotes a moist environment, and permits viewing of the wound
   c. Hydrocolloid dressing: maintains wound humidity, liquifies necrotic debris, and provides a protective cushion
   d. Absorptive dressing: absorbs drainage
6. Antibiotic therapy
7. Skin grafts
8. Growth hormone therapy

Nursing Care of Clients with Pressure Ulcers

A. ASSESSMENT
1. Stage, size, and location
2. Type and amount of exudate
3. Risk factors: immobility, incontinence, malnutrition

B. ANALYSIS/NURSING DIAGNOSES
1. Risk for infection related to disruption of the skin surface
2. Impaired skin integrity related to immobility

C. PLANNING/IMPLEMENTATION
1. Emphasize preventive care as soon as contributing factors are identified
2. Change client's position at least every 1 to 2 hours
3. Use supportive devices (e.g., pillows, heel and elbow pads, cushions, special mattresses or bed) to reduce pressure on bony prominences
4. Encourage activity to enhance circulation
5. Bathe the skin to remove irritants and stimulate circulation
6. Massage around bony prominences, but avoid massaging reddened areas that are already damaged
7. Ensure adequate fluid intake

8. Provide well-balanced diet; emphasize importance of protein, zinc, and vitamins C, A, and B
9. Avoid shearing force by lifting, not dragging, the client during position changes

D. EVALUATION/OUTCOMES
1. Maintains intact skin
2. Consumes diet high in protein, zinc, and vitamins C, A, and B
3. Changes position every hour

▼ BURNS

Data Base
A. Etiology and pathophysiology
1. Thermal, radiation, electrical, and chemical (acids, bases) burns: cause cell destruction and result in depletion of fluid and electrolytes
2. Extent of the fluid and electrolyte loss directly related to extent and degree of the burn
   a. Partial thickness
      (1) Superficial partial-thickness (first-degree) burn affects epidermis causing erythema, edema, and pain; fluid loss slight, especially if less than 15% of body surface is involved
      (2) Deep partial-thickness (second-degree) burn affects epidermis and dermis causing erythema, pain, vesicles with oozing; fluid loss slight to moderate, especially if less than 15% of the body surface is involved
   b. Full-thickness (third-degree) burn affects entire dermis and at times the subcutaneous tissue, resulting in charred or pearly white, dry skin and absence of pain; fluid loss usually severe, especially if more than 2% of the body surface is involved
   c. Full-thickness (fourth degree) burn involves skin, fat, muscle, and bone; areas are charred or burned away
3. Classification of burns
   a. Minor burns: no involvement of hands, face, or genitalia; total partial-thickness burn area does not exceed 15%
   b. Moderate burns: partial-thickness involvement of 15% to 25% of body; but full-thickness burns do not exceed 10% of body area
   c. Major burns: involvement exceeds 25% (if partial-thickness) or 10% (if full-thickness) of body surface; involvement of hands, face, genitalia, or feet; this classification is also used if the client has a preexisting chronic health problem, is under 18 months or over 50 years of age, or has additional injuries

4. Pulmonary injury should be suspected if two of the following factors are present, and expected if three or all four are present:
   a. Hair in nostrils singed
   b. Client was trapped in a closed space
   c. Face, nose, and lips burned
   d. Initial blood sample contains carboxyhemoglobin
5. Percentage of body-surface involvement can be estimated by rule of nines or other burn area chart
6. Curling's ulcer may occur after a burn
   a. The client may complain of gastric discomfort, or there may be profuse bleeding; usually occurs by end of the first week after a burn
   b. Treatment essentially the same as for a gastric ulcer; however, mortality following surgical repair is high because of the client's debilitated state
7. Suppressed immune system involving lymphocytes, immunoglobin production, and changes in neutrophil and macrophage functioning
8. Fluid shifts as a result of an osmotic gradient from vessel damage causing increased intercellular and interstitial volumes and diminished intravascular volume

B. Clinical findings
1. Subjective: extreme anxiety, restlessness; pain (severity depends on type of burn) paresthesia; disorientation
2. Objective
   a. Changes in appearance of skin indicate degree of burn
   b. Hematuria; blood hemolysis with subsequent rise in plasma hemoglobin may occur with full-thickness burns
   c. Elevated hematocrit as a result of fluid loss
   d. Electrolyte imbalance: cellular destruction results initially in hyperkalemia, hyponatremia, and hyperuricemia
   e. Presence of symptoms of hypovolemic shock caused by circulatory failure resulting from seepage of water, plasma, proteins, and electrolytes into burned area
   f. Presence of symptoms of neurogenic shock (symptoms similar to hypovolemic shock) caused by the fright, terror, hysteria, and pain involved in the situation
   g. Evidence of renal impairment (e.g., increased BUN and creatinine levels) if acute tubular necrosis occurs as a result of circulatory collapse

C. Therapeutic interventions
1. Establishment of airway and administration of oxygen; mechanical ventilation as needed

2. IV replacement (electrolyte solutions and colloids such as blood and plasma) to maintain circulation
   a. Volume of fluid replacement is based on percentage of body surface area involved and client's weight (e.g., Parkland/Baxter and Brooke Army formula)
   b. Half of fluid is administered in first 8 hours; second half is administered over next 16 hours
3. Reduction of total IV solutions during second 24 hours depends on the urinary output, blood work, and hemodynamic pressures
4. Foley catheter; monitor the urinary output and specific gravity hourly to observe kidney functioning and determine fluid replacement
5. Insertion of central line to monitor hemodynamic pressures (e.g., CVP, PCWP)
6. Vital signs monitored every 15 minutes
7. Serum electrolytes and blood gases to observe for levels and assist in deciding replacement therapy
8. Tetanus toxoid booster administration; tetanus human immune globulin for passive immunity if not previously immunized
9. Nothing by mouth except mineral water for first 24 to 48 hours; clear liquids as tolerated after 2 days; then high-protein, high-carbohydrate, high-fat, high-vitamin diet as tolerated
10. Maintenance of surgical asepsis
11. Daily hydrotherapy; water temperature should be tepid (100° F [37.8° C])
12. Skin grafting to limit fluid loss, promote healing, and limit contractures
   a. Heterograft (xenograft): skin from animals, usually pigs (porcine xenograft)
   b. Homograft (allographs): skin from another person or cadaver
   c. Autograft: skin from another part of the client's body
      (1) Mesh graft: machine used to mesh skin obtained from a donor site so it can be stretched to cover a larger area of burn
      (2) Postage stamp graft: earlier method of accomplishing the same goal as a mesh graft; a small amount of skin is used to cover a larger area; the donor skin is cut into small pieces and applied to the burn
      (3) Sheet grafting: large strips of skin placed over the burn as close together as possible
      (4) Cultured epithelial autografting is used for massive burn treatment
   d. Synthetic coverings

13. Surgical, mechanical, or enzymatic debridement
14. IV antibiotics (based on C&S) and topical antibiotics (mafenide acetate ointment, silver nitrate solution, and silver sulfadiazine, neomycin sulfate, bacitracin, polymyxin B) to limit infection
15. Narcotics to reduce pain and sedatives to decrease anxiety, given IV or orally because of decreased muscle absorption

Nursing Care of Clients with Burns

A. ASSESSMENT

1. Signs of airway involvement: burns of face, neck, or chest; sooty sputum; or hoarseness
2. Vital signs, arterial blood gases, and breath sounds to establish a baseline for respiratory function
3. Central venous pressure (CVP) or pulmonary capillary wedge pressure (PCWP), urine output, and specific gravity to establish baseline for assessment of circulation
4. Estimated body surface area involvement and severity of burns

B. ANALYSIS/NURSING DIAGNOSES

1. Impaired gas exchange related to damaged pulmonary tissue
2. Pain related to exposed nerve endings
3. Deficient fluid volume related to fluid loss through burn wound and shift of fluid out of intravascular compartment
4. Risk for infection related to disruption of skin
5. Excess fluid volume related to the physiologic response to the stress of injury and IV fluid administration
6. Disturbed body image related to perception of appearance

C. PLANNING/IMPLEMENTATION

1. Neutralize the burn if caused by a chemical (acid, base); flush with water and apply the opposite chemical in a weak form as ordered
2. Monitor vital signs, CVP or PCWP, intake and output (hourly urine output), and specific gravity as ordered; notify the physician if deviations occur or if output falls below 30 ml or rises above 50 ml per hour
3. Maintain patency of the Foley; obtain hourly urines
4. Observe for signs of electrolyte imbalance (calcium, potassium, and sodium) and metabolic acidosis
5. Administer fluid and electrolytes as ordered
6. Monitor respiratory function: characteristics of respirations, breath sounds, and arterial blood gases
7. Administer oxygen as ordered
8. Elevate head of the bed
9. Encourage client to cough, deep breathe, and use incentive spirometer
10. Observe for signs of infection (rising temperature and white blood cell count, odor)
11. Follow principles of infection control (gown, gloves, mask, hair covering) during contact because the client's ability to resist infection is compromised
12. Administer tetanus toxoid as ordered
13. Administer IV and topical antibiotics as ordered
14. Use sterile technique for wound care
15. Apply pressure dressings as ordered to reduce contractures and scarring
16. Support the joints and extremities in a functional position and perform range-of-motion exercises; use beds or mattresses designed to avoid pressure
17. Provide care related to skin graft
    a. Keep donor sites (which are covered with a nonadherent dressing and wrapped in an absorbent gauze) dry; remove absorbent gauze as ordered; nonadherent dressing will separate as healing occurs
    b. Monitor the grafts, which are generally left with a light pressure dressing for approximately 3 days; after the graft has "taken," roll cotton-tipped applicators gently over the graft to remove underlying exudate; allowed to remain, exudate could promote infection, which could prevent the graft from adhering; instruct client to restrict mobility of the affected part
    c. Observe for foul-smelling drainage, temperature elevation, and other signs of infection.
    d. Instruct the client to avoid exposure of the graft and donor sites to the sun
18. Support the client physically and emotionally while turning
19. Keep room temperature warm and humidity high
20. Observe for symptoms of stress ulcer; give ordered drugs to decrease or neutralize HCl
21. Provide small, frequent feedings; diet high in protein, carbohydrates, vitamins, and minerals; moderate in fat, with adequate calories for protein sparing
22. Give medication for pain as ordered and particularly before dressing change
23. Expect the client to express negative feelings and accept them
24. Explain need for staff wearing gowns and masks
25. Give realistic reassurance
26. Encourage participation in self-care
27. Refer client and family to support groups and rehabilitative services

D. EVALUATION/OUTCOMES
1. Maintains respiratory function
2. Maintains fluid balance
3. Remains free of infection
4. Expresses feelings about altered body image

▼ CELLULITIS

Data Base

A. Etiology and pathophysiology
   1. Infection of deep layers of the dermis; spreads along connective tissue planes
   2. Usually caused by streptococcal or staphylococcal organisms
   3. Organism enters tissue through abrasion, bite, trauma, or wound
   4. Erysipelas is an acute infection of superficial dermis and lymphatics caused by beta-hemolytic group A streptococci
B. Clinical findings
   1. Subjective: pain; itching
   2. Objective: swelling; redness, warmth; leukocytosis
C. Therapeutic interventions
   1. IV, IM, or oral antibiotic therapy following cultures of the area
   2. Rest with elevation of extremity
   3. Hot compresses

Nursing Care of Clients with Cellulitis

A. ASSESSMENT
1. Progression of symptoms
2. Signs of inflammation
3. Evidence of trauma
4. Evidence of impaired immune response from history
5. Vital signs and white blood cell count for database

B. ANALYSIS/NURSING DIAGNOSES
1. Risk for infection related to disruption of skin surface
2. Impaired skin integrity related to inflammatory response
3. Pain related to pressure on nerve endings

C. PLANNING/IMPLEMENTATION
1. Monitor vital signs and WBC count for evidence of systemic involvement
2. Use appropriate aseptic technique when cleaning area
3. Use infection control techniques
4. Administer analgesics and antibiotics as ordered
5. Elevate extremity
6. Apply warm compresses as ordered; protect from thermal trauma

D. EVALUATION/OUTCOMES
1. Experiences resolution of inflammatory process
2. Reports relief of pain

▼ CANCER OF THE SKIN

Data Base

A. Etiology and pathophysiology
   1. Most common cancer; slow progression and cure rate high
   2. Exposure to the sun, irritating chemicals, and chronic friction implicated; more common in persons with fair complexions
   3. Types
      a. Basal cell carcinoma: generally located on the face and appears as a waxy nodule that may have telangiectasias visible; the most common type of skin cancer, but metastasis is rare
      b. Squamous cell carcinoma: develops rapidly and may metastasize through local lymph nodes; may develop secondarily to precancerous lesions such as keratosis and leukoplakia and is found most frequently on upper extremities and face, which are exposed to the sun; it appears as a small, red, nodular lesion
      c. Malignant melanoma: most serious type and arises from the pigment-producing melanocytes; the color of the lesion may vary greatly (white, flesh, gray, brown, blue, black); changes in size, color, sensation, or characteristics of a mole suggest the possibility of malignant melanoma; metastasis via blood can be extensive
B. Clinical findings
   1. Subjective: pruritus may or may not be present; localized soreness
   2. Objective: change in color, size, or shape of preexisting lesion; oozing, bleeding, or crusting; biopsy of tumor reveals type of cancer; lymphadenopathy if metastasis has occurred
C. Therapeutic interventions
   1. Surgical excision of the lesion and surrounding tissue
   2. Chemosurgery, which involves the use of zinc chloride to fix the cells before they are dissected by layers
   3. Cryosurgery utilizing liquid nitrogen to destroy the tumor cells by freezing
   4. Radiation (malignant melanoma does not respond well to this mode of treatment)
   5. Electrodesiccation and curettage—mechanical disruption of cells by heat which are cut away with curet

6. Laser light is used to vaporize lesions
7. Chemotherapy
8. Nonspecific immunostimulants such as BCG vaccine

Nursing Care of Clients with Cancer of the Skin

A. ASSESSMENT
1. History of changes in size, color, shape, sensation, or unusual bleeding of lesions
2. Risk factors from history
3. Skin for presence of suspicious lesions, documenting objective and subjective characteristics

B. ANALYSIS/NURSING DIAGNOSES
1. Risk for infection related to damaged skin
2. Disturbed body image related to altered appearance

C. PLANNING/IMPLEMENTATION
1. Instruct the client to examine moles for changes and have those subject to chronic irritation (bra or belt line) removed
2. Encourage to avoid exposure to the sun; use sunscreens with a rating higher than 15 SPF (solar protection factor); wear protective clothing
3. Emphasize continued medical supervision
4. Encourage verbalization; maintain a therapeutic environment
5. Provide care to the client receiving radiation: observe skin for local reaction; avoid use of ointments or powders containing metals
6. Provide care related to specific chemotherapeutic agents (see Pharmacology Related to Neoplastic Disorders)
7. Support natural defense mechanisms of client; encourage intake of nutrient-dense foods with emphasis on fruits, vegetables, whole grains, and legumes, especially those high in the immune-stimulating nutrients selenium and vitamins A, C, and E; betacarotene has been associated with prevention of skin cancer
8. Encourage client to verbalize fears

D. EVALUATION/OUTCOMES
1. Avoids exposure to the sun and known irritants
2. Examines skin lesions regularly and reports changes to physician
3. Verbalizes acceptance of physical appearance after surgical excision of lesions

▼ HERPES ZOSTER (SHINGLES)

Data Base
A. Etiology and pathophysiology
1. Acute viral infection of structures along the pathway of peripheral nerves caused by reactivation of the varicella-zoster virus
2. Occurs in clients who have had chickenpox and are exposed to an affected individual
3. Occurs in immunosuppressed clients who have previously had chickenpox (e.g., leukemia, lymphoma)
4. May involve the eye, leading to keratitis, uveitis, and blindness
B. Clinical findings
1. Subjective: pain; paresthesias; pruritus
2. Objective: painful, pruritic vesicles along the involved nerves; stains made from lesion exudate isolate the organism
C. Therapeutic interventions
1. Administration of acyclovir (Zovirax) or valacyclovir (Valtrex)
2. Medications for pain, relaxation, itching, and prevention of secondary infection
3. Control of pain by blocking the nerve through injection of drugs such as lidocaine or applying medication such as triamcinolone (Kenalog)
4. Antiinflammatory drugs such as systemic or topical steroids

Nursing Care of Clients with Herpes Zoster

A. ASSESSMENT
1. Progression of symptoms from history, includes factors that compromise the immune response (e.g., age, disease, chemotherapy)
2. Presence of characteristic lesion

B. ANALYSIS/NURSING DIAGNOSES
1. Risk for infection related to disruption of skin surface
2. Pain related to irritation of nerve endings

C. PLANNING/IMPLEMENTATION
1. Administer analgesics and other medications as ordered
2. Reduce itching and protect lesions from air by the application of salves, ointments, lotions, and sterile dressings as ordered
3. Protect from pressure by use of air mattress, bed cradle, and light, loose clothing (avoid synthetic and woolen materials and use cotton fabrics)
4. In addition to standard precautions, use airborne and/or contact precautions as indicated
5. Administer antibiotics as ordered
6. Encourage client to avoid scratching and to use gloves at night to limit the possibility of accidental scratching
7. Assist the client to understand the basis for the rash and the itch
8. Allay fears that may be based on old wives' tales about shingles
9. Encourage the client to express feelings
10. Encourage diet rich in nutrient-dense foods such as fruits, vegetables, whole grains, and legumes to improve and maintain nutritional

status and prevent possible drug-induced nutrient deficiencies; encourage intake of vitamin C because it has been reported to stimulate the immune response to viral infection by increasing interferon, which limits viral reproduction in early stages

11. Teach proper hand washing to help prevent spreading of the virus; individuals who have not had chickenpox should not be assigned to provide care

D. EVALUATION/OUTCOMES
1. Experiences an improvement in skin integrity
2. Reports that pain and pruritus have subsided

▼ SYSTEMIC LUPUS ERYTHEMATOSUS (SLE)

Data Base

A. Etiology and pathophysiology
1. Origin unknown; affects the connective tissue and is thought to result from a defect in the body's immunologic mechanisms, genetic predisposition, or environmental stimuli
2. Immune complex deposits in blood vessels, among collagen fibers, and on organs
3. Necrosis of the glomerular capillaries, inflammation of cerebral and ocular blood vessels, necrosis of lymph nodes, vasculitis of the GI tract and pleura, and degeneration of the basal layer of skin
4. More common in females, ages 15 to 40

B. Clinical findings
1. Subjective: malaise; photosensitivity; joint pain
2. Objective: fever; butterfly erythema on the face; erythema of palms; positive lupus erythematosus preparation (LE prep); increased antinuclear antibodies (ANA) in blood; Raynaud's phenomenon; weight loss; evidence of impaired renal, gastrointestinal, cardiac, respiratory, and neurologic functions

C. Therapeutic interventions
1. Corticosteroids and analgesics to reduce pain and inflammation
2. Supportive therapy as major organs become affected
3. Plasmapheresis to remove autoantibodies and immune complexes from the blood
4. Life-threatening SLE may be treated with stem cell transplants

Nursing Care of Clients with Systemic Lupus Erythematosus

A. ASSESSMENT
1. Progression of symptoms from the history
2. Presence of skin lesions

3. Sensitivity to light (photosensitivity)
4. Vital signs for baseline data
5. Heart and lung sounds
6. Abdomen for enlargement of liver and spleen
7. Neurologic status
8. Renal function (review BUN and creatinine analysis results)

B. ANALYSIS/NURSING DIAGNOSES
1. Excess fluid volume related to disease process and corticosteroid therapy
2. Pain related to damage to nerve endings
3. Anxiety related to fear of death

C. PLANNING/IMPLEMENTATION
1. Administer corticosteroids and observe for side effects, teaching client to do the same (see Pharmacology Related to Integumentary System Disorders)
2. Help client and family cope with severity of the disease and its poor prognosis
3. Explain the importance of protecting skin: use of mild soap; avoidance of exposure to sunlight; use of sun-blocking agents
4. Assist client to establish regular program of exercise balanced by rest periods to avoid fatigue
5. Instruct client to alter the consistency and frequency of meals if dysphagia and anorexia exist
6. Encourage diet rich in nutrient-dense foods such as fruits, vegetables, whole grains, and legumes to improve and maintain nutritional status and compensate for nutrient interactions of corticosteroid and other therapeutic medications; emphasize vitamin C because it is essential in the biosynthesis of collagen, and large doses have been found to increase total collagen synthesis
7. Emphasize the need for continued medical follow-up

D. EVALUATION/OUTCOMES
1. Demonstrates a reduction in skin lesions
2. States that pain is reduced
3. Verbalizes fears with family and health care providers

▼ PROGRESSIVE SYSTEMIC SCLEROSIS (SCLERODERMA)

Data Base

A. Etiology and pathophysiology
1. Thought to be caused by an autoimmune defect; occurs in women more frequently than in men
2. Systemic disease that causes fibrotic changes in connective tissue throughout the body

3. May involve the skin, blood vessels, synovial membranes, esophagus, heart, lungs, kidneys, or GI tract
4. CREST syndrome refers to a group of symptoms associated with a poor prognosis: **C**alcium deposits in organs; **R**aynaud's phenomenon; **E**sophageal dysfunction; **S**clerodactyly (scleroderma of the digits); **T**elangiectasia

B. Clinical findings
1. Subjective: articular pain; muscle weakness
2. Objective
   a. Hard skin that eventually adheres to underlying structures; face becomes masklike; body motion restricted
   b. Telangiectases on the lips, fingers, face, and tongue
   c. Dysphagia
   d. Raynaud's phenomenon
   e. Positive LE prep elevated gamma-globulin levels, presence of antinuclear antibodies

C. Therapeutic interventions
1. Corticosteroids
2. Salicylates or analgesics for joint pain
3. Vasodilators for symptoms of Raynaud's phenomenon
4. Physical therapy

Nursing Care of Clients with Scleroderma

A. ASSESSMENT
1. Onset and progression of symptoms from history
2. Skin, particularly of the hands and face
3. Joints for inflammation

B. ANALYSIS/NURSING DIAGNOSES
1. Impaired skin integrity related to disturbance of the skin surface
2. Risk for injury related to pain and altered mobility
3. Anxiety related to prognosis

C. PLANNING/IMPLEMENTATION
1. Support the client and family emotionally; there is no cure at present
2. Use mild soaps and lotions for skin care
3. Instruct client to avoid smoking and exposure to cold
4. Encourage deep-breathing exercises
5. Teach the client the importance of observing for side effects of corticosteroids or other immunosuppressive drugs
6. Monitor function of all vital organs (e.g., cardiac, respiratory, and renal status)

D. EVALUATION/OUTCOMES
1. Maintains skin integrity
2. Verbalizes acceptance of changes in appearance and disease
3. Reports symptoms of vital organ involvement

NEUROMUSCULOSKELETAL SYSTEM

REVIEW OF ANATOMY AND PHYSIOLOGY

Structures and Functions of the Nervous System

Overview
A. Neurons (nerve cells) are basic structural and functional units
B. Central nervous system (CNS): spinal cord and brain
C. Peripheral nervous system (PNS): nerves and ganglia
D. Autonomic nervous system (ANS): sympathetic and parasympathetic
E. Sense organs

Neurons
A. General properties and functions
1. Irritability: response to stimulus
2. Conductivity: conduct electrical energy (nerve impulse); basis for body's rapid communication and integration network
3. Types
   a. Sensory (afferent) neurons: transmit impulses to spinal cord or brain
   b. Motoneurons (motor or efferent neurons): transmit impulses away from brain or spinal cord toward or to muscles or glands
   c. Interneurons: transmit impulses from sensory neurons to motoneurons
4. Neurons cannot be replaced if lost, but neuronal contents are constantly being replenished
B. Structure: well suited to transmitting impulses over distances
1. Cell body contains a nucleus and other cytoplasmic organdies
2. Axon: one fiber per neuron; carries impulse away from cell body
3. Dendrites: several per neuron; carry impulses toward cell body
4. Supportive coverings and sheaths
   a. Neurilemma: sheath of cells (Schwann cells) forming an envelope around axons and some dendrites (myelin sheath); responsible for effective regeneration of a nerve fiber after injury in the peripheral nervous system
   b. Myelin: multiple, dense layers of membrane wrapped around an axon or dendrite; gaps in myelin are called nodes of Ranvier; myelinated nerve fibers transmit nerve impulses more rapidly than nonmyelinated fibers of same diameter
5. Neuronal cell membrane
   a. Pumps: actively transport ions (notably sodium and potassium) between intracellular and interstitial fluid

b. Channels: provide selective pathways for diffusion of specific ions; channels open and close (gating mechanisms) in response to voltage changes and chemicals

c. Receptors: involved in depolarization and repolarization

d. Enzymes: catalyze chemical reactions on the membrane surface

e. Structural proteins: interconnect cells to form tissues and organs; hold cell parts together

6. Synapse

a. Point of contact between axon of one cell and dendrite of another; actual physical gap is called synaptic cleft

b. At the synapse, the axon terminals enlarge to form a terminal button (bouton), which is the information-delivering part of the synapse

c. Some synapses are excitatory and others inhibitory

7. Neuroglia support, defend, and nourish neurons; chief source of GNS tumors; retain the ability to divide; astrocytes provide framework of cells and fibers that suspend neurons and help provide the blood-brain barrier

Brain

A. General considerations

1. Most active of all body organs in energy consumption; has large blood supply and high oxygen consumption

2. Neurons can only utilize glucose for energy metabolism; therefore hypoglycemia can seriously alter brain function and lead to coma

3. Brain cells protected by the blood-brain barrier, a selective filtration system that isolates the brain from substances in the general circulation

B. Regions of brain and their functions

1. Basic tissue types

a. Gray matter: aggregations of neuron cell bodies

b. White matter: composed primarily of tracts of myelinated fibers (axons)

2. Anatomic regions

a. Hindbrain (brainstem): lowermost brain division; formed by enlargement of the spinal cord as it enters the cranial cavity

(1) Medulla: lowest portion of the hindbrain

(a) Conducts impulses between the cord and brain

(b) Contains important reflex centers for heart, blood vessel diameter, respiratory reflexes, vomiting, coughing, and swallowing

(2) Pons: located just above the medulla

(a) Conducts impulses between the cord and various parts of the brain

(b) Contains reflex centers for cranial nerves V, VI, VII, and VIII (trigeminal, abducent, facial, and acoustic)

b. Cerebellum: dorsal appendage of the hindbrain

(1) Exerts synergic control over the skeletal muscles producing smooth, steady, and precise movements

(2) Coordinates skeletal muscle contractions and plays an essential part in producing normal postures and maintaining equilibrium

c. Midbrain: part of the brain located between the pons, which lies below it, and the diencephalon and cerebrum, which lie above it

(1) Integrates and analyzes sensory input from the ears, eyes, and various regions of the cerebral cortex; puts out motor information to lower motor system

(2) Reflex centers for cranial nerves III (oculomotor) and IV (trochlear): pupillary reflexes and eye movements

(3) Pineal body; precise function unknown; may be part of endocrine system, helping to regulate secretion of gonadotropins from the hypophysis cerebri

d. Forebrain

(1) Optic vesicles: develop into the retinas connected to base of the forebrain by their stalks, the optic nerves

(2) Diencephalon: unpaired division of the forebrain; cerebral hemispheres diverge from this structure

(a) Thalamus

• Processes incoming sensory information before distribution to the somatosensory cortex; crudely translates sensory impulses into sensations but does not localize them on a body region

• Processes motor information from the cerebral cortex and cerebellum and projects its analysis back to the motor cortex

• Contributes to the concentrating ability by filtering out distracting sensory input

• Contributes to emotional component of sensations (pleasant or unpleasant)

(b) Hypothalamus: forms floor of third ventricle

• Forms a crucial part of the neural path by which emotions and

other cerebral functions can alter vital, automatic functions such as the heartbeat, blood pressure, peristalsis, and secretion by glands
- Secretes neuropeptides that influence secretion of various important anterior pituitary hormones; for example, TRH and LH-RH regulate the pituitary secretions of TSH and gonadotropic hormones, respectively
- Hypothalamic neurons make ADH and oxytocin, but the posterior pituitary gland secretes them
- Contains appetite center and satiety center
- Serves as a heat-regulating center by relaying impulses to lower autonomic centers for vasoconstriction, vasodilation, and sweating, and to somatic centers for shivering
- Maintains waking state; part of arousal or alerting neural pathway

(c) Corpus callosum: interconnects the two cerebral hemispheres

(d) Optic chiasm: the point of crossing over (decussation) of optic nerve fibers from the nasal half of each retina to the opposite side, where they join optic nerve fibers from the lateral half of the other eye's retina to form the optic tracts

(3) Paired cerebral hemispheres: consists of frontal, parietal, temporal, and occipital lobes and deeper regions of gray matter and fiber tracts

(a) Cerebral cortex is outer layer of gray matter forming folds (convolutions) composed of hills (gyri) and valleys (sulci)

(b) Frontal lobes:
- Influence abstract thinking, sense of humor, and uniqueness of personality
- Control contraction of skeletal muscles and synchronization of muscular movements
- Exert control over hypothalamus; influence basic biorhythms
- Control muscular movements necessary for speech; found only in one cerebral hemisphere

(c) Parietal lobes:
- Translate nerve impulses into sensations (e.g., touch, temperature)
- Interpret sensations; provide appreciation of size, shape, texture, and weight
- Interpret sense of taste

(d) Temporal lobes:
- Translate nerve impulses into sensations of sound and interpret sounds
- Interpret sense of smell
- Control behavior patterns

(e) Occipital area
- Translates nerve impulse into sights and interprets sights
- Provides appreciation of size, shape, and color

(4) Brain and spinal cord coverings

(a) Bony: vertebrae around the cord; cranial bones around the brain

(b) Membranous: called meninges; consist of three layers
- Dura mater: white fibrous tissue, outer layer
- Arachnoid membrane: cobwebby middle layer
- Pia mater: innermost layer; adheres to outer surface of the cord and brain; contains blood vessels

(5) Cord and brain fluid spaces

(a) Subarachnoid space around the brain and cord and extending beyond the cord into the fourth and fifth lumbar vertebrae

(b) Central canal inside the cord

(c) Ventricles and cerebral aqueduct inside the brain; four cavities known as first, second, third, and fourth ventricles

(6) Formation and circulation of the cerebrospinal fluid (CSF)

(a) Formed by plasma filtering from the network of capillaries (choroid plexus) in each ventricle; active transport of plasma also involved

(b) Circulates throughout the ventricles, brain, and subarachnoid space and returns to blood via venous sinuses of the brain

Cranial Nerves: 12 Pairs
See Table 6-5
Spinal cord
A. Location: in the spinal cavity, from the foramen magnum to the first lumbar vertebra

B. Structure
   1. Incompletely divided into right and left symmetric halves
   2. Inner core consists of gray matter shaped like a three-dimensional H
   3. Long columns of white matter surround the cord's inner core of gray matter; namely, right and left anterior, lateral, and posterior columns; composed of numerous sensory and motor tracts (Fig. 6-3, *A* and *B*)
C. Functions
   1. Sensory tracts conduct impulses up cord to brain; motor tracts conduct impulses down cord from brain
   2. Gray matter of cord contains reflex centers for all spinal cord reflexes

Spinal nerves: 31 pairs
A. Branches of the spinal nerves form plexuses or intricate networks of fibers (e.g., brachial plexus), from which nerves emerge to supply various parts of the skin, mucosa, and skeletal muscles
B. All spinal nerves are mixed nerves composed of both sensory dendrites and motor axons

Autonomic nervous system
A. Division of the nervous system: conducts impulses from the brainstem or cord out to visceral effectors: cardiac muscle, smooth muscle, and glandular tissue
B. Consists of two divisions: the sympathetic nervous system and the parasympathetic nervous system
   1. Sympathetic system
      a. Adrenergic fibers secrete norepinephrine

TABLE 6-5   Distribution and function of cranial nerve pairs

Name and number	Distribution	Function
Olfactory (I)	Nasal mucosa, high up along the septum especially	Sense of smell (sensory only)
Optic (II)	Retina of eyeball	Vision (sensory only)
Oculomotor (III)	Extrinsic muscles of eyeball, except superior oblique and external rectus; also intrinsic eye muscles (iris and ciliary)	Eye movements; constriction of pupil and bulging of lens, which together produce accommodation for near vision
Trochlear (IV), smallest cranial nerve	Superior oblique muscle of eye	Eye movements
Trigeminal (V) (or trifacial), largest cranial nerve	Sensory fibers to skin and mucosa of head and to teeth; muscles of mastication (sensory and motor fibers)	Sensation in head and face; chewing movements
Abducent (VI)	External rectus muscle of eye	Abduction of eye
Facial (VII)	Muscles of facial expression; taste buds of anterior two thirds of tongue; motor fibers to submaxillary and sublingual salivary glands	Facial expressions; taste; secretion of saliva
Acoustic (VIII) (vestibulocochlear)	Inner ear	Hearing and equilibrium (sensory only)
Glossopharyngeal (IX)	Posterior third of tongue; mucosa and muscles of pharynx; parotid gland; carotid sinus and body	Taste and other sensations of tongue; secretion of saliva; swallowing movements; function in reflex arcs for control of blood pressure and respiration
Vagus (X) (or pneumogastric)	Mucosa and muscles of pharynx, larynx, trachea, bronchi, esophagus; thoracic and abdominal viscera	Sensations and movements of organs supplied; for example, slows heart, increases peristalsis and gastric and pancreatic secretion; voice production
Spinal accessory (XI)	Certain neck and shoulder muscles (muscles of larynx, sternocleidomastoid, trapezius)	Shoulder movements; turns head; voice production; muscle sense
Hypoglossal (XII)	Tongue muscles	Tongue movements, as in talking; muscle sense

Note: The first letters of the words in the following sentence are the first letters of the cranial nerves, and many generations of anatomy students have used it as an aid to memorizing the names: "On Old Olympus' Towering Tops, A Finn and German Viewed Some Hops." (There are several slightly different versions of the mnemonic.)

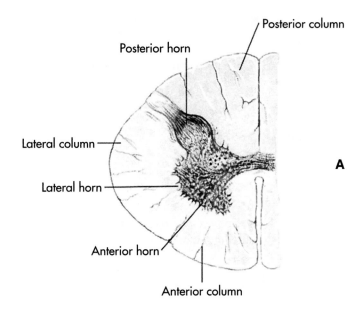

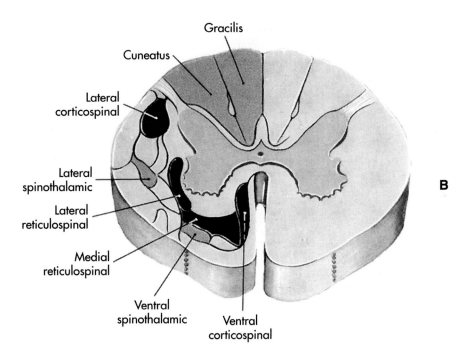

FIGURE 6-3 **A,** Distribution of gray matter (horns) and white matter (columns) in a section of the spinal cord at the thoracic level. **B,** Location in the spinal cord of some major projection tracts. Black areas are descending motor tracts. Shaded areas are ascending sensory tracts. (From Thibodeau GA, Patton KT: *Anatomy and physiology,* ed 4, St. Louis, 1999, Mosby.)

  b. Influences smooth muscle of blood vessels and hairs and sweat glands
2. Parasympathetic system
  a. Cholinergic fibers secrete acetylcholine
  b. Influences digestive tract and smooth muscle to promote digestive gland secretion, peristalsis, and defecation

  c. Influences the heart to decrease rate and strengthen contractility
  d. Vagus nerve is the most significant parasympathetic nerve
C. Autonomic antagonism and summation: sympathetic and parasympathetic impulses tend to produce opposite effects (Table 6-6)

TABLE 6-6   Autonomic functions

Autonomic effector	Effect of sympathetic stimulation (neurotransmitter: norepinephrine unless otherwise stated)	Effect of parasympathetic stimulation (neurotransmitter: acetylcholine)
CARDIAC MUSCLE	Increased rate and strength of contraction (beta receptors)	Decreased rate and strength of contraction
SMOOTH MUSCLE OF BLOOD VESSELS		
Skin blood vessels	Constriction (alpha receptors)	No effect
Skeletal muscle blood vessels	Dilation (beta receptors)	No effect
Coronary blood vessels	Constriction (alpha receptors) Dilation (beta receptors)	Dilation
Abdominal blood vessels	Constriction (alpha receptors)	No effect
Blood vessels of external genitals	Constriction (alpha receptors)	Dilation of blood vessels causing erection
SMOOTH MUSCLE OF HOLLOW ORGANS AND SPHINCTERS		
Bronchioles	Dilation (beta receptors)	Constriction
Digestive tract, except sphincters	Decreased peristalsis (beta receptors)	Increased peristalsis
Sphincters of digestive tract	Constriction (alpha receptors)	Relaxation
Urinary bladder	Relaxation (beta receptors)	Contraction
Urinary sphincters	Constriction (alpha receptors)	Relaxation
Reproductive ducts	Contraction (alpha receptors)	Relaxation
Eye		
Iris	Contraction of radial muscle; dilated pupil	Contraction of circular muscle; constricted pupil
Ciliary	Relaxation; accommodates for far vision	Contraction; accommodates for near vision
Hairs (pilomotor muscles)	Contraction produces goose pimples, or piloerection (alpha receptors)	No effect
GLANDS		
Sweat	Increased sweat (neurotransmitter: acetylcholine)	No effect
Lacrimal	No effect	Increased secretion of tears
Digestive (salivary, gastric, etc.)	Decreased secretion of saliva; not known for others	Increased secretion of saliva
Pancreas, including islets	Decreased secretion	Increased secretion of pancreatic juice and insulin
Liver	Increased glycogenolysis (beta receptors); increased blood sugar level	No effect
*Adrenal medulla**	Increased epinephrine secretion	No effect

*Sympathetic preganglionic axons terminate in contact with secreting cells of the adrenal medulla. Thus the adrenal medulla functions, to quote someone's descriptive phrase, as a "giant sympathetic postganglionic neuron." (From GA Thibodeau, KT Patton: *Anatomy and physiology,* ed 4, St. Louis, 1999, Mosby.)

D. Under conditions of stress, sympathetic impulses to the visceral effectors usually increase greatly and dominate over parasympathetic impulses; however, in some individuals under stress, parasympathetic impulses via the vagus nerve to glands and smooth muscle of the stomach greatly increase, causing increased hydrochloric acid secretion and increased gastric motility

E. Sympathectomy, a surgical procedure that interferes with the nervous system, causes blood vessel dilation resulting in a lowered blood pressure

Nerve impulse conduction

A. General considerations
1. Permits communication between distant body regions
2. Larger nerve fibers and a thicker myelin sheath

produce greater velocity
3. Sodium-potassium pump: transports sodium out and potassium into the cell; requires ATP to work

B. Impulse generation
1. Resting potential: exists when cells are in an unstimulated or resting state
2. Action potential: composed of depolarization and repolarization, propagates itself down the axon or dendrite and is known as the nerve impulse

C. Reflex arcs
1. Two-neuron (monosynaptic) reflex arc: simplest arc possible; consists of at least one sensory neuron, one synapse, and one motoneuron (motor neuron)
2. Three-neuron arc: consists of at least one sensory neuron, one synapse, one interneuron, one synapse, and one motoneuron
3. Complex multisynaptic neural pathways also exist

D. Conduction across synapses
1. Given synapse can transmit only one type of transmitter substance
2. There are 30 different types of neurotransmitters, including
   a. Monoamines (norepinephrine, dopamine, serotonin, acetylcholine); axons that release acetylcholine are called cholinergic; those that release norepinephrine are called adrenergic
   b. Amino acids (gamma-aminobutyric acid [GABA], glutamic acid, glycine, taurine); GABA is the most common inhibitory transmitter in the brain
   c. Neuropeptides (hormone-releasing hormones, enkephalins, and endorphins); some influence hormone levels and some influence perception and integration of pain and emotional experience
   d. Prostaglandins: high levels in brain tissue; some inhibit and some excite; may moderate the action of other transmitters by influencing the neuronal membrane

Sensorineural pathways (from periphery to cerebral cortex)
A. Sensory pathways to the cerebral cortex from the periphery
1. Sensory neuron I: from periphery to the cord or brainstem
2. Sensory neuron II: from cord or brainstem to the thalamus
3. Sensory neuron III: from thalamus to the somatosensory area of cerebral cortex

B. Localization and discrimination of sensations occur when impulses reach the cerebral cortex
C. Most sensory neuron II axons decussate; one side

of the brain registers most of the sensations for the opposite side of the body
D. Impulses related to pain and temperature are conducted up the lateral spinothalamic tracts to the thalamus
E. Impulses related to touch and pressure are conducted to the thalamus by the posterior white columns and the ventral spinothalamic tracts
F. Impulses that result in proprioception or kinesthesia (sense of position of body parts) are conducted over the same pathway as touch and pressure sensations
G. Reticular activating system: conduction by this system is essential for producing and maintaining consciousness

Motoneural pathways (from cerebral cortex to periphery)
A. Final common path (lower motoneurons and somatic motoneurons): consists of anterior horn neurons (motoneurons whose dendrites and cell bodies lie in anterior gray columns of the cord and whose axons extend through the anterior roots of spinal nerves and their branches to terminate in skeletal muscles)
B. Motor pathways from the cerebral cortex to anterior horn cells are classified according to the route by which the fibers enter the cord
1. Pyramidal tracts (corticospinal tracts): axons of neurons whose dendrites and cell bodies lie in the cerebral cortex; necessary for willed movements to occur; hence one cause of paralysis is interruption of pyramidal tract conduction
2. Extrapyramidal tracts: all tracts that conduct between the motor cortex and the anterior horn cells, except the pyramidal tracts; essential for producing large, automatic movements and facial expressions
C. Motor conduction pathway from the primary motor area of the cerebral cortex to skeletal muscles via pyramidal tracts consists of a two-neuron relay; an upper motoneuron conducts impulses from cerebrum to cord and a lower motoneuron (anterior horn cell) conducts from cord to skeletal muscle

Sense organs
A. General considerations
1. Millions of receptors distributed widely throughout the skin and mucosa; muscles, tendons, joints, and viscera are sense organs of body
2. Receptors monitor internal and external environment
3. Stimuli are interpreted and converted to nerve impulses, which are conducted through sensory neurons to the brain
4. Receptors' degrees of depolarization depend on the strength of the stimulus
B. Types of receptors

1. Exteroceptors of skin and mucosa: different receptors for different sensations such as heat, cold, pain, touch, and pressure
2. Proprioceptors of muscles, tendons, and joints: stretching of muscles or tendons during movements initiates stretch reflexes
3. Visceroceptors: pressoreceptors (baroreceptors) respond to stretch in walls of the aorta and carotid arteries, providing the brain with information on blood pressure; oxygen chemoreceptors in the aortic and carotid bodies monitor O_2 levels; carbon dioxide chemoreceptors in the respiratory center (in medulla) help control the rate and depth of respirations
4. Taste
   a. Taste buds consist of groups of receptor cells connected to the facial and glossopharyngeal nerves (VII and IX)
   b. Respond to chemicals: sweet at tongue tip; sour and salt at tip and sides; bitter at back
   c. Olfaction intimately involved in the sense of taste
5. Olfaction
   a. Receptors in epithelium of the nasal mucosa; odors sensed as chemicals interact with receptor sites on sensory hairs of olfactory cells
   b. Olfactory neural pathways utilize cranial nerve I
6. Sight
   a. Coats of the eyeball: outer (sclera proper and cornea); middle (choroid proper, ciliary body, suspensory ligament holding lens, iris); inner (retina)
   b. Cavities and humors of the eyeball: anterior cavity contains aqueous humor; posterior cavity contains vitreous humor
   c. Muscles of the eye
      (1) Extrinsic: attached to outside of eyeball and to bones of orbit; move eyeball in various directions
      (2) Intrinsic: within eyeball; regulate size of pupil and control shape of lens making possible accommodation for near and far objects
   d. Refractory media of the eye: cornea, aqueous humor, vitreous humor, crystalline lens (has greatest refractive power)
   e. Accessory structures of the eye
      (1) Eyebrows and lashes
      (2) Eyelids: lined with mucous membrane (conjunctiva) that continues over surface of eyeball; where lids join, called inner and outer canthi
      (3) Lacrimal apparatus: lacrimal glands, ducts, sacs, and nasolacrimal ducts
   f. Physiology of vision
      (1) Formation of an image on the retina
         (a) Macula lutea: center of the retina that receives and analyzes light only from the center of the visual field; contains the fovea centralis where cones are concentrated
         (b) Refraction: bending of light rays as they pass through the eye
         (c) Accommodation: bulging of the lens for viewing near objects
         (d) Constriction of pupils: occurs simultaneously with accommodation and in bright light
         (e) Convergence of the eyes for near objects so light rays from the object may fall on corresponding points of two retinas; necessary for binocular vision
         (f) Binocular vision: visual fields of the two eyes overlap; although each eye sees some areas of the environment that the other eye cannot, both eyes also see large areas in common; the human brain interprets these overlapping fields in terms of depth (three dimensions)
      (2) Stimulation of the retina: dim light causes breakdown of the chemical rhodopsin present in rods, thereby initiating impulse conduction by the rods; rods considered receptors for night vision, cones receptors for daylight and color vision
      (3) Conduction to visual area in occipital lobe of cerebral cortex by fibers of optic nerves and optic tract
   g. Errors of refraction
      (1) Myopia (nearsightedness): focuses rays anterior to the retina
      (2) Hyperopia (farsightedness): focuses rays posterior to the retina
      (3) Astigmatism: irregular curvature of the surface of the cornea that focuses rays unevenly on the retina
7. Hearing
   a. External ear: consists of the auricle (or pinna), external acoustic meatus (ear opening), and external auditory canal
   b. Middle ear: separated from the external ear by the tympanic membrane; middle ear contains auditory ossicles (malleus, incus, stapes) and openings from the eustachian tubes, mastoid cells, external ear, and internal ear
   c. Inner ear (or labyrinth)

(1) Bony vestibule: contains maculae acusticae; vestibular nerve (branch of eighth cranial [acoustic or vestibulocochlear] nerve) communicates with the maculae acusticae; provides information about equilibrium, position of the head, and acceleration and deceleration

(2) Bony, semicircular canals: contain the membranous semicircular canals in which are located the crista ampullaris, the sense organ for sensations of equilibrium and head movements; vestibular nerve supplies the crista as well as the macula acusticae

(3) Bony cochlea: contains the membranous cochlear duct in which is located the organ of Corti, the hearing sense organ; cochlear nerve (branch of eighth cranial nerve) supplies the organ of Corti

d. Physiology of hearing

(1) Sound waves enter the ear canal and strike the tympanic membrane, causing it to vibrate; these vibrations sequentially move the malleus, incus, and stapes

(2) Movement of the stapes against the oval window into which it fits starts a ripple in the perilymph, which is transmitted to the endolymph inside the cochlear duct and stimulates the organ of Corti

(3) Cochlear nerve conducts impulses from the organ of Corti to the brain; hearing occurs when impulses reach the auditory area in the temporal lobe of the cerebral cortex

e. Interpretation of sounds

(1) Loudness: neurologic or psychologic interpretation of intensity; the greater the intensity, the greater the size of nerve impulses

(2) Pitch: corresponds to frequency; the higher the frequency, the higher the pitch of the sound

(3) Quality: sound rarely represents a pure tone but many frequencies occurring simultaneously

Structures and Functions of the Muscular System

A. Purpose: movement, posture, and heat production

B. Types of muscles and neural control

1. Striated: controlled by voluntary nervous system via somatic motoneurons in spinal and some cranial nerves

2. Smooth: controlled by autonomic nervous system via autonomic motoneurons in autonomic,

spinal, and some cranial nerves; not under voluntary control

3. Cardiac: control is identical to that of smooth muscle

C. Bursa: synovial fluid-filled sac situated in places where friction occurs; facilitates movement of tendons over bone relieving pressure between moving parts

D. Tendons: band of fibrous tissue connecting muscle to bone

E. Ligament: band of fibrous tissue connecting bone to cartilage; supports and strengthens joints

Skeletal muscles

A. Anatomy

1. Typically spindle shaped; muscle fibers coated with fibrous connective tissue (fascia), which binds muscle to surrounding tissues

2. Attach to at least two bones; the bone that moves is called the insertion bone, and that which remains stationary its origin bone

3. Muscle fibers contain myofibrils specialized for contraction; composed of two types of protein myofilaments, actin and myocin

B. Physiology of muscle contraction

1. Basic principles of muscle contraction

a. Contract only if stimulated; a skeletal muscle and its motor nerve function as a physiologic unit; anything that prevents impulse conduction to a skeletal muscle paralyzes the muscle

b. Skeletal muscles almost always act in groups; classified as prime movers, synergists, or antagonists

c. Contraction of a skeletal muscle either shortens the muscle, producing movement, or increases the tension (tone) in the muscle

(1) Tonic contractions: produce muscle tone; do not shorten the muscle to produce movements

(2) Isometric contractions: increase the degree of muscle tone; do not shorten the muscle to produce movements; daily isometric contractions gradually increase muscle strength

(3) Isotonic contractions: the muscle shortens, thereby producing movement

d. Treppe (staircase phenomenon): when a muscle has contracted a few times, subsequent contractions are more powerful

e. Shivering: rapid, repeating, involuntary skeletal muscle contractions caused by hypothalamic temperature regulating center; most of the energy of ATP is converted to heat but a small part goes to muscle contraction

f. Rigor mortis: after death ATP is depleted from muscle fibers and actin associates with myosin, producing rigor mortis; subsequent decomposition of muscle proteins brings about relaxation; the rigor state begins about 6 hours after death and remains until decomposition occurs

2. Energy of muscle contraction
   a. Electrical energy flows into muscle along transverse intracellular tubules associated with sarcoplasmic reticulum
   b. Calcium ions released by electrical energy inactivate troponin, which normally blocks the interaction between actin and myosin
   c. Myosin releases and uses energy from ATP to cause contraction
   d. Creatine phosphate replenishes the supply of ATP as needed; the source of energy is glucose and fatty acids oxidized aerobically to carbon dioxide and water
   e. Anaerobic breakdown of glucose during prolonged and vigorous muscle contraction results in lactic acid buildup associated with fatigue and an aching feeling; this oxygen debt is reversed during rest

3. Neuromuscular junction
   a. Axon terminal forms junction with the sarcolemma of muscle fiber; tiny synaptic cleft separates the presynaptic membrane (axon) from postsynaptic membrane (sarcolemma)
   b. Axon terminals contain tiny sacs, synaptic vesicles; these contain the neurotransmitter acetylcholine; the enzyme cholinesterase, which inactivates acetylcholine, is found in the synaptic cleft
   c. When a nerve impulse reaches the axon terminal, acetylcholine is released from synaptic vesicles into synaptic cleft; it diffuses across the cleft and attaches to receptor sites on sarcolemma; when acetylcholine binds to the receptor site, a channel opens and sodium and potassium ions flow down their concentration gradients; the sarcolemma is depolarized, and electrical energy flows into the muscle fiber; cholinesterase inactivates acetylcholine; additional stimulation of muscle requires release of more acetylcholine

4. Changes in muscle mass
   a. Hypertrophy is physical enlargement of the muscle resulting from the addition of more myofibrils making the muscle swell; muscle fibers do not divide to produce more fibers
   b. Atrophy is a wasting of a muscle resulting from a decrease in myofibrils; results from disuse or disease

Structures and Functions of the Skeletal System

A. Purpose
   1. Provides supporting framework; protects viscera, brain, and hemopoietic system
   2. Bones serve as levers and joints as fulcrums of these levers
   3. Hemopoiesis by red bone marrow: formation of all kinds of blood cells; note that some lymphocytes and monocytes are formed in lymphatic tissue
   4. Mineral storage: calcium, phosphorus, and sodium

B. Skeleton: contains 206 bones divided into the axial and appendicular skeletons

C. Joint: junction or union of two or more bones
   1. Synarthrotic (fibrous): generally nonmovable; no joint cavity or capsule; bones held together by fibrous tissue; e.g., sutures and syndesmoses
   2. Amphiarthrotic (cartilaginous): slightly movable; no joint cavity or capsule; bones held together by cartilage and ligaments; e.g., symphyses pubis
   3. Diarthrotic: freely movable; lined by a thin layer of hyaline cartilage covering the articular surfaces of the joining bones; held together by a fibrous capsule lined with synovial membrane and ligaments
      a. May be ball and socket (as in hip), hinge (as in elbow), condyloid (as at wrist), pivot, gliding, or saddle
      b. Kinds of movement possible at diarthrotic joints
         (1) Flexion: bending one bone on another
         (2) Extension: stretching one bone away from another
         (3) Abduction: moving bone away from body's midline
         (4) Adduction: moving bone toward the body's midline
         (5) Rotation: pivoting bone on its axis
         (6) Internal rotation: turning of a limb toward the midline of the body
         (7) External rotation: turning of a limb away from the midline of the body
         (8) Circumduction: circular movement of a limb
         (9) Supination: forearm movement turning the palm forward
         (10) Pronation: forearm movement turning the back of the hand forward
         (11) Inversion: ankle movement turning the sole of the foot inward
         (12) Eversion: ankle movement turning the sole of the foot outward
         (13) Protraction: moving a part, such as the lower jaw, forward

(14) Retraction: pulling a part back; opposite of protraction

(15) Plantar flexion: pointing toes away from the body

(16) Dorsiflexion: pointing toes toward the body

D. Differences between male and female skeletons
   1. Male skeleton larger and heavier than female skeleton.
   2. Male pelvis deep and funnel shaped with narrow, pubic arch; female pelvis shallow, broad, and flaring with wider pubic arch

E. Age changes in skeleton
   1. From infancy to adulthood, not only do bones grow but their relative sizes change due in part to stimulation of somatotrophic hormone; e.g., the head becomes proportionately smaller, the pelvis relatively larger, the legs proportionately longer
   2. From young adulthood to old age, bone margins and projections change gradually; marginal lipping and spurs occur, thereby restricting movement
   3. Osteoporosis mostly occurs in postmenopausal women; related to decreased hormone production, lack of exercise that stresses skeleton, and inadequate intake of calcium, magnesium, and vitamins A, C, and D

Nature of bone substance

A. Organic matter: makes up about 33% of bone by weight
   1. Cells: osteoblasts (bone-producing cells), osteoclasts (bone-dissolving cells), osteocytes (former osteoblasts embedded in and maintaining bone substance)
   2. Collagen: responsible for tensile strength of bone
   3. Polysaccharides part of ground substance of bone

B. Inorganic matter: makes up about 67% of bone by weight
   1. Apatite salts; make bone hard and are responsible for the high compressional strength of bone
   2. Magnesium and sodium ions are part of bone matrix
   3. Certain radioactive isotopes accumulate in bone and may increase likelihood of bone tumors and leukemia

Bone formation

A. Ossification: the development of or conversion into bone
   1. Intramembranous ossification: occurs in and replaces connective tissue
   2. Endochondral ossification: occurs in and replaces cartilage

3. Cancellous (spongy) bone: the end result of either intramembranous or endochondral ossification
4. Compact bone: the denser type of bone substance that forms later in development through conversion of selected regions of cancellous bone
5. Ossification process
   a. Formation of bone matrix (the intercellular substance of bone), made up of collagen fibers and a cementlike ground substance; the osteoblasts (bone-forming cells) synthesize collagen and cement substance from proteins provided by the diet; exercise and estrogens act to stimulate osteoblasts to form bone matrix
   b. Calcification of bone matrix: calcium salts deposit in the bone matrix

B. Repair of skeleton
   1. When bone is fractured, connective tissue called a callus grows into and around the broken region
   2. Macrophages reabsorb dead and damaged cells
   3. Osteoclasts dissolve bone fragments
   4. Osteoblasts produce new bone substance and fuse bone together
   5. Final bone shape slowly remodeled; the complete process takes several months; much slower than epithelial tissue, which has a higher metabolic rate and richer blood supply

C. Nutrients required for growth, maintenance, and remodeling of bone
   1. Vitamin A: promotes chondrocyte function and synthesis of lysosomal enzymes for osteoclast activity
   2. Vitamin C: promotes synthesis of collagen and bone matrix
   3. Vitamin D: promotes calcium and phosphorus absorption
   4. Calcium: needed to form calcium phosphate and hydroxyapatite
   5. Magnesium: important enzyme activator in the mineralization process
   6. Phosphorus: needed to form calcium phosphate and hydroxyapatite

Review of Physical Principles

A. Lever: rigid bar that moves about a fixed point known as the fulcrum; a small force is applied through a large distance and the other end of the lever exerts a large force over a small distance; related to effective body mechanics
B. Pulleys: can multiply force at the expense of distance; used in traction
C. Center of gravity

1. Position in a body where all the weight is considered to be located; in a human the center of gravity is in the pelvic cavity
2. When bending over the body's center of gravity shifts from a stable position between the legs to an unstable position outside the legs; keeping the legs apart widens the base of support

D. Buoyancy of water: reduces the energy to move muscles or objects against the force of gravity

Principles of physical properties of matter

A. Pascal's principle: when pressure is applied to a fluid in a closed, nonflexible container, it is transmitted undiminished throughout all parts of the fluid and acts in all directions; e.g., brain tumor and hydrocephalus

B. Electromagnetic fields: use of a strong magnetic field (MRI) or high-energy electromagnetic radiation (x-ray, CT scan) to diagnose abnormalities

C. Sound
1. Mechanical vibration that does not occur in a vacuum; propagated best through solids, and through liquids better than gases; e.g., bowel sounds and breath sounds
2. Ultrasonic vibrational frequencies exceeding the upper level of human hearing
   a. Low-intensity ultrasonic waves are used to treat arthritis and bursitis, to break kidney stones, and to help dissolve scars
   b. Sonograms are pictures of the body derived through differential reflection or transmission of sound waves
3. Hearing aids: electronic devices that amplify sounds and assist partially deaf persons to hear
   a. Air-conduction type sends an amplified sound wave into the ear, thus utilizing the person's own middle ear
   b. Bone-conduction type bypasses the middle ear and transmits amplified vibrations to the skull bones, which in turn produce vibrations in the inner ear

REVIEW OF MICROORGANISMS

A. Bacterial pathogens
1. *Clostridium tetani:* large, gram-positive, motile bacillus forming large terminal spores; an obligate anaerobe; causes tetanus (lockjaw)
2. *Neisseria meningitidis:* gram-negative diplococcus; causes epidemic (meningococcic) meningitis

B. DNA viruses: herpes viruses (chickenpox), herpes zoster (shingles), infectious mononucleosis, and cytomegalic inclusion disease

C. RNA viruses: mostly borne by mosquitoes and ticks; cause eastern equine encephalomyelitis, western equine encephalomyelitis, and Venezuelan equine encephalomyelitis

D. Nematode: *Trichinellas spiralis:* a small parasitic nematode; causes trichinosis

 RELATED PHARMACOLOGY

Anticonvulsants (AEDs)

A. Description
1. Modify bioelectric activity at subcortical and cortical sites by stabilizing the nerve cell membrane and/or raising the seizure threshold to incoming stimuli
2. Decrease the occurrence, frequency, and/or severity of convulsive episodes
3. Available in oral and parenteral (IM, IV) preparations

B. Examples
1. Control of tonic-clonic (grand mal) seizures
   a. Carbamazepine (Tegretol): also used for partial seizures
   b. Phenytoin (Dilantin): also used for partial seizures
   c. Phenobarbital (Luminal): may be used
   d. Gabapentin (Neurontin)
   e. Valproic acid (Depakene)
2. Control of absence (petit mal) seizures
   a. Ethosuximide (Zarontin)
   b. Trimethadione (Tridione)
   c. Clonazepam (Klonopin)

C. Major side effects
1. Dizziness, drowsiness (CNS depression)
2. Nausea, vomiting (irritation of gastric mucosa)
3. Skin rash (hypersensitivity)
4. Blood dyscrasias (decreased RBCs, WBCs, platelet synthesis)
5. Phenytoin: ataxia (neurotoxicity); gingival hyperplasia (gum irritation leading to tissue overgrowth); hirsutism (virilism); hypotension (decreased atrial and ventricular conduction)

D. Nursing care
1. Administer with food to reduce GI irritation
2. Instruct client to:
   a. Avoid alcohol and other CNS depressants
   b. Notify physician if fever, sore throat, or skin rash develops
   c. Carry medical alert card
3. Encourage diet rich in nutrient-dense foods such as fruits, vegetables, whole grains, and legumes to improve and maintain nutritional status and prevent possible drug-induced nutrient deficiencies
4. Care for clients receiving phenytoin (Dilantin)
   a. Avoid mixing with other IV infusions
   b. Provide oral hygiene; inspect oral mucosa for infection
   c. Assess for potentiation of anticoagulant effect

d. Assess urine; drug may discolor urine pink to red-brown

e. Assess for therapeutic blood levels (10 to 20 mcg/ml)

f. Assess for tissue necrosis because phenytoin is highly irritating to veins

Osmotic diuretics

A. Description

1. Reduce cerebral edema and intraocular pressure by increasing the osmotic pressure within the vasculature, thus causing fluid to leave the tissues and be excreted in the urine

2. Treat increased intracranial pressure

3. Available in parenteral (IV) preparations

B. Example: mannitol (Osmitrol)

C. Major side effects

1. Headache (dehydration)

2. Nausea (fluid and electrolyte imbalance)

3. Chills (fluid and electrolyte imbalance)

4. Rebound edema when discontinued (fluid and electrolyte imbalance)

5. Fluid/electrolyte imbalances (hyponatremia, hypokalemia resulting from promotion of sodium and potassium excretion)

D. Nursing care

1. Monitor intake and output, daily weight, and serum electrolytes

2. Question administration to clients with congestive heart failure or impaired renal function

3. Elevate head of bed during therapy

4. Assess client for signs of increased intracranial pressure (decreasing pulse rate, widening pulse pressure, increasing systolic pressure, unequal pupils, change in level of consciousness)

Calcium enhancers

A. Description.

1. Calcium ion replacement directly increases serum calcium concentration

2. Vitamin D replacement improves absorption of calcium from intestines

3. Biphosphonates absorb calcium phosphate crystals in bone and may directly block dissolution of hydroxyapatite crystals of bone; inhibit resorption of bone

4. Parathyroid agents decrease bone resorption

5. Hormone replacement therapy (see Osteoporosis and Estrogens in Women's Health)

B. Examples

1. Calcium ion replacement: calcium carbonate . (OsCal); calcium chloride; IV administration only; calcium gluconate

2. Vitamin D replacement: calcitriol (Rocaltrol) and cholecalciferol (Calciferol)

3. Biphosphonates: alendronate (Fosamax), pamidronate (Aredia), risedronate (Actonel)

4. Parathyroid agents: etidronate (Didronel) calcitonin (Miacalcin)

C. Major side effects

1. Nausea, vomiting, renal calculi, muscle flaccidity (hypercalcemia)

2. Constipation (increased serum calcium delays passage of stool in GI tract)

3. Calcium preparations: cardiac disturbances (stimulation of cardiac conduction)

4. Vitamin D: dry mouth; metallic taste (early vitamin D toxicity associated with hypercalcemia)

5. Biphosphonates: bone pain, headache, abdominal pain, nausea,

6. Parathyroid agents; diarrhea; nephrotoxicity and seizures (Didronel); headache, chest pressure, dyspnea (Miacalcin)

D. Nursing care

1. Assess for signs of hypercalcemia and tetany

2. Monitor serum electrolytes during course of therapy

3. Encourage increased fluid intake and acid ash diet to reduce potential of renal calculi and constipation; stress vitamin D and calcium-rich foods such as eggs, cheese, whole-grain cereals, and cranberries; limit milk, fruits, and vegetables

4. Calcium preparations: assess for potentiation of digitalis effect

Antiparkinson agents

A. Description

1. Anticholinergic drugs act at central sites to inhibit cerebral motor impulses and to block efferent impulses that cause rigidity of the musculature

2. Dopaminergic agents supply or cause the release of dopamine required for norepinephrine synthesis and maintenance of the neurohormonal balance at subcortical, cortical, and reticular sites that control motor function

3. COMT inhibitors deter enzymes involved in the breakdown of levodopa, thereby prolonging the duration of action of levodopa in the CNS

4. MAO-B inhibitor exerts a neuroprotective effect

5. Control the symptoms of Parkinson's disease

6. Available in oral and parenteral (IM, IV) preparations

B. Examples

1. Anticholinergic drugs: benztropine mesylate (Cogentin) and trihexyphenidyl HCl (Artane)

2. Dopaminergic agents: levodopa (Dopar), carbidopa-levodopa (Sinemet), bromocriptine (Parlodel)

3. Catecho-o-methyltransferase (COMT) inhibitor: entacapone (Comtan)

4. MAO-B inhibitor: selegiline (Eldepryl)

C. Major side effects

1. Anticholinergic drugs (decrease parasympathetic stimulation)

a. Dry mouth (decreased salivation)

b. Blurred vision (pupillary dilation)

c. Constipation (decreased peristalsis)

d. Urinary retention (decreased muscle tone)

2. Other drugs

a. Orthostatic hypotension (loss of compensatory vasoconstriction with position change)

b. Ataxia (neurotoxicity)

c. CNS disturbances and emotional disturbances (CNS effect)

d. Nausea, vomiting (irritation of gastric mucosa)

D. Nursing care

1. Instruct client to:

a. Avoid discontinuing drug suddenly

b. Understand that treatment controls symptoms but is not a cure

c. Continued health supervision is necessary

d. Take COMT inhibitors in conjunction with dopaminergic agents or no benefit will be derived

2. Offer emotional support; therapy is usually for life

3. Encourage diet rich in nutrient-dense foods such as fruits, vegetables, whole grains, and legumes to improve and maintain nutritional status and prevent possible drug-induced nutrient deficiencies

4. Care for the client receiving anticholinergic drugs

a. Offer sugar-free chewing gum and hard candy to increase salivation

b. May interfere with ability to perform potentially hazardous activities

5. Care for the client receiving levodopa

a. Limit or eliminate vitamin B_6 from diet (e.g., pork, veal, lamb, potatoes, legumes, oatmeal, wheat germ, arid bananas)

b. Inform client regarding dosage and "holiday" periods

6. Care for the client receiving Eldepryl

a. Inform families that Eldepryl may be started early in the course of the disease because neuroprotective actions are expected

b. Use safety precautions because drug can cause orthostatic hypotension

c. Avoid foods containing tyramine such as wine, cheese, and chocolate because this drug is an MAO inhibitor; ingestion of these foods can cause a severe hypertensive crisis

Cholinesterase inhibitors

A. Description

1. Act by:

a. Preventing enzymatic breakdown of acetylcholine at nerve endings, thus allowing accumulation of the neurotransmitter

b. Improving the strength of contraction in all muscles, including those involved with the process of respiration

2. Diagnose and treat myasthenia gravis

3. Available in oral and parenteral (IM, IV) preparations

B. Examples: edrophonium chloride (Tensilon) (used for diagnostic purposes) and neostigmine bromide (Prostigmin)

C. Major side effects

1. Nausea, vomiting (irritation of gastric mucosa)

2. Diarrhea (increased peristalsis)

3. Hypersalivation (increased parasympathetic stimulation)

4. Muscle cramps (increased skeletal muscle contraction);

5. CNS disturbances (CNS effect)

6. Acute toxicity: pulmonary edema and respiratory failure (bronchial constriction)

D. Nursing care

1. Administer medications on time exactly as prescribed; monitor client; dosage is adjusted according to needs

2. Have atropine sulfate available for treatment of overdosage

3. Administer with food to reduce GI irritation

4. Instruct client to:

a. Carry a medical alert card

b. Take medication before meals to improve chewing and swallowing

c. Encourage diet rich in nutrient-dense foods such as fruits, vegetables, whole grains, and legumes to improve and maintain nutritional status and prevent possible drug-induced nutrient deficiencies

Skeletal muscle relaxants

A. Description

1. Central agents act by CNS depression to bring about relaxation of voluntary muscles

2. Peripheral agents block nerve-impulse conduction at the myoneural junction

3. Relieve inappropriate and abnormal muscle contraction

4. Available in oral and parenteral (IM, IV) preparations

B. Examples

1. Carisoprodol (Soma)

2. Cyclobenzapine (Flexeril)

3. Diazepam (Valium)

4. Methocarbamol (Robaxin)

C. Major side effects

1. Dizziness, drowsiness (CNS depression)

2. Nausea (irritation of gastric mucosa)

3. Headache (central antimuscarinic effect)

4. Tachycardia (brain stem stimulation)

D. Nursing care
1. Encourage diet rich in nutrient-dense, foods such as fruits, vegetables, whole grains, and legumes to improve and maintain nutritional status and prevent possible drug-induced nutrient deficiencies
2. Teach client receiving central agents to use safety precautions during initial therapy and to avoid engaging in potentially hazardous activities or using alcohol and other CNS depressants

Nonsteroidal antiinflammatory drugs (NSAIDs)
A. Description
1. Interfere with prostaglandin synthesis
2. Alleviate inflammation and subsequent discomfort of rheumatoid conditions
3. Available in oral and parenteral (IM) preparations
B. Examples
1. Diclofenac (Voltaren)
2. Etodolac (Lodine)
3. Ibuprofen (Motrin)
4. Naproxen (Naprosyn)
5. Salicylates (ASA)
6. Celecoxib (Celebrex)
7. Ketorolac (Toradol)
C. Major side effects
1. GI irritation (local effect)
2. Skin rash (hypersensitivity)
3. Blood dyscrasias (decreased RBCs, WBCs, platelet synthesis)
4. CNS and GU disturbances
D. Nursing care
1. Administer with meals to reduce GI irritation
2. Monitor blood work
3. Assess vital signs
4. Instruct client to report the occurrence of any side effects to the physician
5. Encourage diet rich in nutrient-dense foods such as fruits, vegetables, whole grains, and legumes to improve and maintain nutritional status and prevent possible drug-induced nutrient deficiencies

Antigout agents
A. Description
1. Act by decreasing uric acid formation and increasing its excretion
2. Prevent and arrest gout attacks that are caused by high levels of uric acid in the blood
3. Available in oral and parenteral (IV) preparations
B. Examples
1. Allopurinol (Zyloprim): blocks formation of uric acid within the body
2. Colchicine: decreases uric acid crystal deposits by inhibiting lactic-acid production by leukocytes; used for acute attacks

3. Probenecid (Benemid): prevents formation of tophi by inhibiting the reabsorption of uric acid by the kidneys
C. Major side effects
1. Nausea, vomiting (irritation of gastric mucosa)
2. Blood dyscrasias (decreased RBCs, WBCs, and platelet synthesis)
3. Liver damage (hepatotoxicity)
4. Skin rash (hypersensitivity)
D. Nursing care
1. Administer antiinflammatory drugs (Prednisone, Indocin) in addition to drugs that will lower serum uric acid during the acute phase
2. Increase fluids to discourage the formation of renal calculi
3. Encourage weight reduction if overweight
4. Monitor serum urate levels to determine effectiveness of treatment
5. Administer with meals to reduce GI irritation
6. Instruct client to avoid high-purine foods such as organ meats, anchovies, sardines, and shellfish; encourage diet rich in nutrient-dense foods such as fruits, vegetables, and whole grains, as well as milk, cheese, and eggs; teach the importance of preventing drug-induced nutrient deficiencies

Ophthalmic agents
A. Description
1. Produce a variety of actions; e.g., constriction, dilation, antiinflammatory, antiinfective
2. Diagnose and treat conditions affecting the eyes
3. Available in a variety of topical preparations; drugs having a systemic action are available in oral and parenteral (IM, IV) preparations
B. Examples
1. Miotics: constrict the pupil, pulling the iris away from the filtration angle and improving outflow of aqueous humor
   a. Betaxolol (Betoptic)
   b. Levobunolol (Betagan)
   c. Latanoprost (Xalatan)
2. Mydriatics: dilate pupil (mydriasis) by causing contraction of the dilator muscle of the iris with minimal effect on the ciliary muscle, which lessens the effect on accommodation
   a. Atropine
   b. Tropicamide (Mydriacyl, Tropicacyl)
3. Anticholinergics dilate the pupil (mydriasis) by relaxing the ciliary muscle and the sphincter muscle of the iris; paralyze accommodation (cycloplegia); thus facilitating eye examination
   a. Atropine sulfate
   b. Cyclopentolate (Cyclogyl)
4. Carbonic anhydrase inhibitors: decrease inflow of aqueous humor in control of intraocular pressure

a. Acetazolamide (Diamox)
b. Ethoxzolamide (Cardrase, Ethamide)
5. Osmotic agents: administered systemically to decrease blood osmolality, which mobilizes fluid from the eye to reduce volume of intraocular fluid
    a. Glycerin (Glycerol, Osmoglyn)
    b. Mannitol (Osmitrol)
    c. Urea (Urevert)
6. Other: alpha-adrenergics and prostaglandins
C. Major side effects
    1. Miotics
        a. Twitching of eyelids and brow ache (increased cholinergic stimulation)
        b. Headache (vasodilation)
        c. Conjunctival pain (irritation of conjunctiva)
        d. Contact dermatitis (local irritation)
    2. Anticholinergics (decreased parasympathetic stimulation)
        a. Dry mouth (decreased salivation)
        b. Flushing, fever, and ataxia (CNS effect)
        c. Blurred vision (pupillary dilation)
        d. Skin rash (hypersensitivity)
        e. Tachycardia (decreased vagal stimulation)
    3. Mydriatics
        a. Brow ache, headache, and hypertension (vasoconstrictor effect)
        b. Blurred vision (pupillary dilation)
        c. Tachycardia (increased sympathetic stimulation)
    4. Carbonic anhydrase inhibitors
        a. Diuresis (increased excretion of sodium and water in renal tubule)
        b. Paresthesia (fluid-electrolyte imbalance)
        c. Nausea, vomiting (GI irritation)
        d. CNS disturbances (CNS effect)
    5. Osmotic agents
        a. Headache (cerebral dehydration)
        b. Nausea, vomiting (fluid-electrolyte imbalance)
D. Nursing care
    1. Instruct client regarding proper method of application and need for medical supervision during therapy
    2. Assess for occurrence of side effects and/or worsening of condition
    3. Encourage diet rich in nutrient-dense foods such as fruits, vegetables, whole grains, and legumes to improve and maintain nutritional status and prevent possible drug-induced nutrient deficiencies
    4. Provide care for the client receiving mydriatics: caution that vision will be blurred temporarily; advise that sunglasses will relieve photophobia; caution about engaging in hazardous activities

RELATED PROCEDURES
Computerized Tomography (CT)
A. Definition
    1. Cross-sectional visualization of the head or other body cavity determined by computer analysis of relative tissue density as an x-ray beam passes through
    2. Provides three-dimensional information about location and extent of tumors, infarcted areas, atrophy, and vascular lesions
    3. May be done with intravenous injection of dye for contrast enhancement
B. Nursing care
    1. Obtain informed consent
    2. Explain procedure; inform the client that it will be necessary to lie still and that the equipment is complex but will cause no discomfort; infants and cognitively impaired or anxious clients may need to be sedated
    3. Assess for allergy to iodine, a component of the contrast material
    4. Withhold food for approximately 2 hours before contrast testing; dye may cause nausea in sensitive clients
    5. Remove wigs, clips, and pins before CT of head
    6. Encourage fluids after the procedure

Magnetic Resonance Imaging (MRI)
A. Definition
    1. Uses magnetic fields and radio waves to produce cross-sectional images
    2. Produces accurate images of blood vessels, bone marrow, gray and white brain matter, the spinal cord, the globe of the eye, the heart, abdominal structures, and breast tissue, and can monitor blood velocity
B. Nursing care
    1. Obtain informed consent
    2. Assess ability to withstand confining surroundings because client must remain in the tunnel-like machine for up to 90 minutes; open MRI may be an option for clients who cannot tolerate closed spaces
    3. Instruct client to toilet before test
    4. Have client remove jewelry, clothing with metal fasteners, dentures, hearing aids, and glasses prior to entering scanner
    5. Review history for contraindications: orthopedic hardware; pacemaker; artificial heart valves; or other implants that may be dislodged or malfunction as a result of the magnetic field

Lumbar Puncture
A. Definition: involves the introduction of a needle into the subarachnoid space below the spinal cord, usually between L3 and L4 or L4 and L5

B. Purposes
1. Withdrawal of cerebral spinal fluid for diagnostic purposes or to reduce spinal pressure (normal is 70 to 200 mm H_2O)
2. Measurement of spinal pressure (Queckenstedt's test involves compression of the jugular veins; normally pressure will rise; but if blockage exists, pressure will not change)
3. Injection of dye for diagnostic x-ray examination
4. Injection of medication such as anesthetics
C. Nursing care
1. Explain procedure to the client and obtain an informed consent
2. Assist the client into a position that will enlarge opening between vertebrae
   a. Lying on side with feet drawn up and head lowered to chest; back near edge of mattress
   b. Sitting on side of bed, leaning on overbed table, feet supported on a stool
3. After procedure assist the client into a recumbent position; the client should remain recumbent for a few hours, depending on the physician's orders
4. Label specimens and send to laboratory; note color and amount of fluid
5. Assess immediate response for signs of shock and complications such as CSF leakage, infection, and brain herniation if space occupying lesion is present
6. Administer fluids unless contraindicated

Positron Emission Tomography (PET)

A. Definition
1. Client is given strong radioactive tracers that emit signals; these images from tracers are formed from computer analysis of the emitted photons
2. Useful in determing blood flow, glucose metabolism, and oxygen extraction
3. Effective in diagnosis of CVA, brain tumors, epilepsy; can evaluate progress of Alzheimer's disease, Parkinson's disease, bipolar disorders, and head injuries
B. Nursing care
1. Obtain informed consent
2. Maintain NPO 4 hours before test
3. Explain that client must lie still for about 45 minutes; sedation may be needed
4. Ensure that individual with diabetes has a blood glucose below 150 g/dl

Neurologic Assessment

A. Definition: systematic evaluation of the cranial nerves, motor and sensory functioning, and mental status to detect neurologic abnormalities
1. Critical aspects of a complete neurologic assessment are generally extracted and compose a "neuro checklist," which is used when the nature of the situation does not warrant complete evaluation
2. May include the Glasgow Coma Scale
B. Nursing care
1. Cranial nerves
   a. Olfactory (I): ability to identify familiar odors such as mint or alcohol with eyes closed and one nostril occluded at a time
   b. Optic (II): visual acuity measured by use of Snellen chart or by gross estimation with reading material; gross comparison of visual fields with those of examiner; color perception
   c. Oculomotor (III), trochlear (IV), and abducent (VI): ability of the pupils to react equally to light and to accommodate to varying distances; normal range of extraocular movement (EOM) evaluated by asking the client to follow a finger or object with the eyes; also assess for nystagmus (jerking motion of eyes), particularly when eyes are directed laterally
   d. Trigeminal (V): sensations of the face evaluated by lightly stroking cotton across forehead, chin, and cheeks while the client's eyes are closed; ability to clench the teeth (jaw closure)
   e. Facial (VII): symmetry of the facial muscles as the client speaks or is asked to make faces
   f. Acoustic or vestibulocochlear (VIII): hearing acuity determined by a watch tick or whispered numbers; Weber's test may be performed by holding the stem of a vibrating tuning fork at midline of the skull (should be heard equally in both ears)
   g. Glossopharyngeal (IX) and vagus (X): uvula should hang in midline; swallow and gag reflexes should be intact
   h. Spinal accessory (XI): symmetric ability to turn the head or shrug the shoulders against counterforce of the examiner's hands
   i. Hypoglossal (XII): ability to protrude the tongue without deviation, to left or right, and without tremors
2. Motor function (including cerebellar function)
   a. Balance
      (1) Observation of gait
      (2) Romberg test: positive if the client fails to maintain an upright position with feet together when the eyes are closed
   b. Coordination: ability to touch the finger to the nose when arms are extended or to perform similar tasks smoothly

c. Muscle strength: evaluated by having the client move symmetrical muscle groups against opposition supplied by the examiner

3. Sensory function: bilateral testing of the response to light touch with cotton, sharp versus dull stimuli, vibration of a tuning fork

4. Mental status (cerebral functioning)
   a. Level of consciousness: determined by the response to stimuli (verbal, tactile, or painful)
   b. Orientation to person, place, and time: determined by general conversation and direct questioning
   c. Judgment, memory, and ability to perform simple calculations
   d. Appropriateness of behavior and mood

5. Reflexes
   a. Deep tendon (biceps, triceps, patellar, Achilles reflexes) with a reflex hammer; classification from 0 (absent) to 4+ (hyperactive); 2+ is normal
   b. Plantar: plantar flexion of the foot when the sole is stroked firmly with a hard object such as a tongue blade; abnormal adult response (dorsiflexion of the foot and fanning of the toes) is described as a positive Babinski and is indicative of corticospinal tract disease
   c. Oculocephalic (doll's-eye movements): when head of comatose client is turned to side, eyes move in opposite direction; absence of reflex suggests brainstem injury; contraindicated with a neck injury
   d. Oculovestibular (caloric test): when warm or ice water is instilled into the ear of a comatose client, nystagmus occurs; eyes deviate toward the stimulated ear if ice water is used and away with warm water; absence of reflex suggests brainstem damage; contraindicated if eardrum is perforated

6. Accurately record findings; report any deviations

7. Explain to and reassure the client when the examination must be repeated frequently (q2h)

8. Coordinate other care with q2h neurologic assessments to promote rest between assessments

Glasgow Coma Scale (GCS)

A. Definition: technique of objectifying a client's level of responses; client's best response in each area is given a numerical value, and the three values are totaled for a score ranging from 3 to 15

1. Eye-opening ability: spontaneous (4); to speech (3); to pain (2); no response (1)
2. Motor response: obeys commands (6); localizes pain (5); withdraws (4); abnormal flexing (3); extension (2); no response (1)
3. Verbal response: oriented (5); confused (4); inappropriate words (3); incomprehensible sounds (2); no response (1)

B. Nursing care
   1. Perform the assessment at appropriate intervals to determine current level of changes in client's level of consciousness; usually every 2 to 4 hours
   2. A score of 7 or less indicates coma
   3. Assess other indicators such as vital signs, pupillary reaction, movement of extremities, strength, etc.

Continuous Passive Motion Devices (CPM)

A. Definition: a machine that provides for passive range of motion, most commonly for the knee

B. Purposes
   1. Move joint without weight bearing or straining muscles following orthopedic surgery
   2. Stimulate regeneration of articular tissues

C. Nursing care
   1. Align extremity in padded CPM device
   2. Set foot cradle at the angle ordered by the physician
   3. Adjust device according to length of client's extremity
   4. Set flexion, extension, and speed dials as ordered by the physician; these are generally increased gradually as tolerated to maximize mobility
   5. Demonstrate use of control cord to client

Braces or Splints

A. Purposes
   1. Support and protect weakened muscles
   2. Prevent and correct anatomic deformities
   3. Aid in controlling involuntary muscle movements
   4. Immobilize and protect a diseased or injured joint

B. Nursing care
   1. Keep equipment in good repair (e.g., oil joints, replace straps when worn)
   2. Provide adequate shoes (e.g., in good repair, heels low and wide, high top to hold the heel in the shoe)
   3. Examine the skin daily for evidence of breakdown at pressure points
   4. Check alignment of the braces (e.g., leg brace: joints should coincide with body joints; back brace: upright bars in center of back, brace should grip the pelvis and trochanter firmly, lacing should begin from the bottom)

Mobility: Assistive Devices

A. Purposes
   1. Improve or maintain stability of client with a

lower limb disability to prevent injury
2. Provide security while developing confidence in ambulating
3. Relieve pressure on weight-bearing joints
4. Assist in increasing speed of ambulation with less fatigue
5. Provide for greater mobility and independence
B. Nursing care: use of a cane
   1. Ascertain that the client is able to bear weight on the affected extremity
   2. Ensure that the client is able to use the upper extremity opposite the affected lower extremity
   3. Measure to determine the length of cane required: highest point should be approximately level with the greater trochanter; handpiece should allow 30 degrees of flexion at the elbow with the wrist held in extension
   4. Explain the proper techniques in using a cane
      a. Hold in the hand opposite the affected extremity and close to the body
      b. Advance the cane and the affected extremity simultaneously, and then the unaffected leg
      c. When climbing, step up with the unaffected extremity and then place the cane and the affected lower extremity on the step; when descending, reverse the procedure
   5. Walk on client's affected side
   6. Observe for incorrect use of the cane
      a. Leaning the body over the cane
      b. Shortening the stride on the unaffected side
      c. Inability to develop a normal walking pattern
      d. Persistence of the abnormal gait pattern after cane is no longer needed
C. Nursing care: crutch walking
   1. Ensure proper fit of crutches
      a. Measure the distance from the anterior fold of the axilla to a point 15 cm (6 inches) out from the heel
      b. Axillary bars must be 5 cm (2 inches) below axillae and should be padded
      c. Hand bars should allow almost complete extension of arm with the elbow flexed about 30 degrees when the client places weight on the hands
   2. Ensure that rubber crutch tips are in good condition
   3. Assist in use of proper technique, depending on ability to bear weight and to take steps with either one or both of the lower extremities
      a. Four-point alternate crutch gait
         (1) Right crutch, left foot, left crutch, right foot; always three points of support on floor
         (2) Equal but partial weight bearing on each limb; slow, stable gait

         (3) Client must be able to manipulate both extremities and get one foot ahead of the other
      b. Two-point alternate crutch gait
         (1) Right crutch and left foot simultaneously; always two points of support on the floor
         (2) More rapid version of the four-point gait and requires more balance and strength
      c. Three-point gait
         (1) Advance both crutches and the weaker lower extremity simultaneously, then the stronger lower extremity
         (2) Fairly rapid gait, but requires more balance and strength in the arms and the unaffected lower extremity
         (3) Used when one leg can support the whole body weight and the other cannot take full weight bearing
      d. Swing crutch gaits
         (1) Swing-to gait: place both crutches forward, lift and swing body up to crutches, then place crutches in front of body and continue; always two points of support on floor; requires adequate power in upper arms
         (2) Swing-through gait: place both crutches forward, lift and swing body through crutches, then place crutches in front of body and continue; a difficult gait that necessitates rolling the pelvis forward and arching the back to get center of gravity in front of hips; requires power in trunk and upper extremities, excellent balance, self-confidence, and a bit of daring
   4. Observe for incorrect use of crutches
      a. Using the body in poor mechanical fashion
      b. Hiking hips with abduction gait (common in amputees)
      c. Lifting crutches while still bearing down on them
      d. Walking on ball of foot with foot turned outward and flexion at hip or knee level
      e. Hunching shoulders (crutches usually too long) or stooping with shoulders (crutches usually too short)
      f. Looking downward while ambulating
      g. Bearing weight under arms; should be avoided to prevent injury to the nerves in the brachial plexus; damage to these nerves can cause paralysis and is known as crutch palsy
D. Nursing care: use of a walker
   1. Assist in selecting a walker
      a. Device should be used when the client is not able to ambulate with a cane; partial weight bearing required

b. Measurements for a walker are the same as for a cane
c. Requires strong elbow extensors and shoulder depressors and partial strength in the hands and the wrist muscles to lift the standard walker; 2- and 4-wheeled walkers are available
d. Device cannot be used on steps
2. Assist in ambulating with the walker
a. Lift the device off the floor and place forward a short distance, then advance between the walker
b. Two-wheeled walkers: raise back legs of the device off the floor, roll walker forward, then advance to it
c. Four-wheeled walkers: push device forward on floor and then walk to it
3. Observe for incorrect use of the walker
a. Keeping arms rigid and swinging through to counterbalance the position of the lower extremity
b. Tending to lean forward with abnormal flexion at the hips
c. Tending to step forward with the unaffected leg and shuffle the affected leg up to the walker

Mobility: Wheelchair

A. Purpose
1. Support and move a client on a special chair that has wheels; the client is propelled or propels self
2. Provide mobility for those who cannot ambulate or those who can ambulate but whose ambulation is unsteady, unsafe, or too strenuous
3. Decrease cardiac workload
4. Promote independence and stimulate activities
B. Nursing care
1. Instruct the client that prolonged sitting in one position can cause flexion contractures of the hips and knees and ischial pressure ulcers (encourage the client to change body positions and to use padded cushions and exercises such as push-ups every hour to relieve pressure)
2. Ensure that device is in operating condition (e.g., wheel brakes, arm locks, seat belts, swing foot rests); inform client about accessories (e.g., removable arms, lap boards, extra-long leg panels, battery or motor propulsion)
3. Assist client with transfer; keep wheelchair in close proximity to bed or chair when transferring

Instillation of Eye Medications

A. Purpose: to provide therapeutic effect of medication ordered
B. Nursing care

1. Position the client with the head slightly backward
2. Pull lower eyelid down and instill solution in center of conjunctival sac; ointment applied from inner canthus outward; check order: OD (right eye), OU (both eyes), OS (left eye)
3. Have client close the eyes gently and instruct that they should not be rubbed
4. Apply pressure to the nasolacrimal duct if liquid instillation

Irrigations of the Ear

A. Definition
1. Introduction of fluid into the external auditory canal
2. Usually done for cleansing but can be used to apply antiseptic solutions
B. Nursing care
1. Verify if tympanic membrane is intact
2. Assist the client to a sitting position with the head tilted to affected side for an irrigation to facilitate drainage; for instillations the client should lie on the unaffected side
3. Gently pull up and back on the external ear of an adult, down and forward on a child, to straighten the canal
4. Direct solution into the canal without exerting excessive force; collect returns in a basin
5. Dry the outer ear
6. Record the procedure, type of drainage, etc.

MAJOR DISORDERS OF THE NEUROMUSCULOSKELETAL SYSTEM

▼ TRAUMATIC BRAIN INJURIES

Data Base

A. Etiology and pathophysiology
1. Motor vehicle accidents are the most common cause; can result from assaults, falls, and sport-related accidents
2. Caused by a sudden force to the head
a. Acceleration injury: immobile head struck by moving object
b. Deceleration injury: head is hit by stationary object
c. Deformation injury: force disrupts the integrity of the skull
3. Fractures
a. Linear: simple break in the bone
b. Depressed: break that results in fragments of bone penetrating brain tissue
c. Basilar: occurs over the base of frontal and temporal lobes; ecchymosis is common over areas involved

4. Hemorrhages (secondary brain injury)
   a. Epidural: hematoma forms between the dura and the skull; may result from a laceration of the middle meningeal artery
   b. Subdural: hematoma forms between the dura and arachnoid layers; generally follows venous damage
   c. Intracerebral hematoma
5. Concussion: temporary disruption of synaptic activity; brief loss of consciousness (<5 minutes)
6. Contusions: bruising of brain tissue, with slight bleeding of small cerebral vessels into surrounding tissues at site of impact (coup) or opposite to site (contrecoup) as a result of rebound reaction
   a. Cerebral contusions manifest depending on areas involved
   b. Brainstem contusions result in unresponsiveness
7. Complications include cerebral edema, brain abscess, meningitis, diabetes insipidus

B. Clinical findings
1. Subjective: lethargy; indifference to surroundings; altered sensory function (e.g., visual or auditory)
2. Objective
   a. Signs of increased intracranial pressure (ICP) (see Brain Tumor)
   b. Lack of orientation to time and place
   c. Positive Babinski reflex
   d. Seepage of cerebral spinal fluid from nose or ears; usually indicative of basilar skull fracture

C. Therapeutic interventions
1. Control seizures with anticonvulsants
2. Mechanical ventilation; hyperventilation constricts cerebral vessels lowering ICP
3. Monitor ICP with external catheter such as ventricular catheter or subarachnoid screw
4. Reduce cerebral edema with glucocorticoids and loop diuretics; there is disagreement regarding their efficacy
5. Maintain adequate fluid and electrolyte balance
6. Surgical intervention in cases of depressed skull fractures or hematomas

Nursing Care of Clients with Head Injuries

A. ASSESSMENT
1. Airway and breathing pattern
2. Neurologic status (see Neurologic Assessment and Glasgow Coma Scale)
3. Signs of increased intracranial pressure (see Brain Tumor)
4. Circumstances of injury
5. Presence of glucose in clear drainage from nose or ears, which indicates cerebrospinal fluid

B. ANALYSIS/NURSING DIAGNOSES
1. Risk for aspiration related to loss of gag reflex or inability to expectorate
2. Decreased intracranial adaptive capacity related to increased ICP
3. Risk for disuse syndrome related to long-term immobility
4. Ineffective role performance related to impaired neuromuscular function

C. PLANNING/IMPLEMENTATION
1. Institute neurologic assessments every 15 minutes for several hours, progressing to every hour and then every 4 hours
2. Maintain airway by suctioning as necessary (coughing increases intracranial pressure); use an airway or endotracheal tube
3. Keep the client's head elevated 30 degrees to reduce venous pressure within the cranial cavity
4. Administer glucocorticoids and/or diuretics if ordered
5. Institute seizure precautions; administer anticonvulsants if ordered
6. Monitor for fluid or electrolyte imbalances; diabetes insipidus or syndrome of inappropriate antidiuretic hormone may occur
7. If the client's eyes remain open, protect the corneas with moistened pads, artificial tears, or ointment as ordered
8. Support client's nutritional needs; administer tube feedings or assist with small frequent meals
9. Position the client to prevent pressure ulcers
10. Provide range-of-motion exercises and splints to prevent contractures
11. Provide auditory and tactile stimulation
12. Assist client to avoid activities that increase ICP such as the Valsalva maneuver, lifting, sneezing, and flexion of head
13. Recognize that confusion upon return of consciousness may be a defense against additional stress
14. Utilize hypothermia as ordered to reduce temperature and metabolic demands
15. Encourage client and family to participate in planning and care
16. Provide opportunity for expression of grief

D. EVALUATION/OUTCOMES
1. Maintains a patent airway
2. Improves level of consciousness
3. Remains free from complications of immobility
4. Participates in decisions about administration of care

▼ BRAIN TUMORS

Data Base

A. Etiology and pathophysiology
1. Either benign or malignant; they require intervention, because the skull cannot accommodate the increasing size of the tumor and intracranial pressure rises
2. Classified according to tissue of origin
   a. Meningioma: occurs outside brain from covering meninges; usually benign
   b. Acoustic neuroma and optic nerve spongioblastoma: occur from the cranial nerves
   c. Gliomas: originate in neural tissue; usually malignant and include astrocytoma, glioblastoma, oligodendroglioma
   d. Hemangioblastomas and angiomas: occur from within blood vessels
   e. Metastatic tumors: originate elsewhere in the body, most commonly the lung, breast, kidney, and site of malignant melanoma
B. Clinical findings
1. Subjective: headache that increases when supine or stooping; lethargy; nausea
2. Objective: signs of increased intracranial pressure; abnormal CT scan, MRI, EEG; vomiting; papilledema
3. Symptoms may vary depending on location of tumor
   a. Frontal lobe: personality changes, focal seizures, blurred vision, hemiparesis, altered thought processes
   b. Temporal lobe: seizures, headache, papilledema, receptive aphasia, tinnitus
   c. Parietal lobe: visual loss, motor and sensory focal seizures
   d. Occipital region: focal seizures, visual hallucinations, homonymous hemianopsia
   e. Cerebellar region: loss of coordination, tremors, nystagmus
C. Therapeutic interventions
1. Radiation therapy and/or chemotherapy
2. Surgery for partial or complete removal of the lesion
   a. Craniotomy with removal of lesion and invaded tissue
   b. Stereotactic radiosurgery; employs computer-directed radiation to eradicate tissue
3. Steroids, anticonvulsives, and osmotic diuretics to control symptoms

Nursing Care of Clients with Brain Tumors

A. ASSESSMENT
1. History from client and family to identify behavioral changes, coping skills, and neurologic deficits
2. Neurologic status (see Neurologic Assessment and Glasgow Coma Scale)
3. Unilateral nonreactive and/or dilated pupil progressing to bilateral as intracranial pressure increases
4. Signs of increased intracranial pressure
   a. Decreased level of consciousness
   b. Rapid rise in body temperature; decreased pulse rate; changes in respiratory pattern
   c. Increased systolic pressure; widening pulse pressure
   d. Restlessness
   e. Headache
   f. Weakness or paralysis
   g. Visual and other sensory disturbances; papilledema
   h. Vomiting
   i. Seizures

B. ANALYSIS/NURSING DIAGNOSES
1. Ineffective breathing pattern related to compromised neurologic function
2. Decreased intracranial adaptive capacity related to increased ICP
3. Anxiety related to uncertain prognosis

C. PLANNING/IMPLEMENTATION
1. Perform routine neurologic assessments
2. Provide emotional support for the client and family; refer to additional resources such as clergy and support groups
3. Administer analgesics and antiemetics as ordered
4. Provide small, frequent feedings, supplements, and oral hygiene
5. Provide care for the client requiring brain surgery
   a. Obtain consent for surgery and removal of hair
   b. After surgery keep the client's head elevated 30 degrees
   c. Support respiratory function by encouraging deep breathing, appropriate positioning, and suctioning to maintain the airway
   d. Use strict aseptic technique with ICP monitoring
   e. Observe dressings for cerebrospinal fluid leakage or hemorrhage
   f. Maintain intake and output
   g. Use hypothermia as ordered if the client is febrile; fever increases metabolic needs of the brain
6. Assist client to focus on abilities rather than disabilities
7. Emphasize need for continued health care supervision

D. EVALUATION/OUTCOMES
1. Maintains adequate respiratory function

2. Oriented to person, place, and time
3. Establishes effective communication

▼ CEREBRAL VASCULAR ACCIDENT (CVA, BRAIN ATTACK)

Data Base

A. Etiology and pathophysiology
1. Destruction (infarction) of brain cells caused by a reduction in oxygen supply
   a. Ischemic stroke results when brain tissues are blocked from oxygen supply by thrombus or embolus; 83% of strokes are this type
   b. Hemorrhagic stroke results from bleeding into brain tissue or subarachnoid space
2. Symptoms depend on the area of the brain involved and extent of damage; may be masked or delayed because of compensatory collateral circulation through the circle of Willis
3. Risk factors include hypertension, hyerlipidemia, obesity, smoking, cerebral arteriosclerosis, cerebral aneurysm, atrial fibrillation, advanced age
4. Transient ischemic attacks (TIA) may also occur without causing permanent damage; these usually last 5 to 20 minutes; warning sign of impending stroke

B. Clinical findings
1. Subjective: syncope; headache; changes in level of consciousness; transient paresthesias (with TIAs); mood swings
2. Objective
   a. Convulsions
   b. Hemiplegia on side opposite the lesion (initially flaccid then spastic)
   c. Aphasia: brain unable to fulfill its communicative functions because of damage to input, integrative, or output centers
      (1) Expressive (motor or Broca's) aphasia: difficulty making thoughts known to others; speaking and writing is most affected
      (2) Receptive (sensory or Wernicke's) aphasia: difficulty understanding what others are trying to communicate; interpretation of speech and reading is most affected
      (3) Global aphasia: affects both expression and reception
   d. Dysphagia
   e. Visual changes
      (1) Homonymous hemianopsia: loss of vision in half of the same visual field in both eyes
      (2) Agnosia: disturbance in ability to recog-

nize objects and attach meaning to them
      (3) Ptosis and paralysis of ocular muscles (Horner's syndrome)
   f. Alterations in reflexes
   g. Altered bladder and bowel function
   h. CSF is bloody if cerebral or subarachnoid hemorrhage is present
   i. Abnormal EEG, CT scan, MRI
   j. Cerebral angiography may reveal vascular abnormalities such as aneurysms, narrowing, or occlusions
   k. Signs of increased intracranial pressure (see Brain Tumor)

C. Therapeutic interventions
1. Complete bed rest with sedation as needed
2. Maintenance of oxygenation by oxygen therapy or mechanical ventilation
3. If ischemic type, thrombolytic therapy with recombinant tissue plasminogen activator (rt-PA) within 3 hours of onset intravenously over 1 hour
4. Maintenance of nutrition by the parenteral route or nasogastric feedings if the client is unable to swallow
5. Anticoagulant therapy if thrombus or embolus is present; antiplatelet therapy
6. Antihypertensives and anticonvulsants if indicated
7. Glucocorticoids may be used to reduce cerebral edema and intracranial pressure
8. Surgical intervention for those who have ICP >30 mm Hg, who have rapid deterioration, and who are younger than 70 years
   a. To relieve pressure and control bleeding if hemorrhage is present
   b. Carotid endarterectomy to improve cerebral blood flow when carotid arteries are narrowed by arteriosclerotic patches

Nursing Care of Clients with Cerebral Vascular Accidents

A. ASSESSMENT
1. Adequacy of airway and respiratory function
2. Neurologic status (see Neurologic Assessment and Glasgow Coma Scale)
3. Presence of signs of increased ICP (see Brain Tumors)

B. ANALYSIS/NURSING DIAGNOSES
1. Risk for aspiration related to dysphagia
2. Ineffective cerebral tissue perfusion related to interruption of arterial blood flow
3. Impaired verbal communication related to aphasia
4. Impaired physical mobility related to hemiparesis

5. Powerlessness related to loss of abilities

C. **PLANNING/IMPLEMENTATION**

1. Perform neurologic assessments; note signs of intracranial pressure
2. Assist with lumbar puncture if performed; may be performed if subarachnoid hemorrhage is suspected (see Lumbar Puncture)
3. Monitor vital signs; avoid using affected extremity for BP because it may produce falsely, lowered readings
4. Maintain patency of the airway by positioning, suctioning, and inserting an artificial airway
5. Provide for drainage and expansion of lungs by placing client in a low semi-Fowler's position with head turned to side; provide oxygen as necessary
6. Encourage deep breathing; utilize mechanical ventilation if ordered
7. Involve all members of the health team when planning care
8. Assist client and family to set realistic goals; provide encouragement and praise
9. Accept and explore feelings of fear, anger, and depression; accept mood swings and emotional outbursts
10. Provide frequent oral hygiene; use artificial tears if blink reflex is absent
11. Institute seizure precautions
12. Provide elastic or pneumatic stockings for both legs
13. Prevent pressure ulcers (see Pressure Ulcers)
14. Prevent muscle atrophy and contractures
    a. Provide passive range-of-motion exercises; active range-of-motion and other exercises may be instituted later
    b. Use devices to prevent footdrop, flexion of fingers, external rotation of hips, adduction of shoulders and arms
15. Provide tube feedings if swallowing and gag reflexes are depressed or absent
16. Provide food in a form that is easily swallowed (mechanical soft, puree, thickening products); encourage intake of nutrient-dense foods; when client is capable of chewing, introduce dietary fiber to promote normal bowel function
17. Assist with, feeding (e.g., use a padded spoon handle; feed on the unaffected side of mouth; feed in as close to a sitting position as possible)
18. Encourage the client with speech difficulties to communicate
    a. Be aware of own reactions to the speech difficulty
    b. Evaluate extent of the client's ability to understand and express self
    c. Reinforce what has been learned in speech therapy
    d. Convey that there is a problem with communication, not with intelligence; try to eliminate anxiety related to communication attempts
    e. Avoid pushing to point of frustration
    f. Keep distractions at a minimum, since they interfere with the reception and integration of messages
    g. Speak slowly, clearly, and in short sentences, and do not raise voice
    h. Use alternate means of communication
    i. Involve the client in social interactions
    j. Be alert for clues and gestures when speech is garbled
19. Make a definite transition between tasks to prevent or reduce confusion
20. Attempt to prevent fecal impaction and/or urinary tract problems
    a. Provide adequate fluid intake
    b. Provide a diet with enough roughage for sufficient quantity of bowel content and proper consistency for evacuation; avoid straining at stool because it can raise ICP; administer stool softeners as ordered
    c. Avoid preoccupation with elimination; avoid encouragement of incontinence
    d. Stimulate normal elimination by exercise and activity
    e. Help develop regular bowel and bladder patterns
    f. Respect the individual: provide for privacy and individuality of routine
    g. Utilize physical and psychologic techniques to stimulate elimination
21. Create environment that keeps sensory monotony to a minimum; orient to time and place, increase social contacts, provide visual stimuli, extend environment
22. Provide for self-esteem; encourage wearing own clothes, doing self-care activities, making decisions
23. Help with adjustment to altered body image and self-esteem

D. **EVALUATION/OUTCOMES**

1. Maintains respiratory function
2. Remains alert and oriented
3. Communicates effectively
4. Remains free of complications of immobility
5. Family and client participate in decisions and care

▼ EPILEPSY (SEIZURE DISORDERS)

Data Base

A. Etiology and pathophysiology

1. Abnormal discharge of electric impulses by the nerve cells in the brain from idiopathic or secondary causes resulting in: loss of consciousness; convulsions; motor, sensory, behavioral changes
2. Onset of idiopathic epilepsy generally before age 30; seizures can be associated with brain tumor, CVA, Alzheimer's disease, hypoglycemia, head trauma
3. Types of seizures
   a. Partial seizures (seizures beginning locally)
      (1) Simple: focal motor or sensory effect; no loss of consciousness
      (2) Complex: cognitive, psychosensory, psychomotor, or affective effect; brief loss of consciousness
   b. Generalized seizures (bilaterally symmetric and without local onset)
      (1) Absence (petit mal): brief transient loss of consciousness with or without minor motor movements of eyes, head, or extremities; most common in childhood and adolescence
      (2) Myoclonic: brief, transient rigidity or jerking of extremities, singly or in groups
      (3) Tonic-clonic (grand mal): aura, loss of consciousness, rigidity followed by tonic and clonic movements, interruption of respirations, loss of bladder and bowel control; may last 2 to 5 minutes
      (4) Atonic: involve loss of muscle control; loss of consciousness may be brief
   c. Status epilepticus: prolonged repetitive seizures without recovery between attacks; may result in complete exhaustion and lead to death
B. Clinical findings (tonic-clonic seizures)
   1. Subjective: seizure often preceded by an aura or warning sensation such as seeing spots or feeling dizzy; loss of consciousness during seizure; lethargy following return to consciousness (postictal phase)
   2. Objective
      a. Shrill cry as seizure begins and air is forcefully exhaled
      b. Tonic and clonic movement of the muscles and incontinence
      c. Abnormal EEG
C. Therapeutic interventions
   1. Antiepileptic therapy continued throughout life; diazepam (Valium) given IV to treat status epilepticus
   2. Sedatives used to reduce emotional stress
   3. Neurosurgery is sometimes indicated if seizures are caused by tumors, abscesses, or vascular problems

Nursing Care of Clients with Epilepsy
A. ASSESSMENT
   1. History of type, frequency, and duration of seizures and precipitating factors
   2. Sensations associated with the seizure that may constitute an aura
B. ANALYSIS/NURSING DIAGNOSES
   1. Risk for injury related to lowered level of consciousness
   2. Risk for aspiration related to lowered level of consciousness and excessive secretions
   3. Powerlessness related to unpredictable nature of illness and limitations imposed on activities
C. PLANNING/IMPLEMENTATION
   1. Provide protection from injury during and after the seizure; nothing should be forced into the mouth because this may cause tongue to occlude airway
   2. Help the client with an aura to plan for self-protection before seizure develops
   3. Encourage use of a medical alert tag
   4. Help plan a schedule that provides adequate rest and reduction of stress
   5. Teach the client and family to observe the aura, initial point of seizure, type of seizure, level of consciousness, loss of bladder and bowel control, progression of seizure, and postictal condition
   6. Encourage expression of feelings about illness and necessary changes in lifestyle and self-esteem
   7. Assist client and family to accept the diagnosis and develop some understanding of the disease process
   8. Teach that medication must be taken continuously for the remainder of life under continued medical supervision
   9. Refer for job counseling as necessary
   10. Encourage client and family to attend local epilepsy association meetings
   11. Refer client to state laws regarding driving
   12. Teach about anticonvulsants (see Anticonvulsants in Pharmacology)
D. EVALUATION/OUTCOMES
   1. Remains free from injury
   2. Verbalizes willingness to follow lifelong medication regimen

▼ BELL'S PALSY (FACIAL PARALYSIS)

Data Base
A. Etiology and pathophysiology
   1. Paralysis that occurs on one side of the face as a result of an inflamed seventh cranial (facial) nerve; generally lasts only 2 to 8 weeks but, may last longer in older clients

2. Cause unknown; possible viral link
3. Most common between ages 20 to 50 years

B. Clinical findings
  1. Subjective: facial pain; altered taste; impaired ability to chew and swallow
  2. Objective: distortion of face; drooping of mouth on affected side; difficulty with articulation; diminished blink reflex; upward movement of eyeball when closing eye; increased lacrimation

C. Therapeutic interventions
  1. Prednisone therapy
  2. Heat, massage, and electric stimulation to maintain circulation and muscle tone
  3. Prevention of corneal irritation with eyedrops and use of protective eye shield

Nursing Care of Clients with Bell's Palsy

A. ASSESSMENT
  1. Presence or absence of blink reflex and ability to close the eye
  2. Facial pain; extent of facial paralysis
  3. Nutritional intake and the ability to chew and swallow

B. ANALYSIS/NURSING DIAGNOSES
  1. Pain related to inflammation or compression of facial nerve
  2. Risk for injury related to absent or diminished blink reflex
  3. Disturbed body image related to change in facial appearance

C. PLANNING/IMPLEMENTATION
  1. Teach prevention of corneal irritation by using artificial tears, manually closing the eye, and applying an eye shield
  2. Teach importance of keeping face warm
  3. Teach gentle massage of face; simple exercises such as blowing; institute only when acute phase is over
  4. Encourage ventilation of feelings
  5. Support nutritional status by providing privacy and small, frequent feedings; encourage favoring the unaffected side while eating

D. EVALUATION/OUTCOMES
  1. Maintains corneal integrity
  2. Expresses a positive body image
  3. States pain is reduced

▼ TRIGEMINAL NEURALGIA (TIC DOULOUREUX)

Data Base

A. Etiology and pathophysiology
  1. Incidence higher in women of middle and older age
  2. Disorder of the fifth cranial (trigeminal) nerve characterized by intense knifelike pain along the branches of the nerve
  3. May result from abnormalities of ganglion, tumors, vascular anomalies, or dental infection

B. Clinical findings
  1. Subjective: burning or knifelike pain lasting 1 to 15 minutes, usually in lip, chin, or teeth; pain precipitated by brushing hair, eating, cold drafts
  2. Objective: sudden closure of an eye; twitching of mouth and cheek

C. Therapeutic interventions
  1. Anticonvulsants to relieve and prevent acute attacks
  2. Injection of alcohol into the ganglion (nerve block) to relieve pain for several months or years until nerve regenerates
  3. Injection of baclofen (Lioresal) with anticonvulsants may control symptoms
  4. Surgical intervention
     a. Severing of the sensory root of the nerve, which will cause loss of all sensation in the area supplied by the nerve
     b. Microscopic relocation of arterial loop that may cause vascular compression of trigeminal nerve
  5. Percutaneous radio frequency trigeminal gangliolysis: destroys nerve, providing permanent relief for most clients

Nursing Care of Clients with Trigeminal Neuralgia

A. ASSESSMENT
  1. Descriptions of pain and factors that precipitates attacks
  2. Effect on activities (e.g., eating, shaving, washing the face, brushing the teeth) because of fear of precipitating an attack

B. ANALYSIS/NURSING DIAGNOSES
  1. Fear related to triggering an attack
  2. Pain related to irritation of the trigeminal nerve
  3. Imbalanced nutrition: less than body requirements related to reluctance to chew

C. PLANNING/IMPLEMENTATION
  1. Teach factors to limit triggering an attack, which can result in exhaustion
     a. Avoid foods that are too cold or too hot
     b. Chew foods on unaffected side
     c. Use cotton pads to gently wash face and for oral hygiene
     d. Keep the room free of drafts; avoid jarring
  2. Provide teaching to clients who have sensory loss as a result of treatment
     a. Inspection of the eye several times a day for foreign bodies, which the client will not be able to feel

b. Warm normal saline irrigation of the affected eye two or three times a day is helpful in preventing a corneal infection

c. Dental checkups every 6 months, because caries will not produce pain

3. Teach about anticonvulsants (see Anticonvulsants in Pharmacology) and the need for continued medical supervision

D. EVALUATION/OUTCOMES

1. Reports decreased severity of attacks
2. Consumes nutritionally balanced diet
3. Develops mechanisms to cope with fear

▼ PARKINSON'S DISEASE (PARALYSIS AGITANS)

Data Base

A. Etiology and pathophysiology
1. Progressive disorder in which there is a destruction of nerve cells in the basal ganglia and substantia nigra of the brain, which results in dopamine deficiency and subsequent generalized degeneration of muscular function
2. Incidence highest in elderly; suspected causes include neurotransmitter imbalance (dopamine and acetylcholine), unknown virus, cerebral vascular disease, and chemical or physical trauma

B. Clinical findings
1. Subjective: mild, diffuse, muscular pain; stiffness and rigidity, particularly of large joints; depression; emotional lability may be present, but intelligence is usually not impaired
2. Objective
a. Diminished voluntary motion: increased difficulty in performing usual activities, such as writing, dressing, eating, and walking (e.g., bent posture, difficulty rising from a sitting position, shuffling propulsive gait, loss of rhythmic arm swing when walking)
(1) Bradykinesia: slowness of voluntary movement
(2) Hypokinesia: decreased movement
(3) Akinesia: inability to move
b. Generalized tremor commonly accompanied by "pill-rolling" movements of the thumb against the fingers; nonintention tremors usually reduced by purposeful movements
c. Masklike facial expression with unblinking eyes
d. Low-pitched, slow, poorly modulated, poorly articulated speech
e. Drooling; difficulty in swallowing saliva
f. Various autonomic symptoms (e.g., lacrimation, constipation, incontinence, decreased sexual capacity, excessive perspiration)

g. Dementia and confusion in 25% to 40% of individuals, especially the elderly

C. Therapeutic interventions
1. Medical regimen is palliative rather than curative
2. Pharmacologic intervention (see Antiparkinson Agents in Pharmacology)
3. Physiotherapy to reduce rigidity of muscles and prevent contractures
4. The role of surgical intervention is limited
a. Destruction of thalamus or globus pallidus for intractable tremor and rigidity
b. Transplantation of tissue of adrenal medulla into brain to produce dopamine and transplantation of fetal tissue has been tried

Nursing Care of Clients with Parkinson's Disease

A. ASSESSMENT
1. History of onset and progression of symptoms
2. Observations of tremors, gait, facial expression, and bradykinesia
3. Nutritional status
4. Elimination status
5. Horizontal and vertical blood pressures to identify postural hypotension

B. ANALYSIS/NURSING DIAGNOSES
1. Impaired physical mobility related to neuromuscular degeneration
2. Risk for injury related to postural changes and bradykinesia
3. Chronic low self-esteem related to loss of independence
4. Risk for aspiration related to dysphagia

C. PLANNING/IMPLEMENTATION
1. Provide a safe environment
2. Teach client or family to cut food into small bite-sized pieces or alter the consistency to prevent choking; encourage diet rich in nutrient-dense foods such as fruits, vegetables, whole grains, and legumes to improve and maintain nutritional status and prevent possible drug-induced nutrient deficiencies
3. Suction to maintain an adequate airway (usually advanced stages)
4. Encourage an adequate intake of roughage and fluids to avoid constipation
5. Teach activities to limit postural deformities (e.g., use firm mattress without a pillow, periodically lie prone, keep head and neck as erect as possible, think about posture when walking)
6. Teach activities to maintain gait as normal as possible; utilize cane or walker as necessary
7. Teach and encourage daily physical therapy to limit rigidity and prevent contractures (e.g., warms baths, passive and active exercises)

8. Avoid rushing as stress intensifies symptoms
9. Encourage continuation of medications even though results may be minimal
10. Teach client and family about antiparkinson agents (see Antiparkinson Agents in Pharmacology)
11. Assist in setting achievable goals to improve self-esteem

D. EVALUATION/OUTCOMES
1. Maintains patent airway
2. Participates in daily exercise program
3. Complies with prescribed medical therapy
4. Remains free from injuries

▼ MULTIPLE SCLEROSIS (DISSEMINATED SCLEROSIS)

Data Base
A. Etiology and pathophysiology
1. Randomly scattered patches of demyelination in brainstem, cerebrum, cerebellum, and spinal cord
2. Chronic debilitating, progressive disease with periods of remission and exacerbation
3. Cause unknown; viral and immunologic causes have been implicated
4. Onset in early adult life (20 to 40 years); higher occurrence in females
5. Greater incidence in Caucasians and those living in cold climates
6. Fatigue, stress, and heat tend to increase symptoms
B. Clinical findings
1. Subjective
a. Paresthesia; altered position sense; ataxia
b. Dysphagia
c. Weakness; fatigue
d. Blurred vision; diplopia
e. Altered emotional affect (depression, apathy, or euphoria)
2. Objective
a. Charcot's triad: intention tremor, nystagmus, scanning (clipped) speech
b. Shuffling gait; increased deep tendon reflexes; spastic paralysis
c. Impaired bowel and bladder function
d. Impotence
e. Cognitive loss (advanced stage)
f. Pallor of optic discs; blindness
g. Increased immunoglobulin G (IgG) levels in the CSF
h. MRI indicates demyelination and presence of MS plaques
C. Therapeutic interventions
1. Generally palliative

2. Corticosteroids or ACTH
3. Baclofen is used to control spasticity
4. Interferon beta-1b (Betaseron)
5. Physiotherapy and psychotherapy
6. Carbamazepine for paresthesias and trigeminal neuralgia
7. Immunosuppressive drugs (e.g., cyclophosphamide, azathioprine)

Nursing Care of Clients with Multiple Sclerosis
A. ASSESSMENT
1. History of onset and progression of motor and sensory loss
2. Factors that intensify symptoms
3. Neurologic status (see Neurologic Assessment in Related Procedures)

B. ANALYSIS/NURSING DIAGNOSES
1. Risk for aspiration related to impaired swallowing
2. Impaired physical mobility related to spasticity and muscle fatigue
3. Risk for injury related to unsteady gait, altered sensations, and impaired vision
4. Constipation related to immobility and neuromuscular impairment
5. Urinary retention related to spasticity
6. Hopelessness related to progression of the disease

C. PLANNING/IMPLEMENTATION
1. Incorporate frequent rest periods
2. Avoid hot baths, which can increase symptoms
3. Teach use of assistive devices when carrying out activities of daily living
4. Assist family to understand why client should be encouraged to be active
5. Assist client and family to plan and implement a bowel and bladder regimen
6. Explain the disease process to both client and family in understandable terms
7. Do not encourage false hopes during periods of remission
8. Spend time listening to both client and family; encourage ventilation of feelings
9. Refer client and family to the National Multiple Sclerosis Society
10. Encourage counseling and rehabilitation
11. Explain to client and family that mood swings and emotional alterations are part of the disease process
12. Help client maintain self-esteem
13. Teach how to compensate for problems with gait: walk with feet farther apart to broaden base of support; use low-heeled shoes; use assistive devices when necessary (tripod cane, walker, wheelchair)
14. Teach how to compensate for loss of sensation: use a thermometer to test water temperature; avoid constricting stockings; use protec-

tive clothing in cold weather; change position frequently
15. Teach how to compensate for difficulty in swallowing: take small bites; chew well; use a straw with liquids; eat foods of more solid consistency
16. Provide a diet rich in nutrient-dense foods such as fruits, vegetables, whole grains, and legumes to improve and maintain nutritional status and compensate for nutrient interactions of corticosteroid medications
17. Provide skin care to prevent formation of pressure ulcers; turn frequently
18. Prevent dysfunctional contractures; provide range-of-motion exercises; splints

D. EVALUATION/OUTCOMES
1. Maintains a patent airway
2. Remains free from injury
3. Establishes exercise/activity and rest/sleep routine that avoids fatigue
4. Maintains bowel and bladder function
5. Copes with changes in physical abilities and lifestyle changes

▼ MYASTHENIA GRAVIS

Data Base

A. Etiology and pathophysiology
1. Chronic, progressive, neuromuscular disorder with remissions and exacerbations; there is a disturbance in the transmission of impulses at the myoneural junction resulting in profound weakness
2. Dysfunction thought to be caused by a reduced number of acetylcholine receptors (AChR) and an alteration of the postsynaptic membrane of the muscle end-plate
3. Autoimmune theory: it is believed that complement and antibodies to AChR cause accelerated destruction and blockage of the AChR
4. Highest incidence in young adult females
5. Myasthenic crisis refers to sudden inability to swallow or maintain respirations because of the weakness of the muscles of respiration

B. Clinical findings
1. Subjective: Extreme muscle weakness; becomes progressively worse with use, but disappears with rest; dyspnea; dysphagia (difficulty chewing and swallowing); dysarthria (difficulty speaking); diplopia
2. Objective
   a. Physical: ptosis; strabismus; weak voice (dysphonia); myasthenic smile (snarling, nasal smile)
   b. Diagnostic measures: spontaneous relief of symptoms with administration of subcuta-neous neostigmine (Prostigmin) or IV administration of edrophonium (Tensilon); edrophonium used to distinguish myasthenic crisis from cholinergic crisis (toxic effects of excessive neostigmine)

C. Therapeutic interventions
1. Medications that block the action of cholinesterase at the myoneural junction (see Cholinesterase Inhibitors in Pharmacology)
2. X-ray therapy or surgical removal of the thymus may cause partial remission
3. Corticosteroids, anticholinesterase drugs, or ACTH
4. Tracheostomy with mechanical ventilation as necessary in myasthenic crisis
5. Plasmapheresis and immunosuppressives to reduce circulating antibody titer

Nursing Care of Clients with Myasthenia Gravis

A. ASSESSMENT
1. History of onset and progression of motor and sensory loss; factors that intensify symptoms
2. Neurologic status (see Neurologic Assessment)

B. ANALYSIS/NURSING DIAGNOSES
1. Fatigue related to profound muscle weakness
2. Ineffective airway clearance related to inability to cough or swallow

C. PLANNING/IMPLEMENTATION
1. Administer medications on strict time schedule to prevent onset of symptoms
2. Observe for signs of dyspnea, dysphagia, and dysarthria; may be caused by worsening of myasthenia (myasthenic crisis) or overdose of anticholinergic drugs (cholinergic crisis)
3. Have an emergency tracheostomy set at bedside
4. Plan activity to avoid fatigue based on the individual's tolerance
5. Teach to avoid people with upper respiratory tract infections, because pneumonia may develop as a result of respiratory impairment
6. Encourage use of a medical alert card
7. Avoid administering morphine to clients receiving cholinesterase inhibitors; these drugs potentiate effects of morphine and may cause respiratory depression
8. Provide emotional support and close client contact to allay anxiety
9. Administer tube feedings to avoid aspiration if client has difficulty swallowing
10. Administer artificial tears to keep cornea moist if client has difficulty closing eyes
11. Encourage client and family to participate in planning care

12. Ensure that client understands the signs and symptoms of myasthenic and cholinergic crises
13. Refer client and family to Myasthenia Gravis Foundation and local self-help groups
14. In severe instances anticipate all needs, because the client is too weak to turn, drink, or even request assistance
15. Maintain a patent airway; suction as necessary; provide tracheostomy care; maintain mechanical ventilation as ordered

D. EVALUATION/OUTCOMES
1. Maintains a balance between activity and rest
2. Maintains effective respiratory function
3. Identifies signs and symptoms of crises

▼ GUILLAIN-BARRÉ SYNDROME (POLYRADICULONEURITIS)

Data Base
A. Etiology and pathophysiology
1. Changes in motor cells of spinal cord and medulla with areas of demyelination
2. Cause unknown; thought to be linked to immunologic status; often follows respiratory or gastrointestinal infection; may be linked to cytomegalovirus and Epstein-Barr virus
3. After initial and plateau periods, recovery may take up to a year; although most recover, some experience residual deficits or die of complications
B. Clinical findings
1. Subjective: generalized weakness; paresthesia; muscle pain; diplopia
2. Objective
   a. Paralysis begins in lower extremities; ascends within the body; maximal deficit usually by 4 weeks
   b. Respiratory paralysis
   c. Autonomic neuropathy (e.g., hypertension, tachycardia, diaphoresis)
   d. Abnormal CSF and electrophysiologic studies
C. Therapeutic interventions
1. Intravenous therapy with IgG
2. Plasmapheresis
3. Support of vital functions

Nursing Care of Clients with Guillain-Barré Syndrome
A. ASSESSMENT
1. Respiratory function including airway, respiratory rate, breath sounds, and arterial blood gases
2. Neurologic status (see Neurologic Assessment)
3. History of any recent illness (particularly viral infections)

4. Onset and progression of symptoms
B. ANALYSIS/NURSING DIAGNOSES
1. Impaired spontaneous ventilation related to muscle weakness
2. Ineffective role performance related to lengthy recovery period
3. Impaired physical mobility related to impaired neuromuscular function
C. PLANNING/IMPLEMENTATION
1. Monitor vital signs, breath sounds, and arterial blood gases
2. Maintain airway and keep tracheostomy set at the bedside
3. Monitor functioning of the ventilator and suction as necessary
4. Provide emotional support for the client and family because of the severity of adaptations and lengthy convalescent period
5. Prevent complications of immobility: skin care; range-of-motion exercises; position changes; coughing and deep breathing; antiembolism stockings
6. Refer client and family to Guillain-Barré Foundation for additional information and community resources
D. EVALUATION/OUTCOMES
1. Maintains effective respiratory function
2. Remains free from complications of immobility
3. Discusses feelings with family and other health-team members

▼ AMYOTROPHIC LATERAL SCLEROSIS (ALS)

Data Base
A. Etiology and pathophysiology
1. Progressive, degenerative process involving the corticospinal and anterior horn neurons, with subsequent upper and lower motor neuron effects
2. Occurs more frequently in men than women in the fourth and fifth decades
3. Cause unknown; autoimmune diseases and genetic causes are implicated
4. Death from respiratory complications frequently occurs within 3 to 5 years
B. Clinical findings
1. Subjective: muscular weakness; malaise; fatigue
2. Objective
   a. Fasciculations (irregular spasmodic twitching of small muscle groups); spasticity; atrophy
   b. Difficulty in breathing, chewing, swallowing, speaking
   c. Outbursts of laughter or crying
   d. Abnormal electromyography

C. Therapeutic interventions
1. Physiotherapy to relieve spasticity
2. Supportive respiratory functions
3. Riluzole (Rilutek) to inhibit glutamate accumulation, possibly preventing injury or death of neurons

Nursing Care of Clients with Amyotrophic Lateral Sclerosis

A. ASSESSMENT
1. History of onset and progression of symptoms
2. Neurologic status (see Neurologic Assessment)
3. Respiratory status including rate, depth, and effort

B. ANALYSIS/NURSING DIAGNOSES
1. Impaired spontaneous ventilation related to neuromuscular impairment
2. Anticipatory grieving related to progressive nature of illness
3. Impaired physical mobility related to neuromuscular impairment

C. PLANNING/IMPLEMENTATION
1. Encourage client to remain active as long as possible, employing supportive devices as needed
2. Encourage range-of-motion exercises
3. Monitor swallowing ability; positioning and consistency of diet to prevent aspiration
4. Provide alternate means of communication as speech declines
5. Allow client to discuss feelings about life support while still able to speak
6. Monitor respiratory function; increased fluids, positioning, chest physiotherapy, coughing and deep breathing exercises, and suctioning help prevent complications
7. Support natural defense mechanisms; encourage a diet consisting of nutrient-dense foods, especially those rich in the immune-stimulating nutrients selenium and vitamins A, C, and E
8. Teach the avoidance of situations that may contribute to infection
9. Provide emotional support for the client and family
10. Refer client and family to ALS Association

D. EVALUATION/OUTCOMES
1. Maintains effective respiratory function
2. Discusses feelings with family and other health team members

▼ ARTHRITIS

Data Base
A. Etiology and pathophysiology
1. Rheumatoid arthritis (RA)
a. Altered antibodies (rheumatoid factors) combine with IgG to form complexes that are deposited in synovial membranes; inflammation and destructive changes follow, leading to joint deformity and fusion
b. Systemic effects may include vasculitis, pulmonary fibrosis, and pericardial disease
c. Etiology unclear; apparent genetic predisposition; incidence higher in women
2. Osteoarthritis (OA)
a. Characterized by enzymatic destruction of articular cartilage
b. Considered a noninflammatory joint disease with no systemic effects
c. Cause is unknown; secondary osteoarthritis is linked to damage from overuse, injury, infection, or chemicals.
3. Gouty arthritis (GA)
a. Disorder in purine metabolism, that leads to high levels of uric acid in the blood and the deposition of uric acid crystals (tophi) in tissues, especially joints; followed by an inflammatory response
b. Incidence highest in males; a familial tendency has been demonstrated
c. Renal urate lithiasis (kidney stones) may result from precipitation of uric acid in the presence of a low urinary pH

B. Clinical findings
1. Subjective
a. Joint pain
(1) Insidious onset of asymmetric pain in hips, knees, fingers or spine that increases with weight-bearing activity and is relieved by rest (OA)
(2) Symmetrical pain in small joints of hands and feet; knees, shoulders, hips, elbows, and ankles affected as disease progresses; not relieved by rest (RA)
(3) Sudden onset of asymmetric joint pain usually in metatarsophalangeal joint of the great toe (GA)
b. Morning stiffness: less than 1 hour with OA; more than 1 hour with RA
c. Anorexia, fatigue, and malaise (RA, GA)
2. Objective
a. Decreased range of motion
b. Inflammation (swelling, heat, redness) of involved joints (RA, GA)
c. Deformities
(1) Ulnar drift, Boutonniere deformity, swan-neck deformity, rheumatoid nodules (RA)
(2) Heberden's and Bouchard's nodes (bony hypertrophy) symmetrically occurring on fingers (OA)

(3) Tophi in outer ear, hands, feet, elbows, or knees (GA)
  d. Crepitus when joint is moved (OA)
  e. Fever (RA, GA)
  f. Laboratory findings
    (1) RA: presence of rheumatoid factors (RF), elevated erythrocyte sedimentation rate (ESR), decreased RBC, and positive C-reactive protein and antinuclear antibody (ANA) tests
    (2) GA: elevated serum uric acid
C. Therapeutic interventions
  1. Pharmacologic management
    a. Acetaminophen (OA)
    b. Nonsteroidal antiinflammatory drugs (RA, OA, GA) (see Pharmacology)
    c. Disease modifying agents such as methotrexate hydroxychloroquine, sulfasalazine, gold, azathioprine, and penicillamine (RA)
    d. Antigout agents (see Pharmacology)
    e. Corticosteroids (RA and resistant GA)
    f. Cyclooxygenase 2 inhibitors
  2. Weight loss
  3. Physical therapy to preserve joint function; application of heat/cold
  4. Use of splints and assistive devices
  5. Surgical intervention (RA, OA)
    a. Synovectomy: removal of the enlarged synovial membrane before bone and cartilage destruction occurs
    b. Arthrodesis: fusion of a joint performed when the joint surfaces are severely damaged; this leaves client with no range of motion of affected joint
    c. Reconstructive surgery: replacement of a badly damaged joint with a prosthetic device (see Fracture of the Hip)

Nursing Care of Clients with Arthritis

A. ASSESSMENT
  1. Extent of range of motion of involved joints; presence of bony deformities
  2. History of onset and progression of symptoms, noting degree to which pain interferes with normal activities
  3. Presence of risk factors such as obesity

B. ANALYSIS/NURSING DIAGNOSES
  1. Chronic pain related to joint inflammation
  2. Impaired physical mobility related to joint pain, stiffness, and swelling
  3. Disturbed body image related to visible joint deformity

C. PLANNING/IMPLEMENTATION
  1. Assist with activities that require using affected joints; allow for rest periods
  2. Maintain functional alignment of joints

3. Provide for range-of-motion exercises up to the point of pain, recognizing that some discomfort is always present
4. Relieve discomfort and edema by medications or application of heat/cold
5. Allow ample time to verbalize feelings regarding limited motion and changes in lifestyle; help set realistic goals, focusing on strengths
6. Support client through weight loss program if indicated
7. Encourage client to follow physical therapist's instruction regarding regular exercise program and use of supportive devices to maintain independence
8. Administer and teach about prescribed pharmacologic therapy
9. Provide dietary instructions
  a. Encourage diet rich in nutrient-dense foods such as fruits, vegetables, whole grains, and legumes to improve and maintain nutritional status and compensate for nutrient interactions of corticosteroid and other treatment medications (RA, GA); avoid high-purine foods such as organ meats, anchovies, sardines, and shellfish
  b. Increase fluid intake to 2000 to 3000 ml daily to prevent formation of calculi; alkaline-ash diet to increase the pH of urine to discourage precipitation of uric acid and enhance the action of drugs such as probenicid (GA)
10. Provide care for the client with RA or OA requiring joint replacement (see Nursing Care of Clients with Fractures of the Extremities or Hip)
11. Refer client and family to the Arthritis Foundation

D. EVALUATION/OUTCOMES
  1. Reports reduction in pain
  2. Completes activities of daily living using supportive devices as needed
  3. Accepts and adjusts to deformities

▼ OSTEOMYELITIS

Data Base

A. Etiology and pathophysiology: infection of bone by direct or indirect invasion usually by *Staphylococcus aureus;* may be acute or chronic
  1. Indirect entry: usually in young males; most often occurs in growing long bones; associated with local trauma
  2. Direct entry: not age related; extends from open wound to bone via arterial blood; ischemia results in formation of sequestrum leading to chronic osteomyelitis

B. Clinical findings
1. Subjective: pain and tenderness of bone; malaise; headache
2. Objective: signs of sepsis such as fever; edema and erythema over bone; positive culture from bone biopsy and positive radionucleide bone scan; MRI useful in confirmation of diagnosis
C. Therapeutic interventions
1. Intravenous antibiotic therapy for 4 to 8 weeks followed by oral antibiotics for 4 to 8 weeks
2. Incision and drainage of a bone abscess
3. Sequestrectomy: surgical removal of the dead, infected bone and cartilage

Nursing Care of Clients with Osteomyelitis
A. **ASSESSMENT**
1. History of trauma or infections
2. Involved tissue for signs of inflammation
3. Onset and characteristics of pain
B. **ANALYSIS/NURSING DIAGNOSES**
1. Ineffective tissue perfusion related to infection and tissue destruction
2. Pain related to bone tissue swelling
C. **PLANNING/IMPLEMENTATION**
1. Monitor neurovascular status of involved extremity
2. Administer pain medications and antibiotics as ordered
3. Maintain functional body alignment and promote comfort
4. Use room deodorizer if a foul odor is apparent
5. Allow expression of feelings about long-term confinement
6. Encourage nutrient-dense diet to compensate for impact of long-term antibiotic therapy on nutritional status
D. **EVALUATION/OUTCOMES**
1. Reports reduction in pain
2. Resolves infectious process

▼ OSTEOGENIC SARCOMA

Data Base
A. Etiology and pathophysiology
1. Malignant bone tumor that usually begins in long bones, especially around knee
2. Metastasis to the lungs common and occurs early; prognosis is poor
3. Highest incidence between 10 and 30 years
B. Clinical findings
1. Subjective: pain; malaise
2. Objective: local swelling; weight loss; anemia; elevated serum alkaline phosphatase; neoplastic cells
C. Therapeutic interventions

1. Surgery: wide excision of tumor, reconstructive surgery, bone grafts, amputation of limb
2. Chemotherapy
3. Radiation

Nursing Care of Clients with Osteogenic Sarcoma
A. **ASSESSMENT**
1. Description of onset and progression of symptoms
2. Extent of support system and home environment
B. **ANALYSIS/NURSING DIAGNOSES**
1. Pain related to disease process
2. Risk for injury: pathologic fractures related to decreased integrity of bone
C. **PLANNING/IMPLEMENTATION**
1. Maintain safe environment to decrease risk of pathologic fractures
2. Help client control pain by relaxation, imagery, distraction, and medication
3. Be available for the client and family to discuss fears, concerns, and treatment
4. Encourage diet of nutrient-dense foods, especially those rich in the immune-stimulating nutrients selenium and vitamins A, C, and E, as well as protein
5. Administer care based on therapeutic interventions (see General Nursing Care of Clients with Neoplastic Disorders Receiving Either Chemotherapy or Radiation Therapy, Amputation)
6. Refer client and family to cancer support groups
D. **EVALUATION/OUTCOMES**
1. Reports reduction in pain
2. Remains free from injury

▼ MULTIPLE MYELOMA

Data Base
A. Etiology and pathophysiology
1. Malignant overgrowth of plasma cells and malignant tumor growth in bone and bone marrow; interferes with RBC, WBC, and platelet production
2. Cause unknown; risk factors include exposure to ionizing radiation and occupational chemicals; genetic and viral factors are being studied
3. Occurs primarily in older men
B. Clinical findings
1. Subjective: bone pain; progressive weakness; low back pain
2. Objective
   a. Anemia; platelet deficiency; weight loss; cachexia
   b. Idiopathic bone fractures; punched-out appearance of the bones

c. Presence of Bence-Jones protein in urine

d. Hypercalcemia and hyperuricemia, which may result in renal damage

C. Therapeutic interventions

1. Chemotherapeutic agents, especially melphalan (Alkeran) and prednisone

2. Radiation therapy

3. Autologous or allogeneic bone marrow transplantation

4. Analgesics and narcotics for pain

5. Supportive therapy such as transfusions

Nursing Care of Clients with Multiple Myeloma

A. ASSESSMENT

1. Description of onset and progression of symptoms

2. Signs of myelosuppression

3. Renal function; precipitation of protein, calcium, and uric acid in urine

B. ANALYSIS/NURSING DIAGNOSES

1. Pain related to disease process

2. Risk for injury: pathologic fractures related to decreased integrity of bone

C. PLANNING/IMPLEMENTATION

1. Allow time to express feelings about the disease and related therapies

2. Help control pain by relaxation, imagery, distraction, and use of analgesics

3. Assist with movement to prevent pathologic fractures

4. Increase fluid intake to prevent renal damage

5. Provide care for the client receiving radiation or chemotherapy (see Nursing Care of Clients with Neoplastic Disorders Receiving Either Chemotherapy or Radiation Therapy)

6. Encourage diet high in nutrient-dense foods, especially those rich in the immune stimulating nutrients selenium and vitamins A, C, and E, as well as protein

D. EVALUATION/OUTCOMES

1. Reports decrease in pain

2. Remains free from injury (fractures, renal damage)

▼ INTERVERTEBRAL DISC DISEASE

Data Base

A. Etiology and pathophysiology

1. Protrusion of the nucleus pulposus into the spinal canal with subsequent compression of the cord or nerve roots; usually occurs as a result of trauma

2. Most common site is lumbosacral area (between L4 and L5), but herniation can also occur in the cervical region (between C5 and C6 or C6 and C7)

B. Clinical findings

1. Subjective

a. Lumbosacral disc

(1) Acute pain in lower back, radiating across buttock and down leg (sciatic pain); pain increases with activities that raise intraspinal pressure

(2) Pain on affected side when raising extended leg

(3) Weakness of the foot

b. Cervical disc

(1) Neck pain that may radiate to hand

(2) Weakness of the affected upper extremity

2. Objective

a. Straightening of normal lumbar curve with scoliosis away from affected side (lumbosacral disc)

b. Atrophy of biceps and triceps (cervical disc)

c. Elevated CSF protein

d. Spinal defect on x-ray, myelogram, CT scan, or MRI

C. Therapeutic interventions

1. Bed rest with traction to the lower extremities (lumbosacral disc) or cervical traction (cervical disc)

2. Back brace or support; cervical collar

3. Local application of heat

4. Muscle relaxants, analgesics, antiinflammatory agents

5. Surgical intervention

a. Laminectomy: excision of the ruptured portion of the nucleus pulposus through an opening created by removal of part of the vertebra

b. Discectomy: entire disc and cartilaginous plate are removed

c. Microdiscectomy: utilizes a magnifying lens to facilitate removal of pieces of disc that press on nerve; incision is generally 1 inch

d. Laminotomy: incision into the lamina

e. Spinal fusion: if two or more discs are involved, the affected vertebrae are permanently fused to stabilize the spine

f. Chemonucleolysis: injection of chymopapain to dissolve disc

g. Percutaneous discectomy: disc material is removed through a trocar; laser may be used to destroy damaged disc

Nursing Care of Clients with Intervertebral Disc Disease

A. ASSESSMENT

1. Characteristics of pain

2. Contributing factors such as trauma, obesity, degenerative joint disease, scoliosis

3. Posture and gait alterations

4. Extent of muscle strength and sensory function of involved extremities

B. ANALYSIS/NURSING DIAGNOSES
1. Pain related to compression of nerves
2. Impaired physical mobility related to pain

C. PLANNING/IMPLEMENTATION
1. Administer analgesics and other medications as ordered
2. Use a firm mattress and bed board
3. Make certain that traction and/or braces are correctly applied and maintained and that weights hang freely
4. Use the fracture bedpan to avoid lifting of hips
5. Frequent and extensive back care to relax muscles and promote circulation
6. Support body alignment at all times
7. Use log-rolling method to turn (instruct client to fold arms across chest, bend knee on side opposite the direction of turn, and then roll over)
8. Teach the importance of weight loss, wearing low-heeled shoes, and appropriate body mechanics
9. Increase fluid intake and encourage diet rich in nutrient-dense foods such as fruits, vegetables, whole grains, and legumes to improve and maintain nutritional status and prevent constipation; use stool softeners to prevent straining
10. Provide care for client undergoing a repair or a removal of a disc
    a. Explain that pain may persist postoperatively for some time because of edema
    b. Place bedside table, phone, and call bell within reach to prevent twisting
    c. Observe the dressing for hemorrhage and leakage of spinal-fluid
    d. Observe for adequate ventilation in clients who have undergone a cervical laminectomy
    e. Assess for changes in neurologic function
11. Foster independence
12. Encourage client to perform exercises as prescribed
13. Encourage the client to express feelings and fears

D. EVALUATION/OUTCOMES
1. Reports a reduction in pain
2. Remains free from injury

▼ FRACTURES OF THE EXTREMITIES

Data Base
A. Etiology and pathophysiology
1. Break in bone continuity, accompanied by localized tissue response and muscle spasm
2. Caused by trauma or pathologic fractures as a result of osteoporosis, multiple myeloma, or bone tumors
3. Types
   a. Complete fracture: bone completely separated into two parts; transverse or spiral
   b. Incomplete fracture: only part of width of bone broken
   c. Comminuted fracture: bone broken into several fragments
   d. Greenstick fracture: splintering on one side of bone, with bending of other side; occurs only in pliable bones, usually in children
   e. Simple (closed) fracture: bone broken but skin is intact
   f. Compound (open) fracture: break in skin at the time of fracture with or without protrusion of bone
4. Stages of healing include formation of a hematoma; fibrocartilage formation; callus formation; ossification; consolidation and remodeling of the callus
B. Clinical findings
1. Subjective: pain aggravated by motion; tenderness; neurovascular changes and numbness
2. Objective
   a. Loss of motion; crepitus grating sound heard when affected limb is moved
   b. Edema; ecchymosis
   c. X-ray examination reveals break in continuity of bone
   d. Shortening of extremity caused by change in bone alignment
   e. Muscle spasm
   f. Loss of function
   g. Shock when accompanied by blood loss
C. Therapeutic interventions
1. Traction may be used to reduce the fracture or to maintain alignment of bone fragments until healing occurs
   a. Skin traction: weights attached to adhesive, which is applied to the skin
      (1) Buck's extension: exerts a straight pull on a limb; often used temporarily to immobilize the leg when a client fractures a hip
      (2) Bryant's traction: both lower limbs extended vertically; used to align fractured femurs in young children; rarely used
      (3) Russell traction: balanced traction in which lower leg is supported in a hammock, which is attached to rope and pulleys on a Balkan frame; used to treat fractures of femur (the foot of the bed is usually elevated for countertraction)
   b. Skeletal traction applied to the bone: Steinmann pin or Kirschner's wire inserted through bone and skin with weights attached

to both ends of pin or wire may be used in conjunction with a cast; skeletal tongs and halotraction for cervical fractures

2. Surgical intervention to align the bone (open reduction), often with plates and screws to hold fracture in alignment
3. Manipulation to reduce fracture (closed reduction)
4. Application of cast to maintain alignment and immobilize limb; may be plaster or fiberglass
5. Use of external fixation device when fractures accompany soft tissue injury

Nursing Care of Clients with Fractures of the Extremities

A. ASSESSMENT
1. Ability of client to move extremity
2. Altered appearance of involved body part
3. Factors precipitating injury
4. Neurovascular assessment; soft tissue injury, or edema may compromise circulatory or neurologic functioning

B. ANALYSIS/NURSING DIAGNOSES
1. Risk for peripheral neurovascular dysfunction related to tissue trauma
2. Impaired physical mobility related to cast/traction
3. Risk for infection related to tissue trauma and pin placement
4. Risk for injury (emboli, pressure ulcer) related to immobility

C. PLANNING/IMPLEMENTATION
1. Provide emergency care
   a. Evaluate the client's general physical condition; treat for shock
   b. Splint extremity in position found before moving client; consider all suspected fractures as fractures until x-rayed
   c. Cover open wound with sterile dressing if available
2. Observe for signs of emboli (fat or blood): severe chest pain, dyspnea, pallor, diaphoresis
3. Observe for signs of gas gangrene, which develops 2 to 5 days after deep wound injury
   a. Culture shows *Clostridium perfringens, C. welchii, C. novyi*
   b. Bronzed or blackened wound tissue; necrosis
   c. Crepitus; pallor
4. Assess for compartment syndrome; edema from fracture increases pressure in fascial compartment and capillary perfusion decreases
5. Provide care for a client with a cast
   a. Observe for signs of circulatory impairment: change in skin temperature or color, numbness or tingling, unrelieved pain, decrease in pedal pulse, inability to move toes or fingers, prolonged blanching of toes/fingers after

compression; compartment syndrome is a serious problem caused by compromised circulation to the muscle; ischemia leads to edema, which further compromises circulation
   b. Protect the cast from damage until dry: elevate on pillow; handle with palms of hands only
   c. Promote drying of the cast by leaving it uncovered
   d. Maintain bed rest until the cast is dry and ambulation is permitted
   e. Observe for signs of hemorrhage and measure extent of drainage on cast
   f. Observe for irritation caused by rough cast edges, and pad as necessary for comfort and to prevent soiling
   g. Observe for swelling and notify the physician if necessary
   h. Administer analgesics judiciously and report unrelieved pain
   i. Observe for signs of infection (e.g., elevated temperature, odor from cast, swelling)
6. Provide care for a client in traction
   a. Check that weights are hanging freely and that the affected limb is not resting against anything that will impede the pull of the traction
   b. Maintain in proper alignment
   c. Observe for foot-drop in clients with Russell traction or Buck's extension, because this may indicate nerve damage
   d. Observe for signs of thrombophlebitis, a more common complication of Russell traction because there is pressure on the popliteal space in addition to stress of immobility
   e. Observe skin for irritation and observe site of insertion of skeletal traction for signs of infection; use surgical asepsis when cleansing site of insertion of skeletal traction (an antiseptic ointment may be ordered)
7. Observe for signs of thromboembolytic complications such as DVT and PE: prevent clots by administering ordered anticoagulants, antiembolism devices
8. Encourage high-protein, high-vitamin diet to promote healing; high-calcium diet is not recommended for the client confined to prolonged bed rest, because decalcification of the bone will continue until activity is restored, and a high calcium intake could lead to formation of renal calculi
9. Encourage fluids to help prevent complications of constipation, renal calculi, and urinary tract infection

10. Teach isometric exercises to promote muscle strength and tone for crutchwalking
11. Teach appropriate crutch-walking technique; nonweight bearing (three-point swing-through); weight bearing (four point) progressing to use of cane (see Related Procedures)

D. EVALUATION/OUTCOMES
1. Remains free from infection
2. Maintains neurovascular functioning of extremities
3. Remains free from complications
4. Regains mobility and function after healing

▼ FRACTURE OF THE HIP

Data Base
A. Etiology and pathophysiology
   1. Fractures of head or neck of femur (intracapsular fracture) or trochanteric area (extracapsular fracture)
   2. Incidence highest in elderly females because of osteoporosis and degenerative joint disease
B. Clinical findings
   1. Subjective: pain; changes in sensation
   2. Objective: affected leg appears shorter; external rotation of the affected limb; X-ray examination reveals lack of continuity of bone
C. Therapeutic interventions
   1. Buck's extension or Russell traction as a temporary measure to relieve pain of muscle spasm or if surgery is contraindicated
   2. Closed reduction with hip spica cast in fractures of the intertrochanteric region
   3. Open reduction and internal fixation (ORIF)
   4. Total hip replacement when joint degeneration will not permit internal fixation

Nursing Care of Clients with a Fracture of the Hip
A. ASSESSMENT
1. Shortening and external rotation of leg
2. Degree and nature of pain
3. Neurovascular assessment; 5 Ps—pain, pulselessness, pallor, paresthesias, paralysis
4. Other health problems that may affect recovery

B. ANALASIS/NURSING DIAGNOSES
1. Impaired physical mobility related to pain and structural impairment
2. Risk for peripheral neurovascular dysfunction related to tissue trauma and surgery
3. Risk for injury (emboli) related to tissue trauma and surgery

C. PLANNING/IMPLEMENTATION
1. See Nursing Care of Clients with Fractures of the Extremities

2. Encourage the use of a trapeze or side rails to facilitate movement
3. Use a fracture pan for elimination
4. Provide postoperative care
   a. Inspect dressing and linen for bleeding
   b. Use a trochanter roll to prevent external rotation of hip
   c. Do not turn on affected side unless specifically ordered; place pillow between legs when turning on unaffected side; use pillow to maintain abduction after hip replacement, to prevent dislodging the prosthesis and to prevent contractures
   d. Encourage quadriceps setting exercises
   e. Assist the client to ambulate; first use a walker and eventually progress to a cane; support on unaffected side; follow orders for extent of weight bearing permitted on affected extremity because this will depend on the type of surgery performed and the type of device inserted
   f. Avoid flexing the hip of a client with a total hip replacement; assist to high, straight-backed chair when permitted to sit
   g. Prevent complication of thromboembolism: administer anticoagulants; observe for bleeding; apply antiembolism stockings; encourage dorsiflexion of feet
   h. Prevent pulmonary complications: encourage coughing and deep breathing; explain use of incentive spirometer; assist with frequent position changes

D. EVALUATION/OUTCOMES
1. Maintains alignment of affected leg
2. Demonstrates improved mobility
3. Avoids complications of immobility

▼ SPINAL CORD INJURY

Data Base
A. Etiology and pathophysiology
   1. Sudden impingements on the spinal cord as a result of trauma
   2. Fractures of the vertebrae can cut, compress, or completely sever the spinal cord; the symptoms depend on the location (lumbar, thoracic, cervical) and extent of the damage (complete transection, partial transection, compression) and may be temporary or permanent; the sensation and mobility of areas that are supplied by nerves below the level of the lesion are affected
B. Clinical findings
   1. Subjective: paresthesias or loss of sensation below the level of the injury

2. Objective
   a. Inability to move body below the level of the injury
   b. Early symptoms of spinal shock
      (1) Absence of reflexes below the level of the injury
      (2) Flaccid paralysis (immobility accompanied by weak, soft, flabby muscles) below level of injury
      (3) Hypotonia (caused by disruption of neural impulses) results in bowel and bladder distention
      (4) Inability to perspire in affected parts
      (5) Hypotension
   c. Later symptoms of spinal cord injury
      (1) Reflex hyperexcitability (spastic paralysis): muscles below site of injury become spastic and hyperreflexic
      (2) State of diminished reflex excitability (flaccid paralysis) below site of injury follows the state of reflex hyperexcitability in all instances of total cord damage and may occur in some instances of partial cord damage
      (3) In total cord damage, because both upper and lower motoneurons are destroyed, the symptoms depend totally on location of injury; motor and sensory function loss present at this time is usually permanent
         (a) Sacral region: paralysis (usually flaccid type) of lower extremities (paraplegia) accompanied by atonic (autonomous) bladder and bowel with impairment of sphincter control
         (b) Lumbar region: paralysis of lower extremities that may extend to pelvic region (usually flaccid type) accompanied by a spastic (automatic) bladder and loss of bladder and anal sphincter control
         (c) Thoracic region: same symptoms as lumbar region except paralysis extends to the trunk below level of the diaphragm
         (d) Cervical region: same symptoms as thoracic region except paralysis extends from neck down and includes paralysis of all extremities (quadriplegia); if injury is above C4 there is an absence of independent respirations
      (4) In partial cord damage either the upper or the lower motoneurons, or both, may be destroyed; therefore symptoms depend not only on location but also on type of neurons involved; destruction of lower motoneurons will result in atrophy and flaccid paralysis of involved muscles, whereas destruction of upper motoneurons causes spasticity
      (5) Autonomic dysreflexia: exaggerated autonomic response to factors such as a distended bowel or bladder; leads to severe hypertension, headache, flushed skin, diaphoresis, and nasal congestion
C. Therapeutic interventions
   1. Maintenance of vertebral alignment
      a. Bed rest with supportive devices or with total immobilization
      b. Skeletal traction (Crutchfield tongs, halo device)
      c. Corsets, braces, and other devices when mobility is permitted
   2. Surgery to reduce pain or pressure and/or stabilize spine (e.g., laminectomy, spinal fusion)
   3. Mechanical ventilation as needed
   4. Temperature control via hypothermia
   5. High doses of steroids to reduce inflammatory process at site of injury
   6. Extensive rehabilitation therapy

Nursing Care of Clients with Spinal Cord Injuries

A. ASSESSMENT
   1. Respiratory status
   2. Neurologic status (see Neurologic Assessment)
   3. Abdomen for bladder or bowel distention
   4. Health problems that impact on recovery
   5. Client's coping skills and support systems

B. ANALYSIS/NURSING DIAGNOSES
   1. Impaired spontaneous ventilation related to neuromuscular impairment
   2. Risk for injury related to immobility
   3. Autonomic dysreflexia related to neurologic impairment
   4. Self-care deficit related to paralysis
   5. Impaired urinary elimination related to neurologic impairment
   6. Constipation related to neurologic impairment
   7. Powerlessness related to abrupt change in lifestyle
   8. Risk for caregiver role strain related to chronicity and complexity of therapeutic regimen

C. PLANNING/IMPLEMENTATION
   1. Maintain frequent observation of respiratory and neurologic functioning
   2. Maintain spinal alignment at all times; use the log-rolling method to turn
   3. Maintain surgical asepsis with skeletal traction or spinal surgery
   4. Provide skin care to back and bony prominences
   5. Maintain body parts in a functional position; prevent dysfunctional contractures

6. Institute active and passive range-of-motion exercises as soon as approved; plan for early ambulation; exercises may be performed in water
7. Encourage verbalization and accept feelings
8. Include client in decision-making process; encourage independence when possible
9. Involve client, family, and entire health team in developing a plan of care
10. Help with adjustment to altered body image, lifestyle, and self-concept
11. Set realistic short-term goals so success can be achieved
12. Avoid bumps and bruises; utilize techniques to prevent pressure and examine skin for signs of pressure from positioning, braces, or splints
13. Provide an opportunity to touch, grasp, and manipulate objects of different sizes, weights, and textures to stimulate tactile sensation
14. Protect affected limbs by proper positioning during transfer
15. Teach use of unaffected extremities to manipulate, move, and stabilize affected parts
16. Attempt to establish a scheduled pattern of bowel function
    a. Compare client's bowel habits before illness to current pattern; establish a specific and definite time for bowel movement
    b. Provide a diet with bowel-stimulating properties; with emphasis on fruits, vegetables, cereal grains, and legumes, because these are rich sources of dietary fiber
    c. Encourage sufficient fluid intake: 2000 to 3000 ml per day
    d. Encourage active and passive activities to develop tone and strength of muscles that can be used
    e. Schedule evacuation after a meal to utilize the gastrocolic reflex (peristaltic wave in the colon induced by entrance of food into a fasting stomach)
    f. Determine if there is an awareness of the need to defecate (e.g., feeling of fullness or pressure in the rectum, flatus, borborygmus)
    g. Encourage assumption of a position most near the physiologic position for defecation
    h. Utilize assistive measures to induce defecation by:
       (1) Teach bearing down and contracting abdominal muscles (Valsalva's maneuver should be avoided by people with cardiac problems)
       (2) Teach leaning forward to increase intraabdominal pressure by compressing the abdomen against the thighs
       (3) Digital stimulation

(4) Using suppository if necessary
(5) Using enemas only as a last resort
    i. Provide for adaptation of equipment as necessary (e.g., elevated toilet seat, grab bars, padded backrest)
    j. Teach the family the bowel training program
17. Attempt to establish bladder function
    a. Determine the type of bladder problem
       (1) Neurogenic bladder: any disturbance in bladder functioning caused by a lesion of the nervous system
       (2) Spastic bladder (reflex or automatic): disorder caused by a lesion of spinal cord above bladder reflex center, in the conus medullaris; there is a loss of conscious sensation and cerebral motor control; the bladder empties automatically when the detrusor muscle is sufficiently stretched (about 500 ml)
       (3) Flaccid bladder (atonic, nonreflex, or autonomous): disorder caused by a lesion of the spinal cord at the level of the sacral conus or below; the bladder continues to fill, becomes distended, and periodically overflows; the bladder muscle does not contract forcefully and therefore does not empty except with a conscious effort
    b. Review the client's bladder habits before illness as well as the current pattern of elimination; record output, voiding times, and times of incontinence
    c. Encourage activity
    d. Encourage sufficient fluid intake: 3000 to 4000 ml per 24-hour period, a glass of water with each attempt to void
    e. Restrict fluid after 6 PM to limit amount of urine in bladder during night
    f. Encourage assumption of as normal a position as possible for voiding
    g. Establish a voiding schedule
       (1) Begin trial voiding at the time the client is most often incontinent
       (2) Attempt voiding every 2 hours all day and 2 to 3 times during the night
       (3) Time intervals between voiding should be shorter in the morning than later in the day
       (4) As ability to maintain control improves, lengthen the time between attempts at voiding
       (5) Time of intervals is not as important as regularity
    h. Determine whether there is an awareness of need or act of urination (e.g., fullness or pressure, flushing, chilling, goose pimples, cold sweats)

i. Utilize assistive measures to induce urination by teaching the client to:
   (1) Use Credé maneuver: manual expression of the urine from the bladder with moderate external pressure, downward and backward, from the umbilicus to over the suprapubic area
   (2) Bend forward to increase intraabdominal pressure
   (3) Stimulate "trigger points": areas that, for the individual, will instigate urination (e.g., stroke the thigh, pull pubic hair, touch meatus)
   j. Provide for adaptive equipment as necessary (e.g., elevated toilet seats, commode, urinals, drainage systems)
18. Discuss need for sexual expression and options available; include discussion of penile implants
19. Care for the client experiencing autonomic dysreflexia
   a. Place in a high-Fowler's position
   b. Ensure patency of urinary drainage system
   c. Assess for fecal impaction
   d. Eliminate other potential stimuli such as drafts
   e. Notify physician; administer prescribed antihypertensives
20. When permitted, encourage and support use of tilt table to imitate weightbearing and reduce loss of calcium from bones
21. Refer client to National Spinal Cord Injury Association

D. EVALUATION/OUTCOMES
1. Maintains respiratory functioning
2. Avoids complications of immobility
3. Establishes program to maintain bowel function
4. Establishes program to maintain bladder function
5. Adjusts to changes in lifestyle
6. Functions satisfactorily sexually

▼ AMPUTATION

Data Base
A. Etiology and pathophysiology
   1. Removal of a body part as a result of trauma or surgical intervention
   2. Necessitated by malignant tumor, trauma, arterial insufficiency
B. Clinical findings
   See Osteogenic Sarcoma and Peripheral Vascular Disease
C. Therapeutic interventions
   1. Below-the-knee amputation (BKA) common in peripheral vascular disease; facilitates suc-

cessful adaptation to prosthesis because of retained knee function
   2. Above-the-knee amputation (AKA) necessitated by trauma or extensive disease
   3. Upper extremity amputation usually necessitated by severe trauma, malignant tumors, or congenital malformation

Nursing Care of Clients with Amputations
A. ASSESSMENT
1. Neurovascular status of involved extremity
2. History to determine causative factors and health problems that can compromise recovery
3. Understanding of the surgery
4. Coping skills and support system

B. ANALYSIS/NURSING DIAGNOSES
1. Disturbed body image related to loss of limb
2. Risk for injury related to altered center of gravity, use of assistive devices, prosthesis
3. Chronic pain related to disruption of nerve endings

C. PLANNING/IMPLEMENTATION
1. Provide care preoperatively
   a. Initiation of exercises to strengthen muscles of extremities in preparation for crutch walking
   b. Coughing and deep-breathing exercises
   c. Emotional support for anticipated alteration in body image
2. Monitor vital signs and dressing for signs of hemorrhage
3. Elevate residual limb for 12 to 24 hours to decrease edema; remove pillow after this time to promote functional alignment and prevent contractures
4. Provide residual limb care
   a. Maintain elastic bandage to shrink and shape residual limb in preparation for prosthesis
   b. When wound is healed, wash daily, avoiding the use of oils, which may cause maceration
   c. Apply pressure to end of residual limb with progressively firmer surfaces to toughen area
   d. Encourage client to move the affected limb; keep extended in functional alignment
   e. Place the client with a lower extremity amputation in a prone position twice daily to stretch the flexor muscles and prevent hip flexion contractures
5. Teach client about phantom limb sensation/pain
   a. Phantom sensation: physiologic reaction of the nerves in the area causing an unpleasant feeling that the limb is still there; this response may or may not be precipitated by a psychologic overlay

b. Phantom limb pain: when the unpleasant feelings become painful or disagreeable

c. Characteristics: sensations/pain may be constant or intermittent; varies from mild to severe; pain may be burning, squeezing, shooting; gradually decreases over 2 years

d. Institute care that may help relieve phantom limb phenomenon: have the client look at the residual limb or close eyes and put the limb through range of motion as if the total full extremity were still there; if severe pain continues for long duration, the medical therapy may include:

   (1) Injecting the nerve endings in the residual limb with alcohol to give temporary relief

   (2) Surgical revision of the residual limb

6. Consider the special needs related to an upper extremity amputation

a. Mastery of an upper extremity prosthesis is more complex than that of a lower extremity prosthesis

b. Bilateral shoulder exercises must be done to prepare for fitting the prosthesis

c. Artificial arms cannot be used above the head or behind the back because of the harnessing

d. No artificial hand can duplicate all the fine movements of the fingers and thumb of the normal hand, although the development of electronic limbs does not negate this possibility for the future

e. There is a loss of sensory feedback; therefore visual control must be used at all times (a blind person could not adequately use a functional prosthesis)

7. Support client through fitting, application, utilization, and care of prosthesis

8. Allow expression of emotions; encourage family to participate in care

D. EVALUATION/OUTCOMES

1. Remains safe from injury

2. Verbalizes acceptance of altered body image

3. Maximizes independence

4. Copes with phantom limb sensation/pain

▼ TUMORS OF THE EYE

Data Base

A. Etiology and pathophysiology

1. May be benign or malignant; can form in or metastasize to the eye

2. Retinoblastoma, a congenital malignant neoplasm found in children; spreads easily by extension to the brain

3. Melanoma in the iris and choroid; grows slowly, metastasizes to liver and lungs

B. Clinical findings

1. Subjective: headache; visual complaints

2. Objective

a. Redness and swelling of the conjunctiva; decreased vision

b. Increased intraocular pressure

c. In retinoblastoma, white pupillary reflex, strabismus, retinal detachment

C. Therapeutic interventions

1. Radiation therapy through insertion of radioactive iodine 125 seeds; left in place several days

2. Photocoagulation for small tumors

3. Surgical removal of the eye (enucleation)

Nursing Care of Clients with Tumors of the Eye

A. ASSESSMENT

1. Description of onset and progression of symptoms

2. Visual acuity

3. Client's coping mechanisms and support system

B. ANALYSIS/NURSING DIAGNOSES

1. Disturbed body image related to enucleation

2. Risk for injury related to visual disturbance

C. PLANNING/IMPLEMENTATION

1. Support client and family as they attempt to cope with diagnosis; support adaptation to changes in body image

2. Observe for side effects of medical therapy and attempt to limit their effects

3. Provide care in post-enucleation period

a. Maintain pressure dressings on eye for 1 or 2 days to minimize hemorrhage

b. Watch for signs of meningitis, which occurs as a complication, including headache or pain on operative side

c. Explain that monocularity results in loss of depth perception; activities that require this should be performed cautiously by turning head from side to side

d. Explain that the artificial eye may be inserted when healing is complete, usually 1 to 2 months; instruct about care of eye socket and prosthesis; cleanse eye prosthesis with warm water or saline

4. Support natural defense mechanisms; encourage intake of nutrient-dense foods, especially those rich in the immune-stimulating mineral selenium and vitamins A, C, and E, as well as protein

D. EVALUATION/OUTCOMES

1. Adapts to loss of eye while maintaining a positive body image

2. Remains free from injury

3. Cares for eye socket and prosthesis appropriately

▼ CATARACT

Data Base

A. Etiology and pathophysiology
1. Opacity of the crystalline lens or its capsule
2. Results from injury, exposure to heat, heredity aging, or congenital factors that cause a diminution of sight

B. Clinical findings
1. Subjective: distortion of vision (e.g., haziness, cloudiness, diplopia); photophobia
2. Objective: progressive loss of vision; black pupil appears clouded, progressing to milky white appearance

C. Therapeutic interventions
1. Corrective lenses as eyes become more myopic
2. Surgical intervention to remove the opaque lens.
   a. Surgery most frequently performed in an ambulatory surgery setting
   b. Extracapsular extraction involves removing the anterior capsule and lens through a small incision after the lens has been fragmented through a phacoemulsification technique; most common procedure
   c. Intracapsular extraction involves removal of the entire lens as a unit with a cryoprobe
   d. Intraocular lens implantation usually done at the time of cataract extraction
   e. Corrective lenses following cataract surgery
   f. Antiemetics, analgesics, and stool softeners postoperatively

Nursing Care of Clients with Cataracts

A. **ASSESSMENT**
1. Description of onset and progression of symptoms
2. Visual acuity
3. Characteristics of lens

B. **ANALYSIS/NURSING DIAGNOSES**
1. Disturbed sensory perception (visual) related to clouding of lens
2. Risk for injury related to change in depth perception and decreased visual acuity

C. **PLANNING/IMPLEMENTATION**
1. Provide thorough orientation to environment
2. Place call bell, phone, and other items on unaffected side
3. Avoid glaring lights
4. Provide auditory stimulation such as television, radio, and talking books
5. Remove environmental hazards
6. Provide care after cataract removal
   a. Instruct the client to prevent pressure on eye by avoiding: touching, rubbing, or tightly closing the eyes, sneezing, bending from the waist, or coughing (teach the client to open the mouth when coughing); rapid head movements; straining at stool or lifting; lying on the affected side
   b. Instruct the client to request prescribed analgesics, antiemetics, and stool softeners as required
   c. Reduce the amount of light and encourage the use of sunglasses when the eye patch is removed
   d. Teach signs of increased intraocular pressure (e.g., pain, restlessness, increased pulse rate) and infection (e.g., pain, changes in vital signs)
   e. Explain that vision may be altered but will clear and lenses will help to compensate for distortion

D. **EVALUATION/OUTCOMES**
1. Remains free from injury
2. Demonstrates increased visual acuity

▼ GLAUCOMA

Data Base

A. Etiology and pathophysiology
1. The pressure within the eyeball is higher than normal
2. Primary open-angle glaucoma
   a. Occurs when aqueous fluid does not drain properly from the eye; related to pathologic changes in the trabecular meshwork or Schlemm's canal
   b. The intraocular pressure increases and destroys retinal nerve fibers, causing progressive vision loss in affected areas
   c. Most common type of glaucoma
3. Closed-angle glaucoma or narrow-angle glaucoma
   a. Occurs when the iris lies close to drainage channels, creating a mechanical blockage of the trabecular meshwork that interferes with the exit of aqueous humor from the anterior chamber
   b. Trapped aqueous humor causes the intraocular pressure to rise suddenly
   c. Occurs more commonly in African Americans and people older than 60
4. Low-tension glaucoma
   a. Resembles primary open-angle glaucoma but with normal pressures
   b. There are significant visual field defects and optic nerve cupping as disease progresses

B. Clinical findings
1. Open-angle
   a. Subjective: halos around lights

b. Objective: gradual loss of peripheral vision; increased intraocular pressure (24 to 32 mm Hg) as measured by a tonometer

2. Closed-angle
   a. Subjective: nausea; halos around lights; severe frontal headache
   b. Objective: loss of peripheral vision; steamy cornea; redness and swelling of the conjunctiva; increased intraocular pressure (50 to 70 mm Hg) as measured with a tonometer
3. Low tension
   a. Subjective: headaches
   b. Objective: loss of peripheral vision late in the disease

C. Therapeutic interventions
1. Lowering the intraocular pressure with topical alpha-adrenergics or prostaglandins because they have less side effects than beta blockers formerly used
2. Surgical intervention to facilitate drainage of the aqueous humor
   a. Peripheral iridectomy
   b. Laser iridotomy
   c. Laser trabeculoplasty
   d. Trabeculectomy
   e. Filtering procedures

Nursing Care of Clients with Glaucoma

A. ASSESSMENT
1. Description of onset and progression of symptoms
2. Visual acuity; peripheral vision
3. Characteristics of sclera, pupil, and anterior chamber

B. ANALYSIS/NURSING DIAGNOSES
1. Disturbed sensory perception (visual) related to increased intraocular pressure
2. Risk for injury related to decreased peripheral vision
3. Anxiety related to decreased vision and potential for blindness

C. PLANNING/IMPLEMENTATION
1. Teach the importance of thorough eye examinations including visual field mapping to identify forms of glaucoma
2. Explain the importance of continued use of eye medications as ordered to prevent further visual loss
3. Explain the need for continued medical supervision for observation of intraocular pressure to ensure control of the disorder
4. Teach avoidance of exertion, stooping, straining for a bowel movement, coughing, or heavy lifting because these increase intraocular pressure
5. Instruct reporting severe eye or brow pain and nausea to the physician

D. EVALUATION/OUTCOMES
1. Maintains present level of visual acuity
2. Remains free from injury

▼ DETACHED RETINA

Data Base
A. Etiology and pathophysiology
1. Retina separates from the choroid and vitreous humor seeps behind the retina
2. May result from trauma, the aging process, or cataract surgery; also seen in clients with myopia greater than −6 or diabetes mellitus

B. Clinical findings
1. Subjective: flashes of light; floaters; sensation of a veil in the line of sight
2. Objective: loss of vision; retinal separation noted on ophthalmoscopy

C. Therapeutic interventions
1. Bed rest, with area of detachment in a dependent position to promote healing
2. Tranquilizers for rest and to reduce anxiety
3. Surgical intervention
   a. Cryosurgery: supercooled probe causes retinal scarring to reattach retina
   b. Photocoagulation: laser beam through the pupil produces a retinal burn, which causes scarring of the involved area
   c. Scleral buckling: depressing the sclera to force choroid closer to retina

Nursing Care of Clients with Detached Retina

A. ASSESSMENT
1. Description of onset and progression of symptoms; history to identify contributing factors such as trauma or recent surgery of the eye
2. Visual acuity
3. Status of retina via ophthalmoscopic examination

B. ANALYSIS/NURSING DIAGNOSES
1. Disturbed sensory perception (visual) related to disease process
2. Risk for injury related to decreased vision
3. Anxiety related to decreased vision and potential for blindness

C. PLANNING/IMPLEMENTATION
1. Provide accurate information in a calm voice; client's anxiety is high as a result of the sudden, unexpected vision loss
2. Keep on bed rest in position as ordered
3. Provide a call bell and answer promptly
4. Maintain protective eye patch
5. Instruct client to avoid activities that increase intraocular pressure such as coughing, straining, and stooping

6. Observe for signs of hemorrhage postoperatively (severe pain, restlessness)
7. Diminish lights in the room

D. **EVALUATION/OUTCOMES**
1. Reports improved vision
2. Remains free from injury

▼ OTOSCLEROSIS

Data Base

A. Etiology and pathophysiology
1. Fixation of the stapes caused by the growth of bone, preventing transmission of vibrations
2. Cause unknown, but incidence higher in females; autosomal dominant trait

B. Clinical findings
1. Subjective: loss of hearing; ringing or buzzing in the ears
2. Objective: use of a tuning fork shows bone conduction better than air conduction (Rinne test); presence of spongy bone in the labyrinth

C. Therapeutic interventions
1. Hearing aids to amplify sound
2. Stapedectomy: removal of the diseased portion of the stapes, and replacement with a prosthetic implant to conduct vibrations from the middle to inner ear

Nursing Care of Clients with Otosclerosis

A. **ASSESSMENT**
1. History of onset and progression of symptoms
2. Extent of hearing loss via audiometry
3. Rinne test to evaluate loss of air conduction

B. **ANALYSIS/NURSING DIAGNOSES**
1. Impaired verbal communication related to hearing loss
2. Risk for injury related to hearing loss, vertigo, presence of a graft

C. **PLANNING/IMPLEMENTATION**
1. Position postoperatively according to orders: lying on the operated side facilitates drainage; lying on the nonoperated side helps prevent displacement of graft
2. Instruct client to alter position gradually to prevent vertigo
3. Question about pain, headache, vertigo, or unusual sensations in ear
4. Instruct avoidance of sneezing, blowing nose, swimming, showering, and flying until permitted by physician; if the client must sneeze, instruct to keep mouth open to equalize pressure in ear
5. Explain that because of edema from surgery and the presence of packing, hearing will be diminished but will improve

D. **EVALUATION/OUTCOMES**
1. Reports improved hearing ability
2. Remains free from injury
3. Establishes effective communication

▼ MÉNIÈRE'S DISEASE (ENDOLYMPHATIC HYDROPS)

Data Base

A. Etiology and pathophysiology
1. Chronic, inner ear disease that incapacitates because of sudden, severe attacks of vertigo
2. Caused by endolymph in the vestibular and semicircular canals
3. Incidence highest in males between 40 and 60 years of age

B. Clinical findings
1. Subjective: whirling vertigo; nausea; headache; tinnitus; sensitivity to loud sounds; sensory hearing loss; usually unilateral; aural fullness
2. Objective: vomiting; diaphoresis; nystagmus during attacks; Weber test and auditory testing document unilateral hearing loss

C. Therapeutic interventions
1. Pharmacologic therapy: diuretics; antihistamines; diazepam (Valium)
2. Surgical destruction of the labyrinth or vestibular nerve, which causes deafness
3. Surgical insertion of endolymphatic drainage shunt may relieve symptoms without loss of hearing
4. Low-sodium diet

Nursing Care of Clients with Ménière's Disease

A. **ASSESSMENT**
1. Description of onset and progression of symptoms; situations that seem to precipitate an attack
2. History of allergies or infections that may complicate the disorder
3. Extent of hearing loss via audiometry
4. Weber test to determine auditory loss

B. **ANALYSIS/NURSING DIAGNOSES**
1. Risk for injury related to vertigo
2. Impaired verbal communication related to hearing loss

C. **PLANNING/IMPLEMENTATION**
1. Support emotionally
2. Encourage avoidance of rapid movements to limit the onset of symptoms
3. Teach self-protection from injury during attack (e.g., pull off the road if driving, lie down)
4. Care for the client after a total labyrinthectomy
   a. Maintain bed rest in the presence of severe vertigo

b. Instruct to avoid sudden movements

c. Explain that Bell's palsy may occur post-operatively but usually subsides

5. Teach avoidance of foods high in salt, such as salted meats and fish, cheese, condensed milk, carrots, and spinach

D. EVALUATION/OUTCOMES

1. Reports a reduction in frequency and intensity of vertigo

2. Remains free from injury

3. Establishes effective communication

URINARY/REPRODUCTIVE SYSTEMS

REVIEW OF ANATOMY AND PHYSIOLOGY: URINARY SYSTEM

Functions of the Urinary System

A. Secrete urine

B. Eliminate urine from body

1. Excrete normal and abnormal metabolic wastes

2. Regulate blood pressure and the composition and volume of blood; maintain fluid, electrolyte, and acid-base balance

Structures of the Urinary System

Kidneys

A. Gross anatomy

1. Shaped like lima beans; lie against the posterior abdominal wall, behind the peritoneum at the level of the last thoracic and first three lumbar vertebrae; right kidney slightly lower than the left

2. External structures: hilum, renal capsule

3. Internal structures: cortex, medulla, pyramids, columns, papillae, calyces, pelvis

B. Blood flow in the kidney

1. Kidneys receive 20% of cardiac output during rest; reduced to 2% to 4% during physical or emotional stress

2. Abdominal aorta gives rise to renal arteries, which enter the hilum of each kidney; eventually branch into afferent arterioles, which enter glomerular capillary beds

3. Efferent arterioles leave the glomerular capillary bed; eventually converge into progressively larger veins until leaving the kidney

C. Nephron

1. Anatomic and functional unit of the kidney; approximately 1 million per kidney

2. Functions via principles of filtration, reabsorption, and secretion (Fig. 6-4)

a. Glomerulus: urine formation starts with process of filtration; water and solutes (except cellular elements of blood, albumins, fibrinogen, and other blood proteins) filter out of capillaries through glomerular-capsular membrane and into Bowman's capsule

b. Bowman's capsule: filtrate collects here before flow to the tubules

c. Tubular reabsorption and secretion

(1) Proximal tubule

(a) Reabsorption of glucose and other nutrients mainly by active transport mechanism

(b) Reabsorption of electrolytes from the tubule filtrate to blood in the peritubular capillaries; cations (notably sodium) reabsorbed by active transport, stimulated by aldosterone; anions (notably chloride and bicarbonate) are reabsorbed by diffusion following cation transport

(c) Reabsorption of about 80% of the water from the tubular filtrate to the blood by osmosis

(2) Loop of Henle: establishes osmotic conditions that promote water reabsorption and actively transport chloride ions from the filtrate, thus passively removing sodium ions with the chloride

(3) Distal tubule

(a) Reabsorption of electrolytes, particularly sodium; under the influence of the mineralocorticoid aldosterone

(b) Reabsorption of water into the blood by osmosis; controlled by ADH

(c) Secretion mainly of hydrogen, potassium, and ammonia from the blood in the peritubular capillaries to the tubular filtrate, via active transport mechanism

D. Collecting tubules: final osmotic reabsorption of most of the remaining water in urine occurs; under ADH influence

E. Urine description/composition

1. Amount: 1.5 L per day average; (30 ml per hour)

2. Color: light yellow to dark amber

3. Odor: aromatic; food and drugs alter odor

4. Specific gravity: 1.005 to 1.030 is average; varies greatly depending on fluid intake and the quantity of solutes; lower specific gravity—more dilute the urine; higher specific gravity—more concentrated the urine

5. Urine pH: usually acetic (4.5 to 7.5 is average)

6. Urea: waste product of protein and amino acid metabolism

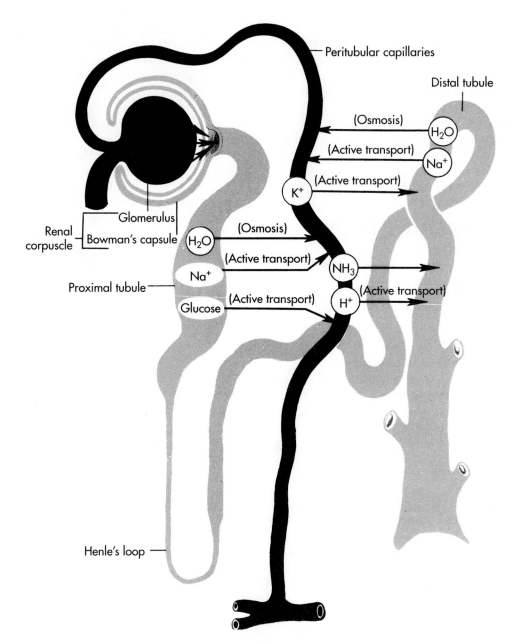

FIGURE 6-4 Diagram showing glomerular filtration, tubular reabsorption, and tubular secretion—the three processes by which the kidneys secrete urine. In the proximal tubule, note that water is reabsorbed from the tubular filtrate and moves into the blood by osmosis (a passive transport mechanism) but that sodium and glucose are reabsorbed mainly by active transport mechanisms. Note also that water and sodium are reabsorbed from the distal tubule. Potassium and hydrogen ions (K^+ and H^+) and ammonia (NH_3), by constrast, are secreted into the tubule from the blood. (From Thibodeau GA, Patton KT: *Anatomy and physiology,* ed 4, St. Louis, 1999, Mosby.)

7. Uric acid: end product of purine metabolism or oxidation in the body
8. Creatinine: waste product of muscle metabolism
9. Ions (electrolytes): potassium, sodium, calcium, chloride
10. Hormones and their breakdown products
11. Abnormal constituents: glucose, protein, red blood cells, ketone bodies, billirubin, calculi

F. Urine volume control
   1. Antidiuretic hormone (ADH): produced in hypothalamus secreted into blood by posterior pituitary gland; secretion stimulated by an increase in the osmotic pressure of extracellular fluid or a decrease in the volume of extracellular fluid; ADH acts on distal and collecting tubules, causing water to osmose from the

tubular filtrate back into the blood; this increased water reabsorption tends to increase the total volume of body fluid by decreasing the urine volume

2. Aldosterone mechanism: stimulates kidney tubules to reabsorb primarily more sodium and secondarily more water

3. Solutes in tubular filtrate: an increase in tubular solutes causes decreased osmosis of water from proximal tubule back into blood and therefore an increase in urine volume (e.g., in diabetes, excess glucose in the tubular filtrate leads to increased urine volume [polyuria, diuresis])

4. Glomerular filtration rate (GFR): usually constant (about 125 ml per minute); in certain pathologic conditions the GFR may change markedly and alter urine volume (e.g., in shock the GFR decreases causing oliguria, a decrease in plasma proteins lowers the colloid oncotic pressure increasing the GFR)

G. Control of amount of blood flow through kidneys
1. Reduced renal blood flow results in renal excretion of the hormone renin
2. Renin interacts with blood proteins producing angiotensin II
3. Angiotensin II causes vasoconstriction and aldosterone secretion, resulting in an increase in blood pressure and renal blood flow

Ureters
A. Location: behind the parietal peritoneum
B. Structure: ureter expands as it enters the kidney to form the renal pelvis; subdivided into calyces, each of which contains renal papillae
C. Function: collect urine secreted by the kidney cells and propel it to the bladder by peristaltic waves

Urinary bladder
A. Location: behind symphysis pubis, below parietal peritoneum
B. Structure: collapsible bag of smooth muscle lined with mucosa arranged in rugae, three openings—two from ureters and one into the urethra
C. Functions: reservoir for urine until sufficient amount accumulated for elimination and expulsion of urine from body by way of urethra

Urethra
A. Location
1. Female: behind the symphysis pubis, anterior to the vagina
2. Male: extends through the prostate gland, fibrous sheet, and penis
B. Structure: musculomembranous tube lined with mucosa; opening to exterior called urinary meatus
C. Functions
1. Female: passageway for expulsion of urine
2. Male: passageway for expulsion of both urine and semen

REVIEW OF ANATOMY AND PHYSIOLOGY: REPRODUCTIVE SYSTEM
Structures of the Male Reproductive System
Glands
A. Main male sex glands (gonads) are the testes
1. Location: in the scrotum, one testis in each compartment (two compartments)
2. Structure: composed of tiny tubules called seminiferous tubules, embedded in connective tissue containing interstitial cells; ducts emerge to enter head of epididymis
3. Functions
a. Seminiferous tubules carry on spermatogenesis, the formation of spermatozoa (male sex cells or gametes)
b. Interstitial cells secrete testosterone, the main androgen, or male hormone; increases protein synthesis, induces growth of secondary sexual characteristics, and promotes development of brain in fetus

B. Accessory glands
1. Seminal vesicles: secrete nutrient-rich fluid estimated to constitute about 30% of semen
2. Prostate gland: secretes estimated 60% of semen; prostatic secretion is alkaline, which increases sperm motility and contains abundance of the enzyme acid phosphatase; therefore blood level of this enzyme increases in metastasizing cancer of prostate
3. Bulbourethral glands (Cowper's): secrete alkaline fluid that lubricates urethra prior to ejaculation

Ducts
A. Epididymis: conducts seminal fluid (semen) from testes to vas deferens; sperm mature while semen is stored prior to ejaculation
B. Vas deferens (seminal ducts): conduct sperm and small amount of fluid from each epididymis to an ejaculatory duct; a vasectomy is the resection of each vas and as a result sperm cannot enter the ejaculatory ducts; it produces sterility, not impotence
C. Ejaculatory ducts: ejaculate semen into urethra
D. Urethra: described under Urinary System

Supporting structures
A. External: scrotum and penis
1. Scrotum: contains testes, epididymis, and first part of seminal duct; allows sperm to develop at 2 to 3 degrees below body temperature, which is ideal for sperm development
2. Penis: contains large vascular spaces that when filled with blood cause erection of penis; contains the urethra
B. Internal: spermatic cords are fibrous tubes located in each inguinal canal; torsion of the testes results

in twisting of these cords, destroys sperm, interrupts blood supply, and can result in cell death and gangrene

Structures of the Female Reproductive System
See Childbearing and Women's Health

REVIEW OF MICROORGANISMS

Bacterial pathogens
A. *Enterobacter aerogenes:* gram-negative bacillus; causes urinary tract infections
B. *Haemophilus ducreyi:* gram-negative bacillus; causes the venereal ulcer called chancroid (soft chancre)
C. *Neisseria gonorrhoeae:* gram-negative diplococcus; causes gonorrhea; transmitted sexually
D. *Pseudomonas aeruginosa:* gram-negative bacillus; infection characterized by blue-green pus; a common secondary invader of wounds, burns, outer ear, and urinary tract; transmitted by catheters and other hospital instruments
E. *Treponema pallidum:* highly motile spirochete; causes syphilis; transmitted sexually

Protozoal pathogen
Trichomonas vaginalis: a flagellated protozoan; causes trichomonas vaginitis; transmitted sexually

Viral pathogens
A. Human immunodeficiency virus (HIV): causes acquired immunodeficiency syndrome (AIDS); transmitted sexually and by blood
B. *Herpesvirus hominus:* causes herpes genitalis; transmitted via genital or oral-genital routes
C. Human papillomavirus (genital or venereal warts): characterized by papillary or cauliflower-like masses in or on the genitourinary structures; may be a precursor to cancer of the cervix

 RELATED PHARMACOLOGY

Kidney-specific antiinfectives
A. Description
   1. Exert an antibacterial effect on renal tissue, including the ureters and bladder
   2. Used to treat local urinary tract infections
   3. Available in oral and parenteral (IV) preparations
B. Examples: nalidixic acid (NegGram), nitrofurantoin (Furadantin, Macrodantin)
C. Major side effects: nausea, vomiting (irritation of gastric mucosa); skin rash (hypersensitivity); CNS disturbances (neurotoxicity); blood dyscrasias (decreased RBCs, WBCs, and platelet synthesis)
D. Nursing care
   1. Administer with meals to reduce GI irritation
   2. Monitor blood work, cultures, and urinary output

   3. Encourage increased fluid intake to promote drug excretion and prevent toxicity
   4. Nalidixic acid: assess for potentiation of anticoagulant effect
   5. Nitrofurantoins: dilute oral suspensions in milk or juice to prevent staining of teeth; instruct client that the urine will appear brown in color

Sulfonamides
See Pharmacologic Control of Infection in this chapter

Urinary spasmolytics
A. Description
   1. Directly affects the smooth muscle of the urinary tract
   2. Used for symptomatic relief of incontinence
B. Examples: flavoxate HCl (Urispas), oxybutynin Cl (Ditropan), tolterodine (Detrol)
C. Major side effects related to anticholinergic effect: tachycardia, palpitations, dry mouth, constipation, drowsiness, blurred vision, urinary retention
D. Nursing care
   1. Do not administer if GI obstruction is present
   2. Administer cautiously to clients with glaucoma
   3. Advise client to avoid driving and other hazardous activities
   4. Monitor urinary output

Androgens
A. Description
   1. Hormones that promote secondary sex characteristics in men and have anabolic properties, which stimulate the building and repair of body tissue
   2. Used in debilitating conditions, inoperable breast cancer, and to restore hormone levels in males; also for treatment of fibrocystic breast disease, dysmenorrhea, and severe postpartum breast engorgement in nonnursing mothers
   3. Available in oral, parenteral (IM, SC), and buccal preparations
B. Examples: danazol (Danocrine), ethylestrenol (Maxibolin), testosterone
C. Major side effects: weight gain, edema (sodium and water retention); acne, changes in libido (androgen effect); hoarseness, deep voice (virilism—androgen effect); nausea, vomiting (irritation of gastric mucosa; hypercalcemia), emotional lability
D. Nursing care
   1. Assess for signs of virilization in females
   2. Encourage a diet high in calories and proteins to aid in building body tissues and low in sodium to limit edema
   3. Administer with meals to reduce GI irritation
   4. Monitor blood pressure during course of therapy
   5. Assess for potentiation of anticoagulant effect

Estrogens
See Related Pharmacology in Childbearing and Women's Health
Progestins
See Related Pharmacology in Childbearing and Women's Health

RELATED PROCEDURES

Urinary catheterization
A. Definitions
  1. Sterile introduction of a catheter through the urethra into the bladder
  2. Intermittent catheterization: a catheter is inserted to drain urine, obtain a urine specimen, or determine a residual volume (amount of urine left in the bladder after voiding)
  3. Retention catheterization: insertion into the bladder of a catheter that remains in place because of the inflation of a balloon; catheter is attached to a collecting bag; the bladder is continually emptied by gravity
B. Nursing care
  1. Explain procedure to client; provide privacy
  2. Position the female client supine with the knees flexed and abducted and the male client supine with the knees slightly abducted
  3. Use sterile technique
  4. Place a sterile fenestrated drape over the external genitalia, exposing meatus
  5. Cleanse the urinary meatus using cotton balls saturated with suitable solution
    a. For female clients separate the labia minora with thumb and forefinger and cleanse from anterior to posterior using one pledget for each stroke (keep labia separated)
    b. For male clients hold the penis between thumb and forefinger and cleanse from meatus to shaft using one pledget for each stroke (retract foreskin during this procedure and replace after procedure)
  6. Insert lubricated catheter into the bladder
    a. For female clients insert approximately 7.5 cm or slightly past the point at which urine returns
    b. For male clients, hold the penis perpendicular to the body and insert catheter 17 to 25 cm or well past the point at which urine returns
  7. Drain urine slowly
    a. Intermittent catheterization: remove catheter when bladder is empty
    b. Retention catheterization: inflate the balloon with sterile solution and place the closed collection system below the level of the bladder

  8. Assist the client to a comfortable position and record data on appropriate records
  9. Ensure patency of catheter: eliminate kinks, dependent loops, and clogs
  10. Wash genital area with soap and water daily and as necessary
  11. Prepare for removal of indwelling catheter by intermittently clamping tubing to restore muscle tone; flaccidity of urinary sphincter may occur following catheterization

Continuous bladder irrigation (CBI)
A. Definitions
  1. Instillation of sterile isotonic solution into the bladder through a triple-lumen catheter: one for instillation of fluid into balloon tip, one for instillation of fluid into bladder, and one for return of fluid and urine from the bladder
  2. Used to prevent occlusion of catheter by clots or to administer direct antibiotic treatment to the bladder
B. Nursing care
  1. Connect catheter port to irrigant via intravenous tubing using sterile technique
  2. Set rate of infusion as per order; order frequently states that flow should be sufficient to keep the drainage pink
  3. Maintain infusion continuously, observing color, clarity, and amount of drainage
  4. Assess for signs of dilutional hyponatremia

MAJOR DISORDERS OF URINARY/REPRODUCTIVE SYSTEMS

See Childbearing and Women's Health for additional disorders of the urinary/reproductive systems in women

▼ URINARY TRACT INFECTIONS (UTI)

Data Base
A. Etiology and pathophysiology
  1. Cystitis is inflammation of the bladder wall usually caused by an ascending bacterial infection (*Escherichia coli* most common)
    a. More common in females due to: shorter urethra, childbirth, anatomic proximity of the urethra to the rectum
    b. Occurs in men secondary to epididymitis, prostatitis, renal calculi
  2. Urethritis is inflammation of the urethra caused by staphylococci, *Escherichia coli*, *Pseudomonas* species, and streptococci
    a. Although inflammatory symptoms are similar to gonorrheal urethritis, sexual contact is not the cause

b. May cause prostatitis and epididymitis
3. Urosepsis is caused by gram-negative bacteria
   a. May result from an indwelling urinary catheter or an untreated urinary tract infection
   b. Can lead to septic shock
B. Clinical findings
   1. Subjective: Urgency; frequency; pain and bearing down on urination
   2. Objective: Nocturia; hematuria; pyuria; bacterial growth evident in urine culture
C. Therapeutic interventions
   1. Identification of causative organism through urine culture
   2. Pharmacologic thearapy with antibiotics, urinary antiseptics, antispasmotics
   3. Diet directed toward altering the properties of urine (e.g., cranberry juice)
   4. Additional fluids to dilute the urine
   5. Warm sitz baths to provide comfort
   6. Urinary dilation and instillation of antiseptic solutions
   7. Treatment for urosepsis: IV therapy with aminoglycosides or beta-lactam antibiotics such as aztreonam (Azactam)

Nursing Care of Clients with Urinary Tract Infections

A. **ASSESSMENT**
   1. Urine for color, clarity, odor, blood, or mucus; presence of dysuria, burning, discharge
   2. Suprapubic area for bladder distention
   3. In males, rectal examination for prostate tenderness or enlargement
B. **ANALYSIS/NURSING DIAGNOSES**
   1. Pain related to inflammation
   2. Urge urinary incontinence related to microbiologic irritation
   3. Impaired urinary elimination related to pathologic processes
C. **PLANNING/IMPLEMENTATION**
   1. Teach the need to seek medical attention at the first sign of symptoms and to take medications as directed
   2. Encourage the intake of additional fluids
   3. Promote physical comfort
   4. Teach preventive measures such as perineal care, avoiding tub baths, voiding after intercourse, wearing cotton underwear
   5. Teach clients at risk for recurrent UTIs that frequent follow-up care with culture and sensitivity testing of the urine is indicated
D. **EVALUATION/OUTCOMES**
   1. Expresses relief of pain on urination
   2. Resumes normal urinary patterns
   3. Describes methods to prevent recurrence of infection

▼ UROLITHIASIS AND NEPHROLITHIASIS

Data Base
A. Etiology and pathophysiology: formation of stones in the urinary tract; stones may be composed of calcium phosphate, uric acid, or oxalate; they tend to recur and may cause obstruction, infection, and/or hydronephrosis
B. Clinical findings
   1. Subjective: severe pain in kidney area radiating down the flank to the pubic area (renal colic), frequency, urgency, nausea; history of prior or associated health problems (e.g., gout, parathyroidism, immobility, dehydration, urinary tract infections)
   2. Objective: diaphoresis, pallor, grimacing, vomiting, hematuria, and pyuria if infection is present
C. Therapeutic interventions
   1. Narcotics and NSAIDs for pain
   2. Antispasmodics to reduce renal colic
   3. Allopurinal or sulfinpyrazone to reduce uric acid excretion
   4. Antibiotics to reduce infection
   5. Intake and output; strain urine
   6. Diet therapy
      a. Large fluid intake to produce dilute urine
      b. Diet altered according to type of stone
         (1) Calcium stones: low-calcium diet (400 mg daily), achieved by eliminating dairy products; if phosphate involvement, limit high-phosphorus foods (e.g., dairy products, meat); if oxalate involvement, avoid oxalate-rich foods (e.g., tea, almonds, cashews, chocolate, cocoa, beans, spinach, rhubarb); because calcium stones have an alkaline chemistry, an acid-ash diet can be used to create an acidic urinary tract, which is less conducive to their formation; encourage whole grains, eggs, cranberry juice, and limit milk, vegetables, fruit; provide riboflavin, vitamins A and C, and folic acid supplements
         (2) Uric acid stones: uric acid is a metabolic product of purines; limit purine foods (e.g., meat [especially organ meats], meat extracts, and to a lesser extent whole grains and legumes); alkaline-ash diet because the stone composition is acid
         (3) Cystine stones (rare): low methionine because methionine is the essential amino acid from which the nonessential amino acid cystine is formed; limit

protein foods (meat, milk, eggs, cheese); alkaline-ash diet, because the stone is an acid composition

7. Surgical intervention if stone is not passed or complications are present (e.g., nephrolithotomy, ureterolithotomy, cystolithectomy)

8. Percutaneous ultrasonic lithotripsy (PUL) a less traumatic alternative to surgery
   a. Nephroscope is inserted through skin into kidney
   b. Ultrasonic waves disintegrate stones that are then removed by suction and irrigation

9. Laser lithotripsy: utilizes lasers with ureteroscope

10. Extracorporeal shock-wave lithotripsy (ESWL): Client is exposed to shock waves that disintegrate stones so that they can be passed with urine; procedure is noninvasive

Nursing Care of Clients with Urolithiasis and Nephrolithiasis

A. ASSESSMENT
1. Vital signs, particularly temperature for baseline data
2. Urine for color, clarity, pH, odor
3. Urine for presence of stones (strain all urine); intake and output

B. ANALYSIS/NURSING DIAGNOSES
1. Urinary retention related to obstruction
2. Pain related to renal colic

C. PLANNING/IMPLEMENTATION
1. Administer analgesics as ordered
2. Permit client to set own pattern of activity; provide periods for undisturbed rest
3. Encourage fluid intake of 3000 to 4000 ml daily
4. Administer antibiotics as ordered to prevent infection
5. Encourage client to remain on diet; teach to read labels on food preparations for the presence of contraindicated additives such as calcium or phosphate
6. Encourage daily weight-bearing exercise to prevent hypercalciuria caused by release of calcium from the bones when not contraindicated
7. Provide care following a nephrolithotomy or percutaneous ultrasonic lithotripsy
   a. Change dressings frequently during the first 24 hours after a nephrolithotomy
   b. Maintain patency of ureteral catheter as well as urethral catheter to prevent hydronephrosis
   c. Encourage use of incentive spirometry and coughing and deep breathing to prevent atelectasis

D. EVALUATION/OUTCOMES
1. States relief of pain
2. Establishes normal urine flow

3. Describes strategies for prevention of stone formation

▼ ACUTE RENAL FAILURE

Data Base
A. Etiology and pathophysiology
   1. Usually follows trauma to the kidneys or overwhelming physiologic stress (e.g., burns, septicemia, nephrotoxic drugs and chemicals, hemolytic blood transfusion reaction, severe shock, renal vascular occlusion) that decreases blood flow to the glomeruli or to the nephrons
   2. Sudden and almost complete loss of glomerular and/or tubular function
   3. May cause death from acidosis, potassium intoxication, pulmonary edema, or infection
   4. May progress from the anuric or oliguric phase through the diuretic phase to the convalescent phase (which can take 6 to 12 months) to recovery of function or may progress to chronic renal failure

B. Clinical findings
   1. Subjective: irritability; headache; anorexia; circumoral numbness; tingling of extremities; lethargy and drowsiness that can progress from stupor to coma
   2. Objective
      a. Sudden dramatic drop in urinary output appearing a few hours after the causative event; oliguria—output less than 400 ml but more than 100 ml/24 hours; anuria—output less than 100 ml/24 hours
      b. Restlessness, twitching, convulsions
      c. Nausea and vomiting
      d. Skin pallor, anemia, and increased bleeding time, which can progress to epistaxis and internal hemorrhage
      e. Ammonia (urine) odor to breath and perspiration, which can progress to uremic frost on skin and pruritus
      f. Generalized edema, hypervolemia, hypertension and increased venous pressure; can progress to pulmonary edema and heart failure
      g. Deep, rapid respirations to compensate for metabolic acidosis
      h. Elevated serum levels of blood urea nitrogen (BUN), creatinine, potassium; decreased serum levels of calcium, sodium, pH, carbon dioxide combining power
      i. Albumin in urine, decreased urine specific gravity

C. Therapeutic interventions
   1. Correct the underlying cause of renal failure

(e.g., treat shock, eliminate drugs and toxins, treat transfusion reactions, restore integrity of urinary tract)
2. Complete bed rest
3. Diet therapy
   a. Calories adequate for maintenance and to prevent tissue breakdown: 2000 to 2500 daily; protein low to moderate according to tolerance: 30 to 50 g; carbohydrate relatively high for energy: 300 to 400 g; fat relatively moderate: 70 to 90 g
   b. Sodium controlled according to serum levels and excretion tolerance: varying from 400 to 2000 mg; potassium controlled according to serum levels and excretion capacities: varying from 1300 to 1900 mg
   c. Water controlled according to excretion: about 800 to 1000 ml
   d. Calcium intake of 1000 mg/day to prevent or delay progression of renal osteodystrophy or demineralization of bone, which results from chronic acidosis and altered vitamin A metabolism; vitamin supplements because of dietary restrictions; calcium supplements only when serum phosphate is under control because of risk of precipitation of calcium phosphate in the kidney; phosphorus intake of less than 600 mg/day to delay progression of renal insufficiency; restriction of milk (1 cup or less per day), meats, poultry, fish, eggs, and cereal grain products; avoid soft drinks and beer
   e. Renal diet low in water-soluble vitamins, iron, and zinc, necessitating daily supplements; dialyzed clients need daily supplements of vitamins B_6 (5 to 10 mg), C (70 to 100 mg), and folic acid (1 mg)
   f. Total parenteral nutrition (TPN) and parenteral intralipid therapy
4. Packed red blood cells, electrolytes, and glucose IV as necessary
5. Exchange resins to decrease serum potassium
6. Antibiotics to reduce possibility of infection
7. Peritoneal dialysis, hemodialysis, or hemofiltration

Nursing Care of Clients with Acute Renal Failure

A. ASSESSMENT
1. Daily weight, fluid balance, electrolytes, BUN, and creatinine levels
2. Signs of hyperkalemia and hyponatremia
3. History of clinical symptoms and potential causative factors

B. ANALYSIS/NURSING DIAGNOSES
1. Fluid volume excess related to inability to secrete urine

2. Altered nutrition related to dietary restrictions and anorexia

C. PLANNING/IMPLEMENTATION
1. Monitor intake and output and hourly urines; assess for signs of overhydration (e.g., pitting, dependent, sacral, or periorbital edema; crackles or dyspnea; headache, distended neck veins, and hypertension)
2. Provide for fluid and electrolyte balance by monitoring, replacing, or limiting fluids and electrolytes as ordered
3. Provide periods of undisturbed rest to conserve energy and oxygen
4. Protect client from injury caused by bleeding tendency, the possibility of convulsions, and a clouded sensorium
5. Observe for early signs and symptoms of complications (e.g., hemorrhage, convulsions, cardiac problems, pulmonary edema, infection)
6. Provide special skin care to prevent breakdown and remove uremic frost
7. Encourage intake of diet as ordered; allow the client as much choice as possible in the selection of food while recognizing that little Variation is possible
8. Support client receiving peritoneal dialysis, hemodialysis, or hemofiltration

D. EVALUATION/OUTCOMES
1. Maintains fluid and electrolyte balance within acceptable limits
2. Adheres to treatment protocols
3. Maintains nutritional status
4. Remains free from injury

▼ CHRONIC RENAL FAILURE

Data Base
A. Etiology and pathophysiology
   1. Occurs as the result of chronic kidney infections, developmental abnormalities, vascular disorders, and destruction of kidney tubules
   2. Ongoing deterioration in renal function results in uremia
B. Clinical findings
   1. Subjective: lethargy; drowsiness; headache; nausea; pruritus
   2. Objective
      a. Oliguria; anuria; vomiting; anemia; hypertension; anasarca; uremic frost
      b. Decreased serum calcium and pH (metabolic acidosis); increased serum phosphate and potassium; X-ray reveals renal osteodystrophy
      c. Kussmaul respirations, mental clouding, convulsions, coma, death

C. Therapeutic interventions
 1. Fluid and sodium restriction
 2. Antihypertensive medications
 3. Recombinant human erythropoietin (Epogen) to manage the anemia
 4. Dietary management
  a. Very low protein (20 g); minimal essential amino acids makes body use its own excess urea nitrogen to synthesize the nonessential amino acids needed for tissue protein production
  b. Controlled electrolytes, especially potassium (1500 mg)
  c. See Acute Renal Failure for additional diet therapy information
 5. Continuous arteriovenous hemofiltration (CAVH); hemofiltration is based on the principle of convection, which is that some elements in plasma fluid are conveyed across a semipermeable membrane as a result of differences in hydrostatic pressure in the system; can use previously established fistulas or externally placed access points without the need for external pumps or dialysis machines; the client's blood pressure is the driving force
 6. Peritoneal dialysis: dialyzing solution is introduced via a catheter inserted in the peritoneal cavity; the peritoneal membrane is used as a dialyzing membrane to remove toxic substances, metabolic wastes, and excess fluid
  a. Intermittent: involves 6 to 48 hours several times a week
  b. Continuous ambulatory peritoneal dialysis (CAPD): involves approximately three or four exchanges a day, 7 days a week, and can be administered at home
 7. Hemodialysis: the client is attached (via a surgically created arteriovenous fistula or graft) to a machine that pumps the blood along a semipermeable membrane; dialyzing solution is on the other side of the membrane, and osmosis and/or diffusion of wastes, toxins, and fluid from the client occurs
 8. Kidney transplant from compatible donor
  a. Human leukocyte antigen (HLA) tests and tissue and blood typing are done to decrease risk of rejection; least risk of rejection occurs if donor and recipient are identical twins
  b. Client's own kidney is not removed unless it is infected or enlarged; new kidney is placed generally in the iliac fossa retroperitoneally and the donor's ureter is attached to the bladder to prevent reflux of urine
 9. Steroids and immunosuppressives (e.g., azathioprine [Imuran]) if a kidney transplant is performed

Nursing Care of Clients with Chronic Renal Failure

A. ASSESSMENT
 1. Data related to urinary elimination patterns; urine for color, consistency, odor, and amount
 2. Neurologic status including attention span, weakness, and neuropathies
 3. Breath for an ammonia odor
 4. Skin for uremic frost or urochromatic pigmentation (bronze pigmentation)
 5. Emotional status of client and significant others

B. ANALYSIS/NURSING DIAGNOSES
 1. Excess fluid volume related to inability to secrete urine
 2. Chronic low self-esteem related to chronic debilitation, loss of function
 3. Disturbed body image related to dependence on technology, anasarca
 4. Risk for injury related to altered sensorium
 5. Infection related to immunosuppression

C. PLANNING/IMPLEMENTATION
 1. Monitor vital signs and intake and output
 2. Provide skin care
 3. Provide care for the client undergoing dialysis
  a. Explain the procedure and answer questions; assure that a staff member will be available at all times
  b. Weigh the client before and after the procedure
  c. Take vital signs before and after and every 15 minutes during the procedure; assess for hypotension and hemorrhage
  d. Use surgical asepsis in preparation of the site (abdomen or area of fistula); if an abdominal catheter is not in place for peritoneal dialysis, have the client void before procedure is started
  e. During peritoneal dialysis keep an accurate flow chart and monitor for signs of respiratory distress and peritonitis; reposition to promote drainage from abdomen; drain abdomen if respiratory distress occurs
  f. During hemodialysis, watch the site for clotting; check clotting time and administer heparin as prescribed by the physician; monitor for patency of internal fistula between treatments by palpating for a thrill and auscultating for a bruit
  g. Check tubes for patency during both procedures
  h. Provide back care to promote comfort and diversional activities to help pass the time because both procedures are long
  i. Refer for nutritional counseling; stress importance of lifelong dietary modifications

4. Provide care for the client undergoing kidney transplantation
   a. Prepare client and family emotionally for possible outcomes of surgery
   b. Maintain patency of drainage tubes, including the Foley catheter; gross hematuria or clots are not expected postoperatively
   c. Monitor fluid and electrolyte balance; initial output is increased because of sodium diuresis; sharp decrease may signal rejection
   d. Monitor weight and vital signs, particularly temperature; isolation may be necessary to prevent infection
   e. Observe client for signs of opportunistic infections such as candidiasis, cytomegalovirus, and *Pneumocystis carinii* pneumonia; teach need to prevent infection by avoiding crowds and using aseptic techniques
   f. Administer steroids and immunosuppressives as ordered to prevent rejection; explain need for lifelong immunosuppressive therapy
   g. Observe for and teach the client signs of rejection: malaise, fever, flank pain or tenderness, decreasing urinary output; serum creatine will increase

D. **EVALUATION/OUTCOMES**
   1. Maintains fluid and electrolyte balance within acceptable limits
   2. Remains free from infection
   3. Adheres to dietary and fluid restrictions
   4. Verbalizes feelings
   5. Describes signs and symptoms of transplant rejection

▼ ADENOCARCINOMA OF THE KIDNEY

Data Base

A. Etiology and pathophysiology
   1. Most common cancer affecting the kidneys; incidence higher in males
   2. Common sites of metastasis include lungs, liver, and long bones
B. Clinical findings
   1. Subjective: may be absent until metastasis occurs; dull back pain; weakness
   2. Objective: weight loss; anemia; elevated temperature; painless hematuria; and enlarged kidney palpable during physical examination
C. Therapeutic interventions
   1. Radical nephrectomy
   2. Partial nephrectomy (heminephrectomy) when neoplasm is bilateral or when only one kidney is functioning
   3. Radiation therapy if tumor is sensitive

4. Chemotherapy; hormonal therapy with medroxyprogesterone (Provera)
5. Palliative care if condition is terminal

Nursing Care of Clients with Adenocarcinoma of the Kidney

A. **ASSESSMENT**
   1. Presence of hematuria, pain
   2. Flank regions for asymmetry
B. **ANALYSIS/NURSING DIAGNOSES**
   1. Anticipatory grieving related to concerns about dying
   2. Pain related to inflammation, pressure
C. **PLANNING/IMPLEMENTATION**
   1. Monitor intake and output; increase fluid intake
   2. Administer analgesics as ordered to alleviate pain
   3. Observe urine for color, amount, and any abnormal components
   4. Support natural defenses of client; encourage intake of foods rich in the immune-stimulating nutrients, especially vitamins A, C, and E, and the mineral selenium.
   5. Care for the client after a nephrectomy
      a. Encourage coughing and deep breathing while splinting the incision
      b. Examine dressing and linen under the client; heavier serosanguinous drainage is expected after a partial nephrectomy than a total nephrectomy
      c. Maintain integrity of the urinary drainage system; avoid kinking of tubes
D. **EVALUATION/OUTCOMES**
   1. States reduction in pain
   2. Discusses feelings related to prognosis
   3. Maintains adequate urine output

▼ GLOMERULONEPHRITIS

Data Base

A. Etiology and pathophysiology
   1. Damage to both kidneys resulting from filtration and trapping of antibody-antigen complexes within the glomeruli; inflammatory and degenerative changes affect all renal tissue
   2. Often follows a streptococcal infection such as tonsillitis
   3. May be acute or chronic; decreases life expectancy if progressive renal damage occurs
   4. Complications include hypertensive encephalopathy, heart failure, infection
B. Clinical findings
   1. Subjective: flank pain; costovertebral tenderness; headache; visual disturbances; malaise;

weakness; fatigue; anorexia; dyspnea resulting from salt and fluid retention

2. Objective: fever; tachycardia; hypertension; oliguria; periorbital and facial edema; urinalysis reveals hematuria, protein, casts; elevated plasma BUN and creatinine; anemia

C. Therapeutic interventions

1. Antibiotics such as penicillin to treat underlying infection
2. Dietary restriction of sodium, fluids, and protein based on clinical status
3. Diuretics and antihypertensives to control blood pressure
4. Rest; regular activity when hematuria and proteinuria resolve

Nursing Care of Clients with Glomerulonephritis

A. **ASSESSMENT**
1. History of recent upper respiratory or skin infections, or invasive procedures
2. Blood pressure for baseline data
3. Urine for blood, protein
4. Presence of dyspnea, edema, neck vein engorgement

B. **ANALYSIS/NURSING DIAGNOSES**
1. Excess fluid volume related to decreased urinary output
2. Fatigue related to pathologic processes

C. **PLANNING/IMPLEMENTATION**
1. Monitor intake and output, daily weight, urine specific gravity
2. Monitor vital signs, particularly temperature; protect from infection
3. Special prophylactic skin care to prevent skin breakdown because of edema
4. Observe for complications such as renal failure, heart failure, and hypertensive encephalopathy
5. Monitor urinalysis, BUN, and creatinine levels
6. Encourage continued medical supervision
7. Refer for case management as needed; the long-term nature of the illness may create economic and familial problems

D. **EVALUATION/OUTCOMES**
1. Maintains fluid balance within acceptable limits
2. Maintains nutritional status
3. Describes signs of complications

▼ BLADDER TUMORS

Data Base

A. Etiology and pathophysiology
1. Occur most frequently in men over 50 years of age
2. Risk factors include smoking, radiation, exposure to certain chemicals over prolonged periods of time, and schistosomiasis
3. Common sites of metastasis include lymph nodes, bone, liver, and lungs

B. Clinical findings
1. Subjective: frequency and urgency of urination; dysuria
2. Objective: painless hematuria, direct visualization by cystoscopic examination with bladder washings

C. Therapeutic interventions
1. Surgical intervention
   a. Resection of tumor
   b. Cystectomy may be partial, resulting in a decreased capacity or radical which requires a diversion
      (1) Ileal conduit: section of the ileum is resected and attached to the ureters; one end of this ileal segment is sutured closed and the other is brought to the skin as an ileostomy to drain urine; technique most widely used to divert urine; appliance needed because urine flow is continuous
      (2) Continent ileal urinary reservoir (Indiana, Florida, and Kock's pouch): similar to an ileal conduit, but involves creation of a nipplelike valve that can be drained by insertion of a catheter
      (3) Nephrostomy: catheter inserted in kidney through an incision
      (4) Ureterostomy: ureters implanted in abdominal wall to drain urine
      (5) Neobladder: the urethra and normal external anatomy is unchanged and a new bladder is created internally
2. Radiation therapy
3. Chemotherapy

Nursing Care of Clients with Bladder Tumors

A. **ASSESSMENT**
1. Abdomen for bladder distention
2. Urine for hematuria

B. **ANALYSIS/NURSING DIAGNOSES**
1. Disturbed body image related to changes in structure and function of urinary system
2. Impaired urinary elimination related to changes in structure and function of urinary system

C. **PLANNING/IMPLEMENTATION**
1. Allow time for the client to verbalize fears of surgery, cancer, death, and body-image alterations
2. Prepare bowel preoperatively with laxatives, antibiotics, and enemas as ordered
3. Assess color and amount of urine; maintain patency of drainage system

4. Care for the client with an ileal conduit
   a. Maintain the urinary drainage bag, which will be fixed around the stoma to collect the continuous flow of urine
   b. Cleanse the skin around the stoma and under the drainage bag with soap and water; inspect for excoriation
   c. After the skin is dry, apply skin adhesive to the area around the stoma and apply collection device
   d. Encourage self-care; teach the client to change the appliance
5. Care for the client with a continent ileal urinary reservoir (Koch's pouch): teach client to insert catheter through nipple valve to drain urine at prescribed times, thus preventing absorption of metabolic wastes from the urine as well as urine reflux into the ureters
6. Expect a variety of psychologic manifestations, such as anger or depression
7. Arrange a visit from a member of an ostomy club
8. Support natural defenses of client; encourage intake of foods rich in the immune-stimulating nutrients, especially vitamins A, C, and E, and the mineral selenium

D. EVALUATION/OUTCOMES
1. Discusses feelings
2. Demonstrates correct care of stoma and appliance

▼ BENIGN PROSTATIC HYPERTROPHY (BPH)

Data Base
A. Etiology and pathophysiology
   1. Slow enlargement of the prostate gland common in men over 40 years of age
   2. Constriction of urethra and subsequent interference in urination
B. Clinical findings
   1. Subjective: frequency, urgency, difficulty initiating stream, feeling of incomplete emptying of bladder after urination
   2. Objective: nocturia, hematuria, decreased force of stream, urinary retention, biopsy reveals hyperplasia rather than malignancy
C. Therapeutic interventions
   1. Relief of acute obstruction by insertion of indwelling or cystostomy catheter
   2. Pharmacologic management
      a. Finasteride (Proscar); inhibits the enzyme 5-alpha reductase, thus blocking the uptake and utilization of androgens by the prostate, reducing glandular hyperplasia

b. Alpha-1-adrenergic receptor blocking agents such as Terazosin (Hytrin)
      c. Urinary antiseptics and antibiotics to prevent infection from stasis of urine
   3. Surgical removal of the prostate
      a. Transurethral (TURP): resectoscope or laser is inserted through urethra
      b. Suprapubic—requires incision of abdomen and bladder
      c. Retropubic—requires abdominal incision
      d. Perineal—requires perineal incision; highest risk for incontinence, impotence, and wound contamination
      e. Continuous bladder irrigation (CBI) after surgery to promote hemostasis and limit clots that block the catheter
   4. Transurethral dilatation of the prostate: reduction of prostatic obstruction of urethra via balloon catheter, stent, or coils

Nursing Care of Clients with Benign Prostatic Hypertrophy
A. ASSESSMENT
1. Rectal examination for enlarged prostate
2. Abdomen for bladder distention
3. Signs indicating impaired renal function as a result of prolonged obstruction

B. ANALYSIS/NURSING DIAGNOSES
1. Urinary retention related to urethral obstruction
2. Urge urinary incontinence related to pathologic processes
3. Sexual dysfunction related to neurovascular changes and altered body image

C. PLANNING/IMPLEMENTATION
1. Encourage increased fluid intake (2400 to 3000 ml/day)
2. Administer antiseptics and antibiotics as ordered to prevent or treat urinary tract infections after urine for culture is obtained
3. Instruct to avoid anticholinergics and antihistamines because they can cause urinary retention
4. Assist the hospitalized client to a standing position to void; moist heat or a warm shower may relax the urinary sphincter
5. Care for the client after a prostatectomy
   a. Observe for signs of hemorrhage (e.g., change in vital signs, nature of drainage, pain, symptoms of shock, frank bleeding)
   b. Maintain patency of the catheter: unobstructed gravity flow, adequate fluid intake, CBI, sterile irrigation as ordered
   c. Monitor output; volume of irrigant must be subtracted from drainage for clients with CBI

d. Administer prescribed stool softeners to prevent straining and pressure on the operative site which can precipitate hemorrhage

e. Maintain suprapubic catheter after suprapubic prostatectomy; change dressings frequently after removal of catheter because of urine leakage

f. Encourage client to express concerns about sexual functioning

g. Provide as much privacy as possible

h. Instruct client to perform perineal exercises to regain urinary control; initially dribbling is common after surgery

D. EVALUATION/OUTCOMES

1. Verbalizes concerns about urinary and sexual functioning

2. Achieves acceptable pattern of urinary elimination

▼ CANCER OF THE PROSTATE

Data Base

A. Etiology and pathophysiology

1. Slow, malignant change in the prostate gland that spreads by direct invasion of surrounding tissues and metastasizes to the bony pelvis and spine

2. Incidence increases with age; family history is an important risk factor

B. Clinical findings

1. Subjective: frequency; urgency; difficulty initiating stream; back, groin, or lower abdominal pain

2. Objective

a. Decreased force of stream, urinary retention

b. Elevated serum acid phosphatase and carcinoembryonic antigen (CEA); increased prostate-specific antigen (PSA); alkaline phosphatase rises with bone metastasis

c. Digital rectal examination reveals enlarged hardened prostate; transurethral ultrasound (TRUS) reveals mass, detects nonpalpable masses; biopsy demonstrates malignancy

C. Therapeutic interventions

1. Type of surgical intervention depends on the extent of the lesion, the client's physical condition, and the client's acceptance of the outcome (impotence follows radical prostatectomy)

2. Radical prostatectomy, done by perineal or retropubic approach, removing the seminal vesicles and a portion of the bladder neck

3. Radiation therapy alone or in conjunction with surgery pre- or postoperatively to reduce lesion and limit metastases; high doses of external-beam radiotherapy and/or seed therapy may be used

4. Diethylstilbestrol (estrogen) may be necessary to reduce the size of an inoperable lesion or postoperatively to limit metastases

5. Orchiectomy may be necessary to limit production of testosterone and thus slow the spread of the disease

Nursing Care of Clients with Cancer of the Prostate

A. ASSESSMENT

1. Progression of urinary symptoms; presence of back pain

2. Rectal examination to palpate prostate for enlargement

3. Presence of metastasis to bone, lungs, liver, or kidneys

B. ANALYSIS/NURSING DIAGNOSES

1. Urinary retention related to urethral obstruction

2. Urge urinary incontinence related to pathologic processes

3. Sexual dysfunction related to neurovascular changes

4. Disturbed body image related to loss of sexual functioning

C. PLANNING/IMPLEMENTATION

1. Provide care similar to the client who has undergone a prostatectomy for benign prostatic hypertrophy (see Benign Prostatic Hypertrophy)

2. Explain to client that development of secondary female characteristics will occur as a result of estrogen therapy and not the surgery

3. Allow time and opportunity for client to express concerns about diagnosis of cancer and impotence; support the client's male image

4. Monitor for evidence of metastasis

5. Provide care for the client receiving radiation (see Nursing Care of Clients with Neoplastic Disorders Receiving Chemotherapy or Radiation)

D. EVALUATION/OUTCOMES

1. Verbalizes concerns regarding sexuality and prognosis

2. Maintains acceptable pattern of urinary elimination

3. Maintains satisfying sexual expression

▼ CANCER OF THE TESTES

Data Base

A. Etiology and pathophysiology

1. Etiology unknown; contributing factors include infection, cryptorchidism, genetics, and hormone levels

2. Leading cause of death from cancer in men 20 to 35 years old
3. Most are germ cell tumors (seminomas, embryonal carcinomas, teratomas, and choriosarcomas)
4. Metastasizes to the retroperitoneal nodes, lungs, and CNS

B. Clinical findings
   1. Subjective: heaviness or dull ache in scrotal area; backache or abdominal pain
   2. Objective
      a. Weight loss; enlarged testes; palpable mass; hydrocele
      b. Elevated tumor markers: alpha-fetoprotein, beta-human chorionic gonadotropin
      c. CT scan of chest and abdomen may reveal metastasis

C. Therapeutic interventions
   1. Orchiectomy (removal of the testis)
   2. Retroperitoneal lymph node dissection (RPLND)
   3. Radiation
   4. Chemotherapy: cysplatin, dactinomycin, vinblastine sulfate

Nursing Care of Clients with Cancer of the Testes

A. ASSESSMENT
   1. Palpation of the testes for enlargement
   2. Evidence of metastasis: back pain, dyspnea, cough, dysphagia, altered mental state, and visual changes

B. ANALYSIS/NURSING DIAGNOSES
   1. Situational low self-esteem related to sterility
   2. Anxiety related to prognosis

C. PLANNING/IMPLEMENTATION
   1. Discuss the possibility of banking sperm before treatment because of risk of sterility
   2. Encourage discussion of feelings
   3. Provide care for the client receiving either chemotherapy or radiation (see Nursing Care of Clients with Neoplastic Disorders Receiving Chemotherapy or Radiation)

D. EVALUATION/OUTCOMES
   1. Verbalizes feelings about sexuality, treatment, and prognosis
   2. Maintains satisfying sexual expression

INFECTIOUS DISEASES

See Infection for additional information

▼ GAS GANGRENE

Data Base

A. Etiology and pathophysiology

1. Caused by an anaerobic gram-positive clostridium (*Clostridium perfringens, C. welchii, C. novyi*) that enters through a deep wound
2. Bacilli colonize in muscle tissue around wound; occurs 2 to 5 days after injury

B. Clinical findings
   1. Subjective: pain; apprehension; anorexia; chills
   2. Objective
      a. Bronzed or blackened wound tissue; crepitus; sweetish, foul-smelling watery exudate; necrosis of muscle tissues
      b. Pallor; diarrhea; vomiting; temperature elevation (may be slight)
      c. Presence of clostridia on culture, low Hgb

C. Therapeutic interventions
   1. Multiple incisions for decompression and drainage
   2. Extirpation and debridement of involved tissue with copious irrigations
   3. Penicillin G, tetracycline, chloramphenicol, or erythromycin, depending on C&S
   4. Amputation
   5. Hyperbaric oxygenation
   6. Whole blood, packed erythrocytes, or plasma transfusions to combat hemolysis and profound anemia
   7. Antitoxin therapy may be started

Nursing Care of Clients with Gas Gangrene

A. ASSESSMENT
Observe for specific signs and symptoms

B. ANALYSIS/NURSING DIAGNOSES
   1. Pain related to inflammatory response
   2. Impaired skin integrity related to disease process
   3. Ineffective peripheral tissue perfusion related to interrupted skin integrity

C. PLANNING/IMPLEMENTATION
   1. Refer to General Nursing Care of Clients at Risk for Infection
   2. Prevent further infection from fecal contamination (organism is found in feces)
   3. Use standard and contact precautions
   4. Monitor fluid, electrolyte, and cardiovascular status

D. EVALUATION/OUTCOMES
   1. Adapts to complications
   2. Remains free from infection

▼ TOXOPLASMOSIS

Data Base

A. Etiology and pathophysiology
   1. Caused by protozoan (*Toxoplasma gondii*), a parasite
   2. Contracted by eating raw meat containing cysts or exposure to contaminated cat feces

3. Most common opportunistic CNS infection of those with AIDS
4. During pregnancy can cause congenital anomalies or death of fetus even though mother may be asymptomatic
5. Leading cause of encephalitis in immunosupressed clients

B. Clinical findings
   1. Subjective: malaise; fatigue; headache
   2. Objective: fever; seizures, cognitive and motor impairment; lymphadenopathy; positive cultures; brain abscesses

C. Therapeutic interventions
   1. Pregnant women and immunosuppressed clients may be treated with pyrimethamine (Daraprim), azithromycin (Zithromax), sulfadiazine (Microsulfon), clindamycin (Cleocin), and leucovorin (Wellcovorin)
   2. Usually no treatment required for otherwise healthy adults

Nursing Care of Clients with Toxoplasmosis

A. **ASSESSMENT**
   Observe for specific signs and symptoms

B. **ANALYSIS/NURSING DIAGNOSES**
   1. Fatigue related to infectious process
   2. Hyperthermia related to pyrogenic activity
   3. Confusion related to encephalitis

C. **PLANNING/IMPLEMENTATION**
   1. Refer to General Nursing Care of Clients at Risk for Infection
   2. Use standard precautions
   3. Encourage a diet rich in nutrient-dense foods
   4. Caution pregnant clients to avoid cleaning cat litter pans or gardening where they may be exposed to cat feces
   5. Teach client about proper handling, preparation, and storage of meat, washing fruits and vegetables, and care of cat litter

D. **EVALUATION/OUTCOMES**
   1. Remains free from infection
   2. Continues with follow-up supervision as necessary

▼ MALARIA

Data Base

A. Etiology and pathophysiology
   1. Caused by a protozoan (*Plasmodium falciparum, P. vivax, P. ovale, P. malariae*) from a bite by an infected *Anopheles* mosquito, through the use of dirty needles, or a transfusion from an infected donor
   2. Parasite enters the bloodstream and invades red blood cells; destruction of red blood cells,

blockage of capillaries, and irreversible damage to the spleen and liver may follow
   3. "Blackwater fever" that causes intravascular hemolysis and hemoglobinuria is a rare complication
   4. Sickle cell trait provides natural resistance

B. Clinical findings
   1. Subjective: malaise; headache; muscle aches; chills; thirst
   2. Objective: high fever; anemia; enlarged spleen; dehydration; renal failure

C. Therapeutic interventions
   1. Antimalarial drugs: for treatment and chemoprophylaxis 1 week before visiting endemic areas and regularly while in the area: pyrimethamine, chloroquine phosphate
   2. Aspirin
   3. Prevention: avoidance of stagnant pools; sprays and protective clothing to prevent mosquito bites

Nursing Care of Clients with Malaria

A. **ASSESSMENT**
   Observe for specific signs and symptoms

B. **ANALYSIS/NURSING DIAGNOSES**
   1. Deficient fluid volume related to diaphoresis/fever
   2. Hyperthermia related to pyrogenic activity
   3. Fatigue related to increased metabolic rate

C. **PLANNING/IMPLEMENTATION**
   1. Refer to General Nursing Care of Clients at Risk for Infection
   2. Monitor fluid and electrolyte balance; maintain hydration
   3. Use therapeutic measures to decrease fever
   4. Maintain bed rest until the fever and other symptoms have ceased
   5. Support natural defense mechanisms of client; encourage intake of nutrient-dense foods with emphasis on fruits, vegetables, whole grains, and legumes, especially those high in the immune-stimulating nutrients selenium and vitamins A, C, and E
   6. If client is receiving quinine, teach to observe for tinnitus, vertigo, and deafness and to take medication with meals to reduce GI irritation

D. **EVALUATION/OUTCOMES**
   1. Continues prophylaxis as necessary
   2. Recognizes that organism is always present in blood

▼ RABIES (HYDROPHOBIA)

Data Base

A. Etiology and pathophysiology

1. Caused by a virus (rhabdovirus) spread by bite of an infected animal; the animal can be a carrier and not be ill with the disease
2. Incubation period is 10 to 50 days in bites of the upper parts of the body, 4 months in bites of the lower parts
3. Bites are usually unprovoked; suspected animals are observed for 10 days
4. Virus spreads from the soft tissue surrounding the wound to the peripheral nerves and ultimately affects the CNS; may cause punctate hemorrhages and neuronal destruction
5. Early treatment with vaccine is necessary as once disease develops it is usually fatal

B. Clinical findings
   1. Subjective
      a. Anxiety; depression; malaise; lethargy; irritability; headaches; stiff neck; photophobia
      b. Thirst; anorexia; nausea
      c. Paresthesia or pain near the bite or in the bitten extremity
      d. Respiratory difficulty such as wheezing, hyperventilation, dyspnea, and spasms
   2. Objective
      a. Hydrophobia: sight, sound, or thought of water triggers painful pharyngeal muscle contractions that expel fluid from mouth
      b. Excessive salivation, frothy drooling, severe difficulty swallowing, choking
      c. Nuchal rigidity, seizures
      d. Apnea; cardiac dysrhythmias
      e. Paralysis; coma

C. Therapeutic interventions
   1. Cleansing of the wound with soap and water
   2. Tracheostomy if severe respiratory embarrassment develops
   3. Sedatives or anesthetics as necessary; phenytoin (Dilantin) used for seizures
   4. Human rabies immune globulin for passive immunity; dose given in the buttock; wound is bathed with the drug
   5. Human diploid cell vaccine is used to induce active immunity; treatment consists of five doses over 4 weeks followed by a sixth dose after 2 months; duck embryo rabies vaccine (DEV) was formerly used requiring a total of 23 doses administered subcutaneously

Nursing Care of Clients with Rabies

A. **ASSESSMENT**
   Observe for specific signs and symptoms
B. **ANALYSIS/NURSING DIAGNOSES**
   1. Impaired swallowing related to symptomatology
   2. Anticipatory grieving related to poor prognosis
   3. Social isolation related to need to reduce stimuli

C. **PLANNING/IMPLEMENTATION**
   1. Refer to General Nursing Care of Clients at Risk for Infection
   2. Avoid contact with the saliva of an infected client
   3. Monitor blood gases, fluid and electrolyte balance, and electrocardiograms
   4. Keep the room dark and quiet to prevent agitation
   5. Monitor the tracheostomy and the need for suctioning
   6. Prevent drafts, which may result in spasms
   7. Allow the family and client to verbalize their feelings

D. **EVALUATION/OUTCOME**
   1. Vaccine prevents nervous system invasion
   2. Avoids contact with potential sources of infection

▼ ROCKY MOUNTAIN SPOTTED FEVER

Data Base
A. Etiology and pathophysiology
   1. Transmitted by a tick infected with *Rickettsia rickettsii*; there may or may not be a history of a tick bite
   2. Sudden onset, with an incubation period of 3 to 17 days
   3. Organism attacks endothelial cells and extends into the vessel walls, causing thrombi, inflammation, and necrosis
B. Clinical findings
   1. Subjective: malaise; insomnia; headache; anorexia; photophobia; joint and muscle discomfort; hearing loss
   2. Objective
      a. Fever; enlarged spleen; hypotension; circulatory collapse; renal collapse
      b. Rash (rose-colored macules); edema; subcutaneous hemorrhage; necrosis
C. Therapeutic interventions
   1. Prompt recognition and treatment vital
   2. Tetracycline or chloramphenicol therapy continued until the client is afebrile for 3 to 5 days
   3. Treatment of symptoms and complications as they develop

Nursing Care of Clients with Rocky Mountain Spotted Fever

A. **ASSESSMENT**
   Observe for specific signs and symptoms
B. **ANALYSIS/NURSING DIAGNOSES**
   1. Impaired nutrition: less than body requirements related to decreased intake
   2. Deficient fluid volume related to diaphoresis/fever

3. Disturbed sensory perception auditory and visual related to disease process

C. **PLANNING/IMPLEMENTATION**
1. Refer to General Nursing Care of Clients at Risk for Infection
2. Assure the family that the client's disturbed emotional responses are associated with the disease
3. Monitor symptoms to determine progression of the disease
4. Assess the cardiovascular status to determine developing circulatory collapse
5. Reassure that hearing loss will last only several weeks
6. Teach prevention such as wearing tick repelents, checking pants legs and animals for the presence of ticks, and removal of ticks
7. Teach individuals to remove ticks with a tweezer to prevent contamination of fingers

D. **EVALUATION/OUTCOMES**
1. Continues with follow-up supervision as necessary
2. Avoids contact with potential sources of infection

▼ LYME DISEASE

Data Base

A. Etiology and pathophysiology
1. Caused by spirochete bacteria *(Borrelia burgdorferi)* transmitted by carrier tick that acquired bacterium from infected host; disease is most often carried by mice, deer, or raccoons; cats, dogs, and horses may also be carriers
2. Tick injects spirochete-laden saliva into blood stream, incubates 3 to 32 days, and then migrates outward, causing a rash
3. Initial rash and flulike symptoms; later neuromusculoskeletal and cardiac symptoms
4. Most common vector-borne illness in the United States
5. Infectious organism can survive in host 10 years or more

B. Clinical findings
1. Subjective: chills; muscle aches; joint pain; headache; dizziness; stiff neck; nausea
2. Objective:
   a. Fever; red-ringed, circular rash (erythema chronicum migrans); swollen joints; lack of coordination; facial palsy; paralysis; dementia
   b. Blood tests include antibody titers, enzyme-linked immunosorbant assay, Western blot assay; a positive result may indicate past or current infection

C. Therapeutic interventions
1. Antibiotics such as penicillin, doxycycline, ceftriaxone sodium (Rocephin)
2. Symptomatic treatment

Nursing Care of Clients with Lyme Disease

A. **ASSESSMENT**
Observe for specific signs and symptoms

B. **ANALYSIS/NURSING DIAGNOSES**
1. Pain related to inflammatory response
2. Fatigue related to disease process

C. **PLANNING/IMPLEMENTATION**
1. Refer to General Nursing Care of Clients at Risk for Infection
2. Assure the family that the client's disturbed emotional responses are associated with the disease
3. Monitor symptoms to determine progression of the disease
4. Question clients with arthritic symptoms about possible exposure
5. Teach clients to:
   a. Avoid tall grass; use chemical repellents; wear light colors to enhance tick identification; wear long sleeves and pants tucked in high boots when walking in areas with tick infestation
   b. Shower and inspect skin
   c. Remove ticks with tweezers, grasping close to skin to avoid breaking mouth parts
6. Advise clients who are at risk to receive vaccine
7. Administer antibiotics as ordered
   a. Early Lyme disease: doxycycline, amoxicillin
   b. Severe symptoms: ceftriaxone (Rocephin), cefotaxime (Claforan), penicillin G

D. **EVALUATION/OUTCOMES**
1. Continues follow-up supervision as necessary
2. Avoids contact with potential sources of infection

▼ TETANUS (LOCKJAW)

Data Base

A. Etiology and pathophysiology
1. Caused by an anaerobic bacillus, *Clostridium tetani,* which is transmitted through an open wound; symptoms from 2 days to 3 weeks after exposure
2. Toxins from the bacillus invade the nervous tissue, and the motor and sensory nerves become hypersensitive, resulting in prolonged contractions and respiratory failure

B. Clinical findings
1. Subjective: irritability; restlessness; pain from muscle spasms

2. Objective: muscle rigidity; spastic contractions of voluntary muscles; trismus (spasm of masticatory muscles); spasms of respiratory tract; grotesque grinning expression (risus sardonicus) caused by spasms of facial muscles

C. Therapeutic interventions
   1. Prompt recognition of potential contamination and treatment vital; tetanus immune globulin (TIG) used to provide temporary passive immunity; tetanus toxoid may also be given in a different site
   2. Once symptoms develop, specific therapy is ineffective; therefore institution of supportive therapy is necessary until toxins are reduced by time
   3. Maintenance of adequate pulmonary ventilation
   4. Debridement of wound to allow exposure to air
   5. Control of muscle spasms
   6. Antibiotics to limit secondary infection; sedation to limit spasms
   7. Maintenance of fluid balance and nutrition via enteral feedings

Nursing Care of Clients with Tetanus

A. **ASSESSMENT**
   Observe for specific signs and symptoms
B. **ANALYSIS/NURSING DIAGNOSES**
   1. Ineffective breathing pattern related to muscle spasms and neurologic impairment
   2. Risk for injury related to muscle spasms and neurologic impairment
C. **PLANNING/IMPLEMENTATION**
   1. Refer to General Nursing Care of Clients at Risk for Infection
   2. Prevent the disease through immunization with tetanus toxoid to provide active immunity; prophylaxis in suspect injuries
   3. Initiate seizure precautions; maintain a quiet environment to decrease excessive stimuli, which may result in seizures
   4. Frequently assess respiratory status; administer oxygen as needed; mechanical ventilation may be required
   5. Frequently suction the airway to maintain patency and promote ventilation; keep an endotracheal tube and tracheostomy set at the bedside
   6. Allow the client and family to verbalize fears and feelings
D. **EVALUATION/OUTCOMES**
   1. Maintains active immunity
   2. Seeks medical assistance with potentially infectious injuries

▼ TYPHOID FEVER

Data Base
A. Etiology and pathophysiology
   1. Caused by the bacterium *Salmonella typhi,* which is carried in human feces and transmitted through sewage, flies, and shellfish; incubation period 3 to 20 days
   2. Bacterium invades the GI tract and localizes in lymph tissue of the intestinal wall (Peyer's patches); these areas may become thrombosed and tissue sloughs off
   3. Hemorrhage, peritonitis, perforation, and hepatitis are serious complications
B. Clinical findings
   1. Subjective: headaches; drowsiness
   2. Objective: fever; bradycardia; rose-colored papules on the abdomen; enlarged spleen and liver; delirium; constipation during the early stage; diarrhea during the late stage
C. Therapeutic interventions
   1. Amoxicillin, sulfamethoxazole and trimethoprim, ciprofloxacin
   2. Corticosteroids the first 4 to 5 days of treatment
   3. Maintenance of fluid balance and nutrition
   4. Symptomatic treatment

Nursing Care of Clients with Typhoid Fever
A. **ASSESSMENT**
   Observe for specific signs and symptoms
B. **ANALYSIS/NURSING DIAGNOSES**
   1. Diarrhea related to disease process
   2. Deficient fluid volume related to fever and diarrhea
   3. Risk for injury related to altered cognition
C. **PLANNING/IMPLEMENTATION**
   1. Refer to General Nursing Care of Clients at Risk for Infection
   2. Maintain safety if delirium is present
   3. Encourage a soft diet rich in high nutrient density and high-calorie foods
   4. Employ methods to decrease the fever
   5. Monitor fluid and electrolytes to prevent imbalance
   6. In addition to standard precautions, use contact precautions if the client is incontinent of feces
   7. Allow the client and family ample time to verbalize emotional reactions and concerns resulting from the illness.
   8. Educate the public to prevent disease through proper sewage treatment
   9. Encourage vaccination programs with booster injections every 3 years in endemic areas
D. **EVALUATION/OUTCOMES**
   1. Maintains active immunity
   2. Practices proper personal hygiene

▼ VIRAL AND BACTERIAL INFECTIOUS GASTROENTERITIS

Data Base

A. Etiology and pathophysioiogy
   1. Gastroenteritis involves inflammation of the stomach and intestines; usually related to contaminated water and food
   2. *Staphylococcus aureus:* caused by a strain that clots plasma (coagulase positive); the most virulent type and causes a variety of infections
      a. Found in unrefrigerated creams, mayonnaise, stuffing, meats, and fish
      b. Usually transmitted to food on the hands of food handlers
      c. Incubation period is 1 to 6 hours after ingestion of contaminated food, with symptoms lasting 24 to 48 hours
   3. *Clostridium botulinum* (botulism): a serious, often fatal form; its exotoxin is the most powerful biologic toxin known
      a. Found in improperly processed foods, mostly canned foods
      b. Blocks neuromuscular transmission in cholinergic nerve fibers by possibly binding with acetylcholine
      c. Incubation period usually 12 to 72 hours after ingestion of contaminated food, but may be as long as 4 to 8 days
   4. Salmonella (salmonellosis): causes a local GI infection in which organisms multiply in the intestines but do not enter blood
      a. Found in inadequately cooked meats
      b. Incubation period usually 10 to 24 hours after ingestion of contaminated food, and symptoms usually last 2 to 3 days
   5. *Clostridium difficile:* spore-forming gram-positive bacteria
      a. Frequent cause of nosocomial infection in clients receiving antibiotic therapy
      b. Toxin can cause pseudomembranous colitis and sepsis
   6. Vancomycin-resistant enterococcus (VRE): gram-positive bacteria normally residing in the GI tract
      a. Frequent cause of nosocomial infection
      b. May resist all microbial agents
B. Clinical findings
   1. Subjective
      a. Nausea, abdominal cramps and pain, malaise
      b. In botulism, diplopia, muscle weakness, dysphasia, and dysphagia
   2. Objective
      a. Diarrhea 1 to 8 hours after ingestion

   b. Vomiting, fever, chills
   c. In botulism, diminished visual acuity, loss of pupillary light reflex, diminished gag reflex
C. Therapeutic interventions
   1. Adequate fluid and electrolytes orally or parenterally
   2. Bed rest
   3. For botulism:
      a. Darkened room
      b. Parenteral feedings to prevent aspiration
      c. Tracheostomy and other supportive measures
      d. Cathartics and cleansing enemas to remove toxins from the body
      e. Trivalent antitoxins as necessary
      f. Gastric lavage
   4. For *C. difficile:*
      a. Discontinuation of antibiotic therapy if implicated as the cause
      b. Administration of metronidazole (Flagyl) or vancomycin for moderate to severe symptoms
      c. Surgical intervention for pseudomembranous colitis may be necessary

Nursing Care of Clients with Infectious Gastroenteritis

A. **ASSESSMENT**
   1. History of ingestion of contaminated foods
   2. Frequency and characteristics of stool
   3. Temperature for baseline data
   4. Presence of nausea and vomiting
   5. For botulism establish neurologic baseline data, especially gag reflex
B. **ANALYSIS/NURSING DIAGNOSES**
   1. Deficient fluid volume related to inadequate intake and fluid loss through diarrhea
   2. Imbalanced nutrition: less than body requirements related to nausea, vomiting, diarrhea
C. **PLANNING/IMPLEMENTATION**
   1. Obtain stool specimen for culture
   2. Offer small amounts of fluids as tolerated; maintain IV fluids
   3. Maintain contact precautions
   4. Monitor clients who are immunocompromised or receiving antimicrobial therapy for profuse water diarrhea indicative of *C. difficile*
   5. Teach the importance of properly storing and cooking foods
   6. For botulism
      a. Prevent aspiration pneumonia by proper positioning; keep suction equipment available at the bedside
      b. Observe neurologic status to determine progression of the disease

   c. Prevent contractures and emboli by the use of range-of-motion exercises

D. EVALUATION/OUTCOMES
1. Reports decreased bowel activity
2. Maintains fluid and electrolyte balance
3. Maintains nutritional status

▼ SYPHILIS

Data Base

A. Etiology and pathophysiology
  1. Caused by the spirochete *Treponema pallidum*
  2. Transmitted primarily during the primary or secondary stages; usually sexually transmitted; may be congenital
  3. Stages
    a. Primary: occurs 10 to 90 days after contact; adaptations generally localized
    b. Secondary: occurs up to 6 months after exposure; a systemic response
    c. Latent: begins after the secondary stage and may last several months to years; client is asymptomatic
    d. Tertiary: may occur 18 to 20 years later
      (1) Gummas (granulomas) attack any organ and cause cardiovascular syphilis (aortitis and thoracic aortic aneurysms) and neurosyphilis
      (2) Rare for an individual to infect another; however, a fetus can be infected

B. Clinical findings
  1. Primary syphilis
    a. Chancre on genitalia, mouth, or anus; serous drainage from chancre
    b. Enlarged lymph nodes
    c. Positive test for syphilis: Venereal Disease Research Laboratory (VDRL), rapid plasma reagin circle card test (RPR-CT), automated reagin test (ART), fluorescent treponemal antibody absorption test (FTA-ABS)
  2. Secondary syphilis
    a. Skin rash on palms and soles of feet, alopecia
    b. Erosions of oral mucous membrane
    c. Fever, enlarged lymph nodes
  3. Latent syphilis: asymptomatic
  4. Tertiary syphilis
    a. Cardiovascular changes: aortitis, aortic aneurysm, stroke
    b. Neurologic changes: personality changes, ataxia, blindness

C. Therapeutic interventions
  1. Penicillin; probenecid to delay excretion of penicillin
  2. Tetracycline or erythromycin if client is allergic to penicillin

Nursing Care of Clients with Syphilis

A. ASSESSMENT
1. Progression of symptoms
2. Genitalia, rectum, and oropharynx for inflammation, lesions, or drainage
3. Regional lymph nodes for enlargement
4. History of allergy to penicillin

B. ANALYSIS/NURSING DIAGNOSES
1. Risk for infection related to knowledge deficit
2. Ineffective sexuality patterns related to fear of transmission of the disease

C. PLANNING/IMPLEMENTATION
1. Provide a supportive, nonjudgmental environment
2. Encourage early screening and educational programs such as STD clinics, hot lines, and workshops
3. Teach about the disease and its transmission; cleansing of the genitals, and condoms help prevent transmission of most STDs
4. Continue to encourage client to identify prior contacts so they can be treated
5. Inform client that the disease must be reported to the health department, but that confidentiality will be maintained
6. Explain need to complete course of antibiotic therapy
7. Tell client to avoid any sexual activity until tests are negative; encourage monogamous relationship

D. EVALUATION/OUTCOMES
1. Avoids sexual contact until follow-up testing indicates transmission will not occur
2. Identifies "safer sex" practices to reduce risk of reinfection

▼ GONORRHEA

Data Base

A. Etiology and pathophysiology
  1. Caused by *Neisseria gonorrhoeae,* a gram-negative diplococcus; Penicillinase-producing *N. gonorrhoeae* is a newer strain resistant to penicillin
  2. Symptoms depend on nature of sexual contact and may appear within a few days after exposure; may remain asymptomatic
  3. When untreated, inflammation subsides in 2 to 4 weeks, but client may become a carrier

B. Clinical findings
  1. Subjective: dysuria, urgency, anal pruritus, lower abdominal discomfort, joint pain, painful defecation
  2. Objective
    a. Purulent penile or vaginal discharge
    b. Fever

c. Urethral or endocervical smear positive for gonococcus; cultures should be obtained from the urethra, endocervix, anal canal, and pharynx

d. If untreated, signs of complications such as salpingitis, infertility, urethral stricture, prostatitis, epididymitis, proctitis, and pharyngitis can occur

C. Therapeutic intervention: CDC recommends ceftriaxone with doxycycline

Nursing Care of Clients with Gonorrhea

A. ASSESSMENT

See Assessment under Nursing Care of Clients with Syphilis

B. ANALYSIS/NURSING DIAGNOSES

See Analysis/Nursing Diagnoses under Nursing Care of Clients with Syphilis

C. PLANNING/IMPLEMENTATION

1. Instruct client to wash hands to prevent conjunctivitis
2. Make arrangements for follow-up culture 2 weeks after therapy is initiated
3. Monitor urinary and bowel elimination
4. Allow time for client to verbalize concerns about potential infertility
5. Identify sexual contacts
6. See Nursing Care of Clients with Syphilis for additional information

D. EVALUATION/OUTCOMES

1. Maintains reproductive functions
2. Identifies "safer sex" practices to reduce risk of reinfection

▼ HERPES GENITALIS

Data Base

A. Etiology and pathophysiology
1. Most commonly caused by herpes simplex type II (herpesvirus hominus type II): may also be caused by type I, which is most often associated with lesions (cold sores) of the mouth
2. Lesions occur 3 to 7 days after infection and may last several weeks
3. When symptoms resolve, virus lies dormant in spinal root ganglia and is capable of repeatedly causing lesions
4. Transmitted through sexual contact when active lesions are present; newborn may be infected during vaginal delivery
5. May cause aseptic meningitis, proctitis, and prostatitis; associated with higher rate of cervical cancer

B. Clinical findings
1. Subjective: dysuria; flulike symptoms; tingling sensation before vesicles appear; genital itching and pain
2. Objective: leukorrhea; vaginal bleeding; vesicles and papules on genitalia; urinary retention; culture reveals herpesvirus type II

C. Therapeutic interventions
1. No cure; acyclovir sodium (Zovirax) reduces healing time and severity of symptoms; not as effective in subsequent episodes
2. Sedation for severe pain
3. Alcohol may be used to dry lesions

Nursing Care of Clients with Herpes Genitalis

A. ASSESSMENT

See Assessment under Nursing Care of Clients with Syphilis

B. ANALYSIS/NURSING DIAGNOSES

1. Impaired skin integrity related to genital lesions
2. Pain related to genital lesions
3. Risk for infection related to knowledge deficit
4. Ineffective sexuality patterns related to fear of transmission of the disease

C. PLANNING/IMPLEMENTATION

1. Provide emotional support to deal with incurable, contagious nature of disease
2. Help client develop stress-reducing strategies; stress precipitates recurrences
3. Encourage increased fluid intake
4. Relieve local discomfort as ordered: analgesics, topical anesthetic agents, sitz baths, application of heat or cold
5. Stress the need to avoid sexual contact when lesions exist; avoid intercourse during the last 6 weeks of pregnancy
6. Advise client to have annual Papanicolaou smears
7. See Planning/Implementation under Nursing Care of Clients with Syphilis for additional information

D. EVALUATION/OUTCOMES

1. Reports relief of dysuria and pain
2. Exhibits intact skin without lesions
3. Abstains from sexual contact when lesions are present

▼ ACQUIRED IMMUNODEFICIENCY SYNDROME (AIDS)

Data Base

A. Etiology and pathophysiology
1. Caused by the human immunodeficiency virus (HIV); a retrovirus; most commonly caused by HIV-1; other strains include HIV-2 and HIV-3

2. HIV infects helper T lymphocytes (T4/CD4 cells), B lymphocytes, macrophages, promyelocytes, fibroblasts, and epidermal Langerhans cells
3. When the T4/CD4 cell count falls below 200/microliter (µL) opportunistic infections are greatest because the immune system is severely depressed
4. Protozoal (*Pneumocystis carinii* pneumonia, toxoplasmosis, cryptosporidiosis), fungal (candidiasis, cryptococcosis, histoplasmosis), bacterial (*Mycobacterium avium-intracellulare* complex, *Mycobacterium tuberculosis* [MTB]), and viral (herpes simplex virus, varicella-zoster virus, cytomegalovirus) infections, and malignancies (Kaposi's sarcoma, B-cell lymphomas, non-Hodgkin's lymphoma) frequently occur with AIDS
5. Classification system for HIV infection according to Centers for Disease Control
   a. T4/CD4 categories
      (1) Category 1: less than or equal to 500 cells/µL
      (2) Category 2: 200 to 499 cells/µL
      (3) Category 3: less than 200 cells/µL
   b. Clinical categories
      (1) Category A: categories B and C have not occurred; asymptomatic HIV infection; persistent generalized lymphadenopathy; acute (primary) HIV infection
      (2) Category B: category C has not occurred; presence of conditions attributed to HIV infection; conditions considered to have a clinical course or require management that is complicated by HIV infection
      (3) Category C: includes all clinical conditions listed as advanced HIV disease or AIDS; once a person is in category C, the person remains in this category
6. The HIV is present in blood, semen, vaginal secretions, blood-tinged saliva, tears, breast milk, and cerebrospinal fluid; transmission occurs through contact with infected blood, semen, and vaginal secretions; the virus is not viable outside the body
7. The adult is considered HIV positive when blood tests reveal the presence of HIV or antibodies to the HIV
8. Once individuals are infected with HIV, they are capable of transmitting the virus
9. Incubation period estimates range from $1/2$ to 10 years and may be longer; the antibodies produced by the body can generally first be detected in the blood in 2 weeks to 3 months or longer after infection; a test that detects the presence of virus within 24 hours of exposure is available

B. Clinical findings
   1. Subjective: anorexia, fatigue, dyspnea, chills, sore throat
   2. Objective
      a. Positive test for HIV antibody: ELISA (enzyme-linked immunosorbent assay), and Western blot
      b. Positive test for presence of HIV itself; polymerase chain reaction (PCR); HIV RNA provides evidence of viral load
      c. Decreased T4/CD4 cells to less than 200/µL
      d. Decreased ratio of T4 cell (helper cell) to T8 cell (suppressor cell)
      e. Night sweats
      f. Enlarged lymph nodes
      g. Wasting syndrome: weight loss exceeding 10% baseline weight, chronic diarrhea for more than 30 days, chronic weakness or constant fever
      h. HIV encephalopathy: memory loss, lack of coordination, partial paralysis, mental deterioration
      i. Presence of associated opportunistic infections and malignancies
   3. Women with AIDS may have gynecologic manifestations (see AIDS in Childbearing and Women's Health)
C. Therapeutic interventions
   1. There is no cure; prevention is the key to control
   2. Pharmacologic therapy: highly active antiretroviral therapy (HART) involves drug combinations
      a. Nucleoside analogue reverse transcriptase inhibitors (NRTIs)
         (1) Interferes with DNA chain
         (2) Examples: zidovudine (AZT, Retrovir), didanosine (ddl, Videx)
         (3) Side effects: peripheral neuropathy, rash
      b. Protease inhibitors (PIs)
         (1) Block virus's ability to break down larger protein molecules into smaller functional units
         (2) Examples: indinavir (Crixivan), ritonavir (Norvir)
         (3) Side effects: nausea, vomiting, diarrhea, abdominal pain, and anorexia (GI irritation); hyperglycemia (diabetes); peripheral paresthesias (neuropathy); headache (dehydration); renal calculi (calcium precipitation); increased liver enzymes (hepatotoxicity)
      c. Nonnucleoside reverse transcriptase inhibitors (NNRTIs)
         (1) Binds to reverse transcriptase and blocks RNA and DNA replication

(2) Examples: delavirdine (Rescriptor), efavirenz (Sustiva), nevirapine (Viramune)

(3) Side effects: transient rash, nausea, diarrhea; hepatotoxicity, nephrotoxicity, depressed bone marrow (Rescriptor)

3. Specific treatment of opportunistic infections
   a. *Pneumocystis carinii:* trimethoprim sulfamethoxazole (Bactrim), pentamidine
   b. Tuberculosis: isoniazid (INH), rifampin (Rifadin), ethambutal (Myambutol)
   c. Fungal infections: nystatin (Mycostatin), amphotericin B (Fungizone), ketoconazole (Nizoral)
   d. Viral infections: acyclovir (Zovirax)
4. Management of symptoms
5. Research to control the disease involves genetic manipulation and vaccines to prevent HIV infection in uninfected individuals
6. Postexposure prophylaxis (PEP) for accidental needle sticks involves treatment with reverse transcriptase inhibitors

Nursing Care of Clients with Acquired Immunodeficiency Syndrome

A. ASSESSMENT
1. Weight and vital signs for baseline
2. Progression of symptoms
3. Presence of lymphadenopathy
4. Skin and mucous membranes for evidence of Kaposi's sarcoma (lesions in epidermis that extend into dermis or extracutaneous lesions) or opportunistic infections
5. Respiratory function (e.g., characteristics of respiration, arterial blood gases, breath sounds)

B. ANALYSIS/NURSING DIAGNOSES
1. Anticipatory grieving related to concerns about dying
2. Risk for infection related to altered immune response
3. Imbalanced nutrition: less than body requirements related to anorexia
4. Chronic low self-esteem related to chronic debilitation

C. PLANNING/IMPLEMENTATION
1. Use standard precautions for all clients, regardless of diagnosis, because the virus can be transmitted before the client shows signs of disease
2. Encourage verbalization of feelings; provide emotional support
3. Refer client and significant others to counselor or support group because client and family must deal with social rejection and death
4. Protect client from secondary infection; assess for signs of opportunistic infections
5. Monitor client receiving zidovudine for blood dyscrasias
6. Teach client taking a protease inhibitor to avoid drinking alcohol (hepatotoxicity) and to drink 8 to 10 glasses of water per day to avoid dehydration
7. Provide frequent rest periods
8. Teach client the importance of:
   a. Complying with prescribed medication dosage regimen; nonadherence has led to emergence of resistant strains
   b. Informing sexual contacts of diagnosis
   c. Avoiding sexual intercourse unless using a condom
   d. Not sharing needles with other individuals
   e. Continuing medical supervision
9. Provide high-calorie, high-protein diet to prevent weight loss; encourage intake of foods rich in the immune-stimulating nutrients, especially vitamins A, C, and E, and the mineral selenium to support natural defense mechanisms; ritonavir and saquinavir should be taken with a high-fat, high-protein meal, indinavir should be taken on an empty stomach

D. EVALUATION/OUTCOMES
1. Avoids opportunistic infections
2. Maintains body weight
3. Completes self-care activities without fatigue
4. Maintains skin integrity
5. Experiences decreased frequency of loose stools
6. Shares feelings with family and health care providers
7. Is aware of community support groups

MEDICAL-SURGICAL NURSING
REVIEW QUESTIONS

Emotional Needs Related to Health Problems

1. A client is admitted to the hospital with metastatic cancer. The client has abdominal pain, a temperature of 100.4° F, and a distended abdomen. The client asks the nurse, "Do you think that I'm going to have surgery?" The statement by the nurse that would best help to establish a therapeutic relationship at this time is:
   1. "Are you afraid to have surgery?"
   2. "Some people with your problem have surgery."
   3. "I really don't know. You'll have to ask your doctor."
   4. "Has someone talked to you about having surgery?"

2. A female client with the diagnosis of Crohn's disease tells the nurse that her boyfriend dates other women. She believes that this behavior causes an increase in her symptoms. In an effort to counsel the client, the nurse should first:
   1. Help her to explore attitudes toward herself
   2. Educate the client's boyfriend about her illness
   3. Suggest that the client should not see her boyfriend for a while
   4. Schedule a counseling session for the client and her boyfriend

3. A 24-year-old college student had a right above-the-knee amputation resulting from trauma sustained in a motor vehicle accident. Upon awakening from surgery the client says, "What happened to me? I don't remember a thing." The nurse's initial response should be:
   1. "Tell me what you think happened."
   2. "You were in a car accident this morning."
   3. "You lost your leg because of a car accident."
   4. "You sound concerned; you'll remember more as you wake up."

4. Three days after an uneventful recovery from an acute myocardial infarction a client is to be moved out of the cardiac unit. The most important nursing function should be to:
   1. Provide a sense of security for the client
   2. Inform the family of the anticipated move
   3. Select a room adjacent to the cardiac unit
   4. Give the prescribed sedative before the move

5. While taking a nursing history from a client the nurse promotes communication by:
   1. Asking "why" and "how" questions
   2. Using broad, open-ended statements
   3. Reassuring the client that there is no cause for alarm
   4. Asking questions that can be answered by a "yes" or "no"

6. The nurse will understand the emotional aspects of ulcerative colitis more readily by recognizing the stress-related functions of the:
   1. Cerebral cortex and thyroid gland
   2. Central nervous system and hypothalamus
   3. Sympathetic nervous system and pancreas
   4. Autonomic nervous system and adrenal glands

7. To give nursing care to a client, the nurse must first:
   1. Understand the client's emotional conflict
   2. Develop rapport with the client's physician
   3. Recognize personal feelings toward this client
   4. Talk with the client's family or significant other

8. A 35-year-old executive secretary is hospitalized for treatment of severe hypertension. The physician orders captopril (Capoten) and alprazolam (Xanax). The client quickly finds fault with the therapeutic regimen and nursing care. The nurse recognizes this behavior is probably a manifestation of the client's:
   1. Denial of illness
   2. Fear of the health problem
   3. Response to cerebral anoxia
   4. Reaction to hypertensive medications

9. After being medicated for anxiety a client who has heart failure says to the nurse, "I guess you are too busy to stay with me." The nurse's best response in this circumstance would be:
   1. "I have to see other clients."
   2. "The medication will help you rest soon."
   3. "You will feel better; I will adjust your oxygen mask."
   4. "I have to go now, but I will come back in 10 minutes."

10. When a physically ill client is being overtly verbally hostile, the most appropriate nursing response would be a:
    1. Verbal defense of the staff's actions
    2. Reasonable exploration of the situation
    3. Silent acceptance of the client's behavior
    4. Complete physical withdrawal from the client

11. The family of a client who is terminally ill is likely to require more emotional nursing care than the client when the client reaches the stage of:
    1. Anger
    2. Denial
    3. Depression
    4. Acceptance

12. A client with a terminal illness reaches the stage of acceptance. The nurse can best help during this stage by:
    1. Allowing the client to cry
    2. Allowing unrestricted visiting
    3. Explaining all that is being done
    4. Being around though not necessarily speaking

13. The nurse is aware that characteristic behavior in the initial stage of coping with dying includes:
    1. Crying uncontrollably
    2. Criticizing medical care
    3. Refusing to receive visitors
    4. Asking for additional medical consultations

14. A client with cancer of the lung says to the nurse, "If I could just be free of pain for a few days, I might be able to eat more and regain strength." In reference to the stages of dying, the client indicates:
    1. Frustration
    2. Bargaining
    3. Depression
    4. Rationalization

15. When reaching the point of acceptance in the stages of dying, a client's behavior may reflect:
    1. Apathy
    2. Euphoria
    3. Detachment
    4. Emotionalism

16. A client who has reached the point of acceptance in the stages of dying appears happy but demonstrates a lack of involvement with the environment. The nurse can best deal with this client by:
    1. Ignoring the client's behavior when possible
    2. Pointing out the reality of the situation to the client
    3. Joining the client in denial because this is a defense
    4. Recognizing and accepting the client's behavior at this point

17. A client asks the nurse, "Should I tell my husband I have AIDS?" The nurse's most appropriate response would be:
    1. "This is a decision you alone can make."
    2. "Do not tell him anything unless he asks."
    3. "You are having difficulty deciding what to say."
    4. "Tell him you feel you contracted AIDS from him."

18. A male physician who is found in a diabetic coma has omitted information about a history of diabetes mellitus from his health record. This pertinent information has most likely been omitted because:
    1. Individuals with diabetes mellitus often have lapses of memory
    2. Physicians with diabetes are not accepted for residency in many hospitals
    3. He needs assistance in developing a more favorable adaptation to this stress
    4. He is unable to handle the psychologic stress related to alterations in body functioning

19. Despite initiation of therapy for pancreatitis, a client continues to be apprehensive and restless. Nursing action should include:
    1. Teaching the importance of rest
    2. Administering antibiotics as ordered
    3. Encouraging the expression of concerns
    4. Explaining that everything will be all right

20. When creating a therapeutic environment for a client who has just had a myocardial infarction, the nurse should provide for:
    1. Short family visits
    2. Telephone communication
    3. Television for short periods
    4. Daily papers in the morning

21. After being scheduled for a colostomy, a client's anxiety is overt and realistic. The most effective way for the nurse to help the client at this point would be to:
    1. Administer a prescribed prn sedative
    2. Encourage the client to express feelings
    3. Explain the procedure and postoperative course
    4. Reassure the client that many people cope with this problem

22. A husband spends most of the day with his wife, who is receiving chemotherapy for inoperable cancer, and asks the nurse how he can continue to help her. The nurse should plan to:
    1. Instruct the husband about the action of the various drugs
    2. Offer the couple a detailed description of the disease process
    3. Assist the couple to maintain open and honest communication
    4. Talk with the husband alone to promote ventilation of feelings

23. Before discharge, a client who had a colostomy for colorectal cancer questions the nurse about resuming activities. The nurse should plan to help the client understand that:
    1. Most sports activities, except for swimming, can be resumed based on the client's overall physical condition
    2. Activities of daily living should be resumed as quickly as possible to avoid depression and further dependency
    3. With counseling and medical guidance, a near normal lifestyle, including complete sexual function, is possible
    4. After surgery, changes in activities must be made to accommodate the physiologic changes caused by the operation

24. During admission a client appears anxious and says to the nurse, "The doctor told me I have lung cancer. My father died from cancer. I wish I had never smoked." The most appropriate response by the nurse would be:
    1. "You are concerned about your diagnosis."
    2. "You are feeling guilty about your smoking."
    3. "Trust your doctor; it's important you have faith."
    4. "There have been improvements in lung cancer therapy."

25. When helping a client with a cerebral vascular accident to develop independence, the nurse should:
    1. Establish long-range goals for the client
    2. Reinforce success in tasks accomplished
    3. Point out errors in performance on which to focus
    4. Demonstrate ways the client can regain independence in activities

26. When helping a client immobilized by the pain of rheumatoid arthritis toward self-reliance and independence, the nurse should approach the problem with:
    1. A series of limited objectives
    2. A positive attitude toward the eventual outcome
    3. The understanding that little can be accomplished
    4. The recognition that a nursing home–type facility is needed

27. The spouse of a client who has had a CVA seems unable to accept the idea that the client must be encouraged to participate in self-care. The nurse may be able to work around these feelings by:
    1. Telling the spouse to let the client do things independently
    2. Allowing the spouse to assume total responsibility for the client's care
    3. Explaining that the nursing staff has full responsibility for the client's activities
    4. Asking the spouse for assistance in planning those activities most helpful to the client

28. A client with hemiplegia is staring blankly at the wall and complains of feeling like half a person. Initially nursing care for this client should be directed at:
    1. Distracting the client from self-pity
    2. Including the client in all decisions
    3. Helping the client explore personal feelings
    4. Preventing the client from developing contractures

29. While receiving a preoperative enema a client starts to cry and says, "I'm sorry you have to do this messy thing for me." The best response by the nurse at this time would be:

    1. "I don't mind it."
    2. "You seem to be upset."
    3. "This is part of my job."
    4. "Nurses get used to this."

30. A client complains that low-salt food is very tasteless. The nurse's best response would be:
    1. "Let's consider some alternatives."
    2. "Salt can be very harmful to your health."
    3. "Ask the doctor if you can splurge occasionally."
    4. "It must be difficult for you, but you'll get used to it."

31. A client who is scheduled to have a hysterectomy starts to sob and says, "I told my husband today that after this operation I will only be half a woman. He reassured me, but I know that was just a front." The most appropriate response by the nurse would be:
    1. "It must be frightening to know that your husband rejects you as a woman."
    2. "You feel this operation will have an effect on how your husband feels about you as his wife?"
    3. "You know of course that this is silly. I wish you would not worry about such irrelevant things. The main thing is that you have to get well quickly."
    4. "I think I'll call your physician who may want to postpone the operation until you and your husband have adjusted better to the outcomes of a hysterectomy."

32. The spouse of a client with a CVA insists on doing everything for the client during visits. After these visits the client seems to be quite depressed. The nurse should assume that the client is probably:
    1. Losing faith in the future
    2. Feeling the loss of independence
    3. Feeling guilty about being a burden
    4. Experiencing the problem that is a natural part of this illness

33. The best approach for the nurse to use when helping a client express anxiety over a scheduled D&C and conization would be to:
    1. Ask, "What are you really upset about?"
    2. Explain that a conization and a D&C are considered minor surgery
    3. Say, "I can tell that something is troubling you. It might help to talk about it."
    4. Tell the client that it is normal to be anxious; everybody is fearful, even though there is no reason to worry

34. After having a transverse colostomy, the client asks what effect the surgery will have on future sexual relationships. The nurse should explain that:
    1. Sexual relationships must be curtailed for several weeks
    2. The client will be able to resume normal sexual relationships
    3. The surgery will temporarily decrease the client's sexual impulses
    4. The partner should be told about the surgery before any sexual activity

35. Immediately after a storm has passed, the rescue team with which the nurse is working is searching for injured people. A victim lying next to a broken natural gas main is not breathing and is bleeding heavily from a wound on the foot. The nurse's first step would be to:
    1. Treat the victim for shock
    2. Start rescue breathing immediately
    3. Apply surface pressure to the foot wound
    4. Remove the victim from the immediate vicinity

36. When a disaster occurs, the nurse may have to treat mass hysteria first. The person or persons to be cared for immediately would be those in:
    1. Panic
    2. Coma
    3. Euphoria
    4. Depression

Growth and Development

37. When planning discharge teaching for a 22-year-old, the nurse should include the potential health problems common in this age group. The nurse can accomplish this by making the client aware of:
    1. Kidney dysfunction
    2. Cardiovascular diseases
    3. Accidents and their prevention
    4. Eye problems, such as glaucoma

38. In meeting the unique teaching needs of an elderly client recently diagnosed with diabetes mellitus, the nurse plans a teaching program based on the principle that learning:
    1. Reduces general anxiety
    2. Is negatively affected by age
    3. Requires continued reinforcement
    4. Necessitates readiness of the learner

39. The occurrence of chronic illness is greatest in:
    1. Older adults
    2. Adolescents
    3. Young children
    4. Middle-aged adults

40. Elderly people have a high incidence of hip fractures because of:
    1. Carelessness
    2. Fragility of bone
    3. Sedentary existence
    4. Rheumatoid diseases

41. When formulating nursing care plans for elderly clients, the nurse should include special measures to accommodate for age-related sensory losses such as:
    1. Difficulty in swallowing
    2. Increased sensitivity to heat
    3. Diminished sensation of pain
    4. Heightened response to stimuli

42. The nurse would expect an elderly client with a hearing loss caused by aging to have:
    1. Copious, moist cerumen
    2. Tears in the tympanic membrane
    3. Difficulty hearing women's voices
    4. Overgrowth of the epithelial auditory lining

Drug-Related Responses

43. Radium is stored in lead containers because:
    1. Radium is a heavy substance
    2. The lead functions as a barrier
    3. Heat is produced as radium disintegrates
    4. Lead prevents disintegration of the radium

44. A systemic drug that may be prescribed to produce diuresis and inhibit formation of aqueous humor is:
    1. Chlorothiazide (Diuril)
    2. Acetazolamide (Diamox)
    3. Bendroflumethiazide (Naturetin)
    4. Demecarium bromide (Humorsol)

45. A client is to be discharged on a diuretic and digitalis. The nurse reviewing the client's diet would be especially careful to look for adequate sources of potassium because:
    1. Potassium is a necessary ion for normal body function
    2. Potassium is a cofactor for several important enzymes
    3. Under conditions of hypokalemia, digitalis exerts toxic effects on the heart
    4. Under conditions of hyperglycemia, digitalis exerts toxic effects on the heart

46. A client complains of fatigue and dyspnea and appears jaundiced. The nurse questions the client about medications taken routinely. In light of the symptoms, the nurse should be most concerned about:
    1. Multivitamin with iron daily
    2. Methyldopa (Aldomet) 250 mg bid
    3. Levothyroxine (Synthroid) 0.15 mg daily
    4. Aspirin 10 grains taken before admission

47. A client is receiving albuterol (Proventil) to relieve severe asthma. The nurse should monitor the client for:
    1. Lethargy
    2. Palpitations
    3. Visual disturbances
    4. Decreased pulse rate

48. Before giving a client digoxin, the nurse should assess the:
    1. Apical heart rate
    2. Radial pulse in both arms
    3. Radial pulse on the left side
    4. Difference between apical and radial pulses

49. The nurse should teach a client to suspect that nitroglycerin SL tablets have lost their potency when:
    1. Sublingual tingling is experienced
    2. The tablets are three or more months old
    3. Pain is unrelieved but facial flushing is increased
    4. Onset of relief is delayed, but the duration of relief is unchanged

50. Evaluation of the effectiveness of nitroglycerine SL is based on:
    1. Relief of anginal pain
    2. Improved cardiac output
    3. A decrease in blood pressure
    4. Dilation of superficial blood vessels

51. The drug the nurse should expect the physician to order if symptoms of warfarin overdose are observed would be:
    1. Heparin
    2. Vitamin K
    3. Protamine sulfate
    4. Iron-dextran (Imferon)

52. The loop diuretics alter active transport systems in the kidney tubules, resulting in increased excretion of sodium and, secondarily, water. The principle explaining the secondary water loss (diuresis) is:
    1. Osmosis
    2. Diffusion
    3. Filtration
    4. Active transport

53. A client receiving hydrochlorothiazide (hydroDIURIL) asks what this drug actually does. The nurse explains that the planned therapeutic effect of the drug is to:
    1. Increase the glomerular filtration rate
    2. Decrease the reabsorption of potassium
    3. Increase the excretion of sodium and chloride
    4. Decrease the amount of fluid reabsorption in Henle's loop

54. When teaching a client receiving prazosin (Minipress) for hypertension why orthostatic hypotension occurs, the nurse knows that this antihypertensive causes vasodilation by:
    1. Depleting acetylcholine
    2. Stimulating histamine release
    3. Blocking the response to norepinephrine
    4. Decreasing adrenal release of epinephrine

55. A client receiving propranolol hydrochloride (Inderal) should be told to expect:
    1. Dizziness with strenuous activity
    2. Acceleration of the heart rate after eating a heavy meal
    3. Flushing sensations for a few minutes after taking the drug
    4. Pounding of the heart for a few minutes after taking the drug

56. A client with a history of arthritis has an acute episode of right ventricular heart failure and is receiving furosemide (Lasix). The physician lowers the client's usual dosage of aspirin. The nurse's explanation for the lower dose is based on the knowledge that:
    1. Aspirin accelerates metabolism of furosemide and decreases the diuretic effect
    2. Aspirin in large doses after an acute stress episode increases the bleeding potential
    3. Competition for renal excretion sites by the drugs causes increased serum levels of aspirin
    4. Use of furosemide and aspirin concomitantly increases formation of uric acid crystals in the nephron

57. When teaching a client about nitroglycerin therapy, the nurse should include the importance of:
    1. Limiting the number of tablets to 4 per day
    2. Discontinuing the medication if a headache develops
    3. Making certain the medication is stored in a dark container
    4. Increasing the number of tablets if dizziness or hypertension occurs

58. When anticipating drug therapy for a client who is experiencing a cardiac arrest because of ventricular fibrillation, the nurse should initially prepare:
    1. Lidocaine HCl (Xylocaine)
    2. Dopamine HCl (Intropin)
    3. Sodium bicarbonate (NaHCO$_3$)
    4. Vasopressin (Pitressin Synthetic)

59. A client asks the nurse why the physician has prescribed captopril (Capoten). The nurse explains it is an effective:
    1. Diuretic
    2. Hypnotic
    3. Tranquilizer
    4. Antihypertensive

60. A client who was recently admitted with the diagnosis of acute myocardial infarction is anxious and the physician orders diazepam (Valium) 50 mg PO prn for nervousness. Before implementing this order, the nurse should:
    1. Assess the apical pulse
    2. Assess the blood pressure
    3. Encourage ventilation of feelings
    4. Clarify the order with the physician

61. The nurse anticipates a nursing diagnosis for a client receiving chemotherapy for the treatment of multiple myeloma to be imbalanced nutrition: less than body requirements, related to chemotherapy. The best intervention to plan is:
    1. Providing low-carbohydrate meals
    2. Explaining the effect of chemotherapy
    3. Encouraging the intake of large meals
    4. Administering ordered antiemetics before meals

62. The physician orders ibuprofen (Motrin) and hydroxychloroquine sulfate (Plaquenil) for an older client's arthritis. The nurse teaches the client about hydroxychloroquine and knows that the information about toxicity was understood when the client states, "I will contact the physician immediately if I develop:
    1. Blurred vision."
    2. Blood in the urine."
    3. Difficulty swallowing."
    4. Feelings of irritability."

63. One week after being hospitalized for an acute myocardial infarction, a client complains of loss of appetite and a nauseous feeling. The nurse should recognize that these symptoms may indicate the:
    1. Adverse effects of Lanoxin
    2. Therapeutic effects of Lasix
    3. Adverse effects of Aldactone
    4. Therapeutic effects of Inderal

64. The nurse is aware that many of the chemotherapeutic agents used in the treatment of cancer cause
   1. Leukocytosis
   2. Bone marrow depression
   3. Decreased sedimentation rate
   4. Increased hemoglobin and hematocrit

65. In addition to a decreased apical rate, the nurse should teach a client to withhold the prescribed digoxin if the client experiences:
   1. Singultus
   2. Chest pain
   3. Blurred vision
   4. Increased urinary output

66. The INR of a client receiving Coumadin has been somewhat unstable when checked in the clinic laboratory. The nurse interviews the client to identify factors contributing to the problem. The nurse should assess the client's:
   1. Use of analgesics
   2. Serum glucose level
   3. Intake of potassium supplements
   4. Compliance with the Coumadin regimen

67. A client is receiving IV heparin sodium and oral warfarin sodium (Coumadin) concurrently for a partial occlusion of the left common carotid artery. The client expresses concern about why both heparin and Coumadin are needed. The nurse's explanation is based on knowledge that the plan:
   1. Allows clot dissolution and prevents new clot formation
   2. Permits the administration of smaller doses of each drug
   3. Immediately provides maximum protection against clot formation
   4. Provides anticoagulant intravenously until the oral drug reaches its therapeutic level

68. A client with a partial occlusion of the left common carotid artery is to be discharged while still receiving Coumadin. When discussing the adverse effects of Coumadin, the nurse should tell the client to consult with the physician if:
   1. Blood appears in urine
   2. Swelling of the ankles increases
   3. The ability to concentrate diminishes
   4. Increased transient ischemic attacks occur

69. A client is receiving an anticoagulant for a pulmonary embolism. The drug that is contraindicated for clients receiving anticoagulants is:
   1. Ferrous sulfate
   2. Acetylsalicylic acid
   3. Isoxsuprine (Vasodilan)
   4. Chlorpromazine (Thorazine)

70. A female client taking medications for a seizure disorder has been placed on Coumadin because of thrombophlebitis. After a weekly prothombin time the client telephones the clinic to find out if the anticoagulant dosage is to be changed. At the same time, the client mentions that she is out of the prescribed barbiturate for sleep, but will get more at the time of her next appointment in three weeks. The nurse tells her to come for a refill immediately because:
   1. She may develop withdrawal symptoms
   2. Absence of sleep may precipitate seizures
   3. Discontinuance of the drug may affect the prothrombin level
   4. Control of seizures is dependent on the combined action of phenytoin (Dilantin) and the sleeping medication

71. Vitamin B$_6$ (pyridoxine) is given with isoniazid (INH) because it:
   1. Enhances tuberculostatic effect of isoniazid
   2. Improves the immunologic response of the client
   3. Provides the vitamin when isoniazid is interfering with natural vitamin synthesis
   4. Accelerates destruction of remaining organisms after inhibition of their reproduction by isoniazid

72. A client is to receive isoproterenol (Isuprel) prn. The nurse administers this drug to:
   1. Produce sedation
   2. Relax bronchial spasm
   3. Decrease blood pressure
   4. Increase bronchial secretions

73. Symptoms of morphine overdose include:
   1. Slow pulse, slow respirations, sedation
   2. Slow respirations, dilated pupils, restlessness
   3. Profuse sweating, pinpoint pupils, and deep sleep
   4. Slow respirations, constricted pupils, and deep sleep

74. When preparing a client's analgesic medication, the nurse should know that meperidine is commonly available for administration as:
    1. Narcan
    2. Darvon
    3. Doriden
    4. Demerol

75. The nurse should be aware that the medication most frequently used to relieve anxiety and apprehension in the client with pulmonary edema is:
    1. Chloral hydrate
    2. Morphine sulfate
    3. Hydroxyzine (Atarax)
    4. Sodium phenobarbital

76. A client is brought to the emergency department in the midst of persistent tonic-clonic convulsions. Diazepam (Valium) is administered, which decreases central neuronal activity and:
    1. Slows cardiac contractions
    2. Relaxes peripheral muscles
    3. Dilates the tracheobronchial structures
    4. Provides amnesia for the convulsive episode

77. The nurse administers alprazolam (Xanax) as ordered to an anxious client who has severe hypertension because it:
    1. Induces sleep
    2. Promotes rest
    3. Reduces hostility
    4. Produces hypotension

78. Levodopa is prescribed for a client with Parkinson's disease. The nurse should know that this drug:
    1. Is poorly absorbed if given with meals
    2. Must be monitored by weekly laboratory tests
    3. Causes an initial euphoria followed by depression
    4. May cause a side effect of orthostatic hypotension

79. When caring for a client who is receiving phenytoin (Dilantin) the nurse plans health teaching and emphasizes meticulous oral hygiene because phenytoin:
    1. Causes hyperplasia of the gums
    2. Increases alkalinity of the oral secretions
    3. Irritates the gingiva and destroys tooth enamel
    4. Increases plaque and bacterial growth at the gum lines

80. Edrophonium HCl (Tensilon) is used for the diagnosis of myasthenia gravis because this drug will cause a temporary increase in:
    1. Symptoms
    2. Consciousness
    3. Blood pressure
    4. Muscle strength

81. After a client with a history of a seizure disorder has received IV heparin sodium for 3 days following open heart surgery, the drug is discontinued. The nurse continues to observe the client closely during the early days of treatment with Coumadin because:
    1. Phenytoin increases the clotting potential
    2. Coumadin affects the metabolism of phenytoin
    3. Coumadin action is greater in clients with seizure disorders
    4. Seizures increase the metabolic degradation rate of Coumadin

82. The physician prescribes phenobarbital sodium (Luminal) for a client who has had a tonic-clonic seizure. The nurse would know that the client understood the teaching about the side effects of phenobarbital when the client states, "I should call the doctor if I develop:
    1. Loss of appetite or persistent fatigue."
    2. Anal itching or dizziness when I stand up."
    3. Diarrhea or a rash on the upper part of my body."
    4. Decreased tolerance to common foods or constipation."

83. Folic acid is often prescribed for a client who is receiving phenytoin (Dilantin) because folic acid:
    1. Improves absorption of iron from foods
    2. Content of common foods is inadequate
    3. Prevents the neuropathy caused by phenytoin
    4. Absorption from foods is inhibited by phenytoin

84. The physician prescribes phenytoin (Dilantin) for a client to control tonic-clonic seizures. The expected effect of this drug is to:
    1. Produce an antispasmodic action on the muscles
    2. Prevent depression of the central nervous system
    3. Control nerve impulses originating in the motor cortex
    4. Alter the permeability of the cell membrane to potassium

85. The effectiveness of carbamazepine (Tegretol) in the management of trigeminal neuralgia is determined by monitoring the client's:
    1. Pain relief
    2. Liver function
    3. Cardiac output
    4. Seizure activity

86. Ceftriaxone (Rocephin) 2.5 g IVPB every 8 hours is ordered for a client with a severe infection. The pharmacy sends a vial labeled 5 g per 10 ml. When preparing the IVPB the nurse should use:
    1. 1 ml
    2. 2.5 ml
    3. 4.5 ml
    4. 5 ml

87. A client is to have mafenide (Sulfamylon) cream applied to burned areas. The nurse should be aware that a serious side effect of Sulfamylon therapy is:
    1. Curling's ulcer
    2. Renal shutdown
    3. Metabolic acidosis
    4. Hemolysis of RBCs

88. The physician orders 20 mEq potassium chloride to be given over an 8-hour period by IV drip in 1000 ml of D5/W to a client after surgery. The IV equipment is calibrated at 20 drops per milliliter. To deliver the correct dosage, the solution must be set to flow at the rate of:
    1. 10 drops/min
    2. 21 drops/min
    3. 34 drops/min
    4. 42 drops/min

89. Whenever quinine is used, the nurse should be alert to symptoms of severe cinchonism, which include:
    1. Deafness
    2. Paresthesias
    3. Difficulty breathing
    4. Painful swollen joints

90. After several days of IV therapy for chloroquine-resistant malaria, the physician replaces the IV injection with quinine sulfate, 2 g per day in divided doses. The nurse should administer this medication after meals to:
    1. Delay its absorption
    2. Minimize gastric irritation
    3. Decrease stimulation of appetite
    4. Reduce its antidysrhythmic action

91. Preparation of a client for a subtotal thyroidectomy may include the administration of potassium iodide solution. This medication is given to:
    1. Decrease the total basal metabolic rate
    2. Maintain the function of the parathyroid glands
    3. Decrease the size and vascularity of the thyroid gland
    4. Ablate the cells of the thyroid gland that produce T_4

92. When teaching a client about antacid therapy, the nurse should include the fact that antacid tablets:
    1. Must be taken 1 hour before meals
    2. Are as effective as the liquid forms
    3. Should be taken only at 4-hour intervals
    4. Interfere with the absorption of other drugs

93. The nurse administers trimethoprim-sulfamethoxazol (Septra) as ordered to combat urinary tract infections. This drug belongs to the group of drugs known as:
    1. Antiseptics
    2. Analgesics
    3. Uricosurics
    4. Antiinfectives

94. A client who has been diagnosed as having Lyme disease is started on doxycycline, a tetracycline. When administering this drug, the nurse should:
    1. Administer medication with meals or a snack
    2. Provide orange or other citrus fruit juice with the medication
    3. Provide medication an hour before milk products are ingested
    4. Offer antacids 30 minutes after administration if GI side effects occur

95. A client has an urticarial response to ampicillin. Diphenhydramine hydrochloride (Benadryl) is administered to:
    1. Destroy histamine in tissues and reverse the urticarial response
    2. Inhibit release of vasoactive substances and dilate tissue capillaries
    3. Compete with histamine for receptors and interfere with vasodilation
    4. Metabolize histamine and inhibit release of substances causing intense itching

96. Before the discharge of a client with Addison's disease, the physician prescribes hydrocortisone and fludrocortisone. The nurse expects hydrocortisone to:
 1. Control excessive loss of potassium salts
 2. Decrease cardiac dysrhythmias and dyspnea
 3. Prevent hypoglycemia and permit the client to respond to stress
 4. Increase amounts of angiotensin II to raise the client's blood pressure

97. The nurse administers desmopressin acetate (DDAVP) to a client with diabetes insipidus. To evaluate the effectiveness of the drug the nurse should monitor the client's:
 1. Pulse rate
 2. Serum glucose
 3. Arterial blood pH
 4. Intake and output

98. A client with tetanus is to continue taking ampicillin after discharge. The nurse should explain the need to:
 1. Take ampicillin with meals
 2. Notify the physician if diarrhea develops
 3. Store the ampicillin in a light-resistant container
 4. Continue the drug until a negative culture is obtained

99. A client will be taking sulfisoxazole (Gantrisin) at home. The nurse instructs the client to:
 1. Increase fluid intake
 2. Strain urine for crystals and stones
 3. Stop the drug if the urinary output increases
 4. Maintain the exact time schedule for drug taking

100. A client with rheumatoid arthritis is receiving aspirin. The nurse should teach the client to report symptoms of salicylate intoxication, which include:
 1. Polyuria
 2. Confusion
 3. Hypertension
 4. Laryngeal spasm

101. Gold salts may be used to treat rheumatoid arthritis. A serious side effect of this drug is:
 1. Kidney damage
 2. Persistent nausea
 3. Pulmonary emboli
 4. Cardiac decompensation

102. A client with rheumatoid arthritis is receiving aurothioglucose, a gold compound. It is most important that the nurse monitor the client for:
 1. Hypertension
 2. Cutaneous lesions
 3. Thrombocytopenia
 4. Elevated blood glucose

103. The physician orders antibiotic therapy for a client receiving chemotherapy because these agents destroy rapidly growing cells in the:
 1. Liver
 2. Blood
 3. Lymph nodes
 4. Bone marrow

104. During chemotherapy for cancer of the lung, the nurse expects the client to develop soreness of the mouth and anus because:
 1. These tissues are poorly nourished because the client is anorectic
 2. The entire GI tract is involved because of the direct irritating effects of chemotherapy
 3. These tissues normally divide rapidly and are damaged by the chemotherapeutic agent
 4. The side effects of the chemotherapeutic agents used tend to concentrate in these body areas

105. A client is to receive leucovorin calcium before receiving methotrexate. This drug is being administered to:
 1. Provide levels of folic acid required by blood-forming organs
 2. Provide the metabolite required for destruction of cancer cells
 3. Provide folic acid, which acts synergistically with antineoplastic drugs to destroy cancer cells
 4. Increase production of phagocytic cells required to remove debris liberated by disintegrating cancer cells

106. While a client is receiving dexamethasone (Decadron) the nurse should test the client's blood glucose level because the drug:
 1. Has a glucose component
 2. Accelerates glucose metabolism
 3. Mobilizes liver stores of glycogen
 4. Lowers the renal threshold for glucose

107. The physician plans to reduce a client's dexamethasone (Decadron) dosage gradually and to continue a lower maintenance dosage. The nurse explains that the reason for the gradual dosage reduction is to allow:
    1. Production of antibodies by the immune system
    2. Return of cortisone production by the adrenal glands
    3. Building of glycogen and protein stores in liver and muscle
    4. Time to observe for return of increased intracranial pressure

108. A client with rheumatoid arthritis has been taking a steroid medication for the past year. A complication of the prolonged use of this medication is:
    1. Leukopenia
    2. Elevated C-reactive protein
    3. Elevated sedimentation rate
    4. Hypochromic, normocytic anemia

109. To assist the medical team in prescribing an effective antibiotic, the most valuable test is the:
    1. Serologic test
    2. Sensitivity test
    3. Susceptibility test
    4. Tissue culture test

110. After receiving streptomycin sulfate for 2 weeks as part of the medical regimen for tuberculosis, the client states, "I feel like I am walking like a drunken seaman." The nurse withholds the drug and promptly reports the problem to the physician because the signs may be a result of the drug's effect on the:
    1. Cerebellar tissue
    2. Peripheral motor end plates
    3. Internal capsule and pyramidal tracts
    4. Vestibular branch of the eighth cranial nerve

111. A client says, "I take baking soda in water when I get heartburn." The nurse suggests an antacid containing aluminum and magnesium hydroxide such as Maalox instead of baking soda. This response is based on the fact that antacids such as Maalox:
    1. Contain little if any sodium
    2. Are readily absorbed by the stomach mucosa
    3. Have no direct effect on systemic acid-base balance when taken as directed
    4. Cause few side effects such as diarrhea or constipation when they are used properly

112. The physician orders ranitidine (Zantac) for a client with peptic ulcer disease. The nurse should teach the client that Zantac is a drug whose main action is to:
    1. Increase gastric motility
    2. Neutralize gastric acidity
    3. Increase histamine release
    4. Inhibit gastric acid secretion

113. A client reports taking calcium carbonate (Tums) frequently. The client should be advised that this practice may lead to:
    1. Diarrhea
    2. Water retention
    3. Rebound hyperacidity
    4. Bone demineralization

Fluid and Electrolytes

114. The percentage of water in the average adult human body is:
    1. 80%
    2. 60%
    3. 40%
    4. 20%

115. The receptors for the regulation of body water through detection of osmotic pressure are located in the:
    1. Blood
    2. Hypothalamus
    3. Kidney tubules
    4. Neurohypophysis

116. The major role in maintaining fluid balance in the body is performed by the:
    1. Liver
    2. Heart
    3. Lungs
    4. Kidneys

117. A nurse administers an intravenous solution of 0.45% sodium chloride. With respect to human blood cells, this solution is:
    1. Isotonic
    2. Isomeric
    3. Hypotonic
    4. Hypertonic

118. The nurse is aware that fluid deficit can most accurately be assessed by:
    1. A change in body weight
    2. The presence of dry skin
    3. A decrease in blood pressure
    4. An altered general appearance

119. Two body systems that interact with the bicarbonate buffer system to preserve the normal body fluid pH of 7.4 are the:
    1. Skeletal and nervous systems
    2. Circulatory and urinary systems
    3. Respiratory and urinary systems
    4. Muscular and endocrine systems

120. The statement that correctly compares blood plasma and interstitial fluid is:
    1. Both contain the same kinds of ions
    2. Plasma exerts lower osmotic pressure than does interstitial fluid
    3. Plasma contains slightly more of each kind of ion than does interstitial fluid
    4. The main cation in plasma is sodium, whereas the main cation in interstitial fluid is potassium

121. The weight of extracellular body fluid is approximately 20% of the total body weight of an average individual. The component of the extracellular fluid that contributes the greatest portion to this amount is the:
    1. Plasma fluid
    2. Interstitial fluid
    3. Fluid in dense tissue
    4. Fluid in body secretions

122. The most important electrolyte of intracellular fluid is:
    1. Sodium
    2. Calcium
    3. Chloride
    4. Potassium

123. The body fluids that make up 40% to 50% of the total body weight are:
    1. Interstitial
    2. Intracellular
    3. Extracellular
    4. Intravascular

124. Ammonia is excreted by the kidney to help maintain:
    1. Osmotic pressure of the blood
    2. Acid-base balance of the body
    3. Low bacterial levels in the urine
    4. Normal red blood cell production

125. The nurse understands that a client with albuminuria has edema caused by a:
    1. Fall in tissue hydrostatic pressure
    2. Rise in plasma hydrostatic pressure
    3. Fall in plasma colloid oncotic pressure
    4. Rise in tissue colloid osmotic pressure

126. When intravenous fluid is allowed to flow into a person by gravity:
    1. Potential energy is converted to kinetic energy
    2. Kinetic energy is converted to potential energy
    3. Chemical energy is converted to kinetic energy
    4. Potential energy is converted to chemical energy

127. A solution containing 1 mole of solute in 1 liter of solution is called:
    1. A molar solution
    2. A normal solution
    3. An isotonic solution
    4. A saturated solution

128. When caring for a client with a portable wound drainage system, the nurse understands that the principle behind its functioning is:
    1. Gravity causes liquids to flow down a pressure gradient
    2. The diameter of the lumen will determine the flow rate of fluid
    3. Siphonage causes fluids to flow from one level to a lower one
    4. Fluids flow from an area of higher pressure to one of lower pressure

129. Larger than normal amounts of acetoacetic acid have been entering the blood as one of the indirect results of a client's insulin deficiency. Like lactic acid and other nonvolatile acids, acetoacetic acid is buffered in the blood chiefly by:
    1. Potassium
    2. Bicarbonate
    3. Carbon dioxide
    4. Sodium chloride

130. The nurse must assess the client with gastric lavage or prolonged vomiting for:
    1. Acidosis
    2. Alkalosis
    3. Loss of oxygen from the blood
    4. Loss of osmotic pressure of the blood

131. The nurse explains to a client that it is not advisable to take bicarbonate of soda regularly. This statement is based on knowledge that bicarbonate of soda can cause:
    1. Gastric distention
    2. Metabolic alkalosis
    3. Chronic constipation
    4. Cardiac dysrhythmias

132. The coronary care unit nurse draws an arterial blood sample to assess a client for acidosis. A normal pH for arterial blood is:
    1. 7.0
    2. 7.30
    3. 7.42
    4. 7.50

133. The nurse must be alert for signs of respiratory acidosis in the client with emphysema because this individual has a long-term problem with oxygen maintenance and:
    1. The carbon dioxide is not excreted
    2. Hyperventilation occurs, even if the cause is not physiologic
    3. There is a loss of carbon dioxide from the body's buffer pool
    4. Localized tissue necrosis occurs as a result of poor oxygen supply to the area

134. A client is in a state of uncompensated acidosis. The nurse would expect the arterial blood pH to be approximately:
    1. 6.9
    2. 7.2
    3. 7.45
    4. 7.48

135. Following extensive, prolonged surgery it is most important that the nurse observe the client for the depletion of the electrolyte:
    1. Sodium
    2. Calcium
    3. Chloride
    4. Potassium

136. The nurse notes that a client's serum potassium level is 5.8 mEq/L. The nurse should first:
    1. Call the laboratory and repeat the test
    2. Call the cardiac arrest team to alert them
    3. Obtain an ECG strip and have lidocaine available
    4. Take the client's vital signs and notify the physician

137. Potassium chloride, 20 mEq, is to be added to the IV solution of a client in diabetic ketoacidosis. The primary purpose for administering this drug is:
    1. Treatment of hyperpnea
    2. Prevention of flaccid paralysis
    3. Replacement of potassium deficit
    4. Treatment of cardiac dysrhythmias

138. A client is admitted with diarrhea, anorexia, weight loss, and abdominal cramps, and a diagnosis of colitis is made. The symptoms of fluid and electrolyte imbalance caused by this condition that the nurse should report immediately are:
    1. Skin rash, diarrhea, and diplopia
    2. Extreme muscle weakness and tachycardia
    3. Development of tetany with muscle spasms
    4. Nausea, vomiting, and leg and stomach cramps

139. When an intestinal obstruction is suspected a client has a nasogastric tube inserted and attached to suction. Critical assessment of this client includes observation for:
    1. Edema
    2. Belching
    3. Dehydration
    4. Excessive salivation

140. A client drank $7^1/_2$ oz of orange juice, 6 oz of tea, and 8 oz of eggnog. The calculated intake would be:
    1. 515 ml
    2. 585 ml
    3. 625 ml
    4. 645 ml

141. The intake and output for a client over an 8-hour period is:
    8 AM: IV with D5W infusing and 900 ml left in bag
    8:30 AM: 150 ml urine voided
    9 AM to 3 PM: 200 ml gastric tube formula and 50 ml water at q3h intervals; no aspirate obtained until final feeding; 25 ml at this time
    8 AM to 4 PM: vitamin solution, 10 ml q4h
    1 PM: 220 ml voided
    3:15 PM: 235 ml voided
    4 PM: IV with 550 ml left in bag
    The nurse calculates the intake and output as:
    1. Intake, 930 ml; output, 650 ml
    2. Intake, 1050 ml; output, 680 ml
    3. Intake, 1080 ml; output, 595 ml
    4. Intake, 1130 ml; output, 630 ml

142. When preparing an IV piggyback medication for a client the nurse is aware that it is essential to:
    1. Use strict sterile technique
    2. Rotate the bag after adding the medication
    3. Use exactly 100 ml of fluid to mix the medication
    4. Change the needle just before adding the medication

143. An IV of 1000 ml 5% dextrose in water to be infused at 125 ml/hr is started on admission to correct fluid imbalance. The infusion set delivers 10 drops per milliliter. To regulate the rate of flow so that the solution would be infused over an 8-hour period, the nurse should set the rate of flow at:
    1. 20 drops per minute
    2. 40 drops per minute
    3. 60 drops per minute
    4. 160 drops per minute

144. The nurse is aware that ascites can be related to:
    1. Portal hypotension
    2. Kidney malfunction
    3. Diminished plasma protein
    4. Decreased production of potassium

145. The nurse is aware that negative nitrogen balance most directly occurs in a client receiving IV administration of 5% dextrose in water because of:
    1. Excessive carbohydrate intake
    2. Lack of protein supplementation
    3. Insufficient intake of water-soluble vitamins
    4. Increased concentration of electrolytes in cells

146. A client who is receiving furosemide (Lasix) and digoxin (Lanoxin) should be observed for symptoms of electrolyte depletion caused by:
    1. Diuretic therapy
    2. Sodium restriction
    3. Continuous dyspnea
    4. Inadequate oral intake

147. The nurse, recognizing that digitalis preparations promote diuresis, should evaluate clients for a depletion of:
    1. Sodium
    2. Calcium
    3. Potassium
    4. Phosphate

148. A serious complication of acute malaria is:
    1. Congested lungs
    2. Impaired peristalsis
    3. Anemia and cachexia
    4. Fluid and electrolyte imbalance

149. The nurse must assess a client experiencing excessive production of antidiuretic hormone for:
    1. Polyuria
    2. Dehydration
    3. Hyponatremia
    4. Hyperglycemia

150. In the emergent phase immediately after a severe burn injury, care is centered on replacement therapy by IV fluids. The nurse should question the physician's order if it is designed to provide:
    1. Water
    2. Potassium
    3. Lactated Ringer's
    4. Plasma expanders

151. While a client is receiving albumin, the planned therapeutic effect will be greater if the infusion is regulated to run:
    1. Rapidly, and fluids are encouraged
    2. Slowly, and fluid intake is restricted
    3. Rapidly, and fluid intake is withheld
    4. Slowly, and fluids are encouraged liberally

152. The nurse administers serum albumin to a client to assist in:
    1. Clotting of blood
    2. Formation of red blood cells
    3. Activation of white blood cells
    4. Maintenance of oncotic pressure

153. The client is receiving 5% dextrose in water at a slow rate. The nurse should be aware that the longest period of time that one bottle can be infused without producing untoward effects would be:
    1. 6 hours
    2. 12 hours
    3. 18 hours
    4. 24 hours

154. A client has an IV infusion. If the IV infusion infiltrates, the nurse should first:
    1. Elevate the IV site
    2. Discontinue the infusion
    3. Attempt to flush the tube
    4. Apply warm, moist soaks

155. When providing teaching about a low-sodium diet the nurse should encourage the client to include:
    1. Celery
    2. Carrots
    3. Tomato juice
    4. Orange juice

156. A client is to receive 2000 ml of IV fluid in 12 hours. The drop factor is 10 gtt/ml. The nurse should regulate the flow so the number of drops per minute is approximately:
    1. 27 to 29
    2. 30 to 32
    3. 40 to 42
    4. 48 to 50

157. A client with esophageal cancer is to receive total parenteral nutrition. A right subclavian catheter is inserted by the physician. The nurse knows that the primary reason for using a central line is that:
1. It prevents the development of phlebitis
2. There is less chance of this infusion infiltrating
3. It is more convenient so clients can use their hands
4. The large amount of blood helps to dilute the concentrated solution

158. When taking the blood pressure of a client who has had a thyroidectomy, the nurse notices the client is pale and has spasms of the hand and notifies the physician. While awaiting the physician's orders, the nurse should prepare for replacement of:
1. Calcium
2. Magnesium
3. Bicarbonate
4. Potassium chloride

159. A client with hypokalemia is placed on a cardiac monitor to evaluate cardiac activity during IV potassium replacement. Before starting the IV, the nurse observes the monitor, which shows:
1. Lowering of the T wave
2. Elevation of the ST segment
3. Shortening of the QRS complex
4. Increased deflection of the Q wave

160. An IV solution containing potassium inadvertently infuses too rapidly. The physician prescribes insulin added to a 10% dextrose in water solution. The rationale for the order is:
1. Potassium moves into body cells with glucose and insulin
2. Increased insulin accelerates excretion of glucose and potassium
3. Glucose and insulin increase metabolism and accelerate potassium excretion
4. Increased potassium causes a temporary slowing of pancreatic production of insulin

161. The nurse suspects hypokalemia is present when a client has:
1. Edema, bounding pulse, confusion
2. Spasms, diarrhea, irregular pulse rate
3. Apathy, weakness, abdominal distention
4. Sunken eyeballs, Kussmaul breathing, thirst

162. Intravenous orders state that the client is to receive 1000 ml of fluid every 8 hours. If the equipment delivers 15 drops/minute, the nurse should regulate the flow at approximately:
1. 15 gtt/min
2. 23 gtt/min
3. 31 gtt/min
4. 60 gtt/min

163. An intravenous piggyback (IVPB) of cefazolin sodium (Kefzol) 500 mg in 50 ml of 5% dextrose in water is to be administered over a 20-minute period. The tubing has a drop factor of 15 drops per milliliter. The nurse should regulate the infusion to run at:
1. 28 gtt/min
2. 38 gtt/min
3. 58 gtt/min
4. 76 gtt/min

Cardiovascular

164. To avoid an error of parallax when taking a client's blood pressure, the nurse should:
1. Use a narrow cuff
2. Read it at eye level
3. Stand close to the manometer
4. Elevate the client's arm on a pillow

165. The nurse explains to a client that the mechanism mediating long-term blood pressure regulation is the:
1. Capillary fluid shifts
2. Fight or flight response
3. Adjustment of urinary output
4. Nervous system baroreceptors

166. When taking a client's apical pulse the nurse should place the stethoscope:
1. Just to the left of the median point of the sternum
2. In the fifth intercostal space at the left midclavicular line
3. Between the sixth and seventh ribs at the left midaxillary line
4. Between the third and fourth ribs and to the left of the sternum

167. The nurse institutes safety precautions for a client receiving oxygen because oxygen:
1. Is flammable
2. Supports combustion
3. Has unstable properties
4. Increases apprehension

168. When instituting oxygen therapy, the nurse recognizes that the method of oxygen administration least likely to increase apprehension in the client is:
    1. Tent
    2. Mask
    3. Cannula
    4. Catheter

169. The nurse identifies a commonality between the strain on a client's heart with prolonged anemia or polycythemia to be:
    1. Pressure
    2. Temperature
    3. Cardiac output
    4. Surface tension

170. A client with pyrexia will most likely demonstrate:
    1. Dyspnea
    2. Precordial pain
    3. Increased pulse rate
    4. Elevated blood pressure

171. The nurse assesses that a client's pulse pressure is decreasing. This would be evaluated by calculating the:
    1. Force exerted against an arterial wall
    2. Difference between the apical and radial rates
    3. Difference between systolic and diastolic readings
    4. Degree of ventricular contraction in relation to output

172. Following open heart surgery a client develops a temperature of 102° F (38.8° C). The nurse notifies the physician because elevated temperatures:
    1. Increase the cardiac output
    2. May indicate cerebral edema
    3. May be a forerunner of hemorrhage
    4. Are related to diaphoresis and possible chilling

173. The nurse should teach clients with peripheral vascular disease to stop smoking because nicotine:
    1. Constricts the superficial vessels, dilating the deep vessels
    2. Constricts the peripheral vessels and increases the force of flow
    3. Dilates the superficial vessels but constricts the collateral circulation
    4. Dilates the peripheral vessels, causing a reflex constriction of visceral vessels

174. With chronic occlusive arterial disease the precipitating cause for ulceration and gangrenous lesions often is:
    1. Emotional stress, which is short lived
    2. Poor hygiene and limited protein intake
    3. Stimulants such as coffee, tea, or cola drinks
    4. Trauma from mechanical, chemical, or thermal sources

175. When obtaining data from a client with thromboangiitis obliterans (Buerger's disease), the nurse would expect the client to demonstrate or report:
    1. Easy fatigue of extremities, continuous claudication
    2. General blanching of skin and intermittent claudication
    3. Intermittent claudication, burning pain after exposure to cold
    4. Burning pain precipitated by cold exposure, fatigue, blanching of skin

176. A simple test for varicose veins is the:
    1. Arteriography
    2. Babinski reflex
    3. Romberg's sign
    4. Trendelenburg test

177. Following a vein ligation and stripping, the client should be positioned:
    1. Flat with the knee gatch engaged
    2. Supine with the legs elevated at 30°
    3. In a semi-Fowler's position with the knees flexed
    4. With the head elevated and the feet against a footboard

178. Prolonged bed rest after surgery appears to promote hemostasis, particularly in the deep veins of the calves. The most likely pathologic result of such hemostasis may be thrombus formation and:
    1. Cerebral embolism
    2. Coronary occlusion
    3. Pulmonary embolism
    4. Dry gangrene of a limb

179. The nurse understands that a pulmonary embolism is a most unlikely complication in the postoperative period following:
    1. Hysterectomy
    2. Prostatectomy
    3. Appendectomy
    4. Saphenous vein ligation

180. To prevent a pulmonary embolus in a client on bed rest, the nurse should:
    1. Limit the client's fluid intake
    2. Encourage deep breathing and coughing
    3. Use the knee gatch when the client is in bed
    4. Teach the client to move the legs when in bed

181. In the postanesthesia unit, while caring for a client who has received a general anesthetic, the nurse should notify the physician if the:
    1. Client pushes the airway out
    2. Client has snoring respirations
    3. Respirations are regular but shallow
    4. Systolic blood pressure drops from 130 to 100 mm Hg

182. Postural changes immediately after spinal anesthesia may result in hypotension because there is:
    1. Dilation of blood vessels
    2. Decreased response of chemoreceptors
    3. Decreased strength of cardiac contractions
    4. Interruption of cardiac accelerator pathways

183. After abdominal surgery a client suddenly complains of numbness in the right leg and a "funny feeling" in the toes. The nurse should first:
    1. Elevate the legs and tell the client to stay in bed
    2. Tell the client to remain in bed and notify the physician
    3. Rub the client's legs to start circulation and cover the client with a warm blanket
    4. Tell the client about the dangers of staying in bed too much and encourage ambulation

184. Following a bilateral lumbar sympathectomy a client has a sudden drop in blood pressure but no evidence of bleeding. The nurse recognizes that this is most likely caused by:
    1. An inadequate fluid intake
    2. The aftereffects of anesthesia
    3. A reallocation of the blood supply
    4. An increased level of epinephrine

185. While convalescing from abdominal surgery a client develops thrombophlebitis. The sign that would indicate this complication to the nurse would be:
    1. Intermittent claudication
    2. Pitting edema of the lower extremities
    3. Severe pain on extension of an extremity
    4. Localized warmth and tenderness of the leg

186. A client is being instructed on the use of elastic stockings. The nurse should teach the client that the stockings should be:
    1. Alternately kept on 2 hours and off 2 hours
    2. Worn only at night when activity is lessened
    3. Put on before getting out of bed in the morning
    4. Left in place until the physician advises otherwise

187. The nurse should be aware that arteriosclerosis of blood vessels leading to the brain may not become evident (until there is an extremely severe blockage or until a stroke occurs) because of collateral blood circulation supplied through the:
    1. Circle of Willis
    2. Jugular vessels
    3. The bicarotid trunk
    4. Hypothalamic-hypophyseal portal system

188. After a client has an endarterectomy the nurse should plan to observe for a change in:
    1. Appetite
    2. Skin color
    3. Bowel habits
    4. Tissue turgor

189. When teaching a client about orthostatic hypotension, the nurse should explain that it can be modified by:
    1. Wearing support hose continuously
    2. Lying down for 30 minutes after taking medication
    3. Avoiding tasks that require high energy expenditures
    4. Sitting on the edge of the bed a short time before arising

190. To assess the effectiveness of a vasodilator administered to lower hypertension, the nurse should take the client's pulse and blood pressure:
    1. Prior to administering the drug
    2. Thirty minutes after giving the drug
    3. Immediately after the client gets out of bed
    4. After a position is maintained for 5 minutes

191. Cholesterol, frequently discussed in relation to atherosclerosis, is a substance that:
    1. May be controlled entirely by eliminating food sources
    2. Is found in many foods, both plant and animal sources
    3. All persons would be better off without because it causes the disease process
    4. Circulates in the blood, the level of which usually decreases when unsaturated fats are substituted for saturated fats

192. When cardiovascular disease is a concern, reduction of the saturated fat in the diet may be desired and substitutes made of polyunsaturated fat. When teaching about this diet the nurse should instruct the client to avoid:
    1. Fish
    2. Corn oil
    3. Whole milk
    4. Soft margarine

193. When teaching a client with a cardiac problem who is on a high-unsaturated fatty acid diet, the nurse should stress the importance of increasing the intake of:
    1. Enriched whole milk
    2. Red meats, such as beef
    3. Vegetables and whole grains
    4. Liver and other glandular organ meats

194. A 2-g sodium diet is prescribed for a client with severe hypertension. The client does not like the diet, and the nurse hears the client tell a friend to bring in some "good home-cooked food." It would be most effective for the nurse to plan to:
    1. Call in the dietitian for client teaching
    2. Wait for the client's family and discuss the diet with the client and family
    3. Tell the client that the use of salt is forbidden, because it will raise the blood pressure
    4. Catch the family members before they go into the client's room and tell them about the diet

195. A client states that anginal pain increases after activity. The nurse should realize that angina pectoris is a sign of:
    1. Mitral insufficiency
    2. Myocardial ischemia
    3. Myocardial infarction
    4. Coronary thrombosis

196. A client asks what the coronary arteries have to do with angina. When determining the answer, the nurse should take into consideration that the coronary arteries:
    1. Supply blood to the endocardium
    2. Carry blood from the aorta to the myocardium
    3. Carry reduced–oxygen-content blood to the lungs
    4. Carry high–oxygen-content blood from the lungs toward the heart

197. The nurse realizes that the pain associated with a coronary occlusion is caused primarily by:
    1. Arterial spasm
    2. Ischemia of the heart muscle
    3. Blocking of the coronary veins
    4. Irritation of nerve endings in the cardiac plexus

198. Nitroglycerin SL is prescribed for anginal pain. When teaching how to use nitroglycerin, the nurse tells the client to place 1 tablet under the tongue when pain occurs and to repeat the dose in 5 minutes if pain persists. The nurse should also tell the client to:
    1. Place 2 tablets under the tongue when intense pain occurs
    2. Swallow 1 tablet and place 1 tablet under the tongue when pain is intense
    3. Place 1 tablet under the tongue 3 minutes before activity and repeat the dose in 5 minutes if pain occurs
    4. Place 1 tablet under the tongue when pain occurs and use an additional tablet after the attack to prevent recurrence

199. When caring for a client after cardiac catheterization, it is most important that the nurse:
    1. Provide for rest
    2. Administer oxygen
    3. Check the ECG every 30 minutes
    4. Check pulse distal to the insertion site

200. During a cardiac catheterization blood samples from the right atrium, right ventricle, and pulmonary artery are analyzed for their oxygen content, Normally:
    1. All contain less CO_2 than does pulmonary vein blood
    2. All contain more oxygen than does pulmonary vein blood
    3. The samples of blood all contain about the same amount of oxygen
    4. Pulmonary artery blood contains more oxygen than the other samples

201. The nurse in the coronary care unit (CCU) should observe for one of the more common complications of myocardial infarction, which is:
    1. Hypokalemia
    2. Anaphylactic shock
    3. Cardiac dysrhythmia
    4. Cardiac enlargement

202. The nurse prepares a client for insertion of a pulmonary artery catheter (e.g., Swan-Ganz catheter). The nurse teaches the client that the catheter will be inserted to provide information about:
    1. Stroke volume
    2. Cardiac output
    3. Venous pressure
    4. Left ventricular functioning

203. The laboratory tests the nurse would expect the physician to order to confirm a diagnosis of myocardial infarction include:
    1. Serum calcium, APPT
    2. Sedimentation rate, ALT
    3. LDH, CK-MB, troponin
    4. Paul-Bunnell, serum potassium

204. During the acute phase following a myocardial infarction, the nurse should make the client's bed by:
    1. Changing the top linen and only the necessary bottom linen
    2. Changing the linen from top to bottom without lowering the head of the bed
    3. Lifting rather than rolling the client from side to side while changing the linen
    4. Sliding the client onto a stretcher, remaking the bed, then sliding the client back to the bed

205. A client is receiving digoxin (Lanoxin) and will continue taking the drug after discharge. The nurse should be primarily concerned with:
    1. Monitoring vital signs and encouraging gradual increase in activities of daily living
    2. Taking the apical pulse before drug administration and teaching the client how to count the pulse
    3. Observing the client for return of normal cardiac conduction patterns and for adverse effects of the drug
    4. Assessing the client for changes in cardiac rhythm and planning activities at home based on tolerance

206. A 72-year-old is admitted with cerebral arteriosclerosis, complicated by polycythemia vera, and heparin q6h is prescribed. If the anticoagulant therapy is effective, the nurse would expect:
    1. A PTT twice the normal value
    2. An absence of ecchymotic areas
    3. A decreased viscosity of the blood
    4. A reduction of confusion and weakness

207. When a client is receiving anticoagulants, the nursing care should include observations for:
    1. Nausea
    2. Epistaxis
    3. Headache
    4. Chest pain

208. A client is receiving Coumadin. The test that would be most specific for calculating the daily dosage of this anticoagulant would be the:
    1. INR
    2. Clotting time
    3. Bleeding time
    4. Sedimentation rate

209. When preparing a client for discharge following surgery for a coronary artery bypass graft, the nurse should teach that there will be:
    1. No further drainage from the incisions after hospitalization
    2. A mild fever and extreme fatigue for several weeks following surgery
    3. Little incisional pain and tenderness after 3 to 4 weeks following surgery
    4. Some increase in edema in the leg used for the donor graft when activity increases

210. The nurse suspects a client is in cardiogenic shock. The nurse understands that this type of shock is:
    1. An irreversible phenomenon
    2. A failure of the circulatory pump
    3. Usually a fleeting reaction to tissue injury
    4. Generally caused by decreased blood volume

211. The nurse assists the physician in treating a client in shock. One modality of treatment that employs the physical law explaining the increased venous return accompanying mild vasoconstriction underlies the use of:
    1. Adrenalin in treating shock
    2. Digoxin to increase cardiac output
    3. Sympathectomy in treating hypertension
    4. Rotating tourniquets in pulmonary edema

212. The nurse finds an injured person, sitting in a chair obviously in shock. The nurse should:
    1. Keep the head elevated; give a stimulant in small sips
    2. Apply tourniquets to three extremities, rotating one every 15 minutes
    3. Surround the body with a warm blanket or chemical heating pads if available
    4. Place the person in the supine position, prevent chilling, and give fluids if possible

213. The adaptations of a client with complete heart block would most likely include:
    1. Nausea and vertigo
    2. Flushing and slurred speech
    3. Cephalalgia and blurred vision
    4. Syncope and low ventricular rate

214. The nurse is aware that the term bradycardia means:
    1. A grossly irregular heartbeat
    2. A heart rate of over 90 per minute
    3. A heart rate of under 60 per minute
    4. A heartbeat that has regular "skipped" beats

215. The nurse would prioritize care and provide treatment first for a client with:
    1. Head injuries
    2. A fractured femur
    3. Ventricular fibrillation
    4. A penetrating abdominal wound

216. While a pacemaker catheter is being inserted, the client's heart rate drops to 38. The drug the nurse should expect the physician to order is:
    1. Atropine sulfate
    2. Digoxin (Lanoxin)
    3. Lidocaine (Xylocaine)
    4. Procainamide (Pronestyl)

217. A client with a bundle branch block is on a cardiac monitor. The nurse would expect to observe:
    1. Sagging ST segments
    2. Absence of P wave configurations
    3. Inverted T waves following each QRS complex
    4. Widening of QRS complexes to 0.12 second or greater

218. The nurse realizes that a pacemaker is used in some clients to serve the function normally performed by the:
    1. AV node
    2. SA node
    3. Bundle of His
    4. Accelerator nerves to the heart

219. A permanent pacemaker is implanted in a client with complete heart block. The nurse observes the cardiac monitor for the presence of a lethal dysrhythmia requiring immediate intervention. This lethal dysrhythmia is known as:
    1. Atrial fibrillation
    2. Sinus tachycardia
    3. Ventricular fibrillation
    4. Second-degree heart block

220. Cardioversion is a procedure used to convert certain dysrhythmias to normal rhythm. In addition to atrial fibrillation, cardioversion is most effective when the client demonstrates:
    1. Ventricular standstill
    2. Ventricular fibrillation
    3. Ventricular tachycardia
    4. Premature ventricular beats

221. The physician has inserted a permanent demand pacemaker in a client. When teaching, the nurse should:
    1. Instruct the client to sleep on two pillows
    2. Encourage the client to reduce the former level of activity
    3. Instruct the client to take the pulse daily and keep accurate records
    4. Inform the client that the pacemaker will function continuously at a set rate

222. To evaluate the effectiveness of a client's demand pacemaker, the nurse ensures that the pulse remains at least:
    1. In a regular rhythm
    2. Above the demand rate
    3. Equal to the pacemaker
    4. Palpable at all pulse sites

223. When ventricular fibrillation occurs in a coronary care unit, the first person reaching the client should:
    1. Administer oxygen
    2. Defibrillate the client
    3. Initiate cardiopulmonary resuscitation
    4. Administer sodium bicarbonate intravenously

224. A client who has a myocardial infarction is in the coronary unit on a cardiac monitor. The nurse observes ventricular irritability on the screen. The nurse should prepare to administer:
    1. Digoxin (Lanoxin)
    2. Furosemide (Lasix)
    3. Lidocaine (Xylocaine)
    4. Levarterenol bitartrate (Levophed)

225. A client is admitted to the coronary care unit with atrial fibrillation and a rapid ventricular response. The nurse prepares for cardioversion. To avoid a potential danger of inducing ventricular fibrillation during cardioversion, the nurse should ensure that the:
    1. Energy level is set at its maximum level
    2. Synchronizer switch is in the "on" position
    3. Skin electrodes are applied after the T wave
    4. Alarm system of the cardiac monitor is functioning simultaneously

226. The nurse observes a client's cardiac monitor and identifies asystole. This dysrhythmia requires nursing attention because the heart is:
    1. Not beating
    2. Beating slowly
    3. Beating irregularly
    4. Beating very rapidly

227. During a cardiac arrest, the nurse and the arrest team must keep in mind the:
    1. Age of the client
    2. Time the client was anoxic
    3. Emergency medications available
    4. Heart rate of the client before the arrest

228. A client is found unconscious and unresponsive. The nurse should first:
    1. Initiate a code
    2. Check for a radial pulse
    3. Give four full lung inflations
    4. Compress the lower sternum 15 times

229. When performing cardiac compression on an adult client, the nurse is aware that it is essential to exert vertical downward pressure, which depresses the lower sternum at least:
    1. 1.3 to 2 cm ($^1/_2$ to $^3/_4$ inch)
    2. 2 to 2.5 cm ($^3/_4$ to 1 inch)
    3. 2.5 to 4 cm (1 to $1^1/_2$ inches)
    4. 4 to 5 cm ($1^1/_2$ to 2 inches)

230. When performing external cardiac compression, the nurse should exert downward vertical pressure on the lower sternum by placing:
    1. The fleshy part of a clenched fist on the lower sternum
    2. The heels of each hand side by side, extending the fingers over the chest
    3. The fingers of one hand on the sternum and the fingers of the other hand on top of them
    4. The heel of one hand on the sternum and the heel of the other on top of it, interlocking the fingers

231. A client has edema during the day, and it disappears at night. The client states it is not painful and is located in the lower extremities. The nurse should suspect:
    1. Lung disease
    2. Pulmonary edema
    3. Myocardial infarction
    4. Right ventricular heart failure

232. The nurse can best assess the extent of edema in an extremity by:
    1. Weighing the client
    2. Monitoring intake and output
    3. Checking for the degree of edema
    4. Performing the Trendelenburg test

233. A client is admitted to the hospital and has edematous ankles. To best limit edema of the feet the nurse should prepare to:
    1. Restrict fluids
    2. Elevate the legs
    3. Apply elastic bandages
    4. Do range-of-motion exercises

234. When taking an admission history of a client with right ventricular heart failure, the nurse would expect the client to complain of:
    1. Dyspnea, edema, fatigue
    2. Fatigue, vertigo, headache
    3. Weakness, palpitations, nausea
    4. A feeling of distress when breathing

235. When assessing the lower extremities of a client with right ventricular heart failure, the nurse expects pitting edema because of the:
    1. Increase in tissue colloid osmotic pressure
    2. Decrease in the plasma colloid osmotic pressure
    3. Increase in the tissue hydrostatic pressure at the arterial end of the capillary bed
    4. Elevation in the plasma hydrostatic pressure at the venous end of the capillary bed

236. The nurse should realize that the client with right ventricular heart failure may develop ascites because of:
    1. Loss of cellular constituents in blood
    2. Rapid osmosis from tissue spaces to cells
    3. Increased pressure within the circulatory system
    4. Rapid diffusion of solutes and solvents into plasma

237. The nurse suggests to an elderly client with heart failure that air conditioning be used in the summer. This suggestion is made because:
    1. The internal body temperature drops below 98.6° F (37° C)
    2. The increased circulation in the skin gives the heart the exercise it needs
    3. The increased circulation in the skin causes excess body heat to radiate away
    4. The heart is relieved of the strain of pumping blood through many miles of blood vessels in the skin

238. When assessing clients with the following medical problems, the nurse would expect pulmonary edema to be associated with:
    1. Mitral stenosis
    2. Pulmonary valve stenosis
    3. Severe arteriosclerosis of the coronary arteries
    4. Calcification and incomplete closure of the tricuspid valve

239. For a client with pulmonary edema the nurse would expect oxygen via nasal cannula to be set at:
    1. 2 L
    2. 6 L
    3. 8 L
    4. 10 L

240. The nurse attempts to allay the anxiety of a client with heart failure because restlessness
    1. Increases the cardiac workload
    2. Interferes with normal respiration
    3. Produces an elevation in temperature
    4. Decreases the amount of oxygen available

241. To help alleviate the distress of a client with heart failure and pulmonary edema, the nurse should:
    1. Elevate the lower extremities
    2. Encourage frequent coughing
    3. Prepare for modified postural drainage
    4. Place the client in an orthopneic position

242. During a teaching session with a client who has experienced an anterior septal myocardial infarction the nurse determines a need for further discussion when the client states:
    1. "I want to stay as pain free as possible."
    2. "I am not good at remembering to take medications."
    3. "I should not have any problems in reducing my salt intake."
    4. "I wrote down my medication information for future reference."

243. Two hours after a cardiac catheterization that was accessed via the right femoral route, an adult client complains of numbness and pain in the right foot. The nurse should:
    1. Call the physician
    2. Check the client's pedal pulses
    3. Take the client's blood pressure
    4. Recognize that this is an expected response

244. A 55-year-old client is admitted with the diagnosis of possible myocardial infarction. The physician orders enzyme studies for the client. The nurse knows the first enzyme to change in the presence of a myocardial infarction is:
    1. ALT
    2. AST
    3. Total LDH
    4. Troponin T

245. When a 70-year-old client with heart failure is transferred from the emergency department to the medical service, the nurse on the unit should first:
    1. Monitor the client's temperature
    2. Interview the client for a health history
    3. Assess the client's heart and lung sounds
    4. Obtain a blood specimen for serum electrolytes

246. When talking with a client with chronic heart failure, the nurse would expect the client to complain about:
    1. Chest pain that decreases with rest
    2. Palpitations in the chest when resting
    3. Frequent coughing with yellow sputum
    4. Edematous ankles and feet in the evening

247. A client has contrast medium injected into the brachial artery so that a cerebral angiogram can be performed. Immediately after the procedure the nurse must assess the client for:
    1. Stability of gait
    2. Presence of a gag reflex
    3. Blood pressure in both arms
    4. Symmetry of the radial pulses

Blood and Immunity

248. A client with upper gastrointestinal bleeding develops a mild anemia. The nurse should expect the client to be treated with:
    1. Dextran
    2. Epogen
    3. Iron salts
    4. Vitamin B_{12}

249. The emergency department nurse is admitting a client following an automobile accident. The client has lost a considerable amount of blood, and early stage hypovolemic shock is suspected. An assessment finding the nurse would expect this client to exhibit is:
    1. A distention of the neck veins
    2. An apical heart rate of 142 bpm
    3. An output of 50 ml urine per hour
    4. A blood pressure of 150/90 mm Hg

250. The physician orders 3 units of whole blood for a client in hypovolemic shock after a gastrointestinal hemorrhage. When administering blood, the nurse first verifies the type and cross-match and then:
    1. Warms the blood to body temperature to prevent chills
    2. Uses an infusion pump to increase the accuracy of the infusion
    3. Draws blood samples from the client before and after each unit is transfused
    4. Runs the blood at a slower rate during the first 5 to 10 minutes of the transfusion

251. During a blood transfusion a client develops chills and headache. The nurse's best action is to:
    1. Lightly cover the client
    2. Notify the physician stat
    3. Stop the transfusion immediately
    4. Slow the blood flow to keep vein open

252. An example of primary prevention activities by the nurse would be:
    1. Prevention of disabilities
    2. Correction of dietary deficiencies
    3. Establishing goals for rehabilitation
    4. Assisting in immunization programs

253. In general, the higher the red blood cell count:
    1. The higher the blood pH
    2. The lower the hematocrit
    3. The greater the blood viscosity
    4. The less it contributes to immunity

254. The nurse understands that the only molecules that do not readily pass through the capillary endothelium are:
    1. Blood gases
    2. Plasma proteins
    3. Glucose and ions
    4. Amino acids and water

255. When caring for a client with an impaired immune system, the nurse recognizes that the blood protein involved is:
    1. Albumin
    2. Globulin
    3. Thrombin
    4. Hemoglobin

256. Antibodies are produced by:
    1. Eosinophils
    2. Plasma cells
    3. Erythrocytes
    4. Lymphocytes

257. Infection with Group A beta-hemolytic streptococci is associated with:
    1. Hepatitis A
    2. Rheumatic fever
    3. Spinal meningitis
    4. Rheumatoid arthritis

258. A client is concerned about contracting malaria while visiting relatives in Southeast Asia. The nurse explains that the best way to prevent malaria is to avoid:
    1. Mosquito bites
    2. Untreated water
    3. Undercooked food
    4. Overpopulated areas

259. The nurse is reviewing the physical examination and laboratory tests of a client with malaria. The nurse understands that an important finding in malaria is:
    1. Leukocytosis
    2. Erythrocytosis
    3. Splenomegaly
    4. Elevated sedimentation rate

260. When caring for a client with malaria, the nurse should know that:
    1. Seizure precautions must be followed
    2. Peritoneal dialysis is usually indicated
    3. Isolation is necessary to prevent cross-infection
    4. Nutrition should be provided between paroxysms

261. When teaching a client about drug therapy against *Plasmodium falciparum*, the nurse should include the fact that:
    1. The infection is controlled
    2. Immunity will prevent reinfestation
    3. The infection can generally be eliminated
    4. Transmission by the *Anopheles* mosquito can occur

262. Blackwater fever occurs in some clients with malaria; therefore, the nurse should observe a client with chronic malaria for:
    1. Diarrhea
    2. Dark red urine
    3. Low-grade fever
    4. Coffee ground emesis

263. When caring for a client who is HIV positive, a primary responsibility of the nurse is to explain how the client can prevent:
    1. AIDS
    2. Social isolation
    3. Other infections
    4. Kaposi's sarcoma

264. When a trauma victim expresses fear that AIDS may develop as a result of a blood transfusion, the nurse should explain that:
    1. Blood is treated with radiation to kill the virus
    2. Screening for the HIV antibodies has minimized this risk
    3. The ability to directly identify HIV has eliminated this concern
    4. Consideration should be given to donating own blood for transfusion

265. A mother with the diagnosis of AIDS states that she has been caring for her little baby even though she has not been feeling well. The nurse should ask her:
    1. If she is breastfeeding the baby
    2. If she has hugged or kissed the baby
    3. When the baby last received antibiotics
    4. How long she has been caring for the baby

266. When providing discharge teaching to the family of a client with AIDS, the nurse should teach the family:
    1. "You need to boil the dishes for 30 minutes after use."
    2. "Let the client eat from paper plates and discard them."
    3. "Wash the dishes in hot soapy water as you usually do."
    4. "Let the dishes soak in hot water overnight before washing."

267. During an AIDS education class, a client states, "Vaseline works great when I use condoms." The nurse recognizes that this statement indicates:
    1. An understanding of safer sex
    2. The ability to assume self-responsibility
    3. Ignorance concerning the transmission of HIV
    4. A lack of information concerning correct condom use

268. A client has a bone marrow aspiration performed. Immediately after the procedure, the nurse should:
    1. Position the client on the affected side
    2. Begin frequent monitoring of vital signs
    3. Cleanse the site with an antiseptic solution
    4. Briefly apply pressure over the aspiration site

269. With Hodgkin's disease the lymph nodes usually affected first are the:
    1. Axillary
    2. Inguinal
    3. Cervical
    4. Mediastinal

270. The highest incidence of Hodgkin's disease is in:
    1. Children
    2. Young adults
    3. Elderly persons
    4. Middle-aged persons

271. A client is to have whole-body radiation for Hodgkin's disease. The nurse's teaching plan should center around the likely occurrence of increased:
    1. Blood viscosity
    2. Susceptibility to infection
    3. Red blood cell production
    4. Tendency for pathologic fractures

272. Fragments of cells in the bloodstream that break down on exposure to injured tissue and begin the chain reaction leading to a blood clot are known as:
    1. Platelets
    2. Leukocytes
    3. Erythrocytes
    4. Red blood cells

273. The nurse understands that thromboplastin, which initiates the clotting process, is found in:
    1. Bile
    2. Plasma
    3. Platelets
    4. Erythrocytes

274. When assessing a wound that exhibits signs of blood coagulation and healing, the nurse understands that the soluble substance that becomes an insoluble gel is:
    1. Fibrin
    2. Thrombin
    3. Fibrinogen
    4. Prothrombin

275. The nurse understands that blood clotting requires the presence of the catalyst:
    1. F^-
    2. Cl^-
    3. Ca^{++}
    4. Fe^{+++}

276. Vitamin K is essential for normal blood clotting because it promotes:
    1. Platelet aggregation
    2. Ionization of blood calcium
    3. Fibrinogen formation by the liver
    4. Prothrombin formation by the liver

277. The increased tendency toward coronary and cerebral thromboses seen in individuals with polycythemia vera is attributable to the:
1. Increased viscosity
2. Fragility of the cells
3. Elevated blood pressure
4. Immaturity of red blood cells

278. A serum bilirubin is performed on a client who is weak, dyspneic, and jaundiced. A bilirubin level above 2 mg/100 ml blood volume could indicate:
1. Hemolytic anemia
2. Pernicious anemia
3. Decreased rate of red blood cell destruction
4. Low oxygen-carrying capacity of erythrocytes

279. As a result of a serious automobile accident, a client is admitted with multiple trauma including a ruptured spleen. A splenectomy is performed because:
1. The spleen is a highly vascular organ
2. It is anatomically adjacent to the diaphragm
3. The spleen is the largest lymphoid organ in the body
4. Rupture of the spleen can cause diseases of the liver

280. In the immediate postoperative period following a splenectomy, the nurse specifically should observe the client for:
1. Shock and infection
2. Intestinal obstruction and bleeding
3. Hemorrhage and abdominal distention
4. Peritonitis and pulmonary complications

281. A client has a splenectomy following a motor vehicle accident. The consideration that is of specific importance after a splenectomy is:
1. Early ambulation
2. Pulmonary embolism
3. Adequate lung aeration
4. Postoperative hemorrhage

282. A client who was exposed to hepatitis A is given gamma globulin to provide passive immunity, which:
1. Increases production of short-lived antibodies
2. Provides antibodies that neutralize the antigen
3. Accelerates antigen-antibody union at the hepatic sites
4. Stimulates the lymphatic system to produce large numbers of antibodies

283. A client with hypothermia is brought to the emergency room. The family should be taught that treatment will include:
1. Core rewarming with warm fluids
2. Ambulation to increase metabolism
3. Frequent oral temperature assessment
4. Gastric tube feedings to increase fluids

284. When it is impossible to determine whether a client has been immunized against tetanus, the preparation of choice used to produce passive immunity for several weeks with minimal danger of allergic reactions is:
1. DTP vaccine
2. Tetanus toxoid
3. Tetanus antitoxin
4. Tetanus immune globulin

285. A client who is suspected of having tetanus asks the nurse about immunizations against tetanus. The nurse explains that the major benefit in using tetanus antitoxin is that it:
1. Stimulates plasma cells directly
2. Provides a high titer of antibodies
3. Provides immediate active immunity
4. Stimulates long-lasting passive immunity

286. A female client has a low hemoglobin level which is attributed to a nutritional deficiency. The foods that the nurse should recommend be increased in the client's diet include:
1. Carrots, beef, and apples
2. Spinach, liver, and raisins
3. Broccoli, pork, and apricots
4. Lima beans, squash, and prunes

287. While being prepared for surgery for a ruptured spleen, a client complains of feeling lightheaded. The client's color is pale and the pulse is very rapid. The nurse assesses that the client may be:
1. Hyperventilating
2. Going into shock
3. Extremely anxious
4. Developing an infection

Respiratory

288. The nurse understands that in the absence of pathology, a client's respiratory center is stimulated by:
1. Oxygen
2. Lactic acid
3. Calcium ions
4. Carbon dioxide

289. The efficacy of the abdominal-thoracic thrust (Heimlich maneuver) to expel a foreign object in the larynx demonstrates the gas volume related to the individual's:
    1. Tidal volume
    2. Vital capacity
    3. Residual volume
    4. Inspiratory reserve volume

290. A client states that the physician said the tidal volume is slightly diminished and asks the nurse what this means. The nurse explains that tidal volume is the amount of air:
    1. Exhaled forcibly after a normal expiration
    2. Exhaled normally after a normal inspiration
    3. Trapped in the alveoli that cannot be exhaled
    4. Forcibly inspired over and above a normal inspiration

291. Air rushes into the alveoli as a result of the:
    1. Relaxation of the diaphragm
    2. Rising pressure in the alveoli
    3. Rising pressure in the pleura
    4. Lowered pressure in the chest cavity

292. A client is scheduled for a pulmonary function test. The nurse explains that during the test the respiratory therapist will ask the client to breathe normally to measure the:
    1. Tidal volume
    2. Vital capacity
    3. Expiratory reserve
    4. Inspiratory reserve

293. Oxygen dissociation from hemoglobin and therefore oxygen delivery to the tissues are accelerated by:
    1. A decreasing oxygen pressure in the blood
    2. An increasing carbon dioxide pressure in the blood
    3. A decreasing oxygen pressure and/or an increasing carbon dioxide pressure in the blood
    4. An increasing oxygen pressure and/or a decreasing carbon dioxide pressure in the blood

294. With an oxygen debt, muscle shows:
    1. Low levels of ATP
    2. High levels of calcium
    3. High levels of glycogen
    4. Low levels of lactic acid

295. A nurse initially will use an Ambu-Bag in the intensive care unit when:
    1. A respiratory arrest occurs
    2. The client is in ventricular fibrillation
    3. The respiratory output must be monitored
    4. A surgical incision with copious drainage is present

296. To facilitate maximum air exchange, a client should be placed in the:
    1. Supine position
    2. Orthopneic position
    3. High-Fowler's position
    4. Semi-Fowler's position

297. A client begins to expectorate blood. The nurse describes this episode as:
    1. Hematuria
    2. Hematoma
    3. Hemoptysis
    4. Hematemesis

298. The position in which a client with dyspnea should be placed is:
    1. Sims'
    2. Supine
    3. Orthopneic
    4. Trendelenburg

299. A client is admitted with suspected atelectasis. When assessing this individual, the nurse would expect:
    1. Slow, deep respirations
    2. Diminished breath sounds
    3. A dry, unproductive cough
    4. A normal oral temperature

300. A client who undergoes a submucosal resection should be observed carefully for:
    1. Periorbital crepitus
    2. Occipital headache
    3. Spitting up or vomiting of blood
    4. White areas of healing sublingually

301. A client is admitted with carbon monoxide poisoning. The nurse understands that the poisonous nature of carbon monoxide results from:
    1. Its tendency to block CO_2 transport
    2. The inhibitory effect it has on vasodilation
    3. Its preferential combination with hemoglobin
    4. The bubbles it tends to form in blood plasma

302. The nurse obtains a laboratory report that shows acid-fast rods in a client's sputum. These are presumed to be:
    1. Influenza virus
    2. *Bordetella pertussis*
    3. Diphtheria bacillus
    4. *Mycobacterium tuberculosis*

303. The nurse must establish and maintain an airway in a client who has experienced a near drowning. The nurse should recognize that one danger of near-drowning in the ocean is:
    1. Alkalosis
    2. Renal failure
    3. Hypervolemia
    4. Pulmonary edema

304. A client is shot in the chest during a holdup and is transported to the hospital via ambulance. In the emergency department chest tubes are inserted, one in the second intercostal space and one at the base of the lung. The nurse understands that the tube in the second intercostal space will:
    1. Remove the air that is present in the intrapleural space
    2. Drain serosanguinous fluid from the intrapleural compartment
    3. Provide access for the instillation of medication into the pleural space
    4. Permit the development of positive pressure between the layers of the pleura

305. To monitor for the complication of subcutaneous emphysema after the insertion of chest tubes, the nurse should:
    1. Assess for the presence of a barrel-shaped chest
    2. Auscultate the breath sounds for crackles and rhonchi
    3. Palpate around the chest tube insertion sites for crepitus
    4. Compare the length of inspiration with the length of expiration

306. During the first 36 hours after the insertion of chest tubes, when assessing the function of the three-chamber, closed-chest drainage system, the nurse notes that the water in the underwater seal tube is not fluctuating. The nurse suspects that the chest tube is occluded. The initial nursing intervention should be to:
    1. Inform the physician
    2. Take the client's vital signs
    3. Encourage the client to cough
    4. Turn the client to the unaffected side

307. An independent nursing measure that would be helpful in preventing the accumulation of secretions in a client who had general anesthesia for surgery would be:
    1. Postural drainage
    2. Cupping the chest
    3. Nasotracheal suctioning
    4. Frequent changes of position

308. After a laryngectomy a client is concerned about improving the ability to communicate. The nurse should arrange for the client to learn more about:
    1. Sign language
    2. Body language
    3. Esophageal speech
    4. An external electronic larynx

309. The nurse would evaluate that after a laryngectomy the teaching about activities and the stoma were understood when the client states, "I should avoid:
    1. Strenuous exercises."
    2. Sleeping with pillows."
    3. All types of water sports."
    4. High-humidity environments."

310. A client who had a coronary bypass graft 6 months ago is admitted for an exacerbation of emphysema. The client has a fever, chills, and difficulty breathing on exertion. Based on the client's history and present status the most accurate nursing diagnosis would be:
    1. Impaired gas exchange
    2. Altered respiratory status
    3. Ineffective airway clearance
    4. Ineffective breathing pattern

311. Before discharge the nurse should teach a client with emphysema who had a coronary bypass graft 6 months ago to:
    1. Take one aspirin every other day
    2. Drink a cup of warm tea before going to bed at night
    3. Wear a scarf or mask over the mouth in cold weather
    4. Take the prescribed bronchodilators on an empty stomach

312. After a thoracotomy and right lower lobe lobectomy the nurse can most accurately detect atelectasis during the client's postoperative period by the presence of:
    1. Bilateral crackles and lethargy
    2. Increased heart rate and cyanosis
    3. Decreased breath sounds and fever
    4. A cough and splinting of the affected side

313. The common factor of puerperal sepsis, scarlet fever, otitis media, bacterial endocarditis, rheumatic fever, and glomerulonephritis is that all:
    1. Are noncontagious, self-limiting infections by spirilla
    2. Can be easily controlled through childhood vaccination
    3. Are caused by parasitic bacteria that normally live outside the body
    4. Result from streptococcal infections that enter via the upper respiratory tract

314. An example of a rapidly acting diuretic that can be administered intravenously to clients with acute pulmonary edema is:
    1. Furosemide
    2. Chlorothiazide
    3. Chlorthalidone
    4. Spironolactone

315. To help a client obtain maximum benefits after postural drainage, the nurse should:
    1. Administer the prn oxygen
    2. Place the client in a sitting position
    3. Encourage the client to cough deeply
    4. Encourage the client to rest for 30 minutes

316. A client with emphysema experiences a sudden episode of shortness of breath. The physician diagnoses a spontaneous pneumothorax. The nurse is aware that the probable cause of the spontaneous pneumothorax is a:
    1. Pleural friction rub
    2. Tracheoesophageal fistula
    3. Rupture of a subpleural bleb
    4. Puncture wound of the chest wall

317. When a spontaneous pneumothorax is suspected in a client with a history of emphysema, the nurse should call the physician and:
    1. Administer 60% O_2 via Ventimask
    2. Place the client on the unaffected side
    3. Give O_2 2 L per minute via nasal cannula
    4. Prepare for IV administration of electrolytes

318. When teaching a client about a spontaneous pneumothorax, the nurse bases the explanation on the understanding that:
    1. The heart and great vessels shift to the affected side
    2. The other lung will collapse if not treated immediately

    3. There is a greater negative pressure within the chest cavity
    4. Inspired air will move from the lung into the pleural space

319. Following a spontaneous pneumothorax, the client becomes extremely drowsy and the pulse and respirations increase. The nurse should suspect:
    1. Hypercapnia
    2. Hypokalemia
    3. An elevated Po_2
    4. Respiratory alkalosis

320. When assessing an individual with a spontaneous pneumothorax, the nurse should expect dyspnea and:
    1. Hematemesis
    2. Unilateral chest pain
    3. Increased chest motion
    4. Mediastinal shift toward the involved side

321. The nurse is aware that when emphysema is present there is a decreased oxygen supply because of:
    1. Pleural effusion
    2. Infectious obstructions
    3. Loss of aerating surface
    4. Respiratory muscle paralysis

322. The nurse administers oxygen at 2 L/minute via nasal cannula to a client with emphysema. The nurse should observe the client closely for:
    1. Cyanosis and lethargy
    2. Anxiety and tachycardia
    3. Hyperemia and increased respirations
    4. Drowsiness and decreased respirations

323. When the alveoli lose their normal elasticity as a result of emphysema, the nurse teaches the client exercises that lead to effective use of the diaphragm because:
    1. Inspiration has been markedly prolonged and difficult
    2. The residual capacity of the lungs has been increased
    3. The client has an increase in the vital capacity of the lungs
    4. Abdominal breathing is an effective compensatory mechanism that is spontaneously initiated

324. While receiving the adrenergic Beta 2 agonist for asthma the client complains of palpitation, chest pain, and a throbbing headache. In view of these symptoms, the most appropriate nursing action would be to:
    1. Withhold the drug until additional orders are obtained from the physician
    2. Tell the client not to worry; these are expected side effects from the medicine
    3. Ask the client to relax; then give instructions to breathe slowly and deeply for several minutes
    4. Reassure the client that these effects are temporary and will subside as the body becomes accustomed to the drug

325. An asthmatic client's pulmonary function studies are abnormal. The nurse should realize that one of the most common complications of chronic asthma is:
    1. Atelectasis
    2. Emphysema
    3. Pneumothorax
    4. Pulmonary fibrosis

326. A client with a long history of asthma is scheduled for surgery. Preoperative teaching should include the fact that the client:
    1. Will be quite prone to respiratory tract infections
    2. Can control and limit asthmatic attacks if desired
    3. Should try to limit coughing, because this causes distention of the chest
    4. Can control anxiety and decrease the severity of postoperative asthma attacks

327. When determining the method of oxygen administration to be used for a specific client, the major concern is:
    1. Level of activity
    2. Facial anatomy
    3. Pathologic condition
    4. Age and mental capacity

328. As a result of fractured ribs, the client may develop:
    1. Scoliosis
    2. Pneumothorax
    3. Obstructive lung disease
    4. Herniation of the diaphragm

329. When a client suffers a complete pneumothorax, there is danger of a mediastinal shift. If such a shift occurs, it may lead to:
    1. Infection of the subpleural lining
    2. Decreased filling of the right heart
    3. Rupture of the pericardium or aorta
    4. Increased volume of the unaffected lung

330. The physician inserts a chest tube in a client who has been stabbed in the chest and attaches it to a closed-drainage system. When caring for the client, the nurse should:
    1. Apply a thoracic binder to prevent tension on the tube
    2. Observe for fluid fluctuations in the waterseal chamber
    3. Clamp the tubing to prevent a rapid decline in pressure
    4. Administer morphine sulfate, because the client will be agitated

331. A client has chest tubes attached to a chest tube drainage system. When caring for this client, the nurse should:
    1. Palpate the surrounding area for crepitus
    2. Clamp the chest tubes when suctioning
    3. Change the dressing daily using aseptic technique
    4. Empty the drainage chamber at the end of the shift

332. Complete lung expansion before the removal of chest tubes is evaluated by:
    1. Return of normal tidal volume
    2. Absence of additional drainage
    3. Decreased adventitious sounds
    4. Comparison of chest radiographs

333. The nurse should position a client recovering from general anesthesia in a:
    1. Supine position
    2. Side-lying position
    3. High-Fowler's position
    4. Trendelenburg position

334. During the immediate postoperative period the nurse should give the highest priority to:
    1. Observing for hemorrhage
    2. Maintaining a patent airway
    3. Recording the intake and output
    4. Checking the vital signs every 15 minutes

335. The nurse reminds a client who has just had a laryngoscopy not to take anything by mouth until instructed to do so. This nursing action would generally be considered:
    1. Inappropriate, because the client is conscious and may be thirsty after being npo
    2. Appropriate, because early eating or drinking after laryngoscopy may result in aspiration
    3. Appropriate, because such clients usually experience painful swallowing for several days
    4. Inappropriate, because the client is likely to be anxious and it is easier to remove the water pitcher

336. A client has a bronchoscopy in ambulatory surgery. To prevent laryngeal edema, the nurse should:
    1. Place ice chips in the client's mouth
    2. Offer the client liberal amounts of fluid
    3. Keep the client in the semi-Fowler's position
    4. Tell the client to suck on medicated lozenges

337. After a bronchoscopy because of suspected cancer of the lung, a client develops pleural effusion. This is most likely the result of:
    1. Excessive fluid intake
    2. Inadequate chest expansion
    3. Extension of cancerous lesions
    4. Irritation from the bronchoscopy

338. As a result of pulmonary tuberculosis, a client has a decreased surface area for gaseous exchange in the lungs. Oxygen and carbon dioxide are exchanged in the lungs by:
    1. Osmosis
    2. Diffusion
    3. Filtration
    4. Active transport

339. Before discontinuing airborne precautions for a client with pulmonary tuberculosis, the nurse must determine that:
    1. The tuberculin skin test is negative
    2. The client no longer has the disease
    3. No acid-fast bacteria are in the sputum
    4. The client's temperature has returned to normal

340. A client has a right pneumonectomy. During surgery the phrenic nerve is accidentally severed. This will:
    1. Produce a partially atonic diaphragm
    2. Limit postoperative pain considerably
    3. Allow the diaphragm to partially descend
    4. Permit greater excursion of the thoracic cavity

341. The nurse expects that the initial treatment for a client who has a leak of the thoracic duct following radical neck surgery would include inserting a:
    1. Gastrostomy tube to drain the fluid, a high-fat diet, and bed rest
    2. Chest tube to drain the fluid, total parenteral nutrition, and bed rest
    3. Rectal tube to prevent distention, a low-fat diet, and increased activity
    4. Nasogastric tube to drain the fluid, a moderate-fat diet, and increased activity

342. Following a radical neck dissection a client has two tubes from the area of the incision connected to portable wound drainage. Inspection of the neck reveals moderate edema even though the drainage systems are functioning. Because of this situation, the nurse should assess the client for:
    1. Loss of the gag reflex
    2. Cloudy wound drainage
    3. Restlessness and dyspnea
    4. Dehiscence of the suture line

343. The factor that would have little influence in predisposing an individual to cancer of the larynx would be:
    1. Air pollution
    2. Poor dental hygiene
    3. Heavy alcohol ingestion
    4. Chronic respiratory infections

344. Immediate postoperative management for a client with a total laryngectomy would include:
    1. Instructing the client to whisper
    2. Placing the client in the orthopneic position
    3. Removing the outer tracheostomy tube prn
    4. Suctioning the tracheostomy tube whenever necessary

345. When suctioning a client with a tracheostomy the nurse must remember to:
    1. Use a new sterile catheter with each insertion
    2. Initiate suction as the catheter is being withdrawn
    3. Insert the catheter until the cough reflex is stimulated
    4. Remove the inner cannula before inserting the suction catheter

346. A thoracentesis is performed. Following the procedure it is most important for the nurse to observe the client for:
    1. Periods of confusion
    2. Expectoration of blood
    3. Increased breath sounds
    4. Decreased respiratory rate

347. A client with a pulmonary embolus is intubated and placed on mechanical ventilation. When suctioning the endotracheal tube, the nurse should:
    1. Apply suction while inserting the catheter
    2. Hyperoxygenate with 100% oxygen before and after suctioning
    3. Use short, jabbing movements of the catheter to loosen secretions
    4. Suction two to three times in quick succession to remove secretions

348. A client has seeds containing radium implanted in the pharyngeal area. When caring for this client, the nurse should:
    1. Have the client void q2h
    2. Maintain the client in isolation
    3. Spend as much time with the client as possible
    4. Use rubber gloves when giving the client a bath

349. The nurse can expect a client who has had a splenectomy to complain of:
    1. Pain on expiration
    2. Pain on inspiration
    3. Shortness of breath
    4. Excessively moist respirations

350. In the first $2^1/_2$ hours following a radical neck dissection, 40 ml of medium red, bloody fluid is obtained from the drainage system. The nurse should:
    1. Take the vital signs, check the dressing, and chart
    2. Reclose the drainage system and check it again in an hour
    3. Reinforce the dressing and observe for bleeding in half an hour
    4. Check the dressing, obtain the vital signs, and immediately notify the surgeon

351. A client should be referred to the pulmonary clinic for suspected tuberculosis when the nurse takes a medical history that includes complaints of:
    1. Chest pain, increased cough, and weight gain
    2. Weight gain, increased cough, and hemoptysis
    3. Unexplained weight loss, nausea, and vomiting
    4. Increased cough, hemoptysis, and night sweats

352. The nurse's responsibility in preventing atelectasis in a client with chest trauma, such as fractured ribs or flail chest, would be to:
    1. Ensure a high fluid intake over 24 hours
    2. Encourage coughing and deep breathing
    3. Defer pain medication the first day after injury
    4. Position the client face down on a soft mattress

353. The arterial blood gases of a client with COPD deteriorate, and respiratory failure is impending. The nurse should first assess the client for:
    1. Cyanosis
    2. Bradycardia
    3. Mental confusion
    4. Distended neck veins

Gastrointestinal

354. The nurse is instructing a group about food preparation. They are told to avoid using products in damaged cans because they might contain the anaerobic spore-forming rod:
    1. *Escherichia coli*
    2. *Clostridium tetani*
    3. *Salmonella typhosa*
    4. *Clostridium botulinum*

355. When teaching an athletic teenager about nutritional intake, the nurse should explain that the carbohydrate food that would provide the quickest source of energy is a:
    1. Glass of milk
    2. Slice of bread
    3. Chocolate candy bar
    4. Glass of orange juice

356. The end products of protein digestion, amino acids, are absorbed from the small intestine by:
    1. Simple diffusion because of their small size
    2. Filtration according to the osmotic pressure direction
    3. Active transport with the aid of vitamin B_6 (pyridoxine)
    4. Osmosis caused by their greater concentration in the intestinal lumen

357. A complete protein, a food protein of high biologic value, is one that contains:
    1. All of the amino acids in sufficient quantity to meet human requirements
    2. All of the essential amino acids in correct proportion to meet human needs
    3. The essential amino acids in any proportion because the body can always fill in the difference needed
    4. Most of the amino acids from which the body will make additional amounts of the essential amino acids needed

358. The statement that is true about the sources of vitamin K is:
    1. Vitamin K is found in a wide variety of foods, so there is no danger of deficiency
    2. Almost all vitamin K sufficient for metabolic needs is produced by intestinal bacteria
    3. Vitamin K is rarely found in dietary food sources, so a natural deficiency can easily occur
    4. Usually vitamin K can easily be absorbed without assistance, so all that is consumed is absorbed

359. Vitamin C is related to tissue integrity and hemorrhagic disease. It controls such disorders by:
    1. Preventing tissue hemorrhage by providing essential blood-clotting materials
    2. Preserving the structural integrity of tissue by protecting the lipid matrix of cell walls from peroxidation
    3. Facilitating adequate absorption of calcium and phosphorus for bone formation to prevent bleeding in the joints
    4. Strengthening capillary walls and structural tissue by depositing cementing material to build collagen from ground substance and thus prevent tissue hemorrhage

360. Energy stored as ATP, ADP, and other high-energy compounds is formed chiefly by:
    1. Peptidation
    2. Respiration
    3. Hydrolysis of fats
    4. Oxidation of glucose

361. A client describes abdominal discomfort following ingestion of milk. The nurse recognizes that this may be the result of a genetic deficiency of the enzyme:
    1. Lactase
    2. Maltase
    3. Sucrase
    4. Amylase

362. One of the main functions of bile is to:
    1. Split protein
    2. Emulsify fats
    3. Help synthesize vitamins
    4. Produce an acid condition

363. The main function of adipose tissue in fat metabolism is synthesizing and:
    1. Releasing glucose for energy
    2. Regulating cholesterol production
    3. Using lipoproteins for fat transport
    4. Storing triglycerides for energy reserves

364. The terms saturated and unsaturated, when used in reference to fats, relate to degree of:
    1. Taste
    2. Color
    3. Density
    4. Digestibility

365. When fat compounds accumulate to abnormal levels in the blood, the diet may be modified as one effort to control them. The foods most affected by such diet therapy would be:
    1. Fruits
    2. Grains
    3. Animal fats
    4. Vegetable oils

366. The breakdown of triglyceride molecules can be expected to produce:
    1. Fatty acids
    2. Ammo acids
    3. Urea nitrogen
    4. Simple sugars

367. Many vitamins and minerals regulate the chemical changes of cell metabolism by acting in a coenzyme role. This means that the vitamin or mineral:
    1. Forms a new compound by a series of complex changes
    2. Is not a part of the enzyme controlling a particular reaction
    3. May be a necessary process present for the reaction to proceed
    4. Prevents unnecessary reactions by neutralizing the controlling enzyme

368. Because fat is insoluble in water, it cannot travel freely in the blood. Therefore the main type of compound formed to serve as a vehicle of transport is:
    1. Lipoprotein
    2. Triglyceride
    3. Phospholipid
    4. Plasma protein

369. Amino acids are involved in total body metabolism building and rebuilding various tissues. Of these, a number are essential amino acids. This means that:
    1. These amino acids can be made by the body because they are essential to life
    2. These amino acids are essential in body processes and the remaining amino acids are not
    3. The body cannot synthesize these amino acids and thus they must be obtained from the diet
    4. After synthesizing these amino acids, the body uses them in key processes essential for growth

370. The food group lowest in natural sodium is:
1. Milk
2. Meat
3. Fruits
4. Vegetables

371. Megadoses of vitamin A are taken by a client. The nurse should question this practice because:
1. This vitamin is highly toxic even in small amounts
2. The liver has a great storage capacity for the vitamin, even to toxic amounts
3. This vitamin cannot be stored, and the excess amount would saturate the general body tissues
4. Although the body's requirement for the vitamin is very large, the cells can synthesize more as needed

372. Most of the work of changing raw fuel forms of carbohydrates to the refined usable fuel glucose is accomplished by enzymes located in the:
1. Mouth
2. Small intestine
3. Large intestine
4. Stomach mucosa

373. Vitamin A is a fat-soluble vitamin produced by humans and other animals from its precursor carotene-provitamin A. One of the main sources of this vitamin is:
1. Oranges
2. Skim milk
3. Tomatoes
4. Leafy greens

374. A client is to have gastric gavage. When the gavage tube is being inserted the nurse should place the client in the:
1. Supine position
2. Mid-Fowler's position
3. High-Fowler's position
4. Trendelenburg position

375. A client expresses aversion to meals and eats only small amounts. The nurse should provide:
1. Nourishment between meals
2. Small portions more frequently
3. Only foods the client likes in small portions
4. Supplementary vitamins to stimulate appetite

376. The term used to most accurately describe a client's lack of interest in food is:
1. Apathy
2. Anoxia
3. Anorexia
4. Dysphagia

377. A flat plate radiograph of the abdomen is ordered. The nurse recognizes that the client should receive:
1. No special preparation
2. A low soapsuds enema
3. Nothing by mouth for 8 hours
4. A laxative the evening before the x-ray

378. Barium salts in the GI series and barium enemas serve to:
1. Fluoresce and thus illuminate the alimentary tract
2. Give off visible light and illuminate the alimentary tract
3. Dye the alimentary tract and thus provide for color contrast
4. Absorb x-rays and thus give contrast to the soft tissues of the alimentary tract

379. As part of the preparation of a client for a sigmoidoscopy, the nurse should:
1. Administer an enema the morning of the test
2. Provide a container for the collection of a stool specimen
3. Withhold all fluids and foods for 24 hours before the examination
4. Explain to the client that a chalklike substance will have to be swallowed

380. Specific nursing responsibility in preparing a client for a sigmoidoscopy and barium enema includes:
1. Giving castor oil the afternoon before
2. Withholding food and fluid for 8 hours
3. Administering soapsuds enemas until clear
4. Ensuring the client's understanding of the procedure

381. The maximum height at which the container of fluid should be held when administering a cleansing enema is:
1. 30 cm (12 inches)
2. 37 cm (15 inches)
3. 45 cm (18 inches)
4. 66 cm (26 inches)

382. During administration of an enema a client complains of intestinal cramps. The nurse should:
1. Give it at a slower rate
2. Discontinue the procedure
3. Stop until cramps are gone
4. Lower the height of the container

383. The nurse explains that visualization of the GI tract after a barium enema is made possible by:
    1. Barium physically coloring the intestinal wall
    2. The high x-ray absorbing properties of barium
    3. The high x-ray transmitting properties of barium
    4. The chemical interaction between barium and the electrolytes

384. A sigmoidoscopy is performed as a diagnostic measure. For this examination, the client may be placed in the position known as:
    1. Sims'
    2. Prone
    3. Lithotomy
    4. Knee-chest

385. During a percutaneous endoscopic gastrostomy (PEG) tube feeding, the observation that indicates that the client is unable to tolerate a continuation of the feeding would be:
    1. A passage of flatus
    2. Epigastric tenderness
    3. A rise of formula in the tube
    4. The rapid flow of the feeding

386. Three days after admission for a cerebral vascular accident, a client has a nasogastric tube inserted and is receiving intermittent feedings. To best evaluate if a prior feeding has been absorbed the nurse should:
    1. Evaluate the intake in relation to the output
    2. Aspirate for a residual volume and reinstill it
    3. Instill air into the stomach while auscultating
    4. Compare the client's body weight to the baseline data

387. Clients receiving hypertonic tube feedings most commonly develop diarrhea because of:
    1. Increased fiber intake
    2. Bacterial contamination
    3. Inappropriate positioning
    4. High osmolarity of the feedings

388. The nurse should administer a nasogastric tube feeding slowly to reduce the hazard of:
    1. Distention
    2. Flatulence
    3. Indigestion
    4. Regurgitation

389. Clients with fractured mandibles usually have them immobilized with wires. The life-threatening problem that can develop postoperatively is:
    1. Infection
    2. Vomiting
    3. Osteomyelitis
    4. Bronchospasm

390. After an incision and drainage of an oral abscess, the client should be instructed to notify the physician if there is:
    1. Foul odor to the breath
    2. Pain and swelling after 1 week
    3. Pain associated with swallowing
    4. Tenderness in the mouth when chewing

391. When assessing a client with cancer of the tongue the specific adaptation the nurse should expect to find is:
    1. Halitosis
    2. Leukoplakia
    3. Bleeding gums
    4. Substernal pain

392. The nurse recognizes that a client has an increased risk of developing cancer of the tongue if there is a history of:
    1. Nail biting
    2. Poor dental habits
    3. Frequent gum chewing
    4. Heavy consumption of alcohol

393. A client with gastroesophageal reflux complains about having difficulty sleeping at night. Appropriate intervention would be:
    1. Sleeping on two or three pillows
    2. Eliminating carbohydrates from the diet
    3. Suggesting a large glass of milk before retiring
    4. Administering antacids such as sodium bicarbonate

394. To limit symptoms of gastroesophageal reflux (GERD), the nurse should advise the client to:
    1. Avoid heavy lifting
    2. Lie down after eating
    3. Increase fluid intake with meals
    4. Wear an abdominal binder or girdle

395. A client with gastric ulcer disease asks the nurse the reason for antibiotic therapy that includes metronidazole (Flagyl). The nurse should explain that antibiotics are prescribed to:
    1. Augment the immune response
    2. Potentiate the effect of antacids
    3. Treat *Helicobacter pylori* infection
    4. Reduce hydrochloric acid secretion

396. Most peptic ulcers occurring in the stomach are in the:
    1. Pyloric portion
    2. Cardiac portion
    3. Esophageal junction
    4. Body of the stomach

397. A client with a peptic ulcer in the duodenum would probably describe the associated pain as:
    1. An ache radiating to the left side
    2. An intermittent colicky flank pain
    3. A gnawing sensation relieved by food
    4. A generalized abdominal pain intensified by moving

398. The basic goal underlying the unique dietary management of gastritis is to:
    1. Provide optimal amounts of all important nutrients
    2. Increase the amount of bulk and roughage in the diet
    3. Eliminate chemical, mechanical, and thermal irritation
    4. Promote psychologic support by offering a wide variety of foods

399. A client is scheduled for a pyloroplasty and vagotomy because of strictures caused by ulcers unresponsive to medical therapy. The nurse reinforces the client's understanding by stating that the vagotomy serves to:
    1. Increase the heart rate
    2. Hasten gastric emptying
    3. Eliminate pain sensations
    4. Decrease secretions in the stomach

400. GI bleeding can be treated medically by infusing medication through an intravenous line. A drug commonly used for this purpose is:
    1. Vasopressin (Pitressin)
    2. Neostigmine (Prostigmin)
    3. Propantheline (Pro-Banthine)
    4. Phytonadione (Aquamephyton)

401. The nurse would expect an antrectomy may be performed if a client has a diagnosis of:
    1. Cataracts
    2. Otosclerosis
    3. Gastric ulcers
    4. Trigeminal neuralgia

402. Following a subtotal gastrectomy for cancer of the stomach a client develops dumping syndrome. The nurse understands that dumping syndrome refers to:

    1. Nausea due to a full stomach
    2. Rapid passage of osmotic fluid into the jejunum
    3. Reflux of intestinal contents into the esophagus
    4. Buildup of feces and gas within the large intestine

403. Two hours after a subtotal gastrectomy the nurse notes that the drainage from the client's nasogastric tube is bright red. The nurse should:
    1. Notify the physician immediately
    2. Clamp the nasogastric tube for one hour
    3. Recognize that this is an expected finding
    4. Irrigate the nasogastric tube with iced saline

404. When caring for a client with a nasogastric tube attached to suction, the nurse should:
    1. Irrigate the tube with normal saline
    2. Use sterile technique when irrigating the tube
    3. Withdraw the tube quickly when decompression is terminated
    4. Allow the client to have small chips of ice or sips of water unless nauseated

405. After a partial gastrectomy is performed, a client is returned to the unit with an IV solution infusing and a nasogastric tube in place. The nurse notes that there has been no nasogastric drainage for $\frac{1}{2}$ hour. There is an order to irrigate the nasogastric tube prn. The nurse should insert:
    1. 30 ml of normal saline and withdraw slowly
    2. 20 ml of air and clamp off suction for 1 hour
    3. 50 ml of saline and increase pressure of suction
    4. 15 ml of distilled water and disconnect suction for 30 minutes

406. A serious danger to which a client with intestinal obstruction is exposed because of intestinal suction is excessive loss of:
    1. Protein enzymes
    2. Energy carbohydrates
    3. Vitamins and minerals
    4. Water and electrolytes

407. The nurse designs a health teaching program specifically for a client who has had a gastrectomy. This plan should include:
    1. A warning to avoid all gas-forming foods
    2. An explanation of the therapeutic effect of a high-roughage diet
    3. Encouragement to resume previous eating habits as soon as possible
    4. A thorough explanation of the dumping syndrome and how to limit or prevent it

408. The nurse should be aware that following a gastrectomy a client may develop pernicious anemia because:
    1. Vitamin B$_{12}$ is only absorbed in the stomach ✗
    2. The hemopoietic factor is secreted in the stomach
    3. The parietal cells of the stomach secrete the intrinsic factor
    4. Chief cells in the stomach promote the secretion of the extrinsic factor

409. After a subtotal gastrectomy a client is returned to the surgical unit. The nurse can best prevent pulmonary complications by:
    1. Keeping a plastic airway in place
    2. Maintaining a consistent oxygen flow rate
    3. Ambulating to increase respiratory exchange
    4. Promoting frequent turning and deep breathing to mobilize secretions ✗

410. The wisest dietary guidelines for an elderly client who has had a subtotal gastrectomy would be:
    1. Increasing intake of dietary roughage
    2. Avoiding oral feedings for a prolonged period
    3. Gradually resuming small, easily digested feedings
    4. Allowing the client to select personally preferred foods

411. Jaundiced clients are susceptible to postoperative hemorrhage because their blood does not clot normally. This is because:
    1. Excess bile salts in the blood inhibit synthesis of prothrombin in the liver
    2. Excess bile salts in the blood inhibit synthesis of vitamin K and prothrombin in the liver
    3. Decreased bile salts in the blood inactivate prothrombinase and prevent formation of thrombin from prothrombin
    4. Lack of bile in the intestine causes inadequate vitamin K absorption, which causes inadequate prothrombin synthesis by the liver

412. The nurse understands that for a client to utilize fat-soluble vitamins, the body must produce:
    1. HCl
    2. Bile
    3. Lipase
    4. Amylase

413. Before scheduling a client for endoscopic retrograde cholangiopancreatography (ERCP), the nurse should assess the client's:
    1. Urine output
    2. Bilirubin level
    3. Serum glucose
    4. Blood pressure

414. A client has an interference in bile utilization caused by cholecystitis. The nurse understands that the ejection of bile into the alimentary tract is controlled by the hormone:
    1. Gastrin
    2. Secretin
    3. Enterocrinin
    4. Cholecystokinin

415. A client with cholelithiasis experiences discomfort after ingesting fatty foods because:
    1. Fatty foods are hard to digest
    2. Bile flow into the intestine is obstructed
    3. The liver is manufacturing inadequate bile
    4. There is inadequate closure of the ampulla of Vater

416. The nurse assesses the client with cholecystitis for the development of obstructive jaundice, which would be evidenced by:
    1. Inadequate absorption of fat-soluble vitamin K
    2. Light amber urine, dark brown stools, yellow skin
    3. Dark-colored urine, clay-colored stools, itchy skin
    4. Straw-colored urine, putty-colored stools, yellow sclerae

417. Before a cholecystectomy the physician orders vitamin K. This is administered because it is used in the formation of:
    1. Bilirubin
    2. Prothrombin
    3. Thromboplastin
    4. Cholecystokinin

418. Following an abdominal cholecystectomy, the nurse should assess for signs of respiratory complications because the:
    1. Incision is in close proximity to the diaphragm
    2. Length of time required for surgery is prolonged
    3. Client's resistance is lowered because of bile in the blood
    4. Bloodstream is invaded by microorganisms from the biliary tract

419. The nurse in the postanesthesia unit notices that after an abdominal cholecystectomy a client has serosanguinous fluid on the abdominal dressing. The nurse should:
    1. Change the dressing
    2. Reinforce the dressing
    3. Apply an abdominal binder
    4. Remove the tape and apply Montgomery straps

420. After a cholecystectomy the client's diet will probably be:
    1. High in protein and calories to promote wound healing
    2. High in fat and carbohydrate to meet energy demands
    3. Low in fat to avoid painful contractions in the area of the wound
    4. Low in protein and carbohydrate to avoid excess calories and help the client lose weight

421. A hormone that stimulates the flow of pancreatic enzymes is:
    1. Enterocrinin
    2. Pancreozymin
    3. Enterogastrone
    4. Cholecystokinin

422. The major digestive changes in fat are accomplished in the small intestine by a lipase from the pancreas. This enzymatic activity:
    1. Synthesizes new triglycerides from the dietary fat consumed
    2. Emulsifies the fat globules and reduces their surface tension
    3. Easily breaks down all the dietary fat to fatty acids and glycerol
    4. Splits off all the fatty acids in about 30% of the total dietary fat consumed

423. Secretin and pancreozymin are hormones secreted by the:
    1. Liver
    2. Adrenals
    3. Pancreas
    4. Duodenum

424. Surgery may be needed to excise a pseudocyst of the pancreas. A pseudocyst of the pancreas:
    1. Is generally a malignant growth
    2. Is filled with pancreatic enzymes
    3. Contains necrotic tissue and blood
    4. Is a pouch of undigested food particles

425. The nurse understands that an acute attack of pancreatitis can be precipitated by heavy drinking because:
    1. Alcohol promotes the formation of calculi in the cystic duct
    2. The pancreas is stimulated to secrete more insulin than it can immediately produce
    3. The alcohol alters the composition of enzymes so they are capable of damaging the pancreas
    4. Alcohol increases enzyme secretion and pancreatic duct pressure and causes backflow of enzymes into the pancreas

426. Following pancreatic surgery, clients are at risk for developing respiratory tract infections because of the:
    1. Length of time required for surgery
    2. Proximity of the incision to the diaphragm
    3. Lowered resistance caused by bile in the blood
    4. Transfer of bacteria from the pancreas to the blood

427. The nurse recognizes that the main role of the liver in relation to fat metabolism is:
    1. Producing phospholipids
    2. Storing fat for energy reserves
    3. Oxidizing fatty acids to produce energy
    4. Converting fat to lipoproteins for rapid transport out into the body

428. The most therapeutic diet for a client recovering from an acute episode of alcoholism would be:
    1. High protein, low carbohydrate, low fat
    2. Low protein, high carbohydrate, high fat, soft
    3. High carbohydrate, low saturated fat, 1800 calories
    4. Protein to tolerance, moderate fat, high calorie, high vitamin, soft

429. The physician orders thiamine chloride and nicotinic acid for a client with alcoholism. The nurse should teach the client that these vitamins are needed for the maintenance of:
    1. Elimination
    2. Efficient circulation
    3. The nervous system
    4. Prothrombin formation

430. Because the detoxification of alcohol damages tissues, a high-calorie diet fortified with vitamins should be encouraged to protect the client's:
    1. Liver
    2. Kidneys
    3. Adrenals
    4. Pancreas

431. The cooked food most likely to remain contaminated by the virus that causes hepatitis A is:
    1. Canned tuna
    2. Broiled shrimp
    3. Baked haddock
    4. Steamed lobster

432. Prophylaxis for hepatitis B includes:
    1. Preventing constipation
    2. Screening of blood donors
    3. Avoiding shellfish in the diet
    4. Limiting hepatotoxic drug therapy

433. In the client with hepatitis B the earliest indication of parenchymal damage to the liver usually is:
    1. A rise in bilirubin
    2. An alteration in proteins
    3. A rise in alanine aminotransferase
    4. An elevation of alkaline phosphatase

434. When caring for a client with hepatitis A the nurse should take special precautions to:
    1. Prevent droplet spread of infection
    2. Use caution when bringing food to the client
    3. Use gloves when removing the client's bedpan
    4. Wear mask and gown before entering the room

435. The type of hepatitis most frequently transmitted by transfusion is:
    1. Hepatitis A
    2. Hepatitis B
    3. Hepatitis C
    4. Hepatitis D

436. A client in a debilitated state is admitted for palliative treatment of cancer of the liver. On admission the objective information that would be most helpful for future monitoring of the client's condition would be:
    1. Diet history
    2. Bowel sounds
    3. Present weight
    4. Pain description

437. The nurse would expect a client with liver cancer to complain of fatigue because a readily available form of energy, although limited in amount, is stored in the liver by conversion of glucose to:
    1. Glycerol
    2. Glycogen

3. Tissue fat
4. Amino acids

438. The nurse would expect a client with cancer of the liver to have difficulty digesting fatty foods because the liver is involved in the production of:
    1. Bile
    2. Lipase
    3. Amylase
    4. Cholesterol

439. A client with cirrhosis of the liver has longstanding poor nutrition, including a protein deficiency. This deficiency leads to:
    1. Decreased bile in the blood
    2. Fat accumulation in the liver tissue
    3. Coagulation of blood in microcirculation
    4. Tissue anabolism and positive nitrogen balance

440. The most therapeutic diet for a client with hepatic cirrhosis would be:
    1. High protein, low carbohydrate, low fat
    2. Low protein, low carbohydrate, high fat, soft
    3. High carbohydrate, low saturated fat, 1200 calories
    4. Low sodium, protein to tolerance, moderate fat, high calorie, high vitamin, soft

441. When caring for a client with ascites the nurse should understand that the portal vein:
    1. Brings blood away from the liver
    2. Enters the superior vena cava from the cranium
    3. Brings venous blood from the intestinal wall to the liver
    4. Is located superficially on the anteromedial surface of the thigh

442. When assessing a client with portal hypertension, the nurse should be alert for indications of:
    1. Liver abscess
    2. Intestinal obstruction
    3. Perforation of the duodenum
    4. Hemorrhage from esophageal varices

443. The nurse is aware that the symptoms of portal hypertension in clients with cirrhosis are chiefly the result of:
    1. Infection of the liver parenchyma
    2. Fatty degeneration of Kupffer cells
    3. Obstruction of the portal circulation
    4. Obstruction of the cystic and hepatic ducts

444. The nurse understands that the ascites seen in cirrhosis results in part from:
    1. The escape of lymph into the abdominal cavity directly from the inflamed liver sinusoid
    2. Increased plasma colloid osmotic pressure due to excessive liver growth and metabolism
    3. The decreased levels of ADH and aldosterone due to increasing metabolic activity in the liver
    4. Compression of the portal veins, with resultant increased back pressure in the portal venous system

445. The physician orders a paracentesis for a client with ascites. Before the procedure, the nurse should instruct the client to:
    1. Empty the bladder
    2. Eat foods low in fat
    3. Remain npo for 24 hours
    4. Assume the supine position

446. The nurse would expect to observe varicose veins when a client has cirrhosis because of:
    1. Increased plasma hydrostatic pressure in veins of the extremities
    2. Toxic irritating products released into the blood from the diseased organs
    3. Ballooning of vein walls from decreased venous pressure and incompetent valves
    4. Decreased plasma protein concentration resulting in the pooling of blood in the venous system

447. The nurse administers Neomycin to a client with hepatic cirrhosis to prevent the formation of:
    1. Bile
    2. Urea
    3. Ammonia
    4. Hemoglobin

448. If intubation is indicated for a client with bleeding esophageal varices, the type of tube most likely to be used would be a(an):
    1. Levin tube
    2. Salem sump
    3. Miller-Abbott tube
    4. Blakemore-Sengstaken tube

449. A client with hepatic cirrhosis begins to develop slurred speech, confusion, drowsiness, and a flapping tremor. With this evidence of impending hepatic coma, the diet would probably be changed to:
    1. 20 g protein, 2000 calories
    2. 70 g protein, 1200 calories
    3. 80 g protein, 2500 calories
    4. 100 g protein, 1500 calories

450. The basic pathophysiologic problem in cirrhosis of the liver causing esophageal varices is:
    1. Ascites and edema
    2. Portal hypertension
    3. Loss of regeneration
    4. Dilated veins and varicosities

451. When assessing a client with liver insufficiency the nurse would expect:
    1. Anuria
    2. Fetor hepaticus
    3. Blepharospasm
    4. Globus hystericus

452. In an effort to prevent hepatic coma in a client with liver dysfunction it may become necessary to:
    1. Give Fleet enemas
    2. Severely restrict dietary protein
    3. Prepare for emergency surgery
    4. Eliminate carbohydrate from the diet

453. The nurse should assess the client with cirrhosis for indications of hepatic coma. One classic sign of hepatic coma is:
    1. Bile-colored stools
    2. Elevated cholesterol
    3. Flapping hand tremors
    4. Depressed muscle reflexes

454. The nurse should assess a client with liver cirrhosis and hepatic coma for:
    1. Icterus
    2. Urticaria
    3. Uremic frost
    4. Hemangioma

455. The laboratory test that would indicate that the liver of a client with cirrhosis is compromised and Neomycin enemas might be helpful would be:
    1. Ammonia level
    2. White blood count
    3. Culture and sensitivity
    4. Alanine aminotransaminase level

456. A client is admitted with anorexia, weight loss, abdominal distention, and abnormal stools. A diagnosis of malabsorption syndrome is made. To meet the client's needs the nurse should:
    1. Allow the client to eat food preferences
    2. Institute IV therapy to improve hydration
    3. Maintain npo status, because food precipitates diarrhea
    4. Encourage consumption of meats at mealtime and high-protein snacks

457. A client is diagnosed as having malabsorption syndrome. Striking clinical improvement should be noted after administration of:
1. Folic acid
2. Vitamin B₁₂
3. Corticotropin
4. A gluten-free diet

458. When planning dietary teaching for a client with malabsorption syndrome the nurse should include the need to avoid:
1. Rice or corn
2. Milk or cheese
3. Fruit or fruit juices
4. Wheat, rye, or oats

459. A typical food combination that can be served to a client with malabsorption syndrome would be:
1. Roast beef, baked potato, carrots, tea
2. Cheese omelet, noodles, green beans, coffee
3. Creamed turkey on toast, rice, green peas, milk
4. Baked chicken, mashed potatoes with gravy, zucchini, Postum

460. A client is diagnosed as having acute appendicitis. This condition is associated with:
1. Poor dietary habits
2. Infection of the bowel
3. Hypertension and resultant edema
4. Compromised circulation to the appendix

461. An 18-year-old is admitted with an acute onset of right lower quadrant pain. Appendicitis is suspected. To determine the etiology of the pain, the client should be assessed for:
1. Urinary retention
2. Gastric hyperacidity
3. Rebound tenderness
4. Increased lower bowel motility

462. A client has an appendectomy and develops peritonitis. The nurse should assess the client for an elevated temperature and:
1. Hyperactivity
2. Extreme hunger
3. Urinary retention
4. Local muscular rigidity

463. The position that is indicated for a client after surgery for a perforated appendix with localized peritonitis is the:
1. Sims' position
2. Semi-Fowler's position
3. Trendelenburg position
4. Dorsal recumbent position

464. Four days after abdominal surgery a client has not passed any flatus and there are no bowel sounds. Paralytic ileus is suspected. In this condition there is an interference caused by:
1. Decreased blood supply
2. Impaired neural functioning
3. Perforation of the bowel wall
4. Obstruction of the bowel lumen

465. The physician has ordered a rectal tube to help a client relieve abdominal distention following surgery. To achieve maximum effectiveness the nurse should leave it in place:
1. 15 minutes
2. 30 minutes
3. 45 minutes
4. 60 minutes

466. A client is to have an enema to reduce flatus. The rectal catheter should be inserted:
1. 2 inches
2. 4 inches
3. 6 inches
4. 8 inches

467. A 93-year-old client with a history of diverticulitis is admitted with severe abdominal pain, anorexia, nausea, vomiting for 24 hours, a markedly elevated temperature, and increased WBCs. The primary reason for performing surgery is most likely that:
1. Surgery is usually indicated for clients with a diagnosis of diverticulitis
2. The symptoms exhibited by the client on admission were life threatening
3. In some instances diverticulitis is difficult to differentiate from carcinoma except surgically
4. The client's age indicated that immediate correction of the potentially fatal condition was needed

468. Vitamins are administered parenterally for clients with an inflamed intestine because:
1. More rapid action results
2. They are ineffective orally
3. They decrease colon irritability
4. Intestinal absorption may be inadequate

469. After many years of coping with colitis, a client makes the decision to have a colectomy as advised by the physician. A significant factor in this decision may have been the knowledge that:
1. Surgical treatment cures ulcerative colitis
2. It would be temporary until the colon heals
3. Ulcerative colitis can progress to Crohn's disease
4. Without surgery the client would be unable to eat table foods

470. When eliciting a health history from a client with colitis the nurse bases the interview on the knowledge that colitis is commonly associated with:
1. Chemical stress
2. Endocrine stress
3. Physiologic stress
4. Psychologic stress

471. To decrease GI irritability, the nurse should teach the client to minimize use of:
1. Table salt and rice products
2. Sugar products and proteins
3. Triglycerides and amino acids
4. Milk products and cola drinks

472. The symptoms that the nurse should expect when assessing a client with colitis are:
1. Leukocytosis, anorexia, weight loss
2. Anemia, hemoptysis, weight loss, abdominal cramps
3. Fever, anemia, nausea and vomiting, leukopenia, diarrhea
4. Diarrhea, anorexia, weight loss, abdominal cramps, anemia

473. The physician orders daily stool examinations for a client with chronic bowel inflammation. These stool examinations are ordered to determine:
1. Ova and parasites
2. Culture and sensitivity
3. Fat and undigested food
4. Occult blood and organisms

474. The most serious complication associated with chronic inflammation of the bowel is:
1. Ileus
2. Bleeding
3. Perforation
4. Obstruction

475. The physician orders a low-residue diet for a client with an acute exacerbation of colitis. The nurse would know that the dietary teaching is understood when the client states, "I can eat:
1. Baked fish, macaroni with cheese, strained carrots, fruit gelatin, and milk."

2. Cream soup, crackers, omelet, mashed potatoes, roll, orange juice, and coffee."
3. Stewed chicken, baked potato with butter, strained peas, white bread, plain cake, and milk."
4. Lean roast beef, buttered white rice with egg slices, white bread with butter and jelly, and tea with sugar."

476. The most important method of preventing amebic dysentery is:
1. Tick control
2. Sewage disposal
3. Killing biting gnats
4. Pasteurization of milk

477. When teaching a client about intussusception, the nurse explains that it is:
1. Kinking of the bowel onto itself
2. A band of connective tissue compressing the bowel
3. Telescoping of a proximal loop of bowel into a distal loop
4. A protrusion of an organ or part of an organ through the wall that contains it

478. When caring for the client with an ileostomy the nurse would:
1. Encourage the client to eat foods high in residue
2. Expect the stoma to start draining on the third postoperative day
3. Anticipate that emotional stress can increase intestinal peristalsis
4. Explain that the drainage can be controlled with daily irrigations

479. If the ileum is removed surgically, the individual may suffer from anemia because:
1. Folic acid is absorbed only in the terminal ileum
2. The hemopoietic factor is absorbed only in the terminal ileum
3. Iron absorption is dependent on simultaneous bile salt absorption in the terminal ileum
4. The trace elements copper, cobalt, and nickel, required for hemoglobin synthesis, are absorbed only in the ileum

480. The sport that should be avoided by a client with an ileostomy is:
1. Skiing
2. Football
3. Swimming
4. Track events

481. When a client has extensive carcinoma of the descending portion of the colon with metastasis to the lymph nodes, the operative procedure that would probably be performed is a(an):
    1. Ileostomy
    2. Colectomy
    3. Colostomy
    4. Cecostomy

482. When receiving an enema, the client should be placed in the:
    1. Sims' position
    2. Back-lying position
    3. Knee-chest position
    4. Mid-Fowler's position

483. The nurse administers neomycin sulfate to a client before colon surgery to:
    1. Destroy intestinal bacteria
    2. Increase the production of vitamin K
    3. Decrease the incidence of any secondary infection
    4. Decrease the possibility of postoperative urinary tract infection

484. Neomycin is especially useful before colon surgery because it:
    1. Will not affect the kidneys
    2. Acts systemically without delay
    3. Is poorly absorbed from the GI tract
    4. Is effective against many organisms

485. The nurse should protect the client's skin surrounding a colostomy opening by using:
    1. Alcohol
    2. Mineral oil
    3. Skin barriers
    4. Tincture of benzoin

486. The primary step toward long-range goals in the rehabilitation of a client with a new colostomy involves the client's:
    1. Mastery of techniques of colostomy care
    2. Readiness to accept an altered body function
    3. Awareness of available community resources
    4. Knowledge of the necessary dietary modifications

487. Neomycin 1 g is ordered preoperatively for a client with a diagnosis of cancer of the colon. The client asks why neomycin is being given. The best response by the nurse would be:

1. "It will decrease your kidney function and lessen urine production during surgery."
2. "It will kill the bacteria in your bowel and decrease the risk of infection after surgery."
3. "It is used to alter the body flora, which reduces the spread of the tumor to adjacent organs."
4. "It is used to prevent you from getting an infection, particularly a bladder infection, before surgery."

488. Postoperatively, if a client's colostomy stoma is viable the nurse would expect the color to be:
    1. Gray
    2. Brick red
    3. Pale pink
    4. Dark purple

489. A client is placed on total parenteral nutrition (TPN) following extensive colon surgery. The purpose of TPN is to:
    1. Provide short-term nutrition after surgery
    2. Assist in providing supplemental nutrition for the client
    3. Provide total nutrition when gastrointestinal function is questionable
    4. Assist people who are unable to eat but have active gastrointestinal function

490. The nurse is aware that the manifestation that is found more in ulcerative colitis than in Crohn's disease (regional enteritis) is:
    1. Inclusion of transmural involvement of the small bowel wall
    2. Correlation with increased malignancy because of malabsorption syndrome
    3. Involvement beginning proximally with intermittent plaques found along the colon
    4. Involvement starting distally with rectal bleeding and spreading continuously up the colon

491. A client with ulcerative colitis has had frequent severe exacerbations over the last several years. The client has had intense pain and severe diarrhea and has recently become cachectic. The therapeutic course that the nurse should expect the physician to explore with this client is:
    1. Intensive psychotherapy
    2. Continued medical therapy
    3. Surgical therapy (colectomy)
    4. Diet therapy (low residue, high protein)

492. When teaching a client to care for a new colostomy, the nurse should advise that the irrigations be done at the same time every day. The time selected should:
    1. Be approximately 1 hour before breakfast
    2. Provide ample uninterrupted bathroom use at home
    3. Approximate the client's usual daily time for elimination
    4. Be about halfway between the two largest meals of the day

493. When teaching a client with a permanent colostomy what might be expected on discharge, the nurse should discuss the:
    1. Need for special clothing
    2. Importance of limiting activity
    3. Periodic dilation of the stoma
    4. Bland, low-residue diet regimen

494. A client who has had a colostomy should follow a diet that is:
    1. Rich in protein
    2. Low in fiber content
    3. High in carbohydrate
    4. As close to normal as possible

495. The solution of choice used to maintain patency of an nasointestinal tube is:
    1. Sterile water
    2. Isotonic saline
    3. Hypotonic saline
    4. Hypertonic glucose

496. A client has a transverse loop colostomy. When inserting a catheter for irrigation, the nurse should:
    1. Use an oil-base lubricant
    2. Instruct the client to bear down
    3. Apply gentle but continuous force
    4. Direct it toward the client's right side

497. If, during a colostomy irrigation, a client complains of abdominal cramps, the nurse should:
    1. Discontinue the irrigation
    2. Lower the container of fluid
    3. Clamp the catheter for a few minutes
    4. Advance the catheter about 2.5 cm (1 inch)

498. When performing a colostomy irrigation, the nurse inserts the catheter into the stoma:
    1. 5 cm (2 inches)
    2. 10 cm (4 inches)
    3. 15 cm (6 inches)
    4. 20 cm (8 inches)

499. When teaching a client to irrigate a colostomy, the nurse indicates that the distance of the container above the stoma should be no more than:
    1. 15 cm (6 inches)
    2. 25 cm (10 inches)
    3. 30 cm (12 inches)
    4. 45 cm (18 inches)

500. A client has surgery for an incarcerated hernia. The physician returns the incarcerated tissue to the abdominal cavity and uses a mesh to reinforce the muscle wall, thereby preventing a future recurrence. This procedure is referred to as a:
    1. Herniotomy
    2. Herniectomy
    3. Hernioplasty
    4. Herniorrhaphy

501. The nurse suspects an elderly client has become impacted when the client states:
    1. "I have a lot of gas pains."
    2. "I don't have much of an appetite."
    3. "I feel like I have to go and just can't."
    4. "I haven't had a bowel movement for 2 days."

502. The assessment by the nurse that indicates the probable presence of a fecal impaction in a client with limited mobility would be:
    1. Tympanites
    2. Fecal liquid seepage
    3. Bright red blood in the stool
    4. Decreased number of bowel movements

503. The nurse administers Phospho-Soda to a client. This cathartic is classified as:
    1. Saline
    2. Emollient
    3. Stimulant
    4. Bulk-forming

504. With the knowledge that a client is accustomed to taking enemas periodically to avoid constipation, the nurse should:
    1. Arrange to have enemas ordered
    2. Have the physician order a daily laxative
    3. Offer the client a large glass of prune juice and warm water each morning
    4. Realize that enemas will be necessary because the normal conditioned reflex has been lost

505. A client with a cerebral vascular accident becomes incontinent of feces. When establishing a bowel training program, the nurse must remember that the most important factor is the:
1. Use of medication to induce elimination
2. Plan to schedule a definite time for attempted evacuations
3. Client's previous habits in the area of diet and use of laxatives
4. Timing of elimination to take advantage of the gastrocolic reflex

506. While helping a client reestablish a regular pattern of defecation, the nurse should base the teaching on the principle that:
1. Inactivity produces muscle atonia
2. The gastrocolic reflex initiates peristalsis
3. Increased fluid promotes ease of evacuation
4. Increased potassium is needed for normal neuromuscular irritability

507. When teaching a client to include more bulk in the diet, the nurse recognizes that the action of bulk to promote defecation is a consequence of the:
1. Irritating effect of fiber on the bowel wall
2. Action of the multiflora of the large intestine
3. Direct chemical stimulation of the colonic musculature
4. Tendency of smooth muscle to contract when stretched

508. Before ligation of hemorrhoids, the nurse should expect the physician will suggest that the client eat a:
1. Bland diet
2. Clear liquid diet
3. High-protein diet
4. Low-residue diet

509. A client with hemorrhoids asks what caused this problem to occur. The nurse explains that it generally results from:
1. Constipation
2. Hypertension
3. Eating spicy foods
4. Poor bowel control

510. A client is scheduled for a hemorrhoidectomy. The nurse should observe the area for the presence of:
1. Pruritus
2. Flatulence
3. Anal stenosis
4. Rectal bleeding

511. Postoperative care for a client who has had a hemorrhoidectomy should include:
1. Occlusive dressings to the area
2. Encouraging showers as needed
3. Administration of stool softeners
4. Administration of enemas to promote defecation

512. A client has been diagnosed as having hepatitis B (HBV). After reviewing the client's health history the nurse, looking for possible situations in which exposure could have occurred, should recognize that the disease was most likely acquired when the client:
1. Had a small tattoo on the arm
2. Helped deliver a baby 2 weeks ago
3. Spent a 2-week vacation in Mexico
4. Attended an ecologic conference in a large urban center

513. A client who is receiving total parenteral nutrition (TPN) complains of nausea, thirst, and a headache. To further assess the situation, the nurse initially should check the client's:
1. Blood glucose
2. Urinary output
3. Blood pressure
4. Oral temperature

514. A bland diet is ordered for a client. When assisting the client with selecting foods from the menu, the nurse should suggest that the client choose:
1. Steamed broccoli
2. Creamed potatoes
3. Raw spinach salad
4. Baked sweet potato

515. A client has severe diarrhea and is extremely dehydrated. The physician orders intravenous therapy, sodium bicarbonate, and an antidiarrheal medication. The nurse is aware that a frequently ordered antidiarrheal drug is:
1. Bisacodyl (Dulcolax)
2. Psyllium (Metamucil)
3. Docusate sodium (Colace)
4. Loperamide HCl (Imodium)

516. A client with hepatitis asks the nurse, "Why don't you give me some medication to help me get rid of this problem?" The nurse's best response would be:
1. "Sedatives can be given to help you relax."
2. "We can give you immune serum globulin."
3. "There are no specific drugs used to treat hepatitis."
4. "Vitamin supplements are frequently helpful and hasten recovery."

517. The nurse has instructed a client with viral hepatitis about the type of diet that should be eaten. The lunch selection that would indicate the client's understanding and compliance with the dietary principles taught is:
    1. Turkey salad, french fries, sherbet
    2. Cheeseburger, taco chips, chocolate pudding
    3. Salad, sliced chicken sandwich, gelatin dessert
    4. Cottage cheese, peanut butter sandwich, milkshake

518. The nurse is reviewing discharge plans with a client who has been hospitalized with hepatitis A. The nurse would recognize that the client understood preventative measures that should be used to reduce the risk of spreading the disease when the client states, "I should:
    1. Wash my hands frequently."
    2. Dispose of my tissues properly."
    3. Launder my clothes separately."
    4. Use sterile dressings and equipment."

519. A 68-year-old female who has a history of arthritis has increased the intake of ibuprofen (Motrin) to try to abate the discomfort. After several weeks on the regimen she becomes increasingly weak and visits her physician. The physician finds she is extremely anemic and admits her to the hospital. When performing an admitting interview, the nurse should expect the client to have a history of:
    1. Constipation
    2. Recent melena
    3. Clay-colored stools
    4. Painful bowel movements

520. An exploratory laparotomy is performed on a client with melena and gastric cancer is discovered. A partial gastrectomy is performed, and a jejunostomy tube is surgically implanted. A nasogastric tube to suction is in place. During the first 24 hours after surgery, the nurse would expect the client's drainage to:

    1. Be green and viscid
    2. Be coffee-ground in nature
    3. Contain some blood and clots
    4. Contain large amounts of frank blood

521. The nurse should teach a client to care for the skin around a colostomy stoma by:
    1. Rinsing the area with peroxide and applying fresh gauze bandages

    2. Applying liberal amounts of petroleum jelly 3 inches around the stoma
    3. Washing with soap and water and then applying a protective ointment or paste

    4. Pouring saline over the stoma and rubbing vigorously to remove hard fecal matter

Endocrine

522. The assessment of a client that would be most indicative of diabetes insipidus is:
    1. Increased blood glucose
    2. Low urinary specific gravity
    3. Elevation of blood pressure
    4. Decreased serum osmolarity

523. To understand diabetes insipidus, the nurse must be aware that an antidiuretic substance important for maintaining fluid balance is released by the:
    1. Adrenal cortex
    2. Adrenal medulla
    3. Anterior pituitary
    4. Posterior pituitary

524. Normally the antidiuretic hormone (ADH) influences kidney function by stimulating the:
    1. Nephron tubules to reabsorb water
    2. Nephron tubules to reabsorb glucose
    3. Glomerulus to withhold the proteins from the urine
    4. Glomerulus to control the quantity of fluid passing through it

525. The administration of corticosteroids to control the symptoms of one disease can cause infections. A rationale that does not support this concept is that corticosteroids:
    1. Prevent the production of leukocytes
    2. Stop antibody production in lymphatic tissue
    3. Promote the growth and spread of enteric viruses
    4. Interfere with the inflammatory response of the body

526. Increased blood concentration of cortisol (hydroxycortisone):
    1. Tends to accelerate wound healing
    2. Blocks gluconeogenesis in the liver
    3. Decreases pituitary secretion of ACTH
    4. Impairs tolerance of stressful situations

527. The nurse knows that most of the hormones present in the body at any given time were secreted from the endocrine glands:
    1. 24 hours ago
    2. 4 to 6 hours ago
    3. 8 to 12 hours ago
    4. More than 72 hours ago

528. Following a head injury a client develops a deficiency of antidiuretic hormone (ADH). Normally secretion of ADH causes:
    1. Serum osmolarity to increase
    2. Urine concentration to decrease
    3. Glomerular filtration to decrease
    4. Tubular reabsorption of water to increase

529. Acromegaly is produced by an oversecretion of:
    1. Testosterone
    2. Growth hormone
    3. Thyroid hormone
    4. Adrenocorticotropin

530. A client who has acromegaly and diabetes mellitus has a hypophysectomy. The nurse recognizes that further teaching about the hypophysectomy is necessary when the client states, "I know I will:
    1. Be sterile for the rest of my life."
    2. Require larger doses of insulin than I did pre-operatively."
    3. Have to take thyroxine or a similar preparation for the rest of my life."
    4. Have to take cortisone or a similar preparation for the rest of my life."

531. Following a hypophysectomy the nurse specifically should observe the client for early signs of:
    1. Urinary retention
    2. Respiratory distress
    3. Bleeding at the suture line
    4. Increased intracranial pressure

532. In an emergency the rapid adjustments made by the body are associated with increased activity of the:
    1. Thyroid gland
    2. Adrenal gland
    3. Pituitary gland
    4. Pancreatic gland

533. A client is scheduled for an adrenalectomy. The nurse should plan to:
    1. Provide a high-protein diet
    2. Administer steroids IM or IV
    3. Collect a 24-hour urine specimen
    4. Withhold all medications for 48 hours

534. A client with Cushing's syndrome may manifest signs of diabetes mellitus because:
    1. The cortical hormones stimulate rapid weight loss
    2. Excessive ACTH secretion damages pancreatic tissue

    3. Tissue catabolism results in a negative nitrogen balance
    4. Glucocorticoids accelerate the process of gluconeogenesis

535. The nurse understands that the cause of Cushing's syndrome is most commonly:
    1. Pituitary hypoplasia
    2. Insufficient ACTH production
    3. Hyperplasia of the adrenal cortex
    4. Deprivation of adrenocortical hormones

536. Glucocorticoids and mineralocorticoids are secreted by the:
    1. Gonads
    2. Pancreas
    3. Adrenal glands
    4. Anterior pituitary

537. When assessing a client with Cushing's syndrome the nurse would expect:
    1. Dehydration and menorrhagia
    2. Buffalo hump and hypertension
    3. Pitting edema and frequent colds
    4. Migraine headaches and dysmenorrhea

538. When assessing a client with Cushing's syndrome, the nurse should expect the client to demonstrate:
    1. Lability of mood
    2. A decrease in the growth of hair
    3. Ectomorphism with a moon face
    4. An increased resistance to bruising

539. In Cushing's syndrome excessive amounts of glucocorticoids and mineralocorticoids will increase the client's:
    1. Urine output
    2. Glucose level
    3. Serum potassium
    4. Immune response

540. A client is to have a bilateral adrenalectomy. Before surgery, steroids are administered to the client. The nurse understands the reason for this is to:
    1. Foster accumulation of glycogen in the liver
    2. Increase the inflammatory action to promote scar formation
    3. Facilitate urinary excretion of salt and water following surgery
    4. Compensate for sudden lack of these hormones following surgery

541. The medication the nurse would expect to administer to a client on the day of a bilateral adrenalectomy and in the immediate postoperative period is:
1. ACTH
2. Regular insulin
3. Pituitary extract (Pituitrin)
4. Hydrocortisone succinate (Solu-Cortef)

542. Until the client is regulated by steroid therapy following an adrenalectomy, the client may show symptoms of:
1. Hypotension
2. Hyperglycemia
3. Sodium retention
4. Potassium excretion

543. A client who has just had an adrenalectomy is told about a death in the family and becomes very upset. After comforting the client, the nurse notifies the physician because the client:
1. Will probably require mild sedation to ensure rest
2. Should have the steroid medication dosage reduced
3. Has a decreased ability to handle stress despite steroid therapy
4. Will have feelings of exhaustion and lethargy as a result of stress

544. A client with Cushing's syndrome is placed on a low-sodium, high-potassium diet because:
1. The use of salt probably contributed to the disease
2. Excess weight will be gained if sodium is not limited
3. The loss of excess salt in the urine requires less renal stimulation
4. Excessive secretions of aldosterone and cortisone cause renal retention of sodium and loss of potassium

545. Hypotension associated with Addison's disease involves a disturbance in the production of:
1. Estrogens
2. Androgens
3. Glucocorticoids
4. Mineralocorticoids

546. The nurse should observe a client with Addison's disease closely for signs of infectious complications because there is a disturbance in:
1. Stress response
2. Respiratory function
3. Electrolyte balances
4. Metabolic processes

547. The emaciation, muscular weakness, and fatigue associated with Addison's disease result from a disturbance in:
1. Fluid balance
2. Electrolyte levels
3. Protein anabolism
4. Masculinizing effects

548. An important nursing intervention specific for a client with Addison's disease is:
1. Encouraging exercise
2. Restricting fluid intake
3. Protecting from exertion
4. Monitoring for hypokalemia

549. Therapy for a client with Addison's disease is aimed chiefly at:
1. Decreasing eosinophils
2. Increasing lymphoid tissue
3. Restoring electrolyte balance
4. Improving carbohydrate metabolism

550. The treatment of a client with Addison's disease includes a high-protein, high-calorie diet with extra salt. As a means of encouraging the client to eat, the nurse explains that:
1. Increased amounts of potassium are needed to replace renal losses
2. Increased protein is needed to heal the adrenal tissue and thus cure the disease
3. Increased vitamins are needed to supply energy to assist in regaining the lost weight
4. Extra salt is needed to replace the amount being lost due to lack of sufficient aldosterone to conserve sodium

551. A client on fludrocortisone therapy for adrenal insufficiency should be taught to consult the physician in the event of:
1. Unpredictable changes in mood
2. Increased frequency of urination
3. Fatigue, particularly in the afternoon
4. Rapid weight gain and dependent edema

552. Glucose is an important molecule in a cell because this molecule is primarily used for:
1. Extraction of energy
2. Synthesis of proteins
3. Building the genetic material
4. Formation of cell membranes

553. The source of glucose for maintaining normal levels when the blood glucose begins to fall is:
    1. Ingested food
    2. Liver glycogen
    3. Gluconeogenesis
    4. Intestinal hydrolysis

554. The fuel glucose is delivered to the cells by the blood for production of energy. The hormone controlling use of glucose by the cell is:
    1. Insulin
    2. Thyroxine
    3. Adrenal steroids
    4. Growth hormone

555. When a client is first admitted with hyperglycemic hyperosmolar nonketotic syndrome (HHNS), the nurse's priority is to provide:
    1. Oxygen
    2. Carbohydrates
    3. Fluid replacement
    4. Dietary instruction

556. Ketone bodies appear in the blood and urine when fats are being oxidized in great amounts. This condition is associated with:
    1. Starvation
    2. Alcoholism
    3. Bone healing
    4. Positive nitrogen balance

557. Oral hypoglycemic agents may be used for clients with:
    1. Ketosis
    2. Obesity
    3. Type 1 diabetes
    4. Some insulin production

558. Diabetic coma results from an excess accumulation in the blood of:
    1. Sodium bicarbonate, causing alkalosis
    2. Ketones from rapid fat breakdown, causing acidosis
    3. Nitrogen from protein catabolism, causing ammonia intoxication
    4. Glucose from rapid carbohydrate metabolism, causing drowsiness

559. The most common cause of diabetic ketoacidosis is:
    1. Emotional stress
    2. Presence of infection
    3. Increased insulin dose
    4. Inadequate food intake

560. The initial treatment of diabetic acidosis will include administration of:
    1. IV fluids
    2. Potassium
    3. NPH insulin
    4. Sodium polystyrene sulfonate (Kayexalate)

561. When a client is in diabetic ketoacidosis the insulin that would be administered is:
    1. Human NPH insulin
    2. Human regular insulin
    3. Insulin lispro injection
    4. Insulin glargine injection

562. A difference between diabetic coma and hyperglycemic hyperosmolar nonketotic syndrome (HHNS) is that clients in diabetic coma experience:
    1. Fluid loss
    2. Glycosuria
    3. Kussmaul respirations
    4. Increased blood glucose

563. A client with untreated type 1 diabetes mellitus may lapse into a coma because of acidosis. This acidosis is directly caused by an increased concentration in the serum of:
    1. Ketones
    2. Glucose
    3. Lactic acid
    4. Glutamic acid

564. A urine specimen for ketones should be removed from a client's retention catheter by:
    1. Disconnecting the catheter and draining it into a clean container
    2. Cleansing the drainage valve and removing it from the catheter bag
    3. Wiping the catheter with alcohol and draining it into a sterile test tube
    4. Using a sterile syringe to remove it from a clamped, cleansed catheter

565. A client has a hypoglycemic reaction to insulin. The assessments that are indicative of this response include:
    1. Pallor, perspiration, tremors
    2. Excessive thirst, dry hot skin
    3. Fruity odor of breath, acetonuria
    4. Anorexia, glycosuria, tachycardia

566. Diabetic acidosis is precipitated by:
    1. Breakdown of fat stores for energy
    2. Ingestion of too many highly acidic foods
    3. Excessive secretion of endogenous insulin
    4. Increased concentrations of cholesterol in the extracellular compartment

567. Of the following factors, the one that would pre-dispose a client to the occurrence of a diabetic ketoacidotic coma is:
    1. Taking too much insulin
    2. Getting too much exercise
    3. Running a fever with the flu
    4. Eating less calories than prescribed

568. Laboratory tests are performed on a client with diabetic ketoacidosis. The nurse should expect the tests to reveal:
    1. Low serum glucose, increased acidity, high carbon dioxide
    2. Low serum glucose, decreased acidity, low carbon dioxide
    3. Elevated serum glucose, normal acidity, high carbon dioxide
    4. Elevated serum glucose, increased acidity, low carbon dioxide

569. The primary use of glucagon is to treat:
    1. Diabetic acidosis
    2. Hyperinsulin secretion
    3. Insulin-induced hypoglycemia
    4. Idiosyncratic reactions to insulin

570. A client's blood gases reflect diabetic acidosis. The nurse should expect:
    1. Increased pH
    2. Decreased Po_2
    3. Increased Pco_2
    4. Decreased HCO_3

571. The nurse knows that glucagon may be given in the treatment of hypoglycemia because it:
    1. Inhibits glycogenesis
    2. Stimulates release of insulin
    3. Increases blood glucose levels
    4. Provides more storage of glucose

572. After administering regular insulin to a client in diabetic ketoacidosis, the IV solution prescribed should eventually contain potassium to replenish potassium ions in the extracellular fluid that are being:
    1. Rapidly lost from the body by copious diaphoresis present during coma
    2. Carried with glucose to the kidneys and excreted in the urine in increased amounts
    3. Quickly used up during the rapid series of catabolic reactions stimulated by insulin and glucose
    4. Moved into the intracellular fluid compartment because of the generalized anabolism induced by insulin and glucose

573. The nursing intervention that should be instituted immediately to relieve the symptoms associated with a client's hypoglycemic reaction include:
    1. Giving 4 oz of fruit juice
    2. Administering 5% dextrose solution IV
    3. Withholding a subsequent dose of insulin
    4. Providing a snack of cheese and dry crackers

574. The best indication that a client with diabetes mellitus is successfully managing the disease after discharge is a:
    1. Reduction in excess body weight
    2. Stabilization of the serum glucose
    3. Demonstrated knowledge of the disease
    4. Compliance with orders for insulin administration

575. The nursing plan includes that before discharge a client with diabetes mellitus will know how to self-administer insulin, adjust the insulin dosage, understand the diet, and test the serum for glucose. The client progresses well and is discharged 5 days following admission. Legally:
    1. The nurse was properly functioning as a health teacher
    2. The visiting nurse should do health teaching in the client's home
    3. A family member also should have been taught to administer the insulin
    4. The physician was responsible and the nurse should have cleared the care with the physician

576. When teaching about diabetes mellitus and diet, it is important that both the client and family understand that the diet for the management of diabetes mellitus:
    1. Should be rigidly controlled to avoid emergencies
    2. Can be planned around a wide variety of commonly used foods
    3. Is based on nutritional requirements that are the same for all clients
    4. Must not include eating any combination dishes and processed foods

577. A client with diabetes mellitus states, "I cannot eat big meals and I prefer to snack throughout the day." The nurse should carefully explain that:
    1. Regulated food intake is basic to control
    2. Salt and sugar restriction is the main concern
    3. Small, frequent meals are better for digestion
    4. Large meals can contribute to a weight problem

578. The nurse plans an evening snack of milk, crackers, and cheese for an average-sized client who is receiving Humulin N insulin. This snack provides:
    1. Encouragement to stay on the diet
    2. Added calories to promote weight gain
    3. Nourishment to counteract late insulin activity
    4. High-carbohydrate nourishment for immediate use

579. An independent nursing action that should be included in the plan of care for a client after an episode of ketoacidosis is:
    1. Observing for signs of hypoglycemia as a result of treatment
    2. Withholding glucose in any form until the ketoacidosis is corrected
    3. Regulating insulin dosage according to the amount of ketones found in the urine
    4. Giving fruit juices, broth, and milk as soon as the client is able to take fluids orally

580. A client with diabetes mellitus has an above-the-knee amputation because of severe peripheral vascular disease. Two days following surgery, when preparing the client for dinner, it is the nurse's primary responsibility to:
    1. Assist the client out of bed into a chair
    2. Check the client's serum glucose level
    3. Place the client in the high-Fowler's position
    4. Ensure that the client's residual limb is elevated

581. The gland that regulates the rate of oxygenation in all the body cells is the:
    1. Thyroid gland
    2. Adrenal gland
    3. Pituitary gland
    4. Pancreatic gland

582. Underproduction of thyroxine produces:
    1. Myxedema
    2. Acromegaly
    3. Graves' disease
    4. Cushing's disease

583. As a result of low levels of T3 and T4 the nurse should expect a client to exhibit:
    1. Irritability
    2. Tachycardia
    3. Cold intolerance
    4. Profuse diaphoresis

584. When assessing a client with hyperthyroidism, the nurse should expect the client to exhibit:
    1. Increased appetite, slow pulse, dry skin
    2. Loss of weight, constipation, listlessness
    3. Nervousness, weight loss, increased appetite
    4. Protruding eyeballs, slow pulse, sluggishness

585. The nurse knows that after radioactive iodine is administered to a client with Graves' disease, the client is:
    1. Not radioactive and can be handled as any other individual
    2. Highly radioactive and should be isolated as much as possible
    3. Mildly radioactive and should be treated with routine safety precautions
    4. Not radioactive but may still transmit some dangerous radiations and must be treated with precautions

586. The nurse, recognizing the need to decrease the size and vascularity of the thyroid gland prior to a thyroidectomy, would expect the physician to order:
    1. Propylthiouracil
    2. Potassium iodide
    3. Potassium permanganate
    4. Liothyronine sodium (Cytomel)

587. To evaluate possible laryngeal nerve injury following a thyroidectomy, the nurse on an hourly basis should:
    1. Ask the client to speak
    2. Ask the client to swallow
    3. Have the client hum a familiar tune
    4. Swab the client's throat to test gag reflex

588. Thyroid crisis (storm) is caused by:
    1. Increased iodine in the blood
    2. Removal of the parathyroid gland
    3. High levels of the hormone triiodothyronine
    4. A rebound increase in metabolism following anesthesia

589. When teaching a client with hyperthyroidism about the diagnostic tests to be done, the nurse should include:
    1. T4 and x-ray films
    2. TSH assay and T3
    3. Thyroglobulin level and Po_2
    4. Protein-bound iodine and SMA

590. The most appropriate diet for a client with Graves' disease would be:
    1. Soft
    2. High-calorie
    3. Low sodium
    4. High-roughage

591. Immediately following a thyroidectomy a client should be monitored for:
    1. Decreased BP
    2. Urinary retention
    3. Signs of restlessness
    4. Signs of respiratory obstruction

592. An accidental removal of the parathyroid glands during a thyroidectomy would cause:
    1. Myxedema
    2. Tetany and death
    3. Hypovolemic shock
    4. Adrenocortical stimulation

593. When a client returns from the postanesthesia care unit following a subtotal thyroidectomy, the nurse should immediately:
    1. Inspect the incision
    2. Instruct the client not to speak
    3. Keep the client supine for 24 hours
    4. Place a tracheostomy set at the bedside

594. On the first postoperative day following a thyroidectomy a client tolerates a full-fluid diet. This is changed to a soft diet on the second postoperative day. The client complains of a sore throat when swallowing. The nurse should:
    1. Reorder the full-fluid diet
    2. Notify the physician immediately
    3. Administer analgesics as prescribed before meals
    4. Provide saline gargles to moisten the mucous membranes

595. The two interbalanced regulatory agents that control overall calcium balance in the body are:
    1. Phosphorus and ACTH
    2. Vitamin A and thyroid hormone
    3. Ascorbic acid and growth hormone
    4. Vitamin D and parathyroid hormone

596. The hormone that tends to decrease calcium concentration in the blood is:
    1. Calcitonin
    2. Aldosterone
    3. Triiodothyronine
    4. Parathyroid hormone

597. Following the removal of the parathyroid glands, calcium is required because the parathyroid hormone tends to:
    1. Decrease blood calcium concentration and relieve tetany
    2. Accelerate bone breakdown with release of calcium into the blood

    3. Increase blood phosphate concentration and decrease calcium levels
    4. Increase calcium absorption into bone and remove calcium from the blood

598. When assessing for complications of hyperparathyroidism, the nurse should monitor the client for:
    1. Tetany
    2. Seizures
    3. Graves' disease
    4. Bone destruction

599. A client is admitted with the diagnosis of primary hyperparathyroidism. The nursing action that should be included in this client's plan of care is the:
    1. Provision of a high-calcium diet
    2. Assurance of a large fluid intake
    3. Institution of seizure precautions
    4. Maintenance of absolute bed rest

Integumentary

600. The temperature of water for a tepid bath should be approximately:
    1. 92° to 94° F
    2. 95° to 97° F
    3. 98° to 100° F
    4. 101° to 103° F

601. Local hot and cold applications transfer temperature to and from the body by:
    1. Radiation
    2. Insulation
    3. Convection
    4. Conduction

602. Cholesterol is important in the human body for:
    1. Blood clotting
    2. Bone formation
    3. Muscle contraction
    4. Cellular membrane structure

603. The client with unresolved edema will most likely develop:
    1. Proteinemia
    2. Contractures
    3. Tissue ischemia
    4. Thrombus formation

604. The darkening of tissue seen in chronic venous insufficiency results from the breakdown of hemoglobin with subsequent formation of:
    1. Heme
    2. Ferric chloride
    3. Ferrous sulfide
    4. Insoluble proteins

605. The nurse realizes that sink faucets in a client's room are considered contaminated because:
    1. They are not in sterile areas
    2. They are opened with dirty hands
    3. Large numbers of people use them
    4. Water encourages bacterial growth

606. The most important aspect of hand washing is:
    1. Time
    2. Soap
    3. Water
    4. Friction

607. A moist sterile dressing placed on a cloth sterile field will be contaminated because of the principle of:
    1. Dialysis
    2. Osmosis
    3. Diffusion
    4. Capillarity

608. When changing a client's postoperative dressing, the nurse is careful not to introduce microorganisms into the surgical incision. This is an example of:
    1. Wound asepsis
    2. Medical asepsis
    3. Surgical asepsis
    4. Concurrent asepsis

609. The nurse is preparing to change a client's dressing. The statement that best explains the basis of surgical asepsis that the nurse will follow in this procedure is:
    1. Keep the area free of microorganisms
    2. Protect self from microorganisms in the wound
    3. Confine the microorganisms to the surgical site
    4. Keep the number of opportunistic microorganisms to a minimum

610. To promote healing of a large surgical incision, a client's physician would most likely order daily doses of
    1. Vitamin A
    2. Mephyton
    3. Ascorbic acid
    4. Vitamin B_{12} complex

611. A disease produced when a *Clostridium* organism enters wounds and produces a toxin causing crepitus is:
    1. Tetanus
    2. Anthrax
    3. Botulism
    4. Gangrene

612. The nurse should assess a client with psoriasis for:
    1. Pruritic lesions
    2. Multiple petechiae
    3. Shiny, scaly lesions
    4. Erythematous macules

613. The nurse should explain to the client with psoriasis that treatment usually involves:
    1. Avoiding exposure to the sun
    2. Topical application of steroids
    3. Potassium permanganate baths
    4. Debridement of necrotic placques

614. When caring for a client with scabies, the nurse should be aware that scabies is:
    1. Highly contagious
    2. A chronic problem
    3. Caused by a fungus
    4. Associated with other allergies

615. The nurse must help the client with pemphigus vulgaris deal with the resulting:
    1. Infertility
    2. Paralysis
    3. Skin lesions
    4. Impaired digestion

616. The assessment that is most indicative of systemic lupus erythematosus (SLE) is:
    1. A butterfly rash
    2. Firm skin fixed to tissue
    3. Muscle mass degeneration
    4. An inflammation of small arteries

617. Although no cause has been determined for scleroderma, it is thought to be caused by:
    1. Autoimmunity
    2. Ocular motility
    3. Increased amino acid metabolism
    4. Defective sebaceous gland formation

618. An elderly client is admitted to the surgical unit from a nursing home for treatment of a pressure ulcer. During the initial physical assessment, the nurse notes that the client is dehydrated and the skin is dry and scaly. The nurse immediately applies emollients to the client's skin and changes the dressing on the pressure ulcer. Legally:
    1. The nurse should have instituted a plan to increase activity
    2. The nurse provided supportive nursing care for the well-being of the client
    3. No treatment should have been instituted for the client until a physician ordered it
    4. Debridement of the pressure ulcer should have been done by the nurse before the dressing was applied

619. An emaciated elderly client develops a large pressure ulcer after refusing to change position for extended periods of time. The family is very upset, blames the nurses, and threatens to sue. The decision in this suit would take into consideration the fact that:
    1. This client should be turned every hour
    2. Nurses are not responsible to the client's family
    3. Pressure ulcers frequently occur in elderly clients
    4. The nurse should uphold the client's right not to be moved

620. The nurse should question clients with basal cell carcinoma about:
    1. Familial tendencies
    2. Their dietary patterns
    3. Their smoking history
    4. Ultraviolet radiation exposure

621. The nurse should assess a client with metastatic melanoma for the presence of:
    1. Oily skin
    2. Nikolsky's sign
    3. Lymphadenopathy
    4. Erythema of the palms

622. The physician suspects that a client with a melanoma also has primary cancerous lesions in the connective tissue. The nurse understands that these lesions are classified as:
    1. Sarcomas
    2. Carcinomas
    3. Collagenomas
    4. Osteoblastomas

623. A client expresses concern about being exposed to radiation therapy because it can cause cancer. When assisting the client to understand the treatment, the nurse should emphasize the:
    1. Dosage of radiation utilized
    2. Extent of the body irradiated
    3. Physical condition of the client
    4. Nutritional environment of the cells

624. When teaching first aid, the nurse should explain that the best first-aid treatment for acid burns on the skin is to flush them with water and then apply a solution of sodium:
    1. Sulfate
    2. Chloride
    3. Hydroxide
    4. Bicarbonate

625. An effective first-aid treatment for an alkali burn is to flush it with water and then with:
    1. A weak acid
    2. A dilute base
    3. A salt solution
    4. An antibiotic solution

626. A client who is to receive radiation therapy for cancer says to the nurse, "My family said I will get a radiation burn." The best response by the nurse would be:
    1. "It will be no worse than a sunburn."
    2. "A localized skin reaction usually occurs."
    3. "Have they had experience with this type of radiation?"
    4. "Daily application of an emollient will prevent the burn."

627. A skin graft that is taken from another portion of a client's own body is known as:
    1. An allograft
    2. A xenograft
    3. An autograft
    4. A homograft

628. A pigskin graft may be applied to burned areas. This graft is known as:
    1. An isograft
    2. An allograft
    3. A homograft
    4. A heterograph

629. The best blood test for the nurse to use to evaluate fluid loss resulting from burns is the:
    1. BUN
    2. Blood pH
    3. Hematocrit
    4. Sedimentation rate

630. When evaluating fluid loss in a burned client, the nurse should recognize that the relationship between body surface area and fluid loss is:
    1. Equal
    2. Unrelated
    3. Inversely related
    4. Directly proportional

631. The medication that the nurse should anticipate administering to a burned client as soon after admission is possible is:
    1. Tetanus toxoid
    2. Gamma globulin
    3. Isoproterenol (Isuprel)
    4. Phytonadione (Aquamephyton)

632. One difficult problem for the nurse to deal with concerning an extensively burned client admitted 3 days ago is:
    1. Severe pain
    2. Maintenance of sterility
    3. Alteration in body image
    4. Frequent dressing changes

633. The condition of an adult with partial-thickness burns over 42% of the body would be considered:
    1. Fair
    2. Poor
    3. Good
    4. Critical

634. A worker is involved in an explosion of a steam pipe and receives a scalding burn to the chest and arms. The burned areas are painful, mottled red, weeping and edematous. These burns would be classified as:
    1. Eschar
    2. Full-thickness burns
    3. Deep partial-thickness burns
    4. Superficial partial-thickness burns

635. During the first few hours after a client is admitted to the burn unit with partial-thickness burns of the trunk and head, the nurse is least concerned with the client developing:
    1. Pain
    2. Leukopenia
    3. Hypovolemia
    4. Laryngeal edema

636. Adequate fluid replacement for a client during the first 24 hours following a burn injury would be indicated by a:

1. Falling CVP readings
2. Urinary output of 15 to 20 ml/hr
3. Slowing of a previously rapid pulse
4. Hematocrit level rising from 50 to 55

637. A client with severe burns is placed on a circulating air bed primarily to:
    1. Increase mobility
    2. Prevent contractures
    3. Limit orthostatic hypotension
    4. Prevent pressure on peripheral blood vessels

638. The nurse should explain to a client whose burns are being treated by the exposure method that:
    1. Bathing will not be permitted
    2. Protective techniques are required
    3. Dressings will be changed every day
    4. Room temperature must be kept at 72° F

639. A severely burned client has been hospitalized for 2 days. Until now recovery has been uneventful, but the client begins to exhibit extreme restlessness. The nurse recognizes that this most likely indicates that the client is developing:
    1. Renal failure
    2. Hypervolemia
    3. Cerebral hypoxia
    4. Metabolic acidosis

640. The most effective first-aid treatment for a client who has been bitten by a raccoon involves:
    1. Administering an antivenin
    2. Maintaining a pressure dressing
    3. Cleansing the wound with soap and water
    4. Applying a tourniquet proximal to the wound

641. The physician performs a colostomy. During the immediate postoperative period nursing care should include:
    1. Withholding all fluids for 72 hours
    2. Limiting fluid intake for several days
    3. Having the client change the colostomy bag
    4. Keeping the skin around the stoma clean and dry

642. The primary nursing diagnosis that is most appropriate for a client with necrotizing fasciitis is:
    1. Deficient fluid volume
    2. Impaired skin integrity
    3. Impaired physical mobility
    4. Impaired urinary elimination

Neuromuscular

643. Coordination of skeletal muscles and equilibrium are controlled by the:
    1. Thalamus
    2. Cerebellum
    3. Hypothalamus
    4. Medulla oblongata

644. Reflex control of respiration occurs in the:
    1. Cerebellum
    2. Hypothalamus
    3. Cerebral cortex
    4. Medulla and pons

645. The nurse should be aware that a common misconception about the autonomic nervous system is that:
    1. Both sympathetic and parasympathetic impulses continually affect most visceral effectors
    2. The autonomic nervous system is regulated by impulses from the hypothalamus and other parts of the brain
    3. Sympathetic impulses stimulate while parasympathetic impulses inhibit the functioning of any visceral effector
    4. Visceral effectors (e.g., cardiac muscle, smooth muscle, glandular epithelial tissue) receive impulses only via autonomic neurons

646. The relay center for sensory impulses is the:
    1. Thalamus
    2. Cerebellum
    3. Hypothalamus
    4. Medulla oblongata

647. Internal organs, such as the bladder and the esophagus, are most directly under the control of the:
    1. Spinal cord
    2. Central nervous system
    3. Peripheral nervous system
    4. Autonomic nervous system

648. Neural impulses travel in one direction because:
    1. Polarization occurs laterally
    2. Axons secrete acetylcholine
    3. Sodium pump does not work in reverse
    4. Cholinesterase acts along the entire axon

649. The terminals of axons supplying skeletal muscle release:
    1. ATP
    2. Epinephrine
    3. Acetylcholine
    4. Cholinesterase

650. An indication of parasympathetic dominance in a client under stress would be:
    1. Constipation
    2. Goose pimples
    3. Excess epinephrine secretion
    4. Increased hydrochloric acid secretion

651. The nurse understands that hemiplegia involves:
    1. Paresis of both lower extremities
    2. Paralysis of one side of the body
    3. Paralysis of both lower extremities
    4. Paresis of upper and lower extremities

652. An overexercised muscle that has an insufficient oxygen supply may become sore from a buildup of:
    1. Acetone
    2. Lactic acid
    3. Butyric acid
    4. Acetoacetic acid

653. Stimulation of the vagus nerve results in:
    1. Tachycardia
    2. Slowing of the heart
    3. Dilation of the bronchioles
    4. Coronary artery vasodilation

654. A feeling of pleasantness or unpleasantness, varying in degree from mild to intense, occurs when sensory impulses reach the:
    1. Thalamus
    2. Basal ganglia
    3. Hypothalamus
    4. Cerebral cortex

655. An arterial anastomosis present at the base of the brain that is important in maintaining the integrity of the cerebral neurons is the:
    1. Volar arch
    2. Circle of Willis
    3. Brachial plexus
    4. Brachiocephalic sinus

656. The medulla has centers for:
    1. Voluntary movement, taste, skin sensations
    2. Control of sexual development, libido, position sense
    3. Fat metabolism, temperature regulation, water balance
    4. Control of breathing, heartbeat, blood vessel diameter

657. A client with a spinal cord injury asks the nurse when walking will be possible. The nurse's reply is based on the knowledge that destroyed nerve fibers in the brain or spinal cord do not regenerate because they lack:
    1. Nuclei
    2. Nissl bodies
    3. A neurilemma
    4. A myelin sheath

658. The fact that a client cannot close the right eye can be explained by nonconduction of:
    1. The 2nd cranial nerve
    2. The 3rd cranial nerve
    3. The 4th cranial nerve
    4. The 7th cranial nerve

659. A client has a dilated right pupil. The nurse understands that this adaptation is related to:
    1. The 2nd cranial nerve
    2. The 3rd cranial nerve
    3. The 4th cranial nerve
    4. The 7th cranial nerve

660. A client's mouth is drawn over to the left. This suggests injury to the:
    1. Left facial nerve
    2. Right facial nerve
    3. Left abducent nerve
    4. Right trigeminal nerve

661. Tendon reflexes, for example, the knee-jerk on the right side of a client's body, are found to be exaggerated. Therefore the nurse is aware that impulses are still being conducted by the:
    1. Basal ganglia
    2. Pyramidal tracts
    3. Upper motoneurons
    4. Anterior horn neurons

662. A physician performs a lumbar puncture. To do this procedure a needle must be inserted into the:
    1. Pia mater
    2. Foramen ovale
    3. Aqueduct of Sylvius
    4. Subarachnoid space

663. Following a cerebrovascular accident a client remains unresponsive to sensory stimulation. The lobe of the cerebral cortex that registers general sensations such as heat, cold, pain, and touch is the:
    1. Frontal lobe
    2. Parietal lobe
    3. Occipital lobe
    4. Temporal lobe

664. A client has a temperature of 99.8° F. This temperature can be converted to:
    1. 36.5° C
    2. 37.0° C
    3. 37.7° C
    4. 38.2° C

665. Cold applications for short periods of time produce:
    1. Local anesthesia
    2. Peripheral vasodilation
    3. Depression of vital signs
    4. Decreased viscosity of blood

666. When caring for an anxious, fearful client an indication of sympathetic nervous system control identifiable by the nurse would be:
    1. Dry skin
    2. Skin pallor
    3. Pulse rate of 60
    4. Constriction of pupils

667. When transporting a client on a stretcher the nurse makes certain that the client's arms do not hang down over the edge. By taking this precaution the nurse prevents injury to the:
    1. Solar plexus
    2. Celiac plexus
    3. Basilar plexus
    4. Brachial plexus

668. A homeless person is brought to the emergency room after prolonged exposure to cold weather. The nurse should assess the client for hypothermia, which would be manifested by:
    1. Stupor
    2. Erythema
    3. Increased anxiety
    4. Rapid respirations

669. A client complains of severe pain 2 days following surgery. The nurse's initial action should be to:
    1. Have the client rest
    2. Take the client's vital signs
    3. Administer the prn analgesic
    4. Determine when the last analgesic was given

670. Impulses initiated by stimulation of pain receptors are conducted by the:
    1. Reticulospinal tracts
    2. Posterior white columns
    3. Lateral spinothalamic tracts
    4. Ventral spinothalamic tracts

671. Electric stimulation by the use of a peripheral nerve implant or dorsal column stimulator is used in intractable pain. The nurse should explain to the client that after surgery:
    1. Tub baths should not be taken
    2. Analgesics will no longer be necessary
    3. The transmitter must be worn externally
    4. The device may interfere with the television remote control

672. A procedure done to relieve intractable pain in the upper torso is a:
    1. Rhizotomy
    2. Rhinotomy
    3. Cordotomy
    4. Chondrectomy

673. Following abdominal surgery a client complains of pain. The first action by the nurse should be to:
    1. Reposition the client
    2. Monitor the vital signs
    3. Administer the ordered analgesic
    4. Determine the characteristics of the pain

674. A client with an inflamed sciatic nerve is to have a conventional transcutaneous electrical nerve stimulation (TENS) device applied to the painful nerve pathway. When operating the TENS unit the nurse should:
    1. Maintain the same dial settings every day
    2. Turn the machine on several times a day for 10 to 20 minutes
    3. Adjust the TENS dial until the client perceives pain relief and comfort
    4. Apply the color-coded electrodes anywhere it is comfortable for the client

675. The nurse assists the physician in performing a lumbar puncture. When pressure is placed on the jugular vein during a lumbar puncture, there is normally a rise in the spinal fluid pressure. This is referred to as:
    1. Homans' sign
    2. Romberg's sign
    3. Chvostek's sign
    4. Queckenstedt's sign

676. To prevent toxoplasmosis, the nurse should instruct clients to avoid:
    1. Contact with cat feces
    2. Working with heavy metals
    3. Ingestion of fresh water fish
    4. Excessive radiation exposure

677. It is most important for the nurse to observe a client with the diagnosis of tetanus for:
    1. Muscular rigidity
    2. Respiratory tract spasms
    3. Restlessness and irritability
    4. Spastic voluntary muscle contractions

678. A characteristic manifestation of rabies includes:
    1. Diarrhea
    2. Memory loss
    3. Urinary stasis
    4. Pharyngeal spasm

679. The nurse is aware that bacteria that produce meningitis may enter the central nervous system via the:
    1. Genitourinary tract
    2. Gastrointestinal tract
    3. Integumentary system
    4. Cranial apertures or sinuses

680. In the postanesthesia care unit the nurse should assess a client who has had a craniotomy for a meningioma and a ventriculoatrial shunt for:
    1. Nausea
    2. Sneezing
    3. Blurred vision
    4. Narrowing pulse pressure

681. The vision cycle in the eye requires vitamin A. Here the vitamin functions as:
    1. An integral part of the retina's pigment called melanin
    2. A part of the rods and cones that controls color blindness
    3. The material in the cornea that prevents cataract formation
    4. A necessary component of rhodopsin (visual purple), which controls light-dark adaptations

682. The nurse is aware that the optic chiasm:
    1. Forms a cavity in which the eyeball is fixed
    2. Receives nerve impulses from the optic tracts
    3. Is a crossing of some optic nerves in the cranial cavity
    4. Is the space posterior to the lens with the consistency of jelly

683. When the ciliary muscles contract they:
    1. Close the eyelids
    2. Cause the pupils to dilate
    3. Focus the lens on near objects
    4. Bring about convergence of both eyes

684. Drugs instilled in the eye are administered by the method known as:
    1. Topical
    2. Injection
    3. Intraocular
    4. Insufflation

685. If a client develops an inflammatory reaction in the eye the drug that will probably be prescribed is:
    1. Cortisone
    2. Neomycin
    3. Nitrofurazone (Furacin)
    4. Acetazolamide (Diamox)

686. The nurse should recognize that further teaching is needed when a client with glaucoma states, "It would be dangerous for me to:
    1. Use any sedatives."
    2. Become constipated."
    3. Use atropine in any form."
    4. Release my emotions by crying."

687. A client with glaucoma should be advised to:
    1. Take laxatives daily
    2. Use eyewashes on a regular basis
    3. Keep an extra supply of eye medication on hand
    4. Have corrective lens prescriptions checked every 3 months

688. When caring for a client with primary closed-angle glaucoma, the nurse should understand that the goal of therapy is:
    1. Dilating the pupil
    2. Resting the eye muscles
    3. Controlling intraocular pressure
    4. Preventing secondary infections

689. The first symptom a client with open-angle glaucoma is most likely to exhibit is:
    1. Constant blurred vision
    2. Sudden attacks of acute pain
    3. Impairment of peripheral vision
    4. A sudden, complete loss of vision

690. A cataract is:
    1. An opacity of the lens
    2. A thin film over the cornea
    3. A crystallinization of the pupil
    4. An increase in the density of the conjunctiva

691. After a client has cataract surgery, the nurse should:
    1. Instruct the client to avoid driving for 2 weeks
    2. Teach the client coughing and deep breathing techniques
    3. Encourage eye exercises to strengthen the ocular musculature
    4. Advise the client to refrain from vigorous brushing of teeth and hair

692. When a client with a detached retina asks about the condition, the nurse should explain that retinal detachment is a:
    1. Consequence of optic-retinal atrophy
    2. Degeneration of the choroid and optic chiasm
    3. Division between the photoreceptor and neural layers of the retina
    4. Separation between the sensory portion of the retina and the pigment layer

693. The goal of surgery for the treatment of a detached retina is to:
    1. Promote growth of new retinal cells
    2. Adhere the sclera to the choroid layer
    3. Graft a healthy piece of retina in place
    4. Create a scar that aids in healing retinal holes

694. The preferred treatment for malignant melanoma of the eye is:
    1. Radiation
    2. Enucleation
    3. Cryosurgery
    4. Chemotherapy

695. The part of the ear that contains the receptors for hearing is the:
    1. Utricle
    2. Cochlea
    3. Middle ear
    4. Tympanic cavity

696. The ear bones that transmit vibrations to the oval window of the cochlea are found in the:
    1. Inner ear
    2. Outer ear
    3. Middle ear
    4. Eustachian tube

697. Nerve deafness would most likely result from an injury or infection that damaged the:
    1. Vagus nerve
    2. Cochlear nerve
    3. Vestibular nerve
    4. Trigeminal nerve

698. A labyrinthectomy can be performed to treat Ménière's syndrome. This procedure results in:
    1. Anosmia
    2. Absence of pain
    3. Reduction of cerumen
    4. Permanent irreversible deafness

699. Otosclerosis is a common cause of conductive hearing loss. With such a partial hearing loss:
1. Stapedectomy is the procedure of choice
2. Hearing aids usually restore some hearing
3. The client is usually unable to hear bass tones
4. Air conduction is more effective than bone conduction

700. A client who complains of tinnitus is describing a symptom that is:
1. Objective
2. Subjective
3. Functional
4. Prodromal

701. Physiologically the middle ear (containing the three ossicles) serves primarily to:
1. Maintain balance
2. Translate sound waves into nerve impulses
3. Amplify the energy of sound waves entering the ear
4. Communicate with the throat via the eustachian tube

702. The nurse should assign a client admitted with delirium tremens to a:
1. One-bed room next to the bathroom
2. One-bed room next to the nurses' station
3. Two-bed room next to the nurses' station
4. Two-bed room at the quiet end of the unit

703. The nurse understands that chlordiazepoxide HCl (Librium) is given to a client experiencing delirium associated with alcohol withdrawal to reduce the client's:
1. Emotional problems
2. Detoxification from alcohol
3. Response to physiologic withdrawal
4. Fluid deficits and electrolyte imbalances

704. The most frequently occurring type of brain tumor is a:
1. Glioma
2. Meningioma
3. Neurofibroma
4. Pituitary adenoma

705. A client is to have a parotidectomy to remove a cancerous lesion. A postoperative complication that may be distressing to the client is:
1. A tracheostomy
2. Frey's syndrome
3. Facial nerve dysfunction
4. An increase in salivation

706. A client who is receiving phenytoin (Dilantin) to control seizures questions the nurse regarding this medication after discharge. The nurse should explain that this medication:
1. Prevents the occurrence of seizures
2. Will probably have to be continued for life
3. Needs to be taken during periods of emotional stress
4. Can usually be stopped after a year's absence of seizures

707. A client with a history of seizures is admitted with a partial occlusion of the left common carotid artery. The client has been taking phenytoin (Dilantin) for 10 years. When planning care for this client it is most important that the nurse:
1. Obtain a history of seizure incidence
2. Place an airway, suction, and restraints at the bedside
3. Ask the client to remove any dentures and eyeglasses
4. Observe the client for increased restlessness and agitation

708. The primary responsibility of a nurse during a client's generalized motor seizure is:
1. Determining if an aura was experienced
2. Inserting a plastic airway between the teeth
3. Clearing the immediate environment for safety
4. Administering the prescribed prn anticonvulsant

709. A client who has a history of seizures is scheduled for an arteriogram at 10 AM and is to have nothing by mouth before the test. The client is scheduled to receive phenytoin (Dilantin) at 9 AM. The nurse should:
1. Omit the 9 AM dose of the drug
2. Give the same dosage of the drug rectally
3. Ask the physician if the drug can be given IV
4. Administer the drug with 30 ml of water at 9 AM

710. Injury to the brain is particularly likely to cause death if it involves the:
1. Pons
2. Medulla
3. Midbrain
4. Thalamus

711. Following head trauma a client complains of hearing ringing noises. The nurse recognizes that this assessment suggests injury of the:
1. Frontal lobe
2. Occipital lobe
3. Sixth cranial nerve (abducent)
4. Eighth cranial nerve (vestibulocochlear)

712. When a client is unconscious, the nurse should expect the person to be unable to:
    1. Hear voices
    2. Control elimination
    3. Move spontaneously
    4. React to painful stimuli

713. A client who has sustained head trauma regains consciousness and is able to move the extremities. This suggests noninvolvement of the:
    1. Parietal lobes
    2. Basal ganglia
    3. Precentral gyrus
    4. Postcentral gyrus

714. A client regains consciousness and has expressive aphasia. As a part of the long-range planning, the nurse should:
    1. Provide positive feedback when the client uses a word correctly
    2. Wait for the client to verbally state needs regardless of how long it may take
    3. Suggest that the client get help at home because the disability is permanent
    4. Help the family to accept the fact that the client cannot participate in verbal communication

715. Soon after being admitted to the hospital for head injuries, a client's temperature rises to 102.2° F (39° C). The nurse recognizes that this suggests injury of the:
    1. Pallidum
    2. Thalamus
    3. Temporal lobe
    4. Hypothalamus

716. When caring for a client who has a possible skull fracture as a result of trauma the nurse should:
    1. Observe the client for signs of brain injury
    2. Check for hemorrhaging from the oral cavity
    3. Elevate the foot of the bed if the client develops symptoms of shock
    4. Observe for symptoms of decreased intracranial pressure and temperature

717. Of the following combinations of symptoms the most indicative of increased intracranial pressure is:
    1. Weak rapid pulse, normal blood pressure, intermittent fever, lethargy
    2. Rapid weak pulse, fall in blood pressure, low temperature, restlessness
    3. Slow bounding pulse, rising blood pressure, elevated temperature, stupor
    4. Slow bounding pulse, fall in blood pressure, temperature below 97° F (36° C), stupor

718. Dexamethasone may be administered to a client after a stroke to:
    1. Improve renal blood flow
    2. Maintain circulatory volume
    3. Reduce intracranial pressure
    4. Prevent the development of thrombi

719. When caring for a client who has sustained a head injury, the nurse should assess for:
    1. Decreased carotid pulses
    2. Bleeding from the oral cavity
    3. Altered level of consciousness
    4. Absence of deep tendon reflexes

720. Two weeks after cranial surgery, a client experiences a change in mental status and is incontinent. Hydrocephalus is suspected. The nurse recognizes that the hydrocephalus is probably related to:
    1. Vasospasm of adjacent cerebral arteries
    2. Ischemic changes in Broca's speech center
    3. Increased production of cerebral spinal fluid
    4. Blocked absorption of fluid from the arachnoid space

721. In the immediate postoperative period the nurse should assess the client for:
    1. Tachycardia
    2. Constricted pupils
    3. Elevated diastolic pressure
    4. Decreased level of consciousness

722. A client has been receiving dexamethasone (Decadron) during the past 3 weeks for control of cerebral edema. The planned effect of the drug is to:
    1. Suppress production of antibodies
    2. Increase elasticity of the ventricle walls
    3. Decreased cerebral capillary permeability
    4. Reduce CSF secretion by the choroid plexus

723. The nurse should be aware that risk factors associated with strokes in the elderly client might include a history of:
    1. Glaucoma
    2. Hypothyroidism
    3. Continuous nervousness
    4. Transient ischemic attacks

724. The nurse is aware that the most common manifestation of a ruptured cerebral aneurysm would be:
    1. Tonic-clonic seizures
    2. Decerebrate posturing
    3. Narrowed pulse pressure
    4. Sudden severe headache

725. A client with a cerebral vascular accident is coma-tose on admission. The nurse would expect this client to:
   1. Exhibit incontinence
   2. Respond with purposeful motions
   3. Have twitching or picking motions
   4. Be unresponsive to painful stimuli

726. One of the primary nursing objectives in a client with a CVA is maintenance of the airway. To achieve this objective the nurse should initially place the client in the:
   1. Prone position
   2. Lateral position
   3. Supine position
   4. Trendelenburg position

727. A client with dysphagia may experience difficulty in:
   1. Writing
   2. Focusing
   3. Swallowing
   4. Understanding

728. A client with a cerebral vascular accident has dysarthria. Initial nursing care requires provision for:
   1. Liquid formula diet
   2. Routine hygienic needs
   3. Prevention of aspiration
   4. Effective communication

729. A client with a cerebral vascular accident has a right hemiplegia. The blood pressure should not be obtained by using this client's right arm because circulatory impairment may:
   1. Produce inaccurate readings
   2. Hinder restoration of function
   3. Precipitate the formation of a thrombus
   4. Cause excessive pressure on the brachial artery

730. Following a cerebral vascular accident a client is confined to bed rest. Forty-eight hours following the CVA the nurse should institute:
   1. Active exercises of all extremities
   2. Passive range-of-motion exercises
   3. Light weight-lifting exercises of the right side
   4. Exercises that would actively capitalize on returning muscle function

731. Urinary retention and overflow, a frequent prob-lem of a client after a stroke, is evidenced by:
   1. Frequent voidings
   2. Oliguria and edema
   3. Continual incontinence
   4. Decreased urine production

732. The nurse would expect a client who has had a cerebral vascular accident involving the right cerebral cortex and cranial nerves and resulting in a left hemiplegia to demonstrate paralysis of the left:
   1. Lower extremity and lower jaw
   2. Arm, left leg, and left side of the face
   3. Arm, left leg, and right side of the face
   4. Upper extremity and left side of the face

733. A client has left hemiplegia. The nurse con-tributes to the client's rehabilitation by:
   1. Beginning active exercises
   2. Making a referral to the physical therapist
   3. Positioning the client to prevent deformity
   4. Not moving the affected arm and leg unless necessary

734. The nurse can best prevent footdrop in a client for whom bed rest has been prescribed by the use of:
   1. Splints
   2. Blocks
   3. Cradles
   4. Sandbags

735. The position of an elderly client with a cerebral vascular accident should be changed at least every:
   1. 2 hours
   2. 3 hours
   3. 4 hours
   4. 6 hours

736. A client with a hemiparesis uses a cane specifi-cally to:
   1. Maintain balance and improve stability
   2. Relieve pressure on weight-bearing joints
   3. Prevent further injury to weakened muscles
   4. Aid in controlling involuntary muscle move-ments

737. For optimum nutrition the nurse may find that a client with a cerebral vascular accident needs assistance with eating. The nurse should:
   1. Request that the client's food be pureed
   2. Feed the client to conserve the client's energy
   3. Have a family member assist the client with each meal
   4. Encourage the client to participate in the feeding process

738. A client is diagnosed as having expressive aphasia. The nurse anticipates that the client will have difficulty with:
    1. Speaking and/or writing
    2. Following specific instructions
    3. Understanding speech and/or writing
    4. Recognizing words for familiar objects

739. As part of the planning of long-term care for a client with expressive aphasia the nurse should:
    1. Help the client accept this disability as permanent
    2. Begin helping the client associate words with physical objects
    3. Wait for the client to verbalize needs regardless of how long it may take
    4. Help family members accept the fact that they cannot verbally communicate with the client

740. When planning nursing care for a client with trigeminal neuralgia (tic douloureux), the nurse should specifically:
    1. Apply iced compresses to the affected area
    2. Be alert to prevent dehydration or starvation
    3. Initiate exercises of the jaw and facial muscles
    4. Emphasize the importance of brushing the teeth

741. The nurse would expect a client with tic douloureux to exhibit:
    1. Multiple petechiae
    2. Unilateral muscle weakness
    3. Excruciating facial and head pain
    4. Uncontrollable tremors of the eyelid

742. To prevent precipitating a painful attack in a client with tic douloureux the nurse should:
    1. Avoid walking swiftly past the client
    2. Keep the client in the prone position
    3. Discontinue oral hygiene temporarily
    4. Massage both sides of the face frequently

743. When developing a teaching plan for a client with trigeminal neuralgia, the nurse should include an explanation that the medication used to treat this disorder is:
    1. Ascorbic acid
    2. Morphine sulfate
    3. Allopurinol (Zyloprim)
    4. Carbamazepine (Tegretol)

744. The nurse would expect a client with trigeminal neuralgia (tic douloureux) to demonstrate:
    1. Prolonged periods of sleep because of anxiety
    2. Hyperactivity because of medications received
    3. Exhaustion and fatigue because of extreme pain
    4. Excessive talkativeness because of anxiety and apprehension

745. To limit triggering the pain associated with trigeminal neuralgia the nurse should instruct the client to:
    1. Drink iced liquids
    2. Avoid oral hygiene
    3. Apply warm compresses
    4. Chew on the unaffected side

746. The nurse should expect a client with an exacerbation of multiple sclerosis to experience:
    1. Double vision
    2. Resting tremors
    3. Flaccid paralysis
    4. Mental retardation

747. A recently hospitalized female client with multiple sclerosis is concerned about her fluctuating physical condition and generalized weakness. The priority nursing intervention for this client would be to:
    1. Have one of her parents stay with her
    2. Space her activities throughout the day
    3. Restrict her activities and encourage bed rest
    4. Teach her the limitations imposed by her disease

748. Clients with myasthenia gravis, Guillain-Barré syndrome, or amyotrophic lateral sclerosis experience:
    1. Progressive deterioration until death
    2. Increased risk of respiratory complications
    3. Deficiencies of essential neurotransmitters
    4. Involuntary twitching of small muscle groups.

749. The incidence of myasthenia gravis is higher in:
    1. Males ages 15 to 35
    2. Children ages 5 to 15
    3. Females ages 20 to 30
    4. Both sexes equally before age 40

750. A client with myasthenia gravis asks the nurse why the disease has occurred. The nurse bases the reply on the knowledge that there is:
    1. A genetic defect in the production of acetylcholine
    2. A reduced amount of neurotransmitter acetylcholine
    3. A decreased number of functioning acetylcholine receptor sites
    4. An inhibition of the enzyme AChE leaving the end plates folded

751. The prognosis for the client with myasthenia gravis is most likely to be:
    1. Excellent with proper treatment
    2. Slowly progressive without remissions
    3. Chronic, with exacerbations and remissions
    4. Poor, with death occurring in a few months

752. During lunch a client with myasthenia gravis who has been prescribed bed rest experiences increased dysphagia. The nurse should:
    1. Call the physician
    2. Administer oxygen
    3. Suction the trachea
    4. Raise the head of the bed

753. Respiratory complications are common in individuals with myasthenia gravis because of:
    1. Narrowed airways
    2. Impaired immunity
    3. Ineffective coughing
    4. Viscosity of secretions

754. A client with myasthenia gravis has been receiving neostigmine (Prostigmin). This drug acts by:
    1. Stimulating the cerebral cortex
    2. Blocking the action of cholinesterase
    3. Replacing deficient neurotransmitters
    4. Accelerating transmission along neural sheaths

755. A client with myasthenia gravis continues to become weaker despite treatment with neostigmine. Edrophonium HCl (Tensilon) is ordered to:
    1. Rule out cholinergic crisis
    2. Promote a synergistic effect
    3. Overcome neostigmine resistance
    4. Confirm the diagnosis of myasthenia

756. Parkinson's disease is caused by:
    1. Disintegration of the myelin sheath
    2. Breakdown of the corpora quadrigemini
    3. Reduced acetylcholine receptors at synapses
    4. Degeneration of the neurons of the basal ganglia

757. When interviewing a client with a tenative diagnosis of Parkinson's disease about the onset of symptoms, the nurse should expect the client to say they occurred:
    1. Suddenly
    2. Overnight
    3. Gradually
    4. Irregularly

758. A female client with the diagnosis of Parkinson's disease asks why she drools. The nurse's best response would be:
    1. "We don't know why this happens."
    2. "There is a paralysis of the throat muscles."
    3. "You have a loss of involuntary movements."
    4. "Muscle rigidity prevents normal swallowing."

759. The nurse would expect a client with Parkinson's disease to exhibit:
    1. A flattened affect
    2. Tonic-clonic seizures
    3. Decreased intelligence
    4. Changes in pain tolerance

760. Levodopa (L Dopa) appears to be useful in treating Parkinson's disease because it can:
    1. Improve myelination of neurons
    2. Increase acetylcholine production
    3. Replace the dopamine in the brain cells
    4. Cause regeneration of injured thalamic cells

761. The most common manifestation of a herniation of a lumbar disc is:
    1. Loss of control of elimination
    2. Pain radiating to the hip and leg
    3. Paralysis of both lower extremities
    4. Overgrowth of tissue on the lower back

762. A client with a herniated nucleus pulposus (HNP) would experience a sudden increase in pain when:
    1. Coughing or sneezing
    2. Sitting on cold surfaces
    3. Standing for extended periods
    4. Lying supine with the knees flexed

763. After microdiscectomy for a herniated lumbar disc the nurse should assess the client for:
    1. Cerebral edema
    2. Spasms of the bladder
    3. Sensory loss in the legs
    4. Pain referred to the flanks

764. After a lumbar laminectomy, the nurse should:
    1. Encourage the client to cough frequently
    2. Logroll the client by utilizing the draw sheet
    3. Assess the client for indications of peritonitis
    4. Instruct the client to bend the knees when turning

765. In contrast to caring for a client with a lumbar laminectomy, when caring for a client with a cervical laminectomy the nurse:
   1. Should maintain the client's head in a flexed position
   2. Has the added responsibility of removing oral secretions
   3. Must keep the client's head at a 45-degree angle from the spine
   4. Should provide range-of-motion exercise early during the postoperative period

766. A nurse finds a victim under the wreckage of a collapsed building. The individual is conscious, breathing satisfactorily, and lying on the back complaining of pain in the back and an inability to move the legs. The nurse should first:
   1. Leave the individual lying on the back with instructions not to move and go seek additional help
   2. Gently raise the individual to a sitting position to see if the pain either diminishes or increases in intensity
   3. Roll the individual onto the abdomen, place a pad under the head, and cover with any material available
   4. Gently lift the individual onto a flat piece of lumber and, using any available transportation, rush to the closest medical institution

767. Following a spinal cord injury the physician indicates that a client is a paraplegic. The family asks the nurse what this means. The nurse explains that:
   1. Upper extremities are paralyzed
   2. Lower extremities are paralyzed
   3. One side of the body is paralyzed
   4. Both lower and upper extremities are paralyzed

768. A client with a spinal cord injury has paraplegia. The nurse recognizes that one major early problem will be:
   1. Bladder control
   2. Nutritional intake
   3. Quadriceps setting
   4. Use of aids for ambulation

769. The nurse should expect the client with a spinal cord injury to have some spasticity of the lower extremities. To prevent the development of contractures, careful consideration must be given to:
   1. Active exercise
   2. Deep massage
   3. Use of a tilt board
   4. Proper positioning

770. A client has paraplegia as a result of a motorcycle accident. Nursing care should include turning the client every 1 to 2 hours primarily to:
   1. Prevent pressure ulcers
   2. Keep the client comfortable
   3. Prevent flexion contractures of the extremities
   4. Improve venous circulation in the lower extremities

771. Following a spinal cord injury a client should be encouraged to drink fluids primarily to prevent:
   1. Dehydration
   2. Skin breakdown
   3. Urinary tract infections
   4. Fluid and electrolyte imbalance

772. A 20-year-old male has injured his neck during a diving accident. He is unresponsive to all stimuli. His vital signs are blood pressure 70/50, pulse 60, and respirations labored. His skin is warm and damp. It is determined that the client has a functional transection of his spinal cord at C7-8 resulting in spinal shock. The nurse would expect to observe:
   1. Spasticity
   2. Incontinence
   3. Flaccid paralysis
   4. Respiratory failure

773. Following a traumatic spinal severance a young client has a great deal of difficulty accepting the paralysis. One day the client has severe leg spasms and says, "My strength is coming back and I will walk again." The nurse's response should be based on the knowledge that:
   1. The nerves are regenerating and motor function is returning
   2. Spinal shock has subsided and the reflexes are now hyperactive
   3. Motor function may be returning now that the edema is subsiding
   4. The client has developed thrombophlebitis and is experiencing pain

774. When a client with a cervical injury complains of a severe headache and nasal congestion, the nurse should assess for:
   1. Suprapubic distention
   2. Increased spinal reflexes
   3. Adventitious breath sounds
   4. A sharp drop in blood pressure

775. A client with quadriplegia is placed on a tilt table daily. Each day the angle of the head of the table is gradually increased. The nurse explains to the client that the tilt table is used to:
    1. Facilitate turning
    2. Prevent pressure sores
    3. Promote hyperextension of the spine
    4. Prevent loss of calcium from the bones

776. The majority of clients with quadriplegia are taught to use adaptive wheelchairs because:
    1. It prepares them for bracing and crutch walking
    2. It assists them in overcoming orthostatic hypotension
    3. They usually are not and never will be functional walkers
    4. They have the strength in the upper extremities for self-propulsion

Skeletal

777. The synovial fluid of the joints minimizes:
    1. Efficiency
    2. Work output
    3. Friction in the joints
    4. Velocity of movements

778. Compact bone is stronger than cancellous bone because of its greater:
    1. Size
    2. Weight
    3. Volume
    4. Density

779. A client with systemic lupus erythematosus questions the nurse as to the source of this disease. The nurse is aware that this is a disease of:
    1. Joints
    2. Bones
    3. Connective tissue
    4. Purine metabolism

780. The risk of osteoporosis is increased when a client:
    1. Receives long-term steroid therapy
    2. Has a history of hypoparathyroidism
    3. Engages in strenuous physical activity
    4. Consumes excessive amounts of estrogen

781. Osteoporosis may be caused by:
    1. Estrogen therapy
    2. Hypoparathyroidism
    3. Prolonged immobility
    4. Excess calcium intake

782. A client with osteoporosis is vulnerable to:
    1. Fatigue fractures
    2. Pathologic fractures
    3. Greenstick fractures
    4. Compound fractures

783. The nurse should encourage a client with osteoporosis to increase the intake of:
    1. Red meat
    2. Soft drinks
    3. Turnip greens
    4. Enriched grains

784. Allopurinol is used to treat gout. The objective of therapy is to:
    1. Increase joint mobility
    2. Decrease synovial swelling
    3. Decrease uric acid production
    4. Prevent crystallization of uric acid

785. One drug that may be prescribed and that has long been known to be of value in the prevention and treatment of acute attacks of gout is:
    1. Colchicine
    2. Hydrocortisone
    3. Ibuprofen (Motrin)
    4. Probenecid (Benemid)

786. Two days after a sprain accompanied by edema the practitioner orders the application of warm compresses. The appropriate temperature range for the compresses should be:
    1. 65° to 79° F (18.0° to 26.1° C)
    2. 80° to 92° F (26.6° to 33.3° C)
    3. 93° to 97° F (34.0° to 36.1° C)
    4. 98° to 105° F (36.6° to 40.5° C)

787. Following a traumatic amputation of a limb, the nursing diagnosis for a client that should receive the lowest priority in the first 24 to 48 hours would be:
    1. Activity intolerance
    2. Ineffective tissue perfusion
    3. Ineffective airway clearance
    4. Deficient knowledge related to stump care

788. To prevent a hip flexion contracture following an amputation of a lower limb the nurse should teach the client to:
    1. Sit in a chair for 30 minutes tid
    2. Lie on the abdomen 30 minutes qid
    3. Turn from side to side every 2 hours
    4. Perform quadriceps muscle setting exercises bid

789. To control edema of the residual limb a week after a client has had an above-the-knee amputation, the nurse should:
    1. Administer the prescribed diuretic
    2. Restrict the client's oral fluid intake
    3. Rewrap the elastic bandage as necessary
    4. Keep the residual limb elevated on a pillow

790. Before ambulation is started, to make walking with crutches easier, the nurse should teach:
    1. Use of the trapeze to strengthen the biceps muscles
    2. The importance of keeping the affected limb in extension and abduction to prevent contractures
    3. Isometric exercises of the hamstring muscles while sitting in a chair until circulatory status is stable
    4. Exercises with or without weights to strengthen the triceps, finger flexors, wrist extensors, and elbow extensors

791. To promote early and efficient ambulation after a client has a midthigh amputation the nurse should:
    1. Keep backrest elevated
    2. Place pillows under the residual limb
    3. Encourage the client to lie on unaffected side
    4. Turn the client to the prone position periodically

792. When a client is allowed to be up after an above-the-knee amputation the nurse should teach the client to:
    1. Keep the hip in extension and alignment
    2. Keep the hip raised with the residual limb elevated
    3. Walk with crutches until the residual limb is completely healed
    4. Lift the shoulder and hip of the affected side when taking a step

793. Rehabilitation of a client scheduled for an amputation should begin:
    1. Before the surgery
    2. During the convalescent phase
    3. On discharge from the hospital
    4. When it is time for a prosthesis

794. Following an above-the-knee amputation of the leg, a client complains of pain in the foot that is no longer there. The nurse understands that phantom limb pain is caused by:

1. Tactile illusions associated with severed blood vessels
2. An unconscious phenomenon to aid with the grieving over the lost body part
3. Hallucinations secondary to emotional symptoms associated with the distress of amputation
4. Sensations in the amputated limb secondary to thalamic localization of stimuli from nerve endings

795. The crutch gait the nurse should teach the client wearing a prosthesis after a single leg amputation is the:
    1. Four-point gait
    2. Three-point gait
    3. Tripod crutch gait
    4. Swing-through crutch gait

796. The principle that the nurse should use when teaching a client the four-point gait is:
    1. Elbows should be maintained in rigid extension
    2. Most of weight should be supported by the axillae
    3. The client must be able to bear weight on both legs
    4. The affected extremity should be kept about 15 cm (6 inches) off the ground

797. Following repair of a fractured shaft of the right femur, a client has been in skeletal traction for 1 week. The client complains of leg discomfort and asks the nurse to release the traction. The nurse's best initial response would be:
    1. "I will remove half of the weights and notify your physician."
    2. "I'll get your pain medication to help relieve your discomfort."
    3. "I have to follow the physician's directions and releasing weights is not ordered."
    4. "I cannot do that because the weights are needed to keep your bone in alignment."

798. A client's leg is set in a long leg cast. Because of the long leg cast, the nurse should observe for signs that indicate compromised circulation such as:
    1. Foul odor
    2. Swelling of the toes
    3. Drainage on the cast
    4. Increased temperature

799. To prepare a client with a long leg cast for crutch walking, the nurse should encourage the client to:
1. Use the trapeze to strengthen the biceps muscles
2. Keep the affected limb in extension and abduction
3. Sit up straight in a chair to develop the back muscles
4. Do exercises in bed to strengthen the upper extremities

800. When a client has paraplegia, the least effective method of preventing contractures of the joints of the lower extremities would be:
1. Changing bed position q2h
2. Maintaining proper bed positions
3. Providing the client with active exercise instructions
4. Passively moving the extremities through ROM several times daily

801. Formation of urinary calculi is a complication that may be encountered by the client with paraplegia. A factor that contributes to this condition is:
1. High fluid intake
2. Inadequate kidney function
3. Increased intake of calcium
4. Accelerated bone demineralization

802. A client who has been immobilized for an extended period questions the need for a tilt table. The nurse explains that the tilt table is used to help:
1. Prevent hypertension
2. Encourage increased activity
3. Encourage circulation to the skin
4. Prevent loss of calcium from long bones

803. A client is placed into a whirlpool tub for range-of-motion exercises. Rehabilitating exercises carried out under water use:
1. Water vapor
2. Water pressure
3. Water temperature
4. Water's buoyant force

804. When assessing a client with a fracture of the neck of the femur, the nurse would expect to find:
1. Adduction with internal rotation
2. Abduction with external rotation
3. Shortening of the affected extremity with external rotation
4. Lengthening of the affected extremity with internal rotation

805. The nurse should explain to a client with a fractured hip that the chief reason for applying traction before surgery is to:
1. Relieve muscle spasm and pain
2. Prevent contractures from developing
3. Keep the client from turning and moving in bed
4. Maintain the limb in a position of external rotation

806. The nurse should know that, following a fracture of the neck of the femur, the desirable position for the limb is:
1. Internal rotation with extension of the knee
2. Internal rotation with flexion of the knee and hip
3. External rotation with flexion of the knee and hip
4. External rotation with extension of the knee and hip

807. Contractures that develop most frequently after fracture of the hip are:
1. Internal rotation with abduction
2. External rotation with abduction
3. Flexion and adduction of the hip with flexion of the knee
4. Hyperextension of the knee joint with foot-drop deformity

808. Aseptic necrosis can occur following a fracture of the head of the femur. The nurse should be aware that this is caused by:
1. Infection at the site of the wound
2. Weight-bearing before fracture is healed
3. Immobilization after reduction of the fracture
4. Loss of blood supply to the head of the femur

809. A frail, eldery client falls and fractures the right hip. To reduce the fracture the client is placed in traction before surgery for a hip pinning. Because the client keeps slipping down in bed, increased countertraction is ordered. The nurse can increase the countertraction by:
1. Elevating the head of the bed
2. Adding more weight to the traction
3. Using a slight Trendelenburg position
4. Tying a chest restraint around the client

810. Intramedullary nailing is used in the treatment of:
1. Slipped epiphysis of the femur
2. Fracture of the shaft of the femur
3. Fracture of the neck of the femur
4. Intertrochanteric fracture of the femur

811. After total hip replacement surgery the nurse should avoid placing the client in the:
    1. Supine position
    2. Lateral position
    3. Orthopneic position
    4. Semi-Fowler's position

812. To prevent circulatory complications after a total hip replacement, the nurse should make sure that the client is:
    1. Turned from side to side q3h
    2. Exercising the ankles and other uninvolved joints
    3. Ambulated as soon as the effects of anesthesia are gone
    4. Permitted to be up in a chair as soon as the effects of anesthesia are gone

813. Nursing care of a client with a fractured hip should include the assessment of pedal pulses. The important characteristics of pedal pulses are:
    1. Contractility and rate
    2. Color of skin and rhythm
    3. Amplitude and symmetry
    4. Local temperature and visible pulsations

814. When monitoring a client for hemorrhage following a total hip replacement, the priority nursing assessment would be:
    1. Checking vital signs q4h
    2. Measuring the girth of the thigh
    3. Examining the bedding under the client
    4. Observing for ecchymosis at the operative site

815. When a client is in the right side-lying position after the insertion of a left hip prosthesis, the nurse ensures that the client has an abduction pillow placed between the thighs and that the entire length of the upper leg is supported. The most important reason for this is to prevent:
    1. Strain on the operative site
    2. Thrombus formation in the leg
    3. Flexion contractures of the hip joint
    4. Skin surfaces from rubbing together

816. When caring for immobilized clients, the nurse should remember to use principles of body mechanics by:
    1. Bending at the waist to provide the power for lifting
    2. Placing the feet apart to increase the stability of the body
    3. Keeping the body straight when lifting to reduce pressure on the abdomen
    4. Relaxing the abdominal muscles and using the extremities to prevent strain

817. When a client with a fractured hip is helped from the bed to a chair after surgery, the nurse encourages the client to bear most of the weight on the unaffected leg before sitting in a chair. This is important because:
    1. There is increased circulation in the lower extremities
    2. This will help maintain strength in the unaffected limb
    3. This is the quickest method of getting the client to and from the bed
    4. This reduces the amount of help necessary to lift the client from the bed to the chair

818. On the first postoperative day following a hip replacement a client asks for assistance onto the bedpan. The nurse should instruct the client to:
    1. Use the elbows and hands to lift the pelvis
    2. Extend both legs and pull on the trapeze to lift the pelvis
    3. Turn gently toward the operative side lifting the pelvis off the bed
    4. Flex the unoperated knee and pull on the trapeze to lift the pelvis

819. When ready to walk with crutches after knee surgery, the client will probably be taught:
    1. Swing-through gait
    2. Two-point crutch walking
    3. Four-point crutch walking
    4. Three-point crutch walking

820. When teaching crutch walking to a client following arthroscopic surgery of the knee, the nurse should instruct the client to place weight on:
    1. The upper arms
    2. The axillary region
    3. Palms of the hands
    4. Both lower extremities

821. In any disaster concerning a number of people, the function that contributes most to saving of lives is sorting, or triage. When determining priority of needs, the people who need immediate care are those with:
    1. Closed fractures of major bones
    2. Partial thickness burns of 10% of the body
    3. Significant penetrating or perforating abdominal wounds
    4. Severe lacerations involving open fractures of major bones

822. Following an open reduction and internal fixation of the hip, the nurse would know that a client understood the discharge teaching when the client states, "I should avoid:
    1. Climbing stairs."
    2. Stretching exercises."
    3. Sitting in a low chair."
    4. Lying prone for over 30 minutes."

823. The primary consideration when caring for a client with rheumatoid arthritis is:
    1. Surgery
    2. Comfort
    3. Education
    4. Motivation

824. The laboratory test that the nurse should refer to in reference to the diagnosis of rheumatoid arthritis is:
    1. Pancreatic lipase
    2. Bence Jones protein
    3. Antinuclear antibody
    4. Alkaline phosphatase

825. To prevent deformities in a client with rheumatoid arthritis, the nurse plans to alternate rest periods with:
    1. Active exercise
    2. Bracing of joints
    3. Passive massage
    4. Isometric exercises

826. A regimen of rest, exercise, and physical therapy is ordered for a client with arthritis. This regimen will:
    1. Prevent arthritic pain
    2. Halt the inflammatory process
    3. Help prevent the crippling effects of the disease
    4. Provide for the return of joint motion after prolonged loss

827. The nurse understands the joints most likely to be involved in a client with osteoarthritis are the:
    1. Hips and knees
    2. Ankles and metatarsals
    3. Fingers and metacarpals
    4. Cervical spine and shoulders

828. A client with rheumatoid arthritis asks the nurse why the physician is going to inject hydrocortisone into the knee joint. The nurse explains that the most important reason for doing this is to:
    1. Relieve pain
    2. Reduce inflammation
    3. Provide physiotherapy
    4. Prevent ankylosis of the joint

829. When planning nursing care for a client with an acute episode of arthritis the nurse should take into consideration the fact that:
    1. Inflammation of the synovial membrane will rarely occur
    2. Bony ankylosis of the joint is irreversible and causes immobility
    3. Complete immobility is desired during the acute phase of inflammation
    4. If redness and swelling of a joint occur, they signify irreversible damage

830. When preparing a teaching plan for a client with osteoarthritis it would be inappropriate for the nurse to include a discussion of:
    1. Heberden's nodes
    2. Degenerative arthritis
    3. Nonankylosing arthritis
    4. Marie-Strümpell disease

831. The nurse should know that a client with rheumatoid arthritis will most often have pain and limited movement of the joints:
    1. When the room is cool
    2. After assistive exercise
    3. In the morning on awakening
    4. When the latex fixation test is positive

832. A client who has intermittently been having painful, swollen knee and wrist joints during the past 3 months is admitted to the hospital for treatment of rheumatoid arthritis. The diet the nurse would expect the physician to order for this client would be:
    1. Salt free and low in fiber
    2. High calorie with low cholesterol
    3. High protein with minimal calcium
    4. Regular diet with vitamins and minerals

833. The medication the nurse would expect to be prescribed to relieve the pain associated with rheumatoid arthritis is:
    1. Xanax, 0.5 mg tid
    2. Aspirin, 0.6 g q4h
    3. Codeine, 30 mg q4h
    4. Meperidine, 30 mg q4h prn

834. To prevent deformities of the knee joints in a client with an exacerbation of arthritis, the nurse should:
    1. Discourage use of the knee joint
    2. Keep the client on a regimen of bed rest
    3. Encourage motion of the joint within limits of pain
    4. Immobilize the joint with pillows for a period of several weeks

835. A client with rheumatoid arthritis has severe pain and swelling of the joints in both hands, Range-of-motion exercises for this client should be:
    1. Passively performed by the nurse
    2. Avoided if any discomfort is present
    3. Preceded by heat or cold application
    4. Gradually increased for aerobic benefits

836. A client with arthritis reports receiving the following dietary suggestions over the years. The recommendation for a daily diet that the nurse should reinforce is the use of:
    1. Wheat germ and yeast
    2. Yogurt and blackstrap molasses
    3. Multiple vitamin supplements in large doses
    4. A variety of meats, fruits, vegetables, milk, cereal grains

837. A client with degenerative arthritis may require a total hip replacement. This surgery is done:
    1. In a laminar airflow room
    2. Using three separate stages
    3. Early in the disease process
    4. With the client in lithotomy position

838. To help prevent further problems with the hands when returning to work as a carpenter, after surgery for carpal tunnel syndrome of the right hand, the client should be instructed to:
    1. Avoid carrying tools with the arms
    2. Learn to hammer with the left hand
    3. Do manual stretching exercises during breaks
    4. Avoid power tools such as cordless screwdrivers

Reproductive and Genitourinary

(For additional questions see Women's Health in Chapter 4, Childbearing and Women's Health)

839. Spermatogenesis occurs:
    1. At the time of puberty
    2. At any time following birth
    3. Immediately following birth
    4. During embryonic development

840. The testes are suspended in the scrotum to:
    1. Protect the sperm from the acidity of urine
    2. Facilitate the passage of sperm through the urethra
    3. Protect the sperm from high abdominal temperatures
    4. Facilitate their maturation during embryonic development

841. The term condylomata acuminata refers to:
    1. Scabies
    2. Herpes zoster
    3. Venereal warts
    4. Cancer of the epididymis

842. Clients who develop general paresis as a complication of syphilis are usually treated with:
    1. Penicillin
    2. Major tranquilizers
    3. Behavior modification
    4. Electroconvulsive therapy

843. The nurse teaches a client that gonorrhea is highly infectious and:
    1. Is easily cured
    2. Occurs very rarely
    3. Can produce sterility
    4. Is limited to the external genitalia

844. When a client is diagnosed as having gonorrhea the nurse should expect the physician to order:
    1. Colistin
    2. Ceftriaxone
    3. Actinomycin
    4. Chloramphenicol

845. The nurse understands that the organism that causes a trichomonal infection is a:
    1. Yeast
    2. Fungus
    3. Protozoan
    4. Spirochete

846. The oral drug that is most likely to be prescribed for treatment of *Trichomonas vaginalis* is:
    1. Penicillin
    2. Gentian violet
    3. Nystatin (Mycostatin)
    4. Metronidazole (Flagyl)

847. When teaching a client how to self-administer a douche, the nurse should instruct the client to direct the douche nozzle toward the:
    1. Left
    2. Right
    3. Sacrum
    4. Umbilicus

848. A female client is very upset with her diagnosis of gonorrhea and asks the nurse, "What can I do to prevent getting another infection in the future?" The nurse is aware that the teaching has been understood when the client states, "My best protection is to:
    1. Douche after every intercourse."
    2. Avoid engaging in sexual behavior."
    3. Insist that my partner use a condom."
    4. Use a spermicidal cream with intercourse."

849. Acute salpingitis is most commonly the result of:
1. Syphilis
2. Abortion
3. Gonorrhea
4. Hydatidiform mole

850. The symptoms observed in a client following radium insertion for cancer of the cervix that are indicative of a radium reaction are:
1. Nausea and vomiting
2. Restlessness and irritability
3. Vaginal discharge and excoriation
4. Pain and elevation of temperature

851. Safety precautions the nurse should employ when radium that had been inserted in the vagina of a client is being removed include:
1. Cleaning radium carefully in ether or alcohol
2. Ensuring that long forceps are available for use
3. Handling the radium carefully wearing foil-lined rubber gloves
4. Charting the date and hour of removal and the total time of treatment

852. The nurse checking the perineum of a client with a radium implant for cervical cancer finds the packing protruding from the vagina. The immediate action to take is to report this situation to the physician at once because the packing:
1. Must be removed
2. Has become radioactive
3. Prevents excessive loss of blood
4. Decreases rectal and bladder trauma

853. When caring for a client who has a radium implant for cancer of the cervix, the nurse should:
1. Restrict visitors to a 10-minute stay
2. Store urine in a lead-lined container
3. Wear a lead apron when giving care
4. Avoid giving IM injections into the gluteal muscle

854. A client has a radium implant for cancer of the cervix. Before discharge the nurse should explain the importance of:
1. Limiting daily fluid intake
2. Continuing a low-residue diet
3. Returning for medical follow-up care
4. Taking daily multivitamin supplements

855. When counseling a client after a vasectomy, the nurse should advise him that:

1. Recanalization of the vas deferens is impossible
2. Some impotency is to be expected for several weeks
3. Unprotected coitus is possible within a week to 10 days
4. It requires at least 15 ejaculations to clear the tract of sperm

856. Torsion of the testes requires immediate surgical correction because:
1. There is no other way to control the pain
2. Irreversible damage occurs after a few hours
3. Swelling is excessive and the testicle may rupture
4. The reduction in testicular blood flow leads to rapid death of sperm

857. With cancer of the prostate it is possible to follow the course of the disease by monitoring the serum level of:
1. Creatinine
2. Blood urea nitrogen
3. Nonprotein nitrogen
4. Prostate-specific antigen

858. A nurse should be aware that benign prostatic hypertrophy (BPH):
1. Is a congenital abnormality
2. Usually becomes malignant
3. Predisposes to hydronephrosis
4. Causes an elevated acid phosphatase

859. A client is diagnosed with herpes genitalis. To prevent cross-contamination the nurse should:
1. Institute droplet precautions
2. Arrange transfer to a private room
3. Wear a gown and gloves when giving direct care
4. Close the door and wear a mask when in the room

860. A client cannot understand how syphilis was contracted because there has been no sexual activity for several days. As part of teaching, the nurse explains that the incubation period for syphilis is about:
1. 72 hours
2. 1 week
3. 2 to 6 weeks
4. 4 months

861. Syphilis is not considered contagious in the:
1. Tertiary stage
2. Primary stage
3. Incubation stage
4. Secondary stage

862. In relation to the public health implications of gonorrhea diagnosed in a 16-year-old, the nurse should be most interested in:
1. Finding the client's contacts
2. Interviewing the client's parents
3. The reasons for the client's promiscuity
4. Instructing the client about birth control measures

863. When teaching a client about the drug therapy for gonorrhea, the nurse should state that it:
1. Cures the infection
2. Prevents complications
3. Controls its transmission
4. Reverses pathologic changes

864. The most important means of maintaining the fluid and electrolyte balance of the body is:
1. Aldosterone
2. The urinary system
3. The respiratory system
4. Antidiuretic hormone (ADH)

865. The reabsorption of water from glomerular filtrate (in the kidney tubules), the flow of water between the intracellular and interstitial compartments, and the exchange of fluid between plasma and interstitial fluid spaces are caused by:
1. Dialysis
2. Osmosis
3. Diffusion
4. Active transport

866. A male client is to have the urethra dilated by the physician. The nurse understands that the structure that encircles the male urethra is the:
1. Epididymis
2. Prostate gland
3. Seminal vesicle
4. Bulbourethral gland

867. When collecting a 24-hour urine specimen, the nurse should:
1. Check if any preservatives need to be added
2. Weigh the client before starting the collection
3. Discard the last voided specimen of the 24-hour period
4. Check the intake and output for the previous 24-hour period

868. A routine urinalysis is ordered for a client. If the specimen cannot be sent immediately to the laboratory, the nurse should:
1. Take no special action
2. Refrigerate the specimen
3. Store on "dirty" side of utility room
4. Discard and collect a new specimen later

869. When a client with a urinary retention catheter in place complains of discomfort in the bladder and urethra, the nurse should first:
1. Notify the physician
2. Milk the tubing gently
3. Check the patency of the catheter
4. Irrigate the catheter with prescribed solutions

870. A client experiences difficulty in voiding after an indwelling urinary catheter is removed. This is probably related to:
1. Fluid imbalances
2. The client's recent sedentary lifestyle
3. An interruption in normal voiding habits
4. Nervous tension following the procedure

871. A client with cancer of the prostate requests the urinal at frequent intervals but either does not void or voids in very small amounts. This is most likely caused by:
1. Edema
2. Dysuria
3. Retention
4. Suppression

872. The nurse can best prevent infection from retention catheters by:
1. Cleansing the perineum
2. Encouraging adequate fluids
3. Irrigating the catheter once daily
4. Cleansing around the meatus periodically

873. When caring for a client with a continuous bladder irrigation, the nurse should:
1. Monitor urinary specific gravity
2. Record urinary output every hour
3. Subtract irrigant from output to determine urine volume
4. Include irrigating solution in any 24-hour urine tests ordered

874. A client has corrective surgery for a bladder laceration. The priority nursing intervention in this client's postoperative period would be:
1. Turning and positioning
2. Range-of-motion exercises
3. Back care three times daily
4. Placing side rails in up position

875. When teaching a female client with recurrent urinary tract infections, the nurse states that women are most susceptible because of:
    1. Inadequate fluid intake
    2. Poor hygienic practices
    3. The length of the urethra
    4. Continuity of the mucous membrane

876. A female has a higher risk of developing cystitis than does a male. This is because of the:
    1. Altered urinary pH
    2. Hormonal secretions
    3. Juxtaposition of the bladder
    4. Proximity of urethra and anus

877. A client in a nursing home is diagnosed with urethritis. Before initiating treatment orders, the nurse should plan to:
    1. Start a 24-hour urine collection
    2. Administer an oil-retention enema
    3. Prepare for urinary catheterization
    4. Obtain a urine specimen for culture and sensitivity

878. When assessing the urine of a client with a urinary tract infection, each specimen of urine should be assessed for:
    1. Clarity
    2. Viscosity
    3. Specific gravity
    4. Sugar and acetone

879. When a client has hematuria, the nurse should observe for:
    1. Diarrhea
    2. Acetone in urine
    3. Symptoms of peritonitis
    4. Gross blood in the urine

880. To prevent recurrent attacks in a client with glomerulonephritis, the nurse should instruct the client to:
    1. Take showers instead of tub baths
    2. Avoid situations that involve physical activity
    3. Continue the same restrictions on fluid intake
    4. Seek early treatment for respiratory infections

881. The immediate objective of nursing care for an overweight, mildly hypertensive client with ureteral colic and hematuria is to decrease:
    1. Pain
    2. Weight
    3. Hematuria
    4. Hypertension

882. When caring for clients with renal calculi, the most important nursing action is to:
    1. Strain all urine
    2. Limit fluids at night
    3. Record blood pressure
    4. Administer analgesics every 3 hours

883. A lithotripsy to break up renal calculi is unsuccessful and nephrolithotomy is performed. A postoperative observation that the nurse should report to the physician would be:
    1. Passage of pink-tinged urine
    2. Intake of 1750 ml in 24 hours
    3. Pink drainage on the dressing
    4. Urine output of 20 to 30 ml per hour

884. A client who is about to have surgery to remove a urinary bladder stone needs education about a:
    1. Cystometry
    2. Cystolithiasis
    3. Cryoextraction
    4. Cystolithectomy

885. On the third postoperative day following a hemi-nephrectomy the nurse notices a large amount of bright red blood coming through the dressing. The nurse should immediately:
    1. Change the dressing
    2. Apply direct pressure
    3. Milk the nephrostomy tube
    4. Note the amount and chart it

886. Diet therapy for renal calculi of calcium phosphate composition would probably be:
    1. Low calcium and phosphorus, acid ash
    2. High calcium and phosphorus, acid ash
    3. Low purine and phosphorus, alkaline ash
    4. High calcium and phosphorus, alkaline ash

887. The pathology report states that a client's urinary calculus is composed of uric acid. The nurse should instruct the client to avoid:
    1. Milk and fruit
    2. Eggs and cheese
    3. Organ meats and extracts
    4. Red meats and vegetables

888. Background knowledge that helps the nurse understand the reasons for a strict 200-mg calcium diet for 3 days with daily urinary calcium tests for a client suspected of having renal calculi is:
  1. Excessive calcium intake has little influence on renal stone formation
  2. The thyroid hormone controls the serum levels of calcium and phosphorus
  3. If calcium excretion is still elevated on the test diet, dietary influences can be ruled out
  4. If calcium excretion is lowered on the test diet, hyperparathyroidism can be identified as the cause of the calculi

889. The diet of choice for a client with renal calculi of calcium oxalate composition would be:
  1. Low in purines, alkaline ash
  2. Low in methionine, acid ash
  3. Low in calcium and oxalate, acid ash
  4. Low in calcium and oxalate, alkaline ash

890. A client has a heminephrectomy and returns from the postanesthesia care unit with a nephrostomy tube and an indwelling catheter. The client's urinary output is 50 ml/hr. The nurse should:
  1. Chart the findings
  2. Encourage oral fluids
  3. Irrigate the nephrostomy tube
  4. Notify the physician immediately

891. A client has been diagnosed as having bladder cancer, and a cystectomy and an ileal conduit are scheduled. Preoperatively, the nurse plans to:
  1. Limit fluid intake for 24 hours
  2. Teach muscle-tightening exercises
  3. Teach the procedure for irrigation of the stoma
  4. Provide cleansing enemas and laxatives as ordered

892. Bladder irritability may follow radiation therapy for cancer of the prostate. A sign of this complication would probably be:
  1. Dysuria
  2. Polyuria
  3. Dribbling
  4. Hematuria

893. The nurse recognizes that the major disadvantage of an ileal conduit is that:
  1. Peristalsis is greatly decreased
  2. Stool continuously oozes from it
  3. Urine continuously drains from it
  4. Absorption of nutrients is diminished

894. After a nephrectomy a client arrives in the postanesthesia unit with a plastic airway in place. When observing the client for signs of hemorrhage, the nurse must be certain to:
  1. Turn the client to observe the dressings
  2. Keep the client's nail beds in view at all times
  3. Observe the client for hemoptysis when suctioning
  4. Report any increase in the client's blood pressure immediately

895. A client has undergone a suprapubic prostatectomy. In addition to a Foley catheter, the nurse should expect the client to have a:
  1. Ureterostomy with gravity drainage
  2. Nephrostomy tube with tidal drainage
  3. Rectal incision and a ureteral catheter
  4. Cystostomy tube and an abdominal incision

896. A client who has just had a suprapubic prostatectomy returns from the postanesthesia care unit and accidentally pulls out the urethral catheter. The nurse should:
  1. Reinsert a new catheter
  2. Notify the physician immediately
  3. Check for bleeding by irrigating the suprapubic tube
  4. Take no immediate action if the suprapubic tube is draining

897. When irrigating an indwelling urinary catheter the nurse should:
  1. Obtain and use sterile equipment
  2. Instill the fluid under high pressure
  3. Warm the solution to body temperature
  4. Aspirate immediately to ensure return flow

898. To obtain an accurate urine output for a client with a continuous bladder irrigation (CBI), the nurse should:
  1. Measure the contents of the bedside drainage bag
  2. Stop the irrigation until the urine output is determined
  3. Subtract the volume of irrigant from the total drainage
  4. Ensure that urine and irrigant drain into two separate bags

899. The nurse understands that metabolic acidosis develops in renal failure as a result of:
1. Inability of renal tubules to secrete hydrogen ions and conserve bicarbonate
2. Inability of renal tubules to reabsorb water to dilute the acid contents of blood
3. Depression of respiratory rate by metabolic wastes causing carbon dioxide retention
4. Impaired glomerular filtration causing retention of sodium and metabolic waste products

900. A client with acute renal failure is to receive a very low-protein diet. This diet is based on the principles that:
1. A high-protein intake ensures an adequate daily supply of all amino acids to compensate for losses
2. Essential and nonessential amino acids are necessary in the diet to supply materials for tissue protein synthesis
3. Urea nitrogen cannot be used to synthesize amino acids in the body, so all the nitrogen for amino acid synthesis must come from the dietary protein
4. If the diet is low in protein and supplies only essential amino acids the reduced amount of metabolic waste products will decrease stress on the kidneys

901. A client with acute renal failure complains of tingling of the fingers and toes and muscle twitching. This is caused by:
1. Acidosis
2. Calcium depletion
3. Potassium retention
4. Sodium chloride depletion

902. A client with acute renal failure becomes confused and irritable. The nurse realizes that this behavior may be caused by:
1. Hyperkalemia
2. Hypernatremia
3. An elevated BUN
4. Limited fluid intake

903. The nurse should monitor a client with chronic renal failure for the occurrence of:
1. Pruritus, impotency, and polyuria
2. Respiratory acidosis, lethargy, and anorexia
3. Glucose intolerance, hypotension, and anemia
4. Azotemia, muscular twitching, and paresthesias

904. A client with chronic renal failure is to be treated with continuous ambulatory peritoneal dialysis (CAPD). The nurse realizes this is done because it:
1. Provides continuous contact of dialyzer and blood to clear toxins by ultrafiltration
2. Exchanges and cleanses blood by correction of electrolytes and excretion of creatinine
3. Decreases the need for immobility of the client because it clears toxins in short intermittent periods
4. Uses the peritoneum as a semipermeable membrane to clear toxins by osmosis and diffusion

905. The purpose of peritoneal dialysis is to:
1. Reestablish kidney function
2. Clean the peritoneal membrane
3. Provide fluid for intracellular spaces
4. Remove toxins and metabolic wastes

906. The main indication for hemodialysis for a client who has chronic renal failure is:
1. Ascites
2. Acidosis
3. Hypertension
4. Hyperkalemia

907. To gain access to a vein and an artery, an external shunt may be used for clients who require hemodialysis. The most serious problem with an external shunt is:
1. Septicemia
2. Clot formation
3. Exsanguination
4. Sclerosis of vessels

908. When caring for a client who has had an arteriovenous shunt inserted for hemodialysis, the nurse should:
1. Cover the entire cannula with an elastic bandage
2. Use strict aseptic technique when giving shunt care
3. Notify the physician if a bruit is heard in the cannula
4. Take the blood pressure every 4 hours from the arm that contains the shunt

909. When assessing a client during peritoneal dialysis, the nurse observes that drainage of the dialysate from the peritoneal cavity has ceased before the required amount has drained out. The nurse should assist the client to:
1. Drink 8 oz of water
2. Turn from side to side
3. Deep breathe and cough
4. Periodically rotate the catheter

910. A client with an invasive carcinoma of the bladder is receiving radiation to the lower abdomen in an attempt to shrink the tumor before surgery. Considering the side effects of radiation the nurse should:
1. Limit the intake of iron and protein
2. Administer enemas to remove sloughing tissue
3. Provide a high-bulk diet to prevent constipation
4. Observe the client's feces for the presence of blood

MEDICAL-SURGICAL NURSING
ANSWERS AND RATIONALES

Emotional Needs Related to Health Problems

1. 1 This statement leaves the way open to learn more about the client's concerns. (2; MR; AS; PS; EH)
  2 This cuts off communication and further discussion is impossible.
  3 Same as answer 2.
  4 Nothing in the statement indicates fear; this response may put the client on the defensive.

2. 1 Because emotional stress can influence the progress of ulcerative colitis, initially the nurse should help the client to explore self-attitudes to aid in better understanding the feelings engendered by the boyfriend's dating others. (2; MR; IM; PS; EH)
  2 Initially the nurse should help the client explore the situation and the feelings it engenders rather than involve the boyfriend.
  3 The client should make the decision about seeing the boyfriend.
  4 Too soon; the client is not ready for a joint counseling session.

3. 3 This is truthful and provides basic information that may prompt recollection of what occurred; it is a good starting point. (2; MR; IM; PS; EH)
  1 This ignores the client's question and tells the client nothing; this avoidance may increase anxiety.
  2 This is too blunt for the initial response to the client's question; the client may not be ready to hear this at this point.
  4 This ignores the client's question; the client has indicated no memory of what happened.

4. 1 A sense of security decreases anxiety and fear, thereby reducing the workload on the heart. (2; CJ; PL; PS; EH)
  2 Although this would be done, the priority is care of the client.
  3 Not always feasible because many progressive care units are not adjacent to the intensive care areas; also, it could promote a feeling of dependency on the critical care unit and actually raise anxiety.

  4 If the client is properly prepared, a sedative should be unnecessary; sedatives are usually not given prophylactically but rather when assessment indicates a need.

5. 2 Open-ended statements provide a milieu in which people can verbalize their problems rather than be placed in a situation of forced response. (1; MR; IM; PS; EH)
  1 This can be threatening to the client, who may not have the answer to these questions.
  3 False reassurance is detrimental to the nurse-client relationship and does not promote communication.
  4 Direct questions do not open or promote communication.

6. 4 The parasympathetic nervous system (a branch of the autonomic nervous system) causes increased GI motility and secretions. The adrenal cortex releases glucocorticoids, which also stimulate the GI tract, increasing the acidity of the secretions. (2; CJ; AN; PS; EH)
  1 They do not affect involuntary muscles of the colon.
  2 Same as answer 1.
  3 The stress function of the pancreas is not directly related to the intestines but is related to glycogen release from the liver. The sympathetic nervous system decreases GI motility.

7. 3 Nurses must actively try to understand their own feelings and prejudices because these will affect the ability to assess a client's behavior objectively. (2; CJ; AS; PS; EH)
  1 Understanding a client's emotional conflict can be accomplished only after dealing with one's own feelings.
  2 The health team members should work together for the benefit of all clients, not just this client.
  4 Information from significant others is beneficial, but only after nurses are able to deal with their own feelings.

8. 2 Clients adapting to illness frequently feel afraid and helpless and strike out at health team members as a way of maintaining control or denying their fear. (2; CJ; AS; PS; EH)

1 There is no evidence that the client denies the existence of a health problem.

3 Although disorders such as cerebral vascular accidents and atherosclerosis, which are associated with hypertension, may lead to cerebral anoxia, there is insufficient evidence to support this conclusion in this situation.

4 Capoten (an antihypertensive) is a renin-angiotensin antagonist that reduces blood pressure and does not cause behavior changes; Xanax reduces anxiety and may cause transient hypotension, not hypertension.

9. 4 The response demonstrates that the nurse cares about the client and will have time for the client's special emotional needs. Such an approach allays anxiety and reduces emotional stress, which is benefical in clients with cardiovascular disease. (1; CJ; IM; PS; EH)

1 This indicates a lack of interest in the client, and interferes with developing an effective nurse-client relationship.

2 This statement does not respond to the client's need and cuts off communication.

3 Same as answer 2.

10. 3 At this time the client is using this behavior as a defense. Quiet acceptance can be an effective interpersonal technique, since it is nonjudgmental. (3; CJ; EV; PS; EH)

1 The nurse may be the target of a broad array of emotions; by focusing on only behaviors that affect the nurse, the full scope of the client's feelings are not considered.

2 During periods of overt hostility, perceptions are altered, making it difficult to evaluate the situation rationally.

4 Withdrawal signifies nonacceptance and rejection.

11. 4 In the stage of acceptance the client frequently detaches the self from the environment and may become indifferent to family members. In addition, the family may take longer to accept the inevitable death than does the client. (3; CJ; PL; PS; EH)

1 Although the family may not understand the anger, dealing with the resultant behavior may serve as a diversion.

2 Denial is often exhibited by both client and family at the same time.

3 During this stage the family is often able to offer emotional support, and sometimes false reassurances, thus fulfilling one of their needs.

12. 4 The nurse's presence communicates concern and provides an opportunity for the client to initiate communication if needed. Silence is an effective interpersonal technique that permits the client to direct the content and extent of verbalizations without the nurse's imposing on the client's privacy. (2; MR; PL; PS; EH)

1 Crying, which is so much a part of depression, usually ceases when the individual reaches acceptance.

2 During acceptance the client may decide not to have visitors, preferring time for personal reflection.

3 Detached from the environment, the client may find the details of various hospital procedures lose significance.

13. 4 Seeking other opinions to disprove the inevitable is a form of denial employed by individuals having illnesses with a poor prognosis. (2; CJ: AS; PS; EH)

1 If the client is crying, the client is aware of the magnitude of the situation and is past the stage of denial.

2 Criticism that is unjust is often characteristic of the stage of anger.

3 This is common during the depression experienced as one moves toward acceptance.

14. 2 Bargaining is one of the stages of dying in which the client promises some type of desirable behavior to postpone the inevitability of death. (1; CJ; AN; PS; EH)

1 Frustration is a subjective experience, a feeling of being thwarted, but not one of the stages of dying.

3 Classified as the fourth stage, depression represents the grief experienced as the individual recognizes the inescapability of fate.

4 Rationalization is a defense mechanism in which attempts are made to justify or explain an unacceptable action or feeling.

15. 3 When an individual reaches the point of being able intellectually and psychologically to accept death, anxiety is reduced and the individual becomes detached from the environment. (3; CJ; AS; PS; EH)

1 Although detached, the client is still concerned and may use this time constructively.
2 Although resigned to death, the individual is not euphoric.
4 At the stage of acceptance, the client is no longer angry or depressed.

16. 4 The client is in acceptance; detachment is a coping mechanism often needed by the client, especially when facing a devastating illness, and should be accepted by the nurse. (1; MR; PL; PS; EH)

1 Ignoring the behavior does not convey a willingness to listen and denies the client's feelings.
2 Coping mechanisms are needed by the client as psychologic protection and must not be taken away until the client is able to replace one for another.
3 The client is past the denial phase and is in acceptance.

17. 3 This promotes an exploration of the client's dilemma; this response encourages further communication. (3; MR; IM; PS; EH)

1 Although this is true, this response is not supportive and abandons the client.
2 It is inappropriate for the nurse to give advice; keeping feelings to self does not promote self-expression.
4 It is inappropriate for the nurse to give advice; the nurse is directing the client to be judgmental.

18. 4 Many people are ashamed or have a distorted body image when they know they have a long-term disorder. (2; CJ; EV; PS; EH)

1 Lapses of memory are not common in diabetes unless advanced vascular changes occur in the brain.
2 Diabetes is not a valid reason for not hiring an individual.
3 This is a judgmental statement; the word "favorable" has individual interpretations.

19. 3 Open communication helps to decrease anxiety. (2; MR; IM; TC; EH)

1 Knowledge itself does not always reduce anxiety.
2 Antibiotics will have no direct effect on the client's anxiety.
4 This is false reassurance.

20. 1 Visits by family members can allay anxiety and consequently reduce emotional stress, an important risk factor in cardiovascular disease. (1; MR; PL; PS; EH)

2 Family, community, or work problems conveyed by phone may cause anxiety; social communications with the family should be permitted.
3 Television programs can cause anxiety or excitement, which would increase the metabolic rate and cardiac output.
4 The client may be disturbed by current news. This would raise the metabolic rate, increasing oxygen demands on the heart.

21. 2 Open communication lines are always important in relieving anxiety and reducing stress, which might interfere with postoperative recovery. (2; MR; IM; PS; EH)

1 This does not acknowledge the client's feelings and therefore does not deal with the source of the anxiety.
3 Learning does not occur when anxiety levels are too high.
4 Reassurances do not allow for open communication and invalidate the emotions experienced by the client.

22. 3 Clients and their families need to maintain honest, open interpersonal contact when a long-term fatal illness is present. (2; MR; PL; PS; EH)

1 The spouse may want to know this, but it will not help meet the general needs of both the client and the spouse.
2 While an understanding of the disease is important, details will not assist the significant other in maintaining an active role in the situation.
4 The spouse should be encouraged to share feelings with the client.

23. 3 There are few physical restraints on activity postoperatively, but the client may have emotional problems resulting from the body image changes. (2; MR; PL; PS; EH)

1 Swimming is not prohibited because water does not harm the stoma.
2 All ADLs cannot be resumed immediately; although independence should be encouraged, many activities require up to 3 months before resumption.
4 No changes in activities are necessary.

24. **1** Recognizes and acknowledges the client's concerns without assuming a specific feeling is involved; allows the client to set the framework for discussion and express self-identified feelings. (2; MR; IM; PS; EH)
 2 This is an assumption by the nurse; the data presented are not specific enough to come to this conclusion.
 3 Avoids the client's concerns and cuts off communication.
 4 Although a true statement, it does not acknowledge the client's concern and cuts off communication.

25. **2** To aid in motivation, the nurse should focus on the positive aspects of the client's progress. (3; CJ; IM; TC; EH)
 1 Short-term attainable goals provide positive reinforcement for the client; goal setting should be done by the client or by the client and the nurse.
 3 This negative reinforcement may result in discouragement.
 4 Having individuals actually perform is more beneficial than telling or showing them what to do.

26. **2** The nurse's positive attitude encourages and motivates the client. (1; CJ; lM; TC; EH)
 1 As many objectives as necessary should be used.
 3 This attitude on the part of the nurse may discourage the client's attempts to attain the highest goals possible.
 4 Same as answer 3.

27. **4** To foster communication and cooperation, family members should be involved in planning and implementing care. (1; MR; IM; PS; EH)
 1 This intervention does not focus on the client's feelings or needs.
 2 The nurse remains responsible; the spouse may promote dependency in the client to satisfy a need to control.
 3 Same as answer 1.

28. **3** Because of the profound effect of paralysis on body image, the nurse should provide the client with an environment that permits exploration of feelings without judgment, punishment, or rejection. (1; CJ; IM; PS; EH)

 1 Attempts to distract the client may be interpreted as denial of the client's feelings and will not resolve the underlying conflict.
 2 This is an important part of nursing care but it is not related to the client's feelings.
 4 Same as answer 2.

29. **2** The nurse should pick up all clues to client anxiety and allow for verbalization. This response recognizes the client's feelings. (1; CJ: IM; PS; EH)
 1 This response negates the client's feelings and presents a negative connotation about the procedure.
 3 This response focuses on the task rather than on the client's feelings.
 4 Same as answer 1.

30. **1** This validates the client's complaint and offers to problem solve with the client. (2; MR; IM; ED; EH)
 2 This response could be frightening.
 3 This suggests that adherence to the prescribed medical regimen is unnecessary.
 4 This is false reassurance.

31. **2** This response reflects and verbalizes the client's feelings in a nonjudgmental way. (1; MR: IM; PS; EH)
 1 The husband did not indicate this; the client's perception is altered by her own feelings.
 3 This demonstrates a lack of acceptance of the client's feelings.
 4 Such feelings are common and need to be verbalized; surgery should not be postponed.

32. **2** Changes in self-image and family role can initiate a grieving process with a variety of emotional responses. (1; CJ; AS; PS; EH)
 1 This cannot be assumed from the situation described unless the client's feelings are elicited.
 3 Same as answer 1.
 4 The ability to cope successfully with an illness varies widely among individuals.

33. **3** This recognizes that the client is upset and by indirect questioning helps facilitate communication. (2; MR; lM; PS; EH)
 1 The client has not verbalized being upset and may be unaware of or unable to verbalize the actual cause of the emotions.
 2 An assumption is being made about the basis for the behavior; this does not focus on the client's feelings.
 4 False reassurance blocks communication.

34. 2 Surgery on the bowel has no direct anatomic or physiologic effect on sexual performance. However, psychologic factors could hamper this function, and the nurse should encourage verbalization. (2; MR; IM; PS; EH)
 1 There is no reason why sexual relationships must be curtailed.
 3 Although it may take several months to resume satisfying sexual relationships, the surgery has no direct physiologic effect.
 4 Although a partner should understand the nature of the surgery, the focus at this time should be on the client.

35. 4 The first action should be to remove the victim from a source of further injury. (2; MR; IM; TC; EH)
 1 Preventing further injury and reestablishing breathing are the priorities.
 2 Breathing is the priority once further injury is avoided.
 3 This wound would be treated after the victim is moved from danger and patency of the airway is verified.

36. 1 People in panic could initiate the panic reaction in those who appear to be in control. (3; CJ: IM; PS; EH)
 2 Comatose individuals will not cause panic in others.
 3 Euphoric individuals would not adversely affect others.
 4 Depressed people will be calm and not affect others.

Growth and Development

37. 3 Accidents are common during young adulthood. (1; CJ; IM; ED; GD)
 1 Kidney dysfunction is not a problem specific to any one stage of growth.
 2 Cardiovascular disease is a common health problem in middle adulthood.
 4 Glaucoma is a common health problem in the older adult.

38. 3 Neurologic aging causes forgetfulness and a slower response time; repetition increases learning. (1; CJ; PL; ED; GD)
 1 This is a general principle applicable to all learning.
 2 Learning occurs but it may take longer.
 4 This is a general principle applicable to all learning.

39. 1 As a result of the normal stresses on the body, the incidence of chronic illness increases in the elderly population. (1; CJ; AN; ED; GD)
 2 Younger individuals have greater physiologic reserves and chronic illnesses are not common.
 3 Same as answer 2.
 4 Same as answer 2.

40. 2 Bones become more fragile with advancing age because of osteoporosis, often associated with lower circulating levels of estrogens or testosterone. (1; CJ; AN; PA; GD)
 1 Carelessness is a characteristic applicable to certain individuals rather than to people within a developmental level.
 3 Although prolonged immobility is associated with bone demineralization, hip fractures also occur in active elderly individuals.
 4 Rheumatoid diseases certainly can affect the skeletal system but do not increase the incidence of hip fractures.

41. 3 This may make an older individual unaware of a serious illness, thermal extremes, or excessive pressure. (2; CJ; PL; TC; GD)
 1 There should be no interference with swallowing in older individuals.
 2 Older individuals tend to feel the cold and rarely complain of the heat.
 4 There is a decreased response to stimuli in the older individual.

42. 3 Generally, female voices have a higher pitch than male voices and the elderly with presbycusis (hearing loss caused by the aging process) have more difficulty hearing these higher-pitched sounds. (2; CJ; AS; PA; GD)
 1 Cerumen becomes drier and harder as a person ages.
 2 There is no greater incidence of tympanic tears caused by the aging process.
 4 The epithelium of the lining of the ear becomes thinner and drier.

Drug-Related Responses

43. 2 Radium atoms are unstable and spontaneously disintegrate. This disintegration produces potentially harmful radiation; lead is a barrier to these radiations. (1; CJ; AN; PA; DR)
 1 Radium is not a heavy substance but an unstable one.
 3 Heat is not produced during spontaneous disintegration; radiation is.
 4 Disintegration of radium occurs in the lead containers.

44. **2** Acetazolamide (Diamox) is a carbonic anhydrase inhibitor that decreases inflow of aqueous humor and controls intraocular pressure in an attack of closed angle glaucoma. (3; CJ; IM; TC; DR)

    1 This diuretic has no effect on the eye.

    3 Same as answer 1.

    4 This strong miotic does not affect the production of aqueous humor.

45. **3** Toxic levels of digitalis overstimulate the vagus nerve, leading to depressed conduction through the AV node (AV block of any degree) as well as SA node depression (sinus bradycardia). In addition, ectopic pacemakers are accelerated leading to multiple premature beats. Such pathologic effects are enhanced by low serum potassium levels from diuretics, vomiting, and nasogastric drainage as well as by chronic arterial hypoxemia and impaired renal function. (2; CJ; AN; TC; DR)

    1 This is true but not specific to the situation described.

    2 Vitamins act as coenzymes.

    4 This is an untrue statement.

46. **2** Methyldopa is associated with acquired hemolytic anemia and should be discontinued to prevent progression and complications. (3; CJ; EV; TC; DR)

    1 This is not associated with red blood cell destruction.

    3 Same as answer 1.

    4 Same as answer 1.

47. **2** Albuterol's sympathomimetic effect causes cardiac stimulation that may cause tachycardia and palpitations. (2; CJ; EV; TC; DR)

    1 Albuterol may cause restlessness, irritability, and tremors, not lethargy.

    3 Albuterol may cause dizziness, not visual disturbances.

    4 Albuterol will cause tachycardia, not bradycardia.

48. **1** Because digoxin slows the heart, the apical pulse should be counted for 1 minute before administration. If the apical rate is below 60 (bradycardia), digoxin should be withheld because its administration could further depress the heart rate. If the heart rate is above 120, digoxin should be withheld because the client may be in digitalis toxicity. (1; CJ; AS; TC; DR)

    2 This is not as accurate as apical pulse; the client may also have an atrial dysrhythmia, which would not be detected with the radial rate alone.

    3 Same as answer 2.

    4 This is the pulse deficit, not an indicator of heart rate.

49. **2** Nitroglycerin tablets are affected by light, heat, and moisture. A loss of potency can occur after 3 months, reducing the drug's effectiveness in relieving pain. A new supply should be obtained routinely. (3; CJ; IM; ED; DR)

    1 This indicates the tablets have retained their potency.

    3 This does not necessarily indicate a loss of potency.

    4 Same as answer 3.

50. **1** Cardiac nitrates relax the smooth muscles of the coronary arteries; so that they dilate and deliver more blood to relieve ischemic pain. (2; CJ; EV; PA; DR)

    2 Although cardiac output may improve because of improved oxygenation of the myocardium, this is not a basis for evaluating the drug's effectiveness.

    3 Although dilation of blood vessels and subsequent drop in BP may occur, this is not the basis for evaluating the drug's effectiveness.

    4 Although superficial vessels dilate, lowering BP and creating a flushed appearance, this is not a basis for evaluating the drug's effectiveness.

51. **2** Warfarin depresses prothrombin activity and inhibits the formation of several of the clotting factors by the liver. Its antagonist is vitamin K, which is involved in prothrombin formation. (3; CJ; PL; TC; DR)

    1 Heparin is an anticoagulant.

    3 Protamine sulfate is the antidote for heparin overdose.

    4 Imferon is an iron supplement, not an antidote for warfarin.

MEDICAL-SURGICAL ANSWERS

52. **1** The presence of excess sodium (a solute) in the nephric tubules effectively decreases the water concentration of the glomerular filtrate and urine; water passively diffuses (osmosis) from the kidney tubule cells into the urine to equalize the water concentration. (2; CJ; AN; PA; DR)

    2 Diffusion is not specific to fluid; osmosis is.

    3 Filtration refers to solutes; none are being passed.

    4 Active transport requires energy; water is passively diffused from the tubule cells to the urine.

53. **3** Hydrochlorothiazide (hydroDIURIL) inhibits sodium reabsorption in the nephron causing an increased excretion of sodium and chloride. (2; MR; IM; ED; DR)

    1 Osmotic diuretics affect the glomerular filtration rate.

    2 Most diuretics cause loss of potassium; however, potassium-sparing diuretics, such as spironolactone, decrease this loss.

    4 Loop diuretics (e.g., furosemide, ethacrynic acid) inhibit the reabsorption of sodium and chloride at the ascending loop of Henle.

54. **3** Prazosin blocks the response to norepinephrine bound to alpha-adrenergic receptors relaxing smooth muscle in peripheral vessels, increasing circulation and decreasing blood pressure. (3; MR; AN; ED; DR)

    1 This is not an action of prazosin.

    2 Same as answer 1.

    4 Prazosin does not affect adrenal release of epinephrine.

55. **1** Because propranolol (Inderal) competes with catecholamines at the beta-adrenergic receptor sites, the normal increase in heart rate and contractility in response to exercise does not occur. This, combined with the drug's hypotensive effect, may lead to dizziness. (3; MR; EV; TC; DR)

    2 This drug does not increase the heart rate, but may cause bradycardia.

    3 This is not a side effect of this drug.

    4 Same as answer 3.

56. **3** Because furosemide (Lasix) and aspirin compete for the same renal excretory sites, salicylate toxicity may occur even with lower dosages. (3; MR; AN; PA; DR)

    1 Aspirin does not affect the metabolism of Lasix.

    2 This response does not take into account the other drug that the client is receiving.

    4 Although furosemide has a hyperuricemic effect similar to that of the thiazide diuretics, it is not potentiated by aspirin.

57. **3** Nitroglycerine is sensitive to light and moisture and must be stored in a dark airtight container. (2; MR; IM; ED; DR)

    1 This medication is usually taken prn. The daily number may be as high as 12 to 15 tablets; if more than three are necessary in a 15-minute period, the doctor should be notified.

    2 This may be an expected side effect and the medication should not be discontinued.

    4 These signs indicate the physician may need to be notified and the dosage may need to be decreased.

58. **4** Vasopressin is the drug of choice for ventricular fibrillation, according to the American Heart Association Advanced Cardiac Life Support (ACLS) guidelines, because it improves the heart's response to defibrillation. (3; CJ; PL; TC; DR)

    1 Lidocaine HCl is used after vasopressin has been administered.

    2 Dopamine HCl is not a first line drug of choice in the management of ventricular fibrillation.

    3 Sodium bicarbonate use is based on blood gas confirmation of the presence of acidosis.

59. **4** Captopril (Capoten) is an antihypertensive because it inhibits conversion of angiotensin I to angiotensin II. (1; CJ; IM; ED; DR)

    1 Capoten is an antihypertensive, not a diuretic; diuretics produce fluid excretion.

    2 Capoten is an antihypertensive, not a hypnotic; hypnotics promote sleep.

    3 Capoten is an antihypertensive, not a tranquilizer; tranquilizers reduce muscle tension and anxiety.

60. **4** Therapeutic doses of diazepam (Valium) are 2 to 10 mg two to four times daily; 50 mg would be an excessive dose. (2; CJ; EV; TC; DR)

    1 The ordered dose is excessive and the order must be questioned; although rapid intravenous injection of diazepam can cause transient hypotension and bradycardia, these usually do not occur with oral doses.

    2 Same as answer 1.

    3 The ordered dose is excessive and should not be given either before or after ventilation of feelings.

61. **4** Antiemetics should be administered prophylactically to decrease nausea and enhance appetite. (2; CJ; PL; TC; DR)
   1 The diet should provide maximum protein and carbohydrates to meet demands related to restoration of body cells and energy.
   2 This would do nothing to alter the client's nutritional status.
   3 Small frequent feedings are more appropriate because they are best tolerated by the individual on chemotherapy.

62. **1** Visual disturbances are a sign of toxicity because retinopathy can occur with this drug. (2; MR; EV; PA; DR)
   2 This is not a sign of toxicity.
   3 Same as answer 2.
   4 Although this may be a side effect, it is not a sign of toxicity

63. **1** Toxic levels of Lanoxin stimulate the medullary chemoreceptor trigger zone, resulting in nausea and subsequent anorexia. (2; CJ; EV; TC; DR)
   2 The therapeutic effect of Lasix is increased urinary output with a reduction in blood pressure.
   3 Adverse effects of Aldactone include diarrhea, rash, pruritus, and hyperkalemia.
   4 The therapeutic effects of Inderal are to limit dysrhythmias and hypertension; nausea and vomiting are not therapeutic effects.

64. **2** Most chemotherapeutic agents interfere with mitosis. The bone marrow consists of rapidly dividing cells, and therefore its activity is depressed. (1; CJ; EV; TC; DR)
   1 Because of bone marrow depression, leukopenia rather than leukocytosis can occur.
   3 The ESR generally increases in the presence of tissue inflammation or necrosis.
   4 If bleeding occurs, the hemoglobin and hematocrit may be decreased because of the decreased number of RBCs.

65. **3** In addition to GI disturbances, visual disturbances such as blurred vision may be evidence of digitalis toxicity. Heart rates over 120 may also indicate toxicity. (2; MR; EV TC; DR)
   1 This is not a symptom of digitalis toxicity.
   2 Same as answer 1.
   4 Same as answer 1.

66. **4** Compliance with the prescribed regimen, which includes taking the drug and having values determined by the laboratory, is necessary for safe and effective warfarin sodium (Coumadin) therapy. The dosage of Coumadin is adjusted according to INR results; if the client fails to take the drug as prescribed, the tests are not reliable in monitoring the response to therapy. (1; CJ; EV; TC; DR)
   1 Although some medications can affect the absorption or metabolism of Coumadin and also should be investigated, this is less likely to be a cause of fluctuations in laboratory values.
   2 This does not affect the absorption of Coumadin.
   3 Same as answer 2.

67. **4** Warfarin anticoagulants are administered orally and take 2 or 3 days to achieve the desired effect on INR. Heparin, which must be administered parenterally, has immediate effects. (3; CJ; PL; TC; DR)
   1 These drugs do not dissolve clots already present.
   2 Because each drug affects a different part of the coagulation mechanism, dosages must be adjusted separately.
   3 This does not account for the reason for the administration of both drugs, because warfarin derivatives will not exert an immediate therapeutic effect.

68. **1** Warfarin derivatives cause an increase in the prothrombin time and INR, leading to an increased risk of bleeding. Any abnormal or excessive bleeding must be reported, because it may indicate toxic levels of the drug. (2; MR; EV; ED; DR)
   2 Edema is not caused by bleeding.
   3 This would not be caused by Coumadin.
   4 TIAs are not caused by bleeding, which is the primary concern in clients receiving anticoagulants.

69. **2** Aspirin can cause a decreased platelet aggregation, increasing the risk of undesired bleeding that may occur with administration of anticoagulants. (1; CJ; AN; TC; DR)
   1 Ferrous sulfate does not affect Coumadin; it is used for RBC development.
   3 Isoxsuprine hydrochloride is a vasodilator; it does not affect bleeding.
   4 Chlorpromazine is a neuroleptic; it does not affect bleeding.

MEDICAL-SURGICAL ANSWERS

70. **3** Barbiturates decrease the body's response to warfarin sodium (Coumadin). As a result there is less suppression of prothrombin; when inhibition caused by barbiturates disappears, hemorrhage can occur. (3; MR; IM; ED; DR)

1 Serious withdrawal symptoms are unlikely in this situation; however, indiscriminate use of the drug should be avoided.

2 Although true, stopping the barbiturate at this time can lead to hemorrhage.

4 Sleeping medications are not used to control seizures, although barbiturates such as phenobarbital may be prescribed for this purpose three or four times a day.

71. **3** INH (isoniazid) often leads to pyridoxine (vitamin B_6) deficiency because it competes with the vitamin for the same enzyme. This is most often manifested by peripheral neuritis, which can be controlled by regular administration of vitamin B_6 (2; CJ; AN; PA; DR)

1 Pyridoxine does not enhance the effect of INH.

2 Vitamin B_6 does not improve immunological status.

4 Pyridoxine does not destroy organisms.

72. **2** Isoproterenol stimulates the beta receptors of the sympathetic nervous system, causing bronchodilation and increased rate and strength of cardiac contractions. (2; CJ; IM; PA; DR)

1 Barbiturates and hypnotics produce sedation.

3 Antihypertensives and diuretics help decrease blood pressure.

4 This is not the action of Isuprel; expectorants mobilize respiratory secretions.

73. **4** Used for its analgesic effects, morphine is a CNS depressant. Its major adverse effect is respiratory depression. It can also cause lethargy, pupillary constriction, depressed reflexes, and it could lead to coma and death. (2; CJ; EV; TC; DR)

1 These symptoms occur to some extent with therapeutic doses because of their effect on the CNS; however, they are not symptoms of an overdose.

2 Overdose causes miosis rather than dilated pupils.

3 Although diaphoresis may accompany hypotension, it is only indirectly related to the drug and is not profuse.

74. **4** Meperidine hydrochloride is the generic name for Demerol. (1; CJ; AN; TC; DR)

1 Naloxone is the generic name for Narcan.

2 Propoxyphene hydrochloride is the generic name for Darvon.

3 Glutethimide is the generic name for Doriden.

75. **2** The exact mode of action of morphine sulfate is unknown. However, it has a rapid onset, lowers blood pressure, decreases pulmonary reflexes, and produces sedation. (3; CJ; AN; TC; DR)

1 Chloral hydrate is a hypnotic but is not appropriate for the acute situation described.

3 Hydroxyzine hydrochloride is generally used to control anxiety associated with less acute situations.

4 Phenobarbital has a slower onset than morphine and does not affect respirations and blood pressure to the same extent as morphine.

76. **2** Valium is a tranquilizer and anticonvulsant used to relax smooth muscles during seizures. (2; CJ; EV; ED; DR)

1 This is not an effect of Valium.

3 Same as answer 1.

4 Same as answer 1.

77. **2** Alprazolam (Xanax) is an anxiolytic. It promotes muscle relaxation, reducing anxiety and facilitating rest. (2; CJ; EV; TC; DR)

1 Drowsiness is a side effect of Xanax, caused by its depression of central nervous system activity.

3 One of the possible adverse reactions to Xanax is hostility.

4 Transient hypotension is a side effect of Xanax.

78. **4** Levodopa is the metabolic precursor of dopamine. It reduces sympathetic outflow by limiting vasoconstriction, which may result in orthostatic hypotension. (2; CJ; EV; TC; DR)

1 Levodopa should be administered with food to minimize gastric irritation.

2 Although periodic tests to evaluate hepatic, renal, and cardiovascular status are required for prolonged therapy, whether these tests should be done on a weekly basis has not been established.

3 Levodopa may produce either symptom, but no established pattern of such responses exists.

79. **1** Gingival hyperplasia is an adverse effect of long-term phenytoin (Dilantin) therapy. The incidence can be decreased by maintaining therapeutic blood levels and meticulous oral hygiene. (3; MR; PL; ED; DR)
   2 Alkalinity is not related to Dilantin or to the gingival hyperplasia caused by Dilantin. The incidence can be decreased by meticulous oral hygiene.
   3 These are not a direct effect of Dilantin.
   4 Plaque and bacterial growth at the gum line are unrelated to Dilantin or to the hyperplasia caused by it. The incidence can be decreased by meticulous oral hygiene.

80. **4** Tensilon, an anticholinesterase drug, causes temporary relief of symptoms of myasthenia gravis in clients who have the disease and is therefore an effective diagnostic aid. (2; CJ; EV; TC; DR)
   1 There is a decrease in symptoms.
   2 Consciousness is not affected.
   3 Hypotension may occur.

81. **2** Warfarin sodium (Coumadin) has been shown to inhibit the metabolism of phenytoin (Dilantin), which results in an accumulation of this drug in the body. (2; CJ; AN; TC; DR)
   1 By potentiating the anticoagulant, phenytoin decreases clotting potential.
   3 This is true only if the client is receiving phenytoin to control the seizure disorder.
   4 They do not have a significant effect on the metabolism of Coumadin.

82. **1** Phenobarbital depresses the CNS, particularly the motor cortex, producing side effects such as lethargy, loss of appetite, depression, and vertigo. (2; MR; EV; ED; DR)
   2 These are not side effects of phenobarbital.
   3 Same as answer 2.
   4 Same as answer 2.

83. **4** Phenytoin inhibits folic acid absorption and potentiates effects of folic acid antagonists. Folic acid is helpful in correcting certain anemias that can result from administration of phenytoin. (Dosage must be carefully adjusted because folic acid diminishes the effects of phenytoin.) (3; CJ; AN; TC; DR)
   1 Although folic acid plays a role in the formation of heme in hemoglobin, its prescription in this case is related to Dilantin.

   2 This situation does not provide data to arrive at this conclusion.
   3 Neurologic side effects include an elevation of the excitability threshold of neurons; neuropathy is not prevented by folic acid.

84. **3** The primary site of action is the motor cortex, where seizure activity is limited by maintaining the sodium ion gradient of neurons. (2; CJ; AN; TC; DR)
   1 This incorrectly describes the pharmacologic action of Dilantin.
   2 Same as answer 1.
   4 Same as answer 1.

85. **1** Carbamazepine (Tegretol) is administered to control pain by reducing the transmission of nerve impulses in clients with trigeminal neuralgia. (2; CJ; EV; PA; DR)
   2 Liver function is monitored to detect an adverse reaction to carbamazepine, not to determine therapeutic effectiveness.
   3 This medication is not given to influence cardiac output.
   4 Tegretol is not administered to clients with tic douloureux for its anticonvulsant properties because seizures are not present with this disorder.

86. **4** Calculate the dosage by using ratio and proportion.
   $$5 \text{ g} : 10 \text{ ml} = 2.5 \text{ g} : x \text{ ml}$$
   $$5x = 25$$
   $$x = 5 \text{ ml} \quad (2; \text{CJ; AN; TC; DR})$$
   1 This dose is too small.
   2 Same as answer 1.
   3 Same as answer 1.

87. **3** Mafenide (Sulfamylon) interferes with the kidneys' role in hydrogen ion excretion, resulting in metabolic acidosis. (3; CJ; EV; PA; DR)
   1 Curling's ulcer does not occur as an adverse effect of this drug.
   2 Renal shutdown does not occur as an adverse effect of this drug.
   4 Hemolysis of RBCs does not occur as an adverse effect of this drug.

88. **4** $\dfrac{1000 \text{ ml} \times 20 \text{ gtt per ml}}{8 \text{ hr} \times 60 \text{ min}} = \dfrac{20,000}{480}$
   = 42 drops/min
   (1; CJ; AN; TC; DR)
   1 This rate would be too slow.
   2 Same as answer 1.
   3 Same as answer 1.

MEDICAL-SURGICAL ANSWERS

89. **1** Signs of cinchonism, such as deafness, tinnitus, headache, dizziness, and nausea, indicate that toxicity caused by excessive quinine has occurred. (3; CJ; EV; TC; DR)

2 Paresthesias do not occur with quinine.

3 Dyspnea does not occur with quinine

4 Painful swollen joints do not occur with quinine.

90. **2** Quinine administered orally can cause gastric irritation, resulting in nausea and vomiting. By administering such a medication immediately after meals the nurse minimizes its irritating effect. (3; CJ; IM; TC; DR)

1 Absorption of the drug is not significantly affected by administration after meals.

3 The appetite is not affected by this drug as long as gastric irritation is avoided.

4 Quinidine sulfate or gluconate, not quinine, is given for its antidysrhythmic effect.

91. **3** Potassium iodide, which aids in decreasing the vascularity of the thyroid gland, decreases the risk of hemorrhage. (2; CJ; IM; PA; DR)

1 Thyroid hormone substitutes will regulate the body's metabolism.

2 Calcium is needed to maintain parathyroid function.

4 Radioactive iodine, not potassium iodide, ablates thyroid tissues.

92. **4** Antacids interfere with absorption of drugs such as anticholinergics, barbiturates; tetracycline, and digoxin. (2; MR; PL; ED; DR)

1 This is false; antacids should be given 1 or 2 hours after meals and at bedtime.

2 Liquid antacids are faster in onset of action.

3 They may be taken as frequently as every 1 to 2 hours without adverse effects.

93. **4** Septra blocks two consecutive steps in bacterial synthesis of essential nucleic acids and protein. (1; CJ; AN; TC; DR)

1 Septra is an antiinfective, not an antiseptic.

2 Septra is an antiinfective, not an analgesic.

3 Septra is an antiinfective; it does not inhibit the reabsorption of uric acid

94. **3** Any product containing aluminum, magnesium, or calcium ions should not be taken in the hours before or after an oral dose, because it decreases absorption by as much as 25% to 50%. (3; CJ; IM; TC; DR)

1 Food interferes with absorption; it should be given 1 hour before or 2 hours after meals or snacks.

2 Citrus juice has no influence on this drug.

4 Antacids will interfere with absorption of this drug.

95. **3** Diphenhydramine hydrochloride (Benadryl), like other antihistamines, competes with histamine at receptor sites. This alleviates the effects of histamine, which include increased dilation and permeability of capillaries (the cause of urticaria). (2; CJ; IM; TC; DR)

1 Benadryl does not destroy histamine; it competes with histamine at receptor sites.

2 Benadryl does not cause these responses; histamine dilates capillaries.

4 Benadryl does not metabolize histamines.

96. **3** Hydrocortisone is a glucocorticoid that has antiinflammatory action and aids in metabolism of carbohydrate, fat, and protein, causing elevation of blood sugar. Thus it enables the body to adapt to stress. (2; CJ; EV; TC; DR)

1 Potassium salts are retained in Addison's disease.

2 Cardiac dysrhythmias are caused by electrolyte imbalances, and dyspnea is caused by hypovolemia and decreased O_2 supply; neither is affected by hydrocortisone.

4 Lack of angiotensin II is not the cause of hypotension in this disorder.

97. **4** DDAVP replaces the ADH, facilitating reabsorption of water and consequent return of normal urine output and thirst. (2; CJ; EV; TC; DR)

1 Although a correction of tachycardia is consistent with correction of dehydration, the client is not dehydrated if the fluid intake is adequate.

2 DDAVP does not alter serum glucose; diabetes mellitus, not diabetes insipidus, results in hyperglycemia.

3 The mechanisms that regulate pH are not affected.

98. **2** Diarrhea is a possible side effect that can be related to a superinfection; it can lead to fluid and electrolyte imbalance. (2; MR; IM; ED; DR)

1 Ampicillin is best absorbed when taken on an empty stomach with water.

3 Although storage in a tight container is necessary, protection from light is not.

4 A culture is generally not repeated unless the client's condition warrants it.

99. **1** To prevent crystal formation, the client should have sufficient intake to produce 1000 to 1500 ml of urine daily while taking this drug. (2; MR; IM; TC; DR)
   2 Straining urine is not indicated when a client is taking a urinary antiinfective.
   3 Urinary decrease is of concern, because it may indicate renal failure. If fluids are encouraged, the client's output should increase.
   4 The drug need not be taken at a strict time daily.

100. **2** Salicylates can cause ototoxicity as well as central nervous system effects such as confusion. (1; MR; EV; TC; DR)
   1 This is not an effect of salicylate intoxication.
   3 Same as answer 1.
   4 Same as answer 1.

101. **1** Gold salts, bound to plasma proteins, are distributed irregularly throughout the body but the highest concentration occurs in the kidneys. The slow excretion of gold salts cannot keep up with their intake; they accumulate in the kidneys, causing damage. (2; CJ; EV; TC; DR)
   2 This is not a side effect associated with gold salts, such as Myochrysine.
   3 Same as answer 2.
   4 Same as answer 2.

102. **3** Adverse reactions include blood dyscrasias, such as eosinophilia, thrombocytopenia, aplastic anemia, and leukopenia, which can be life threatening. (3; CJ; EV; TC; DR)
   1 This is not an adverse reaction to a gold compound.
   2 Although cutaneous lesions can occur, they are not life threatening as thrombocytopenia can be.
   4 Same as answer 1.

103. **4** Prolonged chemotherapy may slow the production of leukocytes in bone marrow, thus suppressing the activity of the immune system. Antibiotics may be required to help counter infections that the body can no longer handle easily. (2; CJ; AN; TC; DR)
   1 The liver does not produce leukocytes:
   2 Although leukocytes are circulating in both blood and lymph, these cells are more mature than those found in the bone marrow and thus more resistant to the effects of chemotherapy.
   3 Same as answer 2.

104. **3** Many chemotherapeutic agents function by interfering with DNA replication associated with normal cellular reproduction (mitosis). The normal rapid mitosis of the stratified squamous epithelium of the mouth and anus result in their being powerfully affected by the drugs. (2; CJ; EV; PA; DR)
   1 The state of nourishment would be applicable to all cells; although anorexia is common, this client may not be anorectic.
   2 This effect is not caused by direct irritation; most agents are administered parenterally.
   4 Chemotherapeutic agents affect the cells that are most rapidly proliferating, which include not only the cells of the GI epithelium but also those of the bone marrow and hair follicles.

105. **1** Methotrexate is a folic acid antagonist that can cause depression of bone marrow. This serious toxic effect is sometimes prevented by administration of folic acid. Some physicians advocate its administration after a course of methotrexate therapy so as not to interfere with methotrexate activity. (3; CJ; AN; TC; DR)
   2 Folic acid is a metabolite and does not destroy cancer cells.
   3 Same as answer 2.
   4 Leucovorin calcium does not increase the production of phagocytes.

106. **3** Dexamethasone (Decadron) increases gluconeogenesis, which may cause hyperglycemia. (3; CJ; EV; TC; DR)
   1 Decadron does not contain a glucose component.
   2 Glucose metabolism is not accelerated by Decadron.
   4 The renal threshold for glucose is not affected by Decadron.

107. **2** Any hormone normally produced by the body must be withdrawn slowly to allow the appropriate organ to adjust and resume production. (2; MR; IM; ED; DR)
   1 Although important, this is not the reason for gradual withdrawal of the drug.
   3 Same as answer 1.
   4 Same as answer 1.

108. 1 Prolonged use of steroids may cause leukopenia as a result of bone marrow depression. (3; CJ; AS; PA; DR)
  2 CRP (**C**-reactive protein) is present in acute inflammatory diseases and necrosis; it is not associated with steroids.
  3 The sedimentation rate is elevated when inflammation is present; it is not associated with steroids
  4 This is the name given to anemias that are characterized by decreased concentration of hemoglobin in erythrocytes; it is not a sequela of the use of steroids.

109. 2 Secretions and drainage are tested to determine the antibiotics to which the organism is particularly sensitive or resistant (sensitivity). (1; MR; AN; PA; DR)
  1 This is a test for antibody content.
  3 This is a test to determine whether a pathogen is virulent.
  4 This is a test for viral activity.

110. 4 Streptomycin is ototoxic and may cause damage to the auditory and vestibular portions of the eighth cranial nerve. (3; LE; EV; TC; DR)
  1 The drug does not adversely affect the cerebellum.
  2 The motor end plates of the peripheral nervous system are not affected.
  3 These cells and tracts of the nervous system are not affected.

111. 3 Sodium bicarbonate is absorbed and can alter the acid-base balance. Antacids are not readily absorbed, so they do not alter acid-base balance. (3; MR; AN; ED; DR)
  1 This is false; aluminum hydroxide and/or magnesium hydroxide preparations do contain sodium
  2 This is false; nonsystemic antacids are insoluble and not readily absorbed.
  4 This is false; these are side effects of nonsystemic antacids.

112. 4 It decreases gastric secretion by inhibiting histamine at H_2 receptors. (3; MR; IM; ED; DR)
  1 It does not affect gastric motility.
  2 It does not affect the pH of gastric secretions already present.
  3 It is an H_2 histamine receptor antagonist.

113. 3 Calcium carbonate's antacid action adds alkalinity neutralizing gastric pH, which in turn stimulates renewed secretion of acid by the gastric mucosa. (2; MR; IM; ED; DR)
  1 This medication causes constipation, not diarrhea.
  2 Calcium carbonate does not contain sodium as do some antacids; thus, it does not promote fluid retention.
  4 This antacid provides a source of calcium that would help prevent bone demineralization.

Fluid and Electrolytes

114. 2 The average adult human body is about 60% water. A newborn infant's body is about 80% water and gradually decreases throughout childhood. (1; CJ; AN; PA; FE)
  1 This is the percent for a newborn infant.
  3 The percent for the elderly may be as low as 40%.
  4 This represents complete dehydration is tissues.

115. 2 The osmoreceptors are located in the hypothalamus. Under conditions of dehydration they stimulate the neurohypophysis to release ADH into the blood. (2; CJ; AN; PA; FE)
  1 Receptors for alterations in osmatic pressure are not located in the blood.
  3 The kidney tubules are the target organ for ADH; they reabsorb more water from the glomerular filtrate.
  4 This is the posterior lobe of the pituitary gland and is the source of antidiuretic hormone (ADH).

116. 4 The kidneys regulate fluid balance by adjusting the amount of fluid reabsorbed from the glomerular filtrate. (2; CJ; AN; PA; FE)
  1 The liver does not play a major role in fluid balance.
  2 The heart is primarily a pump for the movement of blood.
  3 The role of the lungs is minimal.

117. **3** Hypotonic solutions are less concentrated (contain less than 0.85 g of sodium chloride in each 100 ml) than body fluids. (1; CJ; AN; PA; FE)
   1 Isotonic solutions are those that cause no change in the cellular volume or pressure, because their concentration is equivalent to that of body fluid.
   2 This relates to two compounds that possess the same molecular formula but that differ in their properties or in the position of atoms in the molecules; isomers.
   4 This contains more than 0.85 g of sodium chloride in each 100 ml.

118. **1** History must include a determination of the client's weight because dehydration is most readily and accurately measured by serial assessments of body weight; 1 liter of fluid weighs 2.2 pounds. (2; CJ; AS; PA; FE)
   2 Although dry skin may be associated with dehydration, it is not an objective, accurate assessment; dry skin is also associated with aging.
   3 Although hypovolemia will eventually result in a decrease in blood pressure, it is not an accurate, reliable assessment because there are many other causes of hypotension.
   4 This is too general and not an accurate assessment to determine fluid volume deficit.

119. **3** Increased respiration blows off carbon dioxide, which decreases hydrogen; the pH rises (less acidity). Decreased respiration results in carbon dioxide buildup, which increases hydrogen; the pH falls (more acidity). The kidneys either conserve or excrete bicarbonate, which helps to adjust the pH. (1; CJ; AN; PA; FE)
   1 Interaction of these two does not maintain the pH.
   2 Although the circulatory system carries fluids and electrolytes to the kidneys, it does not interact with the urinary system to regulate plasma pH.
   4 Same as answer 1.

120. **1** Blood plasma and interstitial fluid are both part of the extracellular fluid and are of the same ionic composition. (2; CJ; AN; PA; FE)
   2 The osmotic pressure is the same.
   3 The composition is the same.
   4 Ionic composition is the same; the main cation of both would be sodium.

121. **2** Interstitial fluid constitutes about 16% of body weight, which is 10 to 12 L in an adult male of 68 kg (150 lb). (2; CJ; AN; PA; FE)
   1 Plasma is 4% of body weight.
   3 This is part of the intracellular component.
   4 This is derived from extracellular fluid and is calculated as part of the 20% of the total body weight.

122. **4** The concentration of potassium is greater inside the cell and is extremely important in establishing a membrane potential, a critical factor in the cell's ability to function. (2; CJ; AN; PA; FE)
   1 Sodium is the most abundant cation of the extracellular compartment.
   2 Calcium is the most abundant electrolyte in the body; 99% is concentrated in the teeth and bones.
   3 Chloride is an extracellular anion.

123. **2** Approximately 25 of the 40 L of body fluid are in the cells. (3; CJ; AN; PA; FE)
   1 Interstitial fluid makes up 16%.
   3 Extracellular fluid makes up 20%.
   4 Intravascular fluid makes up 4%.

124. **2** The excreted ammonia combines with hydrogen ions in the glomerular filtrate to form ammonium ions, which are excreted from the body. This mechanism helps rid the body of excess hydrogen, maintaining acid-base balance. (2; CJ; AN; PA; FE)
   1 Osmotic pressure is not affected by excretion of ammonia.
   3 Ammonia is formed by the decomposition of bacteria in the urine; ammonia excretion is not related to the process and does not control bacterial levels.
   4 Ammonia excretion does not affect hemopoiesis.

125. **3** Because the plasma colloidal oncotic pressure (COP) is the major force drawing fluid from the interstitial spaces back into the capillaries, a drop in COP caused by albuminuria results in edema. (3; CJ; AN; PA; FE)
   1 Hydrostatic tissue pressure is unaffected by alteration of protein levels; colloidal pressure is affected.
   2 Hydrostatic pressure is influenced by the volume of fluid and the diameter of the blood vessel, not by the presence of protein such as albumin.
   4 The osmotic pressure of tissues is not affected.

126. **1** The fluid in a bottle hung over a person lying down possesses potential energy. When that fluid is allowed to drip into the person intravenously, its potential energy is then converted to kinetic energy (energy of motion). (3; CJ; AN; TC; FE)
2 Energy is not being stored in this action; rather stored energy is converted to energy of motion.
3 No chemical reaction occurs when fluid drips into a vein.
4 No chemical reaction or formation of new substances occurs when fluid drips into a vein.

127. **1** A molar (1 M) solution contains 1 gram-molecular weight of solute per liter of solution. Molarity is not as informative as normality because the latter is based on the actual chemical-combining properties of the substance involved. (3; CJ; AN; PA; FE)
2 A normal (1 N) solution is defined as containing 1 gram-equivalent weight of solute per liter of solution. In human body fluids the milliequivalent (1/1000 of the gram-equivalent) is a more convenient term for expressing concentration, because the gram-equivalent is rather large.
3 This deals with the osmotic pressure of two liquids; isotonic solutions have equal osmotic pressure.
4 A solution holding all the solute it can at a given temperature and pressure is a saturated solution.

128. **4** A portable wound drainage system has negative pressure; fluid flows down the pressure gradient from the client to the collection device. (2; CJ; AN; TC; FE)
1 This is Newton's law of gravity, not the physical principle underlying the functioning of a portable wound drainage system.
2 Although true, this is not what causes the fluid to drain.
3 Siphonage is not the principle underlying the functioning of a portable wound drainage system.

129. **2** Sodium bicarbonate is a base and one of the major buffers in the body. (2; CJ; AN; PA; FE)
1 Potassium is not a buffer; only a base can buffer an acid.

3 Carbon dioxide is carried in aqueous solution as carbonic acid (H_2CO_3); an acid does not buffer another acid.
4 Sodium chloride is not a buffer; it is a salt.

130. **2** Excessive loss of gastric fluid results in excessive loss of hydrochloric acid and can lead to alkalosis; the HCl is not available to neutralize the sodium bicarbonate ($NaHCO_3$) secreted into the duodenum by the pancreas. The intestinal tract absorbs the excess bicarbonate and alkalosis results. (1; CJ; AS; TC; FE)
1 Loss of HCl will move the pH to an alkaline level.
3 Oxygen is not drawn from the blood by gastric lavage.
4 Gastric fluid does not regulate osmotic pressure in the blood; also, the volume of blood would be altered not by loss of gastric fluid but by severe dehydration.

131. **2** Prolonged use of sodium bicarbonate may cause systemic alkalosis as well as retention of sodium and water. (1; CJ: IM; TC; FE)
1 This statement is inaccurate in describing the effects of sodium bicarbonate.
3 Same as answer 1.
4 Same as answer 1.

132. **3** Arterial blood has a narrow pH range of 7.35 to 7.45. Venous blood is more acidic and closer to 7.35 than is arterial blood, which is normally closer to a pH of 7.45. (1; CJ; AS; TC; FE)
1 This is very acidic and needs immediate treatment.
2 This is slightly acidic for both arterial and venous blood.
4 This is alkaline and needs treatment.

133. **1** Retention of carbon dioxide after exhausting the available bicarbonate ions as buffers will cause a lower pH (respiratory acidosis). (1; CJ; AS; PA; FE)
2 Hyperventilation will cause respiratory alkalosis.
3 The loss of carbon dioxide reduces the body's level of carbonic acid, causing respiratory alkalosis.
4 Tissue necrosis results from localized tissue anoxia and will not cause the systemic response of respiratory acidosis; this is caused by excessive carbonic acid resulting from a respiratory insufficiency.

134. 2 The pH of blood is maintained within the narrow range of 7.35 to 7.45. When there is an increase in hydrogen ions, acidosis results and is reflected in a lower pH. (1; CJ; AS; PA; FE)

1 This is too acidotic and may not be compatible with life.
3 This is within the normal range for pH.
4 This is slightly alkaline.

135. 4 Release of adrenocortical steroids (cortisol) by the stress of surgery causes renal retention of sodium and excretion of potassium. (2; CJ; EV; TC; FE)

1 Although sodium may be depleted by nasogastric suction, retention by the kidneys generally balances this loss.
2 This is not depleted by surgery or urinary excretion.
3 Same as answer 2.

136. 4 Vital signs monitor cardiorespiratory status; hyperkalemia causes serious cardiac dysrhythmias. (2; CJ; IM; TC; FE)

1 A repeat laboratory test would take time and probably reaffirm the original results; the client needs immediate attention.
2 The cardiac arrest team is always on alert and will respond when called for a cardiac arrest.
3 These are insufficient interventions.

137. 3 Once treatment with insulin for diabetic ketoacidosis is begun, potassium ions reenter the cell, causing hypokalemia; therefore potassium, along with the replacement fluids, is generally supplied. (2; CJ; AN; TC; FE)

1 Potassium would not correct this.
2 Flaccid paralysis would not occur in diabetic ketoacidosis; potassium replaces that which has reentered the cell after insulin therapy.
4 Knowing the relationship of insulin and potassium, the nurse should recognize that treatment with KCl is prophylactic, aborting any development of dysrhythmias.

138. 2 Potassium, the major intracellular cation, functions with sodium and calcium to regulate neuromuscular activity and contraction of muscle fibers, particularly the heart muscle. In hypokalemia these symptoms develop. (2; CJ; AS; PA; FE)

1 These symptoms do not indicate an electrolyte imbalance.
3 These symptoms would indicate hypocalcemia, which does not generally occur in colitis.

4 Nausea and vomiting might occur with prolonged potassium deficit; however, this is not an early sign; leg and abdominal cramps occur with potassium excess, not deficit.

139. 3 Dehydration is a danger because of fluid loss with GI suction. (2; CJ; EV; TC; FE)

1 Based on the data provided, this symptom is not likely to occur.
2 Same as answer 1.
4 Same as answer 1.

140. 4 Because 1 oz equals approximately 30 ml and the client drank a total of 21.5 oz, 215×30 yields the answer in milliliters. (1; CJ; AN; TC; FE)

1 This is an incorrect calculation; it is too low.
2 Same as answer 1.
3 Same as answer 1.

141. 4

Intake (ml)		Output (ml)	
IV fluid	350	Voiding	
NG tube		8:30 AM	150
feeding	600	1:00 PM	220
Water	150	3:15 PM	235
Vitamin	30	Aspirated	
		stomach	
		contents	25
	1130 ml		630 ml

(3; CJ; IM; TC; FE)

1 This is a miscalculation; too little intake and too much output.
2 Same as answer 1.
3 This is a miscalculation; too little intake and output.

142. 1 Because IV solutions enter the body's internal environment, all solutions and medications utilizing this route must be sterile to prevent the introduction of microbes. (2; CJ; IM; TC; FE)

2 The medication can be mixed with the IV solution in many ways; sterility takes priority.
3 The amount and type of solution depend on the medication; sterility takes priority.
4 The needle does not have to be changed if sterility is maintained.

143. 1 $$\frac{\text{Amount to be infused} \times \text{Drop factor}}{\text{Time of infusion in minutes}}$$

(1; CJ; AN; TC; FE)

2 This is an incorrect calculation; it is too rapid; it would take approximately 4 hours.
3 This is an incorrect calculation; it is too rapid; it would take between 2 and 3 hours to infuse.
4 This is an incorrect calculation; it would infuse too rapidly.

144. 3 The liver manufactures albumin, the major plasma protein. A deficit of this protein will lower the osmotic (oncotic) pressure in the intravascular space, leading to a fluid shift. (3; CJ; AN; PA; FE)
1 The enlarged liver compresses the portal system, causing increased rather than decreased pressure.
2 The kidneys are not the primary source of the pathologic condition. It is the liver's ability to manufacture albumin that maintains the colloid oncotic pressure.
4 Potassium is not produced by the body, nor is its major function the maintenance of fluid balance.

145. 2 IV fluids do not provide proteins required for tissue growth, repair, and maintenance; therefore, tissue breakdown occurs to provide the essential amino acids. (2; CJ; EV; PA; FE)
1 Each liter provides approximately 170 calories, which is insufficient to meet minimal energy requirements; tissue breakdown will result.
3 Weight loss is caused by insufficient intake of nutrients; vitamins will not prevent weight loss.
4 An infusion of 5% dextrose in water may decrease electrolyte concentration because of a fluid shift.

146. 1 Diuretic therapy that affects the loop of Henle generally involves the use of drugs that directly or indirectly increase urinary sodium, chloride, and potassium excretion. (1; CJ; EV; TC; FE)
2 Sodium restriction does not necessarily accompany administration of furosemide (Lasix).
3 Dyspnea does not directly result in a depletion of electrolytes.
4 Unless otherwise ordered, oral intake is unaffected.

147. 3 Potassium is lost with the urine during diuresis. Hypokalemia, in turn, predisposes the client to digitalis toxicity. (1; CJ; EV; TC; DR)
1 This electrolyte is not lost as a result of digitalis-induced diuresis.
2 Same as answer 1.
4 Same as answer 1.

148. 4 Fluid and electrolyte disturbances occur because of fever, profuse diaphoresis, vomiting, and diarrhea. (3; CJ; AS; PA; FE)
1 This symptom is not associated with complications of malaria.
2 Same as answer 1.
3 These symptoms are not associated with complications of malaria.

149. 3 ADH causes increased resorption of water by renal tubules, which dilutes sodium levels causing hyponatremia. (3; CJ; AS; TC; FE)
1 ADH will decrease urine volume.
2 ADH causes fluid retention.
4 ADH does not alter glucose metabolism.

150. 2 Potassium replacement is generally not indicated in the initial management of burns because hyperkalemia results from the liberation of potassium ions from the injured cells. (3; LE; EV; TC; FE)
1 This will be given with colloidal Ringer's solution in various combinations depending on the client's needs.
3 This will be given with colloidal and dextrose solutions in various combinations depending on the client's needs.
4 This will be given with Ringer's and dextrose solutions in various combinations depending on the client's needs.

151. 2 Albumin acts to elevate the BP to normal levels when it is administered slowly and oral fluid intake is restricted. It causes fluid to move from the interstitial spaces into the circulatory system. Administration should not exceed 5 to 10 ml/minute. (2; CJ; IM; TC; FE)
1 Rapid administration could cause circulatory overload; high fluid intake would limit the shift of fluid from the interstitial to the intravascular compartment, interfering with the optimal effects of the drug.
3 Rapid administration could cause circulatory overload; fluid is restricted, not withheld.
4 Fluids are restricted to facilitate the optimal effects of the drug, which shifts fluids from the interstitial spaces to the intravascular compartment.

152. **4** Blood albumin, a protein, establishes the plasma colloid osmotic (oncotic) pressure because of its high molecular weight and size. (2; CJ; AN; PA; FE)
    1 Blood clotting involves blood protein fractions other than albumin; for example, prothrombin and fibrinogen are within the alpha and beta globulin fractions.
    2 Red cell formation (erythropoiesis) occurs in red marrow and can be related to albumin only indirectly; albumin is the blood transport protein for thyroxine, which stimulates metabolism in all cells, including those in red bone marrow.
    3 Albumin does not activate WBCs; white blood cells are activated by antigens and substances released from damaged or diseased cells.

153. **4** After 24 hours there is increased risk of contamination of the solution and the container should be changed. (2; LE; PL; TC; FE)
    1 It is unnecessary to change the bag this often.
    2 Same as answer 1.
    3 Same as answer 1.

154. **2** When an IV infusion is infiltrated, it should be removed to prevent swelling of the tissues and pain. (2; CJ; EV; TC; FE)
    1 Elevation does not change the position of the IV cannula; the infusion must be discontinued.
    3 This would add to the infiltration of fluid.
    4 Soaks may be applied, if ordered, after the IV is removed.

155. **4** Orange juice contains 4 mg sodium/100 g. (2; MR; PL; TC; FE)
    1 Too high in sodium; raw celery contains 126 mg sodium/100 g; cooked celery contains 88 mg sodium/100 g.
    2 Higher in sodium; raw carrots contain 47 mg sodium/100 g; canned carrots contain 236 mg sodium/100 g.
    3 Too high in sodium; tomato juice contains 200 mg sodium/100 g.

156. **1** $\dfrac{\text{Amount to be infused} \times \text{Drop factor}}{\text{Amount of time (in minutes)}}$

$$\frac{2000 \times 10 = 20,000}{12 \times 60 = 720} = 27.77 \text{ drops/minutes}$$

(2; CJ; EV; TC; FE)
    2 This is an incorrect calculation and would result in excessive fluid administration.
    3 Same as answer 2.
    4 Same as answer 2.

157. **4** Unless diluted the highly concentrated solution can cause hyperosmolar diuresis. (1; CJ; AN; TC; FE)
    1 The potential of phlebitis is not the primary reason.
    2 This is not the primary reason; although the infusion at this site is more secure and promotes free use of the arms and hands.
    3 Same as answer 2.

158. **1** These signs may indicate calcium depletion. (2; CJ; PL; TC; FE)
    2 Symptoms associated with hypomagnesemia include tremor, neuromuscular irritability, and confusion.
    3 Symptoms associated with metabolic acidosis include deep rapid breathing, weakness, and disorientation.
    4 Symptoms associated with hypokalemia include muscle weakness and malaise.

159. **1** Hypokalemia causes a flattening of the T wave of the ECG because of its effect on muscle function. (3; CJ; AS; PA; FE)
    2 Hypokalemia causes a depression of the ST segment.
    3 Hypokalemia causes a widening of the QRS complex.
    4 Hypokalemia does not cause a deflection of the Q wave.

160. **1** Potassium follows insulin into the cells of the body, thereby raising the cellular potassium and preventing fatal dysrhythmias. (3; CJ; AN; PA; FE)
    2 Insulin does not cause excretion of these substances.
    3 Potassium is not excreted as a result of this therapy; it shifts into the intracellular compartment.
    4 The potassium level has no effect on pancreatic insulin production.

161. **3** Hypokalemia promotes mental confusion and apathy with poor muscle contractions and weakness; these effects are related to the diminished magnitude of the neuronal and muscle cell resting potentials. Abdominal distention results from flaccidity of intestinal and abdominal musculature. (2; CJ; EV; PA; FE)
    1 These are signs of sodium excess.
    2 These are signs of hyperkalemia.
    4 These are signs of diabetic ketoacidosis.

162. **3** To calculate the rate of fluid infusion:

$$\frac{\text{Amount of fluid to be infused} \times \text{Drop factor}}{\text{Number of hours} \times 60 \text{ minutes}}$$

$$\frac{1000 \times 15}{8 \times 60} = \frac{15000}{480} = 31.25 = 31 \text{ drops/min}$$

(2; CJ; IM; TC; FE)

1 This is an incorrect calculation, resulting in an inadequate administration of fluid.
2 Same as answer 1.
4 This is an incorrect calculation, resulting in an excessive administration of fluid.

163. **2** $\dfrac{50 \text{ ml} \times 15 \text{ drops/min}}{(\text{time in minutes})} = \dfrac{750}{20} = 37.5$

37.5 is rounded to 38. (2; CJ; IM; TC; PE)

1 This rate is too slow; it would take longer than 20 minutes to infuse.
3 This rate is too fast; it would infuse in less than 20 minutes.
4 Same as answer 3

Cardiovascular

164. **2** An improper reading of the level of mercury will be obtained if the reader is not perpendicular to the column. An error of parallax results when an object is displaced by an observer's altered position. (1; CJ; PL; TC; CV)

1 Too narrow a cuff can result in erroneously high readings; not an error of parallax.
3 Standing close to the manometer is not explicit; there may or may not be a resultant error of parallax depending on whether the examiner is perpendicular to the column of mercury.
4 Elevating the arm above the level of the heart will result in erroneously low readings; not an error of parallax.

165. **3** If there is a decrease in urinary output with increased conservation of body fluid, the blood pressure will be increased and vice versa. (3; CJ; AN; PA; CV)

1 These cause a rapid response and have a short-term effect.
2 This may cause a short-term increase, but does not have a long-term effect.
4 Same as answer 1.

166. **2** The heart's apex is between the fifth and sixth ribs at the midclavicular line. It is closest to the chest wall here, so auscultation is easier. (2; CJ; PL; TC; CV)

1 Although it may be possible to auscultate the heart in this area, it is usually easier to do so over the apex.
3 Same as answer 1.
4 Same as answer 1.

167. **2** An open flame or spark from static electricity (e.g., leather-soled shoes, wool, silk, nylon, and Dacron blankets, ungrounded electric appliances) can initiate an explosion and fire in the presence of higher than normal oxygen levels. (1; MR; IM; TC; CV)

1 Oxygen is not flammable; however, it increases the rate of combustion.
3 Oxygen is not unstable.
4 Oxygen does not increase apprehension; by reducing dyspnea and shortness of breath, it usually reduces apprehension.

168. **3** Oxygen via nasal cannula is the most comfortable and least intrusive, because the cannula extends minimally, into the nose. (1; CJ; EV; TC; CV)

1 This method is oppressive, and clients complain of feeling "suffocated" when it is used.
2 Same as answer 1.
4 Same as answer 1.

169. **3** With anemia there is a greater return of blood to the heart from the peripheral vessels; the greater volume of blood returning to the heart stretches it and results in greater cardiac output. With polycythemia the heart must work harder to propel the more viscous blood through the circulatory system. (1; CJ; AS; PA; CV)

1 Pressure is not involved; the terms anemia and polycythemia both refer to the number of cells present in a given volume (viscosity).
2 Temperature is not involved; the terms anemia and polycythemia both refer to the number of cells present in a given volume (viscosity).
4 Surface tension is not involved; the terms anemia and polycythemia both refer to the number of cells present in a given volume (viscosity).

170. **3** The pulse increases to meet increased tissue demands for oxygen in the febrile state. (1; CJ; AS; PA; CV)

1 Fever may not cause difficulty in breathing.
2 Pain is not related to fever.
4 Blood pressure is not necessarily elevated in fever.

171. 3 Pulse pressure is obtained by subtracting the diastolic from the systolic readings after the blood pressure has been recorded. (1; CJ; EV; TC; CV)
  1 This is only a partial factor in determining pulse pressure; it is not the pulse pressure itself.
  2 This is not pulse pressure; it is pulse deficit.
  4 This is not pulse pressure.

172. 1 Temperatures of 102° F (38° C) or greater lead to an increased metabolism and cardiac workload. (1; CJ; AN; TC; CV)
  2 An elevated temperature is not an early sign of developing cerebral edema, although the temperature may rise eventually because of medullary compression.
  3 Fever is unrelated to hemorrhage; in hemorrhage with shock, the temperature decreases.
  4 Although these symptoms are related to an elevated temperature, they are not the reason for notifying the physician.

173. 2 Constriction of the peripheral blood vessels and the resulting increase in blood pressure impair circulation and limit the amount of oxygen being delivered to body cells, particularly in the extremities. (1; CJ; PL; ED: CV)
  1 Nicotine constricts all peripheral vessels, not just superficial ones; its primary action is vasoconstriction; it will not dilate deep vessels.
  3 Nicotine constricts rather than dilates peripheral vessels.
  4 Same as answer 3.

174. 4 Injured tissue cannot heal properly because of cellular deprivation of oxygen and nutrients; ulceration and gangrene may result; diminished sensation decreases awareness of injury. (2; CJ; AS; PA; CV)
  1 Emotional stress does not cause tissue injury; however, because of vasoconstriction, it may prolong healing.
  2 Poor hygiene is only one stress that may cause tissue trauma; protein is not related to this disease.
  3 Caffeine stimulates the cerebral cortex; it does not contribute to ulceration or deprivation of oxygen.

175. 3 Buerger's disease (thromboangiitis obliterans) is characterized by vascular inflammation, usually in the lower extremities, leading to thrombus formation. As a result of impaired circulation, there is burning pain and intermittent claudication. (1; CJ; AS; PA; CV)
  1 These symptoms are not related to thromboangiitis obliterans.
  2 Blanching is not related to thromboangiitis obliterans.
  4 Fatigue and blanching of the skin are not related to thromboangiitis obliterans.

176. 4 The Trendelenburg test evaluates the backflow of blood through defective valves. If, after raising the legs to empty the veins, the client stands and the veins fill from above the site of the suspected varicosity, the diagnosis is supported. (3; CJ; AS; PA; CV)
  1 This is not a simple test that the nurse can perform.
  2 This test is used to determine injury to the pyramidal tract in adults; if present, it is obtained by firmly stroking the lateral aspect of the sole of foot.
  3 This is a test for position sense; the client loses balance when standing erect with feet together and eyes closed.

177. 2 The legs should be elevated to promote venous return by gravity. (1; CJ; IM; PA; CV)
  1 This position increases pressure on the popliteal space, which may interfere with venous return from the legs.
  3 Flexion of the knees and hips with the legs lower than the heart interferes with venous return.
  4 Dorsiflexion of the feet places tension on the suture line and should be avoided; placing the legs lower than the level of the heart will not promote venous return.

178. 3 The pulmonary capillary beds are the first small vessels (capillary beds) that the embolus encounters once it is released from the calf veins. (2; CJ; EV; PA; CV)
  1 This would not occur because the embolus would enter the pulmonary system first.
  2 Same as answer 1.
  4 Dry gangrene occurs when the arterial rather than the venous circulation is compromised.

179. 3 An appendectomy is a relatively simple operation; the client is generally out of bed the
same day. With an ambulatory client there is
less risk of venous stasis, a condition that predisposes the individual to thrombus formation and emboli. (1; CJ; EV; PA; CV)
  1 Although generally ambulated the first day
postoperatively, the client often is hampered
by pain; pelvic surgery increases risk.
  2 The client may or may not be out of bed the
same day depending on the surgical approach.
  4 Vein ligation is performed for varicose veins;
the diseased vein is removed, placing an
additional burden on the deep venous system
and possibly increasing the risk of thrombi.

180. 4 The client who is on bed rest must do exercises such as dorsiflexion of the feet to prevent venous stasis and thrombus formation.
(1; CJ; IM; TC; CV)
  1 Limiting fluid intake may lead to hemoconcentration and subsequent thrombus formation.
  2 This improves pulmonary function rather than
prevents venous stasis.
  3 This actually promotes venous stasis by compressing the popliteal space.

181. 4 A drop in blood pressure, rapid pulse, cold
clammy skin, and oliguria are signs of shock,
which, if not treated promptly, can lead to
death. (1; CJ; EV; TC; CV)
  1 This is an expected response; the client will
push out the airway as the effects of anesthesia subside.
  2 Snoring respirations are common because of
the depressant effects of anesthesia.
  3 Shallow respirations are common because of
the depressant effects of anesthesia.

182. 1 Paralysis of the sympathetic vasomotor nerves
after administration of spinal anesthesia
results in dilation of blood vessels, which
causes a subsequent drop in blood pressure.
(3; CJ; AN; PA; CV)
  2 These receptors are sensitive to pH, oxygen
and carbon dioxide tension; they are not
related to postural hypotension and are not
affected by spinal anesthesia.
  3 The strength of cardiac contractions is not
affected by spinal anesthesia and postural
hypotension.
  4 The cardiac accelerator center neurons in the
medulla regulate heart rate; they are not
related to postural hypotension and are not
affected by spinal anesthesia.

183. 2 Localized sensory changes may indicate nerve
damage, impaired circulation, or thrombophlebitis. Activity should be limited, and
the physician notified. (1; CJ; IM; TC; CV)
  1 Symptoms may indicate a serious problem,
and the physician must be notified.
  3 Rubbing or massaging the legs is contraindicated because of possible dislodging of a
thrombus if present.
  4 Bed rest is indicated to prevent the possibility
of further damage or creation of an embolus.

184. 3 The sympathectomy causes dilation of the
blood vessels in the lower extremities; the
resulting shift in the fixed blood volume lowers
systemic blood pressure. (3; CJ; EV; TC; CV)
  1 Fluid losses associated with surgery may gradually lower BP and are compensated by endocrine and renal mechanisms.
  2 Although anesthesia depresses vital signs,
generally there is not a sudden drop in BP
postoperatively.
  4 Epinephrine would increase BP by stimulating cardiac contractility.

185. 4 Thrombophlebitis is inflammation of a vein
that occurs with the formation of a clot. Signs
include pain (especially on dorsiflexion of the
foot), redness, warmth, tenderness, and edema. (1; CJ; AS; TC; CV)
  1 Intermittent claudication (pain when walking
resulting from tissue ischemia) may occur
with peripheral vascular disease.
  2 Pitting edema does not occur in thrombophlebitis.
  3 Pain occurs on flexion of the foot (Homan's
sign).

186. 3 Support hose apply external pressure on the
veins, preventing the retrograde pressure or
flow that may occur in the standing or sitting
positions; application before arising prevents
the veins from having the opportunity to
become engorged. (1; CJ; IM; TC; CV)
  1 If the feet are permitted to be dependent before the stockings are put on, venous pooling
and edema may occur; application of elastic
stockings at this time can cause tissue trauma.
  2 Because they promote venous return, they do
not need to be worn when the legs are elevated when in bed.
  4 Stockings must be removed so the legs can be
washed and dried at least daily. They usually
need not be worn while in bed with the feet
elevated because gravity prevents venous
pooling.

187. **1** The vessels branching from the circle of Willis provide excellent collateral circulation for the brain; partial blockage of one vessel is compensated by flow through other vessels. (2; MR; AN; PA; CV)
2 These take blood away from the brain.
3 This is not collateral circulation.
4 Same as answer 3.

188. **2** After removal of an arterial obstruction by endarterectomy, adequate circulation may be monitored by observation of skin color, pulses, and skin temperature. (2; CJ; EV; PA; CV)
1 Appetite does not change as a result of vascular surgery.
3 Bowel habits would not be altered after surgery.
4 Turgor would be affected by changes in hydration.

189. **4** Sitting on the edge of the bed before getting up is recommended because it gives the body a chance to adjust to the effects of gravity on circulation in the upright position. (2; MR; PL; PA; CV)
1 Support hose would not be worn continuously and would not prevent hypotension.
2 This would not prevent episodes of orthostatic hypotension.
3 Energetic tasks do not increase hypotension.

190. **4** Change in position causes hypotension; when a position has been maintained for 5 minutes, the blood pressure has probably stabilized. (3; CJ; EV; TC; CV)
1 Assessment before administration will not yield information related to effectiveness.
2 This is too short a tune for determination of the drug's effect.
3 Many antihypertensive agents lower peripheral vascular resistance and may cause orthostatic hypotension and would not reflect the effectiveness of the drug.

191. **4** Cholesterol is a sterol found in tissue; it is attributed in part to diets high in saturated fats. (1; CJ; IM; PA; CV)
1 Cholesterol is also produced by the body.
2 Only animal foods furnish dietary cholesterol.
3 Cholesterol is needed for the synthesis of bile salts, adrenocortical and steroid sex hormones, and provitamin D.

192. **3** Whole milk is high in saturated fat. (1; MR; IM; ED; CV)
1 Most fish have a low fat content.
2 Corn oil is high in unsaturated fat.
4 Soft margarine is high in unsaturated fat.

193. **3** Vegetables and whole grains are low in fat and may reduce the risk of heart disease. (2; MR; IM; ED; CV)
1 Animal-derived products such as milk are high in saturated fats.
2 Meats are high in saturated fats.
4 These are high in cholesterol.

194. **2** Clients' families should be included in dietary teaching; families provide support that promotes compliance. (1; MR; PL; ED; CV)
1 The dietitian is a resource person who can give specific, practical information about diet and food preparation once the client has a basic understanding of the reasons for the diet.
3 Foods high in sodium will also have to be restricted; this teaching is inadequate.
4 The client should be included in own care; the client will ultimately assume the responsibility.

195. **2** Angina pectoris is pain in the chest that is caused by hypoxia of the cardiac muscle. (2; CJ; AS; PA; CV)
1 Mitral insufficiency refers to an incompetent mitral valve; it could be only indirectly related to angina.
3 There is no cell death in angina.
4 A coronary thrombosis is an aggregation of platelets, clotting factors, and blood cellular elements that reduces the lumen of the artery; it may progress to a complete obstruction, resulting in a myocardial infarction.

196. **2** The two coronary arteries are the first branches of the aorta and carry blood with a high oxygen content to the myocardium. (3; CJ; AN; PA; CV)
1 They carry blood with high oxygen content to the myocardium, not to the endocardium.
3 They carry blood with high oxygen content to the myocardium.
4 This is a function of the pulmonary veins.

197. **2** Ischemia causes tissue injury and the release of chemicals, such as bradykinin, that stimulate sensory nerves and produce pain. (2; CJ; AN; PA; CV)
  1 Arterial spasm, resulting in tissue hypoxia and pain, is associated with angina pectoris.
  3 Arteries, not veins, are involved in the etiology of a myocardial infarction.
  4 Tissue injury and pain occur in the myocardium.

198. **3** Anginal pain, which can be anticipated during certain activities, may be prevented by dilating the coronary arteries immediately before engaging in the activity. (2; MR; IM; ED; CV)
  1 One tablet is generally administered at a time; doubling the dosage may produce severe hypotension and headache.
  2 The sublingual form of nitroglycerin is absorbed directly through the mucous membranes and should not be swallowed.
  4 When the pain is relieved, rest will generally prevent its recurrence by reducing oxygen consumption of the myocardium.

199. **4** The pulse should be assessed because the trauma at the insertion site may interfere with blood flow distal to the site. There is also danger of bleeding. (1; CJ; IM; TC; CV)
  1 The client does not usually require additional rest after the initial period of immobilization.
  2 This would be determined on an individual basis; it is not routine.
  3 It is not necessary to check the ECG every 30 minutes following the procedure.

200. **3** Blood samples from the right atrium, right ventricle, and pulmonary artery would all be about the same with regard to oxygen concentration. Such blood contains slightly less oxygen than does systemic arterial blood. (2; CJ; AN; PA; CV)
  1 These contain slightly more carbon dioxide than does blood in the pulmonary vein, which has had some of its CO_2 expelled into the alveoli.
  2 These contain less oxygen than does the pulmonary vein, which will carry oxygenated blood to the circulation.
  4 It contains the same amount as do samples from the right atrium and right ventricle.

201. **3** Myocardial infarction (MI) may cause increased irritability of tissue or interruption of normal transmission of impulses. Dysrhythmias occur in about 90% of clients after MI. (2; CJ; AS; TC; CV)
  1 Hypokalemia may result when clients are taking cardiac glycosides and diuretics; this is a complication associated with therapy, not a pathologic entity related to the MI itself.
  2 Anaphylactic shock is caused by an allergic reaction, not by an MI.
  4 Cardiac enlargement is a slow process and is not a complication that can be observed.

202. **4** The catheter is placed in the pulmonary artery. Information regarding left ventricular function is obtained when the catheter balloon is inflated. (3; MR; IM; ED; CV)
  1 Information on stroke volume, the amount of blood ejected by the left ventricle with each contraction, will not be provided by a pulmonary catheter.
  2 Cardiac output is not usually measured via the pulmonary artery catheter used for continuous monitoring of the client.
  3 Although CVP can be obtained with the pulmonary catheter, it is not as specific as a pulmonary wedge pressure, which reflects pressure in the left side of the heart.

203. **3** LDH, CK-MB and troponin are enzymes released into the blood from cardiac muscle cells when the myocardium is damaged. (1; CJ; AS; PA; CV)
  1 Calcium level will not diagnose MI; there is no test called APPT; APTT assesses blood clotting time.
  2 The sedimentation rate identifies the presence of inflammation or infection but is not specific; ALT identifies tissue destruction but it is more specific for liver injury.
  4 The Paul-Bunnell test identifies heterophilic antibodies in infectious mononucleosis; it would not be specific for myocardial infarction.

204. 1 Until the client's condition has reached some degree of stability after myocardial infarction, routine activities such as changing sheets are avoided so that the client's movements will be minimized and the cardiac workload reduced. (2; CJ; IM; TC; CV)

2 Changing all the linen causes unnecessary movement, which increases oxygen demands and makes the heart work harder.

3 Activity is contraindicated because it increases oxygen consumption and cardiac work load.

4 Any activity is counterproductive to rest; rest must take precedence so the cardiac workload will be reduced.

205. 2 Adverse effects of digoxin include many types of dysrhythmias. An apical pulse rate less than 60 or above 120 contraindicates administration of the drug. Because the client will be taking the medication at home, teach the client how to take an accurate pulse and to contact the physician if the rate falls outside the parameters mentioned. (2; CJ; PL; TC; CV)

1 The client will be assuming responsibility for drug administration at home; teaching is more of a priority than the nurse's assessments at this time.

3 Same as answer 1.

4 Same as answer 1.

206. 1 Desired anticoagulant effect is achieved when the activated partial thromboplastin time is 1.5 to 2 times normal. (2; CJ; EV; TC; CV)

2 Although absence of bleeding suggests that the drug has not reached toxic levels, it does not indicate its effectiveness.

3 This does not affect viscosity.

4 Weakness and confusion are not related to anticoagulant therapy.

207. 2 The high vascularity of the nose, combined with its susceptibility to trauma (e.g., sneezing, nose blowing), makes it a frequent site of hemorrhage. (1; CJ; EV; TC; CV)

1 This symptom is usually not associated with anticoagulant therapy.

3 Same as answer 1.

4 Same as answer 1.

208. 1 Coumadin is ordered day by day, based on the INR of the client. This test provides a standard system to interpret prothrombin times. (2; CJ; PL; TC; CV)

2 Clotting time is the time required for blood to form a clot; it is not used for dosage calculation.

3 Bleeding time is the time required for blood to cease flowing from a small wound; it is not used for Coumadin dosage calculation.

4 Sedimentation rate is a test used to determine the presence of inflammation or infection; it does not indicate clotting ability.

209. 4 The client is up more at home so edema usually increases. (2; MR; IM; ED; CV)

1 Serosanguineous drainage will persist after discharge.

2 These should not be expected and are, in fact, signs of postpericardotomy syndrome.

3 These symptoms will persist longer.

210. 2 Shock may have different etiologies (e.g., hypovolemic, cardiogenic, septic, anaphylactic) but always involves a drop in blood pressure and failure of the peripheral circulation because of sympathetic nervous system involvement. (2; CJ; AN; PA; CV)

1 Shock can be reversed by the administration of fluids, plasma expanders, and vasoconstrictors.

3 It may be a reaction to tissue injury but has many different etiologies (e.g., hypovolemia, sepsis, anaphylaxis).

4 Hypovolemia is only one cause; shock may also be septic, cardiogenic, or anaphylactic; it always involves a drop in blood pressure.

211. 1 Adrenalin is used to treat shock because the induced arterial constriction reduces blood pooling (vessels cannot hold as much blood) and increases venous return and cardiac output. (3; CJ; AN; PA; CV)

2 Digoxin slows and strengthens the heartbeat; it does not cause vasoconstriction.

3 A sympathectomy interferes with autonomic vasoconstriction; it reduces venous return.

4 Tourniquets constrict veins of the extremities and reduce venous return; these are no longer used.

212. 4 This position is useful in treating shock because it promotes gravity-induced venous return. Warmth and fluids are also supportive to the person. (1; CJ; IM; TC; CV)

1 These are not methods used in the treatment of shock.

2 This promotes venous pooling, which compounds shock.

3 Same as answer 1.

213. **4** In complete atrioventricular block, the ventricles take over the pacemaker function in the heart, but at a much slower rate than that of the SA node. As a result there is decreased cerebral circulation, causing syncope. (1; CJ; AS; PA; CV)
1 These symptoms are unrelated to complete heart block.
2 These are symptoms of a cerebrovascular accident.
3 Same as answer 1.

214. **3** Bradycardia refers to a heart rate of less than 60 per minute. It may be a physiologic adaptation to long-term exercise, cardiac disease, or digitalis toxicity. (1; CJ; AN; TC; CV)
1 This condition is described as a dysrhythmia; whereas bradycardia is also considered a dysrhythmia, the rhythm is usually regular.
2 Tachycardia is the term used for rapid heart rates.
4 This is called a bigeminal rhythm.

215. **3** Ventricular fibrillation will cause irreversible brain damage and then death within minutes because the heart is not pumping blood. Defibrillation or CPR until defibrillation is possible must be initiated immediately. (1; CJ; AN; TC; CV)
1 Although this condition requires prompt treatment, a client will live if treatment is withheld for several minutes.
2 Same as answer 1.
4 Same as answer 1.

216. **1** Atropine blocks vagal stimulation of the SA node, resulting in an increased heart rate. (3; CJ; PL; PA; CV)
2 Digoxin (Lanoxin) slows the heart rate; hence it would not be indicated in this situation.
3 Lidocaine hydrochloride (Xylocaine) decreases myocardial sensitivity and would not increase heart rate.
4 Procainamide hydrochloride (Pronestyl) is an antidysrhythmic drug; it would not stimulate the heart rate.

217. **4** Bundle branch block interferes with the conduction of impulses from the AV node to the ventricle supplied by the affected bundle. Conduction through the ventricles is delayed, as evidenced by a widened QRS complex. (3; CJ; AS; PA; CV)

1 Changes in the T waves and/or ST segments usually occur as a result of cardiac damage.
2 P waves, produced when the SA node fires to begin a cycle, are present in bundle branch block.
3 Same as answer 1.

218. **2** The SA node is the heart's natural pacemaker. An electronic pacemaker is used in some persons to supply an impulse that stimulates the heart to more efficient action. (1; CJ; AN; PA; CV)
1 This is modified cardiac muscle, which receives impulses from the SA node and conducts them to the ventricular walls via the bundle of His and Purkinje fibers.
3 This is special cardiac muscle, which receives impulses from the AV node and conducts them to the ventricular walls.
4 Sympathetic fibers to the heart do not act as pacemakers to initiate and regulate the heartbeat.

219. **3** Ventricular fibrillation is a death-producing dysrhythmia because the heart is not functioning as a pump. Immediate action is required or death will occur as a result of anoxia to the brain and other vital organs. (2; CJ; EV; TC; CV)
1 This is not a lethal dysrhythmia.
2 Same as answer 1.
4 This may require intervention and insertion of a pacemaker but is not lethal.

220. **3** Cardioversion involves administration of precordial shock, which is synchronized with the R wave to interrupt the heart rate. It is used for atrial fibrillation, paroxysmal atrial tachycardia (PAT), and ventricular tachycardia when pharmaceutical preparations fail. The heart is stopped by the electric stimulation, and it is hoped that the SA node will take over as pacemaker. (3; CJ; AN; TC; CV)
1 Because there are no R waves, cardioversion would not be done.
2 Same as answer 1.
4 Premature ventricular beats suggest an irritable myocardium and generally respond well to antidysrhythimic agents.

221. **3** A demand pacemaker functions only when the heart rate falls below the set rate of the pacemaker. The client can detect pacemaker malfunctions by monitoring the pulse rate and noting a drop below the set rate. (2; MR; PL; TC; CV)
  1 The client need not alter previous sleeping habits.
  2 Normal activity may be resumed when healing has occurred.
  4 Demand pacemakers function only when the heart rate drops below a predetermined level.

222. **3** Functioning pacemakers initiate impulses when the client's pulse rate falls below the preset rate. (2; CJ; EV; TC; CV)
  1 The client's heart beat may still be irregular.
  2 The client's heart rate may exceed the pacemaker.
  4 The pacemaker affects the rate, not the volume of the pulse.

223. **2** Ventricular fibrillation is a death-producing dysrhythmia and, once identified, must be terminated immediately by precordial shock (defibrillation). This is usually a standing physician's order in a cardiac care unit. (3; CJ; PL; TC; CV)
  1 Oxygen is administered to correct hypoxia; it does not take priority over defibrillation.
  3 CPR is instituted only when defibrillation fails to terminate the dysrhythmia.
  4 Bicarbonate is administered to correct acidosis; it does not take priority over defibrillation.

224. **3** Lidocaine hydrochloride (Xylocaine) decreases the irritability of the ventricles and is used in the treatment of ectopic beats originated by a ventricular focus. (2; CJ; IM; TC; CV)
  1 Digoxin slows and strengthens ventricular contractions; it will not rapidly correct ectopic beats.
  2 Furosemide (Lasix), a diuretic, does not affect ectopic foci.
  4 Levarterenol bitartrate (Levophed) is a sympathomimetic and is not the drug of choice for ventricular irritability

225. **2** The precordial shock during cardioversion must not be delivered on the T wave or ventricular fibrillation may ensue. By placing the synchronizer in the "on" position, the physician presets the machine so it will not deliver the shock on the T wave. (2; CJ; IM; TC; CV)
  1 The energy level may be set from 50 to 400 watts per second.
  3 This will not ensure that the shock is not delivered on the T wave.
  4 Same as answer 3.

226. **1** Asystole refers to the absence of atrial and ventricular contractions, which can cause death within minutes. (2; CJ; AS; TC; CV)
  2 This might be bradycardia (less than 60 beats per minute) or heart block (a partial or complete interruption in transmission of impulses from the sinoatrial node to the ventricles).
  3 The heartbeat has ceased in asystole.
  4 This would be tachycardia if the heart rate was 100 to 150 beats per minute.

227. **2** Irreversible brain damage will occur if a client is anoxic for more than 4 minutes. (1; CJ; IM; TC; CV)
  1 The age of the client does not affect the code.
  3 Although a variety of emergency medications must be available, their administration is ordered by the physician.
  4 Earlier heart rate is of minimal importance. Rhythm is more significant.

228. **1** Help must be obtained immediately. (1; CJ; IM; TC; CV)
  2 The radial pulse is not used.
  3 Before cardiac compression, open the airway, pinch the nose, and give two, rather than four, full lung inflations.
  4 This would not be done until the airway was open, two breaths were given, and reassessment indicated that there was no carotid pulse.

229. **4** The sternum must be depressed at least 3.7 to 5 cm ($1^1/_2$ to 2 inches) to compress the heart adequately between the sternum and vertebrae and to stimulate cardiac pumping action. (3; CJ; IM; TC, CV)
  1 This distance is ineffectual for an adult.
  2 Same as answer 1.
  3 Same as answer 1.

230. **4** This provides the best leverage for depressing the sternum. Thus, the heart is adequately compressed and blood is forced into the arteries. Grasping the fingers keeps them off the chest and concentrates the energy expended in the heel of the hand while minimizing the possibility of fracturing ribs. (1; CJ; IM; PA; CV)
    1 Both hands must be utilized; pressure on the lower portion of the sternum may fracture the xiphoid process, which can injure vital underlying organs.
    2 Pressure spread over two hands may inadequately compress the heart and fracture the ribs.
    3 Application of pressure by the fingers is less effective; this provides inadequate cardiac compression.

231. **4** Right ventricular heart failure causes increased pressure in the systemic venous system, which leads to a fluid shift into the interstitial spaces. Because of gravity, the lower extremities are first affected in an ambulatory client. (2; CJ; AS; TC; CV)
    1 Pulmonary disease would not result in varying degrees of edema.
    2 Pulmonary edema results in severe respiratory distress and peripheral edema.
    3 Myocardial infarction itself does not cause peripheral edema.

232. **3** Edema can be classified on a four-point scale from 1+ (barely detectable) to 4+ (indentation of greater than 10 mm). (2; CJ; AS; TC; CV)
    1 Although assessing fluid balance by weighing a client is important, it does not determine the degree of edema in a specific extremity.
    2 Although monitoring intake and output helps in assessing fluid balance, it does not determine the degree of edema in a specific extremity.
    4 The Trendelenburg test helps assess venous peripheral vascular disease, not the extent of edema.

233. **2** Elevation of an extremity promotes venous and lymphatic drainage by gravity. (1; CJ; PL; PA; CV)
    1 This is a dependent function of the nurse.
    3 Same as answer 1.
    4 This procedure will have little effect on edema.

234. **1** Heart failure is the failure of the heart to pump adequately to meet the needs of the body, resulting in a backward buildup of pressure in the venous system. Adaptations by the body include edema, ascites, hepatomegaly, tachycardia, dyspnea, and fatigue. (1; CJ; AS; PA; CV)
    2 These symptoms are generally not related to a specific disorder.
    3 These symptoms might indicate coronary insufficiency or infarction.
    4 This vague complaint is not specific to HF; it might indicate a variety of pulmonary conditions.

235. **4** In right ventricular heart failure, blood backs up in the systemic capillary beds; the increase in plasma hydrostatic pressure shifts fluid from the intravascular compartment to the interstitial spaces, causing edema. (2; CJ; AN; PA; CV)
    1 This would occur with crushing injuries or if proteins were pathologically shifting from the intravascular compartment to the interstitial spaces.
    2 Although a decrease in colloid osmotic (oncotic) pressure can cause edema, it results from lack of protein intake, not increased hydrostatic pressure associated with right ventricular heart failure.
    3 Increased fluid pressures within the tissue would result in fluid shifts into the intravascular compartment.

236. **3** Failure of the right ventricle causes an increase in pressure in the systemic circulation. To equalize this pressure, fluid moves into the tissues, causing edema, and into the abdominal cavity, causing ascites. (3; CJ; AN; PA; CV)
    1 There is no loss of cellular constituents of blood in right ventricular heart failure.
    2 Ascites is the accumulation of fluid in an extracellular space, not intracellular.
    4 The opposite results when there is an increase in hydrostatic pressure.

237. **4** With air conditioning, blood vessels in the skin remain partially constricted, preventing extensive blood flow through the skin. Such extensive skin blood flow would ordinarily occur in hot weather to promote radiation of heat from the body; however, the heart must then work to pump the blood through many extra miles of blood vessels in the skin. (1; MR; AN; PA; CV)
1 Body temperature is maintained.
2 There is decreased circulation to the skin in a cool environment versus a warm environment, which makes it beneficial to the person with cardiopulmonary problems.
3 Same as answer 2.

238. **1** Mitral stenosis impairs blood flow from the left atrium to the left ventricle. This backs up blood into the pulmonary veins and lungs. The result may be pulmonary edema. (3; CJ; AS; PA; CV)
2 Pulmonic stenosis tends to cause a bulging of the intraventricular septum.
3 Severe arteriosclerosis of the coronary arteries narrows the arterial lumen, which can result in a decreased blood supply to the myocardium causing hypoxia and angina.
4 Tricuspid disease may cause jugular vein distention and hepatic congestion.

239. **2** Six liters provide enough oxygen without adversely altering the client's blood gases, which would cause increased respiratory distress. (2; CJ; PL; TC; CV)
1 This is insufficient.
3 Higher concentrations of oxygen may depress CO_2 and raise O_2 concentrations, interfering with the impetus to breathe.
4 Same as answer 3.

240. **1** Irritability and restlessness increase the metabolic rate, heart rate, and blood pressure. This complicates heart failure. (1; CJ; AN; PA; CV)
2 Restlessness does not directly influence respirations; an increase in cardiac workload would increase respirations.
3 Restlessness alone usually does not elevate the body temperature.
4 Restlessness does not affect oxygen supply.

241. **4** The orthopneic position allows maximum lung expansion because gravity reduces the pressure of the abdominal viscera on the diaphragm and lungs. (2; CJ; IM; PA; CV)
1 Elevation of the extremities should be avoided because it increases venous return, placing an increased workload on the heart.
2 Excessive coughing and mucus production is characteristic of pulmonary edema and does not need to be encouraged.
3 Positioning for postural drainage does not relieve acute dyspnea; furthermore, it increases venous return to the heart.

242. **2** Self-identification of factors that would interfere with the treatment plan clues the nurse that the client may be noncompliant and further teaching is necessary. (2; MR; EV; PA; CV)
1 This statement is an appropriate response related to teaching concerning self-care after a myocardial infarction.
3 Same as answer 1.
4 Same as answer 1.

243. **2** These symptoms are associated with compromised arterial perfusion; a thrombus is a complication of a femoral arterial cardiac catheterization and must be suspected in the absence of a pedal pulse in the extremity below the entry site. (2; CJ; EV; TC; CV)
1 A circulatory assessment should be conducted first; the physician may or may not need to be notified immediately concerning the results of the assessment.
3 Unnecessary; the symptoms indicate a local peripheral problem, not a systemic or cardiac problem.
4 These symptoms are not expected.

244. **4** Troponin T (cTnT) has an extraordinary high specificity for myocardial cell injury. Cardiac troponins elevate sooner and remain elevated longer than many of the other enzymes that reflect myocardial injury. (2; CJ; AS; PA; CV)
1 ALT (alanine aminotransferase) is found predominantly in the liver; it is found in lesser quantities in the kidneys, heart, and skeletal muscles; it is used primarily to diagnose and monitor liver, not heart, disease
2 AST (serum aspartate aminotransferase) also known as SGOT (serum glutamic-oxaloacetic transaminase) is elevated 8 hours after a myocardial infarction.
3 Total LDH (lactate dehydrogenase) levels elevate 24 to 48 hours after a myocardial infarction.

245. 3 With heart failure (HF) the left ventricle is not functioning effectively, which is evidenced by an increased heart rate and crackles associated with pulmonary edema. (3; CJ; AS; PA; CV)

1 Unnecessary; although an infection would complicate heart failure, there are no signs that indicate this client has an infection.
2 This is done after vital signs and breath sounds are obtained and the client is stabilized.
4 Inappropriate for immediate monitoring; this would be done after vital signs and clinical assessment.

246. 4 Decreased cardiac output causes fluid retention, which results in dependent edema. (2; CJ; AS; PA; CV)

1 This is indicative of cardiac ischemia.
2 This is indicative of cardiac dysrhythmias.
3 This is indicative of an infectious process in the respiratory tract; pink, frothy sputum is associated with pulmonary edema.

247. 4 Trauma to the artery can interfere with circulation to the accessed extremity; most easily assessed by checking the pulse bilaterally. (2; CJ; EV; TC; CV)

1 The client is prescribed bed rest after the procedure, so gait is not assessed.
2 The gag reflex is not affected by the test.
3 Blood pressure should not be taken in the affected arm; the increase in pressure may initiate bleeding.

Blood and Immunity

248. 3 Iron is needed in the formation of hemoglobin. (2; CJ; PL; TC; BI)

1 Dextran is a plasma volume expander; it does not affect erythrocytes.
2 The client's anemia is caused by gastrointestinal bleeding, not the process of RBC production.
4 Vitamin B_{12} is a water-soluble vitamin that must be supplemented when an individual has pernicious anemia.

249. 2 In the early stages of hypovolemic shock, tachycardia is a compensatory mechanism to try to increase blood flow to body organs. (1; CJ; AS; PA; BI)

1 This is a sign of fluid volume excess.
3 Urine output would be decreased below 30 ml/hour because a decreased blood volume would cause a decreased glomerular filtration rate.
4 The blood pressure would be decreased because of the decreased blood volume.

250. 4 A slow rate provides time to recognize a transfusion reaction that is developing before too much blood is administered. (2; LE; AM; TC; BI)

1 Warming the blood to body temperature will cause clotting and hemolysis.
2 An infusion pump will cause RBC damage; the blood should flow by gravity.
3 Blood samples may be drawn after a transfusion, but this is not routinely done; they would not be drawn before the transfusion was started.

251. 3 Chills, headache, nausea, and vomiting are all signs of a transfusion reaction. (2; LE; EV; TC; BI)

1 The infusion must be stopped before treatment of the symptoms begins.
2 The physician should be notified after the transfusion is stopped.
4 Slowing the infusion will continue the reaction; it may lead to kidney damage.

252. 4 Immunization programs prevent the occurrence of disease and are considered primary interventions. (2; CJ; AN; PA; BI)

1 This is a tertiary intervention.
2 This is a secondary intervention.
3 Same as answer 1.

253. 3 Viscosity, a measure of a fluid's internal resistance to flow, is increased as the number of red cells suspended in plasma increases. (1; CJ; AN; PA; BI)

1 The number of cells does not affect the blood pH.
2 The hematocrit would be higher.
4 RBCs do not affect immunity.

254. 2 Plasma proteins do not easily pass through the capillary endothelium; however, the leakage through the capillary endothelium is important and results in edema if not corrected (one of the lymphatic system's functions is to return "leaked" plasma proteins to blood). (1; CJ; AN; PA; BI)

1 Blood gases (oxygen and carbon dioxide) pass through capillary endothelium easily.
3 Glucose and ions pass through the capillary endothelium easily.
4 Amino acids and water pass through the capillary endothelium easily.

255. **2** The gamma globulin fraction in the plasma is the fraction that, includes the antibodies. (1; CJ; AN; PA; BI)
   1 Albumin helps regulate fluid shifts by maintaining plasma oncotic pressure.
   3 Thrombin is involved in clotting.
   4 Hemoglobin carries oxygen.

256. **2** In active immunity, plasma cells provide antibodies in response to a specific antigen. (3; CJ; AN; PA; BI;)
   1 Eosinophils are involved in phagocytosis of antigen-antibody complexes.
   3 Erythrocytes (red blood cells) carry oxygen in the bloodstream.
   4 Not all lymphocytes are involved with antibody production

257. **2** Antibodies produced against group A beta-hemolytic streptococci sometimes interact with antigens in the heart's valves, causing damage and symptoms of rheumatic heart disease; early recognition and treatment of streptococcal infections has limited the occurrence of rheumatic heart disease. (2; CJ; AS; PA; BI)
   1 Hepatitis A, an inflammation of the liver, is caused by the hepatitis A virus (HAV), not by bacteria.
   3 The most common causes of meningitis, an infection of the membranes surrounding the brain and spinal cord, include *Streptococcus pneumoniae, Neisseria meningitides,* and *Haemophilus influenzae.*
   4 Rheumatoid arthritis is thought to be an autoimmune disease; it is not caused by microorganisms such as beta-hemolytic streptococci.

258. **1** Malaria is caused by the protozoan *Plasmodium falciparum,* which is carried by mosquitoes. (1; MR; IM; TC; BI)
   2 Ingestion of untreated water will not enable protozoa to enter the bloodstream.
   3 Ingestion of contaminated food will not facilitate the entry of protozoa into the bloodstream.
   4 Exposure to crowds will not enable the protozoa to enter the bloodstream.

259. **3** Parasites invade the erythrocytes, subsequently dividing and causing the cell to burst. The spleen enlarges from the sloughing of red blood cells. (3; MR; AS; PA; BI)
   1 WBCs (leukocytes) are not increased in number.
   2 RBCs (erythrocytes) are not increased in number.

4 Malaria is an infestation, not an infection or inflammation.

260. **4** Maintaining adequate nutritional and fluid balance is essential to life and must be accomplished during periods when intestinal motility is not too excessive so that absorption can occur. (2; CJ; PL; TC; BI)
   1 Although shaking chills may occur, seizures do not generally occur.
   2 Peritoneal dialysis is not generally used in the treatment of malaria.
   3 Infection may occur only through direct serum contact or a bite from an infected *Anopheles* mosquito.

261. **3** Quinine sulfate is used in malaria when the plasmodia are resistant to the less toxic chloroquine. However, a new strain of *Plasmodium,* resistant to quinine, must be treated with a combination of quinine (quick acting), pyrimethamine, and sulfonamide (slow acting). (2; CJ; IM; ED; BI)
   1 The aim of therapy is to eliminate the asexual erythrocytic parasite, which is responsible for the symptoms, not to control them.
   2 Reinfestation can occur with a different species or strain of *Plasmodium.*
   4 This would not occur if drug therapy is successful.

262. **2** *Plasmodium falciparum* in persons who have chronic malaria can cause hemoglobinuria, intravascular hemolysis, and renal failure as a result of destruction of red blood cells. (3; CJ; AS; PA; BI)
   1 This symptom is unrelated to the development of blackwater fever.
   3 Same as answer 1.
   4 Same as answer 1.

263. **3** The client has a weakened immune response; instructions regarding rest, nutrition, and avoiding unnecessary exposure to people with infections help reduce the risk of infection. (1; MR; IM; ED; BI)
   1 Although the onset of AIDS may be delayed, it represents the extreme of the continuum caused by HIV infection.
   2 The client may experience social isolation as a result of society's fears and misconceptions; these are beyond the client's control.
   4 Although Kaposi's sarcoma is related to HIV infection there are no specific measures to prevent its occurrence.

264. **2** Although blood is screened for the antibodies, there is a period between the time a potential donor is infected and the time when antibodies are detectable; there is still a risk but it is minimal. (2; MR; IM; ED BI)
1 There is no current method of destroying the virus in a blood transfusion.
3 The screening tests involve identification of the antibody, not the virus itself; the virus can be identified by the polymerase chain reaction test but is not part of normal screening.
4 Although many people consider autotransfusion for elective procedures, a trauma victim does not have this option.

265. **1** Epidemiologic evidence has identified breast milk as a source of HIV transmission. (2; MR; AS; TC; BI)
2 These behaviors are not believed to transmit HIV.
3 This is unrelated to modes of transmission of HIV.
4 HIV transmission does not occur from this type of contact.

266. **3** A person cannot contract HIV by eating from dishes previously used by an individual with AIDS; normal care is adequate (2; MR; IM; ED; BI)
1 This is unnecessary.
2 This is unnecessary; it may make the client feel different and create a feeling of isolation.
4 Same as answer I.

267. **4** Vaseline (petroleum jelly) breaks down the properties of condoms and would increase the risk of condom failure. (2; CJ; EV; ED; BI)
1 Using Vaseline instead of a water-soluble lubricant shows a lack of knowledge about condom use, a form of safer sex.
2 Although the person is attempting to be responsible, there is a lack of knowledge and the behavior is unsafe.
3 Condom use shows the client has some understanding about the transmission of HIV.

268. **4** Brief pressure is generally enough to prevent bleeding. (2; CJ; IM; TC; BI)
1 Complications are rare; no special positioning is required.
2 Complications are rare; frequent monitoring is unnecessary.
3 The site is cleansed before aspiration.

269. **3** Painless enlargement of the cervical lymph nodes is often the first sign of Hodgkin's disease, a malignant lymphoma of unknown etiology. (3; CJ; AS; PA; BI)
1 Axillary enlargement occurs after cervical.
2 Inguinal enlargement occurs later.
4 Mediastinal involvement follows after the disease progresses.

270. **2** For reasons unknown, Hodgkin's disease occurs most frequently between 15 and 30 years of age. (2; CJ; AS; PA; BI)
1 It is less common in children.
3 It is uncommon in later years.
4 It is uncommon during middle years.

271. **2** Radiation exposure may lead to depression of the bone marrow, with subsequent insufficient WBCs to combat infection. (2; MR; PL; ED; BI)
1 There is no increase in the number of cells, therefore viscosity is not increased.
3 Red blood cell production is decreased by radiation.
4 Bone structure is not affected by treatment; pathologic fractures may occur in response to disease.

272. **1** Platelets (thrombocytes) adhere to the intima of damaged vessels within seconds after injury, releasing substances that promote hemostasis. (2; CJ; AN; PA; BI)
2 Leukocytes play no role in clotting; they protect the body against microorganisms.
3 Erythrocytes are red blood cells; they carry oxygen and play no role in coagulation.
4 Red blood cells play no role in clotting; they carry oxygen to all body cells.

273. **3** Thromboplastin is a substance released by platelets that initiates the clotting process by converting prothrombin to thrombin. (2; CJ; AN; PA; BI)
1 Bile does not contain thromboplastin.
2 Plasma does not produce thromboplastin.
4 RBCs do not produce thromboplastin.

274. **3** Fibrinogen is a soluble plasma protein that becomes the insoluble gel, fibrin, during the clotting process. (3; CJ; AN; PA; BI)
1 Fibrin is the insoluble gel formed from fibrinogen by the action of thrombin.
2 Thrombin is needed to convert fibrinogen to fibrin; it is also needed in platelet aggregation.
4 Prothrombin is the precursor of thrombin.

275. **3** Calcium acts as a catalyst to convert pro-thrombin to thrombin. Thrombin accelerates the formation of insoluble fibrin from the soluble fibrinogen. (3; CJ; AN PA; BI)

1 Fluorine is a gas of the halogen group and is not involved in clotting; sodium fluoride helps harden tooth enamel.

2 Chloride is an extracellular anion that helps regulate osmotic pressure and combines with hydrogen to form hydrochloric acid; it is not involved with clotting.

4 Iron is essential for synthesis of hemoglobin; it is not involved in clotting.

276. **4** Vitamin K, synthesized by the bacterial flora of the intestine, promotes the liver's synthesis of prothrombin, an important blood-clotting factor. (3; CJ; AN; PA; BI)

1 Vitamin K does not promote platelet aggregation.

2 Vitamin K does not affect calcium ionization.

3 Vitamin K does not promote fibrinogen formation.

277. **1** Polycythemia vera results in pathologically high concentrations of erythrocytes in the blood; increased viscosity promotes the tendency toward thrombosis. (2; CJ; AN; PA; BI)

2 The fragility of blood cells does not affect the viscosity of the blood.

3 Hypertension is usually related to narrowing or sclerosing of arteries, not to increased number of blood cells.

4 There is an increased number of RBCs in polycythemia; their immaturity is not related to the increased viscosity.

278. **1** An elevated plasma bilirubin level could indicate an increased rate of red blood cell destruction (bilirubin is a product of free hemoglobin metabolism); the individual may have a hemolytic anemia (e.g., sickle cell anemia, glucose 6-phosphate dehydrogenase deficiency). (2; CJ; AN; PA; BI)

2 This does not involve the destruction of red blood cells with subsequent liberation of bilirubin.

3 A decreased amount of bile pigment would be liberated.

4 Oxygen-carrying ability is reflected by hemoglobin.

279. **1** Because of its great blood supply and general fragility, the spleen, when ruptured, must be removed to prevent possible hemorrhage, septicemia, or peritonitis. (2; CJ; AN; TC; BI)

2 This is not the reason for performing a splenectomy.

3 This does not explain the reason for its removal.

4 Although rupturing of the spleen may cause hemorrhage, septicemia, or peritonitis, it does not cause liver disease.

280. **3** Because the spleen has such vascularity, hemorrhage may occur and result in abdominal distention. (3; CJ; AS; TC; BI)

1 Although an elevated temperature is common, it is usually not the result of infection; the incidence of infection is not higher after a splenectomy, except in children, and it would not occur in the immediate postoperative period.

2 The incidence of obstruction is not higher than for other abdominal surgery.

4 The incidence is not higher after splenectomy than after other abdominal surgery.

281. **3** Postoperative pain will cause splinting, shallow breathing, and underaeration of the lung's left lower lobe because of close proximity of the spleen to the diaphragm. (3; CJ; PL; PA; BI)

1 This would be true of any surgery and is not specific to a splenectomy.

2 Same as answer I.

4 Same as answer 1.

282. **2** Gamma globulin, an immune globulin, contains most of the antibodies circulating in the blood. When injected into an individual, it prevents a specific antigen from entering a host cell. (2; CJ; EV; TC; BI)

1 This does not stimulate antibody production.

3 This does not affect antigen-antibody function.

4 Same as answer 1.

283. **1** Core rewarming with heated oxygen and administration of warmed PO or IV fluids is the preferred method of treatment. (2; MR; AN; PA; BI)

2 The victim would be too weak to ambulate; ambulation would expend energy.

3 Oral temperatures are not the most accurate assessment of core temperature because of environmental influences.

4 Warmed oral feedings are advised; gastric gavage would be unnecessary.

284. **4** Tetanus immune globulin (TIG) provides antibodies against tetanus; it is used if the client has never received tetanus toxoid, which confers active immunity (the body makes its own antibodies in response to the antigen). (3; CJ; IM; PA; BI)

1 DTP vaccine—diphtheria and tetanus toxoid combined with pertussis vaccine—produces active, not passive, immunity; in addition, DTP is not usually given to adults, Td is used.

2 Administration of this substance would produce active immunity.

3 Although this substance provides passive immunity, the risk of a hypersensitivity reaction is high and therefore TIG is preferred.

285. **2** Tetanus antitoxin provides antibodies, which confer immediate passive immunity. (3; MR; IM; PA; BI)

1 Antitoxin does not stimulate production of antibodies.

3 It provides passive, not active, immunity.

4 Passive immunity, by definition, is not long lasting.

286. **2** These foods are high in iron, which is necessary to build red blood cells. (1; MR; IM; ED; BI)

1 Although iron is contained in these foods, they are not the best recommended source for iron.

3 Same as answer 1.

4 Same as answer 1.

287. **2** When the spleen ruptures, internal loss of blood may be profound resulting in shock. (2; CJ; AS; TC; BI)

1 The nurse can assess hyperventilation if the client's breathing patterns are observed.

3 Although anxiety can cause hyperventilation resulting in lightheadedness, the data do not indicate that the client is anxious.

4 These symptoms are not inclusive enough to indicate infection.

Respiratory

288. **4** The respiratory center in the medulla responds primarily to increased carbon dioxide concentration in the blood. (1; CJ; AN; PA; RE)

1 Oxygen is normally not the primary stimulus to breathing; it functions as a primary stimulus in individuals who have chronic hypercapnia.

2 This is not a stimulant; it is a byproduct of muscular activity.

3 These are not stimulants for respiration; they are involved in transmission of neural impulses.

289. **3** The residual volume is the amount of air remaining in the lungs after maximum exhalation. (2; CJ; AN; PA; RE)

1 This is normally under the individual's control. The force exerted by the abdominal thrust surpasses that which the individual is voluntarily capable of exerting.

2 Same as answer 1.

4 Same as answer 1.

290. **2** Tidal volume (TV) is defined as the amount of air exhaled normally after a normal inspiration. (2; MR; AN; PA; RE)

1 This is the expiratory reserve volume (ERV).

3 This is the residual volume (RV).

4 The volume of air that can be forcibly inspired over and above a normal inspiration is the inspiratory reserve volume (IRV).

291. **4** Thoracic pressure is reduced because thoracic volume is increased as the diaphragm descends. (3; CJ; AN; PA; RE)

1 Contraction of the diaphragm causes inspiration.

2 Rising pressure in the alveoli and the intrapleural space or relaxation of the diaphragm expel air from the alveoli.

3 Same as answer 2.

292. **1** The tidal volume is the amount of air inhaled and exhaled while breathing normally. (2; MR; AS; PA; RE)

2 This is air that can be forcibly expired after deep inspiration.

3 This is the maximum amount of air that can be expired after expiration of the tidal volume.

4 This is the maximum amount of air that can be inspired following the inspiration of the tidal volume

293. **3** The lower the Po_2 and the higher the Pco_2 the more rapidly oxygen dissociates from the oxyhemoglobin molecule. (3; CJ; AN; PA; RE)

1 It must be associated with an increase in carbon dioxide pressure.

2 It must be associated with a decrease in oxygen pressure.

4 Oxygen dissociations would be decreased in this situation.

294. **1** With an oxygen debt, a muscle would show primarily low levels of oxygen and low levels of ATP caused by the low levels of aerobic respiration and high levels of lactic acid formation. (3; CJ; AS; PA; RE)
     2 Low levels of calcium are present.
     3 Low levels of glycogen are present.
     4 High levels of lactic acid are present.

295. **1** An Ambu-bag is a piece of equipment that can be compressed at regular intervals by hand for temporary ventilation of the client in respiratory arrest. (1; CJ; PL; TC; RE)
     2 Ventricular fibrillation requires immediate defibrillation.
     3 The Ambu-bag is used to ventilate a client, not to measure respiratory output.
     4 Wound drainage systems, not an Ambu-bag, may be used for gross incisional drainage.

296. **2** The orthopneic position is a sitting position that permits maximum lung expansion for gaseous exchange, because the abdominal organs do not provide pressure against the diaphragm and gravity facilitates the descent of the diaphragm. (2; CJ; lM; PA; RE)
     1 This position does not permit the diaphragm to descend by gravity, and pressure of the abdominal organs against the diaphragm limits its movement.
     3 This position does not maximize lung expansion to the same degree as the orthopneic position.
     4 Same as answer 3.

297. **3** Hemoptysis is expectoration of blood-stained sputum derived from the lungs, bronchi, or trachea. (1; CJ; AS PA RE)
     1 Hematuria refers to blood in the urine.
     2 Hematoma refers to a local accumulation of blood in the tissues.
     4 Hematemesis refers to vomiting of blood.

298. **3** Orthopneic position refers to sitting up and leaning slightly forward, which drops the diaphragm, allowing the lungs more room for expansion. (1; CJ; IM; PA; RE)
     1 Horizontal positions do not allow the gravitational effect on the diaphragm and thus do not maximize air exchange.
     2 Same as answer 1.
     4 The Trendelenburg position forces the diaphragm up, interfering with lung expansion.

299. **2** Because atelectasis involves collapsing of alveoli distal to the bronchioles, breath sounds would be diminished in the lower lobes. (2; CJ; AS; PA; RE)
     1 A client would have rapid, shallow respirations to compensate for poor gas exchange.
     3 Atelectasis results in a loose, productive cough.
     4 Atelectasis results in an elevated temperature.

300. **3** After a submucosal resection (SMR), hemorrhage from the area is frequently detected by vomiting of blood that has been swallowed. (2; CJ; AS; TC; RE)
     1 Crepitus would be caused by leakage of air into tissue spaces; it is not usually a complication of SMR.
     2 Headaches in the back of the head would not be a complication of a submucosal resection.
     4 The area under the tongue is not involved in this surgery.

301. **4** Carbon monoxide binds with hemoglobin more avidly than does oxygen. The progressive results are dyspnea, asphyxia, and death. (2; CJ; AN; PA; RE)
     1 Carbon monoxide does not block carbon dioxide transport; it binds with hemoglobin.
     2 Carbon monoxide inhibits oxygen transport, not vasodilation.
     3 Carbon monoxide does not form bubbles in the blood plasma; bubbles in tissues are caused by increased nitrogen, as in decompression sickness.

302. **4** This is the acid-fast causative organism of tuberculosis. (1; CJ; AN; PA; RE)
     1 This is not an acid-fast organism.
     2 Same as answer 1.
     3 Same as answer 1.

303. **4** This may occur because of the high osmotic pressure of the aspirated ocean water. (3; CJ; AS; TC; RE)
     1 Hypoxia and acidosis may occur after a near-drowning.
     2 This is not a sequela of near drowning.
     3 Hypovolemia occurs because fluid is drawn into the lungs by the hypertonic salt water.

304. **1** Air rises and is removed via a tube inserted in the upper intrapleural space. (2; CJ; AN; PA; RE)

    2 This is accomplished by the tube placed at the base of the lung; fluid flows toward the base via gravity.

    3 Medication will not be instilled into the intrapleural space in this situation.

    4 This would cause, not prevent, a pneumothorax.

305. **3** Subcutaneous emphysema occurs when air leaks from the intrapleural space through the thoracotomy or around the chest tubes into the soft tissue; crepitus is the crackling sound heard when tissues containing gas are palpated. (3; CJ; EV; TC; RE)

    1 This is related to prolonged trapping of air in the alveoli associated with emphysema, a chronic obstructive pulmonary disease.

    2 Unnecessary to determine crepitus; crackles and rhonchi occur within the lung; subcutaneous emphysema occurs in the soft tissues.

    4 This is unrelated to subcutaneous emphysema, which involves gas in the soft tissues from a pleural leak.

306. **3** Coughing raises intraabdominal and intrathoracic pressures which promote drainage from the chest tube; once the drainage tube is patent the fluctuation in the water column will resume; a lack of fluctuation because of lung reexpansion is unlikely 36 hours after a traumatic open chest injury. (3; CJ; IM; TC; RE)

    1 Unnecessary at this time; the chest tube is occluded and nursing intervention should be attempted first.

    2 This may be done eventually, but this is not the priority at this time.

    4 This would compromise aeration of the unaffected lung.

307. **4** This minimizes pooling of respiratory secretions and maximizes chest expansion, which aids in the removal of secretions; this maintains the airway and is an independent nursing function. (2; CJ; PL; PA; RE)

    1 This is part of pulmonary therapy that requires a physician's order.

    2 Same as answer 1.

    3 This will remove secretions once they accumulate, not prevent their accumulation.

308. **3** This is one method for the client to communicate following a laryngectomy; speech is produced by expelling swallowed air across constricted tissue in the pharyngoesophageal segment. (2; MR; PL; ED; RE)

    1 This is used for individuals who wish to communicate with someone who is deaf.

    2 Although this may be an adjunct to verbal speech, it should not be the primary means of communication.

    4 This is an alternative method used if a client cannot learn esophageal speech or for a short period of time during the early postoperative period.

309. **3** Water sports pose a severe threat; should water enter the stoma, the client will drown. (3; CJ; EV; TC; RE)

    1 This is not harmful; as long as there is no obstruction, adequate oxygen will be available because the respiratory rate will increase.

    2 Pillows are not contraindicated, although care should be taken not to occlude the airway by any bedding while asleep.

    4 Humidity is desirable and helpful in keeping secretions liquified.

310. **1** With a history of emphysema and probable respiratory infection the alveolar-capillary membrane is thickened, impairing diffusion of O_2 and CO_2. (3; CJ; AN; PA; RE)

    2 There is no nursing diagnosis called altered respiratory status.

    3 If the client has a respiratory infection and is unable to expectorate tenacious respiratory secretions, this nursing diagnosis would be appropriate; however, at this time there are no data to support this diagnosis.

    4 Rate, rhythm, and characteristics of breathing would have to be altered to support this nursing diagnosis; at this time there are no data to support this diagnosis.

311. **3** This helps warm the air, preventing bronchospasm. (3; MR; IM; ED; RE)

    1 This requires a physician's order and is used to prolong the clotting time, not prevent infection.

    2 Not recommended unless decaffeinated; tea contains caffeine, a stimulant, which may interfere with sleep.

    4 Bronchodilators cause gastrointestinal irritation and should not be taken on an empty stomach.

312. **3** Atelectasis refers to the collapse of alveoli; breath sounds over the area are diminished; fever may occur because retained secretions provide a medium for bacteria and the development of an infection. (3; CJ; AS; PA; RE)
1 These symptoms are associated with heart failure, not atelectasis.
2 This is not specific to atelectasis; the heart rate may be increased for many reasons; cyanosis is a very late sign of hypoventilation precluding early intervention.
4 A cough is caused by irritation of the upper airway, while atelectasis involves the alveoli; splinting is most often associated with inflammation of the pleural lining, not atelectasis.

313. **4** Streptococcal organisms are present on the skin, mucous membranes, and in the environment at all times. The most frequent portals of entry are the respiratory tract and breaks in the skin. (2; CJ; AN; PA; RE)
1 All are caused by streptococci.
2 Vaccinations are not available for most of these conditions; there is an antitoxin for scarlet fever, but antibiotics are now used.
3 Bacteria are not classified as parasites.

314. **1** Furosemide (Lasix) acts on the loop of Henle by increasing the excretion of chloride and sodium. (2; CJ; AN; TC; RE)
2 Although used in the treatment of edema and hypertension, this drug is not as potent as furosemide.
3 Same as answer 2.
4 This is a potassium-sparing diuretic; it is less potent than thiazide diuretics.

315. **3** Coughing is needed to raise secretions for expectoration. (1; MR; IM; TC; RE)
1 Oxygen will not mobilize the secretions.
2 A sitting position will allow secretions to remain in the lungs unless coughing is encouraged.
4 Rest should be encouraged only after coughing to bring up secretions mobilized by postural drainage.

316. **3** The etiology of a spontaneous pneumothorax is commonly the rupture of blebs on the lung surface. Blebs are similar to blisters. (2; CJ; AS; PA; RE)
1 Pleural friction rub would result in pain on inspiration, not a pneumothorax.
2 A tracheoesophageal fistula would cause aspiration of food and saliva, resulting in respiratory distress.
4 The client had no history of trauma.

317. **3** Oxygen is supplied to prevent anoxia but cannot be given in higher concentrations because, in an individual with emphysema, a low Po_2 (not high Pco_2) is the only respiratory stimulus. (2; CJ; IM; TC; RE)
1 This concentration is too high for a client with emphysema because it precipitates carbon dioxide narcosis.
2 This might increase the risk of mediastinal shift and interfere with expansion of the unaffected lung.
4 This dependent action would require orders as to specific electrolytes.

318. **3** As a person with a tear in the lung inhales, air moves through that opening into the intrapleural space. This creates a positive pressure and causes partial or complete collapse of the lung. (3; CJ; AN; PA; RE)
1 Mediastinal shift occurs toward the unaffected side.
2 This is not an impending problem.
4 There is loss of intrathoracic negative pressure.

319. **1** A pneumothorax results in decreased surface area for gaseous exchange. If the unaffected pleural regions cannot compensate, carbon dioxide builds up in the blood (hypercapnia). The client becomes drowsy and may lose consciousness. The body attempts to compensate by increasing the respiratory and pulse rates and by the renal retention of bicarbonate. (3; CJ; AS; TC; RE)
2 Hypokalemia causes extreme muscle weakness, abdominal distention, and changes in the ECG pattern.
3 Carbon dioxide builds up in the blood, and the Po_2 is lowered because of the decreased surface area for gaseous exchange.
4 Acidosis occurs with elevated Pco_2.

320. **2** Sudden chest pain occurs on the affected side; it may also involve the arm and shoulder. (2; CJ; AS; PA; RE)
1 Bloody vomitus is unrelated to pneumothorax.
3 Decreased chest motion would occur because of failure to inflate the involved lung.
4 The shift toward the unaffected side is caused by pressure from the pneumothorax.

321. **3** Destruction of the alveolar walls leads to diminished surface area for gaseous exchange and an increased CO_2 level in the blood. (2; CJ; AN; PA; RE)

1 Pleural effusion occurs when there is seepage of fluid into the intrapleural space; this does not occur with emphysema.

2 Infectious obstructions occur in conditions in which microorganisms invade lung tissue; emphysema is not an infectious disease.

4 Muscle paralysis may occur in diseases affecting the neurologic system; emphysema does not affect the neurologic system; therefore it is not a neurologic disease.

322. **4** Clients with COPD (chronic obstructive pulmonary disease) respond only to the chemical stimulus of low oxygen levels. Administration of high concentrations of oxygen will eliminate the stimulus to breathe, leading to decreased respirations and lethargy. (3; CJ; EV; TC; RE)

1 Cyanosis is caused by excessive amounts of reduced oxyhemoglobin; because oxygen is being administered, cyanosis may be reduced.

2 Rising carbon dioxide levels cause lethargy rather than anxiety.

3 High concentrations of oxygen will eliminate the stimulus to breathe, so the respiratory rate would decrease.

323. **2** Loss of elasticity causes difficult exhalation, with subsequent air trapping. Clients who have emphysema are taught to use accessory abdominal muscles and to breathe out through pursed lips to help keep the air passages open until exhalation is complete. (2; CJ; AN; PA; RE)

1 Expiration is difficult because of air trapping and poor elasticity.

3 There will be decreased vital capacity.

4 Diaphragmatic breathing is a learned mechanism that is beneficial.

324. **1** These drugs cause increased heart contraction (positive inotropic effect) and increased heart rate (positive chronotropic effect). If toxic levels are reached, side effects occur and the drug should be withheld until the physician is notified. (3; CJ; IM; TC; RE)

2 This is false reassurance and a false statement; the drug will have to be withheld until the physician is notified.

3 Controlled breathing may be helpful in allaying a client's anxiety; however, the drug may be producing side effects and should be withheld.

4 Same as answer 2.

325. **2** As a result of the narrowed airways, exhalation is difficult, leaving air trapped in the lung. Distention of alveolar walls to accommodate this volume leads to emphysema. (2; CJ; AS; PA; RE)

1 Atelectasis is the collapse of lung tissue.

3 Pneumothorax is the term that describes the collapse of a lung.

4 Pulmonary fibrosis is a condition in which fibrous connective tissue spreads over normal lung tissue.

326. **1** Hypersecretion of the mucous glands provides an excellent warm, moist medium for microorganisms. (2; MR; lM; ED; RE)

2 Asthma is not a disease that is voluntarily controlled.

3 Coughing must be encouraged; it prevents retention of mucus, which is an excellent medium for microorganisms. Excessive secretions also limit gaseous exchange.

4 Anxiety is not willfully controlled.

327. **3** There are several modes for the administration of oxygen. Selection is based on the disease and the client's adaptation. Oxygen administration is a particular concern for many clients. (2; CJ; AN; TC; RE)

1 Although consideration may be given to activity, selection is based on the pathologic condition and therapeutic needs.

2 Although anatomy may be one factor considered, selection depends on the therapeutic effect relative to the client's disease and needs.

4 Although these will be taken into consideration, the ultimate decision is based on the pathologic condition and therapeutic needs.

328. **2** The ribs may penetrate the pleura and lung, allowing air to fill the pleural space and collapse the lung. (1; CJ; AS; PA; RE)

1 Scoliosis involves altered vertebral alignment, not the ribs.

3 This does not occur.

4 Same as answer 3.

329. 2 Pressure within the pleural cavity causes a shift of the heart and great vessels to the unaffected side. This not only decreases the capacity of the unaffected lung but also impedes the filling of the right side of the heart and leads to a decreased cardiac output. (3; CJ; AN; PA; RE)

    1 Infection is not caused by a mediastinal shift.

    3 This complication might occur in severe chest trauma, not in mediastinal shift.

    4 The volume of the unaffected lung may decrease because of pressure from the shift.

330. 2 Fluctuations occur with normal inspiration and expiration until the lung is fully expanded. If these fluctuations do not occur, the chest tube may be clogged or kinked; coughing should be encouraged. (1; CJ; EV; TC; RE)

    1 The binder does not prevent tension on the tube; it would be contraindicated, because it limits thoracic expansion.

    3 The tube should be clamped only if ordered or if an air leak is suspected.

    4 The client may not be agitated; morphine depresses respirations and is usually avoided.

331. 1 Leakage of air into the subcutaneous tissue is evidenced by a crackling sound when the area is gently palpated. This is referred to as crepitus. (1; CJ; MS; EV; TC)

    2 Although hemostats should be readily available for any client with chest tubes in the event of a break in the drainage system, clamping the tube would not be otherwise necessary.

    3 To minimize the risk of pneumothorax, the dressing is not routinely changed.

    4 The system is kept closed to prevent the pressure of the atmosphere from causing a pneumothorax; drainage levels are marked on the drainage chamber to measure output.

332. 4 Chest x-ray films or radiographs reveal the degree to which the lung fills the pleural cavity and also the presence of any mediastinal shift. (3; CJ; EV; PA; RE)

    1 This would be an indicator of expansion of both lungs, and would not be specific to expansion of the affected side.

    2 The chest tubes may have minimal drainage; this is not an indicator.

    3 These are not normal chest sounds and do not indicate the degree of lung expansion.

333. 2 Turning the client to the side promotes drainage of secretions and prevents aspiration, especially when the gag reflex is not intact. This position also brings the tongue forward, preventing it from occluding the airway in the relaxed state. (1; CJ; IM; TC; RE)

    1 The risk of aspiration is increased when this position is assumed by a semialert client.

    3 This increases the risk of aspiration; this position may flex the neck in an individual who is not alert, interfering with respirations.

    4 This position is not generally used for a postoperative client because it interferes with breathing.

334. 2 Maintenance of a patent airway is always the priority, because airway obstruction impedes breathing and may result in death. (3; CJ; AN; TC; RE)

    1 This is important in the client's postoperative care; however, oxygenation is the priority.

    3 Same as answer 1.

    4 Same as answer 1.

335. 2 Oral intake should not be attempted until return of the gag reflex. (1; MR; EV; TC; RE)

    1 This is not a correct statement; there are additional factors that must be considered.

    3 Although some slight irritation may occur following this test, there is usually no painful sequela.

    4 Same as answer 2.

336. 3 With the head elevated, rather than horizontal or dependent, fluid will not collect in the interstitial spaces around the trachea. (2; CJ; PL; TC; RE)

    1 This may cause aspiration if the gag reflex has not returned.

    2 Same as answer 1.

    4 Same as answer 1.

337. 3 Cancerous lesions in the pleural space increase the osmotic pressure, causing a shift of fluid to that space. (2; CJ; AN; PA; RE)

    1 Excessive intake is normally balanced by increased urine output.

    2 Inadequate chest expansion results from pleural effusion and is not the cause of it.

    4 A bronchoscopy does not involve the pleural space.

338. 2 The respiratory membrane, consisting of the alveolar and capillary walls, is extremely thin. This thinness facilitates exchange of respiratory gases without the need for additional energy. (1; CJ; AN; PA; RE)

1 Osmosis is diffusion of water through a selective membrane.

3 Filtration is a process to prevent passage of certain-sized particles.

4 This mechanism is utilized when energy is required to move matter against a concentration gradient.

339. 3 The absence of bacteria in the sputum indicates that the disease can no longer be spread by the airborne route. (2; CJ; EV; PA; RE)

1 Once an individual has been infected, the test will always be positive.

2 Treatment is over an extended period; eventually the client may not have an active disease, but still remains infected.

4 This is not evidence that the disease will not be transmitted.

340. 1 The phrenic nerve stimulates the diaphragm; accidental severance of one phrenic nerve would result in partial paralysis of the diaphragm. (2; CJ; AN; PA; RE)

2 Because the phrenic nerve stimulates the diaphragm, its effect on postoperative pain would be negligible.

3 The diaphragm would ascend, not descend.

4 There is less excursion because the nerve has been severed.

341. 2 A chest tube drains the leaking chyle from the thoracic area; TPN provides nutrition, boosts immune defenses, and decreases thoracic duct flow; bed rest is recommended because lymphatic flow increases with activity. (2; CJ; PL; PA; RE)

1 A gastrostomy tube will not drain fluid from the thoracic area; a high-fat diet is contraindicated but bed rest is recommended.

3 This has no relationship to the drainage of chyle from the thoracic area; a low-fat diet and bed rest are recommended.

4 The nasogastric tube does not drain fluid from the thoracic area; a fat-poor diet and bed rest are recommended; a low-fat diet of medium chain triglycerides will reduce the production and flow of chyle.

342. 3 The client has a high risk for airway obstruction, and restlessness and dyspnea indicate hypoxia. (2; CJ; AS; TC; RE)

1 This is unimportant; the pharyngeal opening is sutured closed and a tracheal stoma is formed; the trachea is anatomically separate from the esophagus.

2 Cloudy drainage may indicate infection, which would not be an immediate postoperative complication.

4 Edema is unlikely to cause dehiscence early in the postoperative period.

343. 2 Inadequate dental hygiene may predispose a person to oral infections but would be only remotely involved in laryngeal neoplasms because of the anatomical relationship of the oral cavity and the larynx. (3; CJ; AS; PA; RE)

1 Irritation by air pollutants may initiate a tissue change that can lead to malignancy.

3 Alcohol is an irritant that may initiate a tissue change that results in a malignant neoplasm.

4 Tissue alterations caused by repeated microbiologic stress may result in a malignant neoplasm.

344. 4 Secretions are increased because of alterations in structure and function. A patent airway must be maintained. (2; CJ; IM; TC; RE)

1 Whispering can put tension on the suture line; initially nonverbal and written forms of communication should be encouraged.

2 The orthopneic position may cause neck flexion and block the airway.

3 The outer tube is not removed because the stoma may close.

345. 2 During suctioning of a client, negative pressure (suction) should not be applied until the catheter is ready to be drawn out because, in addition to the removal of secretions, oxygen is being depleted. (2; CJ; IM; TC; RE)

1 The sterility of the catheter can be maintained during one suctioning session; a new sterile catheter should be used for each new session of suctioning.

3 A cough reflex may be absent or diminished in some clients; the catheter should be inserted approximately 12 cm (4 to 5 inches) or just past the end of the tracheostomy tube.

4 The inner cannula is not removed during suctioning; it may be removed during tracheostomy care.

346. 2 Expectoration of blood is an indication that the lung itself was damaged during the procedure; a pneumothorax or hemothorax may occur. (2; CJ; EV; TC; RE):
1 Increased lung expansion should improve cerebral oxygenation and decrease confusion if present.
3 Increased breath sounds are anticipated as the lung is closer to the chest wall after the fluid in the pleural space is removed.
4 A decreased rate may indicate improved gaseous exchange and is not evidence that the client is in danger.

347. 2 Suctioning also removes oxygen, which can cause cardiac dysrhythmias; the nurse should try to prevent this by hyperoxygenating the client before and after suctioning. (2; CJ; IM; PA; RE)
1 To prevent trauma to the trachea, suction should only be applied while removing the catheter.
3 This kind of movement could cause tracheal damage.
4 Suction only as needed; excessive suctioning irritates the mucosa, which increases secretion production.

348. 2 During radiation therapy with radium implants the client is placed in isolation so that exposure to radiation by family and staff will be decreased. (1; MR; IM; TC; RE)
1 This is unnecessary.
3 Excess exposure to radiation is hazardous to personnel.
4 Rubber gloves will not protect the nurse from radiation.

349. 2 Because of the location of the spleen, expansion of the thoracic cavity during inspiration causes pain at the operative site. (2; CJ; AS; PA; RE)
1 Pain does not occur on expiration, for the lungs deflate and decrease pressure on the operative site.
3 Because limited activity decreases oxygen consumption, shortness of breath is not a common complaint.
4 This is not to be expected; accumulation of secretions can be avoided by coughing and deep breathing.

350. 4 80 to 120 ml of drainage is expected in the first 24 hours postoperatively; this is an excessive amount of drainage in 2½ hours and the surgeon should be notified immediately. (3; CJ; IM; TC; RE)
1 The surgeon should be notified; drainage is excessive.
2 Same as answer 1.
3 Same as answer 1.

351. 4 These are the classic signs of tuberculosis. (2; CJ; AS; PA; RE)
1 Weight gain is not associated with tuberculosis.
2 Same as answer 1.
3 Nausea and vomiting are not associated with tuberculosis.

352. 2 Atelectasis with impaired gas exchange is a major complication when clients use shallow breathing to avoid pain. (1; CJ; PL; TC; RE)
1 Excessive fluids should be avoided.
3 Pain medication is essential in diminishing or eliminating pain when breathing.
4 The face down position may diminish breathing for both lungs and is contraindicated.

353. 3 Decreased oxygen to the vital centers in the brain results in restlessness and confusion. (2; CJ; AS; PA; RE)
1 This would be a late sign of respiratory failure.
2 Tachycardia, not bradycardia, would occur as a compensatory mechanism to increase oxygen to body cells.
4 This occurs with fluid volume excess and pulmonary edema.

Gastrointestinal

354. 4 This is the organism that causes botulism. (1; CJ; AN; ED; GI)
1 This is a normal inhabitant of the intestines; it is not anaerobic.
2 This is an anaerobic organism that causes tetanus.
3 *Salmonella*, a gram-negative rod, is not anaerobic.

355. 4 Orange juice has a higher proportion of simple sugars, which are readily available for conversion to energy. (3; MR; PL; TC; GI)

1 Milk contains fat and protein, which require a longer digesting time, and lactose, which is a disaccharide.

2 Bread contains carbohydrates, which require a longer time to digest because they must be converted to simple sugars.

3 Candy bars do not contain the high proportion of simple sugars found in orange juice; they also contain fat, which takes longer to digest.

356. 3 Amino acids are absorbed into the blood in the intestinal capillaries with the aid of vitamin B_6 via the energy-dependent system, active transport. (2; CJ; AN; PA; GI)

1 Proteins are fairly large molecules; they do not passively diffuse.

2 This refers to movement across a semipermeable membrane; it does not apply to proteins.

4 Same as answer 2.

357. 2 Complete proteins contain sufficient amounts of all essential amino acids and are of animal origin. (2; CJ; AN; PA; GI)

1 Not all but rather the essential amino acids are needed during growth.

3 Sufficient amounts of all essential amino acids must be present.

4 The body cannot make the essential amino acids; they must be present in foods ingested.

358. 2 Vitamin K is synthesized by intestinal bacteria but is also found in liver, egg yolks, cheese, tomatoes, and green leafy vegetables. (2; CJ; AN; PA; GI)

1 Vitamin K is found in a small variety of foods.

3 It is found in enough foods so that a natural deficiency usually does not occur.

4 Vitamin K is not easily absorbed; it is fat soluble and requires bile salts for its absorption.

359. 4 Vitamin C is an intercellular cement substance. (3; CJ; AN; PA; GI)

1 This is the function of vitamin K.

2 This is the function of vitamin A.

3 This is the function of vitamin D.

360. 4 The aerobic oxidation of glucose occurring in the mitochondrion produces 38 moles of ATP for every mole of glucose oxidized. (2; CJ; AN; PA; GI)

1 This is the formation of peptide bonds.

2 This activity involves gaseous exchange.

3 The digestion, not hydrolysis, of fats is involved.

361. 1 Milk and milk products are not tolerated well because they contain lactose, a sugar that is converted to galactose by lactase. Lactose intolerance is common in those of Afro-American heritage. (3; CJ; AS; PA; GI)

2 This enzyme assists in the digestion of maltose, which is not a milk sugar.

3 This enzyme assists in the digestion of sucrose, which is not a milk sugar.

4 This enzyme assists in the digestion of starch, which is not a milk sugar.

362. 2 The salts in bile act as detergents to break large fat droplets into smaller ones (emulsification), providing a larger surface area for the enzymatic action of fat-splitting enzymes (lipases). (1; CJ; AN; PA; GI)

1 Bile does not act on proteins.

3 Bile does not help synthesize vitamins; it emulsifies fat and thus assists in absorption of fat soluble vitamins.

4 Bile does not have an acid pH.

363. 4 A triglyceride is composed of three fatty acids and a glycerol molecule. When energy is required, the fatty acids are mobilized from adipose tissue for fuel. (2; CJ; AN; PA; GI)

1 This is not the function of adipose tissue; its main function is storage.

2 This is not a function of adipose tissue; cholesterol is produced in the liver.

3 This is not the function of adipose tissue in fat metabolism.

364. 3 Saturated fats found in animal tissue are more dense than unsaturated fats, which are found in vegetable oils. (3; CJ; AN; PA; GI)

1 This characteristic of food has no bearing on fat content.

2 Same as answer 1.

4 The denseness of fat has nothing to do with digestibility.

365. 3 Animal fats are high in dense saturated fats. (1; CJ; PL; TC; GI)

1 Fruits do not contain saturated fats.

2 Grains do not contain saturated fats.

4 Vegetable oils contain unsaturated fats.

366. 1 Because triglycerides are made up of fatty acids bonded (esterified) to glycerol, their breakdown releases fatty acids as well as glycerol. (1; CJ; AN; PA; GI)
2 Triglycerides do not contain amino acids.
3 Triglycerides do not contain urea nitrogen.
4 Triglycerides do not contain simple sugars.

367. 3 A coenzyme is a nonprotein substance that, in the presence of a suitable enzyme, serves as a catalyst in chemical changes. (1; CJ; AN; PA; GI)
1 It doesn't form a new compound; it facilitates the process involved.
2 The vitamin or mineral is part of the process when functioning as a coenzyme.
4 The coenzyme does not neutralize the enzyme.

368. 1 Lipoproteins are simple proteins combined with lipid to facilitate circulation of fat in the blood. (2; CJ; AN; PA; GI)
2 Triglycerides are part of lipoproteins.
3 Phospholipids are incorporated in lipoproteins.
4 Plasma proteins do not contain fat.

369. 3 These amino acids are needed to maintain life and are not produced by the body. (1; CJ; AN; PA; GI)
1 The essential amino acids cannot be made by the body.
2 All amino acids are needed for metabolism; however, arginine and histidine are necessary for growth, but not during adulthood.
4 The body does not synthesize these amino acids; they must be ingested in the diet.

370. 3 Fruits contain less natural sodium than do other foods. (2; CJ; AN; PA; GI)
1 Milk is higher in natural sodium than is fruit.
2 Meat is higher in natural sodium than is fruit.
4 Vegetables are higher in natural sodium than is fruit.

371. 2 Vitamin A is a fat-soluble vitamin that accumulates in the body and is not significantly excreted even if extremely large amounts are ingested. After prolonged ingestion of extremely large doses, toxic effects (irritability, increased intracranial pressure, fatigue, night sweats, severe headache) can occur. (2; CJ; IM; TC; GI)
1 Vitamin A is toxic only after prolonged large dosages.
3 Vitamin A can be stored in the liver.
4 Vitamin A cannot be synthesized by the body.

372. 2 Pancreatic amylase (which enters the small intestine at the sphincter of Oddi) and sucrase, lactase, and maltase (which are released by epithelial cells covering the villi in the small intestine) are responsible for carbohydrate digestion. (3; CJ; AN; PA; GI)
1 Because ptyalin is present in saliva, some starch digestion occurs in the mouth.
3 Digestion of carbohydrates is completed before their arrival in the large intestine, which is concerned primarily with fluid reabsorption.
4 Limited carbohydrate digestion occurs in the stomach; pepsin begins the digestion of proteins.

373. 4 Deep green and yellow vegetables contain large quantities of the pigments alpha-, beta-, and gamma-carotene; beta-carotene is the major chemical precursor of vitamin A in human nutrition. (1; CJ; AN; PA; GI)
1 Oranges are considered a good source of both vitamin C and potassium.
2 Levels of vitamin A are higher in whole milk than in skim milk.
3 Tomatoes are a good source of vitamin C.

374. 3 The high-Fowler's position promotes optimal entry into the esophagus aided by gravity. (3; CJ; IM; TC; GI)
1 This position does not take full advantage of the effect of gravity.
2 Same as answer 1.
4 This is opposite to the desired position.

375. 2 Small meals are not as psychologically overwhelming and do not upset the stomach as easily. They are therefore better tolerated. (1; CJ; PL; TC; GI)
1 If no attempts are made to decrease portions at regular mealtimes, aversion will usually persist.
3 This does not ensure adequate nutrition; if the portion size is decreased, frequency must be increased.
4 Administration of vitamins is a dependent nursing function; vitamins do not stimulate appetite.

376. 3 Anorexia refers to loss of appetite. (1, CJ; AS; PA; GI)
1 Apathy refers to lack of concern or emotion.
2 Anoxia refers to lack of oxygen.
4 Dysphagia refers to difficulty in swallowing.

377. **1** A flat plate film of the abdomen visualizes abdominal organs as they are. (2; CJ; PL; TC; GI)

2 No bowel preparation is indicated.

3 The client may eat and drink as tolerated.

4 Same as answer 2.

378. **4** Barium salts used in a GI series and barium enemas coat the inner lining of the GI tract and then absorb x-rays passing through. They thus outline the surface features of the tract on a photographic plate. (1; CJ; IM; PA; GI)

1 Barium does not fluoresce.

2 Barium has no light-emitting properties.

3 Barium does not have properties of a dye.

379. **1** To permit adequate visualization of the mucosa during the sigmoidoscopy, the bowel must be cleansed with a nonirritating enema before examination. (1; CJ; IM; TC; GI)

2 Stool should be eliminated from the colon by an enema before the examination.

3 Because only the lower bowel is being visualized, keeping the client NPO is unnecessary and debilitating; clear liquids and a laxative may be given the day before to limit fecal residue.

4 The client does not drink such a substance in preparation for a sigmoidoscopy.

380. **4** To promote understanding and allay anxiety, all diagnostic tests should be explained to the client. (2; MR; IM; TC; GI)

1 Preparations for tests may vary depending on the client's condition.

2 Same as answer 1.

3 Same as answer 1.

381. **1** If the height of the enema fluid container above the anus is increased, the force and rate of flow also increase. If the container is raised excessively, damage to the mucosa may result and the procedure will be much more difficult for the client to tolerate. (2; CJ; IM; TC; GI)

2 The enema container can be held this high above the anus only if a high cleansing enema is to be given.

3 This would be too high and could cause mucosal injury.

4 Same as answer 3.

382. **3** Administration of additional fluid when a client complains of abdominal cramps adds to discomfort because of additional pressure. By clamping the tubing a few minutes the nurse allows the cramps generally to subside and the enema can be continued. (2; MR; EV; TC; GI)

1 Slowing the rate decreases pressure but does not reduce it entirely.

2 Cramps are not a reason to discontinue the enema entirely; temporary clamping of the tubing usually relieves the cramps and the procedure can be continued.

4 This will reduce the flow of the solution, which will decrease pressure but not reduce it entirely.

383. **2** Because the soft tissues of the GI tract lack sufficient quantities of x-ray–absorbing atoms (as are naturally present in the dense calcium salts of bone), an x-ray–absorbing coating of barium is used for radiologic studies. (3; CJ; AN; PA; GI)

1 Barium does not color the intestinal wall.

3 Barium absorbs x-rays.

4 Barium does not interact with electrolytes.

384. **4** This position maximally exposes the rectal area and facilitates entry of the sigmoidoscope. (2; MR; IM; TC; GI)

1 The Sims' position does not expose the rectal area to the same extent as the knee-chest position does but can still be used for a sigmoidoscopy if the client is unable to maintain the knee-chest position.

2 Although prone refers to a face-down position, the rectal area is not exposed.

3 The lithotomy position is appropriate for gynecologic examinations.

385. **3** A rise in the level of formula within the tube indicates a full stomach. (1; CJ; EV; PA; GI)

1 Passage of flatus reflects intestinal motility, which does not pose a potential problem.

2 Epigastric tenderness is not necessarily caused by a full stomach.

4 A rapid inflow is the result of positioning the container too high or using a feeding tube with too large a lumen.

386. 2 The presence of 50 ml or more of undigested formula may indicate impaired absorption; the volume of the next feeding may need to be reduced or the feeding postponed to reduce the risk of aspiration. (2; CJ; EV; TC; GI)

1 This evaluates fluid balance and is best performed over a 24-hour period.

3 This is a method for evaluating placement.

4 Although weighing the client regularly is important to evaluating overall nutritional progress, it cannot provide information about absorption of a particular feeding.

387. 4 The increased osmolarity (concentration) of many formulas draws fluid into the intestinal tract, which would cause diarrhea; such feedings may need to be diluted initially until the client develops tolerance. (1; CJ; AN; TC; GI)

1 Formulas frequently have reduced fiber content, causing problems with constipation.

2 Bacterial contamination is not a factor if feedings are administered as recommended by the manufacturer.

3 Inappropriate positioning may increase the risk of aspiration, but does not cause diarrhea.

388. 4 Because the cardiac sphincter of the stomach is slightly opened to admit the nasogastric tube, rapid feeding could result in regurgitation. (2; CJ; IM; TC; GI)

1 Distention can be diminished by avoiding the instillation of air with the feeding.

2 The speed of feeding does not cause flatulence, but the administration of air may.

3 Indigestion is not hazardous to the client.

389. 2 Vomiting may result in aspiration of vomitus, because it cannot be expelled; this could cause pneumonia or asphyxia. (2; CJ; EV; TC; GI)

1 This is not a life-threatening problem.

3 Same as answer 1.

4 Same as answer 1.

390. 2 Pain and swelling should subside before 1 week postoperative. Continued pain may indicate infection. (2; MR; EV; TC; GI)

1 The breath may have an odor because of dried blood in the oral cavity; this is to be expected during the postoperative period.

3 Painful swallowing may occur because of generalized trauma resulting from surgery and is to be expected.

4 Tenderness is expected during the postoperative period.

391. 2 Leukoplakia are white thickened patches that tend to fissure and to become malignant; ulcerations in the mouth or on the tongue may indicate cancer. (2; CJ; AS; PA; GI)

1 Halitosis would not be an early sign or specific to cancer of the mouth.

3 Bleeding gums occur in gingival diseases.

4 Pain associated with cancer of the tongue would not radiate to the substernal area.

392. 4 Heavy alcohol ingestion predisposes an individual to the development of oral cancer. (2; CJ; AS; PA; GI)

1 Nail biting has no effect on the development of oral cancer.

2 Dental hygiene does not affect the development of oral cancer.

3 Gum chewing is not a contributing factor to development of oral cancer.

393. 1 Sleeping on pillows raises the upper torso and prevents reflux of the gastric contents. (1; MR; IM; ED; GI)

2 This would have no effect on the reflux of gastric contents.

3 Increasing the content of the stomach before lying down would aggravate the symptoms associated with a gastroesophageal reflux.

4 The effect of antacids is not long lasting enough to promote a full night's sleep; sodium bicarbonate is not recommended as an antacid.

394. 1 Heavy lifting increases intraabdominal pressure, allowing gastric contents to move up through the lower esophageal sphincter (regurgitation) causing heartburn (pyrosis). (3; MR; IM; ED; GI)

2 This encourages regurgitation and should be avoided.

3 Increasing fluids with meals increases gastric volume, causing distention and reflux.

4 Constrictive garments such as belts, binders, and girdles increase intraabdominal pressure and could lead to reflux.

395. 3 Approximately 2/3 of clients with peptic ulcer disease have been found to have *Helicobacter pylori* infecting the mucosa and interfering with its protective function. (2; MR; IM; ED; GI)

1 Antibiotics do not affect immunity.

2 Antibiotics do not increase the effect of antacids.

4 Antibiotics do not affect acid secretion.

396. **1** Almost all peptic ulcers in the stomach develop along the lesser curvature of the antral (pyloric) region. About 85% of all peptic ulcers occur within the first 2 cm of the duodenum. These regions are most exposed to acid conditions. (2; CJ; AS; PA; GI)
  2 This is less exposed to gastric secretions.
  3 This is less exposed to gastric secretions; however, erosion may occur after repeated episodes of gastric reflux.
  4 Same as answer 2.

397. **3** The act of eating allows the hydrochloric acid in the stomach to work on and be neutralized by food rather than irritate the intestinal mucosa. (2, CJ; AS; PA; GI)
  1 This symptom is not specific to duodenal ulcers.
  2 This may indicate renal colic.
  4 This is a generalized symptom not specific to duodenal ulcers.

398. **3** Irritation of the mucosa may cause increased bleeding or perforation and therefore should be avoided. (2; CJ; AN; TC; GI)
  1 All clients' diets should be nutritionally balanced; this is not specific to this client's problem.
  2 Bulk and roughage may irritate the mucosa and should be decreased.
  4 Psychologic support is not the primary goal; efforts should be made to include foods that are psychologically beneficial, but do not include foods that are irritating to the mucosa.

399. **4** The vagus nerve stimulates the stomach to secrete hydrochloric acid. When it is severed, this neural pathway is interrupted and there will be a decrease in stomach secretions. (2; MR; IM; ED; GI)
  1 The portion of the vagus nerve that was severed innervated the stomach, not the heart; therefore the heart rate would not be affected.
  2 The vagus nerve controls hydrochloric acid secretion, not gastric emptying; emptying is determined by the nature of foods being digested.
  3 The vagus nerve is not a sensory nerve.

400. **1** Pitressin is a vasoconstrictor that can be used to control GI bleeding. (3; CJ; PL; TC; GI)
  2 Neostigmine inhibits cholinesterase, permitting acetylcholine to function; it is used primarily for myasthenia gravis.

  3 Pro-Banthine is a gastrointestinal anticholinergic; it decreases motility but has no effect on bleeding.
  4 Aquamephyton is vitamin K; it promotes formation of prothrombin in the liver; although this action would be helpful, it would take too long to be of value in an emergency situation.

401. **3** The antrum is responsible for gastrin production, which stimulates hydrochloric acid secretion; its removal reduces HCl secretion and thus reduces irritation of the gastric mucosa. (3; CJ; AS; TC; GI)
  1 Removal by means of a laser beam, cryotechnique, or surgery is used when cataracts occur.
  2 A stapedectomy, mobilization of the stapes, or a prosthetic implant would be used with otosclerosis.
  4 A resection of the fifth cranial nerve would be done in trigeminal neuralgia.

402. **2** When high-osmotic fluid passes rapidly into the small intestine, it causes hypovolemia. This results in a sympathetic response with tachycardia, diaphoresis, and dizziness. The symptoms are also attributed to a sudden rise and subsequent fall in blood sugar. (2; CJ; AN; PA; GI)
  1 The stomach is not full; its contents rapidly empty into the jejunum.
  3 This could occur with intestinal obstruction; dumping syndrome is associated with increased motility originating in the jejunum. Reflux would need reverse peristalsis.
  4 This is usually associated with paralytic ileus; dumping syndrome leads to increased intestinal motility.

403. **3** Nasogastric drainage is expected to be bright red at first and gradually darken within the first 24 hours after surgery. (3; CJ; AS; TC; GI)
  1 Bloody drainage is expected this soon after surgery and the physician does not need to be notified.
  2 Nasogastric suction must be working and the tube must remain patent to prevent stress on the suture line.
  4 The nasogastric tube is only irrigated if the physician orders it because of the danger of injury to the suture line; generally saline at room temperature would be ordered.

404. 1 To ensure continued suction, the patency of the tube should be maintained. Normal saline is used to prevent fluid and electrolyte disturbances during irrigation. (1; CJ; PL; TC; GI)

   2 The stomach is not considered a sterile body cavity, so medical asepsis is indicated.

   3 Care must be taken to avoid traumatizing the mucosa.

   4 Ice chips and water represent fluid intake, which must be approved by the physician; being hypotonic in nature, such intake may lower the serum electrolytes.

405. 1 Physiologic normal saline is used in gastric irrigation to prevent electrolyte imbalance. Because of the fresh gastric sutures, slow and gentle irrigation should be performed. Most surgeons, however, prefer gastric instillations. (1; CJ; IM; TC; GI)

   2 The purpose of irrigation is to maintain the patency of the tube for gastric decompression; with disconnection from suction a buildup of secretions and air can occur or the tube can become blocked by viscous drainage.

   3 Increasing the pressure may cause damage to the suture line.

   4 Same as answer 2.

406. 4 Fluid and electrolytes are lost through intestinal decompression; on a daily basis about one-fifth of the total body water is secreted into and almost completely reabsorbed by the GI tract. (1; CJ; EV; TC; GI)

   1 Because the client is kept NPO, there would be no stimulus to cause enzymes to be secreted into the GI tract.

   2 IV dextrose supplies some carbohydrates as a source of energy; it would not be drawn from storage by intestinal decompression.

   3 Because the client is being kept NPO, vitamins and minerals are not entering the GI tract and therefore are not lost.

407. 4 Symptoms of dumping syndrome occur to some degree in about 50% of all individuals who have undergone a gastrectomy. They include weakness, faintness, heart palpitations, and diaphoresis. It is therefore important to explain to the client that such symptoms can be minimized by resting after meals in the semi-Fowler's position, eating small meals, and omitting concentrated and highly refined carbohydrates. (2; MR; PL; ED; GI)

   1 Gas-forming foods affect the intestines, not the stomach.

   2 Modification of roughage is part of the management of intestinal rather than gastric disorders.

   3 Eating habits must be modified to prevent rapid emptying of the stomach.

408. 3 Pernicious anemia is caused by a lack of vitamin B_{12}. Intrinsic factor, produced by the parietal cells of the gastric mucosa, is necessary for B_{12} absorption. (3; CJ; EV; PA; GI)

   1 B_{12} is absorbed in the ileum.

   2 The intrinsic factor is secreted by the stomach; the hemopoietic factor is the combination of B_{12} and intrinsic factor.

   4 Chief cells secrete the enzymes of the gastric juice.

409. 4 To promote drainage of different lung regions, clients should turn every 2 hours. Deep breathing inflates the alveoli and promotes fluid drainage. (2; CJ; IM; TC; GI)

   1 The airway will be expelled once the gag reflex returns.

   2 Oxygen administration is a dependent function and is not generally required unless there is an underlying cardiac or respiratory disease.

   3 During physical effort, individuals with abdominal incisions often revert to shallow breathing.

410. 3 Small frequent feedings are tolerated best after a subtotal gastrectomy. (1; CJ; PL; TC; GI)

   1 Roughage may be irritating to the GI tract after surgery.

   2 As soon as edema subsides, the individual is generally given small amounts of fluid and then the diet is gradually progressed.

   4 Recuperation from gastric surgery may take up to 3 months; allowing only food preferences does not ensure inclusion of nutrients necessary for recovery.

411. 4 Vitamin K is a fat-soluble vitamin and needs bile salts for its absorption from the upper segment of the small intestine. It is a catalyst in the carboxylation of glutamine to prothrombin. (3; CJ; AN; PA; GI)

   1 Bile salts do not inhibit the synthesis of prothrombin.

   2 The liver does not synthesize vitamin K; the intestine does.

   3 Bile salts do not affect prothrombinase (thromboplastin).

412. **2** Bile, a natural antioxidant, helps stabilize the vitamins and prevents destruction by oxygen. In addition, it is a transport vehicle for fat through the intestinal wall. (3; CJ; AN; PA; GI)
1 This is stomach acid.
3 This is the digestive enzyme for lipids.
4 This is the digestive enzyme for starch.

413. **2** ERCP involves the insertion of a cannula into the pancreatic and common bile ducts during an endoscopy. The test is not performed if the client's bilirubin is greater than 3 to 5 mg/dl because cannulization may cause edema, which would increase obstruction of bile flow. (2; CJ; AS; PA; GI)
1 This is not directly related to this test.
3 Same as answer 1.
4 Same as answer 1.

414. **4** Cholecystokinin is a widely distributed hormone whose functions include stimulation of gallbladder contraction and the release of pancreatic enzymes. (2; CJ; AN; PA; GI)
1 Gastrin stimulates the secretion of gastric juice.
2 Secretin promotes the production of bile by the liver and the secretion of pancreatic juice.
3 Enterocrinin stimulates the secretion of intestinal juice (succus entericus).

415. **2** When bile does not mix with foods in the intestine, emulsification of fats cannot occur and fat digestion is retarded. Stomach motility is also reduced, because increased stomach peristalsis depends on fat digestion in the small intestine. (2; CJ; AN; PA; GI)
1 Once emulsified by bile, fatty foods are readily broken down by digestive enzymes.
3 The production of bile is unaffected.
4 Obstruction would cause discomfort. Bile and pancreatic secretions enter the duodenum through the ampulla of Vater. With obstruction, edema and spasm occur, blocking the flow of enzymes and causing pain.

416. **3** These symptoms result from failure of bile to enter the intestines, with subsequent backup into the biliary system and diffusion into the blood. The bilirubin is carried to all body regions, including the skin (itching) and kidneys (excretion of bile-colored urine). The absence of bilirubin in the intestine results in clay-colored stools. (3; CJ; AS; PA; GI)

1 Signs refer to objective findings of an examiner; the signs of inadequate absorption of vitamin K include ecchymosis, hematuria, and other bleeding.
2 The urine would be dark, reflecting increased serum bilirubin levels, and the stools would not be brown because the bile pigments would not be present in the GI tract.
4 If bile levels in the bloodstream are high, there would be bile in the urine, causing it to have a dark color.

417. **2** Vitamin K is necessary in the formation of prothrombin to prevent bleeding. It is a fat-soluble vitamin and is not absorbed from the GI tract in the absence of bile. (1; CJ; AN; TC; GI)
1 Bilirubin is the bile pigment formed by the breakdown of erythrocytes.
3 Thromboplastin converts prothrombin to thrombin during the normal coagulation process.
4 Cholecystokinin is the hormone that stimulates contraction of the gallbladder.

418. **1** The location of the incision results in pain on inspiration or coughing. The subsequent reluctance to cough and deep breathe facilitates respiratory complications from retained secretions. (2; CJ; AS; PA; GI)
2 This surgery does not take a prolonged period of time.
3 Bile does not impair inflammatory or immune responses.
4 A cholecystectomy is usually performed to treat cholelithiasis or cholecystitis; there is generally an inflammatory, not an infectious, process.

419. **2** The nurse should anticipate drainage and reinforce the surgical dressing as needed, (1; CJ; IM; TC; GI)
1 Changing a dressing at this time unnecessarily increases the risk of infection.
3 An abdominal binder is rarely ordered and it would interfere with assessment of the dressing at this time.
4 Montgomery straps are utilized when frequent dressing changes are anticipated; they are not appropriate at this time.

420. 1 Protein and calories provide energy, both of which are necessary for tissue building. (1; CJ; PL; TC; GI)

    2 A high-fat diet is contraindicated because fat requires bile to be absorbed.

    3 The gallbladder has been removed and painful contractions should not occur; dietary fat intake depends on individual tolerance.

    4 This is inadequate for tissue repair.

421. 2 This is the unique function of pancreozymin, which is secreted by the duodenal mucosa. It particularly affects the production of amylase. (1; CJ; AN; PA; GI)

    1 Enterocrinin increases intestinal juice secretion.

    3 Enterogastrone lessens gastric secretion and motility.

    4 Cholecystokinin stimulates the flow of bile from the gallbladder.

422. 4 Lipase is a pancreatic enzyme that aids in the digestion of fat. (3; CJ; AN; PA; GI)

    1 Lipase does not synthesize triglycerides.

    2 This is the function of bile.

    3 Lipase does not break down all dietary fat.

423. 4 The duodenum secretes several digestion-related hormones, including secretin, which elicits bicarbonate secretion from the pancreas, and pancreozymin, which elicits enzyme secretion from the pancreas. It also brings about gallbladder contraction and secretion of bile; in this function it is known as cholecystokinin. (2; CJ; AN; PA; GI)

    1 The liver produces bile, which aids in the digestion of fat, but does not produce any hormones.

    2 The adrenals produce glucocorticoids, mineralocorticoids, and epinephrine.

    3 The pancreas produces the hormone insulin.

424. 3 A pseudocyst of the pancreas is an abnormally dilated space that contains blood, necrotic tissue, and enzymes and is surrounded by connective tissue. (3; CJ; AN; PA; GI)

    1 This is an incorrect definition of a pseudocyst.

    2 Same as answer 1.

    4 Same as answer 1.

425. 4 Alcohol stimulates pancreatic enzyme secretion and an increase in pressure in the pancreatic duct. The backflow of enzymes into the pancreatic interstitial spaces results in partial digestion and inflammation of the pancreatic tissue. (2; CJ; AN; PA; GI)

    1 Although blockage of the bile duct with calculi may precipitate pancreatitis, this is not associated with alcohol.

    2 Alcohol does not deplete insulin stores; the demand for insulin is unrelated to pancreatitis.

    3 Although the volume of secretions increases, the composition remains unchanged.

426. 2 An incision close to the diaphragm (as in surgery of the pancreas) causes a great deal of pain when the client coughs and deep breathes. These clients tend to take shallow breaths, leading to inadequate expansion of the lungs, the accumulation of secretions, and infection. (1; CJ; AN; PA; GI)

    1 This is unrelated to the development of respiratory infections.

    3 The elevation of serum bilirubin in the blood does not affect the immune mechanisms.

    4 Pancreatitis is usually an inflammatory, not an infectious, process.

427. 4 In the liver a simple protein combines with a lipid to form a lipoprotein. Lipoproteins circulate freely in the blood and can be utilized easily and quickly in various metabolic processes. (3; CJ; AN; PA; GI)

    1 The liver does not produce phospholipids.

    2 Fat is stored in adipose tissue.

    3 The liver does not oxidize fat.

428. 4 Protein helps correct severe malnutrition; moderate fat limits need for bile; a high-calorie, high-vitamin diet prevents tissue breakdown. (2; CJ; AS; PA; GI)

    1 A diet high in protein, carbohydrates, and calories is needed to improve nutritional status.

    2 A high-protein diet is essential in repairing tissues and restoring nutritional status.

    3 This diet does not offer enough fat or calories.

429. 3 Thiamine and nicotinic acid help convert glucose for energy and therefore influence nerve activity. (1; CJ; AN; PA; GI)

    1 These vitamins do not affect elimination.

    2 These vitamins are not related to circulatory activity.

    4 Vitamin K, not thiamine and niacin, is essential for the manufacture of prothrombin in the liver.

430. **1** The liver detoxifies alcohol and is the organ most often damaged in chronic alcoholism. The high-calorie diet prevents tissue breakdown, which produces additional amino acids and nitrogen. (1; CJ; AN; PA; GI)
    2 These organs are not involved in detoxification of alcohol.
    3 Same as answer 2.
    4 This organ is not involved in detoxification of alcohol.

431. **4** The temperature during steaming is never high enough or sustained long enough to kill organisms. (2; CJ; IM; ED; GI)
    1 Processing destroys the organisms.
    2 Because of the extremely high temperature, broiling sufficiently destroys the virus.
    3 Baking would destroy the organisms.

432. **2** Contracting hepatitis B through blood transfusions can be prevented by screening donors and testing the blood. (2; CJ; PL; TC; GI)
    1 This does not prevent transmission of hepatitis B.
    3 Same as answer 2.
    4 Same as answer 2.

433. **3** This is an enzyme, also known as glutamic-pyruvic transaminase, that is released early in the course of liver damage. (3; CJ; AS; PA; GI)
    1 This is not an early sign of liver damage.
    2 Same as answer 1.
    4 Same as answer 1.

434. **3** The virus is present in the stool of clients with hepatitis A, so special handling is required. The virus may also be present in the urine and in the nasotracheal secretions. (2; CJ; PL; TC; GI)
    1 Hepatitis A is not usually transmitted via the air.
    2 Bringing food to a client requires no precautions; however, disposable utensils should be used because the client's nasotracheal secretions contain the virus.
    4 Same as answer 1.

435. **3** Hepatitis C, formerly called non-A, non-B hepatitis, is caused by an RNA virus that is transmitted parenterally. The incubation period is 5 to 10 weeks. (2; CJ; AN; PA; GI)

    1 Hepatitis A, also known as infectious hepatitis, is caused by an RNA virus that is transmitted via the fecal-oral route. The incubation period is 2 to 6 weeks.
    2 Hepatitis B is transmitted parenterally, sexually, and by direct contact with infected body secretions. The incubation period is 1 to 6 months. It is not the major cause of posttransfusion hepatitis.
    4 Hepatitis D is a complication of hepatitis B.

436. **3** Weight is valuable objective information that can be helpful in determining the development or extent of ascites. (1; CJ; AS; TC; GI)
    1 Diet history will not help in monitoring a client's condition.
    2 Bowel sounds are objective data but do not help monitor the liver.
    4 Pain is subjective.

437. **2** The liver stores carbohydrates as glycogen, which is a polymer of glucose. (1; CJ; AS; PA; GI)
    1 Glycerol, a byproduct of lipids, combines with three fatty acids to form a triglyceride.
    3 Fat is not stored in the liver.
    4 These are not a ready form of energy; combinations of amino acids form protein.

438. **1** Fatty acids are insoluble and must combine with bile to form water-soluble substances. (1; CJ; AN; PA; GI)
    2 Lipase is a pancreatic enzyme.
    3 Amylase, which digests starch, is found in saliva and pancreatic juice.
    4 This is a component of bile. It is produced in the liver and stored in the gallbladder, but it is not the component of bile that emulsifies fats.

439. **2** Lipoproteins, a combination of a fat and a simple protein, have not been formed because of poor protein intake. Therefore fat accumulates in the liver. (3; CJ; AN; PA; GI)
    1 Elevations of bile in the blood occur because hepatic ducts are obstructed by the enlarged liver.
    3 Individuals with cirrhosis of the liver are likely to have bleeding tendencies (rather than clotting) because of the decreased synthesis of prothrombin.
    4 Deficiency of protein results in the breakdown of tissue (catabolism) and a negative nitrogen balance.

440. **4** Low sodium controls fluid retention, blood pressure, and consequently edema; low protein controls ammonia formation in proportion to the liver's ability to detoxify ammonia in forming urea; moderate fat and high calories and vitamins help repair a long-standing nutritional deficit. (2; CJ; PL; PA; GI)

  1 High-protein diets are contraindicated because of the damaged liver's inability to detoxify ammonia.
  2 Because protein is required for tissue regeneration, restriction is based on the liver's ability to detoxify ammonia; a high-fat diet is avoided because of the related cardiovascular risks and the related demand for bile.
  3 Regeneration of tissue requires a high-calorie diet; 1200 calories is too low.

441. **3** The hepatic portal vein carries blood from the capillary beds of the viscera (small and large intestinal walls, stomach, spleen, pancreas, gallbladder) to the sinusoids of the liver. The hepatic veins drain the liver sinusoids into the inferior vena cava. (2; CJ; AN; PA, GI)

  1 The portal vein takes blood to the liver; the hepatic veins drain the liver sinusoids into the inferior vena cava.
  2 Enters the superior vena cava from the capillary beds of the viscera.
  4 Same as answer 2.

442. **4** The elevated pressure within the portal circulatory system causes elevated pressure in areas of portal systemic collateral circulation (most importantly, in the distal esophagus and proximal stomach). Hemorrhage is a possible complication. (2; CJ; AS; TC; GI)

  1 Liver abscesses may occur as a complication of intestinal infections; they are not related to portal hypertension.
  2 This is not related to portal hypertension; it may be caused by manipulation of the bowel during surgery, peritonitis, neurologic disorders, or organic obstruction.
  3 Perforation of the duodenum is usually caused by peptic ulcers; it is not a direct result of portal hypertension or cirrhosis.

443. **3** With obstruction of the portal vein there is an increase in pressure in the abdominal veins, which empty into the portal system. These veins develop collaterals to circumvent the obstruction. The collaterals are usually in the paraumbilical, hemorrhoidal, and esophageal areas. (1; CJ; AN; PA; GI)

  1 Although hepatitis A may predispose to the development of cirrhosis, which in turn causes portal hypertension, most often it does not.
  2 Kupffer cells are part of the reticuloendothelial system, which helps prevent infection and does not primarily affect venous pressure.
  4 Obstruction of these ducts blocks flow of bile, causing obstructive jaundice.

444. **4** In cirrhosis of the liver, fibrous scarring within the liver parenchyma, most often from alcohol toxicity, compresses the portal veins and causes a backup of blood and increased pressure within the portal system. Fluid seeps into the abdominal cavity (ascites), mainly from the surface of the liver. (2; CJ; AN; PA; GI)

  1 Lymph does not escape from the liver sinusoids.
  2 Plasma osmotic (oncotic) pressure is decreased because of decreased albumin production.
  3 Secretion of ADH and aldosterone increases as renal blood flow decreases.

445. **1** The bladder must be empty to decrease the chance of puncturing it during the paracentesis. (1; MR; IM; TC; GI)

  2 This is not necessary.
  3 Same as answer 2.
  4 This is usually performed in the Fowler's position to assist the flow of fluid by gravity.

446. **1** The increased plasma hydrostatic pressure in the extremities resulting from heart failure or liver cirrhosis, possibly combined with a genetic weakness in the vein walls, may lead to varicose veins. (3; CJ; AS; PA; GI)

  2 Toxins are not responsible for varicose veins.
  3 Distention of venous walls occurs as a result of increased rather than decreased pressure.
  4 Decreased plasma protein causes fluid to move out of the vascular compartment into the interstitial spaces.

447. 3 Neomycin destroys intestinal flora, which breaks down protein and in the process gives off ammonia. Ammonia at this time is poorly detoxified by the liver and can build up to toxic levels. (2; CJ; IM; TC; GI)
 1 Bile levels may be elevated because of biliary obstruction by the enlarged liver but are unaffected by Neomycin.
 2 Urea is a byproduct of protein metabolism formed in the liver as it detoxifies ammonia. The production of urea is hampered by severe liver damage and is unaffected by Neomycin.
 4 Hemoglobin formation is not influenced by the administration of Neomycin.

448. 4 This tube includes an esophageal balloon that on inflation exerts pressure, which retards hemorrhage. (2; CJ; PL; TC; GI)
 1 This is used for gastric decompression; gavage, or lavage; it has one lumen.
 2 This is used for gastric decompression, it has two lumens, one for decompression; and one for an air vent.
 3 This is used for intestinal decompression.

449. 1 Because the liver is unable to detoxify ammonia to urea, protein intake should be further restricted when coma is inevitable. (2; CJ; PL; PA; GI)
 2 This relatively high intake of protein will increase blood ammonia levels.
 3 Same as answer 2.
 4 Same as answer 2.

450. 2 Cirrhosis of the liver results in the development of extensive scar tissue within the liver structure; such scar tissue contracts around hepatic blood vessels, impeding blood flow and raising the pressure in the hepatic portal system. The physiologic response to slowly developing portal circulatory obstruction is the growth of collateral vessels linking portal veins with esophageal veins; as destruction progresses, the collaterals become so large that they bulge into the esophageal lumen and are called esophageal varices. (2; CJ; AS; PA; GI)
 1 Ascites and edema are the result of the pathophysiologic process in the liver, not the cause; the fluid is present in the interstitial spaces and abdominal cavity as a result of portal hypertension and decreased plasma protein.

 3 The liver regenerates; but in the case of cirrhosis, scar tissue is formed.
 4 The varicosities are the result of increased portal pressure.

451. 2 The client's breath has a sweet odor because the liver is not metabolizing the amino acid methionine. (2; CJ; AS; PA; GI)
 1 Anuria is characteristic of renal failure.
 3 This refers to spasm of the eyelid associated with anxiety or cranial nerve pathology; it is unrelated to liver disease.
 4 A sensation of a lump in the throat is associated with acute anxiety; it is unrelated to liver disease.

452. 2 Because protein breakdown gives off ammonia, which cannot be detoxified by the liver, protein should be eliminated from the diet. (1; CJ; IM; TC; GI)
 1 A Fleet enema would not affect ammonia levels, which are associated with hepatic coma; a Neomycin enema would limit intestinal bacteria, which breaks down protein, giving off ammonia.
 3 No surgical intervention would affect ammonia levels associated with hepatic coma.
 4 Carbohydrates are unrelated to protein breakdown and rising ammonia levels; eliminating carbohydrates would have no effect.

453. 3 An accumulation of nitrogenous wastes in hepatic coma affects the nervous system. Flapping tremors and generalized twitching occur in the second stage of this disease. (2; CJ; AS; PA; GI)
 1 Stool is often clay colored because of biliary obstruction by a cirrhotic liver.
 2 Elevated cholesterol levels are not necessarily present.
 4 As encephalopathy progresses to coma, all reflexes are absent.

454. 1 Bile deposits will impart a yellowish tinge (jaundice or icterus) to the skin, often first observed in the sclerae. (2; CJ; AS; PA; GI)
 2 Urticaria (or hives) is generally characteristic of an allergic response.
 3 Uremic frost is characteristic of renal failure.
 4 Hemangioma is a benign lesion composed of blood vessels.

455. **1** Increased ammonia levels indicate that the liver is unable to detoxify protein byproducts. Neomycin reduces the amount of ammonia-forming bacteria in the intestines. (3; CJ; AS; PA; GI)

 2 White blood cells may indicate infection; however, this would have no relationship to the need for Neomycin enemas.

 3 Culture and sensitivity testing would identify the presence of a microorganism and the medication that would be effective in its eradication; it would not be indicated in cirrhosis.

 4 Alanine aminotransferase (ALT), also called serum glutamic-pyruvic transaminase (SGPT), is a test to assess for liver disease but has no relationship to the need for Neomycin enemas.

456. **4** The diet should be high in protein and calories, low in fat, and gluten free for individuals with malabsorption syndrome. Protein is needed for tissue rebuilding. (2; MR; IM; TC; GI)

 1 The client may prefer foods high in gluten, which would potentiate malabsorption.

 2 IV therapy is a dependent function and does not provide all the necessary nutrients.

 3 Diarrhea is caused by malabsorption, which accounts for the poor nutritional status; once the diarrhea is corrected, it is essential to compensate by providing a nutritious diet.

457. **4** Gluten, a cereal protein, appears to be responsible for morphologic changes of the intestinal mucosa in individuals with nontropical sprue (adult celiac disease). (2; CJ; EV; TC; GI)

 1 Folic acid, along with antimicrobial agents, is used to treat tropical sprue; it causes dramatic improvement.

 2 Vitamin B_{12} may be administered if macrocytic anemia or achlorhydria develops; however, it does not correct the major pathology.

 3 The use of corticosteroids may be advantageous with either form of sprue; however, this does not produce the same effect as the specific treatment already described.

458. **4** Gluten is found in rye, wheat, and oat products. (1; MR; PL; ED; GI)

 1 Gluten is not found in these foods; they do not have to be avoided.

 2 Same as answer 1.

 3 Same as answer 1.

459. **1** These foods are low in gluten. (3; CJ; IM; TC; GI)

 2 Flours used in the production of noodles are high in gluten.

 3 Flours used in the production of bread are high in gluten.

 4 Postum is a cereal drink high in gluten.

460. **4** When circulation to the appendix is interfered with by a fecalith or foreign body, inflammation occurs. (2; CJ; AN; PA; GI)

 1 Diet patterns do not predispose the individual to the development of appendicitis.

 2 Bowel infections are rare and do not predispose the individual to the development of appendicitis.

 3 Hypertension may cause generalized edema; local edema would not occur.

461. **3** Rebound tenderness is a classic subjective sign of appendicitis. (1; CJ; AS; PA; GI)

 1 Urinary retention does not cause acute lower right quadrant pain.

 2 Hyperacidity causes epigastric, not lower right quadrant, pain.

 4 There is generally decreased bowel motility distal to an inflamed appendix.

462. **4** Muscular rigidity over the affected area is a classic sign of peritonitis. (1; CJ; AS; TC; GI)

 1 Malaise, rather than hyperactivity, is often associated with peritonitis.

 2 Nausea is a common occurrence with peritonitis.

 3 Urinary retention may occur following surgery as a complication of anesthesia.

463. **2** The semi-Fowler's position aids in drainage and prevents spread of infection throughout the abdominal cavity. (2; CJ; IM; TC; GI)

 1 The Sims' position is generally used for administration of enemas or rectal examination; it would not be helpful in draining the area.

 3 The Trendelenburg position would contribute to the spread of infection throughout the abdominal cavity.

 4 The dorsal recumbent position would not allow for localization of drainage.

MEDICAL-SURGICAL **ANSWERS**

464. 2 Paralytic ileus occurs when neurologic impulses are diminished, as from anesthesia, infection, or surgery. (1; CJ; EV; PA; GI)
1 Interference in blood supply would result in necrosis of the bowel.
3 Perforation of the bowel would result in pain and peritonitis.
4 Obstruction of the bowel lumen would initially cause increased peristalsis and bowel sounds.

465. 2 A rectal tube promotes maximum benefits in 30 minutes. This allows adequate time for gas to escape. (2; CJ; IM; TC; GI)
1 Fifteen minutes is not adequate time to permit removal of flatus.
3 After 30 minutes the release of flatus would be minimal.
4 Same as answer 3.

466. 2 A rectal catheter should be inserted approximately 4 inches to pass the rectal sphincters. (1; CJ; IM; TC; GI)
1 A catheter inserted just 2 inches will not be passed beyond the rectal sphincters.
3 Deep insertion may damage the intestinal mucosa.
4 Same as answer 3.

467. 1 The client's status requires immediate intervention; to delay treatment may prove dangerous because symptoms indicate possible perforation. (3; CJ; AN; TC; GI)
2 Diverticulitis can in most cases be treated by diet, rest, and antibiotic therapy.
3 This is not true with the diagnostic techniques presently available.
4 Age is not the factor; the symptoms indicate possible peritonitis.

468. 4 Because the mucosa of the intestinal tract is damaged, its ability to absorb vitamins taken orally is greatly impaired. (2; CJ; IM; PA; GI)
1 Although this is true, the risks associated with IV administration will outweigh the benefits.
2 Vitamins are effective orally unless there is disease involving the GI tract that hampers absorption.
3 IV vitamins do not decrease colonic irritability.

469. 1 When the diseased bowel is removed, the client's symptoms cease. (3; MR; AN; TC; GI)
2 Surgical removal of a body part is not temporary, but permanent.

3 Ulcerative colitis does not progress to Crohn's disease; clients with ulcerative colitis have an increased risk for colorectal cancer.
4 This is not a true statement.

470. 4 Personality and psychologic stresses cause pathologic changes that influence the development of ulcerative colitis. (2; CJ; AS; PA; GI)
1 Although this may be another causative factor, psychologic stress is more commonly associated with this disease.
2 Same as answer 1.
3 Same as answer 1.

471. 4 Milk and the caffeine in cola are chemically irritating to the intestinal mucosa. They also promote secretion of gastric juice. (2; MR; IM; ED; GI)
1 These foods do not irritate the bowel and need not be restricted.
2 This is too general; except for those that contain lactose sugars, products containing sugar generally are not irritating to the mucosa; protein also is not irritating.
3 These are absorbed slowly and are not irritating.

472. 4 The inflammatory process tends to increase peristalsis, causing cramping and diarrhea with subsequent weight loss. As ulceration occurs, loss of blood leads to anemia. (2; CJ; AS; PA; GI)
1 Leukocytosis or increased leukocytes in the blood are not common in this disease.
2 Hemoptysis (coughing up blood from the respiratory tract) is not a related symptom.
3 Fever may or may not be a symptom and leukopenia (deficiency in number of leukocytes) does not occur.

473. 4 Occult blood in the stool could indicate active bleeding; the stool should also be examined for microorganisms to detect early infections that could easily become systemic by spread through the damaged intestinal mucosa. (2; CJ; AN; PA; GI)
1 There is no indication that parasites are present; the situation does not warrant this examination.
2 This situation does not warrant culturing.
3 This situation does not warrant these examinations.

474. 3 As a result of chronic irritation, the colon becomes thin and may perforate. (2; CJ; AS; TC; GI)
1 Paralytic ileus may be a complication of surgical interventions involving the intestines or of perforation.
2 Bleeding may vary from a small amount to hemorrhage; this is not the most serious complication.
4 Obstruction rarely occurs, but if it does it is not the most serious complication.

475. 4 This is a low-residue diet and is necessary in the acute phase of ulcerative colitis to prevent irritation of the colon. (3; MR; EV; ED; GI)
1 Milk contains lactose, which is irritating to the colon; contraindicated in colitis.
2 The juice in this diet contains cellulose, which is not absorbed and irritates the colon; cream soup contains lactose, which is irritating to the colon.
3 Same as answer 1.

476. 2 *Entamoeba histolytica*, the organism that causes amebic dysentery, is transmitted through excreta. (1; CJ; PL; PA; GI)
1 This is not a tick-borne disease.
3 This organism is not transmitted by gnats.
4 This organism is not transmitted via milk.

477. 3 Intussusception is the telescoping or prolapse of a segment of the bowel within the lumen of an immediately connecting part. (1; MR; IM; ED; GI)
1 Volvulus is a twisting of the bowel onto itself.
2 Adhesions are bands of scar tissue that can compress the bowel.
4 Herniation is the term that describes protrusion of an organ through the wall that contains it.

478. 3 Emotional stress of any kind can stimulate peristalsis and thereby increase the volume of drainage. (2; CJ; PL; PA; GI)
1 The client should be encouraged to eat a diet as normal as possible.
2 The stoma will start to drain within the first 24 hours after surgery.
4 Ileostomy drainage is liquefied and continuous, so irrigations are not indicated.

479. 2 Vitamin B_{12} (extrinsic factor) combines with intrinsic factor, a substance secreted by the parietal cells of the gastric mucosa, forming hemopoietic factor. Hemopoietic factor is only absorbed in the ileum, from which it travels to bone marrow and stimulates erythropoiesis. (3; CJ; EV; PA; GI)
1 Folic acid is not absorbed in the terminal ileum.
3 Iron absorption does not occur in the ileum.
4 Trace elements are not absorbed in the ileum.

480. 2 Trauma to the abdominal wall and to the stoma should be avoided, so contact sports are contraindicated. (1; CJ; PL; TC; GI)
1 Trauma to the abdominal wall is a minimal risk in this sport.
3 Same as answer 1.
4 Same as answer 1.

481. 3 The location of the tumor will usually indicate whether a colostomy, creation of an opening proximal to the tumor between the colon and the skin surface, is needed. (1; CJ; AN; TC; GI)
1 An ileostomy is the creation of an opening between the ileum and the skin surface; it would not be done.
2 A colectomy is the surgical removal of a portion of the colon, with creation of an anastomosis; it is generally used in less extensive carcinoma.
4 A cecostomy is the creation of an opening between the cecum and the skin surface; it is usually a temporary procedure.

482. 1 To take advantage of the anatomic position of the sigmoid colon and the effect of gravity, the client should be placed in a left Sims' position for the enema. (2; CJ; IM; TC; GI)
2 This position does not facilitate the flow of fluid into the sigmoid colon by gravity.
3 Same as answer 2.
4 Same as answer 2.

483. 1 Neomycin Sulfate is poorly absorbed from the GI tract and is therefore used for sterilization of intestines prior to bowel surgery. (1; CJ; IM; TC; GI)
2 Because intestinal bacteria are destroyed, there is a decreased production of vitamin K.
3 Oral administration of neomycin primarily affects intestinal bacteria.
4 Because it is poorly absorbed from the GI tract, Neomycin Sulfate does not affect urinary tract infections.

484. 3 Because Neomycin is poorly absorbed from the GI tract, most remains in the intestines and exerts its antibiotic effect on the intestinal mucosa. In preparation for GI surgery the level of microbial organisms will be reduced. (1; CJ; AN; TC; GI)

1 Neomycin is nephrotoxic.
2 Because it is poorly absorbed from the GI tract, the systemic effect is minimal.
4 Neomycin is mainly effective in suppression of intestinal bacteria.

485. 3 A skin barrier provides a coating that creates a barrier to gastrointestinal enzymes and protects against allergic reactions to the tape on the appliance. (2; CJ; IM; TC; GI)

1 Alcohol tends to dry out the skin and mucous membranes, leading to irritation and breakdown.
2 Mineral oil is not an effective skin protectant and would interfere with adherence of any appliance.
4 This contains alcohol which is drying and leads to skin irritation.

486. 2 The client must be ready to accept changes in body image and function; this acceptance will facilitate mastery of the techniques of colostomy care, special diets, and optimal use of community resources. (2; MR; AN; PS; GI)

1 Specific knowledge can be imparted only when an individual is ready to learn; it requires acceptance of a new body image.
3 Same as answer 1.
4 Same as answer 1.

487. 2 Factual answer; neomycin provides preoperative intestinal antisepsis. (2; MR; IM; ED; GI)

1 The desired effect of this drug is unrelated to kidney function; nephrotoxicity is a side effect.
3 It will not prevent metastasis of tumor to other areas.
4 This is not the purpose of administering this medication.

488. 2 This describes the stoma that has adequate vascular perfusion. (3; CJ; AS; PA; GI)

1 Indicates inadequate perfusion of the stoma.
3 Same as answer 1.
4 Same as answer 1.

489. 3 When GI absorption is inadequate, total parenteral nutrition (TPN) is the nutritional therapy of choice because it provides needed nutrients. (2; CJ; AN; PA; GI)

1 TPN is usually used in chronic or long-term therapy, not for short-term therapy.
2 TPN is used for total, not supplemental, nutrition.
4 Not the indication for TPN; a feeding tube would be used.

490. 4 In ulcerative colitis, pathology is usually in the descending colon (left side); in Crohn's disease, it is primarily in the terminal ileum, cecum, and ascending colon on the right side. (3; CJ; AN; PA; GI)

1 Ulcerative colitis, as the name implies, affects the colon, not the small intestine.
2 There is no direct correlation of colitis with malignancy of the bowel, although psychologic, environmental, genetic, and nutritional factors, as well as preexisting disease, appear to be influential in malignancy.
3 Involvement is in the distal portion of the colon, not the proximal portion.

491. 3 If medical management has failed, this is the next logical choice because it removes the affected intestine. (2; CJ; PL; ED; GI)

1 Psychotherapy might improve the client's ability to cope with the disease, but it will not solve the physical problems.
2 This has already been tried over an extended period of time and has failed.
4 This is part of the medical management that has been tried and has failed.

492. 2 Ample time in the bathroom must be ensured for the actual irrigation process and fecal returns, which may not be immediate. (3; MR; PL; ED; GI)

1 The availability of adequate time takes precedence; this would not use the gastrocolic reflex that would occur after eating.
3 This is important, but the availability of adequate time takes precedence.
4 Same as answer 1.

493. **3** The stoma of a colostomy must be dilated with a lubricated, gloved finger to prevent strictures and subsequent obstruction. (2; MR; IM; ED; GI)
1 Clothing need not be special but should be nonconstricting.
2 Once healing has occurred, activity is not limited.
4 Diet should be as close to normal for the individual as possible; gas-forming foods should be avoided.

494. **4** Although foods that produce gas are generally avoided, the diet of an individual with a colostomy should be as close to normal as possible for optimal physiologic and psychologic adaptation. (2; CJ; PL; PA; GI)
1 A high-protein diet is important until healing occurs; but a balanced diet generally meets nutritional needs for protein.
2 There is no need to limit fiber; it provides bulk necessary for unconstipated stools.
3 Because absorption of nutrients is unaffected, there is no need to increase carbohydrate intake.

495. **2** Isotonic saline most closely resembles normal body fluids; it will not cause an imbalance by pulling extra fluids and electrolytes out of the circulation. (1; CJ; IM; TC; GI)
1 Hypotonic solutions would allow absorption of fluid into the circulation, resulting in dilution of electrolytes and possible circulatory overload.
3 Same as answer 1.
4 Hypertonic solutions would draw fluids out of the circulation into the GI tract; glucose provides a medium for bacterial growth.

496. **4** A transverse colostomy is an opening created in the transverse colon. The rectal tube should be pointed to the proximal intestine to evacuate the bowels. (2; CJ; IM; TC; GI)
1 A water-soluble lubricant is generally used to facilitate insertion.
2 There are no sphincters so bearing down is unnecessary.
3 Continual force may traumatize the mucosa; lack of nerve endings diminishes sensation.

497. **3** The rapid rate of enema administration or ostomy irrigation often causes cramping. Additional fluid leads to more discomfort. Cramping will generally subside if the enema tubing is clamped for a few minutes; the procedure can then be continued. (2; CJ; IM; TC; GI)
1 Discontinuing the irrigation could lead to ineffective evacuation of the colon.
2 Lowering the container will decrease the rate of flow, but fluid will continue to enter the colon if the container remains above the stoma.
4 Indiscriminate advancing of the catheter can injure the mucosa and does not affect cramping.

498. **2** This is far enough to direct the flow of solution into the bowel. (3; CJ; IM; TC; GI)
1 This is inadequate; fluid may leak back around the catheter.
3 An insertion of 6 inches may cause trauma to the mucosa.
4 An insertion of 8 inches may cause trauma to the mucosa.

499. **3** A colostomy irrigation is much like a tap water enema. The solution must be held high enough to allow it to flow into the bowel but not so high that it flows rapidly, or it can cause cramping or mucosal injury. (2; CJ; IM; ED; GI)
1 This does not represent maximum height permitted and may not ensure flow of solution into the bowel.
2 Same as answer 1.
4 This is too high and could cause intestinal trauma.

500. **3** Hernioplasty involves not only the reduction of a hernia but also an attempt to change or strengthen the structure to prevent recurrence. (2; CJ; AN; PA; GI)
1 Analysis of the word shows that it means an opening cut into the hernia; it does not refer to repair of a hernia.
2 There is no such word; hernias are not cut out. They are reduced and the area reinforced to prevent recurrence.
4 Herniorrhaphy is surgical repair of a hernia.

501. **3** Because of the presence of feces in the colon, a client with a fecal impaction has the urge to defecate but is unable to. (1; CJ; AS; TC; GI)
   1 Flatulence may occur as a result of immobility, not just obstruction.
   2 Anorexia may occur with an impaction but may also be caused by other conditions.
   4 The frequency of bowel movements varies for individuals; it may be normal for this individual not to have a BM for several days.

502. **2** When the bowel is impacted with hardened feces, there is often seepage of liquid feces around the obstruction and thus uncontrolled diarrhea. (1; CJ; AS; PA; GI)
   1 The bowel may become distended if completely obstructed, but this is a late symptom if it occurs at all.
   3 This is indicative of lower GI bleeding.
   4 There are often frequent liquid bowel movements in the presence of an impaction.

503. **1** Phospho-Soda is a saline cathartic, increasing the osmotic pressure within the intestine so that body fluids are drawn into the bowel, stimulating bowel stretching, peristalsis, and defecation. (3; CJ; IM; TC; GI)
   2 Emollients have a detergent action, softening the stool by facilitating its absorption of water.
   3 Stimulants irritate the mucosa so that peristalsis is increased.
   4 Bulk-forming laxatives are cellulose derivatives that remain in the intestinal tract and absorb water; they cause bulk, which stimulates peristalsis.

504. **3** Prune juice and warm water can be administered prophylactically by the nurse to promote defecation. Prune juice irritates the bowel mucosa, stimulating peristalsis. Increased fiber in the diet may also improve intestinal motility. (2; CJ; IM; TC; GI)
   1 The routine use of enemas should be avoided because they promote dependency and can result in electrolyte imbalance.
   2 The routine use of laxatives promotes dependency.
   4 Same as answer 1.

505. **2** Bowel training is a program for the development of a conditioned reflex that controls regular emptying of the bowel. The key to success in a conditioning program is adherence to a strict time for evacuation based on the client's individual schedule. (3; CJ; PL; TC; GI)
   1 The indiscriminate use of laxatives can result in dependency.
   3 Although this should be considered, the cerebrovascular accident affects the responses of the client by altering motility, peristalsis, and sphincter control despite adherence to previous habits.
   4 The passage of food into the stomach does stimulate peristalsis but is only one factor that should be considered when planning a specific time for evacuation.

506. **2** Because stomach distention after eating results in contractions of the colon (gastrocolic reflex) promoting defecation, establishing some regularity of meals that include adequate bulk or fiber will help establish routine patterns of defecation. (2; CJ; IM; ED; GI)
   1 Although increased fluid intake and activity facilitate elimination, in general they do not help establish a pattern.
   3 Same as answer 1.
   4 Increased potassium is not needed for normal elimination.

507. **4** Fiber absorbs water, swells, and consequently stretches the bowel wall, promoting peristalsis, mass movements, and defecation. Smooth muscle tends to contract when stretched because of the reflex activity of stretch receptors. (3; MR; IM; ED; GI)
   1 Bulk caused by fiber does not irritate the bowel wall.
   2 Bacterial action is not involved in the process by which bulk stimulates defecation.
   3 There is no chemical stimulation.

508. **4** A low-residue diet limits stool formation. (1; MR; PL; PA; GI)
   1 Bland diets are usually employed in the management of upper, not lower, GI disturbances.
   2 Although a clear diet is low in residue, it does not meet normal nutritional needs.
   3 A high-protein diet is indicated postoperatively to promote healing.

509. **1** Constipation and prolonged standing may cause this problem. (1; MR; IM; ED; GI)

2 Hypertension does not contribute to the development of hemorrhoids.

3 Spicy foods may irritate hemorrhoids but do not cause them.

4 Bowel control is unrelated to the development of hemorrhoids.

510. **4** Rectal bleeding is a common problem when hemorrhoids are present. (1; CJ; AS; TC; GI)

1 Pruritus is not a symptom that can be observed.

2 Flatulence is unrelated to hemorrhoids.

3 Anal stenosis is not a complication of hemorrhoids.

511. **3** The client must be advised to avoid straining and constipation; stool softeners are widely used. (2; CJ; IM; TC; GI)

1 Light dressings of witch hazel may be used to promote drainage and healing.

2 Baths are advised to promote healing and cleaning of the area.

4 Enemas may be ordered several days after surgery if the client has not had a bowel movement.

512. **1** Any situation in which a needle is inserted under the skin is a potential source of hepatitis. (2; CJ; AS; PA; GI)

2 The normal incubation period is 6 weeks to 6 months.

3 Having visited an area with possible poor sanitation or contaminated water supply is irrelevant for this type of hepatitis B is not transmitted in this manner.

4 Presence in areas congested by people is not relevant because hepatitis B is not transmitted in this manner.

513. **1** The client is exhibiting classic symptoms of hyperglycemia, and simple serum glucose monitoring evaluated by test tape or a glucose monitoring machine would help guide the nurse's next action. (3; CJ; EV; TC; GI)

2 This would be a useless assessment; urinary output must be evaluated in relation to intake.

3 This may be a secondary action to assess for overhydration; if headache alone were present, rather than the classic signs of hyperglycemia, taking the blood pressure might be the initial action.

4 Unnecessary; the symptoms do not indicate infection.

514. **2** This is the only vegetable listed that is included in a standard bland diet; this vegetable is low in fiber. (3; MR; IM; PA; GI)

1 This vegetable contains more fiber than creamed potatoes.

3 Same as answer 1.

4 Same as answer 1.

515. **4** This drug is a piperidine derivative that acts directly on the intestinal muscles to decrease peristalsis. (2; CJ; AN; TC; GI)

1 This drug is a laxative, not an antidiarrheal; it increases motor activity of the gastrointestinal tract.

2 This is not an antidiarrheal but a bulk laxative that promotes an easier expulsion of feces.

3 This drug corrects constipation, not diarrhea; water and fat are increased in the intestine, permitting easier expulsion of feces.

516. **3** Supportive drug therapy is used for concomitant problems, not the hepatitis. (3; CJ; IM; ED; GI)

1 Although a true statement, sedatives are given only prn and do not treat the hepatitis.

2 This is used only during the incubation period.

4 Vitamins are used as adjunctive therapy and will not eliminate the hepatitis.

517. **3** The diet should be high in carbohydrates with moderate protein and fat content. (3; MR; EV; ED; GI)

1 This is too high in fat.

2 This is too high in both fat and protein.

4 This is too high in protein.

518. **1** Hepatitis A microorganisms are transmitted via the anal-oral route; handwashing, particularly after toileting, is the most important precaution. (1; MR; EV; TC; GI)

2 Hepatitis A microorganisms exit through the rectum, not the respiratory system.

3 This will not deter the spread of the virus; handwashing is necessary.

4 The client with hepatitis does not need to use sterile dressings or equipment.

MEDICAL-SURGICAL ANSWERS

519. **2** A reduction in the number of RBCs may have been precipitated by bleeding; ibuprofen (Motrin) irritates the gastrointestinal mucosa and can cause mucosal erosion resulting in bleeding; melena (tarry stools) results from degradation of hemoglobin in the digestive process. (2; CJ; AS; PA; GI)
  1 This is unrelated to the data presented in the situation; constipation is usually related to immobility, a low-fiber diet, and inadequate fluid intake.
  3 This is related to biliary problems, not gastrointestinal bleeding.
  4 This is related to hemorrhoids, not gastrointestinal bleeding.

520. **3** This is an expected response during the first 24 hours after a gastric resection because of oozing of blood and blood coagulation. (3; CJ; EV; TC; GI)
  1 These are normal characteristics of gastric contents, which would be altered after gastric surgery.
  2 Coffee ground material results from blood that has been digested by the gastric acid; gastric bleeding with a nasogastric tube in place will be red because gastric acids will not have time to act on the blood.
  4 This would indicate hemorrhage and is unexpected.

521. **3** Using soap and water and ointment helps maintain skin integrity and reduces infection. (2; MR; PL; ED; IT)
  1 Plain water is adequate unless peroxide is specifically prescribed by the physician.
  2 Applying an ointment to this extent is contraindicated because it would interfere with adherence of the appliance.
  4 Vigorous rubbing may be irritating and may promote conditions that contribute to infection.

Endocrine

522. **2** Because water is not being reabsorbed, urine is dilute, resulting in a low specific gravity. (1; CJ; AS; PA; EN)
  1 Diabetes insipidus is not a disorder of glucose metabolism; blood levels are not affected.
  3 Loss of fluid may actually lower blood pressure.
  4 As fluid is lost from the vascular compartment, serum osmolarity increases.

523. **4** Antidiuretic hormone (ADH), from the posterior pituitary, promotes water uptake by the kidney tubules; the result is decreased urinary output—an antidiuretic effect. (3; CJ; AN; PA; EN)
  1 The adrenal cortex does not produce ADH; the antidiuretic effect from the aldosterone that is secreted by the adrenal cortex is a secondary osmotic effect of sodium reabsorption and not a direct antidiuretic effect (as is caused by ADH).
  2 The adrenal medulla does not produce ADH.
  3 The anterior pituitary does not produce ADH.

524. **1** The antidiuretic hormone aids the body in retaining fluid by causing the nephrons to reabsorb water. (2; CJ; AN; PA; EN)
  2 Reabsorption of glucose is not affected, only the reabsorption of water.
  3 The glomeruli are not affected.
  4 Same as answer 3.

525. **3** These agents are classified as antiinflammatory or immunosuppressive. Glucocorticoids interfere with the body's response to microorganisms but do not directly promote the spread of enteroviruses. (1; CJ; AN; PA; EN)
  1 Immunosuppressant action causes bone marrow depression, which decreases the number of WBCs.
  2 They interfere with antibody production.
  4 They interfere with the release of enzymes responsible for the inflammatory response.

526. **3** ACTH is released in response to decreased blood levels of cortisol. The ACTH then stimulates release of more adrenocortical hormone. (3; CJ; AN; PA; EN)
  1 Cortisol has antiinflammatory properties, which delay wound healing.
  2 As a glucocorticoid it increases gluconeogenesis in the liver.
  4 Cortisol assists the body in adapting to stress.

527. **2** Endocrine gland secretions (hormones) are inactivated by the liver and other tissues fairly rapidly; continuous hormonal secretion by the endocrine glands is regulated by immediate feedback controls, and the body's metabolism is always close to being suitable to the body's immediate needs. (2; CJ; AN; PA; EN)
  1 This time interval does not represent secretory patterns of the endocrine glands.
  3 Same as answer 1.
  4 Same as answer 1.

528. 4 Reabsorption of sodium and water in the tubules decreases urinary output and retains body fluids. (3; CJ; AN; PA; EN)
1 The opposite is true.
2 Same as answer 1.
3 There is no effect on filtration with ADH; ADH increases reabsorption in the tubules.

529. 2 Somatotropin promotes growth by accelerating amino acid transport into cells. Oversecretion after full growth and epiphyseal closure results in acromegaly, with enlargement of bones and overlying soft tissue in the feet, hands, lower jaw, and cheeks. This growth hormone also increases blood glucose levels. (2; CJ; AN; PA; EN)
1 Oversecretion of testosterone would affect secondary sexual characteristics.
3 This causes hyperthyroidism; it is not produced by the hypophysis.
4 Excessive secretions of adrenocorticotropic hormones produce Cushing's syndrome.

530. 2 The hypophysis (pituitary) does not directly regulate insulin release. This is controlled by serum glucose levels. Because somatotropin release will stop after the hypophysectomy, any elevation of blood glucose caused by somatotropin will also stop. (1; MR; EV; TC; EN)
1 This effect may be expected after a hypophysectomy because follicle-stimulating hormone and follicle-stimulating hormone releasing factor will no longer be present to stimulate spermatogenesis.
3 Thyroid-stimulating hormone will not be present; extrinsic thyroxine will have to be taken.
4 ACTH, which stimulates glucocorticoid secretion by the adrenal glands, is absent and cortisone will have to be administered.

531. 4 Because the pituitary gland is located in the brain, edema following surgery may result in increased intracranial pressure. (3; CJ; EV; TC; EN)
1 This may follow any surgery because of the effects of anesthesia and is not a specific occurrence following cranial surgery.
2 Although this may be the result of pressure on the medulla caused by increased intracranial pressure, it is not an initial sign of increased ICP.
3 This may occur with any surgery, not just a hypophysectomy.

532. 2 The adrenal glands, stimulated by the sympathetic nervous system, secrete epinephrine during stressful situations. The ensuing alarm reaction involves rapid adjustment of the body to meet the emergency situation. (1; CJ; AN; PA; EN)
1 There may be modification in secretion of thyroid hormones, but it is not directly related to meeting emergency situations.
3 There may be modification in secretion of pituitary hormones, but it is not directly related to meeting emergency situations.
4 There may be modification in secretion of pancreatic hormones, but it is not directly related to meeting emergency situations.

533. 2 Steroid therapy is usually instituted preoperatively and continued intraoperatively to prepare for the acute adrenal insufficiency that follows surgery. (2; CJ; PL; PA; EN)
1 The diet must supply ample, not high, protein and potassium; however, it must be low in calories, carbohydrates, and sodium to promote weight loss and reduce fluid retention.
3 A 24-hour urine specimen is unnecessary.
4 Glucocorticoids must be administered preoperatively to prevent adrenal insufficiency during surgery.

534. 4 Excess glucocorticoids cause hyperglycemia and signs of diabetes mellitus may develop. (3; CJ; AN; PA; EN)
1 Adrenocortical hormones cause sodium retention and subsequent weight gain.
2 ACTH affects the adrenal cortex, not the pancreas.
3 Although muscle wasting is associated with excessive corticoid production, this will not cause diabetes mellitus.

535. 3 Hyperplasia of the adrenal cortex leads to increased secretion of cortical hormones, which causes signs of Cushing's syndrome. (3; CJ; AS; PA; EN)
1 This malfunction of the pituitary would result in Simmond's disease (panhypopituitarism), which has symptoms similar to Addison's disease.
2 ACTH stimulates production of adrenal hormones. Inadequate ACTH would result in addisonian symptoms.
4 Cushing's syndrome results from excessive cortical hormones.

536. 3 Glucocorticoids (e.g., cortisone) and miner-alocorticoids (e.g., aldosterone) are secreted by the adrenals. (1; CJ; AN; PA; EN)
1 The gonads secrete testosterone (primarily in males) and estrogen and progesterone (primarily in females).
2 The pancreas secretes insulin and glucagon.
4 The anterior pituitary (adenohypophysis) regulates secretions such as STH, FSH, LH, LTH, TSH, and ACTH; it also secretes prolactin and endorphins.

537. 2 Cushing's syndrome results from excess adrenocortical activity. Signs include slow wound healing, buffalo hump, hirsutism, weight gain, hypertension, acne, moon face, thin arms and legs, and behavioral changes. (3; CJ; AS; PA; EN)
1 Menorrhagia (excessive menstrual bleeding) and dehydration do not occur; menses may cease or be scanty because of virilization; water balance is maintained by mineralocorticoid production.
3 Pitting edema does not occur except when heart failure is present and severe. There is no increase in frequency of colds because the ability to adapt to pathogens is not affected.
4 Menses may become irregular or scanty, and headaches are not caused by this syndrome.

538. 1 Excess adrenocorticoids cause emotional lability, euphoria, and psychosis. (2; CJ; AS; PA; EN)
2 Increased secretion of androgens results in hirsutism.
3 Although a moon face is associated with corticosteroid therapy, ectomorphism is a term for tall, thin, genetically determined body type and is not related to adaptations to Cushing's syndrome.
4 Capillary fragility results in multiple ecchymotic areas.

539. 2 As a result of increased cortisol levels, clients experience increased blood glucose. (2; CJ; AS; PA; EN)
1 Increased mineralocorticoids will decrease urine output.
3 Sodium is retained by the kidneys but potassium is excreted.
4 The immune response is suppressed.

540. 4 Adrenal steroids help an individual adjust to stress. Unless received from external sources, there would be no hormone available to cope with surgical stresses after an adrenalectomy. (3; CJ; AN; TC; EN)
1 Glucose stores (glycogen) will be utilized after surgery to adapt to surgery. Insulin is the hormone that facilitates conversion of glucose to glycogen.
2 Steroids do not increase inflammatory reactions.
3 Steroids would result in fluid retention, not loss.

541. 4 Hydrocortisone succinate (Solu-Cortef) is a glucocorticoid. A client undergoing bilateral adrenalectomy must be given adrenocortical hormones so that adjustment to the sudden lack of these hormones that occurs with this surgery can take place. (3; CJ; PL; TC; EN)
1 Because the adrenal glands are removed, ACTH will have no target gland on which to act.
2 Insulin is produced by the pancreas, and its function is not altered by this surgery.
3 Because the surgery involves the adrenals, not the pituitary gland, secretion of pituitary hormones will not be affected.

542. 1 After an adrenalectomy, adrenal insufficiency causes hypotension because of fluid and electrolyte alterations. (3; CJ; EV; TC; EN)
2 Hypoglycemia may be a problem stemming from the loss of glucocorticoids.
3 Hyponatremia may occur because of the lack of mineralocorticoid production.
4 Potassium ions may be retained because of the lack of mineralocorticoids.

543. 3 Clients with adrenocortical insufficiency who are receiving steroid therapy usually require increased amounts of medication during periods of stress, because they are unable to produce the excess needed by the body. (2; CJ; EV; TC; EN)
1 Although sedation may be prescribed, the major concern is the regulation of glucocorticoids in the presence of emotion or physiologic stress.
2 Increased stress requires increased glucocorticoids.
4 Although these symptoms may occur and may be minimized by an increase in glucocorticoids, the primary reason for an adjustment in dosage is to assist the body's ability to adapt to stress.

544. 4 Clients with Cushing's syndrome must limit their intake of salt and increase their intake of potassium. The kidneys are retaining sodium and excreting potassium. (3; CJ; IM; ED; EN)

1 An excessive secretion of adrenocortical hormones in Cushing's syndrome, not increased or high sodium intake, is the problem.

2 Although sodium retention causes fluid retention and weight gain, the need for increased potassium must also be considered.

3 Because of steroid therapy, excess sodium may be retained rather than excreted.

545. 4 Mineralocorticoids such as aldosterone cause the kidneys to retain sodium ions. With sodium, water is also retained, elevating blood pressure. Absence of this hormone thus causes hypotension. (2; CJ; AN; PA; EN)

1 Estrogen is a female sex hormone produced by the ovaries; it does not affect blood pressure.

2 Androgens are produced by the adrenal cortex; they have an effect similar to that of the male sex hormones; they do not affect blood pressure.

3 The major effect of glucocorticoids such as hydrocortisone is on glucose, not on sodium and water metabolism; absence of this hormone would not cause significant hypotension.

546. 1 Because of diminished glucocorticoid production, there is a decreased response to stress. (2; CJ; PL; TC; EN)

2 The respiratory system is not affected.

3 There is hyponatremia and hyperkalemia in this disorder; however, these do not alter the defense against infection.

4 Glucocorticoids are involved with metabolism; however, this does not directly affect susceptibility to infection.

547. 3 Glucocorticoids help maintain blood sugar and liver and muscle glycogen content. A deficiency of glucocorticoids causes hypoglycemia, resulting in breakdown of protein and fats as energy sources. (3; CJ; AN; PA; EN)

1 These three symptoms are not related to fluid balance.

2 Emaciation results from diminished protein and fat stores and hypoglycemia, not from an alteration in electrolytes.

4 Masculinization does not occur in this disease.

548. 3 Exertion, either physical or emotional, places additional stress on the adrenal glands, which may precipitate an addisonian crisis. (2; CJ; IM; TC; EN)

1 Low levels of adrenocortical hormones will cause fatigue, and exercise may result in crisis because of increased metabolic demands.

2 This is contraindicated because of the risk for hypovolemia.

4 The nurse should assess for hyperkalemia and hyponatremia.

549. 3 Lack of mineralocorticoids causes hyponatremia, hypovolemia, and hyperkalemia. Dietary modification and administration of cortical hormones is aimed at correcting these electrolyte imbalances. (1; CJ; PL; TC; EN)

1 There is no disturbance in the eosinophil count.

2 Lymphoid tissue does not change in this disease.

4 Although glucocorticoids are involved in metabolic activities, including carbohydrate metabolism, the primary aim of therapy is to restore electrolyte imbalance. Lack of electrolyte balance is life threatening.

550. 4 Lack of mineralocorticoids (aldosterone) leads to loss of sodium ions in the urine and subsequent hyponatremia. (1; MR; IM; ED; EN)

1 Potassium intake is not encouraged; hyperkalemia is a problem because of insufficient mineralocorticoids.

2 This disease is caused by idiopathic atrophy of the adrenal cortex; tissue repair of the gland is not possible.

3 Vitamins are not directly energy producing.

551. 4 Fludrocortisone acetate (Florinef) has a strong effect on sodium retention by the kidneys, which leads to fluid retention (weight gain and edema). (1; MR; IM; ED; EN)

1 Mood swings frequently occur with fludrocortisone therapy; this is not an indication of a problem.

2 Fluid retention and hence decreased urination may occur.

3 Fatigue may occur with adrenal insufficiency and is not related to cortisoned therapy.

552. **1** Glucose catabolism is the main pathway for cellular energy production. (2; CJ; AN; PA; EN)

  2 Glucose is not used directly for this process; ATP is the energy source.

  3 Same as answer 2.

  4 Same as answer 2.

553. **2** Ingested glucose not used immediately for energy needs is stored in the liver as glycogen and broken down when the blood glucose level falls (glycogenolysis). (1; CJ; AN; PA; EN)

  1 Not all foods provide glucose; ingested glucose may meet immediate needs but must be converted to glycogen for storage; glycogen is converted to glucose as needed.

  3 This is formation of glucose from protein or fat.

  4 This is digestion.

554. **1** Insulin functions by facilitating the transport of glucose through the cell membrane and increasing the deposits of glycogen in muscle. Both cellular glucose and muscle glycogen can be utilized for energy. (1; CJ; AN; PA; EN)

  2 Thyroxine stimulates the rate of oxygen consumption and thus the rate at which carbohydrates are burned; it is not the main controlling hormone.

  3 Adrenal steroids stimulate glyconeogenesis.

  4 Growth hormone accelerates protein anabolism and stimulates growth.

555. **3** As a result of osmotic pressures created by increased serum glucose, the cells become dehydrated; the client must receive fluid and then insulin. (3; CJ; AN; PA; EN)

  1 Oxygen therapy is not necessarily indicated.

  2 Carbohydrates would increase the blood glucose, which is already high.

  4 Although dietary instruction may be appropriate if the problem is related to dietary noncompliance, such instruction is inappropriate during the crisis.

556. **1** In starvation there are inadequate carbohydrates available for immediate energy and stored fats are used in excessive amounts. (1; CJ; AS; PA; EN)

  2 There is no fat in alcohol; no fat oxidation occurs.

  3 This does not require the use of great amounts of fat; calcium is deposited to form callus.

  4 This does not require the use of great amounts of fat.

557. **4** Oral hypoglycemics may be helpful when some functioning of the beta cells exists, as in type 2 diabetes. (1; CJ; PL; PA; EN)

  1 Rapid-acting regular insulin is needed to reverse ketoacidosis.

  2 Obesity as a symptom does not offer enough information to determine the status of beta-cell function.

  3 Clients with type 1 diabetes have no functioning beta cells.

558. **2** Ketones are given off when fat is broken down for energy. (1; CJ; AN; PA; EN)

  1 Although rarely used, sodium bicarbonate may be administered to correct the acid-base imbalance resulting from ketoacidosis; acidosis is caused by excess acid, not excess base bicarbonate.

  3 Diabetes does not interfere with removal of nitrogenous wastes.

  4 Carbohydrate metabolism is hampered in the diabetic.

559. **2** Infection increases the body's metabolic rate, and insulin is not available for increased demands. (2; CJ; AS; PA; EN)

  1 Although emotional stress will affect glucose levels, diabetic ketoacidosis will rarely result.

  3 Increased insulin dose will lead to insulin coma (hypoglycemia) if diet is not increased as well.

  4 This would result in insulin.

560. **1** IV fluids are given to combat dehydration in acidosis and to keep an IV line open for administration of medications. When the electrolyte levels have been evaluated, potassium may be added if needed. (2; CJ; IM; TC; EN)

  2 In acidosis potassium ions initially shift from intracellular to extracellular fluids, which results in hyperkalemia; as acidosis is corrected, hypokalemia may occur and then potassium may be administered.

  3 This is an intermediate-acting insulin; rapid-acting insulin is indicated in an emergency.

  4 This is not indicated; abnormally high serum potassium levels will revert once dehydration is corrected.

561. **2** Regular insulin is rapid acting and should be used for diabetic coma. (2; CJ; IM; TC; EN)

1 This is intermediate-acting insulin; it is not indicated for use in an emergency.

3 This is too short acting and must be administered concurrently with a longer acting insulin or sulfonyluria.

4 This is a long-acting insulin that is not indicated in an emergency.

562. **3** Kussmaul respirations occur in diabetic coma as the body attempts to correct a low pH caused by accumulation of ketones (ketoacidosis); HHKS affects people with type 2 diabetes who still have some insulin production; the insulin prevents the breakdown of fats into ketones. (3; CJ; EV; PA; EN)

1 Fluid loss is common to both because elevated blood glucose ultimately leads to polyuria.

2 Glycosuria is common to both conditions.

4 Hyperglycemia is common to both conditions.

563. **1** The ketones produced excessively in diabetes are acetoacetic acid, beta-hydroxybutyric acid, and acetone. The major ketone, acetoacetic acid, is an alphaketoacid that lowers the blood pH, resulting in acidosis. (3; CJ; AS; PA; EN)

2 Glucose is not an acid; it does not change the pH.

3 Lactic acid is produced as a result of muscle contraction; it is not unique to diabetes.

4 This is a product of protein metabolism.

564. **4** The urinary catheter and drainage bag should always remain a closed sterile system; urine should be drawn only from the catheter, not the collection bag. (1; CJ; IM; TC; EN)

1 The system should remain closed so that there will be fewer microorganisms entering the urinary system.

2 This would not yield a fresh specimen indicating present acetone levels.

3 The system should remain closed so that there will be a decreased possibility of urinary system infection.

565. **1** Because the brain requires a constant supply of glucose, hypoglycemia triggers the response of the sympathetic nervous system, which causes these symptoms. (2; CJ; EV; TC; EN)

2 These symptoms are consistent with dehydration, which is often associated with hyperglycemic states.

3 These are associated with hyperglycemia; these symptoms are caused by the breakdown of fats as a result of inadequate insulin supply.

4 Hypoglycemia causes the compensatory mechanism of hunger. Because blood glucose is low, the renal threshold is not exceeded, and there is no glycosuria.

566. **1** In the absence of insulin, which facilitates the transport of glucose into cells, the body breaks down proteins and fats to supply energy; ketones, a byproduct of fat metabolism, accumulate causing metabolic acidosis (pH below 7.35). (2; CJ; AN; PA; EN)

2 The pH of food ingested has no affect on the development of acidosis.

3 The opposite is true.

4 Cholesterol level has no affect on the development of acidosis.

567. **3** The stress of an infection increases metabolism and the production of glucocorticoids, resulting in an elevated blood glucose. (3; CJ; AN: PA; EN)

1 This would result in an insulin coma (hypoglycemia).

2 Same as answer 1.

4 Same as answer 1.

568. **4** In the absence of insulin, glucose cannot enter the cell or be converted to glycogen, so it remains in the blood. Breakdown of fats as an energy source causes an accumulation of ketones, which results in acidosis. The lungs, in an attempt to compensate for lowered pH, will blow off CO_2 (Kussmaul respirations). (3; CJ; EV; PA; EN)

1 Hyperglycemia and a low CO_2-combining power would be present.

2 Hyperglycemia and increased acidity would be present.

3 High acidity and a low CO_2-combining power would be present.

569. **3** Glucagon is an insulin antagonist produced by the alpha cells in the islets of Langerhans. It causes the breakdown of glycogen and protein to glucose. (2; CJ; AN; PA; EN)

1 Acidosis occurs when there is a high serum glucose level; therefore glucagon is not indicated.

2 Diabetes mellitus involves a decreased insulin production.

4 Glucagon is not indicated in idiosyncratic reactions to insulin.

570. **4** The bicarbonate-carbonic acid buffer system helps maintain the pH of the body fluids; in metabolic acidosis there is a decrease in bicarbonate because of an increase of metabolic acids. (3; CJ; AS; PA; EN)
1 The pH is decreased.
2 The Po_2 is not decreased in diabetic acidosis.
3 The Pco_2 may be decreased by the body's attempt to eliminate CO_2 to compensate for a low pH.

571. **3** Glucagon, an insulin antagonist produced by the alpha cells in the islets of Langerhans, leads to the conversion of glycogen to glucose in the liver. (2; CJ; IM; TC; EN)
1 It stimulates glycogenolysis, the conversion of glycogen to glucose.
2 It is an insulin antagonist.
4 It does not stimulate the storage of glucose but rather is released by the conversion of glycogen to glucose.

572. **4** Insulin stimulates cellular uptake of glucose and also stimulates the membrane-bound pump for sodium and potassium ions, leading to the influx of potassium into cells. The resulting hypokalemia is offset by parenteral administration of potassium. (3; CJ; AN; PA; EN)
1 Hypokalemia may be caused by the movement of potassium back into the cells as dehydration is reversed.
2 Hypokalemia may occur because the potassium moves back into the cells as dehydration is reversed.
3 Anabolic reactions are stimulated by insulin and glucose administration; potassium is drawn into the intracellular compartment, necessitating a replenishment of extracellular potassium.

573. **1** Liquids containing simple carbohydrates are most readily absorbed and thus increase blood sugar quickly. (1; CJ; IM; TC; EN)
2 Although a solution of 50% dextrose may be given if the client is comatose, 5% dextrose does not supply sufficient carbohydrates.
3 This will not alter the current situation.
4 Complex carbohydrates and protein take longer to elevate blood glucose, so they should be administered after simple carbohydrates.

574. **2** A combination of diet, exercise, and medication is necessary to control the disease; the interaction of these therapies is reflected by the serum glucose. (2; MR; EV; TC; EN)
1 Weight loss may occur with inadequate insulin.
3 Acquisition of knowledge does not guarantee its application.
4 Insulin alone is not enough to control the disease.

575. **1** The Nurse Practice Act states that the nurse will do health teaching and administer nursing care supportive to life and well-being. (1; LE; EV; ED; EN)
2 The teaching was essential before discharge.
3 The client is responsible for self-care.
4 Health teaching is an independent function of the nurse.

576. **2** Each client should be given an individually devised diet selecting commonly used foods from the American Diabetic Association diet; family members should be included in the diet teaching. (2; MR; PL; ED; EN)
1 Rigid diets are difficult to comply with; substitutions should be offered.
3 Nutritional requirements are different for each individual depending on many factors, such as activity level, degree of compliance, and physical status.
4 Seasonings in processed foods do not affect the management of diabetes mellitus.

577. **1** An understanding of the diet is imperative for compliance. A balance of carbohydrates, proteins, and fats usually apportioned over three main meals and two between-meal snacks needs to be tailored to the client's specific needs, with due regard for activity, diet, and therapy. (2; MR; IM; ED; EN)
2 Although restriction of calories and concentrated sweets is essential, a total dietary regimen must be followed to ensure adequate nutrition and control of the disease.
3 This is true; however, indigestion is not the basis for the client's problems.
4 Total caloric intake, rather than the distribution of meals, is the major factor in weight gain.

578. **3** The protein in milk and cheese may be slowly converted to glucose (gluconeogenesis), providing the body with some glucose during sleep while the Humulin N insulin is still acting. (2; CJ; PL; PA; EN)
1 The purpose of an evening snack is to cover for insulin activity during sleep.
2 The client's physical size does not indicate a need to gain weight.
4 The foods chosen are rich in protein and will be utilized slowly.

579. **1** During treatment for acidosis the client may develop hypoglycemia; careful observation for this complication should be made by the nurse, even without an order. (2; CJ; EV; TC; EN)
2 Withholding all glucose may cause insulin shock; monitoring glucose is indicated to prevent this.
3 The regulation of insulin depends on the physician's orders for coverage.
4 Whole milk and fruit juices contain large amounts of carbohydrates, which are contraindicated in this period immediately following ketoacidosis.

580. **2** Because the client has severe diabetes, it is essential that the blood glucose level be determined before meals to evaluate the success of control of diabetes and the possible need for insulin coverage. (3; CJ; EV; PA; EN)
1 To prevent flexion contractures of the hip, the client should not sit in a chair for a prolonged time.
3 Raising the head of the bed flexes the hips, which could result in hip flexion contractures.
4 This could result in a hip flexion contracture.

581. **1** The thyroid gland produces thyroxine (T4) and triiodothyronine (T3), which help regulate oxidation in all body cells. (1; CJ; AN; PA; EN)
2 The primary regulator is the thyroid; the adrenals influence metabolism of carbohydrates in times of stress.
3 The pituitary gland is involved in secondary regulation because it secretes TSH, which stimulates thyroid production of thyroxine and triiodothyronine.
4 The pancreas regulates glucose metabolism by secretion of insulin.

582. **1** Myxedema is the severest form of hypothyroidism. Decreased thyroid gland activity means reduced production of thyroid hormones. (2; CJ; AN; PA; EN)
2 This results from excess growth hormone in adults once the epiphyses are closed.
3 This results from an excess, not a deficiency, of thyroid hormones.
4 This results from excess glucocorticoids.

583. **3** Decreased production of thyroid hormones lowers metabolism, which leads to decreased heat production and cold intolerance. (2; CJ; AS; PA; EN)
1 Lethargy, rather than irritability, is expected.
2 Decreased metabolism requires less oxygen, so the pulse rate is generally slower.
4 The skin is dry and coarse, not moist.

584. **3** Excessive thyroid hormones increase the metabolic rate, causing nervousness, weight loss, increased appetite, heat intolerance, and tachycardia. (2; CJ; AS; PA; EN)
1 Although the appetite is increased, moist skin and a rapid pulse rate are associated with hyperthyroidism; a slow pulse rate and dry skin accompany hypothyroidism because of a decreased metabolic rate.
2 Although loss of weight is associated with hyperthyroidism, constipation and listlessness occur with hypothyroidism because of a decreased metabolic rate.
4 Exophthalmos is common in hyperthyroidism; however, the pulse rate is rapid and the client is nervous and hyperactive.

585. **3** An individual treated for a thyroid problem by intake of radioactive iodine (^{131}I) becomes mildly radioactive, particularly in the region of the thyroid gland, which preferentially absorbs the iodine. Such clients should be treated with routine safety precautions. (2; CJ; EV; TC; EN)
1 Because radioactive iodine is internalized, the client becomes the source of radioactivity.
2 The amount of radioactive iodine used is not enough to cause high radioactivity.
4 Same as answer 1.

586. 2 This adds iodine to the body fluids, exerting negative feedback on the thyroid tissue and decreasing its metabolism and vascularity. (1; CJ; PL; TC; EN)

1 This drug interferes with production of thyroid hormone but causes increased vascularity and size of the thyroid.

3 This is a topical antiseptic.

4 This is a synthetic thyroid hormone; its use is contraindicated because there is already an excessive production of thyroid hormone.

587. 1 If the laryngeal nerves are injured bilaterally during surgery, the vocal cords will tighten, interfering with speech. If one cord is affected, hoarseness develops. This can be evaluated simply by having the client speak every hour. (2; CJ; EV; TC; EN)

2 This ability is not influenced by laryngeal nerve damage.

3 Same as answer 2.

4 Same as answer 2.

588. 3 Thyroid trauma, thyroid surgery, or psychologic stress in a client with hyperthyroidism may lead to the release of abnormally high levels of thyroid hormones. This intensifies all symptoms of hyperthyroidism—thyroid storm or crisis (increased pulse, elevated temperature, restlessness, vomiting, and often death). (2; CJ; AN; PA; EN)

1 Iodine would bind with thyroxine, decreasing the potential crisis.

2 Tetany occurs from this inadvertent surgical excision.

4 Anesthesia would depress metabolism, not increase it.

589. 2 A decreased TSH assay together with an elevated T3 (triiodothyronine) level may indicate hyperthyroidism. (2; CJ; IM; ED; EN)

1 X-ray results would not indicate thyroid disease, and elevation of T4 (thyroxine) might indicate hyperthyroidism. However, this could be a false reading because of the presence of thyroid-binding globulin (TBG) and is inadequate for diagnosis when used alone.

3 Po_2 is not specific to thyroid disease, and the thyroglobulin level is most useful to monitor for recurrence of thyroid carcinoma or response to therapy.

4 The results with the sequential multichannel autoanalyzer (SMA 12) are not specific to thyroid disease; the protein-bound iodine test is not definitive because it is influenced by the intake of exogenous iodine.

590. 2 Because of the individual's increased metabolic rate, a high-calorie diet is needed to meet the energy demands of the body and prevent weight loss. (1; CJ; PL; TC; EN)

1 Modification of the consistency is unnecessary.

3 Sodium is not restricted because clients with hyperthyroidism perspire heavily and lose sodium.

4 GI motility is increased and does not require the additional stimulus of increased roughage.

591. 4 The first and most important observation should be for respiratory obstruction. If this occurs, treatment must be instituted immediately. (3; CJ; EV; TC; EN)

1 The blood pressure is not significantly affected by this type of surgery; however, surgery itself can have an influence on it. If the BP significantly increases, other symptoms of thyroid crisis (storm) would be present.

2 This would be a later concern; retention would not occur in the immediate postoperative period.

3 This could result from the anesthesia; however, it is not life threatening and usually passes.

592. 2 Parathyroid removal eliminates the body's source of parathyroid hormone which increases blood calcium. The resulting low body fluid calcium affects muscles, including the diaphragm, resulting in dyspnea, asphyxia, and death. (1; CJ; EV; PA; EN)

1 Loss of the thyroid gland would upset thyroid hormone balance and might cause myxedema.

3 The parathyroids are not involved in regulating plasma volume; the pituitary and adrenal glands are

4 The parathyroids do not regulate the adrenal glands.

593. 4 Thyroid surgery sometimes results in accidental removal of the parathyroid glands. A resultant hypocalcemia may lead to contraction of the glottis, causing airway obstruction; edema also causes obstruction. (2; CJ; IM TC; EN)

1 The airway takes priority.

2 Speaking is important to determine the status of the laryngeal nerve.

3 The client should be maintained in a semi-Fowler's position to maximize respiratory excursion.

594. 3 Soreness is to be expected. A progression to a soft diet will provide nutrients needed for healing and energy and will stimulate the return of bowel activity. Analgesics as ordered will reduce soreness during meals. (1; CJ; IM; PA; EN)

1 This is not a nursing function.

2 Soreness is to be expected; this is not an emergency necessitating medical action.

4 The soreness is not because of drying; humidified air might help reduce soreness, but it would not help the client eat the soft diet.

595. 4 Parathyroid hormone increases blood calcium by accelerating calcium absorption from the intestine and kidneys and releasing calcium from bone. Vitamin D promotes calcium absorption from the intestine. (2; CJ; AN; PA; EN)

1 Phosphorus and ACTH do not interact to regulate calcium levels. Phosphorus is a component of bone; ACTH stimulates the adrenal cortex to secrete the corticosteroid hormones.

2 Vitamin A and thyroid hormone do not interact to regulate calcium levels. Vitamin A is essential for function of epithelial cells and visual purple; calcitonin lowers serum calcium.

3 Ascorbic acid (vitamin C) and growth hormone do not interact to regulate calcium levels. Vitamin C promotes collagen production and formation of bone matrix; growth hormone controls the rate of skeletal growth.

596. 1 Calcitonin, a thyroid gland hormone, prevents the reabsorption of calcium by bone. It also inhibits the release of calcium from bone. The net result is lowered serum calcium levels. (1; CJ; AN; PA; EN)

2 Aldosterone regulates fluid and electrolyte balance by promoting the retention of sodium and water and the excretion of potassium.

3 Calcitonin lowers serum calcium levels; the other thyroid hormones (thyroxine and tri-iodothyronine) control the body's metabolic rate.

4 Parathyroid hormone promotes the intestinal absorption of calcium and mobilizes calcium from the bones to increase blood calcium levels.

597. 2 Parathyroid hormone increases osteoclastic activity, resulting in breakdown of bone substance and release of calcium into the blood. (2; CJ; AN; TC; EN)

1 It increases blood calcium and will thereby prevent tetany.

3 Blood calcium levels increase as do blood phosphate levels.

4 The hormone calcitonin, released by the thyroid gland, increases the incorporation of calcium into the bones.

598. 4 Hyperparathyroidism causes calcium release from the bones, leaving them porous and weak. (2; CJ; AS; TC; EN)

1 Tetany is the result of low calcium; in this condition serum calcium is high.

2 Seizures are caused by increased neural activity, a condition not related to this disease.

3 Graves' disease is the result of increased thyroid, not parathyroid, activity.

599. 2 Fluids help prevent the formation of renal calculi associated with high levels of serum calcium. (3; CJ; TC; EN)

1 Additional calcium intake could raise already high levels of serum calcium.

3 Seizures are associated with low, not high, levels of serum calcium.

4 Rest is contraindicated because bone destruction is accelerated.

Integumentary

600. 3 The temperature range for tepid applications is approximately body temperature. (2; CJ; IM; TC; IT)

1 This temperature is too cool to be considered tepid.

2 Same as answer 1.

4 This temperature is too hot to be considered tepid.

601. 4 Conduction is the conveyance of energy such as heat, cold, or sound by direct contact. (1; CJ; AN; PA; IT)

1 Direct contact is not necessary to convey heat by radiation.

2 This refers to retention of heat, not its transfer.

3 This is the transfer of heat by air circulation (e.g., by fans or open windows).

602. **4** Cholesterol is an absolutely essential structural and functional component of most cellular membranes. That it is associated with atherosclerotic plaques does not detract from its essential functions in membrane structure and steroid hormone metabolism. (2; CJ; AN; PA; IT)

1 Cholesterol is not necessary for blood clotting; calcium and vitamin K are.
2 Cholesterol is not essential for bone formation; calcium, phosphorus, and calciferol are.
3 Cholesterol is not involved in muscle contraction; potassium, sodium, and calcium are.

603. **3** Oxygen perfusion is impaired during prolonged edema, leading to tissue ischemia. (2; CJ; AN; PA; IT)

1 This is not a complication resulting from long-term edema.
2 Same as answer 1.
4 Same as answer 1.

604. **3** The release of iron from hemoglobin as erythrocytes disintegrate in tissue results in ferrous sulfide formation, causing darkening of the tissues. (3; CJ; AN; PA; IT)

1 Heme constitutes the pigment portion of the hemoglobin molecule, which gives blood its red color; it does not cause the darkening of tissue associated with chronic venous insufficiency.
2 Ferric chloride is used as a reagent; it is also used topically as an antiseptic and as an astringent; it is not related to discoloring of tissue related to chronic venous insufficiency.
4 Proteins are not insoluble.

605. **2** Unwashed hands are considered contaminated and are used to turn on sink faucets. The use of foot pedals or a paper towel barrier prevents recontamination of washed hands. (3; CJ; AN; PA; IT)

1 They are not considered contaminated for this reason; areas cannot be sterile.
3 It has nothing to do with the number of people; it is related to being touched by contaminated hands.
4 Although bacterial growth is facilitated in moist environments, this is not why sinks are considered contaminated.

606. **4** Soap helps by reducing the surface tension of water, but friction is necessary for the removal of microorganisms. (2; CJ; IM; TC; IT)

1 Although this aspect of hand washing is important, without friction it has minimal value.
2 Although soap reduces surface tension, without friction it has minimal value.
3 Although water flushes some microorganisms from the skin, without friction it has minimal value.

607. **4** The absorption of fluids by gauze results from the adhesion of water to the gauze threads. The surface tension of water causes contraction of the fiber, pulling fluid up the threads. (3; CJ; EV; TC; IT)

1 This is separation of substances in solution utilizing their differing rates of diffusion through a membrane.
2 This refers to movement of water through a semipermeable membrane.
3 This is movement of molecules from high to low concentration.

608. **3** Intact skin is the first line of defense against entry of microorganisms. A surgical incision is a portal of entry so a technique that requires the absence of all microorganisms (surgical asepsis) is essential. (3; CJ; AN; TC; IT)

1 Wound asepsis is incorrect terminology.
2 Medical asepsis utilizes clean technique to minimize the spread of microorganisms; when there is a break in the skin, this is insufficient.
4 Concurrent disinfection refers to measures initiated to control the spread of infection while an infection is present; concurrent asepsis is incorrect terminology.

609. **1** Surgical asepsis means that the defined area contains no microorganisms. (2; CJ; AN; PA; IT)

2 This would apply to personal protective equipment and medical asepsis.
3 Same as answer 2.
4 This would apply to medical asepsis.

610. **3** Vitamin C (ascorbic acid) plays a major role in wound healing. It is necessary for the maintenance and formation of strong collagen, the major protein of most connective tissues. (2; CJ; PL; PA; IT)

1 Vitamin A is important for the healing process; however, vitamin C cements the ground substance of supportive tissue.
2 Phytonadione (e.g., Mephyton) is vitamin K, which plays a major role in blood coagulation.
4 Vitamin B_{12} is needed for RBC synthesis and a healthy nervous system.

611. 4 *Clostridium welchii (C. perfringens)* is a spore-forming bacterium that produces a toxin that decays muscle, releasing a gas; it is one of the major causative agents for gas gangrene. (1; CJ; AS; PA; IT)

1 *Clostridium tetani* enters the body via puncture of the skin and affects the nervous system; gas gangrene does not occur with this organism.
2 This disease is caused by *Bacillis anthracis*, not *Clostridium*.
3 *Clostridium botulinum* contaminates food that is then ingested, causing botulism.

612. 3 Psoriasis is characterized by dry, scaly lesions that occur most frequently on the elbows, knees, scalp, and torso. (1; CJ; AS; PA; IT)

1 Pruritus, if present at all, is generally mild.
2 Petechiae are not characteristic.
4 Macules are erythematous flat spots on the skin as in measles; no scales are present.

613. 2 Steroids are applied locally and the lesion is usually covered with plastic (or Saran Wrap) at night to reverse the inflammatory process. (2; MR; IM; TC; IT)

1 Solar rays are used in the treatment of psoriasis.
3 Potassium permanganate is an antiseptic astringent used on infected, draining, or vesicular lesions.
4 The plaques are not necrotic and therefore do not require debriding.

614. 1 Scabies is caused by the itch mite *(Sarcoptes scabiei)*, the female of which burrows under the skin to deposit eggs. It is intensely pruritic and is transmitted by direct contact or in a limited way by soiled sheets or undergarments. (2; CJ; AS; PA; IT)

2 Scabies is an acute infection.
3 It is caused by the itch mite, a parasite.
4 It is an infectious disease and is unrelated to allergies.

615. 3 Pemphigus is primarily a serious disease characterized by large vesicles called bullae. Although potentially fatal, it can be relatively controlled by steroid therapy. (2; MR; IM; PA; IT)

1 Pemphigus is a disease of the skin.
2 Same as answer 1.
4 Same as answer 1.

616. 1 The connective tissue degeneration of SLE leads to involvement of the basal cell layer, producing a butterfly rash over the bridge of the nose and in the malar region. (2; CJ; AS; PA; IT)

2 This occurs in scleroderma and may advance until the client has the appearance of a living mummy.
3 This occurs in muscular dystrophy, which is characterized by muscle wasting and weakness.
4 This occurs in polyarteritis nodosa, a collagen disease affecting the arteries and nervous system.

617. 1 Scleroderma is an immunologic disorder characterized by inflammatory, fibrotic, and degenerative changes. (3; CJ; AN; PA; IT)

2 This is not involved in the development of scleroderma.
3 Same as answer 2.
4 Same as answer 2.

618. 2 According to the Nurse Practice Act, a nurse may independently treat human responses to actual or potential health problems. (3; LE; EV; TC; IT)

1 Activity parameters must be prescribed by the physician.
3 Providing supportive care is an independent, not dependent function of the nurse.
4 Surgical wound debridement is performed by the physician.

619. 1 Reasonablty prudent behavior in dealing with a client such as this is to change the client's position at least every hour to relieve pressure on tissues and promote circulation. The nurse is negligent in not doing this. (2; LE; AN; TC; IT)

2 The family is included in the health team.
3 Although pressure ulcers may occur, nursing care must include preventive measures.
4 When a capable client refuses necessary health care despite explanation, the client's rights must be respected but a document absolving health professionals of liability must also be signed.

620. **4** Basal cell carcinoma, the most common type of skin cancer, is most closely linked to solar ultraviolet radiation. (1; CJ; AS; PA; IT)

1 Although skin type is a genetically determined risk factor, it cannot be altered and it is influenced by solar ultraviolet radiation.
2 Diet is not a risk factor.
3 Smoking is not a risk factor.

621. **3** Lymphadenopathy occurs in clients with malignancies that have metastasized. (2; CJ; AS; PA; IT)

1 Skin is generally dry and itchy.
2 Nikolsky's sign occurs in clients with pemphigus.
4 Erythema of the palms is not a symptom of melanoma.

622. **1** A sarcoma is defined as a malignant tumor whose cells resemble those of the supportive (connective) tissues of the body. (3; CJ; AN; PA; IT)

2 Carcinoma refers to a malignant neoplasm of epithelial tissue.
3 Although collagen is the substance used to form the connective tissue, the term collagenoma is incorrect.
4 Osteoblastomas are benign tumors of the bone.

623. **1** Radiation in controlled doses is therapeutic. When uncontrolled or in excessive amounts, it is carcinogenic. (1; MR; IM; ED; IT)

2 Therapeutic doses are helpful in whatever areas are being treated.
3 Physical status does not affect the outcome of radiation therapy.
4 The nutritional status of the cells does not influence radiation's effect.

624. **4** Application of a solution of sodium bicarbonate (a mild alkali) after a thorough flushing with water is the best way to treat acid-splashed skin, because the alkali will neutralize residual acid on the skin. (2; MR; IM; ED; IT)

1 Sodium sulfate is a neutral salt, which would serve no immediate first-aid benefit.
2 Sodium chloride is a neutral salt, which would serve no immediate first-aid benefit.
3 Although sodium hydroxide is an alkali and would neutralize acid, it is too strong and can also cause burns.

625. **1** This first-aid treatment will chemically neutralize residual alkali still on the skin. It will not reverse the chemical burns already caused by the alkali but will minimize additional chemical change. (1; CJ; IM; TC; IT)

2 A weak base will not neutralize alkaline substances.
3 This is a neutral substance; it will not neutralize a base.
4 This would not affect the pH.

626. **2** Radiodermatitis occurs 3 to 6 weeks after the start of treatment. (2; MR; IM; ED; IT)

1 The word *burn* should be avoided because it may increase anxiety.
3 This response does not address the client's concern.
4 Emollients are contraindicated; they may alter the calculated x-ray route and injure normal tissue.

627. **3** An autograft is one taken from an uninjured area of the same person's body. (2; CJ; AN; PA; IT)

1 An allograft is skin taken from the same species.
2 A xenograft (heterograft) is skin taken from a different species.
4 A homograft is skin taken from the same species.

628. **4** A heterograft (xenograft) involves the grafting of tissues from a different species. (2; CJ; AN; PA; IT)

1 This type of graft does not exist.
2 An allograft is skin taken from the same species.
3 A homograft is skin taken from the same species.

629. **3** An increased hematocrit level indicates hemoconcentration secondary to fluid loss. (2; CJ; AS; PA; IT)

1 This may be used to indicate dehydration from burns, but interpretation can be complicated by other conditions accompanying burns that also cause elevation of the BUN.
2 The pH level reflects acid-base balance.
4 The sedimentation rate is not used as an indicator of fluid loss; it indicates the presence of an inflammatory process.

630. **4** As the amount of tissue involved increases, there is greater extravasation of fluid into the tissues. Thus the relationship of fluid loss to body surface is directly proportional. Several formulas (e.g., the Evans, the Baxter, the Brooke Army Hospital) are used to estimate fluid loss based on percent of body surface burned. (2; CJ; AN; PA; IT)
 1 This is incorrect; the relationship is proportional.
 2 Same as answer 1.
 3 Same as answer 1.

631. **1** *Clostridium tetani* can develop in partial- and full-thickness burns that contain dead tissue. (2; CJ; PL; PA; IT)
 2 Although gamma globulin provides passive immunity against certain infectious agents, it is not specifically indicated in the treatment of burns.
 3 Isuprel is an adrenergic drug used in the treatment of bronchospasm and heart block.
 4 This drug is indicated for hypoprothrombinemia caused by the deficiency of vitamin K; it is not related to burns.

632. **1** The severe pain experienced by the client during debridement of burns places an emotional strain on the relationship. (2; CJ; AN; PS; IT)
 2 Maintaining sterility is not a problem if the nurse understands surgical asepsis.
 3 According to Maslow, basic needs of survival and safety take precedence over higher-level needs. Pain becomes all encompassing, and the nurse must help the client cope with it.
 4 This answer is not complete. The frequency with which the nurse must perform tasks is not the problem; rather it is the pain associated with debridement and the nurse's inability to eliminate the pain.

633. **4** A partial-thickness burn over 30% of the body is considered critical. Shock, infection, electrolyte imbalance, and respiratory distress are life-threatening complications that can occur. (1; CJ; AS; PA; IT)
 1 Burns involving less than 30% of the body surface of older children and adults under 50 years of age are generally less severe; the condition would be rated accordingly.
 2 Same as answer 1.
 3 Same as answer 1.

634. **3** In deep partial-thickness burns, destruction of the epidermis and upper layers of the dermis and injury to deeper portions of the dermis occur. (3; CJ; AS; PA; IT)
 1 Eschar, a dry leathery covering of denatured protein, occurs with full-thickness burns.
 2 In full-thickness burns, total destruction of the epidermis, dermis, and some underlying tissue occurs.
 4 In superficial partial-thickness burns, the epidermis is destroyed or injured and a portion of the dermis may be injured.

635. **2** The leukocyte count would not be affected in the first few hours. (2; CJ; AN; TC; IT)
 1 Pain is present in partial-thickness burns because the sensory nerves are not damaged.
 3 Replacement of fluids and electrolytes is essential in all burned clients.
 4 Inhalation of hot air can cause laryngeal edema and would be a concern.

636. **3** The pulse rate is one indicator of optimum vascular fluid volume; the pulse rate decreases as intravascular volume normalizes. (2; CJ; EV; PA; IT)
 1 This would indicate hypovolemia.
 2 This indicates inadequate kidney perfusion; if adequate, output should be above 30 ml/hr.
 4 This would indicate hypovolemia and hemoconcentration.

637. **4** The circulating air bed disperses body weight over a larger surface, which reduces pressure against the capillary beds allowing for tissue perfusion. (2; CJ; PL; TC; IT)
 1 These beds are used for clients who are immobile; they do not increase mobility.
 2 This bed will have no effect on the development of contractures.
 3 This bed will have no effect on the development of orthostatic hypotension.

638. **2** Medical and surgical aspesis are essential for prevention of infection with the exposure method. (2; CJ; IM; ED; IT)
 1 Bathing will be performed in a large tank tub.
 3 Dressings are not used with the exposure method.
 4 Clients are more comfortable with room temperatures of 85° F.

639. 3 Extreme restlessness in a severely burned client usually indicates cerebral hypoxia. (3; CJ; AS; PA; IT)

1 With renal failure the client would become progressively confused and lethargic, not restless.

2 At this stage the client would be hypovolemic rather than hypervolemic.

4 With metabolic acidosis the client would be lethargic.

640. 3 Infection is caused by viral contact with the dermal layer of skin; cleansing the wound with soap and water helps remove superficial contaminants. (3; CJ; IM; TC; IT)

1 Antivenins are not effective against microbiological stresses.

2 A pressure dressing will not prevent infection.

4 Application of a tourniquet may impair circulation and will not prevent infection.

641. 4 If the area is not kept both clean and dry, drainage from the colostomy can quickly cause a breakdown of the skin around the stoma. This, in combination with a warm moist surface, also predisposes the individual to infection. (1; CJ; PL; TC; IT)

1 Although oral fluids are withheld until peristalsis returns, it is essential that parenteral fluids be administered to replace the losses incurred by surgery.

2 Same as answer 1.

3 The client is often unable to accept the altered body image and must be given time to adjust before participating actively in care of the colostomy.

642. 2 Necrotizing fasciitis destroys subcutaneous tissue and fascia and predisposes the client to infection and sepsis. (1; CJ; AN; TC; IT)

1 Although ultimately this diagnosis could be made, it is not the primary diagnosis.

3 Same as answer 1.

4 Necrotizing fasciitis is a problem of the integument, not the urinary system.

Neuromuscular

643. 2 The cerebellum coordinates muscular activity and promotes balance. The other brain regions govern motor, sensory, and higher integrative functions. (1; CJ; AN; PA; NM)

1 This controls conscious recognition of pain, temperature, and crude touch and pressure.

3 This is involved in temperature regulation; it controls and integrates the autonomic nervous system; it is the intermediary between the

nervous and endocrine systems; it is associated with feelings of rage and aggression.

4 This controls the heartbeat, blood pressure, and reflexes such as vomiting and coughing.

644. 4 One of the centers for reflex control of respiration is in the medulla. Another important reflex respiratory center is in the pons. The other brain regions—cerebral cortex, hypothalamus, and cerebellum—may influence respiration but not so directly as the centers in the medulla and pons. (1; CJ; AN; PA; NM)

1 This is the center for coordination and equilibrium.

2 This controls and integrates the higher autonomic functions; it influences respiration but not so directly as the centers in the medulla and pons.

3 This is the center of control for all conscious functions.

645. 3 Although sympathetic impulses usually control most visceral effectors in times of stress, parasympathetic fibers likewise stimulate increased gastric contractions and increased peristalsis. Sympathetic fibers also inhibit organs such as the bladder and cause relaxation of this organ. (3; CJ; AN; PA; NM)

1 This statement is accurate.

2 Same as answer 1.

4 Same as answer 1.

646. 1 The thalamus receives sensory impulses from the spinothalamic tract and relays them to the cerebral cortex. (3; CJ; AN; PA; NM)

2 The cerebellum is involved in motor activity and coordination.

3 The hypothalamus relays messages between the cortex and autonomic centers.

4 The medulla contains the vital respiratory, cardiac, and vasomotor centers.

647. 4 The autonomic nervous system regulates visceral effectors and maintains internal equilibrium. (2; CJ; AN; PA; NM)

1 The spinal cord transmits impulses from the periphery to the brain and from the brain to the periphery; it also integrates reflexes.

2 The CNS is concerned with overall control; it consists of the brain and spinal cord.

3 The peripheral nervous system conveys information from peripheral receptors to the central nervous system and information from the CNS to muscles and glands.

648. 2 Only axon terminals secrete acetylcholine, so never impulse propagation occurs in one direction only: from axon terminal to dendrite or cell body of the next neuron, or from axon terminal to effector organ (muscle or gland). (2; CJ; AN; PA; NM)
1 Polarization refers to the resting potential of the neuron when one side of the membrane is negatively charged and the other side positively charged.
3 This refers to the active movement of sodium ions into the cell and back across the membrane to the opposite side, which promotes transmission of this impulse but does not affect the direction of the impulse.
4 Cholinesterase acts only at the synapse, inactivating acetylcholine at the myoneural junction.

649. 3 Axon terminals release acetylcholine at the myoneural junctions. As acetylcholine contacts the sarcolemma, it stimulates the muscle fiber to contract. (1; CJ; AN; PA; NM)
1 ATP is not produced by axons; it is a nucleotide that gives off energy when it loses a phosphate radical.
2 Epinephrine is produced by the adrenal medulla and released by axons of the autonomic nervous system.
4 Cholinesterase is released by muscle cells to inactivate acetylcholine.

650. 4 Parasympathetic nerves increase peristalsis and secretion of gastric hydrochloric acid. (2; CJ; AS; PA; NM)
1 The parasympathetic nervous system increases intestinal motility, which would result in diarrhea.
2 Goosebumps (piloerection), caused by contraction of the musculi arrectores pilorum, are under sympathetic control; vasoconstriction is also under sympathetic control.
3 Epinephrine is a sympathomimetic.

651. 2 Hemiplegia is paralysis of one side of the body. (2; CJ; AN; PA; NM)
1 Paresis is a weakness or partial paralysis.
3 Paraplegia is the paralysis of both lower extremities and the lower trunk.
4 This is quadriparesis.

652. 2 The ache in muscles that have been vigorously worked without adequate oxygen supply is caused in part by the buildup of lactic acid. During rest the lactic acid is oxidized completely to carbon dioxide and water, providing ATP for further muscular contraction. (1; CJ; AN; PA; NM)
1 Acetone is not a product of muscle contraction; it is a ketone body and a byproduct of acetoacetic acid metabolism.
3 Butyric acid is not a product of muscle contraction; it is a fatty acid occurring in feces, urine, and perspiration.
4 Acetoacetic acid is not a product of muscle contraction; it is a ketone body resulting from incomplete oxidation of fatty acids. It is also produced by the metabolism of lipids and pyruvates.

653. 2 Vagal stimulation slows the heart. The vagus is the principal nerve of the parasympathetic portion of the autonomic nervous system, and its axon terminals release acetylcholine. The response of the viscera to acetylcholine varies, but in general the organ is in a relaxed state. (3; CJ; AS; PA; NM)
1 This is an action of the sympathetic nervous system (accelerator nerve) caused by the release of norepinephrine.
3 Stimulation of the sympathetic nervous system dilates bronchioles in the lungs; the vagus nerve constricts them.
4 There are no parasympathetic fibers to the coronary blood vessels; sympathetic impulses dilate these vessels.

654. 1 The thalamus associates sensory impulses with feelings of pleasantness and unpleasantness; therefore it is partly responsible for emotions. The cortical limbic system is also involved in expression of emotions. (3; CJ; AN; PA; NM)
2 This is located in the cerebrum and controls all conscious functions.
3 This controls body temperature and serves as a neural pathway.
4 This is the outer layer of the cerebrum and controls mental functions.

655. **2** The arteries communicating (anastomosing) at the base of the brain are referred to as the circle of Willis. (2; CJ; AN; PA; NM)
1 This is an anastomosis of blood vessels that is located in the palm of the hand.
3 This is a nerve communication network in the region of the neck and axilla.
4 This is a single large branch of the aorta.

656. **4** The medulla, part of the brainstem just above the foramen magnum, is concerned with vital functions. (2; CJ; AN; PA; NM)
1 Voluntary movements are mediated through the somatomotor area of the frontal cerebral lobe. The opercular-insular area of the parietal cerebral lobe is concerned with taste sensations.
2 Sexual development and libido are controlled by the hypothalamus (through releasing hormones) and the pituitary at puberty; proprioceptors are located around muscles, tendons, and joints.
3 Temperature and water balance are controlled by the hypothalamus; fat metabolism is unrelated to the medulla.

657. **3** The Schwann cells that comprise the neurilemma of peripheral nerve fibers (dendrites and axons) are capable of supporting nerve fiber regeneration. (2; CJ; AN; PA; NM)
1 These are not involved in regeneration.
2 Same as answer 1.
4 The myelin sheath, produced peripherally by Schwann cells and centrally by oligodendrocytes, is not involved directly in the regenerative process.

658. **4** Lesions affecting the seventh cranial (facial) nerve cause paralysis of the eyelids. (3; CJ; AS; PA; NM)
1 The optic nerve is concerned with vision; lesions result in visual field defects and loss of visual acuity.
2 The oculomotor nerve is concerned with pupillary constriction and eye movements; lesions result in ptosis, strabismus, and diplopia.
3 The trochlear nerve is concerned with eye movements; lesions result in diplopia, strabismus, and head tilt to the affected side.

659. **2** The third cranial (oculomotor) nerve contains autonomic fibers that innervate the smooth muscle responsible for constriction of pupils. (3; CJ; AS; PA; NM)
1 The optic nerve is concerned with vision; lesions result in visual field defects and loss of visual acuity.
3 The trochlear nerve is concerned with eye movements; lesions result in diplopia, strabismus, and head tilt to the affected side.
4 The facial nerve is concerned with facial expressions; lesions result in loss of taste and paralysis of the facial muscles and the eyelids (lids remain open).

660. **1** The facial nerve (seventh cranial) has motor and sensory functions. The motor function is concerned with facial movement, including smiling and pursing the lips. Nonconduction of the 7th nerve will cause drooping on the side of the problem. (3; CJ; AS; PA; NM)
2 Nonconduction of the facial nerve on the right side would cause that side of the face to droop.
3 Nonconduction of the left abducent nerve would prevent abduction of the left eye.
4 Nonconduction of the trigeminal nerve would cause problems in mastication.

661. **4** Anterior horn neurons are also known as lower motoneurons. Their cell bodies are located in the anterior gray columns and are part of the reflex arc. (3; CJ; EV; PA; NM)
1 Basal ganglia are islands of gray matter in each cerebral hemisphere; they are not part of the reflex arc.
2 Pyramidal tracts are motor nerve pathways from the brain that pass down the spinal cord to motor cells in the anterior horn; they are not part of the reflex arc.
3 Upper motoneurons are neurons in the cerebral cortex that conduct impulses to the spinal cord or the motor nuclei of the cerebral nerves.

662. **4** This is the space between the arachnoid and the pia mater. It is filled with cerebrospinal fluid. (2; CJ; IM; TC; NM)
1 This is the innermost of the three meninges covering the brain and spinal cord.
2 This is an opening in the atrial septum in the fetal heart.
3 This is the cerebral aqueduct, between the third and fourth ventricles, in the midbrain.

663. **2** Sensory impulses from temperature, touch, and pain travel via the spinothalamic pathway to the thalamus and then to the postcentral gyrus of the parietal lobe, the somatosensory area. (1; CJ; AN; PA; NM)
  1 This is the area of abstract thinking and muscular movements.
  3 This is the area where nerve impulses are translated into sight.
  4 This is the area where nerve impulses are translated into sound.

664. **3** $C° = \frac{5}{9}(F° - 32)$
        $C = \frac{5}{9}(99.8 - 32)$
        $C = \frac{5}{9}(67.8)$
        $C = 37.7$ (2; CJ; AN; PA; NM)
  1 36.5° C = 97.7° F
  2 37.0° C = 98.6° F
  4 38.2° C = 100.8° F

665. **1** Cold reduces the sensitivity of receptors for pain in the skin. In addition, local blood vessels constrict, limiting the amount of interstitial fluid and its related pressure and discomfort. (2; CJ; EV; TC; NM)
  2 Local blood vessels constrict.
  3 Local cold applications do not depress vital signs.
  4 Local cold applications increase blood viscosity.

666. **2** The sympathetic nervous system constricts the smooth muscle of blood vessels in the skin when a person is under stress. (1; CJ; AS; PA; NM)
  1 The sympathetic system stimulates rather than inhibits secretion by the sweat glands.
  3 The parasympathetic system (vagus nerve) slows the pulse, and the sympathetic increases it.
  4 This is not under sympathetic control; the parasympathetic system constricts the pupils.

667. **4** The brachial plexus is a maze of nerves extending from the axilla to the neck in the shoulder area; trauma to the arm may also injure this plexus. (1; CJ; AN; TC; NM)
  1 The solar plexus, also known as the celiac plexus, is where the splanchnic nerves terminate; it is unrelated to the arms.
  2 The celiac plexus (solar plexus) is where the splanchnic nerves terminate; it is unrelated to the arms.
  3 The basilar plexus is a venous plexus over the basilar part of the occipital bone; it is unrelated to the arms.

668. **1** This may occur with hypothermia because of slowed cerebral metabolic processes. (3; CJ; AS; TC; NM)
  2 Pallor, not erythema, would be present as a result of peripheral vasoconstriction.
  3 Drowsiness occurs; the client is unable to focus on anxiety-producing aspects of the situation.
  4 Respirations would be lowered.

669. **2** Immediately before administration, an assessment of vital signs is necessary to determine whether any contraindications to analgesia exist (e.g., hypotension, a respiratory rate of 12 or less). (3; CJ; EV; PA; RE)
  1 Pain prevents both psychologic and physiologic rest.
  3 Before administration, the nurse must check the physician's orders, the time of the last administration, and the client's vital signs.
  4 Before determining the time of the last dose, the nurse should obtain the client's vital signs; the client's status must be evaluated further.

670. **3** Pain and temperature sensations enter the posterior horns of the spinal cord, cross to the contralateral side, and travel upward via the spinothalamic tracts to the thalamus. There they synapse with other sensory neurons for transmission to the cortex. (3; CJ; AN; PA; NM)
  1 These are descending motor tracts. The lateral tracts facilitate impulse transmission to the skeletal muscles; the medial tracts inhibit transmission to the skeletal muscles.
  2 This is the location of the fasciculus gracilis, which is involved with pressure sensation.
  4 These are ascending tracts. They conduct impulses of crude touch, pain, and temperature.

671. **3** Electrodes are attached to sensory nerves or over the dorsal column; a transmitter is worn externally and, by electric stimulation, may be used to interfere with the transmission of painful stimuli as needed. (3; MR; IM; ED; NM)
  1 Clients may bathe when the transmitter is disconnected.
  2 The client may need analgesics in conjunction with the transmitter.
  4 The device should not interfere with a remote control apparatus.

MEDICAL-SURGICAL ANSWERS

672. **1** A rhizotomy is the resection of posterior nerve roots to eliminate nerve impulses associated with severe pain from the thoracic area (as in lung cancer). (3; CJ; IM; TC; NM)
2 A rhinotomy is an incision into the nose.
3 A cordotomy is the surgical interruption of pain-conducting pathways in the spinal cord.
4 A chondrectomy is the surgical excision of a cartilage.

673. **4** The exact nature of the pain must be determined to distinguish whether this is pain caused by the surgery or is from some other cause. (1; CJ; AS; PA; NM)
1 This should be done later but the first action would be to determine the nature of the pain.
2 Same as answer 1.
3 Prescribed analgesics would be given after determining the exact nature of the pain.

674. **3** The voltage or current is adjusted on the basis of the client's degree of pain relief and comfort levels. (2; CJ; EV; TC; NM)
1 This could be unsafe.
2 This is true of the pain suppressor TENS unit; not the conventional units.
4 The electrodes should be applied either on the painful area or immediately below or above the area.

675. **4** If there is no obstruction, pressure on the jugular vein causes increased intracranial pressure (Queckenstedt's sign). This, in turn, causes an increase in spinal fluid pressure. (3; CJ; AS; PA; NM)
1 Homans' sign is calf pain elicited by dorsiflexion of the foot if thrombophlebitis is present.
2 Romberg's sign is failure to maintain balance when the eyes are closed; indicates cerebellar pathology.
3 Chvostek's sign is twitching elicited by tapping the angle of the jaw if hypocalcemia is present.

676. **1** *Toxoplasma gondii,* a protozoan, can be transmitted by exposure to infected cat feces or ingestion of undercooked contaminated meat. (1; MR; IM; PA; NM)
2 Toxoplasmosis is not related to heavy metals.
3 *Toxoplasma gondii* is a parasite of warm-blooded animals; fish are not considered the source of contamination.
4 Toxoplasmosis is not related to radiation.

677. **2** Toxins from the bacillus invade nervous tissue; respiratory spasms may result in respiratory failure. (3; CJ; AS; PA; NM)
1 Muscular rigidity can occur; this generalized condition is not life threatening.
3 These symptoms are not life threatening.
4 Voluntary muscles may contract because of toxins from the bacillus; however, this is not life threatening.

678. **4** Painful pharyngeal spasms when swallowing or even looking at water are responsible for the use of the term *hydrophobia* to refer to rabies. (3; CJ; AS; PA; NM)
1 The central nervous system is affected; diarrhea is not a concern.
2 Memory is not affected by this disease.
3 Urinary stasis is not a potential problem; catheterization can be employed.

679. **4** Infections of cranial structures can cause meningitis because bacteria travel by direct anatomical route to the meninges and cerebral spinal fluid (CSF). (1; CJ; AN; PA; NM)
1 This part of the body does not come into contact with CSF.
2 Same as answer 1.
3 Same as answer 1.

680. **3** This is a sign of increasing intracranial pressure, which may follow a craniotomy. (3; CJ; EV; TC; NM)
1 Vomiting without nausea occurs with increased intracranial pressure.
2 Sneezing is not related to either the craniotomy or the shunt.
3 The pulse pressure widens with increased intracranial pressure.

681. **4** Vitamin A is used in the formation of retinene, a component of the light-sensitive rhodopsin molecule. (1; CJ; AN; PA; NM)
1 Melanin is a pigment of the skin.
2 Vitamin A does not influence color vision, which is centered in the cones.
3 The cornea is a transparent part of the anterior portion of the sclera; a cataract is an opacity of the normally transparent crystalline lens. Vitamin A does not prevent cataracts.

682. **3** The optic chiasm is the point of crossover of some optic nerve fibers in the cranial cavity at the base of the brain. The optic tracts conduct nerve impulses from the optic chiasm to other brain regions. (2; CJ; AN; PA; NM)
   1 The orbit is the cavity in which the eyeball is fixed.
   2 Optic tracts conduct nerve impulses from the optic chiasm.
   4 This is the vitreous body.

683. **3** The contraction permits the lens to return to its normal bulge, decreasing focal length and allowing focus on near objects. (3; CJ; AN; PA; NM)
   1 The ciliary muscles are intrinsic (within the eyeball); the third cranial nerve (oculomotor), an extrinsic nerve, controls some movements of the eyelid.
   2 In this case the ciliary muscles would relax.
   4 The rectus and oblique muscles of the eye are involved in convergence.

684. **1** Eye medications are applied directly to the eye. (1; CJ; IM; TC; NM)
   2 This route is not used for ocular medications.
   3 Intraocular drugs are given by an ophthalmologist for severe infections.
   4 Same as answer 2.

685. **1** Cortisone, a steroid, stabilizes lysosomal membranes, inhibiting the release of proteolytic enzymes during inflammation. This antiinflammatory drug also maximizes vasoconstrictor effects. (2; CJ; PL; TC; NM)
   2 An inflammatory process does not necessarily have to have a microbial etiology. This drug would only indirectly decrease inflammation.
   3 Same as answer 2.
   4 This is not an antiinflammatory drug; it decreases secretion of aqueous humor, decreasing intraocular pressure in glaucoma.

686. **1** Sedatives have no effect on the intraocular pressure. (2; MR; EV; ED; NM)
   2 Additional teaching is not necessary; this should be avoided as it would raise the intraocular pressure.
   3 Same as answer 2.
   4 Same as answer 2.

687. **3** Because continued use of eyedrops is indicated, an extra supply should always be available. (2; MR; IM; ED; NM)

   1 Although it is important to avoid constipation because straining may increase intraocular pressure, laxatives should not be taken on a routine basis.
   2 Eyewashes (collyria) have no effect on the disease.
   4 Corrective lenses do not need to be checked this frequently.

688. **3** Glaucoma is a disease in which there is increased intraocular pressure resulting from narrowing of the aqueous outflow channel (canal of Schlemm). This can lead to blindness, caused by compression of the nutritive blood vessels supplying the rods and cones. (1; CJ; AN; PA; NM)
   1 Pupil dilation increases intraocular pressure because it narrows the canal of Schlemm.
   2 Intraocular pressure is not affected by activity of the eye.
   4 Although secondary infections are not desirable, the priority is to maintain vision.

689. **3** Open-angle glaucoma has an insidious onset, with increased intraocular pressure causing pressure on the retina and blood vessels in the eye. Peripheral vision is decreased as the visual field progressively diminishes. (2; CJ; AS; PA; NM)
   1 This may occur with untreated acute angle closure glaucoma.
   2 Pain occurs in acute angle closure, not open-angle glaucoma.
   4 Occlusions of the central retinal artery would cause a sudden loss of vision.

690. **1** A cataract is a clouding of the crystalline lens or its capsule. (2; CJ; AS; PA; NM)
   2 This is not included in the pathophysiology related to cataracts.
   3 Same as answer 2.
   4 Same as answer 2.

691. **4** Activities such as rigorous brushing of hair and teeth cause increased intraocular pressure and may lead to hemorrhage in the anterior chamber. (2; MR; IM; TC; NM)
   1 This is unnecessary; clients are usually permitted to drive before this time.
   2 Coughing and deep breathing can increase intraocular pressure.
   3 Weakening of the eye musculature is not related to cataracts.

692. **4** Retinal detachment is a separation between the sensory retina and the retinal pigment epithelium. These layers are not attached by any special structures and can separate as a result of various pathologic processes. (3; MR; AN; PA; NM)

1 This statement does not explain the disease process involved.
2 Same as answer 1.
3 Same as answer 1.

693. **4** Scar formation seals the hole and promotes attachment of the two retinal surfaces. (3; CJ; AN; TC; NM)

1 The retina is part of the nervous system; it does not regenerate or grow new cells.
2 The sclera is not involved; the retina adjoins and is nourished by the choroid.
3 This is not the treatment used; treatment includes the formation of a scar by the use of lasers or surgical "buckling."

694. **2** Malignant melanoma of the eye is an intraocular tumor that metastasizes rapidly; therefore enucleation (removal of the eye) is the treatment of choice. (2; CJ; IM; TC; NM)

1 This is only palliative at best.
3 Same as answer 1.
4 Same as answer 1.

695. **2** The dendrites of the cochlear nerve terminate on the hair cells of the organ of Corti in the cochlea. (1; CJ; AN; PA; NM)

1 The utricle is a membranous sac that communicates with the semicircular canals of the ear.
3 The middle ear contains bones (malleus, incus, stapes).
4 This is the part of the middle ear that contains the auditory ossicles; it is the area between the tympanic membrane and the bony labyrinth.

696. **3** The bones in the middle ear transmit and amplify air pressure waves from the tympanic membrane to the oval window of the cochlea, which is in the inner ear. The tympanic membrane separates the outer from the middle ear. (2; CJ; AN; PA; NM)

1 The organ of Corti, cochlea, and semicircular canals are in the inner ear.
2 The outer ear consists of the pinna and outer ear canal.
4 This connects the middle ear and nasopharynx; it helps maintain the balance of air pressure.

697. **2** Because the organ of hearing is the organ of Corti, located in the cochlea, nerve deafness would most likely accompany damage to the cochlear nerve. (2; CJ; AS; PA; NM)

1 The vagus nerve would affect voice production.
3 The vestibular nerve would affect balance.
4 The trigeminal nerve would affect chewing movements.

698. **4** The labyrinth is the inner ear and consists of the vestibule, cochlea, semicircular canals, utricle, saccule, cochlear duct, and membranous semicircular canals. A labyrinthectomy is performed to alleviate the symptom of vertigo but results in deafness, because the organ of Corti and cochlear nerve are located in the inner ear. (2; CJ; EV; TC; NM)

1 Anosmia is loss of the sense of smell and would not be affected by surgery to the ear.
2 There is no pain associated with Ménière's syndrome.
3 Ménière's syndrome is not related to cerumen production.

699. **2** With a partial hearing loss the auditory ossicles have not yet become fixed; as long as vibrations occur a hearing aid may be beneficial. (2; CJ; AN; PA; NM)

1 When what is heard is useless or if there is total hearing loss then this procedure may be performed.
3 Although the bass tones are particularly affected, all tones are affected.
4 With conduction hearing loss, bone conduction is more effective than air conduction.

700. **2** A subjective symptom such as ringing in the ears can be felt only by the client. (2; CJ; AS; PA; NM)

1 An objective symptom refers to signs that can be assessed through direct physical examination.
3 This term is not generally used to describe a symptom; a functional disease is one in which there is an alteration in the ability to perform as intended without physiologic changes.
4 *Prodromal* refers to symptoms that are early indications of a developing disease; there is insufficient information to decide this from the situation described.

701. **3** The middle ear contains the three ossicles—malleus, incus, and stapes—which, with the tympanic membrane and oval window, form an amplifying system. (2; CJ; AN; PA; NM)
1 The inner ear contains both the organ of hearing (the cochlea) and the organ of balance (the vestibule).
2 The pressure of sound waves is amplified in the middle ear and transmitted to the cochlea (part of the inner ear), where it is detected by the organ of Corti and transmitted along the acoustic nerve.
4 Normally the eustachian tube, which connects the middle ear and nasopharynx, is closed and flat to prevent organisms from entering the middle ear; however, it allows air into the middle ear and thus equalizes pressure on both sides of the eardrum.

702. **2** Proximity to the nurses' station is vital. The client must be observed frequently, because behavior is unpredictable. (1; CJ; IM; TC; NM)
1 The client may be unable to ambulate safely to the bathroom; this choice does not indicate proximity of the room to the nurses' station.
3 Sharing a room with another client would disturb the other client.
4 Sharing a room with another client would disturb the other client; a room far from the nurses' station would prevent close observation.

703. **3** Librium is an antianxiety agent ordered to reduce the response to psychomotor stimuli. (2; CJ; AN; TC; NM)
1 Emotional problems are masked, not resolved, by antianxiety agents.
2 Detoxification is a slow process that still occurs but the symptoms are modified.
4 Fluid and electrolyte balance is unaffected by this drug.

704. **1** Gliomas account for about 45% of all brain tumors. (3; CJ; AS; PA; NM)
2 Meningioma, which occurs in the meninges of the brain, accounts for about 20% of all brain tumors.
3 Neurofibroma is a tumor of nerve tissue but is more common in the peripheral nervous system.
4 An adenoma is a tumor involving glandular tissue; it may occur in the pituitary gland.

705. **3** The facial nerve may be damaged during surgery. Drooping of the area results from loss of muscle tone. (2; CJ; AS; PA; NM)
1 A tracheostomy may not be performed; it is not a complication but rather a preventive measure.
2 This is also called auriculotemporal syndrome; it may follow infection and suppuration of the parotid gland; it is not a surgical complication.
4 The parotid is a salivary gland; its removal would decrease salivation.

706. **2** Seizure disorders are usually associated with marked changes in the electrical activity of the cerebral cortex, requiring prolonged or lifelong therapy. (2; MR; IM; ED; NM)
1 Seizures may occur despite drug therapy; the dosage may need to be adjusted.
3 A therapeutic blood level must be maintained through consistent administration of the drug.
4 Absence of seizures would probably result from medication effectiveness rather than from correction of the pathophysiologic condition.

707. **1** Phenytoin (Dilantin) is an anticonvulsant most effective in controlling tonic-clonic seizures. Data collection before planning nursing care for a client with a seizure disorder should always include a history of seizure incidence (type and frequency). (3; CJ; PL; TC; NM)
2 Although protection is important, restraints and airway insertion during a seizure often cause injury as a result of violent muscle contractions and should not be used.
3 Although these may be removed during a seizure, the client's normal routines should be respected.
4 Increased restlessness may be evidence of the prodromal phase in some individuals, but symptoms vary so widely that the history of the client should be obtained.

708. **3** A seizure is generally self-limiting; the nurse's responsibilities include protecting the client from injury and assessing the characteristics of the seizure. (1; CJ; IM; TC; NM)

1 During a seizure the client loses consciousness and would be unable to discuss any aura experienced.

2 Nothing should be forced into the client's mouth when the teeth are clenched during a seizure; this could damage the teeth or cause an airway occlusion if improperly placed.

4 Anticonvulsants are given on a regular basis, not prn, to achieve therapeutic levels; diazepam (Valium) may be given IV in an emergency to control status epilepticus.

709. **3** To achieve the anticonvulsant effect, therapeutic blood levels of phenytoin must be maintained. If the client is not able to take the prescribed oral preparation, the physician should be questioned about alternate routes of administration. (2; CJ; IM; TC; NM)

1 Omission would result in lowered blood levels, possibly below the necessary therapeutic level to prevent a seizure.

2 The route of administration cannot be altered without physician approval.

4 The client is being kept NPO.

710. **2** The medulla contains the vital respiratory, cardiac, and vasomotor centers. (1; CJ; AN; PA; NM)

1 The pons conducts impulses; it contains reflex centers for cranial nerves V, VI, VII, VIII (trigeminal, abducent, facial, vestibulocochlear).

3 The midbrain deals with sensory input from the eyes and ears.

4 The thalamus relays sensory impulses to the cerebral cortex.

711. **4** The eighth cranial nerve has two parts—the vestibular nerve and the cochlear nerve. Sensations of hearing are conducted by the cochlear nerve. (1; CJ; AS; PA; NM)

1 The frontal lobe is concerned with thinking, skeletal muscle tone, and biorhythms.

2 The occipital lobe is concerned with sight, particularly shape and color.

3 Cranial nerve VI (abducent) is concerned with abduction of the eye.

712. **2** An unconscious individual loses voluntary control of the sphincters surrounding the urethra and anus. (2; CJ; AS; PA; NM)

1 This cannot be assumed; hearing is often the last sense to be lost.

3 Motion (although often purposeless) is possible in coma.

4 Unconscious clients may react to various degrees of pain.

713. **3** The precentral gyrus is the most posterior convolution of the frontal lobe and the primary motor area. Other gyri also contain motor neurons. (3; CJ; AN; PA; NM)

1 The parietal lobes translate nerve impulses into sensations such as taste, touch, and temperature.

2 The basal ganglia are islands of gray matter within the cerebral hemispheres; one activity with which they are concerned is muscle tone.

4 The postcentral gyrus is the primary sensory area of the cerebral cortex; it is unrelated to motor activity.

714. **1** It is important to help the client who has expressive aphasia regain maximum communicative abilities early during the hospital stay; this action provides reinforcement. (2; CJ; PL, PS; NM)

2 This approach may increase client frustration and anxiety.

3 Although expectations should be realistic, improvements are possible and should be encouraged.

4 Some abilities do return, and therefore the client should be encouraged to participate.

715. **4** The hypothalamus connects with the autonomic area for vasoconstriction, vasodilation, and perspiration and with the somatic centers for shivering; therefore it is an important area for regulating body temperature. (1; CJ; AN; PA; NM)

1 The pallidum is part of the basal ganglia; it is also called the globus pallidus. Together with the putamen, it comprises the lenticular nucleus; it is concerned with muscle tone, which is required for specific body movements.

2 The thalamus receives all sensory stimuli, except taste, for transmission to the cerebral cortex; it is also involved with emotions and instinctive activities.

3 The temporal lobe is concerned with auditory stimuli; it may also be involved with the sense of smell.

716. 1 Head injuries can cause trauma to the brain and the client should be observed for signs of increased intracranial pressure (e.g., headache, dizziness, visual disturbances). (2; CJ; PL; TC; NM)

2 This is not indicated in this situation.

3 Elevating the lower extremities should be avoided because it will increase intracranial pressure.

4 The intracranial pressure may increase after trauma because of bleeding and edema.

717. 3 Increased intracranial pressure places tension on the brain stem, causing signs such as increased systolic blood pressure, slow bounding pulse, elevated temperature, and changes in respiratory patterns. (2; CJ; AS; PA; NM)

1 These combinations of symptoms are not found when vital brain centers are subjected to increased pressure.

2 Same as answer 1.

4 Same as answer 1.

718. 3 As an antiinflammatory agent, dexamethasone (Decadron) helps prevent cerebral edema, which generally peaks between day 3 and 5 after a cerebral vascular accident (CVA); this medication may also be used following a ruptured cerebral aneurysm. (1; CJ; AN; PA; NM)

1 This drug is not given for this purpose.

2 This is not the reason for giving this drug; although blood volume may increase because dexamethasone causes sodium retention, this is not beneficial to a client after a CVA.

4 Same as answer 1.

719. 3 An altered level of consciousness, as determined by the Glasgow Coma Scale, precedes other changes, such as vital sign alterations. (2; CJ; AS; TC; NM)

1 Carotid circulation is not altered.

2 This would not occur in this situation.

4 Spinal reflexes generally remain intact.

720. 4 Residual blood from the ruptured aneurysm may have blocked the arachnoid villi, interrupting the flow of cerebrospinal fluid (CSF), causing hydrocephalus to occur. (3; CJ; AN; PA; NM)

1 Vasospasm is a protective adaptation during the active bleeding process; it does not cause hydrocephalus.

2 Broca's center is not directly affected; if it were, there is no relationship to the development of hydrocephalus.

3 The production of CSF is not increased in this situation; increased production may result when there is a tumor of the choroid plexus.

721. 4 This is a sign of increasing intracranial pressure, which may follow a craniotomy. (3; CJ; EV; TC; NM)

1 Bradycardia, not tachycardia, would occur.

2 The pupils will dilate, not constrict.

3 The systolic, not the diastolic, pressure would be elevated.

722. 2 Decadron is a corticosteroid that acts on the cell membrane to prevent the normal inflammatory responses as well as stabilize the blood-brain barrier. (3; CJ; EV; TC; NM)

1 This is not an effect of corticosteroid therapy.

3 Same as answer 1.

4 Same as answer 1.

723. 4 TIAs are temporary neurologic deficits related to cerebral hypoxia; about one third of the people who have TIAs will have a CVA within 2 to 5 years. (2; CJ; AS; PA; NM)

1 This is not a risk factor associated with a CVA.

2 Same as answer 1.

3 Same as answer 1.

724. 4 Bleeding into the enclosed cavity of the skull creates pressure, causing pain. (3; CJ; AS; PA; NM)

1 Seizures are not directly related to the hemorrhage; they result from abnormal electrical charges that may eventually develop as a consequence of tissue ischemia.

2 This indicates caudal deterioration with damage to the midbrain and pons.

3 As pressure increases, widening of the pulse pressure occurs because of compression of vasomotor centers.

725. 1 A comatose client loses voluntary control of elimination. (1; CJ; AS; PA; NM)

2 Because cerebral functioning is depressed, purposeful or voluntary movement is absent.

3 Twitching motions may be evidence of abnormal cerebral electrical activity; such seizure-like activity is often present in comatose individuals.

4 Because there are different levels of coma, the individual may respond to intense stimuli such as pain.

726. 2 Absence of a gag reflex is common after a CVA. To prevent aspiration, the client is positioned on the side to allow gravity to drain mucus in the nasopharyngeal area away from the trachea. (2; CJ; IM; TC; NM)

1 Chest expansion is hindered in the prone position.

3 This position allows the tongue to occlude the airway and encourages the aspiration of secretions if the gag reflex is not intact.

4 This position interferes with respiration and leads to increased intracranial pressure.

727. 3 Dysphagia is difficulty in swallowing. (1; CJ; AS; PA; NM)

1 Writing is unrelated to dysphagia.

2 Focusing with the eyes is unrelated to dysphagia.

4 Understanding information is unrelated to dysphagia.

728. 4 Clients with dysarthria have difficulty communicating verbally, and alternate means may be indicated. (2; CJ; PL; TC; NM)

1 This is an important aspect of care but not related to dysarthria.

2 Same as answer 1.

3 Same as answer 1.

729. 1 The paralyzed side has decreased muscle tone, which may lower blood pressure readings; tissue damage may also occur. (2; CJ; IM; TC; NM)

2 The return of function to the affected extremity is not influenced by taking blood pressure; if it occurs, it is because of resolution of inflammation or resorption of blood in the area of the infarct.

3 Taking blood pressure does not precipitate the formation of thrombi.

4 There is no difference when pressure is exerted on the brachial artery in either arm.

730. 2 Passive ROM exercises prevent the development of deformities and yet do not require any energy expenditure by the client who is confined to bed. Instituting ROM exercises is an independent nursing function. (2; CJ; PL; TC; NM)

1 Bed rest is prescribed to decrease oxygen demands; active exercises markedly increase oxygen consumption.

3 Same as answer 1.

4 Same as answer 1.

731. 1 Atony permits the bladder to fill without being able to empty. As pressure builds within the bladder, the urge to void occurs and just enough urine is eliminated to relieve the pressure and the urge to void. The cycle is repeated as pressure again builds. Thus small amounts are voided without emptying the bladder. (3; CJ; AS; TC; NM)

2 These might be signs of renal failure.

3 Continual incontinence would not occur if urine were retained.

4 The total amount of urine produced and voided would be unchanged.

732. 3 Cerebral damage on one side of the cortex causes alterations on the opposite side, because three-fourths of the fibers originating in the cortex decussate (cross over) in the medulla before extending down the spinal cord. When there is cranial nerve damage, the same side of the body is affected, because the cranial nerves do not decussate but leave the cranial cavity by way of the small formina in the skull. (3; CJ; AS; PA; NM)

1 Hemiplegia refers to paralysis of one side of the body and affects both extremities; the right side of the face, not just the jaw, would be involved.

2 Facial muscles on the same side as the cerebral lesion are paralyzed because they are innervated by the cranial nerves, which originate above the points where the spinal nerves decussate.

4 Same as answer 1.

733. **3** To prevent deformity after a CVA, the client should be repositioned frequently and passive ROM exercises should be instituted. (2; CJ; IM; TC; NM)

1 Active exercises require a physician's order; active exercises are impossible with paralyzed limbs.

2 The nurse must directly assist the client; periodic visits by the physical therapist are insufficient.

4 This would increase deformities and atrophy.

734. **1** Various types of splints or boots are available to keep the foot in a position of dorsiflexion. (1; CJ; IM; TC; NM)

2 Blocks elevate the frame of the bed and have no effect on position of the feet.

3 Cradles keep linen off the client's abdomen and legs but do nothing to position the feet.

4 Sandbags help prevent lateral movement of an extremity or the head.

735. **1** Change of position at least every 2 hours helps prevent the respiratory, urinary, and cutaneous complications of immobility. (1; CJ; PL; TC; NM)

2 Too protracted a period in one position increases the potential for respiratory, urinary, and neuromuscular impairment; prolonged physical pressure increases the possibility of skin breakdown.

3 Same as answer 2.

4 Same as answer 2.

736. **1** Hemiparesis creates instability. Using a cane provides a wider base of support and, therefore, greater stability. (1; CJ; AN; TC; NM)

2 Involvement of these joints is not mentioned; therefore this is unnecessary.

3 Activity should not injure but strengthen weakened muscles.

4 The use of a cane would not prevent involuntary movements if they were present.

737. **4** As part of the rehabilitative process after a CVA, clients must be encouraged to participate in their own care to the extent that they are able and to extend their abilities by establishing short-term goals. (2; CJ; IM; TC; NM)

1 A client with a CVA may or may not have dysphagia; altering the consistency of food without the need to do so may make it less palatable.

2 Making the client feel helpless discourages independence.

3 This is unrealistic; family members may not be available because of other responsibilities.

738. **1** Damage to Broca's area, located in the posterior frontal region of the dominant hemisphere, causes problems in the motor aspect of speech. (1; CJ; AN; PA; NM)

2 This would be associated with receptive aphasia, not expressive aphasia; receptive aphasia is associated with disease of Wernicke's area of the brain.

3 Although difficulty in writing may be associated with expressive aphasia, understanding speech would be associated with receptive aphasia.

4 Same as answer 2.

739. **2** Clients with expressive aphasia must be encouraged to associate words with objects so that communication is regained. (2; CJ; PL; TC; NM)

1 Speech can usually be improved through therapy.

3 To avoid frustration, the client's needs should be anticipated.

4 Despite difficulty speaking, individuals with expressive aphasia can understand what is said to them.

740. **2** The pain may prevent the client from ingesting anything by mouth. (2; CJ; PL; TC; NM)

1 Hot or cold foods or compresses should be avoided because they may trigger a painful attack.

3 Exercises may precipitate an attack.

4 This would initiate an acute attack of trigeminal neuralgia; often clients must limit oral hygiene to rinsing the mouth.

741. **3** Tic douloureux, also referred to as trigeminal neuralgia, is an inflammation of the fifth cranial (trigeminal) nerve, which innervates the midline of the face and head. (3; CJ; AS; PA; NM)

1 Petechiae are minute subcutaneous hemorrhages; they are not present in this disorder.

2 Pain, not weakness, occurs in this disease.

4 The oculomotor (or third, not the fifth) cranial nerve innervates the eyelid.

742. **1** The nurse should avoid walking swiftly past the client because drafts or even slight air currents can initiate pain. (3; CJ; PL; TC; NM)

2 The client may assume any position of comfort, but pressure on the face while in the prone position may trigger an attack.

3 Although the procedure for oral hygiene may be altered, it is necessary to prevent infection.

4 Massaging may trigger an attack and should be avoided.

743. **4** Carbamazepine (Tegretol) is a nonnarcotic analgesic, anticonvulsive drug used to control pain in trigeminal neuralgia and to abort future attacks. It sometimes eliminates the need for surgery. (3; MR; PL; TC; NM)

1 Ascorbic acid is vitamin C. This vitamin is utilized when the body is subject to stress as occurs with pain and may be used as an adjunct to more specific therapy.

2 Morphine is a narcotic analgesic that will relieve severe pain but will not prevent its recurrence; prolonged frequent use is contraindicated because of possible addiction.

3 Allopurinal is used in the treatment of gout.

744. **3** Severe constant pain, emotional stress, muscle tensing, and diminished nutritional intake can lead to exhaustion and fatigue. (3; CJ; AS; PA; NM)

1 Because clients are apprehensive and have pain, prolonged periods of sleep usually do not occur.

2 Pain medications do not normally cause hyperactivity.

4 The client may be very quiet for fear of precipitating an attack.

745. **4** The client may be able to avoid stimulating the involved trigeminal nerve and thus prevent pain by chewing on the unaffected side. (2; MR; PL; ED; NM)

1 Food that is too hot or too cold can precipitate pain.

2 Although oral hygiene may initiate pain, it cannot be avoided. It can be modified to include rinsing the mouth or using a soft swab instead of tooth brushing.

3 Warm compresses may precipitate pain.

746. **1** Diplopia and nystagmus are experienced by clients with multiple sclerosis as a result of demyelination. (1; CJ; AS; PA; NM)

2 Clients experience intention tremors, not resting tremors; resting tremors occur with Parkinson's disease.

3 Clients experience spastic paralysis as upper motoneurons are involved.

4 Although emotional affect and speech are affected, intelligence remains intact.

747. **2** Spacing activities will encourage maximum functioning within the limits of strength and fatigue. (2; MR; PL; TC; NM)

1 This probably is unnecessary if client is closely observed by nursing staff.

3 Bed rest and limited activity may lead to muscle atrophy and calcium depletion.

4 Strengths rather than limitations should be stressed; this is more appropriate as client is moving toward discharge.

748. **2** As a result of muscle weakness the vital capacity is reduced, leading to increased risks of respiratory complications; impaired swallowing can also lead to aspiration. (3; CJ; AS; TC; NM)

1 Although ALS is progressive, clients with myasthenia gravis may be stable with treatment and clients with Guillain-Barré syndrome may experience a complete recovery.

3 None of these diseases are caused by a lack of neurotransmitters.

4 Twitching is not expected with myasthenia gravis or Guillain-Barré syndrome.

749. **3** Myasthenia gravis is a degenerative disease that occurs slightly more often in females during young adulthood. (2; CJ; AN; PA; NM)

1 Myasthenia gravis does not occur more often in males.

2 Myasthenia gravis is not a disease that is common in childhood.

4 Myasthenia gravis does not affect males and females equally.

750. **3** One of the pathologic changes is electron-microscopic evidence of fewer AChR sites; also, antibodies cause destruction and blockade at the acetylcholine receptor sites. (3; CJ; IM; PA; NM)

1 There is no genetic defect in the production of acetylcholine; rather than a genetic cause, it is believed that myasthenia gravis has an autoimmune etiology.

2 Although the defect is at the neuromuscular junction, it is not a decrease in acetylcholine, but in the receptor sites.

4 This enzyme is inhibited by anticholinesterase drugs used to treat myasthenia gravis, leaving more acetylcholine available to the damaged or decreased acetylcholine receptors.

751. **3** Myasthenia gravis is a chronic degenerative disorder with exacerbations that are precipitated by emotional stress, ingestion of alcohol, and physical stress such as infection. (2; CJ; AN; PA; NM)
  1 The prognosis is not excellent; there is no cure.
  2 The disease is characterized by exacerbations and remissions.
  4 The disease is chronic; death does not occur within a short period but usually after the muscles of respiration are affected.

752. **4** Raising the head of the bed allows gravity to assist in the swallowing of food, thus decreasing the chance for aspiration. (2; CJ; IM; TC; NM)
  1 Alerting the physician to the problem is necessary, but only after client safety is ensured.
  2 Oxygen will not assist in the management of dysphagia or the prevention of aspiration.
  3 Unless the client has aspirated this is unnecessary; the problem is the weakness of the musculature and the difficulty in propelling food down the esophagus into the stomach.

753. **3** Weakened muscles result in ineffective coughing; secretions are retained and provide a medium for bacterial growth. (2; CJ; AN; PA; NM)
  1 Airways are not narrowed.
  2 Immune mechanisms are not directly impaired.
  4 Viscosity of secretions depends on fluid intake and humidity.

754. **2** Neostigmine, an anticholinesterase, inhibits the breakdown of acetylcholine, thus prolonging neurotransmission. (3; CJ; AN; TC; NM)
  1 Neostigmine's action is at the myoneural junction, not the cerebral cortex.
  3 Neostigmine prevents neurotransmitter breakdown but is not a neurotransmitter.
  4 Neostigmine's action is at the myoneural junction, not the sheath.

755. **1** Tensilon improves muscle strength in myasthenic crisis; weakness persists if symptoms are caused by cholinergic crisis, which can result from toxic levels of neostigmine. (3; CJ; EV; TC; NM)
  2 Tensilon is not used for synergistic effects; the duration of effect is brief.
  3 This is the same type of drug as neostigmine; no resistance is indicated.
  4 The diagnosis has already been established and treatment initiated.

756. **4** Parkinson's disease involves destruction of the neurons of the substantia nigra, caudate nucleus, and globus pallidus of the basal ganglia. The cause of this destruction is unknown. (2; CJ; AN; PA; NM)
  1 This pathologic condition is associated with multiple sclerosis.
  2 This condition would result in auditory and visual problems; it is not associated with Parkinson's disease.
  3 This condition is believed to be associated with myasthenia gravis.

757. **3** The onset of this disease is not sudden but insidious with a prolonged course and gradual progression. (2; CJ; AS; PA; NM)
  1 The onset is slow and gradual.
  2 Same as answer 1.
  4 The onset is not irregular; there is a gradual, regular progression of symptoms.

758. **3** This is the best response to the client's question; the client with this disease cannot execute automatic involuntary movements and has difficulty swallowing saliva. (2; MR; IM; PA; NM)
  1 It is known that bradykinesia and muscular weakness cause difficulty in swallowing saliva.
  2 There is no true paralysis or loss of sensation with this disease.
  4 Muscular rigidity occurs with this disease but is not the cause of drooling.

759. **1** Destruction of the neurons of the basal ganglia results in decreased muscle tone. The masklike appearance and monotonous speech patterns can be interpreted as flat. (2; CJ; AS; PA; NM)
  2 These are not associated with Parkinson's disease.
  3 This is not associated with Parkinson's disease.
  4 Same as answer 3.

760. **3** Levodopa (L Dopa) is the precursor of dopamine. It is converted to dopamine in the brain cells, where it is stored until needed by axon terminals; it functions as a neurotransmitter. (2; CJ; AN; TC; NM)
  1 This is not an action of L Dopa.
  2 Same as answer 1.
  4 This is not an action of L Dopa; neurons do not regenerate.

761. **2** Because of pressure on the sciatic nerve, pain radiating to the hip and leg is common. (1; CJ; AS; PA; NM)
    1 This is not associated with a ruptured nucleus pulposus.
    3 Although weakness (paresis) may occur, paralysis is not common.
    4 Same as answer 1.

762. **1** These actions, as well as lifting and straining, cause an increase in the intraspinal pressure, resulting in pain. (3; CJ; AS; PA; NM)
    2 This does not affect the intraspinal pressure.
    3 Although pain may increase as a result of compression of the vertebrae, the increase is gradual, not sudden.
    4 Flexing the knees and hips relieves pressure and pain.

763. **3** Inflammation from the trauma of surgery could lead to injury of the nerve root, with consequent motor or sensory dysfunction. (2; CJ; EV; TC; NM)
    1 Cerebral edema does not occur.
    2 Urinary retention rather than spasticity may develop if pressure on the nerve root occurs as a result of edema or bleeding.
    4 Pain is usually experienced at the operative site and in the legs as a result of edema around the cord.

764. **2** Logrolling maintains the alignment of the vertebral column. (2; CJ; IM; TC; NM)
    1 Coughing will increase the pressure of the cerebrospinal fluid surrounding the spinal cord and intensify the pain; incentive spirometry and turning should be used to prevent respiratory complications.
    3 Peritonitis is not a danger because the abdominal cavity is not opened.
    4 Extreme flexion of the knees is avoided postoperatively because it alters intervertebral pressure.

765. **2** Sore throat and oral secretions are additional problems of the client after cervical laminectomy. (3; CJ; PL; TC; NM)
    1 To prevent strain on the operative site, flexion of the head is avoided.
    3 The head of the bed may be only slightly elevated after a cervical laminectomy.
    4 Limited range of motion occurs after both operations.

766. **1** To avoid additional spinal cord damage, the victim must be moved only with great care. Moving a person whose spinal cord has been injured could cause irreversible paralysis. (2; CJ; IM; TC; NM)
    2 A back injury is suspected; therefore the person should not be moved.
    3 A back injury precludes changing the person's position.
    4 A flat board would be indicated; however, one rescuer could not move the person alone.

767. **2** Both legs and generally the lower part of the body are paralyzed in paraplegia. (1; MR; IM; PA; NM)
    1 There is no term to describe this condition; all parts below an injury are affected.
    3 This is hemiplegia.
    4 This is quadriplegia.

768. **1** Because of the location of the micturition reflex center (in the sacral region of the spinal cord), bladder function may be impaired with lower spinal cord injuries. (2; CJ; AS; PA; NM)
    2 This client's ability to ingest, digest, or metabolize is not affected; therefore, nutrition is less of a problem than bladder control.
    3 These exercises require motor control, which the client does not have.
    4 Because there is no voluntary control over the lower extremities, mobility is usually accomplished through the use of a wheelchair rather than ambulation.

769. **4** Correct positioning prevents the client from assuming incorrect positions, which could result in contracture formation. (1; CJ; PL; TC; NM)
    1 Because the client is paralyzed, active exercises are not possible.
    2 Deep massage may dislodge thrombi that have formed as a result of venous stasis.
    3 The tilt board is used primarily to prevent orthostatic hypotension or bone demineralization.

770. 1 Pressure ulcers easily develop when a particular position is maintained; the body weight, directed continuously in one region, restricts circulation and results in tissue necrosis. (1; CJ; AN; TC; NM)

2 Clients often state that they are comfortable and wish to remain in one position.

3 Proper positioning with supportive devices and ROM are more effective measures to prevent contractures.

4 Because turning is usually done laterally, the circulation to the lower extremities is not dramatically affected.

771. 3 Clients with early spinal cord damage experience an atonic bladder, which is characterized by the absence of muscle tone, an enlarged capacity, no feeling of discomfort with distention, and overflow with a large residual. This leads to urinary stasis and infection. High fluid intake limits urinary stasis and infection by diluting the urine and increasing urinary output. (2; CJ; IM; PA; NM)

1 Dehydration is not a major problem after spinal cord injury.

2 Pressure-relieving devices and interventions are most essential in preventing skin breakdown.

4 A fluid and electrolyte imbalance is not a major problem after spinal cord injury.

772. 3 Spinal shock is immediate after a transection of the spinal cord; it usually lasts from 1 to 6 weeks and results in flaccid paralysis of all skeletal muscles. (3; CJ; AS; PA; NM)

1 This occurs after spinal shock has subsided.

2 During the acute phase, retention of urine and feces occurs as a result of decreased tone of the bladder and bowel; thus incontinence is unusual.

4 Respirations are labored, but spontaneous breathing continues, indicating that the level of injury is below C4 and respirations are not affected.

773. 2 Muscles are flaccid during spinal shock but develop spasticity with recovery; these movements are entirely involuntary. (2; CJ; AN; PA; NM)

1 Once nervous tissue is transected, it does not regenerate and paralysis therefore remains.

3 Although edema may be subsiding, motor function will not return if the cord is transected; paralysis remains below the level of the lesion.

4 Although thrombophlebitis could occur, the client would not have any sensation of pain.

774. 1 These are symptoms of autonomic dysreflexia, which is commonly precipitated by a distended bladder. (2; CJ; AS; TC; NM)

2 These are not associated with autonomic dysreflexia.

3 Same as answer 2.

4 Blood pressure rises suddenly with autonomic dysreflexia.

775. 4 During prolonged inactivity bone resorption proceeds faster than bone formation, and lack of therapeutic weight bearing on bone results in demineralization. A tilt table provides gradual progressive weight bearing, which counters these effects. (3; CJ; IM; ED; NM)

1 Lateral turning is possible and necessary if a client is immobile, but a tilt table does not make this possible.

2 The tilt table is used for scheduled periods in physical therapy; the nursing care required to prevent pressure ulcers must be consistently performed frequently throughout all shifts.

3 The tilt table does not cause hyperextension of the spine; the spine remains in functional body alignment.

776. 3 Clients with quadriplegia do not have and never will have the muscle innervation, strength, or balance needed for ambulation. (2; MR; AN; TC; NM)

1 Bracing and crutch walking require muscle strength and coordination that an individual with quadriplegia does not have.

2 Orthostatic hypotension can be prevented by any upright positioning and does not necessarily require a wheelchair.

4 Quadriplegia refers to paralysis of all four extremities.

Skeletal

777. 3 Synovial fluid minimizes friction at joints by providing lubrication for the moving parts. (2; CJ; AN; PA; SK)

1 Synovial fluid increases the efficiency of joint movements.

2 Synovial fluid increases work output.

4 Synovial fluid increases the speed of movements.

778. **4** The greater density of compact bone makes it stronger than cancellous bone. Compact bone forms from cancellous bone by the addition of concentric rings of bone substance to the marrow spaces of cancellous bone; the large marrow spaces are reduced to haversian canals. (1; CJ; AN; PA; SK)
   1 Overall size does not determine strength.
   2 Weight alone is not a factor.
   3 Volume is not related to strength.

779. **3** Systemic lupus erythematosus is a chronic, autoimmune, systemic disease with inflammatory and degenerative changes in the body's connective tissue. (3; CJ; AN; PA; SK)
   1 It is connective tissue throughout the organs of the body that is affected, not joints.
   2 Bones are not the focus of this disease.
   4 Purine metabolism is affected in gout.

780. **1** Increased levels of steroids will accelerate bone demineralization. (2; CJ; AS; PA; SK)
   2 Hyperparathyroidism, not hypoparathyroidism, accelerates bone demineralization.
   3 Weight bearing that occurs with strenuous activity promotes bone integrity by preventing bone demineralization.
   4 Estrogen promotes deposition of calcium into bone.

781. **3** Prolonged immobility results in bone demineralization because there is decreased bone production by osteoblasts and increased resorption by osteoclasts. (3; CJ; AS; PA; SK)
   1 Estrogen helps prevent bone demineralization.
   2 Hypoparathyroidism decreases mobilization of calcium from the bones and thus serum calcium is lowered.
   4 Decreased calcium intake or absorption may precipitate osteoporosis.

782. **2** Pathologic fractures occur as a result of minimal injury to an already weakened bone; osteoporosis causes this weakening. (2; CJ; AN; PA; SK)
   1 Fatigue fractures occur when muscles are so fatigued that they no longer act as shock absorbers to protect the bone, a condition not related to osteoporosis.
   3 Greenstick fractures occur in soft bones, usually just in children.
   4 Compound fractures refer to the protrusion of the bone fragments through the skin. This is not related to osteoporosis.

783. **3** Turnip greens are high in calcium, but not in phosphorus. (3; MR; IM; ED; SK)
   1 High levels of nitrogen from protein breakdown may increase calcium resorption from bone to serve as a buffer of the nitrogen.
   2 Soft drinks that are high in phosphorus may interfere with calcium absorption from the GI tract.
   4 Enriched grains that are high in phosphorus may interfere with calcium absorption from the GI tract.

784. **3** Allopurinol interferes with the final steps in uric acid formation by inhibiting the production of xanthinoxidase. (1; CJ; AN; PA; SK)
   1 This drug prevents the formation of uric acid.
   2 Allopurinol has no effect on swelling of the synovial membranes.
   4 Same as answer 1.

785. **1** Colchicine decreases the formation of lactic acid, which may promote the deposition of uric acid in the joints. It also decreases the inflammatory response. (2; CJ; AN; PA; SK)
   2 Hydrocortisone is an antiinflammatory; it is not used to treat gout.
   3 Ibuprofen is a nonsteroidal antiinflammatory agent; it does not prevent the formation of uric acid.
   4 Benemid acts to inhibit the resorption of urate in the kidneys and, therefore, decreases uric acid in the blood; it is not useful in the treatment of acute gout but rather of chronic gout.

786. **4** Warm compresses (at or slightly above body temperature) dilate blood vessels, increasing blood flow to the area and decreasing edema. (3; CJ; IM; TC; SK)
   1 This temperature is too cool to increase blood flow to the area.
   2 Same as answer 1.
   3 Same as answer 1.

787. **4** Not a priority at this point; it will assume priority as the client progresses. (2; MR; AN; TC; SK)
   1 This diagnosis has a higher priority than deficient knowledge at this stage following a traumatic amputation.
   2 An important diagnosis because an amputation creates a potential for pulmonary emboli.
   3 An important diagnosis because respiratory complications related to anesthesia and immobility are likely.

788. 2 The hips are in extension when the client is prone; this keeps the hips from flexing. (2; MR; IM; PA; SK)

1 This promotes flexion and contracture formation.

3 In the left side-lying position the right hip will be flexed, promoting contracture formation.

4 This is not related to the prevention of hip-flexion contractures.

789. 3 Elastic bandages compress the residual limb, preventing edema and promoting stump shrinkage and molding; the bandage must be rewrapped when it loosens. (1; CJ; PL; TC; SK)

1 This would have a systemic effect on fluid balance; edema of the residual limb is a localized response to inflammation.

2 Same as answer 1.

4 Prolonged immobilization of the residual extremity in one position can lead to a flexion contracture of the hip.

790. 4 Preparing muscles that will do the work in crutch walking is imperative. (2; MR; IM; ED; SK)

1 The biceps are not the major muscles required for crutch walking.

2 Contractures of the limb will not have a great influence on the ability to use crutches.

3 Strengthening the hamstring muscles will not assist in the use of crutches.

791. 4 Flexion contracture of the hip can be prevented by routinely placing the client in a prone position to extend the hip. (2; CJ; IM; TC; SK)

1 This can cause flexion of the hip, which will result in a hip contracture and affect balance.

2 Same as answer 1.

3 Lying in this position does not allow for full extension of the hip.

792. 1 This position offsets the development of hip deformities resulting from contractures. It also maintains the correct center of gravity when the client is upright. (2; MR; IM; ED; SK)

2 This promotes flexion contracture of the hip.

3 A prosthesis may be applied early in the postoperative period but requires a rigid dressing (cast) to prevent edema; ambulation can be facilitated by the use of a walker, crutches, parallel bars, or cane.

4 This may alter the center of gravity and cause a loss of balance.

793. 1 Rehabilitation should begin immediately; this includes preoperative discussion of the nature of the operation and rehabilitation techniques. (2; CJ; PL; TC; SK)

2 This is too late; valuable rehabilitation time has been wasted.

3 Same as answer 2.

4 Same as answer 2.

794. 4 The neural endings that innervated the limb are still intact and may be stimulated within the residual limb. (2; CJ; AN; PA; SK)

1 Severed blood vessels are not involved in phantom limb pain.

2 Although an individual must grieve over a lost body part, the grieving is unrelated to the phantom limb pain.

3 Although phantom limb pain is an hallucinatory-type experience, it is not part of a psychotic process.

795. 1 A four-point gait provides for weight bearing on all points that touch the floor and maximum support during ambulation. (2; MR; IM; ED; SK)

2 A three-point gait is used when one extremity cannot bear weight.

3 Same as answer 2.

4 A swing-through gait does not simulate ambulation; it is used when the individual can bear weight but lacks the muscular control needed for ambulation without an assistive device.

796. 3 In the four-point gait the client brings the left crutch forward first, followed by the right foot; then the right crutch is brought forward, followed by the left foot. Thus both legs must be able to bear some weight. (3; CJ; IM; ED; SK)

1 Although the arms are extended to allow the hands to bear weight, the elbows are not maintained in this position.

2 Pressure on the axillae may damage nerves in the area.

4 Both extremities must be able to bear weight.

797. 4 This response explains why the traction may not be released; a continuous pull must be maintained. (2; MR; IM; TC; SK)

1 Reducing the weight requires a physician's order; removing half the weights will not maintain the bone in alignment.

2 This ignores the client's request to release the traction; further assessment is needed.

3 Although this is a true statement, it does not provide the rationale as to why the weights cannot and should not be released.

798. 2 Constriction of circulation decreases venous return and increases pressure within the vessels. Fluid then moves into the interstitial spaces, causing edema. (1; CJ; EV; PA; SK)

1 This would indicate infection.
3 Same as answer 1.
4 Same as answer 1.

799. 4 In crutch walking the client uses the triceps, trapezius, and latissimus muscles. A client who has been in bed may need to implement an exercise program to strengthen these shoulder and upper arm muscles before initiating crutch walking. (1; MR; IM; PA; SK)

1 This activity does not strengthen muscles used in crutch walking.
2 Keeping the leg in abduction alters the center of gravity, which impedes ambulation.
3 Back muscles are not used in crutch walking.

800. 3 The paraplegic client is unable to exercise the lower extremities actively. (3; MR; IM; TC; SK)

1 Changing a position involves moving the extremities. Contractures develop as a result of prolonged immobility.
2 The use of pillows, splints, and other supportive devices helps maintain alignment and prevent the shortening of muscle fibers associated with contractures.
4 Passive ROM helps maintain joint mobility and muscle tone.

801. 4 Calcium that has left the bones as a response to prolonged inactivity enters the blood and may precipitate in the kidneys, forming calculi. (2; CJ; AN; PA; SK)

1 Increased fluid intake is helpful in avoiding this condition by preventing urinary stasis.
2 Calculi may develop despite adequate kidney function; kidney function may be impaired by the presence of calculi and the high incidence of urinary tract infections associated with urinary stasis or repeated catheterizations.
3 Calcium intake is usually limited to prevent the increasing risk of calculi.

802. 4 Calcium leaves the long bones during periods of prolonged bed rest. The tilt table places the client in an upright position, which provides for weight bearing. (2; MR; AN; TC; SK)

1 The tilt table is used to prevent orthostatic hypotension by gradually allowing an individual who has been immobilized to adjust to an upright position.
2 The client is carefully strapped to the table so that mobility is actually impaired to ensure safety.
3 Although the pressure on bony prominences is altered, the use of the tilt table is not frequent enough to prevent the development of pressure ulcers.

803. 4 Rehabilitating exercises carried out underwater minimize strain on the body. The buoyant force of the water makes the limbs easier to move. (2; CJ; AN; PA; SK)

1 Vapors are produced above water as a result of evaporation; they do not facilitate exercise.
2 Exercises are carried out near the surface of the water where the water pressure would have little effect.
3 Water temperature would not assist movement.

804. 3 As a result of contracting and pulling of the muscles on the two portions of bone, there is a characteristic shortening of the femur with external rotation of the extremity. (3; CJ; AS; PA; SK)

1 Lateral motion of the leg does not occur; the leg externally rotates.
2 Lateral motion of the leg does not occur.
4 The extremity externally rotates as the muscles contract; shortening, not lengthening, occurs.

805. 1 Traction is frequently used in the treatment of a fractured hip to align the bones (reduction of fracture). If such traction were not employed, the muscles would go into spasm, shifting the bone fragments and causing pain. (2; MR; IM; ED; SK)

2 Traction is usually a temporary measure before surgery; contractures result from a shortening of the muscles by prolonged immobility.
3 Although the affected extremity must be properly aligned, turning and moving the client is still necessary.
4 External rotation is contraindicated and prevented by the use of sandbags or trochanter rolls.

806. 1 A fracture in the neck of the femur will cause shortening of the femur and external rotation. To correct this malalignment, the client's leg should be extended and maintained in slight internal rotation. (3; CJ; PL; TC; SK)

2 To reduce the fracture, it is necessary to maintain the leg in extension, counteracting the contraction of the quadriceps, which may cause overriding of bone fragments.

3 To reduce the fracture, it is necessary to maintain the leg in extension, counteracting the contraction of the quadriceps that may cause overriding of bone fragments. External rotation of the thigh as a result of muscle contraction tends to misalign the bone fragments; therefore slight internal rotation or functional alignment is preferred.

4 External rotation of the thigh as a result of muscle contraction tends to misalign the bone fragments; therefore slight internal rotation or functional alignment is preferred.

807. 3 This type of contracture frequently occurs when the client lies in bed with knees bent and thighs not abducted. (2; CJ; AS; PA; SK)

1 This does not describe a contracture.

2 Same as answer 1.

4 Although footdrop is a problem for all clients confined to bed, hyperextension of the knee is not normally possible.

808. 4 After a fracture, if blood supply is cut off or impaired, necrosis of the bone may occur from lack of oxygen and nutrient perfusion. (3; CJ; AN; PA; SK)

1 Aseptic indicates that infection is not present.

2 Early weight bearing at the fracture site might result in trauma to bone; circulation would not be impaired.

3 Immobilization does not cut off circulation to the bone; it may cause contractures.

809. 3 Elevating the foot of the bed uses gravity and the client's weight for countertraction. (2; CJ; IM; PA; SK)

1 This would not increase countertraction.

2 This would increase traction rather than countertraction.

4 This would have no effect on countertraction.

810. 2 Intramedullary nails are used to maintain bone alignment and provide support along the femur's length. (3; CJ; AN; TC; SK)

1 Because this orthopedic problem does not affect the shaft of a long bone; an intramedullary nailing device is not appropriate.

3 Same as answer 1.

4 Same as answer 1.

811. 3 This position involves hip flexion greater than 90°; this puts stress on the operative site and could dislodge the prosthesis. (3; CJ; PL; TC; SK)

1 This is acceptable because little stress is placed on the operative site.

2 Same as answer 1.

4 Same as answer 1.

812. 2 Ankle movement, particularly dorsiflexion of the foot, allows muscle contraction, which compresses veins, reducing venous stasis and risk of thrombus formation. (2; CJ; PL; TC; SK)

1 The client must be turned at least every 2 hours to help prevent the complications of immobility; 3 hours is too long to keep a client in one position.

3 The client is generally not allowed out of bed until at least 1 day postoperatively.

4 This is too soon and sitting is contraindicated because hip flexion can cause displacement of the prosthesis.

813. 3 Assessment of the pedal pulse should include the strength of the pulse. Symmetry, the correspondence of homologous parts on opposite sides of the body, indicates whether the pulses are equal. (2; CJ; AS; TC; SK)

1 Contractility is not a characteristic of pulse but of the heart; rate is not measured with pedal pulses.

2 Color of skin is not a pulse characteristic; rhythm relates to radial and apical pulses, not pedal pulses.

4 Local temperature is not a characteristic of the pedal pulse; pulsations are not visible in pedal pulses.

814. 3 Because of the recumbent position, drainage may flow under the client and not be noticed. (2; CJ; EV; TC; SK)

1 This should be done more frequently; however, the site is a more reliable indicator of hemorrhage.

2 The girth of the thigh is not an indicator of hemorrhage.

4 Dressings impede accurate assessment.

815. 1 This supports the site; the involved leg must be maintained in alignment, avoiding adduction. (1; CJ; PL; TC; SK)

2 The pillow will not affect venous return, which relates to thrombus formation.

3 Adduction, not flexion, contractures are of most concern after surgery.

4 Although friction is decreased when skin does not interface with skin, this is not the reason for separating the thighs and lower limbs.

816. 2 Placing the feet apart creates a wider base of support and brings the center of gravity closer to the ground. This improves stability. (1; CJ; IM; TC; SK)

1 Bending at the waist should be avoided because it strains the lower back muscles; the power for lifting should be supplied by the muscles of the thighs and buttocks.

3 Pressure on the abdomen is prevented by tightening the abdominal and gluteal muscles to form an internal girdle; keeping the body straight does not reduce strain on the abdominal musculature.

4 Relaxing the abdominal muscles with physical activity increases strain on the abdomen.

817. 2 Weight bearing on the uninvolved leg helps maintain its muscle tone while limiting the stress on the involved extremity. (3; MR; IM; TC; SK)

1 When the legs are in a dependent position, venous return is reduced.

3 Speed is not important when ambulating.

4 This is an unacceptable rationale for care.

818. 4 The pelvis is elevated by actions involving the unaffected upper extremities and unoperated leg. (2; MR; IM; ED; SK)

1 It is impossible to lift the pelvis with this movement.

2 Lifting with the arms requires strength; use of both heels puts pressure on the operative hip.

3 The client should not turn on the operative side immediately after surgery.

819. 4 The three-point gait, which requires considerable arm strength, is used when a limb cannot bear weight. The affected leg and crutches are advanced together, and the strong leg swings through. (3; MR; IM; ED; SK)

1 This is used for individuals who cannot move their lower extremities; it does not simulate normal ambulation.

2 This requires weight bearing on both feet.

3 Same as answer 2.

820. 3 To prevent nerve damage in the axillary area, the palms should bear all the weight. (1; MR; IM; ED; SK)

1 This is unsafe and next to impossible to perform.

2 Pressure in the axillary area causes nerve damage to the brachial plexus.

4 Weight bearing on the affected lower extremity is initially contraindicated.

821. 4 This group would succumb quickly to severe blood loss if dressings as indicated were not applied. (3; MR; PL; TC; SK)

1 These individuals could wait for treatment per the triage routine.

2 Same as answer 1.

3 These clients must wait for treatment per triage protocol; they require extended care not available in emergency situations.

822. 3 Excessive flexion of the hip can cause dislocation. (2; MR; EV; ED; SK)

1 Climbing stairs does not cause undue stress on the operative site.

2 This would be encouraged as long as no extremes of position are used.

4 This would be encouraged because it prevents hip flexion contractures.

823. 2 Because pain is an all-encompassing and often demoralizing experience, the client should be kept as pain free as possible. (2; CJ; PL; TC; SK)

1 Surgery is used to correct deformity and facilitate movement; relief of pain is the priority.

3 Concentration on learning something is difficult when a client is in severe pain; relief of pain is the priority.

4 Motivation is difficult when a client is in severe pain; relief of pain is the priority.

824. 3 An antinuclear antibody test (ANA) may be positive in clients with autoimmune disorders such as rheumatoid arthritis and systemic lupus erythematosus. (1; CJ; IM; PA; SK)

1 Pancreatic lipase is an enzyme that catalyzes the breakdown of lipids; this is a test used to diagnose pancreatic problems.

2 Bence Jones protein is a urine test helpful in diagnosing multiple myeloma.

4 Alkaline phosphatase is a blood test to determine phosphorus activity; it is generally used in diagnosing liver and biliary tract disorders and identifying periods of active bone growth or metastasis of cancer to bone.

825. **1** Active exercises, alternated with periods of rest, offer the best chance at avoiding the joint deformities associated with rheumatoid arthritis because they move the involved joint through its full range of motion. (2; MR; PL; PA; SK)

2 Immobilization of joints by bracing would promote the formation of contractures and deformities.

3 Massage affects the muscles, not the joints, and would do little to prevent deformities.

4 Isometric exercise will promote muscle, not joint function.

826. **3** ROM exercises must be instituted to maintain mobility of joints. However, overuse may prevent resolution of the inflammation. (1; CJ; AN; TC; SK)

1 Pain may persist but cannot be allowed to legitimize inactivity.

2 Activity will not prevent the inflammatory process; it may aggravate it.

4 Severely damaged joints may require prosthetic replacement.

827. **1** Osteoarthritis affects the hips and knees first because they are the weight-bearing joints and undergo the most stress. (2; CJ; AS; PA; SK)

2 Although these are weight-bearing joints, normal motion is not as great as in the hips and knees; thus there is less degeneration.

3 Although the distal interphalangeal joints are frequently affected, the remaining interphalangeal joints and metacarpals are not.

4 These are not weight-bearing joints.

828. **2** Steroids have an antiinflammatory effect that can reduce arthritic pannus formation. (3; MR; AN; TC; SK)

1 Pain relief is a secondary result of the antiinflammatory action of steroids.

3 Injection of a drug is not physiotherapy.

4 Ankylosis refers to fusion of joints. It is only indirectly influenced by steroids, which exert their major effect on the inflammatory process.

829. **2** Ossification of cartilage, particularly of the spine, causes fixation of the involved joints. (3; CJ; PL; TC; SK)

1 Inflammation and thickening of the synovial membrane are characteristic of arthritis.

3 Although rest is essential, complete immobility would result in a loss of joint motion.

4 Redness and swelling are symptoms of local inflammation; they do not indicate irreversible damage.

830. **4** Marie-Strümpell disease is synonymous with rheumatoid spondylitis, not osteoarthritis, which involves fixation of joints (usually vertebral). (3; MR; PL; ED; SK)

1 Heberden nodules are the bony or cartilaginous enlargements of the distal interphalangeal joints that are associated with degenerative arthritis.

2 As the cartilage of the joints degenerates, there are hypertrophic changes of the bone edges, which eventually replace the articular cartilage.

3 Ankylosis occurs in rheumatoid arthritis, not in hypertrophic or degenerative arthritis.

831. **3** Inactivity over an extended time increases stiffness and pain in joints. (1; CJ; PL; PA; SK)

1 This is not a factor; cold packs may decrease joint discomfort.

2 Assistive exercises help maintain joint mobility.

4 The latex fixation test is positive when the rheumatoid factor is found in blood serum; this factor is present in many conditions, including rheumatoid arthritis, aging, narcotic addiction, and SLE.

832. **4** There are no dietary restrictions, but iron and vitamins should be encouraged to normalize any underlying nutritional deficiencies. (2; CJ; PL; TC; SK)

1 These nutritional restrictions are not indicated.

2 A high-calorie diet would increase the client's weight; this is contraindicated because it would increase the strain on weight bearing joints.

3 A normal protein intake should fulfill nutritional needs; there is no need to restrict calcium.

833. **2** Because of its antiinflammatory effect, aspirin is useful in treating arthritis symptoms. (1; CJ; IM; TC; SK)

1 Xanax is an antianxiety, not an antiinflammatory, agent.

3 Narcotics should be avoided because they promote drug dependency and do not affect the inflammatory process.

4 Same as answer 3.

834. 3 Exercise of involved joints is important to maintain optimal mobility and prevent build-up of calcium deposits. (3; MR; IM; TC; SK)

1 Immobilization causes loss of joint mobility and contractures.
2 Same as answer 1.
4 Same as answer 1.

835. 3 Heat and cold reduce inflammation and discomfort. (3; CJ; IM; TC; SK)

1 This will depend on the client's tolerance.
2 Avoiding exercise will increase the destructive effects of immobility.
4 Exercises are necessary to prevent contractures and permanent joint damage; aerobic exercises may be too strenuous and accelerate joint destruction.

836. 4 There is no special diet for arthritis. A balanced diet, consisting of foods from all levels of the food pyramid, is essential in maintaining nutrition. (2; MR; IM; ED; SK)

1 Limiting the diet to particular foods does not provide all essential nutrients.
2 Same as answer 1.
3 If nutritional intake is adequate, large doses of multivitamins are unnecessary.

837. 1 Laminar air flow decreases the risk of bone infection, because potentially contaminated air continuously flows away from the sterile field, decreasing the concentration of airborne pathogens. (3; MR; IM; TC; SK)

2 The procedure is performed at one time.
3 Surgery is generally considered when destruction of the femoral head and acetabulum is extensive.
4 The lithotomy position is used for gynecologic procedures; the side-lying position is generally used for hip surgery.

838. 3 Manual stretching exercises will assist in keeping the muscles and tendons supple and pliable, reducing the traumatic consequences of repetitive activity. (2; MR; IM; PA; SK)

1 The problem is not caused by carring articles in the arms but by repetitive-type trauma.
2 This would not be a satisfactory alternative for a skilled carpenter.
4 The use of power tools would not be a problem.

Reproductive and Genitourinary

839. 1 Primitive sex cells, called spermatogonia, are present in newborn males. At puberty these cells mature and form spermatozoa (spermatogenesis). (2; CJ; AN; PA; RG)

2 Spermatogenesis does not occur until puberty.
3 Spermatogonia or primitive sex cells are found at this time.
4 Only immature cells are found during this period.

840. 3 Sperm cells are very fragile and can be destroyed by heat, resulting in sterility. (2; CJ; AN; PA; RG)

1 Sperm do not move through the urine; they are found in semen.
2 Sperm are motile, achieving this by motion of their flagella; they move from the epididymis to the vas deferens to the ejaculatory ducts to the urethra.
4 During this period the testes are not suspended.

841. 3 *Condylomata acuminata* are variably sized cauliflower-like warts occurring principally on the genitals or the anogenital skin or mucosa of both females and males; they are transmitted by sexual activity. (3; CJ; AN; PA; RG)

1 Scabies is an infestation of the skin by *Sarcoptes scabiei* (itch mite).
2 Herpes zoster is an acute vesicular skin infection caused by the varicella zoster virus.
4 *Condylomata acuminata* are warts occurring on the genitals or the anogenital skin or mucosa of both males and females; the epididymis is part of the male reproductive system and is an internal structure.

842. 1 Massive doses of penicillin may limit CNS damage if treatment is started before neural deterioration from syphilis occurs. (3; CJ; PL; TC; RG)

2 Tranquilizers are used to modify behavior, not to treat general paresis.
3 Paresis is not a behavior and is therefore not suitably treated with behavior modification.
4 Electroconvulsive therapy is used in the treatment of certain psychiatric disorders.

843. 3 In males the inflammatory process associated with the infection may lead to destruction of the epididymis. In females the gonorrheal infection causes destruction of the tubal mucosa and eventually tuboovarian abscesses. (1; MR; IM; ED; RG)

1 Gonorrhea has become more difficult to treat because many gonococci have become penicillin resistant.
2 Gonorrhea is a common sexually transmitted disease.
4 *Neisseria gonorrhoeae* will invade internal structures, particularly the epididymis in males and the fallopian tubes in females.

844. 2 Ceftriaxone (Rocephin) inhibits the synthesis of bacterial cell walls. It is effective against *Neisseria gonorrhoeae*, a gram-negative diplococcus. (2; CJ; PL; TC; RG)
1 Colistin sulfate is effective against most gram-negative enteric pathogens such as *Escherichia coli*.
3 Actinomycin is an antineoplastic agent.
4 Chloramphenicol is a broad-spectrum antimicrobial agent; however, it can cause bone marrow depression, so its use is limited to severe infections that do not respond to less toxic drugs.

845. 3 *Trichomonas vaginalis* is a protozoan that favors an alkaline environment. (3; CJ; AN; PA; RG)
1 A yeast is a unicellular, usually oval, nucleated fungus; it does not cause trichomonal infections.
2 A fungus is a simple parasitic plant; it does not cause trichomonal infections.
4 A spirochete is a motile spiral-shaped bacterium; it does not cause trichomonal infections.

846. 4 Metronidazole (Flagyl) is a potent amebicide. It is extremely effective in eradicating the protozoan *Trichomonas vaginalis*. (3; CJ; PL; TC; RG)
1 Penicillin is administered for its effect on bacterial, not protozoal, infections.
2 Gentian violet is a local antiinfective that is applied topically and may cause discoloration of the skin; it is particularly effective against *Candida albicans*.
3 Nystatin is an antifungal used for infections caused by *Candida albicans*.

847. 3 This is the anatomic direction of the vaginal tract in the back-lying position. (2; MR; IM; ED; RG)
1 The vaginal tract may be injured when the douche nozzle is not directed with consideration of normal anatomy.
2 Same as answer 1.
4 Same as answer 1.

848. 3 The nurse's best response is one that is realistic; once people become sexually active they usually remain sexually active; a condom, although not 100% effective, is the best protection against gonorrhea in a sexually active person. (2; MR; EV; TC; RG)
1 Douching has no proven protective effect against sexually transmitted disease; excessive douching can actually alter the natural environment of the vagina and may even promote an ascending infection.

2 Although this is the best way to prevent a sexually transmitted disease, it is not the most realistic response to a sexually active person.
4 Spermicidal cream has no protective effect against sexually transmitted diseases.

849. 3 Gonorrhea frequently is an ascending infection and affects the fallopian tubes. (2; CJ; AS; PA; RG)
1 Syphilis, if untreated, may spread to the nervous system via the blood; it does not usually cause ascending infection of the fallopian tubes.
2 Abortion should not cause inflammation of the fallopian tubes.
4 This is not an infection, it is an aberrant growth; it would not cause inflammation of the fallopian tubes.

850. 4 Pain and elevated temperature may indicate toxic effects. Excessive sloughing of tissue can cause hemorrhage or infection. (2; CJ; EV; TC; WH)
1 These are expected side effects of internal radiotherapy.
2 These are associated with need to maintain position, not with radium itself.
3 These are expected side effects of internal radiotherapy.

851. 2 Radium must be handled with long-handled forceps because distance helps limit exposure. (2; CJ; IM; TC; WH)
1 A nurse is not responsible for cleaning radium implants.
3 Foil-lined rubber gloves do not provide adequate shielding from the gamma rays emitted by radium.
4 The amount and duration of exposure are important in assessing the effect on the client; however, this will not affect safety during removal.

852. 4 Radium, a radioactive isotope, is used to destroy or delay the growth of malignant cells; packing maintains the insert in its correct placement to maximize the effect on cancerous tissue and minimize the effect on normal tissue. (2; CJ; AN; TC; WH)
1 The packing must be readjusted or replaced to protect normal tissue from damage from the radium implant.
2 This is not true.
3 There should be no active bleeding with radium implants although there may be cellular sloughing.

853. **1** Time, distance, and shielding are the important factors in determining the amount of radiation the visitor receives. Restriction of each visitor to a 10-minute stay minimizes the risk of exposure. Many institutions will not allow visitors while an implant is in place. (3; CJ; IM; TC; WH)

2 The urine is not radioactive, so no precautions are indicated.

3 Lead aprons are effective shields against x-rays but not against rays emitted by internal sources of radiation.

4 Radium implants will not affect the location of IM injections.

854. **3** Before discharge it is important for the nurse to instruct the client to follow through with medical care at specified intervals. (2; MR; PL; ED; WH)

1 Fluids are not reduced unless other cardiac or renal pathology is present.

2 A low-residue diet is indicated to avoid pressure from a distended colon only when the implant is in place; the radium implant is removed before discharge.

4 If diet is adequate, multivitamins are unnecessary.

855. **4** Some spermatozoa will remain viable in the vas deferens for a variable time after vasectomy. (3; MR; IM; ED; RG)

1 Although it is considered a permanent form of sterilization, there has been some success in reversing the procedure.

2 The procedure does not affect sexual functioning.

3 Precautions must be taken to prevent fertilization until absence of sperm in the semen has been verified.

856. **2** When the testes are twisted, a decrease in their blood supply occurs. This can result in gangrene. (3; CJ; AN; TC; RG)

1 Pain can be alleviated through the use of medication.

3 Although edema occurs, the testes do not rupture.

4 Sperm are continually produced, so their destruction is not the concern.

857. **4** The PSA is an indication of cancer of the prostate; the higher the level, the greater the tumor burden. (2; CJ; EV; TC; RG)

1 Elevated creatinine levels may be caused by impaired renal function as a result of blockage by an enlarged prostate but do not indicate that metastasis has occurred.

2 Elevated BUN levels may be caused by impaired renal function as a result of blockage by an enlarged prostate but do not indicate that metastasis has occurred.

3 Nonprotein nitrogen refers to waste products from metabolism of protein and includes urea, creatinine, uric acid, and ammonia.

858. **3** Inability to empty the bladder, as a result of pressure exerted by the enlarging prostate on the urethra, causes a backup of urine into the ureters and finally the kidneys (hydronephrosis). (2; CJ; AS; PA; RG)

1 BPH develops over the client's life span; it is not congenital.

2 It is uncommon for BPH to become malignant.

4 This level is elevated in prostatic carcinoma.

859. **3** The exudate from herpes virus type 2 is highly contagious; gown and gloves provide a barrier, a concept related to medical asepsis. (2; CJ; IM; TC; RG)

1 The organism is not in respiratory tract secretions; the organism is present in the exudate from active lesions.

2 This is unnecessary.

4 This is not an airborne infectious disease.

860. **3** Although the usual incubation period of syphilis is about 3 weeks, clinical symptoms may appear as early as 9 days or as long as 3 months after exposure. (2; MR; IM; PA; RG)

1 The normal incubation period is 21 days.

2 Same as answer 1.

4 Same as answer 1.

861. **1** The tertiary stage is noncontagious; tertiary lesions contain only small numbers of treponemes; fatal cases involve the aorta, CNS, or eye. (3; CJ; AN; PA; RG)

2 The primary stage lasts 8 to 12 weeks; the chancre is teeming with spirochetes, and the individual is contagious.

3 The incubation stage lasts 2 to 6 weeks; spirochetes proliferate at entry site, and the individual is contagious.

4 The duration of the secondary stage is variable (about 5 years); skin and mucosal lesions contain spirochetes, and the individual is highly contagious.

862. **1** Gonorrhea is a highly contagious disease transmitted through sexual intercourse. The incubation period varies, but symptoms usually occur 2 to 10 days after contact. Early effective treatment prevents complications. (1; MR; AS; TC; RG)

2 The parents may be unaware that their child has gonorrhea.

3 Contracting venereal disease is not necessarily indicative of promiscuity.

4 Most birth control measures do not protect against the transmission of sexually transmitted disease.

863. **1** Ceftriaxone with doxycycline is specific for *Neisseria gonorrhoeae* and eradicates the microorganism; other treatment regimens are available for resistant strains. (1; MR; IM; ED; RG)

2 If the disease progresses before diagnosis is made, complications such as sterility, valve damage, or joint degeneration may occur.

3 Transmission is not controlled; the organism is eliminated.

4 If tubal structures, valves, or joints degenerate, the pathologic changes will not be reversed by antibiotic therapy.

864. **2** The kidneys are ultimately responsible for maintaining fluid and electrolyte balance by excretion or retention based on body's needs. (2; CJ; AN; PA; RG)

1 Aldosterone will cause retention of sodium ions by the nephrons and subsequent fluid retention.

3 The lungs eliminate water and carbon dioxide only if excess carbonic acid is present; their role in fluid and electrolyte balance is less extensive than the kidneys'.

4 Antidiuretic hormone has a direct effect on the nephrons, resulting in water retention.

865. **2** Osmosis is the diffusion of water through a selectively permeable membrane. Such membranes include cellular membranes and capillary walls. Osmosis occurs in the kidney tubules and in all capillary beds. (1; CJ; AN; PA; RG)

1 Dialysis is the diffusion of small molecules, other than water, down their concentration gradients through a selectively permeable membrane.

3 Diffusion is the process by which particulate matter in a fluid moves from an area of greater concentration to an area of lesser concentration.

4 Active transport is the movement of molecules against a concentration gradient and requires energy input; osmosis and diffusion are passive processes.

866. **2** The prostate gland is a tubuloalveolar gland shaped like a ring, with the urethra passing through its center. (1; CJ; AN; PA; RG)

1 The epididymis lies along the top and sides of the testes.

3 The seminal vesicles are on the posterior surface of the bladder.

4 This gland lies below the prostate.

867. **1** Depending on the purpose of the collection, a preservative to prevent breakdown of the specimen may be necessary. (2; CJ; IM; TC; RG)

2 This is not necessary.

3 The last specimen should be collected as close as possible to the end of the 24-hour period and added to the urine collected.

4 This is not necessary, nor is the measurement of each voiding during the 24-hour collection, unless the client is on intake and output.

868. **2** Refrigeration retards the growth of bacteria and may preserve the specimen for several hours. (2; CJ; IM; TC; RG)

1 Growth of bacteria will alter the pH and the glucose and protein levels in the urine; it must be refrigerated to retard growth.

3 Same as answer 1.

4 This represents an unnecessary waste of time, effort, and money.

869. **3** Catheter patency ensures drainage and prevents bladder distention and other complications. Therefore patency of a catheter should be established before notifying the physician. (1; CJ; IM; TC; RG)

1 Assessment is necessary before consultation with the physician.

2 Patency of the catheter should be assessed first. Milking the tubing may be necessary if the catheter is clogged. Milking a catheter is usually required when the drainage is viscous rather than liquid.

4 Irrigation is avoided if possible because of the associated risk of infection.

MEDICAL-SURGICAL ANSWERS

870. **3** An indwelling catheter dilates the urinary sphincters, keeps the bladder empty, and short-circuits the normal reflex mechanism based on bladder distention. When the catheter is removed, the body must adapt to functioning once again. (2; CJ; AN; PA; RG)
1 Although this could cause difficulty in voiding, there are no data presented to draw this conclusion.
2 This would not cause this problem.
4 Same as answer 1.

871. **3** An enlarged prostate constricts the urethra, interfering with urine flow causing retention. When the bladder fills and approaches capacity, small amounts can be voided but the bladder never empties completely. (2; CJ; AN; PA; RG)
1 Edema does not cause the client to void frequently in small amounts because of decreased production of urine.
2 Dysuria is painful or difficult urination that is not part of the client's symptoms.
4 The urge to void is caused by stimulation of the stretch receptors as the bladder fills with urine; in suppression little or no urine is produced.

872. **4** Cleansing the urinary meatus and adjacent skin removes accumulated bacteria, limiting the possible introduction of microbes into the urinary tract. (3; CJ; PL; TC; RG)
1 Although cleansing the perineal area is helpful, it is actually the organisms closest to the meatus that gain entry to the urinary tract first.
2 Although encouraging fluids helps prevent urinary stasis and subsequent infection, the most common source of infection is microorganisms from around the meatus.
3 Irrigations require opening the closed drainage system and allowing the entry of microorganisms; this increases the risk of infection.

873. **3** The total amount of irrigation solution instilled into the bladder is eliminated with urine and therefore must be subtracted from the total output to determine the volume of urine excreted. (2; CJ; IM; TC; RG)
1 An accurate specific gravity cannot be obtained when irrigating solutions are being instilled into the bladder.
2 Hourly outputs are indicated only if there is concern about renal failure or oliguria.
4 Twenty-four hour urine tests would not be accurate if the client were receiving continuous irrigations.

874. **1** Frequent position changes are important to ensure proper urinary drainage; gravity promotes flow, which prevents obstruction. (2; CJ; AN; TC; RG)
2 Range of motion would be of minimal importance, because the client would be able to move without limitation.
3 Back care is necessary but is not the priority.
4 This is not a priority unless the client is sedated.

875. **3** The length of the urethra is shorter in females than in males; therefore microorganisms have a shorter distance to travel to reach the bladder. The proximity of the meatus to the anus in females also increases this incidence. (2; MR; AS; PA; RG)
1 Fluid intake may be adequate in both males and females and would not account for the difference.
2 Hygienic practices can be poor in males or females; however, the anatomic length of the urethra in females predisposes them to infection.
4 Mucous membranes are continuous in both males and females and would not make a difference.

876. **4** Because the female urethra is closer to the anus than in the male, it is at greater risk of becoming contaminated. (1; CJ; AN; PA; RG)
1 Urinary pH is within the same range in both males and females.
2 Hormonal secretions have no effect on the development of bladder infections.
3 The position of the bladder is the same in males and females.

877. **4** The causative organism should be isolated before starting antibiotic therapy. (1; CJ; PL; TC; RG)
1 This test will not determine the infective organisms causing the problem.
2 The bowel is not affected by the diagnosis; enemas are not required.
3 Catheterization is not a routine procedure for urethritis.

878. **1** Cloudy urine usually indicates purulent drainage associated with infection. (2; CJ; AS; PA; RG)
2 Viscosity is a subjective characteristic that would not be measurable.
3 Specific gravity yields information related to fluid balance.
4 Sugar and acetone are not affected by urinary tract infections.

879. **4** Changes in the amount of blood in the urine may indicate progressive increases in kidney damage. (2; CJ; AS; PA; RG)
   1 This is unrelated to hematuria.
   2 This is unrelated to hematuria; it is associated with breakdown of adipose tissue.
   3 Same as answer 1.

880. **4** Hemolytic streptococci, common in throat infections, can initiate an immune reaction that damages the glomerulus. (2; MR; IM; ED; RG)
   1 Baths have been linked to urethritis, not glomerulonephritis.
   2 Moderate activity is helpful in preventing urinary stasis.
   3 Any fluid restriction is moderated as the client improves; fluid is allowed to prevent urinary stasis.

881. **1** Sharp, severe pain (renal colic) radiating toward the genitalia and thigh is caused by ureteral distention. (2; CJ; AN; TC; RG)
   2 Although the client is overweight and weight loss would be desirable, it is a long-term goal.
   3 Although this may occur, blood loss is usually not massive.
   4 Hypertension is not specific to urinary calculi.

882. **1** Urine is strained to determine whether any calculi or calcium gravel has been passed. (1; CJ; IM; TC; RG)
   2 Fluids should be encouraged to promote dilute urine and facilitate passage of the calculi.
   3 Blood pressure assessment is of no particular importance to the client with kidney stones.
   4 Administration of analgesics is based on the physician's order.

883. **4** Output should be about 50 ml/hr with an intake of at least 1200 ml per 24 hours. (2; CJ; EV; TC; RG)
   1 Some blood, tinting the urine pink, is expected, but not bright red drainage.
   2 This intake is adequate; however, a higher intake is usually preferred.
   3 Drainage may be pink; bright red drainage should be reported.

884. **4** Cystolithectomy refers to the removal of bladder stones. (3; MR; PL; ED; RG)
   1 Cystometry is the process of measuring the bladder's pressure and capacity.

2 Cystolithiasis denotes the presence of stones in the bladder.
   3 Cryoextraction refers to the use of subfreezing temperatures in the removal of tissue; generally used in cataract extraction.

885. **2** A large amount of bright red blood indicates hemorrhage; immediate pressure should compress vessels which will limit blood flow. (2; CJ; MS; IM; TC)
   1 This is unsafe; it will not correct the problem.
   3 This is unsafe.
   4 This is unsafe as a first action; charting would be done later.

886. **1** Calcium and phosphorus are components of these stones and should therefore be avoided. Also an acid environment is not favorable to their development. (1; CJ; PL; TC; RG)
   2 Diets high in calcium must be avoided.
   3 This diet is indicated for clients with gout.
   4 Same as answer 2.

887. **3** Uric acid stones are controlled by a low-purine diet. Foods high in purine, such as organ meats and extracts, should be avoided. (3; MR; IM; ED; RG)
   1 Calcium stones are controlled by a low-calcium, low-phosphate diet; milk, fruits, and vegetables need not be avoided with uric acid stones.
   2 Cystine, not uric acid, stones are controlled by a low-methionine diet, which excludes meat, milk, eggs, and cheese from the diet.
   4 Only organ meats must be avoided; vegetables need not be controlled.

888. **3** This is a low calcium intake and continued high excretion levels would then have to be from other than a dietary source; recurrent infections and inadequate fluids contribute most to formation of calculi; most stones are calcium or oxalate in nature. (3; CJ; AN; TC; RG)
   1 Calcium intake through the diet may affect the blood calcium levels.
   2 Parathyroid hormone controls the serum calcium levels.
   4 This is not conclusive evidence that parathyroidism is the cause.

MEDICAL-SURGICAL ANSWERS

889. **3** Calcium oxalate renal stones can be prevented by adhering to a diet low in calcium and oxalate and high in acid ash. (2; CJ; PL; TC; RG)
1 Purines are catabolized to uric acid and must be avoided in gout.
2 Methionine is an essential amino acid and must be included in the diet.
4 The diet should be high in acid, not alkaline, ash to control production of these stones.

890. **1** An output of 50 ml/hr is adequate; when output drops below 30 ml/hr it may indicate renal failure and the physician should be notified. (2; CJ; IM; PA; RG)
2 Contraindicated; the client would probably still be under influence of anesthesia and have no gag response.
3 This is unnecessary and would require a physician's order.
4 The physician should be notified if hourly output drops below 30 ml.

891. **4** Preoperative cleansing of the bowel is mandated before surgical resection and formation of a urinary conduit. (1; CJ; PL; TC; RG)
1 Fluids should not be restricted until after midnight of the operative day.
2 Muscle-tightening exercises have no effect on this procedure
3 The stoma of an ileal conduit is not irrigated.

892. **1** Dysuria, nocturia, and urgency are all signs of an irritable bladder after radiation therapy. (2; CJ; EV; PA; RG)
2 This is not an indication of bladder irritability.
3 Same as answer 2.
4 Same as answer 2.

893. **3** The ureters are implanted in a segment of the ileum, and urine drains continually because there is no sphincter. (2; CJ; EV; PA; RG)
1 Ileal conduits are not neurologically innervated; therefore no peristalsis exists.
2 No feces are present in an ileal conduit.
4 Nutrients are not normally absorbed from urine.

894. **1** Because of the anatomic position of the incision, drainage would flow by gravity and accumulate under the client lying in the supine position. (2; CJ; EV; TC; RG)
2 Nail beds would indicate peripheral perfusion, not early hemorrhage.
3 Respiratory hemorrhage is not common after kidney surgery.

4 Blood pressure decreases in hemorrhage, and pulse increases.

895. **4** A suprapubic prostatectomy involves an abdominal incision to gain access to the prostate through the bladder. Postoperatively the client has a suprapubic cystotomy tube to instill a GU irrigant to dilute the urine and limit clot formation as well as a Foley catheter under tension to limit bleeding and drain urine. (2; CJ; PL; PA; RG)
1 The ureters are not involved in this surgery.
2 The kidneys are not involved in this surgery.
3 An incision is made in the lower abdomen; a ureteral catheter is not used.

896. **2** The catheter must be reinserted by the physician to ensure bladder emptying, maintain pressure at the operative site, and prevent hemorrhage. (2; CJ; IM; TC; RG)
1 Because of the danger of further trauma to the urethra and surgical site, the surgeon should insert the catheter.
3 Irrigations require a physician's order.
4 In addition to urinary drainage, the balloon of the urethral catheter exerts pressure against the prostate to help control bleeding and should be reinserted.

897. **1** The bladder is a sterile body cavity. Any time a solution or catheter is introduced into the urinary meatus, strict surgical asepsis is required. (2; CJ; IM; TC; RG)
2 Excessive pressure can traumatize the lining of the urinary tract.
3 The solution is generally administered at room temperature.
4 This would only be done if the fluid did not return by gravity; the negative pressure exerted during aspiration may cause trauma.

898. **3** Continuous bladder irrigation requires a three-way indwelling catheter so that the irrigant infuses through one port and both urine and irrigant drain out together through another port; the third port allows for inflation of the balloon that keeps the catheter in the bladder. (2; CJ; IM; TC; RG)
1 The bedside drainage bag contains both irrigant and urine.
2 The purpose of CBI is to prevent obstruction of the catheter; stopping the irrigation would increase the risk of obstruction.
4 Both urine and irrigant mix in the bladder and drain from the same port.

899. **1** Bicarbonate buffering is limited, hydrogen ions accumulate, and acidosis results (3; CJ; AN; PA; RG)

2 The fluid balance does not significantly alter the pH.

3 The rate of respirations increases in metabolic acidosis to compensate for a low pH.

4 The retention of sodium ions is related to fluid retention and edema rather than to acidosis.

900. **4** The amount of protein permitted in the diet (usually below 50 g) depends on the extent of kidney function; excess protein causes a rise in urea, which should be avoided; adequate calories are also provided to prevent tissue catabolism that also results in an increase in metabolic waste products. (3; CJ; AN; TC; RG)

1 The diet used in managing renal failure is low in protein because the kidneys are unable to eliminate the waste products from the body.

2 The body is able to synthesize the nonessential amino acids.

3 Urea is a waste product of protein metabolism; the body is able to synthesize the nonessential amino acids.

901. **2** In renal failure, as the glomerular filtration rate decreases, phosphorus is retained. As hyperphosphatemia occurs, calcium is excreted. Calcium depletion (hypocalcemia) causes tetany. (2; CJ; AN; PA; RG)

1 The symptoms described are not characteristic of this condition.

3 Same as answer 1.

4 Same as answer 1.

902. **3** An elevated blood urea nitrogen, indicating uremia, is toxic to the central nervous system and causes mental cloudiness, confusion, and loss of consciousness. (1; CJ; AS; PA; RG)

1 Hyperkalemia is associated with muscle weakness, irritability, nausea, and diarrhea.

2 Hypernatremia is associated with firm tissue turgor, oliguria, and agitation.

4 If decreased fluid intake results in dehydration, it can cause fatigue, dry skin and mucous membranes, and rapid pulse and respiratory rates.

903. **4** These adaptations result from excess nitrogenous wastes, altered fluid and electrolyte balance, and altered regulatory functions. (2; CJ; AS; PA; RG)

1 Oliguria occurs because of extensive nephron damage.

2 Metabolic, not respiratory, acidosis occurs because of the kidneys' inability to excrete hydrogen and regulate sodium and bicarbonate.

3 Hypotension does not occur; the blood pressure is normal or elevated as a result of increased total body water.

904. **4** Diffusion moves particles from an area of greater to an area of lesser concentration; osmosis moves fluid from an area of lesser to an area of greater concentration of particles. (2; CJ; AN; PA; RG)

1 The principle of ultrafiltration involves a pressure gradient, which is associated with hemodialysis, not peritoneal dialysis.

2 Peritoneal dialysis cleanses the peritoneal cavity directly and the blood indirectly.

3 Dialysate does not clear toxins in a short time; exchanges may occur four or five times a day.

905. **4** Peritoneal dialysis uses the peritoneum as a selectively permeable membrane for diffusion of toxins and wastes from the blood into the dialyzing solution. (1; CJ; AN; PA; RG)

1 Peritoneal dialysis acts as a substitute for kidney function; it does not reestablish kidney function.

2 The dialysate does not clean the peritoneal membrane; the semipermeable membrane allows toxins and wastes to pass into the dialysate within the abdominal cavity.

3 Fluid in the abdominal cavity does not enter the intracellular compartment.

906. **4** Protein breakdown liberates cellular potassium ions, leading to hyperkalemia, which can cause cardiac dysrhythmia and standstill. The failure of the kidneys to maintain a balance of potassium is one of the main indications for dialysis. (2; CJ; PL; TC; RG)

1 Ascites occurs in liver disease and is not an indication for dialysis.

2 Dialysis is not the usual treatment for acidosis. This usually responds to administration of alkaline drugs.

3 Dialysis is not a treatment for hypertension; this is usually controlled by antihypertensive medication and diet.

907. 3 Because an external shunt provides circulatory access to a major artery and vein, special safety precautions must be taken to prevent disconnection of the cannulas. Disconnection can cause unimpeded excessive blood loss and death. Clamps should be carried at all times by the client in case this emergency should arise. (3; CJ; EV; TC; RG)

1 Although a potential complication, this does not pose the same immediate threat to life as does exsanguination.

2 Same as answer 1.

4 Same as answer 1.

908. 2 Insertion of an arteriovenous shunt represents a break in the first line of defense against infection, the skin. An infection of an arteriovenous shunt can be avoided by strict aseptic (sterile) technique. (1; CJ; IM; TC; RG)

1 An elastic bandage would interfere with examination of the site.

3 Expected; bruit is auscultated by virtue of the increased arterial pressure in the area.

4 To prevent damage to the shunt, blood pressure should not be measured in the affected arm.

909. 2 Turning from side to side will change position of the catheter, thereby freeing the drainage holes, which may be obstructed. (3; CJ; IM; TC; RG)

1 Taking fluids into the gastrointestinal tract does not influence drainage of dialysate from the peritoneal cavity.

3 This improves pulmonary ventilation and helps in maintaining comfort but does not improve flow of dialysate from the catheter.

4 The position of the catheter should only be changed by the physician.

910. 4 Radiation may damage the bowel mucosa, causing bleeding. (2; CV; EV; PA; RG)

1 Iron and protein may need to be increased to promote RBC production and tissue healing.

2 Enemas are contraindicated with lower abdominal radiation because of the damaged intestinal mucosa.

3 Diarrhea, not constipation, occurs with radiation.

BIBLIOGRAPHY

Foundations of Nursing Practice

Ackley BJ, Ladwig GB: *Nursing diagnosis handbook: a guide to planning care,* ed 5, St. Louis, 2002, Mosby.

Balzer-Riley J: *Communication in nursing,* ed 4, St. Louis, 2000, Mosby.

Brent NJ: *Nurses and the law: a guide to principles and application,* ed 2, Philadelphia, 2001, WB Saunders.

Chernecky C et al: *Real-world nursing survival guide: drug calculations and drug administration,* Philadelphia, 2002, WB Saunders.

Dochterman JM, Grace HK: *Current issues in nursing,* ed 6, St. Louis, 2001, Mosby.

Gordon M: *Manual of nursing diagnosis,* ed 10, St. Louis, 2002, Mosby.

Huber D: *Leadership and nursing care management,* ed 2, Philadelphia, 2000, WB Saunders.

Johnson M, Maas ML, Moorhead S: *Nursing outcomes classification,* ed 2, St. Louis, 2000, Mosby.

Lancaster J: *Nursing issues in leading and managing change,* ed 2, St. Louis, 1999, Mosby.

McCloskey JC, Bulechek GM: *Nursing interventions classifications,* ed 3, St. Louis, 2000, Mosby.

McCuistion LE, Gutierrez K: *Real-world nursing survival guide: pharmacology,* Philadelphia, 2002, WB Saunders

National League for Nursing: Nursing's role in patient rights, Pub No 11-1671, New York, 1997, The League.

Niven N: *Health psychology for health care professionals,* ed 3, Philadelphia, 2000, Churchill Livingstone.

Ogden SJ: *Radcliff & Ogden's calculation of drug dosages,* ed 6, St. Louis, 1999, Mosby.

Redman BK: *The practice of patient education,* ed 9, St. Louis, 2001, Mosby.

Psychiatric/Mental Health Nursing

Aguilera DC: *Crisis intervention: theory and methodology,* ed 8, St. Louis, 1998, Mosby.

American Nurses Association: *Scope and standards of psychiatric-mental health clinical nursing practice,* Washington, DC, 2000, The Association.

American Psychiatric Association: *Diagnostic and statistical manual of mental disorders (DSM-IV-TR),* ed 4, Washington, DC, The Association.

Dubowitz H, DePanfilis D: *Handbook for child protection practices,* Thousand Oaks, Calif, 2000, Sage Publications, Inc.

Erickson E: *Childhood and society,* New York, 1963, W.W. Norton.

Haber J et al: *Comprehensive psychiatric nursing,* ed 5, St. Louis, 1997, Mosby.

Keltner NL, Folks DG; *Psychotropic drugs,* ed 3, St. Louis, 2001, Mosby.

Keltner NL, Schwecke LH, Bostrom CD: *Psychiatric nursing,* ed 3, St. Louis, 1999, Mosby.

Stuart GW, Laraia MT: *Principles and practice of psychiatric nursing,* ed 7, St. Louis, 2001, Mosby.

Sundeen SJ et al: *Nurse-client interaction: implementing the nursing process,* ed 6, St. Louis, 1998, Mosby.

Varcarolis EM: *Foundations of psychiatric mental health nursing,* ed 4, Philadelphia, 2001, WB Saunders.

Childbearing and Women's Health Nursing

Biancuzzo M: *Breastfeeding the newborn: clinical strategies for nurses,* St. Louis, 1999, Mosby.

Blackburn ST: *Maternal, fetal and neonatal physiology: a clinical perspective,* ed 2, Philadelphia, 2003, WB Saunders.

Gilbert ES, Harmon JS: *Manual of high risk pregnancy and delivery,* ed 2, St. Louis, 1998, Mosby.

Lowdermilk DL, Perry SE, Bobak IM: *Maternity and women's health care,* ed 7, St. Louis, 2000, Mosby.

Matteson PS: *Women's health during the childbearing years,* St. Louis, 2001, Mosby.

Schlef C: *Mosby's maternal-newborn patient teaching guides,* St. Louis, 1999, Mosby.

Thureen PJ et al: *Assessment and care of the well newborn,* Philadelphia, 1999, WB Saunders.

Tucker SM: *Pocket guide to fetal monitoring and assessment,* ed 4, St. Louis, 2000, Mosby.

Pediatric Nursing

Ball JW: *Mosby's pediatric patient teaching guides,* St. Louis, 1998, Mosby.

Betz CL, Sowden L: *Mosby's pediatric nursing reference,* ed 4, St. Louis, 2000, Mosby.

Engel JK: *Pocket guide to pediatric assessment,* ed 4, St. Louis, 2002, Mosby.

Hazinski MF: *Manual of pediatric critical care,* St. Louis, 1999, Mosby.

Langton H: *The child with cancer: family centered nursing care,* Philadelphia, 2000, WB Saunders.

Miller S, Fioravanti J: *Pediatric medications: a handbook for nurses,* St. Louis, 1997, Mosby.

Wong DL, Hess CS: *Wong and Whaley's clinical manual of pediatric nursing,* ed 5, 2000, Mosby.

Wong DL et al: *Wong's essentials of pediatric nursing,* ed 6, St. Louis, 2001, Mosby.

Medical/Surgical Nursing

Barker E: *Neuroscience nursing,* ed 2, St. Louis, 2002, Mosby.

Burden N etal: *Ambulatory surgical nursing,* ed 2, Philadelphia, 2001, WB Saunders.

Carrougher GJ: *Burn care and therapy,* St. Louis, 1998, Mosby.

Chernecky C, Macklin D, Murphy-Ende K: *Real-world nursing survival guide: fluids & electrolytes,* Philadelphia, 2002, WB Saunders.

Chernecky C et al: *Real-world nursing survival guide: ECGs and the heart,* Philadelphia, 2002, WB Saunders.

Clark JF, Queener SF, Karb VB: *Pharmacologic basis of nursing practice,* ed 6, St. Louis, 2000, Mosby.

Conover MB: *Pocket guide to electrocardiography,* ed 4, St. Louis, 1998, Mosby.

Darovic GO: *Hemodynamic monitoring: invasive and noninvasive clinical applications,* ed 3, Philadelphia, 2002, WB Saunders.

Ebersole PE, Hess P: *Geriatric nursing and healthy aging,* St. Louis, 2001, Mosby.

Edelman CL, Mandle CL: *Health promotion throughout the lifespan,* ed 5, St. Louis, 2002, Mosby.

Emergency Nurses Association; *Sheehy's emergency nursing: principles and practice,* ed 4, St. Louis, 1998, Mosby.

Gahart BL, Nazareno AR: *Intravenous medications 2002: a handbook for nurses and allied health professionals,* St. Louis, 2002, Mosby.

Gutierrez K, Peterson PG: *Real-world nursing survival guide: pathophysiology,* Philadelphia, 2002, WB Saunders.

Heitz UE, Horne MM: *Pocket guide to fluid, electrolyte, and acid-base balance,* ed 4, St. Louis, 2001. Mosby.

Jarvis C: *Physical examination and health assessment,* ed 3, Philadelphia, 2000, WB Saunders.

Kinney M et al: *Andreoli's comprehensive cardiac care,* ed 8, St. Louis, 1996, Mosby.

Kirton C, Talotta D, Zwolski K: *HIV/AIDS nursing handbook,* St. Louis, 2001, Mosby.

Langford RW, Thompson JM: *Mosby's handbook of diseases,* ed 2, St. Louis, 2000, Mosby.

Lewis SL et al: *Medical-surgical nursing: assessment and management of clinical problems,* ed 5, St. Louis, 2000, Mosby.

McCaffery M, Pasero C: *Pain: clinical manual,* ed 2, St. Louis, 1999, Mosby.

Meeker MH, Rothrock JC: *Alexander's care of the patient in surgery,* ed 11, St. Louis, 1999, Mosby.

Pagana KD, Pagana TJ: *Mosby's manual of diagnostic and laboratory tests,* ed 2, St. Louis, 2002. Mosby.

Perry AG, Potter PA: *Clinical nursing skills and techniques,* ed 5, St. Louis, 2002, Mosby.

Phipps WJ, Sands JK, Marek JF: *Medical-surgical nursing: concepts and clinical practice,* ed 6, St. Louis, 1999, Mosby.

Potter PA: *Pocket guide to health assessment,* ed 5, St. Louis, 2002, Mosby.

Potter PA, Perry AG: *Fundamentals of nursing,* ed 5, St. Louis, 2001, Mosby.

Seidel HM et al: *Mosby's guide to physical examination,* ed 4, St. Louis, 1999, Mosby.

Skidmore-Roth L: *Mosby's 2002 nursing drug reference,* St. Louis, 2002, Mosby.

Thibodeau GA, Patton KT: *Anatomy & physiology,* ed 4, St. Louis, 1999, Mosby.

Thibodeau GA, Patton KT: *The human body in health and disease,* ed 3, St. Louis, 2002, Mosby.

Thompson JM et al: *Mosby's clinical nursing,* ed 5, St. Louis, 2002, Mosby.

Tucker SM et al: *Patient care standards: collaborative practice planning guides,* ed 7, St. Louis, 2000, Mosby.

Urden LD, Stacy KM: *Priorities in critical care nursing,* ed 3, St. Louis, 2000, Mosby.

Williams SR: *Basic nutrition and diet therapy,* ed 11, St. Louis, 2001, Mosby.

Winningham M, Preusser B: *Critical-thinking in the medical-surgical setting: a case study approach,* ed 2, St. Louis, 2001, Mosby.

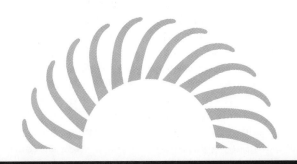

Comprehensive Tests

COMPREHENSIVE TESTS

The questions in the two comprehensive examinations have been developed to reflect the current NCLEX-RN CAT. For you to achieve maximum learning from this experience we have divided each Comprehensive Test into two sections. Part A contains 75 questions, which is the minimum number of questions every candidate must answer. Part B contains 190 questions, which when added to Part A, totals 265 questions, the maximum number of questions for the examination. You should allow about 1 minute per question and complete the total examination (Parts A and B) at one sitting, taking a 15-minute break at the end of Part A. This will reflect the testing session of the present computerized NCLEX-RN.

In Comprehensive Test 1 we recommend that you review the answers and rationales for each part as you complete it. In Comprehensive Test 2 we recommend that you wait until you have completed both parts before checking the answers and rationales. We have made these recommendations so that Test 1 continues and reinforces your immediate learning and Test 2, while reinforcing learning, better reflects the actual situation you will experience when taking the computerized NCLEX-RN.

To help you analyze your mistakes on the comprehensive examinations and to provide a data base for making study plans, worksheets have been included. These sheets are designed to aid you in identifying and recording errors in the way you process information and to help you identify and record gaps in knowledge. Follow the directions that appear on p. 819, using a separate worksheet for each examination. As you review material in class notes or this review book, pay special attention to correcting your most common problems and identifying the topics you need to review. It might be helpful to set priorities; review the most difficult topics first so that you will have time to review them more than once. The worksheets can be used to focus your future study.

Remember, if you study the subject matter, the knowledge you gain will provide you with the ability to answer questions, regardless of the medium used to ask the question, because the required knowledge of the subject matter does not change.

The comprehensive test questions are classified by level of difficulty and by five categories: (1) critical thinking and professional decision making, (2) phases of the nursing process, (3) clinical area, (4) client need, and (5) category of concern. Full descriptions of these categories and their subclassifications are presented in Chapter 1, pp. 2-5.

ANSWERS AND RATIONALES FOR COMPREHENSIVE TEST QUESTIONS

To enhance your study and review:

- First, find the parentheses containing a number and five pairs of letters following the correct answers.
- Use the number to determine the difficulty level of the question. The number 1 signifies that more than 75% of the students answering the question answered it correctly; 2 signifies that between 50% and 74% of the students answering the question answered it correctly; and 3 signifies that between 25% and 49% of the students answering the question answered it correctly.
- The first pair of letters is the abbreviation for the critical thinking/professional decision making abilities tested by the question: (CJ) clinical judgment; (LE) legal and ethical accountability; (MR) managerial responsibilities.
- The second pair of letters is the abbreviation for the step in the nursing process tested by the question: (AS) assessment; (AN) analysis; (PL) planning; (IM) implementation; (EV) evaluation.
- The third pair of letters is the abbreviation for the clinical area tested by the question: (MS) medicine/surgery; (CW) childbearing and women's health; (PE) pediatrics; (MH) mental health/psychiatry.
- The fourth pair of letters is the abbreviation for the area of client need tested by the question: (PA) physiologic and anatomic equilibrium; (TC) therapeutic care; (ED) education and health promotion; (PS) psychosocial and emotional equilibrium.
- The fifth pair of letters is the abbreviation for the specific area of content or, as we call it, the category of concern tested by the question.

The categories of concern used in **medical/ surgical** and **pediatric nursing** include (BI) blood and immunity; (CV) cardiovascular; (DR) drug-related responses; (EH) emotional needs related to health problems; (EN) endocrine; (FE) fluid and electrolyte; (GI) gastrointestinal; (GD) growth and development; (IT) integumentary; (NM) neuromuscular; (RG) reproductive and genitourinary; (RE) respiratory; (SK) skeletal.

The categories of concern used in **childbearing and women's health nursing** include (DR) drug-related responses; (EC) emotional needs related to childbearing and women's health; (HC) healthy childbearing; (HN) high-risk neonate; (HP) high-risk maternal-fetal conditions affecting childbearing; (NN) normal neonate; (RC) reproductive choices; (RP) reproductive problems; (WH) women's health.

The categories of concern used in **mental health/psychiatric nursing** include (AX) anxiety, somatoform, and dissociative disorders; (CS) crisis situations; (DD) dementia, delirium, and other cognitive disorders; (BA) disorders first evident before adulthood; (ED) emotional problems related to physical health and childbearing; (MO) disorders of mood; (PR) disorders of personality; (DR) drug-related responses; (ES) eating and sleep disorders; (PD) personality development; (SD) schizophrenic disorders; (SA) substance abuse; (TR) therapeutic relationships.

USING YOUR ANALYSIS OF THE QUESTIONS TO DEVELOP A FOCUS FOR STUDY

The question analysis gives you an opportunity to review the questions on the Comprehensive Test that you answered incorrectly. For each question on the Comprehensive Test, this book tells you why the correct answer is correct and why each of the other options is incorrect. The rationale for the correct answer includes in parentheses the specific areas critical thinking/professional decision making, measured by the question; that is, the difficulty level, the type of nursing behavior, clinical area, and client need. Also included is the category of concern for the question. These categories of concern identify the specific content area within the broad clinical area covered by the question; they provide the basis for developing your own personal focus of study.

Use the Focus for Study Worksheets that are included with the answers and rationales for each of the Comprehensive Tests as you look over the list of questions you missed. You will also need to refer to the questions on the Comprehensive Test. By identifying the topic of each question and its category of concern, you can identify those areas in which you missed the greatest number of questions. The category of concern is given in the parentheses following the rationale for the correct answer. This information provides the basis for your focus of study.

The worksheet has seven columns across the top of the page. The first column contains a list of the categories of concern used in this book. The other six columns, entitled pathophysiology (basic science), pharmacology, nutrition, diagnostic studies, physical care, and emotional care, are empty.

To develop a meaningful focus of study, simply follow these directions.

1. In the Comprehensive Test, reread each question you missed.
2. In the Answers and Rationales section, read the correct answer and the rationale for that answer.
3. Read the answer you chose and the reason your answer was incorrect.
4. Identify the category of concern for the question by looking at the last set of two letters in the parentheses following the correct rationale.
5. Find these same two letters in the category of concern column on the worksheet.
6. Now your professional judgment comes into action. Look at the question you missed and decide if the subject matter being questioned best fits under the general heading of pathophysiology (basic science), pharmacology, nutrition, diagnostic studies, physical care, or emotional care.
7. Write the number of this question in the box that intersects both the category of concern column and the general heading row. Make your numbers small so that you can enter the numbers of all applicable questions in the appropriate box. Do this for every question you answered incorrectly.
8. After you complete this process, you will be able to identify the areas of knowledge where you missed the most questions. These gaps, requiring additional study, may be in a topic area, a category of concern, or both. You may want to go over those questions you missed along with the answers and rationales again to be sure you understand why you answered incorrectly and to identify the specific information you need to study.

It is important that you take the time to complete the worksheets carefully. The resulting information will assist you in identifying areas of strength and weakness and help you to use your study time effectively.

The topics that the worksheets demonstrate need further study can be found in the index of most nursing textbooks or in the review section of this book. You can therefore use whatever text or resource material is available to you and with which you are already familiar.

Although the questions in the comprehensive examination reflect the NCLEX-RN in its current computerized assistive testing (CAT) format, you should keep the following in mind. If you review the subject matter, the knowledge you gain will provide you with the ability to answer questions regardless of the medium used to ask the question. Remember, if you know the material, you can handle any question.

You may wish to check out additional review material such as *Mosby's Review Questions for NCLEX-RN* or *Mosby's NCLEX-RN Review of Nursing, an interactive CD-ROM.* If you want additional simulated testing situations check out *Mosby's Assess Test* and our online products *Mosby's NCLEX-RN CAT* and *Mosby's Assess Test Online.*

COMPREHENSIVE TEST 1: PART A

1. To assess the neurovascular status of an extremity casted from the ankle to the thigh the nurse should:
   1. Palpate the femoral artery of the affected leg
   2. Assess the affected leg for a positive Homan's sign
   3. Compress and release the toenails of the affected foot
   4. Instruct the client to flex and extend the knee of the affected leg

2. A client is scheduled for a left modified radical mastectomy. Before the consent form is signed, the nurse should plan to reinforce that this surgery involves removal of:
   1. About one third of the left breast
   2. The mammary tissue of the left breast
   3. The breast, axillary nodes, and pectoral or superior apical nodes
   4. The breast, pectoralis minor and major muscles, and dissection of axillary contents

3. On the first postoperative day after a left modified radical mastectomy it is essential that the nursing care plan include:
   1. Changing the pressure dressing as necessary
   2. Having someone from Reach to Recovery visit the client
   3. Keeping the left arm and shoulder immobile until drainage ceases
   4. Placing the client in a semi-Fowler's position with left arm and hand elevated

4. A client who had stage II breast cancer has received a mastectomy and chemotherapy. She is now scheduled for radiation on an outpatient basis. The nurse should:
   1. Assess the radiated site daily for redness or irritation
   2. Rinse the radiated site once a day with an antibacterial solution
   3. Encourage the client to wear a breast prosthesis between treatments
   4. Instruct the client to apply lotion twice daily to the skin at the radiated site

5. A client's problem with ineffective control of type 1 diabetes is pinpointed as a sudden fall in the blood glucose level followed by rebound hyperglycemia. This is known as:
   1. Diabetic ketoacidosis
   2. Somogyi phenomenon
   3. Diabetic hypoinsulinemia
   4. Hyperosmolar nonketotic coma

6. To avoid lipodystrophy in a client on insulin therapy the nurse should teach the client to:
   1. Exercise regularly
   2. Rotate injection sites
   3. Use the Z-track technique
   4. Avoid massaging the injection site

7. A client with type 1 diabetes mellitus asks, "Why can't I take insulin by mouth? I have a cousin who takes pills." The nurse's response should be based on the fact that:
   1. The cousin does not have true diabetes mellitus
   2. Oral hypoglycemics predispose diabetics to lipodystrophies
   3. Insulin if taken by mouth is destroyed by the gastric juices that are always present
   4. Oral hypoglycemics and insulin are the same, but oral agents are used for mild diabetes

8. The statement by a client with type 2 diabetes mellitus that reveals additional teaching about the ADA diet is needed is:
   1. "I can eat all the dietetic fruit that I want."
   2. "I can have a lettuce salad whenever I want it."
   3. "I know that 50% of my diet should be carbohydrate."
   4. "I need to reduce the amounts of saturated fats in my diet."

9. When reviewing an ADA diet a client with type 2 diabetes mellitus expresses a dislike for sweet potatoes. The nurse teaches the client that a safe equivalent would be:
   1. White bread
   2. A cup of milk
   3. A slice of avocado
   4. Mayonnaise on salad

10. A client recently beginning a regimen of haloperidol (Haldol) is observed pacing and shifting weight from one foot to another. The nurse recognizes that this may indicate:
    1. Akathisia
    2. Parkinsonism
    3. Tardive dyskinesia
    4. Acute dystonic reaction

11. A client continually talks about delusional material. It would be most therapeutic for the nurse to:
    1. Ask the client to explain the delusion
    2. Allow the client to maintain the delusion
    3. Encourage the client to focus on reality issues
    4. Explain to the client why the thoughts are not true

12. An infant is born with a myelomeningocele. When answering the parents' questions the nurse should recognize that this condition is a:
    1. Herniation of brain and meninges through a defect in the base of the skull
    2. Fusion failure of the vertebral arches without herniation of cord or meninges
    3. Saclike cyst of meninges filled with spinal fluid that protrudes through a defect in the spine
    4. Saclike cyst of meninges, containing a portion of spinal cord and fluid, that protrudes through a defect in the spine

13. Immediate nursing care for an infant with a myelomeningocele should include:
    1. Placing the infant prone with the legs adducted
    2. Applying sterile, moist gauze dressings to the sac
    3. Immediately changing the diaper when it is moist
    4. Placing the infant in reverse Trendelenburg position

14. Pitocin augmentation is ordered for a client after a period of ineffective labor contractions. If strong contractions occur lasting 90 seconds or longer, the nurse should:
    1. Stop the infusion and turn the client on her side
    2. Apply a fetal monitor to verify length of contractions
    3. Continue the infusion and notify the client's physician
    4. Continue the infusion but give oxygen to prevent fetal hypoxia

15. A client in labor is 8 cm dilated, has a desire to push, and is becoming increasingly uncomfortable. She requests pain medication. The nurse should:
    1. Help her to take panting breaths
    2. Transfer her to the delivery room
    3. Assist her out of bed to the bathroom
    4. Give meperidine HCl (Demerol) as ordered

16. A newborn receives an intramuscular injection of vitamin K. The purpose of the injection is to:
    1. Maintain normal intestinal flora count
    2. Promote proliferation of intestinal flora
    3. Stimulate vitamin K production in the baby
    4. Provide protection until intestinal flora is established

17. A new mother asks the nurse how to care for her baby's umbilical cord. The nurse should teach the mother to:
    1. Keep the area moist with normal saline
    2. Expect a moderate amount of drainage
    3. Apply a sterile 2 × 2 dressing twice a day
    4. Sponge-bathe the baby until the cord falls off

18. A client complains of nausea, dyspnea, and right upper quadrant pain unrelieved by antacids. The pain occurs most often after eating in fast-food restaurants. The diet that would be most appropriate for this client would be:
    1. Low fat
    2. Low cholesterol
    3. Soft textured and bland
    4. High protein and kilocalories

19. Preoperatively a client is given meperidine (Demerol) and hydroxyzine (Vistaril). The Vistaril is given to:
    1. Inhibit peristalsis
    2. Promote unconsciousness
    3. Limit the development of dysrhythmias
    4. Reduce the amount of needed narcotics

20. After an abdominal cholecystectomy a client has a T-tube attached to a collection device. On the day of surgery at 10:30 PM 300 ml of bile is emptied from the collection bag. At 6:30 AM the next day the bag contains 60 ml of bile. The nurse's intervention should be guided by the knowledge that:
    1. The T-tube may need to be irrigated
    2. The bile is now draining into the duodenum
    3. There may be a mechanical problem with the T-tube
    4. Suction needs to be reestablished in the portable drainage system

21. A 39-year-old divorced man has a history of gambling and unstable employment. He is in legal difficulties for embezzling money from his boss and is required to obtain counseling. During an intake interview at a psychiatric clinic he says, "I have never been paid what I am worth." The problem that would pose the greatest difficulty in assisting this client to develop insight would be his:
    1. Grandiosity related to his abilities
    2. Feelings of boredom and emptiness
    3. Anger toward those in authority positions
    4. Tendency to project responsibility for his difficulties

22. When working with a client who has the diagnosis of borderline personality disorder with antisocial behavior, the nurse would expect the client to be:
    1. Retiring and devious
    2. Engaging and rejecting
    3. Suspicious and withdrawn
    4. Self-destructive and perfectionistic

23. A client is diagnosed with borderline personality disorder with antisocial behavior. A realistic short-term goal would be, the client will:
    1. Explore job possibilities with the nurse
    2. Acknowledge resentment of authority figures
    3. Initiate discussion of feelings of being victimized
    4. Spend 15 minutes twice a day discussing problems with the nurse

24. A client with the diagnosis of borderline personality disorder with antisocial behavior is hospitalized. His history includes problems with his relationship with his ex-wife, children, and employer from whom he has stolen money. He is presently facing criminal charges. Behavior that would indicate that the client is ready for discharge with continued care in a clinic would be:
    1. Expression of feelings of resentment toward his employer
    2. Discussion of plans for each of the possible outcomes of his trial
    3. Expression of remorse over the outcome of his marriage and his relationship with his children
    4. Discussion of his decision to file a grievance against his boss after he is discharged from the hospital

25. An adolescent who is pregnant comes to the clinic at 10 weeks' gestation. The nutrition interview indicates that her dietary intake consists mainly of soft drinks, candy, french fries, and potato chips. This diet is considered inadequate because the:
    1. Caloric content of this diet will make her gain too much weight
    2. Ingredients in soft drinks and candy can be teratogenic in early pregnancy
    3. Nutritional composition of the diet places her at risk for a low birth weight infant
    4. Salt in this diet will contribute to the development of pregnancy-induced hypertension

26. At 34 weeks' gestation the nurse identifies a client's BP as 166/100, her urine is +3 for albumin, and she complains of a mild headache and occasional blurred vision. Her baseline BP was 100/62. The nurse recognizes that this client is exhibiting signs of:
    1. Eclampsia
    2. Mild preeclampsia
    3. Severe preeclampsia
    4. Essential hypertensive disease

27. A client with severe pregnancy-induced hypertension is hospitalized. To ensure her physical safety the nurse should first:
    1. Decrease environmental stimuli
    2. Administer sedatives as ordered
    3. Place her on seizure precautions
    4. Strictly monitor her intake and output

28. The nurse should assist a client with glaucoma to accept the need for treatment of the disease because:
    1. Total blindness is inevitable
    2. Lost vision cannot be restored
    3. Surgery will only temporarily help the problem
    4. There is usually restriction in the use of both eyes

29. Following an amputation, the nurse can help a client prepare the residual limb for a prosthesis by encouraging the client to:
    1. Abduct the residual limb when ambulating
    2. Dangle the residual limb off the bed frequently
    3. Soak the residual limb in warm water twice a day
    4. Periodically press the end of the residual limb against a pillow

30. A client with bronchial asthma has difficulty breathing because of:
    1. A too rapid expulsion of air
    2. Spasms of the bronchi, which trap the air
    3. Hyperventilation due to an anxiety reaction
    4. An increase in the vital capacity of the lungs

31. The physician orders daily sputum specimens to be collected from a client. It is most appropriate for the nurse to collect this specimen from the client:
    1. After activity
    2. Before meals
    3. On awakening
    4. Before a respiratory treatment

32. A client is found to be allergic to dust. The teaching plan for this client should include the fact that:
1. Housework must be done by someone else
2. Damp-dusting the house will help limit dust particles in the air
3. The condition must be accepted because dust cannot be limited
4. The house must be redecorated because the environment must be dust-free

33. Following surgery a client is extubated in the postanesthesia unit. The nurse would know that acute respiratory distress is occurring when the client demonstrates:
1. Restlessness and confusion
2. Anxiety and constricted pupils
3. Decreased pulse and respirations
4. Cyanosis and clubbing of the fingers

34. When assessing a child with croup, the nurse would expect to find:
1. Expiratory stridor, crackles
2. Laryngospasm, barking cough
3. Bronchospasm, whooping cough
4. Productive cough, inspiratory stridor

35. The physician orders magnesium sulfate that is twice the usual adult dose for a client with pregnancy-induced hypertension. The physician insists that it is the desired dose and directs the nurse to administer the medication. The nurse should:
1. Give the dose and observe the client closely
2. Withhold the dose and notify the nursing supervisor
3. Give the dose and document the situation on the chart
4. Administer the usual dose and notify the chief of obstetrics

36. The therapeutic effect of magnesium sulfate for a client with preeclampsia would be demonstrated by:
1. Increased urinary output
2. Increased blood pressure
3. Decreased respiratory rate
4. Decreased uterine irritability

37. A nursing action to be included in the plan of care for a child with acute glomerulonephritis is:
1. Encouraging fluids
2. Checking the pupils
3. Measuring abdominal girth
4. Maintaining seizure precautions

38. A child with acute glomerulonephritis is receiving hydralazine (Apresoline). The nurse evaluates that the drug is effective when assessment reveals that the client has:
1. An increase in energy
2. A decrease in hematuria
3. An increase in urinary output
4. A decrease in baseline blood pressure

39. A child with acute glomerulonephritis requests a snack. The most therapeutic selection of food would be:
1. A banana
2. Applesauce
3. Orange juice
4. Chicken broth

40. An adolescent is admitted to the psychiatric unit with the diagnosis of anorexia nervosa. The nurse recognizes that the primary gain a client with anorexia achieves from this disorder is:
1. Reduction of anxiety via control over food
2. Separation from parents via hospitalization
3. Release from school responsibilities via illness
4. Parental overattentiveness via massive weight loss

41. In addition to being underweight, other physical characteristics of the adolescent with anorexia nervosa would include:
1. Pyrexia
2. Tachycardia
3. Heat intolerance
4. Secondary amenorrhea

42. The initial treatment of an adolescent with anorexia nervosa would most specifically include:
1. Family psychotherapy sessions
2. Separation from family members
3. Correcting electrolyte imbalances
4. Medications to reduce her anxiety

43. During the first trimester a pregnant client complains of frequently feeling nauseated. The nurse should teach that nausea and vomiting may best be reduced by:
1. Eating small but frequent meals
2. Eating a pat of butter before rising
3. Taking small sips of soda bicarbonate mixture when nauseated
4. Drinking large amounts of hot or cold tea until nausea subsides

44. When a client has a history of COPD, the nurse should be aware of complications involving:
1. Kidney function
2. Cardiac function
3. Joint inflammation
4. Peripheral neuropathy

45. The purpose of the water in the water seal chamber of a chest tube drainage system is to:
1. Prevent entrance of air into the pleural cavity
2. Foster removal of chest secretions by capillarity
3. Facilitate emptying bloody drainage from the chest
4. Decrease the danger of sudden change in pressure in the tube

46. Following a resection of a lower lobe of the lung, a client has excessive respiratory secretions. In addition to encouraging the client to cough, independent nursing care should also include:
1. Postural drainage
2. Turning and positioning
3. Administration of an expectorant
4. Percussion and vibration techniques

47. The physician plans a cystectomy and an ileal conduit for a male client with an invasive carcinoma of the bladder. After an ileal conduit is described, the client focuses his concern on the odor being offensive. The best response by the nurse would be:
1. "Tell me more about what you are thinking."
2. "This is a problem, but the surgery is necessary."
3. "There are products available to help limit this problem."
4. "Most people having this surgery have this same concern."

48. According to Piaget's theory of cognitive development, a 6-month-old infant should be demonstrating:
1. Early traces of memory
2. Beginning sense of time
3. Repetitious use of reflexes
4. Beginning of object permanence

49. A client in labor is placed on an internal fetal monitor and should be told that while she is on the monitor she:
1. Should detach the monitor leads when using the toilet
2. May feel free to assume any position that is comfortable for her

3. Must maintain a side-lying position to ensure more accurate monitoring
4. Must maintain a supine position to avoid dislodging the internal electrode

50. It is suspected that a newborn may be developing respiratory distress when the nurse observes:
1. Flaring nares
2. Acrocyanosis
3. Respirations of 48/min
4. Abdominal respirations

51. On the third postpartum day a woman who is breastfeeding complains of tight, swollen breasts. The nurse explains that engorgement of the breasts on the third postpartum day is due largely to:
1. An overabundance of milk
2. Ineffective nursing of the baby
3. Lack of adequate breast support
4. Venous and lymphatic congestion

52. When a client sustains a deep partial-thickness burn because of a severe sunburn, the best first-aid measure to use is:
1. Cool, moist towels
2. Dry, sterile dressings
3. Analgesic sunburn spray
4. Vitamin A and D ointment

53. A person sustains deep partial-thickness burns but refuses to seek medical attention. This person should be advised to go to the hospital or a physician if:
1. Blisters appear
2. Edema and redness occur
3. A low-grade fever develops
4. The urinary output decreases

54. When assessing elderly clients the nurse should be aware that normal aging will usually not affect their:
1. Sense of taste or smell
2. Gastrointestinal motility
3. Muscle or motor strength
4. Ability to handle life's stresses

55. According to Kübler-Ross, individuals with serious health problems would most likely seek other medical opinions during the stage of:
1. Anger
2. Denial
3. Bargaining
4. Depression

56. After surgery a client has a urinary catheter. When planning for the client's safety needs in relation to this device, the nurse should:
    1. Empty the bag every 6 hours
    2. Keep the system closed at all times
    3. Maintain slight tension on the tubing
    4. Attach the bag to the siderail of the bed

57. A transurethral resection of the prostate is performed. After surgery, the client's nursing care should include:
    1. Changing the abdominal dressing
    2. Maintaining patency of the cystostomy tube
    3. Observing for hemorrhage and wound infection
    4. Maintaining patency of a three-way Foley catheter

58. A client is to receive 800 ml of IV fluid every 8 hours. The drop factor of the tubing is 10 gtt/ml. The nurse should set the flow to provide:
    1. 20 gtt/min
    2. 17 gtt/min
    3. 13 gtt/min
    4. 10 gtt/min

59. A client who has been hearing voices is receiving a neuroleptic medication for the first time. The client takes the cup of water and pill and stares at them. The most therapeutic response by the nurse would be:
    1. "You have to take your medicine."
    2. "This is medication that your doctor ordered."
    3. "Is there some reason you don't want to take your medicine?"
    4. "This is medicine that your doctor wants you to have. Drink it."

60. After a therapy session with the psychologist a client tells the nurse that the therapist is uncaring and impersonal. The nurse could best respond:
    1. "Your therapist is really very good."
    2. "Do you think the rest of the staff is caring?"
    3. "The therapist is there to help you; try to cooperate."
    4. "You have strong feelings about your therapy session and your therapist."

61. A client has a kidney transplant. After the client is transferred from the postanesthesia care unit to the intensive care unit, the nurse should monitor the urinary output every:
    1. Hour
    2. Half hour
    3. Two hours
    4. Quarter hour

62. The most important test used to determine if a transplanted kidney is working is:
    1. Renal scan
    2. Serum creatinine
    3. White blood cell count
    4. Twenty-four hour output

63. Three weeks after a kidney transplant a client develops leukopenia. The nurse should be aware that this leukopenia is probably caused by:
    1. Bacterial infection
    2. High creatinine levels
    3. Rejection of the kidney
    4. Antirejection medications

64. A small underdeveloped child has been passing loose, bulky, foul-smelling stools and is diagnosed as having cystic fibrosis. The nurse knows that this child's failure to grow is primarily due to:
    1. Impaired digestion and absorption because of the lack of pancreatic enzymes
    2. Dyspnea and shortness of breath, which cause anorexia and disinterest in food
    3. Increased bowel motility and diarrhea, which lead to inadequate absorption of nutrients
    4. Pulmonary obstruction, which has caused an oxygen deficit and inadequate tissue nourishment

65. A child is diagnosed with cystic fibrosis. The nurse evaluates that the parents understand the dietary regimen for their child when they say they will:
    1. Restrict fluids during mealtimes
    2. Discontinue using salt when cooking
    3. Provide high-calorie foods between meals
    4. Eliminate milk and milk products from the diet

66. A parent of a child with cystic fibrosis expresses concern about the child's frailty and low weight. The nurse's most appropriate reply would be:
    1. "Digestive enzymes will be given to help your child digest food."
    2. "Your child's appetite will improve once respiratory therapy is initiated."
    3. "Your child's coughing and shortness of breath prevent adequate chewing of food."
    4. "Your child can't tolerate unstrained foods yet. I suggest that you return to baby foods for a while."

67. During the first well-baby visit after discharge from the hospital the mother informs the nurse that the baby has difficulty feeding and tires easily. The nurse should be aware that:
    1. Feeding problems are fairly common in newborns
    2. Poor sucking is insignificant in the absence of cyanosis
    3. Poor sucking and swallowing may be early indications of a heart defect
    4. Many babies retain mucus that may interfere with feeding for several days

68. When assessing a child with tetralogy of Fallot the nurse should monitor for:
    1. Clubbing of fingers
    2. Slow, irregular respirations
    3. Subcutaneous hemorrhages
    4. Decreased red blood cell count

69. Buck's extension is often ordered initially for clients with fractures of the femur primarily to:
    1. Prevent soft tissue edema
    2. Reduce the need for cast application
    3. Prevent damage to the surrounding nerves
    4. Reduce muscle spasms around the fracture site

70. A client has a total hip arthroplasty. After surgery the nurse should:
    1. Log roll the client when turning
    2. Elevate the affected limb on a pillow
    3. Keep an abduction pillow between the legs at all times
    4. Place a trochanter roll along the entire extremity

71. The client in a psychiatric unit that needs immediate therapeutic intervention from the nurse would be a:
    1. Fifty-year-old woman who is pacing back and forth across the dayroom and picking fights with other clients
    2. Forty-five-year-old man who sits quietly in the corner of the room watching the movements of other clients
    3. Twenty-five-year-old man who is making sounds and actions like a machine gun in front of the nurse's station
    4. Thirty-three-year-old woman who wanders aimlessly around the unit saying, "I just don't know what to do. I feel so lost."

72. A client with the diagnosis of major depression is tearful and refuses to eat. It would be most therapeutic for the nurse to:

    1. Sit next to the client without speaking
    2. Encourage the client to come for a walk
    3. Provide the client with quiet thinking time
    4. Remove potentially dangerous articles from the client's room

73. A person with a history of alcoholism states, "I have been drinking since last Friday to celebrate my son's graduation from college." This is an example of the defense mechanism of:
    1. Denial
    2. Projection
    3. Identification
    4. Rationalization

74. When evaluating whether the environment is conducive to psychologic safety for a confused client with dementia, the nurse should determine if:
    1. There is passive acceptance
    2. All the client's needs are met
    3. Realistic limits and controls are set
    4. The physical environment is kept in order

75. A client who uses ritualistic behavior taps other clients on the shoulders three times while going through the ritual. The nursing diagnosis that would be most appropriate for this client would be:
    1. Ineffective coping
    2. Impaired adjustment
    3. Disturbed personal identity
    4. Disturbed sensory perception

COMPREHENSIVE TEST 1: PART B

76. Following surgery for a colostomy, the most effective way of helping a client accept the colostomy would be to:
    1. Begin to teach self-care of the colostomy immediately
    2. Provide literature containing factual data about colostomies
    3. Contact a member of a support group to come and speak with the client
    4. Point out the number of important people who have had colostomies

77. Given a choice, the child with autism would usually enjoy playing with a:
    1. Cuddly toy
    2. Large red block
    3. Small yellow block
    4. Playground merry-go-round

78. A client comes to the clinic and is 6 months pregnant. Her blood pressure is 150/86 and she has gained 2.27 kg (5 lbs) in the last 2 weeks. The nurse should:
1. Take the client's temperature and pulse
2. Prepare the client for a vaginal examination
3. Give the client another appointment in 2 weeks
4. Test the client's urine for the presence of albumin

79. The nurse prepares for the possibility of magnesium sulfate toxicity by having at the bedside:
1. Nalline
2. Oxygen
3. Calcium gluconate
4. Suction equipment

80. A client is scheduled for extensive head and neck surgery, and although the physician has explained the surgery, the client is still quite anxious. Nursing intervention should be directed toward:
1. Attempting to discover what is bothering the client
2. Elaborating on what the physician has already told the client
3. Teaching the client to use the suction equipment preoperatively
4. Planning for postoperative communication, because a tracheostomy is likely

81. A client who is recovering from an acute episode of colitis is placed on a high-protein diet. The nurse should teach the client that this diet will primarily:
1. Repair tissues
2. Slow peristalsis
3. Correct the anemia
4. Improve muscle tone

82. Nursing management for a client with an acute episode of bronchial asthma should be directed toward:
1. Curing the condition permanently
2. Raising mucus secretions from the chest
3. Limiting pulmonary secretions by decreasing fluid intake
4. Convincing the client that the condition is emotionally based

83. The nurse administers beclomethasone (Vanceril) by inhalation to a client with asthma. The purpose of this therapy is to:
1. Promote rest and relaxation
2. Diminish respiratory bacteria
3. Stimulate smooth muscle relaxation
4. Reduce inflammatory cell responses

84. At delivery a mother observes a nevus vasculosus on her newborn's midthigh and becomes extremely upset. The nurse can best respond by telling her:
1. "The area will spread and then regress."
2. "This is a superficial area that will fade in a few days."
3. "This mark will not grow or fade, but will be covered by clothes."
4. "Surgical removal will be necessary as soon as the infant is older."

85. When a new mother refuses to look at her baby who has a severe birth defect, the nursing approach that would be most therapeutic would be to:
1. Explain to the family why she needs to be distracted
2. Gently tell her that she should stop blaming herself for the child's handicap
3. Reinforce the explanation of the handicap and allow time for the mother to discuss her fears
4. Wait until she has sufficiently recovered from the stress of delivery before bringing the baby to her again

86. When teaching a class about parenting, the nurse asks the participants what they do when their toddlers have a temper tantrum. The nurse should recognize that one woman understands the basis for temper tantrums when she states she:
1. Ignores and isolates her child until the behavior improves
2. Disciplines her child by restricting a favorite food or activity
3. Allows her child to choose between two reasonable alternatives
4. Partially gives in to her child before the tantrums become excessive

87. If interrupted in the performance of the ritual, a client with an obsessive-compulsive disorder would most likely react with:
1. Anxiety
2. Hostility
3. Withdrawal
4. Aggression

88. When working with clients with psychiatric problems a primary goal is the establishment of a therapeutic nurse-client relationship. The major purpose of this relationship is to:
1. Increase the client's nonverbal communication
2. Provide an outlet for suppressed hostile feelings
3. Assist the client to acquire more effective behavior
4. Provide the client with someone to help make decisions

89. An African-American woman is diagnosed with primary hypertension. She asks, "Is hypertension a disease of black people?" The nurse should respond:
    1. "Black men and women comprise a higher-risk population."
    2. "The highest-risk population is older white men and women."
    3. "The prevalence of hypertension is about equal for women of all races."
    4. "The prevalence of hypertension is higher for black women than for black men."

90. The physician prescribes a 2 gram sodium diet and a diuretic for a client with hypertension. The nurse explains that diuretics reduce blood pressure by:
    1. Promoting vasodilation
    2. Promoting smooth muscle relaxation
    3. Reducing the circulating blood volume
    4. Blocking the sympathetic nervous system

91. Clients receiving diuretics should be encouraged to eat:
    1. Apples
    2. Broccoli
    3. Cherries
    4. Cauliflower

92. A 20-year-old male college student comes to the college health clinic complaining of feeling increasingly anxious, a loss of appetite, and an inability to concentrate. Also, his grades have dropped considerably. An appropriate response by the nurse would be:
    1. "With whom have you shared your feelings of anxiety?"
    2. "What have you identified as the cause of your anxiety?"
    3. "It must be difficult for you; how long has this been going on?"
    4. "Sounds like you're having problems adjusting; let's talk about it."

93. When a client attempts suicide, an immediate short-term goal during this crisis situation would be to:
    1. Strengthen coping skills
    2. Restore psychologic balance
    3. Learn problem-solving techniques
    4. Recognize why suicide was attempted

94. A 3½-year-old child is admitted to the hospital for an appendectomy. To best prepare the child for the hospital experience the nurse should use:
    1. A diagram
    2. A storybook
    3. Puppet play
    4. Medical play

95. The nurse should be aware that a preschooler's concept of death includes the belief that it is:
    1. Not a permanent condition
    2. The result of certain illnesses
    3. Something that happens in the hospital
    4. Something that eventually happens to everyone

96. A client is admitted to the hospital with a diagnosis of chronic renal failure. When assessing this client, the nurse should monitor for the occurrence of:
    1. Pruritus, impotency, and polyuria
    2. Respiratory acidosis, lethargy, and anorexia
    3. Glucose intolerance, hypotension, and anemia
    4. Azotemia, muscular twitching, and paresthesias

97. During her sixth month of pregnancy a woman comes to the prenatal clinic for the first time. As part of the obstetrical workup a complete blood count and a urinalysis are performed. The nurse is aware that further assessment is required if the laboratory findings indicate:
    1. Glucose trace
    2. Specific gravity 1.020
    3. Hemoglobin 10 g/100 ml
    4. White blood cells 9000/mm

98. Two hours after an uneventful labor a client's uterus is 4 fingerbreadths above the umbilicus, the BP is 80/40, and the TPR is 98/100/22. After catheterization the fundus remains firm and 4 fingerbreadths above the umbilicus. The nurse should:
    1. Notify the client's physician immediately
    2. Palpate the client's fundus every two hours
    3. Recheck the client's vital signs again in 30 minutes
    4. Catheterize the client again in 1 hour for a residual urine

99. During labor and delivery a client receives spinal anesthesia. Twenty-four hours after delivery the woman complains of a headache. The nurse recognizes this is a reaction to the anesthesia when the client states:
    1. "My headache improves when I sit up."
    2. "My headache gets better as soon as I walk a while."
    3. "My head hurts worse when I am resting flat in the bed."
    4. "My head hurts worse when I am sitting up feeding the baby."

100. A client has a history of myxedema. When performing a physical assessment the nurse would expect the client's skin to be:
1. Dry and flaky
2. Flushed and dry
3. Warm and moist
4. Smooth and silky

101. After an open reduction and internal fixation of a fractured hip, assessment of the affected leg should include:
1. Condition of the pin and site
2. Mobility of the knee and ankle
3. Pedal pulse and mobility of toes
4. Femoral pulse and body temperature

102. A client with myxedema has surgery. When administering narcotics the nurse should know that:
1. Tolerance to the drug develops more readily
2. Narcotics may interfere with the thyroid hormone
3. Sedation will have a paradoxical effect causing hyperactivity
4. One-third to one-half the usual dose of the narcotic should be prescribed

103. When caring for a child with spasmodic croup, the assessment that requires immediate nursing intervention is the:
1. Irritability
2. Hoarseness
3. Barking cough
4. Rapid respirations

104. When preparing a child with asthma for discharge, the nurse must emphasize to the family that:
1. A cold, dry environment is best for the child
2. Limits should not be placed on the child's behavior
3. When the child is asymptomatic, the health problem is gone
4. Medications must be continued even if the child is asymptomatic

105. Parents of a child with croup ask why their child is receiving humidified oxygen. The nurse should teach the parents that this will:
1. Decrease edema and liquefy secretions
2. Provide a mode for giving inhalant drugs
3. Increase the surface tension of the respiratory tract
4. Provide an environment free of pathogenic organisms

106. The test that would be done immediately to confirm the diagnosis of meningitis in a child is:
1. Blood cultures
2. Lumbar puncture
3. Meningomyelogram
4. Peripheral skin smears

107. When caring for a client following a left pneumonectomy for cancer, the nurse should palpate the client's trachea at least once a day because:
1. The position may indicate mediastinal shift
2. Nodular lesions may demonstrate metastasis
3. Tracheal edema may lead to an obstructed airway
4. The cuff of the endotracheal tube may be overinflated

108. A complete blood count, urinalysis, and x-ray examination of the chest are ordered for a client prior to surgery. The client asks why these tests are done. The nurse's best reply would be:
1. "I don't know; the doctor ordered them."
2. "Don't worry, these tests are strictly routine."
3. "They are done to identify other health risks."
4. "They determine whether it's safe to proceed with surgery."

109. A client is scheduled for an abdominal resection. The first priority of preoperative nursing care should be directed toward:
1. Alleviating the client's anxiety
2. Recording accurate vital signs
3. Maintaining proper nutritional status
4. Teaching and answering all questions

110. An infant is to be discharged after insertion of a ventriculoperitoneal shunt. Discharge planning for the parents should include teaching them to observe for the most common complication of this type of surgery, which is:
1. Violent involuntary muscle contractions
2. Excessive fluid accumulation in the abdomen
3. Eyes with sclerae visible above the irises
4. Fever accompanied by decreased responsiveness

111. When teaching parents to pump the valve of a ventriculoperitoneal shunt, the nurse should include the fact that the primary purpose of this procedure is to:
1. Keep the tubing of the shunt patent
2. Increase absorption of cerebrospinal fluid
3. Drain excessive cerebrospinal fluid rapidly
4. Divert the cerebrospinal fluid from the ventricles

112. When helping a new mother develop her parenting role, the nurse should:
    1. Do things for the baby in the mother's presence
    2. Demonstrate baby bathing and care before discharge
    3. Provide enough time for her and the baby to be together
    4. Find out what she knows about babies and proceed from there

113. A newborn develops a cephalhematoma. The nurse should plan to explain to the mother that:
    1. The swelling may cross a suture line
    2. The soft sac will bulge when the infant cries
    3. It will resolve spontaneously in 3 to 6 weeks
    4. This condition is unusual with vaginal delivery

114. The physician orders famotidine (Pepsid) for a client with dyspepsia. The nurse should teach that this drug acts by:
    1. Lowering the stress level
    2. Neutralizing gastric acidity
    3. Decreasing gastric motor activity
    4. Diminishing gastric secretions in the stomach

115. The nurse should recognize that a chronic loss of a small amount of blood over a long period of time often results in:
    1. Iron depletion
    2. Shock syndrome
    3. Pernicious anemia
    4. Thrombocytopenia

116. A client with severe gastritis vomits a large amount of blood and a lavage is performed. A room temperature irrigating solution is used to produce:
    1. Coagulation of blood
    2. Neutralization of acids
    3. Constriction of blood vessels
    4. Stimulation of the vagus nerve

117. After emergency surgery a client requires a blood transfusion. If an allergic reaction to the transfusion occurs, the nurse's first intervention should be to:
    1. Call the physician immediately
    2. Stop the blood and infuse saline
    3. Slow the rate of the blood transfusion
    4. Relieve the symptoms with an ordered antihistamine

118. Upon entering a room the nurse finds a new mother looking at her newborn who is lying in the bassinet with the eyes wide open. In response to this infant's behavior the nurse:
    1. Turns on the lights in the room
    2. Positions the baby on the abdomen
    3. Begins the baby's physical assessment
    4. Encourages the mother to talk to her baby

119. The postpartum nurse notes that a client is gravida 1 and para 1. Her blood type is B negative and her baby's blood type is O positive. The nurse is aware that the client's plan of care should include:
    1. Obtaining an order for RhoGAM
    2. Observing for ABO incompatibility
    3. Determining the father's blood type
    4. Immediate typing and crossmatching of her blood

120. While changing her baby's diaper a client expresses concern about a small spot of red vaginal discharge on the diaper. The nurse should:
    1. Explain this is a normal finding
    2. Assess for other signs of bleeding
    3. Obtain an order for vaginal cultures
    4. Apply a urine specimen bag to the perineum

121. When assessing a client with hyperthyroidism the nurse would expect:
    1. Constipation, dry skin, and weight gain
    2. Lethargy, weight gain, and forgetfulness
    3. Weight loss, exophthalmos, and restlessness
    4. Weight loss, protruding eyeballs, and lethargy

122. A client with a small nodule of the thyroid gland is to have a subtotal thyroidectomy. The nurse should understand that:
    1. The entire thyroid gland is removed
    2. A small part of the gland is left intact
    3. One parathyroid gland is also removed
    4. A portion of the thyroid and four parathyroids are removed

123. When assessing for the presence of affective behaviors associated with major depression, the nurse should monitor the client for:
    1. Confusion
    2. Indigestion
    3. Forgetfulness
    4. Hopelessness

124. The most therapeutic approach when dealing with a client with a major depression shortly after admission to the hospital would be:
1. Setting up a routine of therapy sessions
2. Introducing the client to one other client
3. Encouraging interaction with others in small groups
4. Employing an attitude of concern that is not intrusive

125. A person who is hospitalized for alcoholism becomes boisterous and belligerent. It would be most appropriate for the nurse to:
1. Place the client in restraints to prevent accidental self-injury
2. Sedate and place the client in a quiet, controlled environment
3. Allow the client to use up excess energy by playing cards and visiting
4. Set firm limits on the client's behavior and enforce adherence to them

126. A client with a history of alcohol abuse says to the nurse, "Drinking is a way out of my depression." The management strategy that would probably be most effective for the client at this stage of therapy would be:
1. A self-help group
2. Psychoanalytic therapy
3. Visits with a religious advisor
4. Talking with an alcoholic friend

127. The nurse explores the possibility of joining Narcotics Anonymous (NA) with a client who has a history of narcotic abuse. This is based on the concept that NA is helpful in treating addictive behavior because:
1. Greater change will take place within the group
2. Group members are supportive of each other's problems
3. Group members share a common background and history
4. Addictive problems are always dealt with more effectively in a group

128. The most important nursing action after a cardiac catheterization would be to:
1. Provide a bed cradle
2. Check for a pulse deficit
3. Elevate the head of the bed
4. Assess the groin for bleeding

129. A client with heart failure is on a drug regimen of lanoxin (Digoxin) and furosemide (Lasix). The client dislikes oranges and bananas. Therefore, the nurse should encourage the intake of:
1. Apples
2. Grapes
3. Apricots
4. Cranberries

130. A hospitalized client comments to the nurse, "Well I guess my sex life is over." The most appropriate response by the nurse would be:
1. "I'm sorry to hear that."
2. "Why do you say that?"
3. "Oh, you have a lot of good years left."
4. "Have you asked your doctor about that?"

131. A hospitalized client hurriedly approaches the nurse saying that it sounds like there is a roaring fire in the bathroom. In reality the roommate has just turned the shower on full force. The term that best describes this experience is:
1. Illusion
2. Delusion
3. Dissociation
4. Hallucination

132. The nurse is aware that newborns acquiring a herpes simplex virus type 2 infection often exhibit deficits in:
1. Visual clarity
2. Renal function
3. Long bone growth
4. Glucose metabolism

133. A newborn weighing 5 pounds 6 ounces is delivered by cesarean delivery and admitted to the newborn nursery. The nurse would assess the respiratory rate as normal if it ranged between:
1. 20 and 40 per minute
2. 30 and 50 per minute
3. 60 and 80 per minute
4. 70 and 90 per minute

134. When assessing a newborn, a finding that indicates a need for follow-up care would be:
1. Babinski reflex is positive
2. Hips are abducted 30 degrees
3. Umbilical cord has three vessels
4. Head circumference is 33 centimeters

135. A client is to be discharged with her newborn, who was just circumcised. The nurse, planning discharge instructions on postcircumcision care, should include telling the mother to:
    1. Apply diapers loosely
    2. Withhold formula for 8 hours
    3. Expect some bleeding for 48 hours
    4. Cleanse the site with alcohol daily

136. A client with the diagnosis of bipolar disorder, manic phase is argumentative, domineering, and exhibitionisitic. This client is found running up and down the hall naked by another client who reports this incident to this nurse. To intervene most effectively in the situation, the nurse should initially:
    1. Assess the client's behavior in a nonthreatening manner
    2. Ask the client the reason for running down the hall naked
    3. Gather several staff members and approach the client together
    4. Contact the client's physician for seclusion and medication orders

137. A 2-year-old child is admitted to the hospital with meningitis. To identify possible increasing intracranial pressure, the nurse should monitor the child for:
    1. Restlessness, anorexia, rapid respirations
    2. Vomiting, seizures, complaints of head pain
    3. Anorexia, irritability, subnormal temperature
    4. Bulging fontanels, decreased blood pressure, elevated temperature

138. A 65-year-old client is admitted to a nursing home with the diagnosis of dementia. When assessing this client's mental status, the question that would best test the ability for abstract thinking would be:
    1. "Can you give me today's complete date?"
    2. "How are a television set and a radio alike?"
    3. "What would you do if you fell and hurt yourself?"
    4. "Can you repeat the following numbers: 8, 3, 7, 1, 5?"

139. An elderly client with dementia is admitted to a nursing home. The client is confused, agitated, and at times unaware of the presence of others. To help this client initially adapt to the unit, the best nursing approach would be to:
    1. Initiate a program of planned interaction
    2. Explain the nature and routines of the unit
    3. Provide for the continuous presence of staff
    4. Explore in depth the reasons for the admission

140. An elderly man with dementia is admitted to a nursing home. His wife appears frail, tired, and angry when she first visits her husband. She remarks to the unit nurse in a sarcastic tone, "Let's see what you can do with him." The nurse's most therapeutic response to this comment would be:
    1. "It must have been very difficult to care for him."
    2. "I don't understand what you mean by that comment."
    3. "We know how to care for clients such as your husband."
    4. "It's too bad you didn't get some help to care for him at home."

141. Because of the involvement of the ocular muscles, a common early symptom of myasthenia gravis that the nurse should assess for is:
    1. Tearing
    2. Blurring
    3. Diplopia
    4. Nystagmus

142. A test that might be performed on a client to help confirm the diagnosis of myasthenia gravis involves the use of the drug:
    1. Prednisolone
    2. Disodium EDTA
    3. Phenytoin (Dilantin)
    4. Edrophonium (Tensilon)

143. A client is receiving neostigmine bromide (Prostigmin) for control of myasthenia gravis. In the middle of the night the nurse finds the client weak, unable to move, and barely breathing. Signs that would identify the problems as being related to neostigmine bromide are:
    1. Distention of the bladder
    2. High-pitched, gurgling bowel sounds
    3. Fine tremor of the fingers and eyelids
    4. Rapid pulse with occasional ectopic beats

144. The family of a client with myasthenia gravis asks the nurse whether the client will be an invalid. Recognizing the individuality of response to myasthenia gravis, the nurse's best response would be:
    1. "Deformities will occur, but people with myasthenia will not become invalids."
    2. "With continuous treatment the progression of the disease can usually be controlled."
    3. "The progression is slow, so people with myasthenia will spend their younger life with few problems."
    4. "There will be periods when bed rest will be necessary and times when fairly normal activity will be possible."

145. The diversional activity that would best meet the nursing objectives for a client with myasthenia gravis during periods of remission would be:
1. Hiking
2. Swimming
3. Sewing classes
4. Watching television

146. A mother whose newborn infant son has a cleft lip and palate asks how to feed her baby, since he cannot suck properly. The nurse demonstrates how feedings are to be given and states:
1. "Since he tires easily, it is best to have him lying in bed while he is being fed."
2. "He should be held in a horizontal position and fed slowly to avoid aspiration."
3. "Give him brief rest periods and frequent burpings during feedings to expel swallowed air."
4. "Try using a soft nipple with an enlarged opening so that he can get the milk through a chewing motion."

147. A client in her fourth month of pregnancy calls the nurse and indicates that her husband just told her he has genital herpes. When teaching about sexual activity, the nurse should include the fact that:
1. It will be necessary to refrain from all sexual contact during pregnancy
2. The use of condoms by her husband during sexual activity will be required
3. Sexual abstinence should be practiced during the last 6 weeks of a pregnancy
4. Meticulous cleaning of the hands and vaginal area after intercourse is essential

148. Early in the ninth month of pregnancy, a client experiences painless vaginal bleeding and is admitted to the hospital. The nursing care plan for this client should include:
1. Administering vitamin K to promote clotting
2. Performing a rectal examination to determine cervical dilation
3. Administering an enema to prevent contamination during delivery
4. Placing her in a semi-Fowler's position to increase cervical pressure

149. A preterm infant is delivered. One of the criteria the nurse should use in assessing gestational age of the infant is:
1. Breast bud size
2. Fingernail length
3. The presence of reflex stability
4. The presence of simian creases

150. The initial nursing action after the birth of a preterm baby with an Apgar score of 8 should be to:
1. Check, clamp, and dress the umbilical cord
2. Assist the physician with resuscitative measures
3. Obtain a footprint and apply an identification band.
4. Quickly dry the baby and place in a controlled, warm environment

151. About 1 hour after birth, the nurse would expect a baby to be:
1. Crying and cranky
2. Hyperresponsive to stimuli
3. Relaxed and sleeping quietly
4. Intensely alert with eyes wide open

152. When caring for clients with atherosclerosis, the nurse should understand that atherosclerosis is:
1. Development of atheromas in the myocardium
2. A mobilization of free fatty acid from adipose tissue
3. Development of fatty deposits within the intima of the arteries
4. A loss of elasticity in and thickening and hardening of the arteries

153. The nurse's initial approach to creating a therapeutic environment for any client should give priority to:
1. Providing for the client's safety
2. Accepting the client's individuality
3. Promoting the client's independence
4. Explaining everything that is being done for the client

154. During the day a nurse puts side rails up on the bed of a 73-year-old client who has had surgery for a fractured hip specifically:
1. As a safety measure because of the client's age
2. Because all clients over 65 years of age should use side rails
3. To be used as handholds and to facilitate the client's mobility in bed
4. Because elderly people are often disoriented for several days after anesthesia

155. A 4½-year-old child is brought to the emergency department with a fractured tibia. The nurse knows that in children of this age the most frequently encountered type of fracture is classified as:
1. Greenstick
2. Transverse
3. Compound
4. Comminuted

156. Based on an understanding of normal preschool behavior during hospitalization, the nurse tells the parents of a $4^1/_2$-year-old child that their child will probably:
    1. Refuse to cooperate with the nurses during their absence
    2. Demonstrate despair if they do not visit at least once a day
    3. Cry when they leave and return but not during their absence
    4. Be unable to relate to children in the playroom if there are other parents present

157. When caring for preschoolers, the nurse should understand that they think of death as:
    1. An end to life
    2. A reversible separation
    3. Something that happens to old people
    4. A persona who takes one away from the family

158. A client is being scheduled for a vacuum aspiration to terminate an unwanted pregnancy. The teaching plan should include telling her that:
    1. It is a lengthy procedure that will cause no pain
    2. Both she and her husband must sign the consent
    3. An elevated temperature of 100.4° F or more should be reported immediately
    4. She will experience a heavy menstrual flow for 1 to 2 weeks following the procedure

159. A client asks for and receives instruction regarding birth control methods. She elects to use a diaphragm along with a spermicide. The nurse is aware that a disadvantage to the use of the diaphragm is:
    1. If used alone it has a failure rate of 50%
    2. It is physically uncomfortable when in place
    3. It can lead to thrombus formation and pulmonary embolus
    4. Its insertion and removal is sometimes found to be objectionable

160. Sputum smears for the acid-fast bacillus (AFB) are positive, and the client is placed in isolation. The nurse should anticipate the need to instruct the family to:
    1. Avoid contact with objects in the room
    2. Limit contact with nonexposed family members
    3. Put on a gown and gloves before going into the room
    4. Wear a high-efficiency particulate respirator when visiting

161. A 2-year-old child who has been on bed rest because of a diagnosis of meningitis is now allowed out of bed. When the nurse suggests going to the playroom, the child, shaking the head vigorously from side to side, states, "No! Won't!" However the child is also trying to climb out of the crib at the same time. The nurse interprets this to mean that the child is:
    1. Attempting to assert independence
    2. Eager to resume normal play activities
    3. Unsure of the difference between yes and no
    4. Confused because of increased intracranial pressure

162. The nurse should explain to the client that sodium restriction is an effective therapeutic tool in the treatment of heart failure because its restriction:
    1. Allows excess tissue fluid to be excreted
    2. Helps to control food intake and thus weight
    3. Aids the weakened heart muscle to contract and improves cardiac output
    4. Helps to prevent the potassium accumulation that occurs when sodium intake is higher

163. When assisting a client to ambulate following repair of a fractured right hip, the nurse should be standing:
    1. Behind the client
    2. In front of the client
    3. On the client's left side
    4. On the client's right side

164. A young preschool boy has been on bed rest since he was admitted to the hospital. However, as he begins to feel better, he becomes interested in playing. Based on his developmental level and activity restriction, the nurse should provide him with:
    1. Television viewing time
    2. Squeaky stuffed animals
    3. Little cars and a shoebox garage
    4. Simple three- or four-piece wooden puzzles

165. A baby is Rh positive and the mother is Rh negative. The baby is to receive an exchange transfusion. The nurse knows that the baby will receive Rh-negative blood because:
    1. It is the same as the mother's blood
    2. It is neutral and will not react with the baby's blood
    3. It eliminates the possibility of a transfusion reaction occurring
    4. Its RBCs will not be destroyed by maternal anti-Rh antibodies

166. An emergency tracheotomy is performed on a child with croup and the child is receiving humidified air via trach collar. When caring for this child, the nurse should suction the tracheotomy routinely and if the child:
    1. Tells the nurse of difficulty in breathing
    2. Becomes restless, diaphoretic, and cyanotic
    3. Has severe substernal retractions and stridor
    4. Becomes restless, pale, or the pulse increases

167. When caring for a client with a spinal cord injury, during the initial postinjury period the initial responsibility of the nurse is to:
    1. Prevent urinary tract infections
    2. Prevent contractures and atrophy
    3. Avoid flexion or hyperextension of the spine
    4. Prepare the client for vocational rehabilitation

168. Three days after birth, a newborn is slightly jaundiced. The nurse knows that this is due primarily to:
    1. Immature liver function
    2. An inability to synthesize bile
    3. The mother's high hemoglobin level
    4. High hemoglobin and low hematocrit levels

169. During phototherapy the nurse should apply eye patches to the newborn's eyes to:
    1. Be sure the eyes are closed
    2. Prevent injury to conjunctiva and retina
    3. Reduce overstimulation from bright lights
    4. Limit excessive rapid eye movements and anxiety

170. When performing a developmental appraisal on a 6-month-old infant, the observation that would be most important to the nurse in light of a diagnosis of hydrocephalus would be:
    1. Head lag
    2. Inability to sit unsupported
    3. Presence of the Babinski reflex
    4. Absence of Moro, tonic neck, and grasp reflexes

171. When assessing an infant with hydrocephalus, the nurse should be especially alert for the signs of increasing intracranial pressure, such as:
    1. Depressed fontanel, bulging eyes, irritability
    2. High shrill cry, decreased skin turgor, elevated fontanels
    3. Dilated scalp veins, depressed and sunken eyeballs, decreased BP
    4. Bulging fontanel, "sunset" eyes, projectile vomiting not associated with feeding

172. In the immediate postoperative period following a gastrectomy, the client's nasogastric tube is draining a light-red liquid. The nurse should expect this drainage for:
    1. 1 to 2 hours
    2. 3 to 4 hours
    3. 10 to 12 hours
    4. 24 to 48 hours

173. Parenteral preparations of potassium are administered slowly and cautiously to prevent:
    1. Acidosis
    2. Cardiac arrest
    3. Psychotic-like reactions
    4. Edema of the extremities

174. Management of the dumping syndrome is best accomplished by planning to maintain the client on a:
    1. Low-residue, bland diet
    2. Fluid intake below 500 ml
    3. Small frequent feeding schedule
    4. Low-protein, high-carbohydrate diet

175. Care of a client on the evening of surgery following a below-the-knee amputation should include:
    1. Applying a binder for support
    2. Elevating the stump on a pillow
    3. Ambulating the client in the room
    4. Assisting the client out of bed to a chair

176. A pregnant client complains of constipation. The nurse should explain that constipation frequently occurs during pregnancy because of:
    1. Changes in the metabolic rate
    2. Pressure of the growing uterus on the anus
    3. The slowing of peristalsis in the gastrointestinal tract
    4. Increased intake of milk as recommended during pregnancy

177. The nurse should be aware that the transitional phase of labor has probably begun when the client:
    1. Complains of pain in the back
    2. Assumes the lithotomy position
    3. Perspires and has a flushed face
    4. States that her pains have lessened

178. Shortly following delivery a client says she feels that she is bleeding. While checking the fundus, the nurse notes a steady trickling of blood from the vagina. The nurse's first action should be to:
    1. Call the physician immediately
    2. Check the client's BP and pulse
    3. Hold the fundus firmly and gently massage it
    4. Take no action, since this is a common occurrence

179. A major objective of nursing care for clients with acute lymphocytic leukemia on chemotherapeutic protocols is to:
1. Check their vital signs every 2 hours
2. Prevent their engaging in physical activity
3. Have them avoid contact with infected persons
4. Reduce unnecessary stimuli in their environment

180. Understanding the side effects of vincristine, the nurse plans a diet for the client receiving vincristine that is:
1. Low in fat with regular fluids
2. High in both roughage and fluids
3. High in iron with decreased fluids
4. Low in residue with increased fluids

181. A client's platelet count is very low. The nurse should monitor the client's urine for the presence of:
1. Casts
2. Leukocytes
3. Erythrocytes
4. Lymphocytes

182. A child with leukemia is to receive irradiation of the spine and skull. The nurse explains that this treatment is used mainly because:
1. Radiation will retard growth of cells in bone marrow of the cranium
2. Radiation will decrease cerebral edema and prevent increased intracranial pressure
3. Leukemic cells invade the nervous system more slowly, but the usual drugs are ineffective in the brain
4. Neoplastic drug therapy without radiation is effective in most cases, but this is a precautionary treatment

183. The father of a child who is dying of cancer asks the nurse if he should tell his 7-year-old son that his sister is dying. The nurse should reply:
1. "A child of his age cannot comprehend the real meaning of death, so don't tell him until the last moment."
2. "Your son probably fears separation most and wants to know that you will care for him, rather than what will happen to his sister."
3. "Why don't you talk this over with your doctor, who probably knows best what is happening in terms of your daughter's prognosis?"
4. "Your son probably doesn't understand death as we do but fears it just the same. He should be told the truth to let him prepare for his sister's possible death."

184. The nurse finds a $4\frac{1}{2}$-year-old hospitalized child crying and shouting at his teddy, "There! You bad boy! Don't be mad at my brother! Go to the hospital!" An understanding of preschooler development leads the nurse to believe that this behavior represents that the child:
1. Thinks the parents love the brother more
2. Is mad at the brother and wishes he were sick
3. Misses the brother and wishes that they could be together
4. Thinks that being sick is related to bad thoughts about the brother

185. Developmentally, a gross motor skill the nurse should expect a 3-year-old child to perform is:
1. Riding alone on a small bicycle
2. Skipping and hopping on alternate feet
3. Standing on one foot for a few seconds
4. Jumping rope by lifting both feet simultaneously

186. Considering the purpose, operation, and complications associated with mechanical ventilators, the nurse should:
1. Regulate PEEP according to the rate and depth of the client's respirations
2. Deflate the cuff on the endotracheal tube for 5 to 10 minutes every 1 to 2 hours
3. Assess the need for suctioning when the high-pressure alarm of the ventilator is activated
4. Adjust the temperature of fluid in the humidification chamber depending on the volume of gas delivered

187. After the chest catheters are attached to a closed drainage system, the nurse should:
1. Check that the fluid in the water seal compartment rises with expiration
2. Ensure the security of the connections from the client to the drainage unit
3. Ensure that there is vigorous bubbling in the wet suction control compartment
4. Empty the drainage container, measure and record the amount, and send a sample for analysis every 24 hours

188. On the birthday of a hospitalized client with schizophrenia, the client's mother brings a gift in a plastic bag and leaves saying, "I'm too busy to visit today." The gift is an unwrapped expensive sweater with the price tags on. The client becomes agitated and tearful. The nurse recognizes this exchange is an example of:
1. Projective behavior
2. Manipulative behavior
3. The mother's rejection
4. A double bind message

189. A client with schizophrenia has been experiencing hallucinations. The nurse should expect that they would be more frequent when:
    1. Trying to rest
    2. Playing sports
    3. Watching television
    4. Interacting with others

190. The nurse determines that a person with schizophrenia, paranoid type, is improving when the client:
    1. Stays away from other clients
    2. Has better organized delusions
    3. Express negative feelings freely
    4. Experiences thoughts that are less disruptive

191. During the first prenatal visit of a woman who is 5 months pregnant the nurse becomes aware that the client has a history of pica. The most appropriate nursing action is to:
    1. Seek a psychological referral for the client
    2. Make sure her diet is nutritionally adequate
    3. Obtain an order for multivitamin supplements
    4. Inform her of the danger this poses to her baby

192. During an 8-month prenatal visit a client complains of discomfort with Braxton Hicks contractions. The nurse should instruct her to:
    1. Lie down until they stop
    2. Time them for at least 1 hour
    3. Walk around until they subside
    4. Take 10 grains of aspirin for the discomfort

193. A client is admitted to the hospital in active labor. After an amniotomy the nurse should expect:
    1. Increased fetal heart rate
    2. Diminished vaginal bleeding
    3. Less discomfort with contractions
    4. Progressive dilation and effacement

194. During the postpartal period the nurse identifies that a client's rubella titer is negative. The nurse should plan to:
    1. Check for allergies to penicillin
    2. Alert the nursing staff in the newborn nursery
    3. Obtain an order for immunization at discharge
    4. Assure the client that she has an active immunity

195. An infant with hydrocephalus has a ventriculoperitoneal (VP) shunt surgically inserted. Nursing care during the first 24 hours involves:
    1. Sedating the infant frequently for pain
    2. Placing the infant in a high-Fowler's position
    3. Positioning the infant on the side that has the shunt
    4. Monitoring the infant for increasing intracranial pressure

196. An elderly individual is hospitalized for weight loss and dehydration because of nutritional deficits. The nurse recognizes that in the elderly:
    1. Daily fluid intake must be markedly increased
    2. Financial resources are usually unrelated to nutritional status
    3. Except for decreased caloric needs, the nutritional needs are unchanged
    4. The individual's diet should be high in carbohydrates and low in proteins

197. Calcium EDTA (edetate calcium disodium) is to be used intravenously as the chelating agent for a child with plumbism (lead poisoning). It is most important for the nurse to recognize that this drug therapy requires that the nurse:
    1. Test the stool for occult blood (Hematest)
    2. Monitor for adequate hydration and urine output
    3. Assess the diet because no "junk food" is allowed
    4. Administer medication at night to reduce the associated pain

198. The nurse explains to a client with arthritis that the prescribed steroid medication should be taken with meals because:
    1. It will decrease gastric irritation
    2. It will serve as a reminder to take the drug
    3. The presence of food will enhance absorption
    4. The medication is ineffective in an acid medium

199. The priority nursing intervention on admission of a primigravida in labor is:
    1. Auscultating the fetal heart
    2. Taking an obstetrical history
    3. Asking the client when she ate last
    4. Ascertaining if the membranes are ruptured

200. A pregnant woman in active labor is placed on an external monitor. The nurse notes that during each contraction the fetal heart decelerates as the contraction peaks. The nurse should:
    1. Notify the physician because there may be head compression
    2. Place the client in a knee-chest position to avoid cord compression
    3. Put the client in a semi-Fowler's position to prevent compression of the vena cava
    4. Continue to observe for return of fetal heart rate to baseline when contraction ends

201. To give effective nursing care to a client with the diagnosis of obsessive-compulsive disorder, the nurse must first recognize that the client:
1. Should be prevented from performing the ritual
2. Needs to realize that the ritual serves no purpose
3. Must immediately be diverted when performing the ritual
4. Does not want to repeat the ritual, but feels compelled to do so

202. A client is admitted for treatment of an obsessive-compulsive disorder that is interfering with activities of daily living. The nurse should anticipate a drug order for:
1. Cogentin (benztropine)
2. Symmetrel (amantadine)
3. Anafranil (clomipramine)
4. Benadryl (diphenhydramine)

203. A client with an obsessive-compulsive disorder performs a specific ritual. The nurse allows the client ample time to perform the ritual because:
1. Without consistency of limit-setting, change will not occur
2. To deny this activity may precipitate increased levels of anxiety
3. This behavior is viewed as a result of anger turned inward on the self
4. Successful performance of independent activities enhances self-esteem

204. A client is admitted with a diagnosis of chronic adrenal insufficiency. Because of this condition, it would be unwise to place this client in a room:
1. With an elderly client who has a CVA
2. With a middle-aged client who has pneumonia
3. Next to a 17-year-old client with a fractured leg
4. That is private and away from the nurses' station

205. A client with adrenal insufficiency complains of weakness and dizziness on arising from bed in the morning. The nurse realizes that this is most probably caused by:
1. A lack of potassium
2. Postural hypertension
3. A hypoglycemic reaction
4. Increased extracellular fluid volume

206. When teaching about a diet appropriate for someone with Addison's disease, the nurse should teach the client to:
1. Add a little extra salt to food
2. Limit intake to 1200 calories
3. Restrict the daily intake of fluids
4. Omit protein foods at each meal

207. When observing a client for cortisone overdose, the nurse should be particularly alert for:
1. Hypoglycemia
2. Severe anorexia
3. Anaphylactic shock
4. Behavioral changes

208. A 12-month-old is admitted with a diagnosis of failure to thrive. The infant's weight is below the third percentile and development is retarded. Based on this assessment, the behaviors that might also support the possibility of parental neglect would include the fact that the child is:
1. Stiff, unpliable, and uncomforted by touch
2. Cuddly, responsive to touch, and wants to be held
3. A poor eater, sleeps soundly, and is easily satisfied
4. Responsive to adults, rarely cries, but shows little interest in the environment

209. The nurse observes that an infant has head control, can roll over, but cannot sit up without support or transfer an object from one hand to another. Based on these facts, the nurse would conclude that the infant is developmentally at age:
1. 2 to 3 months
2. 3 to 4 months
3. 4 to 6 months
4. 6 to 8 months

210. When selecting a toy for a 5-month-old infant, the nurse should avoid giving the infant:
1. Brightly colored mobiles
2. Snap toys, large snap beads
3. Small rattles that the infant can hold
4. Soft, stuffed animals that the infant can hold

211. A somatoform disorder is:
1. A psychosomatic reaction to stress
2. A conscious defense against anxiety
3. A psychologic defense against stress
4. An unconscious means to control conflict

212. During a group therapy session some members accuse a client of intellectualizing to avoid discussing feelings. The client asks if the nurse agrees with the others. The nurse's best response would be:
1. "It seems that way to me, too."
2. "You seem to need my opinion."
3. "I'd rather not give my personal opinion."
4. "What is your perception of my behavior?"

213. A client is admitted to the postanesthesia care unit after an abdominal hysterectomy. The observation that should be reported to the physician immediately is:
1. An apical pulse of 90
2. A decreased urinary output
3. Increased drainage from the nasogastric tube
4. Serosanguinous drainage on the perineal pad

214. Fluid shifts are a great danger to the client with partial- and full-thickness burns. The nurse should initially expect to observe:
1. A rise in blood volume
2. Decreased capillary permeability
3. A loss of sodium and an increase in blood potassium
4. Increased fluid shifts and irreversible shock after 2 hours

215. IV fluid replacement therapy is important for the client with severe burns. An expected intake and output in the first 24 hours would be:
1. Intake, 8000 ml; output, 480 ml
2. Intake, 3000 ml; output, 2400 ml
3. Intake, 6000 ml; output, 1200 ml
4. Intake, 12,000 ml; output, 4500 ml

216. A male client with the diagnosis of bipolar disorder is admitted and placed in a room with another client. The history of the client with the bipolar disorder demonstrates recent periods of hyperactivity and combativeness. Later that evening a commotion is heard, and this client is found beating the other client. Legally:
1. A client who is known to have been combative should have been sedated
2. A client with bipolar disorder who is in contact with reality does not require supervision
3. Knowing that the client was frequently combative, close observation by the nursing staff was indicated
4. The admitting office should not have put a client with a history of combativeness in a two-bedded room

217. While the nurse is talking to a hypermanic client, the client's conversation becomes embarrassingly vulgar. The nurse should respond to the client's behavior by:
1. Tactfully teasing the client about the use of such vulgarity
2. Restricting the client's contact with staff until this symptom passes
3. Asking the client to limit the use of vulgarity while continuing the conversation
4. Discreetly refusing to talk to the client when the client is speaking in this manner

218. When there is only one person to perform cardiopulmonary resuscitation, the ratio of ventilations to cardiac compressions is:
1. 1:5
2. 1:10
3. 2:15
4. 4:15

219. A client with a history of acute myocardial infarction complains about the lack of salt in the food. The nurse should explain that the salt must be limited to:
1. Prevent any rise in blood pressure from the tissue edema
2. Produce a diuretic effect and reduce the circulating blood volume
3. Reduce the amount of edema present, which interferes with the heart action
4. Prevent the further accumulation of fluid and increasing workload of the heart

220. A client has a diagnosis of acute cholecystitis with biliary colic. In addition to pain in the right upper quadrant, the nurse should expect the client to have:
1. Melena and diarrhea
2. Vomiting of coffee-ground emesis
3. An intolerance to foods high in lipids
4. Gnawing pain when the stomach is empty

221. Following a cholecystectomy the client should be assessed for signs of bleeding or hemorrhage. These observations are made because:
1. Prostaglandins are released at the surgical site
2. The inflammatory process interferes with platelet formation
3. Diaphragmatic excursion places pressure on the suture line
4. Blood clotting may be hindered by lack of vitamin K absorption

222. A client has a T-tube in place following a cholecystectomy and a choledochostomy. A T-tube is inserted primarily to:
    1. Drain bile from the cystic duct
    2. Keep the common bile duct patent
    3. Prevent abscess formation at the surgical site
    4. Provide a port for contrast dye in a cholangiogram

223. When caring for a client 8 hours following the surgical creation of a colostomy, the observation that would be considered normal is:
    1. The presence of hyperactive bowel sounds
    2. The absence of drainage from the colostomy
    3. A dusky-colored, edematous-appearing stoma
    4. Bright bloody drainage from the nasogastric tube

224. On admission of a client to the labor and delivery unit the nurse asks the client about her marital status. The client refuses to answer and becomes very agitated, telling the nurse to leave. The nurse should:
    1. Have this information to complete the client's history
    2. Refer the client to a social service organization for help
    3. Question the family about the marital status of the client
    4. Have restricted questions to those relevant to the situation

225. A 5-week-old infant is admitted to the hospital with a tentative diagnosis of congenital heart defect. The infant tires easily and has difficulty breathing and feeding. The best position in which to place this infant would be:
    1. Supine with the knees flexed
    2. Orthopneic with pillows for support
    3. Prone with the head supported by pillows
    4. Side-lying with the head and chest elevated

226. A female client is admitted in a depressed state. The client's family reports that she has been agitated and has had difficulty sleeping. The client frequently tells the nurse, "Soon I will be dead." The nurse repeatedly tells the client this is not true and urges the client to forget about it and to go into the TV room and talk with the other clients. The client becomes more agitated and ultimately has to be sedated. The situation may have been altered if the nurse recalled that:
    1. The client's delusions should be accepted without rebuff or argument
    2. Clients should be given antidepressants before incidents such as this develop
    3. The client's sleeplessness and agitation should have been treated as symptoms
    4. Clients need to be encouraged and often gently pushed into relating to other clients

227. When a client is taking lithium carbonate, it is vital that the nursing staff carefully monitor:
    1. Serum levels
    2. Daily weights
    3. Leukocyte counts
    4. Psychomotor activity

228. Nutritional management is most important for the pregnant woman with cardiac problems. The nurse should advise these clients to eat a balanced diet with:
    1. Moderate fats
    2. Limited protein
    3. Increased sodium
    4. Controlled calories

229. A new father tells the nurse that he is anxious about feeling like a father. The priority in planning to meet the father's needs would be to:
    1. Encourage the father's participation in a fathering class
    2. Provide time for the father to be alone with and get to know the baby
    3. Provide a demonstration on diapering, feeding, and bathing the baby
    4. Provide the opportunity to ask questions after viewing a film about a new baby

230. On a 6-week postpartum visit, a new mother tells the nurse she wants to feed her baby a whole milk (cow's milk) formula after 2 months, because she will be returning to work. The nurse should plan to teach her that whole milk does not meet this infant's nutritional requirements because it is low in:
    1. Fat and calcium
    2. Vitamin C and iron
    3. Thiamin and sodium
    4. Protein and carbohydrates

231. When a client has a transfusion reaction because of incompatible blood, the nurse should assess the client for:
    1. Dyspnea
    2. Cyanosis
    3. Backache
    4. Bradycardia

232. As a result of a transfusion reaction, a client suffers kidney damage. When determining kidney damage, the most significant clinical response that the nurse should assess is:
1. Polyuria
2. Hematuria
3. Decreased urinary output
4. Acute pain over kidney area

233. A client with acute renal failure complains of nausea, pain in the abdomen, diarrhea, and muscular weakness. The nurse notes an irregularity in pulse and signs of pulmonary edema. These are probably manifestations of:
1. Calcium excess
2. Potassium excess
3. Sodium deficiency
4. Calcium deficiency

234. To control uremia in a client with renal failure, the nurse should teach the client to limit the intake of:
1. Fluid
2. Protein
3. Sodium
4. Potassium

235. When caring for a client who is receiving peritoneal dialysis, the nurse should:
1. Position the client from side to side if fluid is not draining properly
2. Notify the physician if there is a deficit of 200 ml in the drainage fluid
3. Maintain the client in a flat, supine position during the entire procedure
4. Remove the cannula at the end of the procedure and apply a dry, sterile dressing

236. Children with special needs have the same needs as other children without any special needs, although their means of satisfying these needs may be limited. These limitations frequently cause:
1. Rejection
2. Frustration
3. Overcompensation
4. Emotional disability

237. A nursing assessment of a client recently admitted to an alcohol-detoxification unit would probably reveal:
1. Lethargy and hypotension
2. Hypotension and agitation
3. Nausea, hypertension, and loss of appetite
4. Hypertension, bradycardia, and hyperactivity

238. After a weight gain of 5 pounds in the last week and a pronounced rise in blood pressure, a client, 38 weeks pregnant, is admitted to the high-risk prenatal unit for control of her symptoms. Appropriate nursing care for this client would include:
1. Administering calcium gluconate
2. Providing a dark, quiet room with minimal stimuli
3. Preparing her for an immediate cesarean delivery
4. Instituting IV therapy to facilitate renal emptying

239. When assessing a client who has been beaten and raped, the emergency department nurse is aware that a potential nursing diagnosis for this client at this time would be:
1. Disturbed thought processes related to fear of the attacker
2. Social isolation related to embarrassment over the sexual attack
3. Ineffective coping related to difficulty assimilating the situation
4. Interrupted family processes related to the husband's feelings about the attack

240. The physician orders oxygen therapy via nasal cannula (nasal prongs) at two L per minute for an elderly client with heart failure. A priority nursing action would be to:
1. Maintain the client on bedrest
2. Investigate if the client has COPD
3. Determine if the client is a mouth breather
4. Obtain the appropriate size cannula for the client

241. The physician orders oropharyngeal suctioning as needed for a client in a coma. The nurse prepares to suction when assessment reveals:
1. Drainage of mucus and saliva from the mouth
2. The presence of a gurgling sound with each breath
3. Development of cyanosis in the nailbeds of the fingers
4. The presence of a dry cough at increasingly frequent intervals

242. When assessing a client with varicose veins, the nurse should expect:
1. Discolored toenails
2. Complaints of leg fatigue
3. Localized heat in the calves
4. Reddened areas on the legs

243. In response to a question about varicose veins, the nurse relates that they tend to develop as a result of:
    1. Repeated venous inflammatory episodes
    2. Increased hydrostatic pressure in the veins
    3. Valves obstructing the flow of blood to the heart
    4. Hereditary weakness in the surrounding leg muscles

244. Clients with AIDS are at special risk for fungal and protozoan infections primarily because of the:
    1. Autoimmune nature of the disease
    2. Destruction of T4 cells by the AIDS virus
    3. High-risk sexual behaviors and practices
    4. Invasion of the vital organs by the AIDS virus

245. A client with the diagnosis of AIDS is receiving pentamidine 300 mg IVPB once daily. While receiving a course of therapy, it is most important that the client be monitored for the common side effect of:
    1. Hypotension
    2. Leukocytosis
    3. Fluid retention
    4. Electrolyte depletion

246. A client with AIDS is to receive aerosolized pentamidine. Before administering this drug the nurse detects a bilateral wheeze on auscultation. At this time it would be best for the nurse to:
    1. Administer medication over at least 20 minutes and auscultate after completion
    2. Instruct the client how to use the aerosol mouthpiece and assist with the treatment
    3. Hold the pentamidine and contact the physician, because a bronchodilator may be indicated
    4. Administer oxygen 15 minutes before the medication and document the client's response to the therapy

247. Ritalin is prescribed for a 7-year-old child for an attention deficit disorder with hyperactivity. When discussing this child's treatment with the parents, the school nurse emphasizes the fact that it would be important for them to:
    1. Tutor their child in the subjects that are troublesome
    2. Monitor the effect of the medication on their child's behavior
    3. Point out to their child that the behavior can be controlled if desired
    4. Avoid imposing too many rules because they would frustrate their child

248. Preoperative teaching for a client who is to have cataract surgery should include the importance of:
    1. Remaining flat for 3 hours
    2. Eating a soft diet for 2 days
    3. Breathing and coughing deeply
    4. Avoiding bending from the waist

249. A client receiving hemodialysis has an external shunt for circulatory access. A nursing diagnosis concerned with a life-threatening complication associated with external cannulas would be:
    1. Risk for infection
    2. Impaired skin integrity
    3. Altered tissue perfusion
    4. Risk for injury, hemorrhage

250. A male client receiving hemodialysis has surgery to create an arteriovenous fistula. Before discharge the nurse discusses care at home with the client and his wife. The nurse recognizes that further teaching is required when the wife says:
    1. "I must touch the shunt several times a day to feel for the bruit."
    2. "I have to take his blood pressure every day in the arm with the fistula."
    3. "He will have to be very careful at night not to lie on the arm with the fistula."
    4. "We really should check the fistula every day for signs of redness and swelling."

251. A pale, listless, and tired 14-month-old child, who has had a poor appetite, is diagnosed with acute nonlymphoid leukemia and admitted to the hospital. In addition to the symptoms reported by the mother, the nurse would expect the child to have:
    1. Oliguria
    2. Hypoblastemia
    3. Inability to swallow
    4. Depressed bone marrow

252. Special nursing care for infants born with a genetic disability should include:
    1. Teaching the infants to nipple-feed
    2. Helping the parents learn about their children
    3. Frequent handling and rocking to keep them from crying
    4. Preventing aspiration of formula by frequently bubbling them

253. To prevent a secondary bladder infection in a client who has just had a suprapubic prostatectomy, the nurse should:
1. Observe for signs of uremia
2. Attach the catheter to suction
3. Clamp off the connecting tubing
4. Change the dressings frequently

254. Following a suprapubic prostatectomy, a client complains of pain in the operative area. The initial response of the nurse should be to:
1. Administer the prescribed analgesic
2. Encourage intake of fluids to dilute urine
3. Inspect the drainage tubing for occlusion
4. Measure and record the vital signs before administering an analgesic

255. When discussing weight loss with an obese individual with Ménière's disease, it would be most therapeutic if the nurse suggests that the client:
1. Limit intake to 900 calories a day
2. Enroll in an exercise class at the local high school
3. Get involved in diversionary activities when there is an urge to eat
4. Keep a diary of all foods eaten each day, making certain to list everything

256. A young child is to receive a liquid iron preparation. The nurse should teach the mother to:
1. Administer this at least an hour before meals
2. Explain that loose stools are common with iron
3. Have the child take the diluted iron preparation through a straw
4. Avoid giving the child orange or other citric juices with the iron preparation

257. When attempting to meet the emotional needs of a 4-year-old child receiving daily injections, the nurse should:
1. Provide the child with a doll and other equipment and observe what happens
2. Allow the child to play with a large needle and syringe and encourage acting out
3. Encourage the child to draw pictures about what is happening and the associated feelings
4. Explain the procedures to the child in simple terms at least one hour before they are scheduled

258. In addition to the usual problems associated with receiving multiple transfusions, the child with anemia has an increased risk of developing:

1. Serum hepatitis
2. Allergic response
3. Pulmonary edema
4. Hemolytic reaction

259. The school nurse should be aware that children with attention deficit problems may be learning disabled. This means that they:
1. Will probably not be self-sufficient as an adult
2. Have intellectual deficits that interfere with learning
3. Experience perceptual difficulties that interfere with learning
4. Are usually performing two grade levels below their age norm

260. The nurse would recognize that a home health aide caring for a paralyzed client understands the teaching about avoiding pressure ulcers when priority is given to:
1. Inspecting the client's skin once a day
2. Applying cream daily to the client's skin
3. Having the client sit on a rubber cushion
4. Applying a hot water bottle to the client's reddened areas

261. The occurrence of a pattern of behavior that uses physical symptoms in response to stress can be reduced if the nurse:
1. Provides client teaching regarding medical care
2. Teaches the family how to decrease stress at home
3. Assists the client in developing new coping mechanisms
4. Decreases anxiety by limiting discussion of problems with the client

262. When assessing the oral cavity of a client with *Pneumocystis carinii* pneumonia, the nurse notes areas of white plaque on the tongue and palate. At this time the nurse should:
1. Instruct the client to use meticulous oral hygiene at least once daily
2. Scrape an area of one of the lesions and send the specimen for a biopsy
3. Document the presence of the lesions, describing their size, location, and color
4. Realize these lesions are almost universally found in clients with AIDS and require no special treatment

263. Three days after surgery for cancer of the colon the client is able to look at the colostomy. The nurse introduces care of the colostomy. The nurse should teach the client to care for the skin around the stoma by:
    1. Applying liberal amounts of Vaseline for 3 inches around the stoma
    2. Rinsing the area with peroxide and then applying fresh gauze bandages
    3. Washing with soap and water and then applying a protective ointment or paste
    4. Pouring saline over the stoma and rubbing vigorously to remove hard fecal matter

264. Before discharge a client with a colostomy questions the nurse about resuming prior activities. The nurse should plan to teach that:
    1. Most sport activities, except for swimming, can be resumed based on overall physical condition
    2. Activities of daily living should be resumed as quickly as possible to avoid depression and further dependency
    3. With counseling and medical guidance, a near normal lifestyle including complete sexual function is possible
    4. After surgery, changes in lifestyles must be made to accommodate the physiological changes caused by the operation

265. After surgical clipping of a cerebral aneurysm, the client develops the syndrome of inappropriate secretion of antidiuretic hormone. Manifestations of excessive levels of antidiuretic hormone (ADH) are:
    1. Increased BUN and hypotension
    2. Hyperkalemia and poor skin turgor
    3. Hyponatremia and decreased urine output
    4. Polyuria and increased specific gravity of urine

COMPREHENSIVE TEST 1: PART A

ANSWERS AND RATIONALES

1. 3 Capillary refill based on the blanch test is an excellent assessment for neurovascular integrity; immediate refill is expected. (2; MR; EV; MS; PA; CV)

  1 Palpation of pulses distal to the injury (popliteal and pedal) would be more appropriate than palpation of the femoral artery.
  2 The pain associated with the Homan's sign indicates thrombophlebitis, not the compromise of blood flow or innervation.
  4 Flexion and extension of the affected knee would be impossible with this cast.

2. 3 These structures are removed when a modified radical mastectomy is performed. (3; MR; PL; CW; PA; WH)

  1 This describes a partial mastectomy.
  2 This describes a simple mastectomy.
  4 This describes a radical mastectomy.

3. 4 This promotes drainage from the operative site via gravity, preventing edema. (2; CJ; PL; CW; PA; EH)

  1 The pressure dressing remains in place for several days to prevent bleeding and accumulation of fluids.
  2 Because of shortened hospital stays Reach to Recovery visits may be made at any time during the hospital stay, but basic physiological needs must be met first.
  3 Nontherapeutic; use of the arm in ADL assists in preventing lymphedema.

4. 1 Radiation is damaging to the skin and may cause it to become sensitive and friable. (2; MR; EV; CW; PA; WH)

  2 A radiation site should be washed only with water.
  3 A prosthesis can irritate delicate, irradiated skin and should be avoided until the irradiated area has healed.
  4 A radiation site should be washed only with water; lotion may contain compounds that alter the direction of x-rays.

5. 2 This is a paradoxical situation in which sudden falls in blood glucose are followed by rebound hyperglycemia; this can result from insulin therapy. (1; CJ; AS; MS; PA; EN)

  1 This is only associated with hyperglycemia; there is no sudden hypoglycemia initially.
  3 An insulin deficiency would result in hyperglycemia and ketoacidosis.
  4 This occurs with hyperglycemia and hyperosmolarity, usually in clients who have non–insulin-dependent diabetes mellitus.

6. 2 Fibrous scar tissue can result from repeated injections; the impurities in insulin are thought to cause this response. (2; MR; PL; MS; ED; EN)

  1 Exercise is unrelated to lipodystrophy; exercise reduces blood sugar, which lowers the insulin requirements.
  3 Insulin should be administered into subcutaneous tissue; Z-track technique is used with an intramuscular injection.
  4 Gentle pressure around the injection site after insulin administration promotes absorption.

7. 3 To be effective, insulin must be administered subcutaneously, where it can be absorbed; gastric juices destroy insulin taken by mouth. (2; CJ; IM; MS; PA; EN)

  1 The other person has noninsulin-dependent diabetes mellitus, also known as type 2 diabetes mellitus.
  2 Oral hypoglycemics are not related to lipodystrophy; repeated injections of insulin cause lipodystrophies.
  4 Oral hypoglycemics are not insulin; they either increase insulin secretion from the islet cells of the pancreas or increase the insulin sensitivity of extrapancreatic tissues.

8. 1 Needs further teaching; dietetic fruit is not sugar free and must be calculated in the exchange diet. (3; MR; EV; MS; ED; EN)

  2 Lettuce is considered a free food in the food exchange diet recommended by the ADA.
  3 The American Diabetes Association (ADA) suggests that the caloric intake should be 50% carbohydrate, 20% protein, and 30% fat.
  4 Saturated fats should be limited to 10% of the fat intake; 90% should be unsaturated fats.

9. **1** In the exchange diet, sweet potatoes are a bread substitute. (3; MR; PL; MS; TC; EN)
   2 Sweet potatoes are a bread exchange, whereas 1 cup of skim or nonfat milk is a milk exchange.
   3 Sweet potatoes are a bread exchange, whereas a slice of avocado is a fat exchange.
   4 Sweet potatoes are a bread exchange, whereas 1 teaspoon of mayonnaise is a fat exchange.

10. **1** Monitor for akathisia (restlessness or desire to keep moving); this can occur within 6 hours of first dose; this side effect is noted with many neuroleptics as well as with clients who take Haldol. (3; LE; EV; MH; PA; DR)
    2 This syndrome resembles Parkinson's disease with the masklike facies, characteristic tremor, and shuffling gait.
    3 This most severe, largely irreversible, extrapyramidal symptom occurs after years of treatment with phenothiazines.
    4 These reactions are characterized by severe, bizarre muscle contractions and would have occurred in the first few days of treatment.

11. **3** Discussing reality-based issues helps decrease delusional and hallucinatory activity by reducing feelings of isolation and competing for sensory awareness. (1; MR; IM; MH; PS; SD)
    1 This would support and reinforce the delusions and tend to validate them; nurse must foster reality.
    2 Same as answer 1.
    4 Inappropriate; judgmental response; this would decrease client's trust and increase anxiety.

12. **4** This is a description of a myelomeningocele, a serious neural tube defect that causes paralysis of the lower extremities. (2; MR; AN; PE; PA; NM)
    1 This is a description of an encephalocele, in which a portion of the brain, not the spinal cord, is involved.
    2 This is a description of a spina bifida occulta; this requires no intervention, since there is no break in the skin or protrusion of any structure.
    3 This is a description of a meningocele; usually not incapacitating, since the spinal cord and nerves are not involved.

13. **2** This is done to prevent drying and breakage of the sac, since any opening greatly increases the risk of infection to the central nervous system. (2; CJ; PL; PE; PA; NM)
    1 The legs are abducted to counteract subluxation, since the child is unable to position legs.
    3 Diapering is contraindicated until the defect is repaired; the diaper may irritate the sac and cause rupture, predisposing to infection.
    4 The baby is generally placed in low Trendelenburg's position to reduce pressure on the affected area.

14. **1** Discontinuing the Pitocin lessens uterine stimulation and decreases intrauterine pressure; continuing the Pitocin could lead to fetal hypoxia, placental separation, or uterine rupture; turning the client on the side increases O_2 perfusion. (2; LE; EV; CW; TC; HC)
    2 Unnecessary; Pitocin would not be administered until client was already on a monitor.
    3 Infusion must be stopped to prevent further stimulation and increasing intrauterine pressure.
    4 Infusion must be stopped to prevent increasing intrauterine pressure; O_2 may be administered.

15. **1** This is the appropriate breathing technique for the transitional phase; it prevents client from pushing too early. (2; MR; IM; CW; PA; HC)
    2 Client is not fully dilated and is not ready to deliver.
    3 This is unsafe; the client is in advanced labor; infant may be delivered in a hazardous area.
    4 Meperidine HCl (Demerol) cannot be used in the late stage of labor; infant would be born with respiratory depression.

16. **4** Normal intestinal flora, which synthesizes vitamin K, is initially absent in the newborn. (1; CJ; AN; CW; PA; NN)
    1 There is no intestinal flora in the newborn; the GI tract is sterile.
    2 Intestinal flora is promoted by the ingestion of formula, not vitamin K.
    3 An injection of vitamin K does not stimulate further production of this vitamin; the bacterial flora of the intestine stimulates the production of vitamin K.

17. 4 This is done instead of immersing the baby in a tub of water, since the moisture will retard drying of the cord and delay its falling off. (2; MR; PL; CW; PA; NN)

1 Drying is desirable because this leads to more rapid falling off of the cord; moisture promotes bacterial growth.

2 Any drainage is indicative of infection; base of cord should be dry.

3 Keeping cord covered delays drying and falling off of cord.

18. 1 The presence of fat in the duodenum stimulates painful contractions of the gallbladder to release bile; fat should therefore be avoided. (3; CJ; AN; MS; PA; GI)

2 Although a low-cholesterol diet will limit stone formation, it will not limit pain.

3 A reduction in spices and bulk will not limit pain; fat intake must be reduced.

4 Although this diet might be desirable as long as the protein is not high in saturated fat, it will not limit pain; a high-calorie diet would not generally be ordered.

19. 4 Vistaril potentiates the CNS-depressant effect of narcotics. (2; CJ; PL; MS; PA; DR)

1 Preoperatively, Vistaril is given to potentiate the effect of the preoperative sedative.

2 Although Vistaril potentiates the sedative effect of narcotics, it does not produce unconsciousness.

3 Vistaril is not used for this purpose.

20. 3 This amount of drainage is inadequate; 1000 ml of bile is expected in 24 hours via this surgically implanted tube; the presence of a mechanical obstruction (tube compression or kinking) should be determined. (3; CJ; EV; MS; PA; GI)

1 Unlikely; this also is not within the purview of nursing.

2 Unlikely; common bile duct edema takes several days to subside.

4 A T tube drains by gravity, not suction.

21. 4 The development of insight is impeded by a client's unwillingness or inability to face his own contribution to a problem. (3; CJ; AN; MH; PS; PR)

1 Grandiosity is often a cover for feelings of inadequacy, which are threatening to the client; feelings usually disappear with insight.

2 These feelings are common in clients with borderline personality disorders; unrelated to development of insight.

3 It is not the anger itself, but how the anger contributes to interpersonal difficulty, that the client must recognize.

22. 2 Clients with borderline personality disorders initially tend to be engaging and establish intense relationships, which they then test for signs of rejection; they tend to make others feel they are not helpful and never could be. (3; CJ; AS; MH; PA; PR)

1 These clients may be manipulative, but they are rarely devious or retiring.

3 These clients have a pronounced intolerance for being alone and are usually quite social.

4 Although clients with this disorder may show some self-destructive behavior, they are not perfectionistic.

23. 4 This goal helps establish a mutual relationship, which individuals with borderline personality disorders have difficulty maintaining on an ongoing basis. (2; MR; AN; MH; TC; PR)

1 Exploration of this topic in a meaningful manner can only occur after an ongoing relationship is established.

2 Difficulty with authority figures often results from their poor impulse control and a tendency to act out rather than discussing problems; establishing a working relationship must precede this goal, which is more long-term.

3 Feeling victimized is a frequent theme in clients with this disorder; however, they rarely have the insight to initiate discussion of these feelings and usually show resistance when the topic is discussed.

24. 2 Since his legal difficulties were a precipitating event for hospitalization, if the client can realistically examine the possible outcomes of the trial, then some benefit has been gained from the therapy. (3; CJ; EV; MH; TC; PR)

1 The client has been freely expressing resentment and victimization by his employer and authority figures; this would not show improvement or insight.

3 The client has been discussing his problems since admission, so this would not indicate the development of insight into his own behavior.

4 This would indicate unrealistic planning and not demonstrate the development of insight into his own behavior.

25. 3 There is no indication of proper nutrition, especially proteins; an adequate caloric intake may also be missing; both factors are necessary for normal birth weight. (2; CJ; EV; CW; PA; HP)

1 The caloric content of these foods is not high if small amounts are consumed; in addition, the weight gain of the client may not be reflective of an adequate weight gain in the developing fetus.
2 There are no data to support this.
4 Salt does not contribute to the development of pregnancy-induced hypertension.

26. 3 Severe pregnancy-induced hypertension (PIH) or preeclampsia develops suddenly with a blood pressure of 160/100 or higher, albumin +3 or more, headache, and blurred vision. (1; CJ; AS; CW; PA; HP)

1 This is characterized by convulsions.
2 In mild PIH or preeclampsia the systolic pressure is 30 mm Hg above baseline and the diastolic is 15 mm Hg above baseline; albumin may be +1 or +2; headaches and blurred vision are not present.
4 The blood pressure is chronically elevated in chronic hypertension; her baseline blood pressure was 100/62.

27. 3 This client can immediately become eclamptic and convulse; seizure precautions are necessary to protect her from injuring herself and the fetus. (2; CJ; PL; CW; TC; HP)

1 This is important, but the client's safety should first be ensured by placing her on seizure precautions.
2 Administering sedatives will help to reduce nervous system irritability; it will not ensure safety if the client convulses.
4 This will be required when the client is placed on magnesium sulfate therapy.

28. 2 Retinal damage caused by the increased intraocular pressure of glaucoma is permanent and is progressive if the disease is not controlled. (2; MR; PL; MS; PA; NM)

1 Blindness may be prevented if treatment is early.
3 Surgery can open up drainage and permanently reduce pressure.
4 One eye may be affected, and there is no restriction in the use of the eyes.

29. 4 The client is usually instructed to do this to toughen the limb for weight bearing. This process is begun by pushing the residual limb against increasingly harder surfaces. (1; MR; IM; MS; PA; NM)

1 Abduction of the residual limb does not maintain normal alignment and should be avoided; it does not prepare the residual limb end for a prosthesis.
2 Dangling the residual limb does not help prepare it for a prosthesis and may impede venous return, which would prolong healing.
3 This would macerate the residual limb and hinder the use of a prosthesis.

30. 2 Asthma involves spasms of the bronchi and bronchioles as well as an increased mucus production. This decreases the size of the lumina, interfering with inhalation and exhalation. (2; CJ; AN; MS; PA; RE)

1 This is not a mechanism involved in asthma, in which there is interference with both inhalation and exhalation.
3 The client cannot hyperventilate because of mucosal edema, bronchoconstriction, and secretions, all of which cause airway obstruction. Emotional stress is only one of many precipitating factors, such as allergens, temperature changes, odors, and chemicals.
4 There will be a decrease in the vital capacity.

31. 3 During sleep, mucus secretions in the respiratory tract move slowly toward the throat. On awakening, increased ciliary motion raises such secretions more vigorously; this facilitates expectoration and the collection of sputum specimens. (1; CJ; PL; MS; PA; RE)

1 Although activity mobilizes secretions, there may not be any secretions present at the time of activity; sputum is most plentiful upon arising.
2 Sputum may leave an unpleasant taste in the mouth, which could interfere with appetite.
4 Sputum would more likely be collected after a respiratory treatment, because this mobilizes secretions due to positive pressure.

32. 2 Although dust cannot be avoided completely, use of a damp cloth helps eliminate the amount of airborne particles that might be inhaled. (2; MR; PL; MS; ED; RE)

1 This is unrealistic.
3 This is untrue; there are ways to limit the amount of airborne particles.
4 Redecorating will not eliminate dust; it is a part of our environment.

33. **1** Inadequate oxygenation of the brain may produce restlessness or behavioral changes. The pulse and respiration rates increase as a compensatory mechanism for hypoxia. (2; CJ; EV; MS; PA; RE)
  2 The pupils dilate with cerebral hypoxia.
  3 The pulse and respiration rates increase with hypoxia.
  4 Clubbing of the fingers, the result of increased vascularization, is an adaptation to prolonged hypoxia.

34. **2** A predominant clinical sign of croup is reactive spasms of the laryngeal muscles, which produces partial respiratory obstruction. The cough is tight, with a barking metallic sound. (2; CJ; AS; PE; PA; RE)
  1 Children with croup experience inspiratory rather than expiratory stridor.
  3 Children with croup experience spasm of the larynx rather than the bronchi; whooping cough (pertussis) is a separate communicable disease.
  4 The cough of croup is tight and nonproductive.

35. **2** To follow the physician's order would result in an act of negligence that could endanger the client; if the dosage is not changed after questioning the physician, the nurse should contact the supervisor. (2; LE; EV; CW; TC; EC)
  1 The dose should be withheld because it could result in respiratory depression and endanger both the woman and the fetus.
  3 The nurse would be at risk for negligence, since giving this medication can endanger the woman and fetus.
  4 The nurse does not have an order for the usual dose and should notify the nursing supervisor before calling the chief of obstetrics.

36. **1** Effective MgSO$_4$ therapy reduces edema, thus leading to increased urinary output. (1; CJ; EV; CW; PA; DR)
  2 The goal of this therapy is to reduce blood pressure.
  3 This is a toxic effect of MgSO$_4$; not an effective response.
  4 Uterine irritability would be monitored if MgSO$_4$ was being given to halt premature labor; this client is receiving MgSO$_4$ for severe pregnancy-induced hypertension.

37. **4** Cerebral edema from hypertension or cerebral ischemia may occur and cause convulsions. (3; CJ; PL; PE; TC; RG)
  1 Normal fluid intake is maintained; forcing fluids may lead to an increase in blood pressure and edema.
  2 Glomerulonephritis will not alter pupillary action.
  3 This is appropriate for nephrosis, in which the child has hypoalbuminemia that causes fluid to shift from plasma to the abdominal cavity.

38. **4** Hydralazine is a vasodilator that acts directly on vascular smooth muscle, reducing blood pressure. (2; CJ; EV; PE; PA; DR)
  1 Hydralazine does not affect energy level.
  2 Hematuria persists for months and is not directly affected by hydralazine.
  3 Hydralazine decreases blood pressure; increased urinary output signifies effectiveness of steroid therapy.

39. **2** Applesauce provides nutrition without large additional amounts of potassium and sodium. (2; CJ; PL; PE; PA; RG)
  1 Bananas contain additional potassium, which is contraindicated.
  3 Orange juice contains additional potassium, which is contraindicated.
  4 Chicken broth is high in sodium, which increases fluid retention.

40. **1** The client controls anxiety by maintaining a childlike body build and by demonstrating a mastery over her food intake. (2; CJ; AN; MH; PS; EA)
  2 Families of anorectic persons are usually fused (very close), so separation from parents would not be a desirable gain.
  3 Anorectic persons generally excel in academic areas and receive attention and praise as the perfect child; they would not gain from having this source of attention removed.
  4 Maintenance of an immature body build, not the resulting overattention of parents, is the primary gain.

41. **4** This occurs because of the endocrine imbalance resulting from starvation; it is thought that severe starvation damages the hypothalamus. (2; CJ; AS; PE; PA; EN)
  1 Many of these clients have lowered body temperature.
  2 These clients have bradycardia.
  3 These clients are cold intolerant.

42. 3 Starvation or poor nutrition can lead to electrolyte imbalances, which are life threatening. (2; CJ; PL; PE; PA; FE)
   1 This will be a later therapy.
   2 This may be done at a later time; it is more important to correct life-threatening electrolyte imbalances.
   4 Same as answer 2.

43. 1 Alteration in hormones during pregnancy may cause a sluggish GI tract; large meals remain in the stomach for long periods, causing nausea and vomiting. (2; MR; IM; CW; ED; HC)
   2 This is not a treatment for nausea; may relieve symptoms of heartburn because digestion of fat is slower and utilization of HCl helps prevent regurgitation.
   3 This is not recommended during pregnancy, since it may cause an electrolyte imbalance.
   4 Ingestion of large amounts of any substance, combined with prolonged emptying of the stomach during pregnancy, may increase nausea; small sips of fluid are recommended.

44. 2 As a result of COPD, there is increased pressure in the pulmonary circulation. The right side of the heart hypertrophies (called cor pulmonale), and right ventricular heart failure may ensue. (2; CJ; AN; MS; PA; RE)
   1 This system is not as closely related to the pulmonary system as the cardiac system is; kidney problems do not usually occur.
   3 The skeletal system is not truly related to the pulmonary system; joint inflammation does not occur.
   4 Peripheral nerves are not as closely related to the pulmonary system as the cardiac system is; peripheral neuropathy does not occur.

45. 1 Atmospheric pressure is greater than the pressure inside the pleural space. If a chest tube were not attached to a drainage system closed by a water seal, air would enter the pleural space and collapse the lung (pneumothorax). (2; CJ; AN; MS; TC; RE)
   2 Capillarity is the tendency of cohesive liquid molecules to rise in a tube; this is not the purpose of water in a chest tube drainage system.
   3 This is the purpose of the drainage collection chamber and suction working together, not the water seal chamber.
   4 The concern is not primarily for pressure within the tube itself but to prevent atmospheric pressure from collapsing the lung.

46. 2 Turning and positioning prevent pooling of secretions in the lung and maximize lung expansion. (3; MR; IM; MS; PA; RE)
   1 This is a dependent nursing function.
   3 Same as answer 1.
   4 Same as answer 1.

47. 1 Focuses on the client and the client's concerns; provides an opportunity for further verbalization of feelings. (2; MR; IM; MS; PS; EH)
   2 Although true, this response could increase anxiety and may cut off communication.
   3 This moves the focus away from the client and minimizes the client's concerns.
   4 Same as answer 3.

48. 4 The concept of object permanence begins to develop around 6 months of age. (3; CJ; AS; PE; ED; GD)
   1 This occurs between 13 and 24 months.
   2 Same as answer 1.
   3 This occurs during the first several months of life.

49. 2 Since electrodes are internally placed (on the fetal scalp, not on the mother's abdomen), position does not affect the monitor. (2; MR; IM; CW; TC; HP)
   1 Constant monitoring provides continuous ongoing assessment of fetal status; there is no reason to detach the leads.
   3 It is not the position, but the internal placement of electrodes on the fetal scalp, that ensures accurate monitoring.
   4 This position can cause hypotension because the gravid uterus will cause decreased venous return and lead to reduced cardiac output.

50. 1 According to the Silverman-Anderson Index for respiratory function, flaring of the nares indicates some respiratory distress. (3; CJ; AS; CW; PA; NH)
   2 Acrocyanosis (blue color of hands and feet) is common in all newborns at birth because of decreased circulation to extremities.
   3 The normal respiratory rate for neonates ranges between 30 and 60; therefore 48 is normal and indicates no distress.
   4 These are normal in the neonate; respiratory function is largely a matter of diaphragmatic contraction; expansion of the rib cage is limited in the neonate.

51. **4** This occurs prior to lactation; it is an exaggeration of venous and lymphatic circulation caused by prolactin. (2; MR; AN; CW; PA; HC)
    1 Engorgement occurs before lactation or milk production.
    2 Effective breastfeeding does not prevent engorgement; a lag between the production of milk and efficiency of the ejection reflex often causes engorgement.
    3 This does not cause engorgement, but good support may relieve some of the discomfort.

52. **1** This will decrease edema, minimize pain, and will not adhere to the skin. (2; CJ; IM; MS; PA; IT)
    2 Dry dressings, when removed, could further damage the burn site.
    3 Although pain is temporarily alleviated, removal of the spray would be necessary prior to medical treatment; removal could cause further injury.
    4 Ointments are contraindicated on burns because they have an oil base.

53. **4** Decreasing urinary output indicates insufficient replacement of fluid lost through the burned area. (2; MR; PL; MS; PA; IT)
    1 This would be expected with deep partial-thickness burns.
    2 Same as answer 1.
    3 Same as answer 1.

54. **4** How people cope with stress remains fairly constant throughout life. (2; CJ; PL; MS; ED; EH)
    1 There are decreases in the senses of taste and smell as people age.
    2 GI motility decreases slightly with aging; sedentary lifestyles and lack of dietary fiber compound the situation.
    3 Motor or muscle strength decreases with aging.

55. **2** Denial includes feelings that the physician has made a mistake and the client seeks additional opinions. (2; CJ; AS; MS; PS; EH)
    1 Anger follows denial; behavior will be hostile and critical; seeking multiple medical opinions is a form of denial.
    3 Bargaining occurs after anger; the client may verbally or secretly promise something in return for wellness or a prolonged life; seeking multiple medical opinions is a form of denial.

    4 Depression occurs after bargaining; the client feels sadness and despair and may be withdrawn; seeking multiple medical opinions is a form of denial.

56. **2** A closed, sterile drainage system reduces the likelihood of introducing microorganisms into the bladder. (2; CJ; PL; MS; PA; RG)
    1 The bag is usually emptied at the end of each shift (usually q8h) or if it becomes full.
    3 Tension on the tubing should be avoided because it could injure the delicate mucous membranes of the urinary tract.
    4 Unsafe; if the side rail were put down abruptly, it could pull out the catheter.

57. **4** Patency promotes bladder decompression, which prevents distention and bleeding; continuous flow of irrigant through the bladder limits clot formation and promotes hemostasis. (2; CJ; IM; MS; PA; RG)
    1 There is no abdominal incision because the resection is performed via the urethra.
    2 Not associated with a transurethral resection of the prostate (TURP); a cystostomy tube is a catheter placed directly into the bladder through a suprapubic incision.
    3 Although hemorrhage could occur, there is no wound to observe because the surgery was performed via the urethra.

58. **2** Multiply the amount to be infused (800) by the drop factor (10) and divide the result by the amount of time in minutes (8 hours × 60 minutes):

    $$\frac{800 \times 10}{8 \times 60} = \frac{8000}{480} = 16.66 = 17 \text{ gtt/min}$$

    (1; CJ; AN; MS; TC; FE)
    1 This would be 3 drops of fluid/minute too much.
    3 This would be 4 drops of fluid/minute too little.
    4 This would be 7 drops of fluid/minute too little.

59. **4** This presents reality and simply states expected behavior. (2; MR; IM; MH; PS; SD)
    1 An authoritarian, not a therapeutic, response; the client does not have to take medication orally.
    2 This does not tell the client what behavior is expected.
    3 This assumes the client does not want to take medication, whereas the client may just not understand what to do.

60. **4** The use of reflection assists client to express feelings, which is the major goal of therapy. (2; MR; AS; MH; PS; TR)
   1 This is a defensive response by the nurse that tends to cut off communication and limit the expression of feelings.
   2 This response avoids discussing the client's expression of feelings.
   3 Same as answer 1.

61. **1** Hourly output is critical when assessing kidney function; decreasing urinary output is a sign of rejection. (2; CJ; AS; MS; TC; RG)
   2 This is too short an interval to assess urinary output; it should be monitored hourly.
   3 This is too long an interval to assess urinary output following kidney transplant; it should be monitored hourly.
   4 Same as answer 2.

62. **2** Serum creatinine concentration, a test of renal function, measures the kidney's ability to excrete metabolic wastes; creatinine, a nitrogenous product of protein breakdown, is elevated in renal insufficiency. (2; CJ; EV; MS; PA; RG)
   1 Although this would be considered, it is not as definitive as serum creatinine.
   3 White blood cell count (WBC) does not measure kidney function; white blood cells are usually depressed because of immunosuppressive therapy to prevent rejection.
   4 Same as answer 1.

63. **4** Immunosuppressives such as azathioprine (Imuran) and cyclosporine (Sandimmune) are given to prevent rejection and depress the WBCs. (2; CJ; AN; MS; PA; BI)
   1 Elevated WBC would be associated with bacterial infection; leukopenia is associated with immunosuppressive therapy.
   2 High creatinine levels do not cause leukopenia; elevated creatinine levels are caused by kidney failure.
   3 Rejection of the kidney does not cause leukopenia; signs of rejection include decreased urine output, elevated serum creatinine, hypertension, and edema.

64. **1** Obstruction of the pancreatic duct and the absence of enzymes (trypsin, amylase, and lipase) to aid digestion and absorption lead to severe wasting of tissues and failure to thrive. (2; CJ; AN; PE; ED; GI)

   2 Despite dyspnea and shortness of breath, these children have voracious appetites; the difficulty lies with poor digestion and malabsorption in the small intestine.
   3 Increased bowel motility and diarrhea are not associated with cystic fibrosis.
   4 The pulmonary disease process leads to localized respiratory dysfunction, not retarded physical growth.

65. **3** The caloric intake should be two to three times the normal intake, since there is such poor absorption in the small intestine. (3; MR; EV; PE; ED; GI)
   1 Fluids are encouraged to liquefy bronchial secretions, which have become thickened as a result of copious amounts of mucus.
   2 Salt is added to the diet to compensate for excessive sodium losses in saliva and perspiration.
   4 Whole milk may not be tolerated because of its high fat content; skim milk or other milk products should be substituted.

66. **1** Because the pancreatic ducts are blocked and fibrotic, oral pancreatic enzymes must be given to make the nutrients digestible and absorbable. (3; MR; IM; PE; PA; GI)
   2 Children with cystic fibrosis have good, even voracious, appetites despite respiratory impairment.
   3 Chewing of food is adequate despite coughing and shortness of breath; undernourishment results from inadequate nutrient absorption.
   4 It is not the consistency of the foods that leads to poor absorption, but the lack of enzymes from the pancreatic duct.

67. **3** Compromised heart functioning in the infant often results in cyanosis and fatigue while sucking and swallowing because of decreased cardiac output. (2; CJ; AN; PE; PA; CV)
   1 Untrue; when a feeding problem persists in a newborn, it is generally an indication of some pathology.
   2 Poor sucking is never insignificant; it may be indicative of many problems, such as CNS involvement or immaturity.
   4 Generally the infants are free from mucus within 24 to 48 hours after birth.

68. **1** Hypoxia leads to poor peripheral circulation; clubbing occurs as a result of tissue hypertrophy and additional capillary development in the fingers. (1; CJ; AS; PE; PA; CV)
  2 The respirations are generally rapid to compensate for O_2 deprivation.
  3 This is not an adaptation of children with tetralogy of Fallot.
  4 These children have polycythemia.

69. **4** Buck's extension traction is used to reduce the fracture, align the bone, and temporarily reduce muscle spasm. (2; CJ; AN; MS; PA; SK)
  1 Edema occurs because of tissue trauma and would not be prevented by Buck's extension.
  2 A fractured hip is repaired via internal fixation; a cast is unnecessary.
  3 Damage has already occurred at the time of trauma and is not prevented by Buck's extension.

70. **4** This ensures abduction of the leg to maintain position of the prosthesis and avoid dislocation. (2; CJ; PL; MS; PA; SK)
  1 This is not necessary as long as abduction of the limb is maintained.
  2 This causes flexion of the hip; it is only done if ordered by the physician.
  3 Rolls at the ankle can cause damage to the peroneal nerve along the external malleolus.

71. **1** This client is demonstrating increased agitation and poses an immediate threat to the safety of other clients; the behavior requires immediate nursing intervention to prevent injury to self or others. (3; CJ; PL; MH; TC; CS)
  2 Although the client may be suspicious, data given do not indicate that this represents a danger to the self or others; controlling the agitated client is the priority.
  3 Although the client is probably hallucinating, there is no immediate threat to the self or others; controlling the agitated client is the priority.
  4 Although anxious, this client does not represent a threat to self or others; controlling the agitated client is the priority.

72. **1** This offers support without putting pressure on client to perform. (1; MR; IM; MH; PS; MO)
  2 Nontherapeutic; client is depressed and does not have the energy to walk; this type of depression is not alleviated by activity.
  3 This limits further assessment and may imply rejection.
  4 Not enough data to support conclusion of possibility of suicide; staying with the client is a more appropriate intervention.

73. **4** Rationalization is an unconscious defense mechanism whereby a person finds logical reasons for behavior or feelings while ignoring the illogical or unacceptable real reasons. (1; CJ; AN; MH; PS; SA)
  1 Denial is an unconscious defense mechanism whereby intolerable situations or events are not acknowledged.
  2 Projection is an unconscious defense mechanism whereby an individual attributes or blames personal inadequacies on others.
  3 Identification is an unconscious defense mechanism whereby an individual assumes the characteristics, traits, posture, and achievements of another person or group.

74. **3** Clients out of control find comfort and security in an environment that provides it, since this reduces the need for their own regulation. (2; CJ; EV; MH; TC; DD)
  1 This could allow dangerous behaviors to occur without interference or interruption, which could be threatening to the client.
  2 No environment can meet all of any client's needs.
  4 Order does not in itself provide for psychologic safety.

75. **1** Ineffective coping is the impairment of a person's adaptive behaviors and problem-solving abilities in meeting life's demands; ritualistic behavior fits under this category as a defining characteristic. (2; CJ; AN; MH; TC; PR)
  2 Not enough information is available to use this nursing diagnosis in this situation.
  3 Same as answer 2.
  4 Same as answer 2.

ANSWERS AND RATIONALES
COMPREHENSIVE TEST 1:
PART B

76. **3** Clients who have radical changes in their body image as a result of surgery are usually best able to relate to someone who has faced the same stress and successfully adapted. (2; MR; IM; MH; PS; EP)
1 Clients cannot learn to do colostomy care until they psychologically accept the presence of the colostomy.
2 This would provide information but do little to aid acceptance.
4 This would do little to aid acceptance.

77. **4** The rhythmic movement of the merry-go-round provides soothing and nonthreatening comfort to the autistic child, who cannot reach out to the environment. (3; CJ; IM; MH; PS; BA)
1 The autistic child rejects cuddling and anything that feels cuddly.
2 The child would prefer a mechanical object over a colored block.
3 Same as answer 2.

78. **4** Albumin in the urine is a sign of pregnancy-induced hypertension, as are an elevated BP and a weight gain of more than 1 kg (2.2 lbs) per week. (3; CJ; AS; CW; PA; HP)
1 BP and weight are more relative; changes in the pulse rate and temperature are not associated with pregnancy-induced hypertension.
2 These signs indicate pregnancy-induced hypertension; treatment of this does not require vaginal examination.
3 The signs indicate that pregnancy-induced hypertension may be present; the client may be seen more frequently than every 2 weeks.

79. **3** The antagonist of magnesium sulfate is calcium gluconate, and it needs to be at the bedside. (2; CJ; PL; CW; TC; DR)
1 This is a narcotic antagonist.
2 This would be ineffective if the action of magnesium is not reversed.
4 This is not related to the toxic effect of magnesium sulfate; it may be necessary if the client convulses.

80. **1** Various aspects of hospitalization and diagnosis could cause the client anxiety. The nurse should determine what disturbs the client most. (2; MR; PL; MH; PS; EP)
2 An anxious client will not be receptive to learning.
3 This may cause the client unnecessary anxiety.
4 A tracheostomy may not be performed, depending on the extent of the surgery and edema.

81. **1** The affected areas of the intestine are in need of repair. Protein is required in the building and repairing of tissues. (3; MR; PL; MS; ED; GI)
2 Increased protein will not significantly affect peristalsis.
3 Anemia may result from chronic bleeding; it usually is corrected, however, with increased iron and normal intake of protein.
4 Protein is given to promote healing; once tissues are repaired, muscle tone may improve.

82. **2** In addition to dilation of bronchi, treatment is aimed at expectoration of mucus. Mucus interferes with gas exchange in the lungs. (2; CJ; PL; MS; PA; RE)
1 This is an unrealistic goal; asthma is a chronic illness.
3 Increased fluid intake helps liquefy secretions.
4 Asthma has a psychogenic factor but this does not imply emotions are the only etiology; there is an interaction between the psyche and the soma.

83. **4** This drug reduces inflammation and the inflammatory response in bronchial walls. (2; CJ; AN; MS; PA; RE)
1 Beclomethasone does not directly promote rest and relaxation.
2 Beclomethasone is not an antibiotic.
3 Beclomethasone does not stimulate smooth muscle relaxation.

84. **1** This is the usual pattern that a nevus vasculosus follows. (2; MR; IM; CW; ED; EC)
2 This is false; a nevus vasculosus involves the dermal and subdermal layers.
3 This is false; a nevus vasculosus grows and fades. Saying it will be covered by clothes gives little reassurance.
4 Surgical removal is not recommended.

85. **3** This approach allows for ventilation of feelings and clarifies explanations that probably were not heard or understood because of anxiety. (3; MR; IM; MH; PS; CS)
    1 This prevents the client from facing the problem, thereby increasing her feelings of loss of control.
    2 This closes off communication by not allowing free expression of grief.
    4 This supports avoidance of the reality of the situation; it does not help the problem.

86. **3** The parent's action gives her child more control by allowing the child to make a decision. It also shows an understanding of what the toddler can and cannot do safely. (3; MR; EV; PE; ED; GD)
    1 Although tantrums as attention-getting devices largely must be ignored, ignoring the child will produce feelings of isolation and insecurity.
    2 Boredom, hunger, and insecurity can lead to additional frustration and anger.
    4 This could lead to the development of more manipulative tactics, since the action brought a degree of success initially.

87. **1** Since the compulsive ritual is used to control anxiety, any attempt to prevent the action would greatly increase the anxiety. (3; CJ; EV; MH; PS; PR)
    2 Underlying hostility is considered to be part of the disorder itself; not a reaction to an interruption of the ritual.
    3 This is not a pattern of behavior associated with this disorder.
    4 This would be possible only if the anxiety reached panic levels and caused the person to express anger overtly.

88. **3** The therapeutic nurse-client relationship provides an opportunity for the client to try out different behaviors in an accepting atmosphere and ultimately to replace pathologic responses with more effective ones. (2; CJ; AN; MH; TC; TR)
    1 Verbal communication, not nonverbal communication, is the objective of the therapeutic relationship.
    2 The nurse, although accepting of the client's hostile feelings, uses the therapeutic relationship to redirect hostile feelings into more acceptable behaviors.
    4 The nurse provides the support and acceptance that encourages clients to make their own decisions.

89. **1** Although all races are affected by hypertension, African-Americans comprise a higher-risk population than Caucasian-Americans; the reason is unknown. (2; CJ; AN; MS; ED; CV)
    2 False statement; blacks of both sexes have a higher prevalence than whites of both sexes.
    3 False statement; black women are more frequently affected by hypertension than white women.
    4 False statement; black men have a higher risk than black women.

90. **3** Diuretics block sodium reabsorption and promote fluid loss, decreasing blood volume and reducing arterial pressure. (1; MR; IM; MS; ED; DR)
    1 Direct relaxation of arteriolar smooth muscle is accomplished by vasodilators, not diuretics.
    2 Vasodilators, not diuretics, act on vascular smooth muscle.
    4 Drugs that act on the nervous system, not diuretics, inhibit sympathetic vasoconstriction.

91. **2** Most diuretics are potassium depleting; broccoli provides 267 mg of potassium per 100 g. (2; CJ; IM; MS; PA; GI)
    1 Apples provide 80 to 110 mg of potassium per 100 g of fruit.
    3 Cherries provide 191 mg of potassium per 100 g of fruit.
    4 Cauliflower provides 206 mg of potassium per 100 g.

92. **3** This action recognizes feelings and attempts to collect more data. (1; MR; AS; MH; PS; TR)
    1 Irrelevant; this will not collect data about the extent of the anxiety.
    2 Anxiety is most often a response to a vague, nonspecific threat; the client would not be able to answer this question.
    4 It is too early to identify the cause of anxiety; crisis intervention with anxious clients requires a more structured approach than "let's talk."

93. **2** The primary goal is to help the person through the immediate crisis and restore a balance so that therapy can be initiated. (2; MR; AN; MH; PS; CS)
    1 Part of the treatment plan after the immediate crisis is controlled.
    3 Part of the long-range treatment plan after the immediate crisis is controlled.
    4 Same as answer 1.

94. 4 This allows the child to manipulate unfamiliar equipment; this action would tend to reduce the stress of hospitalization. (2; MR; IM; PE; ED; GD)
1 This is appropriate for school-age children and adolescents.
2 Storytelling is more appropriate for the school-age child.
3 Although appropriate play for a 3-year-old child, it is somewhat limited because it does not give the child an opportunity to handle unfamiliar hospital equipment.

95. 1 Preschoolers do not have the cognitive ability to understand that death is irreversible. (2; CJ; AN; PE; ED; NM)
2 Preschoolers are unable to make logical connections between cause and effect.
3 If a family member died in the hospital, this might be true; however, this is not a predominant belief.
4 Preschoolers do not have an understanding of the inevitability of death.

96. 4 These adaptations result from excess nitrogenous wastes, altered fluid and electrolyte balance, and altered regulatory functions. (2; CJ; AS; MS; PA; RG)
1 Oliguria occurs because of extensive nephron damage.
2 Metabolic acidosis occurs because of the kidney's inability to excrete hydrogen ions and manufacture bicarbonate.
3 Hypotension does not occur; the blood pressure is normal or elevated as a result of increased total body water.

97. 3 This reading suggests a true anemia rather than pseudoanemia, which occurs because the plasma volume increases more than the red blood cells during pregnancy. (2; CJ; EV; CW; PA; HC)
1 Not unusual during pregnancy; lowered renal threshold for glucose exists during pregnancy.
2 This is within the normal range of 1.010 to 1.030.
4 This is within the normal range of 4800 to 10,000/mm.

98. 1 The increased height of the uterus may result from accumulation of blood in the uterus from internal hemorrhaging; vital signs may be indicative of impending shock. (2; CJ; EV; CW; TC; HP)
2 Client needs immediate medical intervention; she may be hemorrhaging.
3 Same as answer 2.
4 Same as answer 2.

99. 4 A headache as a result of low spinal anesthesia usually occurs 24 to 72 hours after administration; headache worsens when client assumes an upright position. (2; CJ; EV; CW; PA; HC)
1 This type of headache will worsen when the head is elevated.
2 This type of headache will worsen when the client is ambulatory.
3 A headache in response to spinal anesthesia improves when the client is lying flat.

100. 1 This is an alteration in the integumentary system caused by decreased function of sebaceous glands; there is evidence of paucity of thyroid hormones T3 and T4, which control BMR and alter function of almost every body system. (2; CJ; AS; MS; PA; EN)
2 The skin would not be flushed, although dryness occurs in hypothyroidism.
3 Occurs with hyperfunction of the thyroid and an increase in BMR.
4 Same as answer 3.

101. 3 This assesses neural and circulatory integrity distal to the surgical site. (1; CJ; EV; MS; TC; SK)
1 No pin is present because an internal fixation was performed.
2 This assessment may cause flexion of the hip, which is contraindicated.
4 Although body temperature is routinely assessed, the femoral artery is not because it is not involved and is not distal to the surgical site.

102. 4 Because of lowered metabolism, the usual adult dose of narcotic could result in overdose. (3; CJ; PL; MS; PA; EN)
1 Hypothyroidism does not alter tolerance.
2 Narcotics do not affect the thyroid hormone; lowered BMR prolongs time for drug detoxification and elimination.
3 Untrue; narcotics will cause excessive sedation, not hyperactivity.

103. 4 Rapid respirations may be a sign of impending airway obstruction. (2; CJ; AS; PE; PA; RE)

    1 Unless irritability is accompanied by severe restlessness, symptomatic care should be given.

    2 Unless accompanied by signs of respiratory embarrassment, this needs no immediate intervention.

    3 This may sound ominous but it is not a sign of respiratory embarrassment.

104. 4 The bronchodilator and antispasmodic medications must be continued to prevent attacks; it is the medications that are keeping the child asymptomatic. (2; MR; PL; TC; RE)

    1 This is untrue; some environmental moisture is necessary for these children.

    2 Consistent limits should be placed on the child's behavior regardless of the disease; a chronic illness does not remove the need for limit setting.

    3 The child's symptoms are being controlled by medications that are necessary to keep the child asymptomatic.

105. 1 Cool mist helps reduce inflammation of the larynx, trachea, and bronchi; the moisture in the mist helps loosen secretions for easier expectoration. (1; MR; AN; PE; ED; RE)

    2 Inhalant drugs are administered through nebulizers.

    3 The mist has no effect on surface tension of the respiratory tract.

    4 This is not the purpose of humidified oxygen.

106. 2 A culture of CSF obtained would reveal the presence of a causative organism (e.g., pneumococcus, tubercle bacillus, meningococcus, or streptococcus). (2; CJ; AN; PE; PA; NM)

    1 This is not a definitive test, although advisable; occasionally it will prove positive when a CSF culture is negative.

    3 This is used to detect the presence of abnormalities by the injection of a contrast medium into the subarachnoid space; it does not identify the organism.

    4 This would demonstrate the presence of bacteria on the skin, not identify organisms in the cerebrospinal fluid.

107. 1 After a pneumonectomy the mediastinum may shift toward the remaining lung, or the remaining lung could shift toward the empty space, depending on the pressure within the empty space. Either of these shifts would cause the trachea to move from its normal midline position. (The trachea is palpated above the suprasternal notch.) (3; CJ; EV; MS; PA; RE)

    2 Metastatic lesions would not appear rapidly.

    3 Tracheal edema cannot be assessed through palpation; edema is not a concern when the endotracheal tube is in place.

    4 The cuff of the endotracheal tube cannot be assessed through palpation of the trachea.

108. 3 Certain diagnostic tests (e.g., CBC, urinalysis, chest x-ray examination) are done preoperatively to rule out the existence of health problems that could increase the risks involved with surgery. (3; MR; IM; MS; ED; RE)

    1 Lack of knowledge without a statement of plans to obtain the information suggests incompetence on the part of the nurse.

    2 Feelings would not be dispelled by this response; it also blocks further communication.

    4 This is false information; surgery poses a risk despite test results.

109. 1 Anxiety experienced by a preoperative client can be a disruptive force affecting the client's ability to adapt psychologically and physiologically. For other nursing measures to be effective, it must be alleviated. (2; CJ; PL; MS; PS; EH)

    2 Vital signs must be recorded, for they will serve as a baseline in postoperative assessment; however, reduction of anxiety is the first priority.

    3 Diet is limited prior to surgery so residue in the intestines will be decreased.

    4 Learning is hampered by high anxiety levels.

110. 4 These are associated with infection, the greatest postoperative hazard for children with shunts for hydrocephalus. (2; MR; PL; PE; ED; NM)

    1 This may occur as a result of an infected shunt; however, it is not the most common complication.

    2 The peritoneum absorbs cerebrospinal fluid adequately; ascites is not a problem.

    3 These occur with progressively increasing intracranial pressure, usually before shunt insertion; it is considered a sign, not a symptom, of infection.

111. **1** Periodic pumping of the valve ensures the patency of the tubing and allows the fluid to move through. (2; MR; IM; PE; ED; NM)
    2 Pumping the shunt does not affect the absorption of cerebrospinal fluid.
    3 Bleeding results if cerebrospinal fluid is drained too rapidly.
    4 This is the purpose of the shunt itself; pumping the valve only keeps the tubing patent.

112. **3** Parenting can begin only when the baby and mother get to know each other. To promote normal development, the nurse should provide time for parent-child interaction. (2; MR; PL; CW; ED; HC)
    1 This may make the mother feel incompetent and retard her mothering.
    2 Time must be provided for the mother with the baby to return demonstrations and ask questions.
    4 This is ineffective; knowledge does not ensure good mothering. Time with the infant is more important.

113. **3** Cephalhematoma is a collection of blood between the skull bone and its periosteum as the result of trauma. It resolves spontaneously in 3 to 6 weeks. (3; CP; PL; PE; ED; CV)
    1 Caput succedaneum, rather than cephalhematoma, crosses the suture line.
    2 A cephalhematoma is a hard, indurated area that remains immobile even when the infant cries.
    4 This is trauma caused by pressure of the head against the birth canal, which occurs in vaginal delivery.

114. **4** Cimetidine inhibits histamine at H_2 receptor sites in the stomach, inhibiting gastric acid secretion. (1; MR; AN; MS; PA; DR)
    1 Cimetidine does not affect stress levels.
    2 Cimetidine inhibits rather than neutralizes gastric secretion.
    3 Same as answer 2.

115. **1** Intermittent or continuous loss of a small amount of blood over extended periods may lead to depleted hemosiderin (stored iron); hypochromic microcytic anemia results. (2; CJ; AS; MS; PA; BI)
    2 Shock results from acute blood loss, which can occur when as little as 10% of the body's total amount of blood is lost.

3 This is caused by lack of the intrinsic factor, not slow or rapid blood loss.
    4 A platelet decrease indicates reduced blood clotting capacity, not blood loss.

116. **3** This removes blood from the stomach and produces vascular constriction, which helps control bleeding by limiting blood flow to the area. (2; CJ; AN; MS; PA; GI)
    1 Lavage does not cause clotting.
    2 Neutralization of acid by water irrigation would take time; antacids could be instilled to alter the pH.
    4 This is not the purpose of lavage for gastric hemorrhage.

117. **2** Prevents additional infusion of allergen to avoid anaphylaxis or kidney damage; the vein can be kept open by running the primary bottle of normal saline. (2; LE; EV; MS; PA; BI)
    1 Stop the blood first; a physician should then be notified.
    3 The allergic reaction would continue and may intensify unless blood is stopped.
    4 This is not an initial action.

118. **4** A quiet, alert state is an optimum time for infant stimulation. (3; CJ; IM; CW; PS; NN)
    1 Bright lights are disturbing to newborns and may impede mother-child interaction.
    2 This position places the baby at risk for SIDS and does not increase the opportunity for stimulation.
    3 A good time for mother-infant interaction; physical examination can be delayed.

119. **1** RhoGAM will prevent sensitization from Rh incompatibility that may arise between Rh-negative mother and Rh-positive infant. (2; CJ; PL; CW; PA; HP)
    2 No ABO incompatibility exists; it could if mother was O positive and baby had type B blood.
    3 Unnecessary; only the mother and baby's Rh factors are relevant at this time.
    4 Because the baby is O no ABO incompatibility exists and neither mother nor child would require a transfusion; this is the mother's first pregnancy, so no RH incompatibility would be present.

120. **1** This is a normal temporary finding related to the influence of maternal hormones. (2; MR; IM; CW; PA; NN)
2 Unnecessary; this is unrelated to problems with bleeding.
3 Unnecessary; this finding is not related to infection.
4 Unnecessary; this finding is unrelated to elimination.

121. **3** These symptoms are associated with hyperthyroidism; weight loss and restlessness are caused by increased metabolic rate, and exophthalmos results from accumulation of fluid behind the eyeball. (1; CJ; AS; MS; PA; EN)
1 These signs are associated with hypothyroidism; frequent loose stools, warm moist skin, and weight loss occur with hyperthyroidism.
2 The client has hyperthyroidism; these are signs of hypothyroidism; hyperactivity, weight loss, and short attention span occur with hyperthyroidism.
4 Although weight loss and protruding eyeballs occur with hyperthyroidism, lethargy occurs with hypothyroidism.

122. **2** The remaining thyroid tissue may provide enough hormone for normal function. (2; CJ; AN; MS; PA; EN)
1 The entire gland is not removed; a small portion is left with the hope that it will provide enough hormone for normal function.
3 The parathyroids are not removed.
4 Same as answer 3.

123. **4** Feelings of hopelessness are symptomatic of depression; the individual feels unable to find any solution to problems and thus feels overwhelmed. (2; CJ; AS; MH; PS; MO)
1 Confusion is not common, since these individuals are in contact with reality.
2 Indigestion is not an affective behavior.
3 Forgetfulness is not common, although the ability to concentrate may be disrupted.

124. **4** This approach allows the client to control the pace of the development of the nurse-client relationship. (3; CJ; PL; MH; TC; MO)
1 It is too early to set a routine of therapy sessions; the first thing to establish is a trusting nurse-client relationship.
2 Depressed clients are unable to move into relationships with other clients.
3 Depressed clients are unable to move into group situations.

125. **2** The client is out of control and is dangerous to the self and others; safety requires sedation and a controlled environment. (2; CJ; IM; MH; TC; SA)
1 Restraining a disturbed, belligerent client can cause severe injury because the restraints will increase anxiety and acting out.
3 The client's attention span would be too short for either of these activities.
4 Any measures directed at verbally or physically correcting the client's behavior would be to no avail.

126. **1** Members of self-help groups, particularly Alcoholics Anonymous, are living with the problem themselves; therefore problem identification and self-responsibility are emphasized and manipulation limited. (1; MR; PL; MH; TC; SA)
2 Long-term therapy tends to increase anxiety until resolution occurs; commitment and duration of therapy render it a poor choice for chemical abusers.
3 This would not be a management strategy; depending on the client's feelings about religion, this could be traumatic.
4 Depends on the friend's drinking status; this could be helpful or harmful; situational variables make this a poor choice.

127. **2** Although members of the group may become impatient with each other's problems at times, the group is usually supportive, members share common goals, and the opportunity is available to test out new patterns of behavior. (2; CJ; PL; MH; TC; SA)
1 This statement is too universal; the rate and amount of change are individually based variables.
3 Not true; people with addictive problems come from varied backgrounds.
4 This statement is too universal; although many clients function well in a group, some clients cannot.

128. **4** Most complications following cardiac catheterization involve the puncture site; included are localized hemorrhage and hematomas, as well as thrombosis of the femoral artery. (1; CJ; EV; MS; TC; CV)
    1 This is not necessary following cardiac catheterization.
    2 This is important but secondary to assessment of the femoral puncture site.
    3 The client should remain supine to avoid postural hypotension and disturbance of the insertion site.

129. **3** Lasix is calcium and potassium depleting; apricots have more than 440 mg of potassium per 100 g. (2; MR; IM; MS; ED; FE)
    1 Apples have about 80 to 110 mg of potassium per 100 g.
    2 Grapes have only about 80 to 160 mg of potassium per 100 g, depending on the variety.
    4 Cranberries have only about 65 mg of potassium per 100 g.

130. **2** This explores the meaning of the statement and allows further expression of concern. (2; MR; AS; MH; PS; CS)
    1 This does not allow explanation of feelings and cuts off communication.
    3 Lacks both empathy and understanding; this also cuts off communication.
    4 Shirks responsibility; the client may be embarrassed to ask the physician and needs the nurse to act as facilitator in initiating the communication.

131. **1** The client misperceived the running shower for a roaring fire; an illusion is a misperception of an actual stimulus. (2; CJ; AN; MH; PS; CS)
    2 A delusion is a fixed false belief that is unrelated to a stimulus.
    3 The situation does not demonstrate any dissociation, since there is no disturbance in integrative functions of the client.
    4 A hallucination is a false perception without any actual stimulus.

132. **1** These infants may have retinal dysplasia. (2; CJ; AN; CW; PA; HN)
    2 This does not affect renal function.
    3 This does not affect long bone growth.
    4 This does not affect glucose metabolism.

133. **2** This is a normal respiratory rate for a newborn. (1; CJ; AS; CW; PA; NN)
    1 Too slow; normal rate is 30 to 50.
    3 Too fast; normal rate is 30 to 50.
    4 Same as answer 3.

134. **2** This is limited hip abduction and is indicative of a congenital hip dysplasia. (2; CJ; AS; CW; PA; HN)
    1 This is a normal newborn reflex.
    3 This is a normal finding.
    4 This is a normal measurement for a term newborn.

135. **1** Applying the diaper loosely for 2 or 3 days lessens pressure on the penis. (1; MR; PL; CW; PA; NN)
    2 Baby can be fed as usual; no anesthesia is used in a circumcision.
    3 Bleeding is not expected; baby should be monitored for any signs of hemorrhage.
    4 Contraindicated; this would be painful and irritating to the wound.

136. **1** The nurse cannot rely on another client's observations to make an assessment and nursing diagnosis. (2; CJ; AS; MH; TC; MO)
    2 Ineffective; the client would probably be unable to answer.
    3 Incorrect; the nurse would be intervening without first assessing the client; this could be threatening if the client is not out of control.
    4 Incorrect; the nurse would be intervening without first assessing the client.

137. **2** Since cranial sutures are closed by this age, increased pressure could cause headache; irritation of cerebral tissue would cause seizures, and pressure on vital centers would cause vomiting. (2; CJ; AS; PE; TC; NM)
    1 Pressure on the respiratory center results in a decreased respiratory rate.
    3 The inflammatory process of meningitis would elevate the temperature; the other two symptoms are possible.
    4 Blood pressure would be elevated in the toddler with closed fontanels because of increased intracranial pressure.

138. **2** This forces the client to find a common characteristic of two things, an ability that is the criterion for abstract thinking. (3; CJ; AS; MH; TC; DD)
    1 This tests orientation, not abstract thinking.
    3 This tests judgment, not abstract thinking.
    4 This tests short-term memory, not abstract thinking.

139. 3 The constant presence of staff members will give the client support and provide an opportunity for the staff to distract and continually reassure him. (2; MR; PL; MH; PS; DD)
  1 Although this intervention has value as a general measure, it is not immediate enough to decrease the client's present level of anxiety.
  2 This is a temporary measure, since it is unlikely the client will comprehend or remember explanations.
  4 The client does not have the capacity to explore concerns; in fact it can be counterproductive and anxiety producing.

140. 1 Acknowledgment of the client's behavior will help lower the spouse's anxiety, reduce guilt, and encourage discussion of feelings. (2; MR; IM; MH; PS; DD)
  2 Lack of understanding by the nurse can be interpreted as uncaring and incite the spouse to make more angry remarks.
  3 Pretentious and insensitive remark; this implies the spouse did not know how to care for the client.
  4 Insensitive; this implies poor judgment on the spouse's part.

141. 3 In myasthenia gravis the sensitivity of the end plates at the postsynaptic junction to acetylcholine is reduced, interfering with muscle contraction. Inadequate contraction of the ocular muscles results in double vision (diplopia). (2; CJ; AS; MS; PA; NM)
  1 This is not a symptom of myasthenia gravis.
  2 Same as answer 1.
  4 Nystagmus is a common symptom of multiple sclerosis.

142. 4 Tensilon is an anticholinesterase compound that drastically increases muscle strength when administered to an individual with myasthenia gravis. (2; CJ; AS; MS; PA; DR)
  1 Prednisolone is a steroid; it is not used to diagnose this disease.
  2 Disodium EDTA is a calcium-chelating agent that is not used in the treatment of myasthenia gravis.
  3 Dilantin is an anticonvulsant; it is not used to test for myasthenia.

143. 2 Neostigmine bromide (Prostigmin) is an anticholinergic that increases the peristaltic activity of the intestines. The result is hyperactive bowel sounds. (2; JC; EV; MS; PA; DR)
  1 Bladder distention is not associated with neostigmine.
  3 These are not side effects associated with neostigmine.
  4 Bradycardia and hypotension may occur with neostigmine.

144. 4 The response should be kept as optimistic as possible while still being realistic. (2; MR; IM; MS; ED; NM)
  1 This is false reassurance; the client's status will depend on individual response.
  2 Medication does not affect progression of the disease; it only treats the symptoms.
  3 The individual response varies; this gives false reassurance.

145. 2 Swimming would help keep the muscles supple, without requiring fine motor activity. (2; CJ; AN; MS; ED; NM)
  1 This might prove too rigorous for the client.
  3 Sewing requires fine motor activity and would be difficult for the client.
  4 Sedentary activities are not helpful in maintaining muscle tone.

146. 3 The congenital defect prevents the infant from creating a tight seal with the lips to promote sucking. As a result the infant swallows large amounts of air when feeding. The mother should be taught to provide frequent rest periods and to bubble the infant often to expel the excess air in the stomach. (2; MR; IM; PE; ED; GI)
  1 Infants with cleft lip and palate should be held upright during feedings.
  2 Same as answer 1.
  4 Newborn infants cannot chew.

147. 3 Abstinence 4 to 6 weeks prior to delivery is the best way to avoid contracting the virus and having an outbreak prior to delivery. (3; MR; AN; CW; ED; WH)
  1 Abstinence is necessary only when disease symptoms are present in the partner and during the last 4 to 6 weeks.
  2 Since the herpesvirus is smaller than the pores of a condom, this kind of protection has limited effectiveness.
  4 Washing is not enough to prevent contraction of this virus; contact has already been made.

148. **4** Placing the expectant mother in a semi-Fowler's position forces the heavy uterus to put temporary pressure on the blood vessels at the site of the separating placenta. This controls bleeding to some extent. (2; CJ; PL; CW; TC; HP)
   1 There is no indication that the clotting mechanism is disturbed.
   2 This is contraindicated when placenta previa is suspected; it may further dislodge the placenta.
   3 This is contraindicated in any client admitted with vaginal bleeding.

149. **1** The size of the breast bud is an indication of gestational age. Small, underdeveloped nipples reflect prematurity. (3; CJ; AS; CW; ED; HN)
   2 This is not related to gestational age.
   3 This is not a good indication of gestational age; reflexes may be impaired in full-term infants also.
   4 This is not present in normal newborns; it is a clinical manifestation of Down syndrome.

150. **4** Cold stress produces hypoxia and acidemia. Because of physiologic factors, such as lack of brown fat, the preterm infant is more vulnerable to cool temperatures. (2; CJ; IM; CW; TC; HN)
   1 These are not a priority; keeping the baby warm is more important.
   2 This would only be necessary if the infant had an Apgar of 0 to 3.
   3 Same as answer 1.

151. **4** This is the first period of reactivity. The newborn is alert and awake. (3; CJ; AN; CW; ED; NN)
   1 This is untrue; after the initial cry, the baby will settle down and become quiet and alert.
   2 This occurs after the first sleep.
   3 First sleep usually occurs more than 1 hour after delivery.

152. **3** Atherosclerosis begins with the accumulation of fatty deposits (plaques) within the inner lining (intima) of the arteries, leading to a narrowing of the lumen. Later the plaques enlarge, cause greater occlusion, and harden by deposition of calcium (atheroarteriosclerosis), eventually increasing the work of the heart. (2; CJ; AN; MS; PA; CV)

   1 Atheromas develop within the intima of arteries, not in the cardiac muscle.
   2 Although atheromas or plaques are deposited from circulating fat, mobilization from adipose storage is not a prerequisite.
   4 This is arteriosclerosis.

153. **2** Each person is unique. The nurse should avoid making the client feel dehumanized. (2; CJ; PL; MH; PS; TR)
   1 Although safety is a priority, it is not the initial need.
   3 This would be a later nursing action.
   4 It is important that the client understand what is happening; however, individuality must be considered first.

154. **3** Devices such as side rails can help clients increase their mobility by facilitating movement in bed. Side rails are immovable objects and provide a handhold for leverage when changing positions. (3; CJ; IM; MS; TC; SK)
   1 The need to use side rails for safety must be evaluated for each individual based on the mental and physical status and hospital regulations.
   2 Same as answer 1.
   4 Same as answer 1.

155. **1** Ossification is incomplete in childhood; children's bones can flex to about a 45-degree angle before breaking; when the bone is angulated beyond these 45 degrees, the compressed side bends and the torsion side breaks (greenstick fracture). (2; CJ; AN; PE; ED; SK)
   2 This is usually a complete fracture seen in blunt trauma; occurs in adults where bone ossification is complete.
   3 This is seldom seen, especially in children.
   4 Rarely seen in children; small fragments of bone are broken from the fracture site and lie in surrounding tissue.

156. **3** Preschoolers generally have learned to cope with parents' absence; however, emotions associated with separation are difficult to hide when parents arrive or leave; anger at being left may also account for emotional outburst. (2; MR; EV; PE; ED; EH)
   1 Preschoolers have great social behavior and will probably be most cooperative.
   2 Preschoolers have learned to cope with parents' absence.
   4 They have good social skills with peers even when parents are present.

157. 2 Preschoolers view death only as a separation; they believe the deceased will return to life; this is part of their fantasy world. (2; CJ; AN; PE; ED; EH)
   1 Preschoolers do not understand this; they view death as a separation, or possibly a kind of sleep, and expect the deceased to return or wake up.
   3 The preschooler does not yet have the understanding that older people are more likely to die.
   4 The preschooler believes that the separation was initiated by the deceased, not by another force.

158. 3 The elevated temperature may be indicative of the presence of infection; if so, the abortion should not be done until the infection clears. (2; MR; PL; CW; ED; RC)
   1 The procedure is a short one; there is some pain or discomfort.
   2 Not universally true; the woman's signature is all that is required in most states.
   4 A light menstrual flow is expected for several days.

159. 4 This is a complaint of some women that must be considered. (2; CJ; AN; CW; ED; RC)
   1 Failure rate is 4% to 35% when used alone; effectiveness increases with the use of a spermicide.
   2 There have been no complaints documented.
   3 These can be side effects of oral contraceptives.

160. 4 Tubercle bacilli are transmitted through airborne droplets; therefore, respiratory isolation with an Ultra-Filter mask is necessary. (2; MR; PL; MS; TC; RE)
   1 Transmission occurs through the airborne route, not via fomites.
   2 Contact does not have to be limited as long as isolation precautions are employed.
   3 Transmission occurs through the airborne route; gowns and gloves are unnecessary.

161. 1 Child is exhibiting normal behavior for this developmental level; most toddlers will say "no" as a means of asserting their independence. (1; CJ; EV; PE; ED; GD)

   2 Although the child may be eager to resume normal play activity, the behavior described is related to the child's assertion of independence.
   3 Incorrect; the child is attempting to assert independence; will say "no" even if meaning yes.
   4 This does not indicate confusion; child's behavior is typical of 2-year-old children; they will say no to most things as a means of asserting their independence.

162. 1 A lowered concentration of extracellular sodium brings about a decrease in the release of ADH. This leads to increased excretion of urine. (2; CJ; AN; MS; ED; CV)
   2 The sodium restriction does not control the volume of food intake; weight is controlled by a low-calorie diet and by prevention of fluid retention.
   3 The resulting elimination of excess fluid reduces the workload of the heart but does not improve contractility.
   4 Potassium is inefficiently retained by the body; an adequate intake of potassium is needed.

163. 3 When ambulating a client, the nurse walks on the client's stronger or unaffected side. This provides a wide base of support and therefore increases stability during the phase of ambulation that calls for weight bearing on the affected side as the unaffected limb moves forward. (3; CJ; IM; MS; TC; SK)
   1 This tends to change the center of gravity from directly above the feet and may cause instability.
   2 Same as answer 1.
   4 The nurse should stand on the client's stronger or unaffected side.

164. 3 This allows an active 4-year-old to move within restrictions and encourages use of the imagination. (3; CJ; IM; PE; ED; GD)
   1 Unless carefully selected, many shows are inappropriate and uninteresting for a 4-year-old.
   2 Although a 4-year-old may still cling to a security toy, it would not allow for expenditure of energy.
   4 This may provide the child with rest, but this activity is too simple for this age child and will not promote development.

165. **4** Giving Rh-positive cells would lead to further hemolysis; Rh-negative cells are not attacked by maternal antibodies. (3; CJ; PL; CW; PA; HN)

 1 This would be irrelevant because the blood cells usually do not come from the mother.

 2 This is not really neutral; it is only a temporary safeguard from further hemolysis.

 3 A reaction to other antigens in the cross-matched blood could still occur.

166. **4** These are some of the first signs of hypoxia; the airway must be kept patent to promote oxygenation. (3; CJ; IM; PE; PA; RE)

 1 The client will not be able to communicate verbally after a tracheotomy.

 2 These are late signs of hypoxia; suctioning should have been done well before this time.

 3 These are late signs of respiratory difficulty; suctioning and other measures should have been done well before this time.

167. **3** The priority of care at this time is to protect the spine from strain to prevent additional damage to the traumatized area while it heals. (3; CJ; IM; MS; PA; NM)

 1 Infection usually results from prolonged immobility; although important, it is not the immediate priority.

 2 Although an important aspect of care, it is not the priority item in the immediate postinjury period.

 4 Survival and safety take priority; vocational rehabilitation will assume greater importance after the client's condition stabilizes.

168. **1** Jaundice occurs because of the normal physiologic breakdown of fetal red blood cells and the immaturity of the infant's liver. (1; CJ; AS; CW; ED; NN)

 2 Conjugation and excretion, not synthesis of bile, are compromised because of the immature liver.

 3 This is unrelated to the infant's hemoglobin level; the mother and baby have separate circulations.

 4 Babies usually have high hemoglobin and high hematocrit levels.

169. **2** Eye patches are applied to prevent drying of the conjunctiva, injury to the retina, and alterations in biorhythms. (2; CJ; IM; CW; TC; NN)

 1 The baby will automatically close the eyes in response to bright lights and application of a patch.

 3 The baby should be exposed to bright lights periodically so normal rhythms will become established.

 4 These movements are automatic during sleep phases and will not be affected by eye patches.

170. **1** Head lag in an infant 6 months old is abnormal and is frequently a sign of cerebral damage. (3; CJ; AS; PE; ED; NM)

 2 The ability to sit unsupported is achieved at 7 to 8 months.

 3 The Babinski reflex is normally present until 2 years of age.

 4 The tonic reflex and grasp reflex usually disappear at 2 and 3 months, respectively.

171. **4** Increased intracranial pressure results in pressure exerted against the cranium. This is especially evident in areas with less confinement, such as the fontanel (which bulges), the orbits (which are pushed forward so the eyelids are pulled taut and upper lids are above the irises [sunset eyes]), and the brain (vomiting center stimulated regardless of activity of eating). (2; CJ; AS; PE; PA; NM)

 1 The fontanel will show signs of increased fluid volume in the skull and therefore bulge.

 2 Decreased skin turgor is not a sign associated with increased intracranial pressure.

 3 The eyeballs will show signs of increased fluid volume in the skull and be pushed forward, pulling the lids taut; systolic pressure is elevated and diastolic is the same or lower, creating a widening pulse pressure.

172. **3** The trauma of surgery normally results in some seeping or oozing of blood into the remaining gastric area, which is being immediately suctioned out of the body via the nasogastric tube. (3; CJ; EV; MS; TC; GI)

 1 The trauma of surgery will result in some blood loss, which will continue until coagulation takes place; this is too short a time for this to occur.

 2 Same as answer 1.

 4 If light-red liquid is still draining 24 to 48 hours after surgery, it is abnormal; the physician should be notified.

173. **2** Too rapid administration can result in hyper-kalemia, which can cause a long refractory period in the cardiac cycle and result in cardiac dysrhythmias and arrest. (3; CJ; IM; MS; TC; FE)

1 This statement is too general; there is no indication of whether it is respiratory acidosis or metabolic acidosis. Metabolic acidosis can cause hyperkalemia.

3 These reactions do not occur in hyperkalemia.

4 Hyperkalemia usually causes nausea, vomiting, and diarrhea, which may result in dehydration; in this instance fluid would shift from interstitial spaces to the intravascular compartment. With edema the fluid shift is in the opposite direction.

174. **3** Small feedings reduce the amount of bulk passing into the jejunum and therefore reduce the fluid shifting into the jejunum. (2; MR; PL; MS; PA; GI)

1 Although a diet high in roughage may be avoided, a low-residue, bland diet is not necessary.

2 Total fluid intake does not have to be restricted; however, fluids should not be taken immediately before, during, or after a meal because they promote rapid stomach emptying.

4 Concentrated sweets pass rapidly out of the stomach and increase fluid shifts; consequently the diet should be low in carbohydrates. Protein is needed to promote tissue repair.

175. **2** The stump is elevated for the first 24 hours after surgery to reduce edema and is then placed flat on the bed to reduce hip flexion contractures. (2; CJ; IM; MS; PA; SK)

1 The dressing applied in the OR should not be disturbed at this time.

3 Too soon; the stump is elevated in bed for the first 24 hours.

4 Same as answer 2.

176. **3** The growing uterus exerts pressure on the mesentery, slowing peristalsis; more water is reabsorbed from the colon and constipation results. (2; MR; AN; CW; ED; HC)

1 The metabolism increases but does not affect the bowel.

2 The growing uterus tends to exert pressure on the bladder; it is way above the anus.

4 Milk is not constipating.

177. **3** As cervical dilation nears completion, labor is intensified with an increase in pain and energy expenditure. (2; CJ; AN; CW; PA; HC)

1 Back pain usually indicates a posterior-lying position of the infant.

2 The client is usually very restless and thrashes about, assuming no particular position.

4 Pain is increased, since contractions are more frequent and intense, and they last longer.

178. **3** A relaxed uterus is the most frequent cause of bleeding in the early postpartum period. The uterus can be returned to a state of firmness by intermittent gentle fundal massage. (2; MR; EV; CW; PA; HC)

1 Immediate action is directed toward the client's safety; the physician is called if uterine massage does not control bleeding.

2 Assessment of the uterus and massage take priority; then the vital signs are checked.

4 Steady bleeding is neither common nor normal and must be attended to immediately.

179. **3** Infection from lowered resistance is a constant threat from the disease and from the immunosuppressant drugs, both of which affect white blood cells. (2; CJ; IM; PE; TC; DR)

1 Although vital signs need to be checked to assess for changes in pulse or BP, unless there is other clinical evidence of bleeding, q 2-hour readings are not needed.

2 The client needs to maintain the physical activity that can be tolerated.

4 Clients need stimuli appropriate for their developmental level except when acutely ill from drug therapy.

180. **2** Constipation from an adynamic ileus can be prevented with high-fiber foods and liberal fluids. These will keep the stool bulky and soft, promoting evacuation. (3; MR; PL; PE; PA; DR)

1 Roughage and fluids are recommended to help minimize the constipation associated with vincristine.

3 Treatment of constipation, a common side effect of vincristine, calls for roughage and fluids.

4 Vincristine causes constipation; roughage and fluids are needed.

181. **3** Low platelet count predisposes to bleeding, which may be evident in the urine. Red blood cells are seen microscopically in the sediment. (2; CJ; EV; PE; PA; BI)
    1 Casts are seen in the urine in some kidney disorders.
    2 White blood cells occur in the urine when there is a urinary tract infection.
    4 Lymphocytes are not normally found in the urine.

182. **3** The protective blood-brain barrier initially screens leukemic cells from the CNS. However, in advanced stages leukemic infiltration occurs. The chemotherapeutic agents, also screened out by the blood-brain barrier, are ineffective. (3; MR; IM; PE; ED; NM)
    1 Radiation destroys leukemic cells.
    2 Radiation does not decrease cerebral edema.
    4 Irradiation of the cranium is needed because chemotherapy does not pass the blood-brain barrier.

183. **4** Children at early school age are not yet able to comprehend death's universality and inevitability, but fear it, often personifying death as a bogeyman or death angel. They need an opportunity to prepare for this. (2; MR; IM; MH; PS; CS)
    1 A child this age needs to know the seriousness of the illness and that recovery may not be possible.
    2 Children of this age interpret death as separation and punishment; they fear this in addition to death itself.
    3 This response only avoids the question.

184. **4** The magical and egocentric thinking of preschoolers results in the belief that their sickness is a punishment for bad thoughts. (2; CJ; EV; PE; ED; EH)
    1 The egocentric thinking of the preschooler would not lead him to think like this.
    2 This is not indicative of his current behavior.
    3 More likely he will feel that he has gotten sick because he has bad feelings toward his sibling.

185. **3** This can be expected; usually accomplished by 3 years of age. (2; CJ; AS; PE; ED; GD)
    1 This requires balance that is not present until 4 or 5 years of age; the 3-year-old child can usually ride a tricycle.

    2 This is usually accomplished at 5 years of age.
    4 This is not accomplished until later in the school-age years.

186. **3** The high-pressure alarm signifies increased pressure in the tubing or respiratory tract; obstruction is usually caused by excessive secretions. (3; CJ; EV; MS; TC; RE)
    1 This is a dependent function of the nurse.
    2 High-volume low-pressure cuffs make this unnecessary; would also decrease the effectiveness of the ventilator and compromise respiratory status.
    4 Incorrect; the temperature can remain constant, usually about 5° F to 10° F below normal body temperature.

187. **2** The system must remain airtight (closed) to prevent collapse of the lung. (3; CJ; IM; MS; TC; RE)
    1 The water will rise with inspiration and fall with expiration and is known as tidaling.
    3 It should bubble but not vigorously; vigorous bubbling will not increase the suction but it will cause the fluid to evaporate more rapidly.
    4 The system is kept closed; a record of drainage is kept by marking the outside of the container or chamber.

188. **4** This is a type of communication whereby two conflicting messages, such as love and rejection, arc sent simultaneously, and the receiver is unable to sort out which message is the real one. (2; CJ; AN; MH; PS; SD)
    1 This behavior was not demonstrated during the exchange.
    2 Same as answer 1.
    3 Rejection is only one of the messages of the exchange, since it was delivered with a gift that demonstrated remembering and caring.

189. **1** Hallucinations most often occur when there is diminished sensory stimulation competing for attention. (2; CJ; AS; MH; PS; SD)
    2 Although this may stimulate delusional thoughts, it frequently competes for sensory attention and therefore diminishes hallucinations.
    3 Same as answer 2.
    4 Same as answer 2.

190. **4** The presence of loose, disruptive association defects is one of the cardinal symptoms of schizophrenia, and their lessening would demonstrate improvement. (3; CJ; EV; MH; PS; SD)
    1 This behavior could represent withdrawal from reality and would not necessarily signal improvement.
    2 Paranoid delusions are usually well organized and on the surface often seem logical.
    3 Most clients with schizophrenia are able to express negative feelings freely because there is poor control by the ego.

191. **2** The primary concern in the practice of pica is that other intake will be nutritionally inadequate. (2; CJ; PL; CW; PA; HC)
    1 Pica does not indicate a psychological/emotional disturbance.
    3 This is not necessary if nutrition is adequate.
    4 If not toxic to the mother, it is generally not fetotoxic.

192. **3** Ambulation decreases Braxton Hicks contractions. (2; MR; IM; CW; PA; HC)
    1 Braxton Hicks contractions increase when client is resting.
    2 These contractions are not indicative of true labor and need not be timed.
    4 Aspirin may be harmful to the fetus because it can hemolyze red blood cells.

193. **4** An amniotomy allows for more effective pressure of the fetal head on the cervix, enhancing dilation and effacement. (2; CJ; EV; CW; PA; HC)
    1 This does not directly affect the fetal heart rate.
    2 Vaginal bleeding may increase because of the progression of labor.
    3 Discomfort may become greater because contractions usually increase after an amniotomy.

194. **3** A negative rubella titer indicates inadequate immunity, and immunizations are safely given in the immediate postpartal period. (2; CJ; PL; CW; TC; HC)
    1 Penicillin will not affect the client's immunity status.
    2 The mother's negative rubella titer does not affect the infant.
    4 A client with a negative titer has no immunity to rubella.

195. **4** The shunt may obstruct and lead to an accumulation of cerebrospinal fluid (CSF), raising intracranial pressure, which leads to brainstem hypoxia. (3; CJ; AS; PE; PA; NM)
    1 Sedation is contraindicated to allow determination of level of consciousness (LOC).
    2 Positioning infant flat helps prevent complications resulting from too rapid reduction of intracranial fluid.
    3 Infant is positioned off shunt to prevent pressure on valve and incisional area.

196. **3** A well-balanced diet with fewer calories because of decreased activity needs is suggested for elderly individuals. (2; CJ; AN; MS; PA; GD)
    1 Fluid needs do not increase in the elderly.
    2 Limited financial resources are one cause of malnutrition in the elderly.
    4 There should be a balance among the four food groups; protein is needed for tissue repair; high carbohydrates would provide excessive calories, which could result in obesity.

197. **2** Urinary output must be sufficient to carry away lead and metabolized chelating agent; in addition, EDTA can damage kidney tissue. (2; CJ; EV; PE; TC; DR)
    1 Calcium EDTA is not irritating to intestinal mucosa because it is excreted by the kidneys.
    3 A regular diet with some "junk food" is permitted.
    4 Calcium EDTA does not cause pain when given intravenously.

198. **1** The presence of food limits the irritating effect of steroids on the gastric mucosa. (2; MR; PL; MS; PA; DR)
    2 It may help the client remember to take the medication, but it is not the reason for taking it with meals.
    3 Food does not increase or decrease absorption of steroids.
    4 The medication is not affected by acid media.

199. **1** Determining fetal well-being supersedes all other measures; if fetal heart rate (FHR) is absent or persistently decelerating, immediate intervention is required. (2; CJ; AS; CW; PA; HC)
    2 Important, but determination of fetal well-being is the priority.
    3 Same as answer 2.
    4 Same as answer 2.

200. **4** This may occur with head compression, but is perfectly normal if FHR returns to baseline at end of contraction. (2; CJ; AS; CW; PA; HC)
   1 Needs no medical intervention; this is a normal occurrence as long as FHR returns to baseline at end of contraction.
   2 Cord compression is a common occurrence; no intervention is necessary if FHR returns to normal baseline at end of contraction.
   3 This position would increase pressure on vena cava.

201. **4** The repeated thought or act defends the client against even higher, more severe levels of anxiety. (2; CJ; PL; MH; PS; PR)
   1 To deny the client the ritual may precipitate panic levels of anxiety.
   2 The client already recognizes that the ritual serves little purpose.
   3 Same as answer 1.

202. **3** Anafranil potentiates the effects of serotonin (antiobsessional effect) and norepinephrine in the CNS; it diminishes obsessive-compulsive behaviors. (2; CJ; AN; MH; PA; AX)
   1 This is an antiparkinsonian agent, not an antianxiety.
   2 Same as answer 1.
   4 This is an antihistamine, not an antianxiety agent.

203. **2** The repeated thought or act defends the client against severe anxiety; the client does not want to perform the ritual but feels compelled to do so to keep anxiety at a controllable level. (2; MR; AN; MH; PS; AX)
   1 No limits are being set by the nurse's action.
   3 This causes depression and is unrelated to ritualistic behavior.
   4 Rituals are not activities that enhance self-esteem; they control anxiety.

204. **2** Exposure to infection or cold, or overexertion of a client with chronic adrenocortical insufficiency (Addison's disease) can cause circulatory collapse. (2; CJ; PL; MS; TC; EN)
   1 This would be an appropriate room assignment.
   3 Same as answer 1.
   4 Same as answer 1.

205. **3** Deficiency of the glucocorticoids causes hypoglycemia in the client with Addison's disease. Signs of hypoglycemia include nervousness; weakness; dizziness; cool, moist skin; hunger; and tremors. (3; CJ; AS; MS; PA; EN)
   1 Hypokalemia is evidenced by nausea, vomiting, muscle weakness, and dysrhythmias.
   2 Weakness with dizziness on arising is called postural hypotension, not hypertension.
   4 This would be evidenced by edema, increased BP, and crackles.

206. **1** Because of diminished mineralocorticoid secretion, clients with Addison's disease are prone to development of hyponatremia. Therefore the addition of salt to the diet is advised. (3; MR; IM; MS; ED; EN)
   2 Caloric intake is determined on an individual basis; diet is not necessarily restricted to 1200 calories.
   3 Fluids are not restricted in Addison's disease.
   4 Protein is not omitted from the diet; ingestion of essential amino acids is necessary for normal metabolism.

207. **4** Development of mood swings and psychosis is possible from an overdose of glucocorticoids due to fluid and electrolyte alterations. (2; CJ; EV; MS; PA; DR)
   1 This is not a sign of glucocorticoid overdose.
   2 Same as answer 1.
   3 Same as answer 1.

208. **1** These children have difficulty reaching out to the environment and tend to be withdrawn. They frequently get little response from the parents and do not learn how to respond to others. (2; MR; AS; PE; PS; EH)
   2 The infant with failure to thrive is usually nonresponsive or only poorly responsive to human contact.
   3 These children show little satisfaction and are very difficult to comfort.
   4 These children do not respond readily to human contact.

209. **3** Head control and rolling over are achieved at 4 and 5 months, respectively. Transferring objects from one hand to another and sitting unsupported are achieved at 7 and 8 months. (2, CJ; AS; PE; ED; GD)
   1 The ability to roll over is achieved by approximately 5 months of age.
   2 Same as answer 1.
   4 Transferring objects from hand to hand is usually achieved in approximately 7 months.

210. **2** Fine motor coordination is inadequately developed to manipulate snap toys. (3; CJ; PL; PE; ED; GD)
   1 These are appropriate to stimulate visual attention.
   3 The voluntary grasp will allow the child to hold the toy and the rattling sound will stimulate the auditory system.
   4 These stimulate the sense of touch, and, since voluntary grasp appears at about 3 to 4 months, they would be handled satisfactorily.

211. **4** The individual cannot resolve the conflict consciously because of emotional pressure pulling in both directions. As anxiety increases, the unconscious seeks a solution. The conversion selected usually resolves the initial conflict by making action impossible, thus removing the need to select one or the other choice. (3; CJ; AN; MH; PS; AX)
   1 There are no physical changes involved with this unconscious resolution of a conflict.
   2 The conversion of anxiety to physical symptoms operates on an unconscious level.
   3 A conversion reaction is a psychologic response to stress, not a defense against it.

212. **2** This helps the client identify behavior and feelings in a nonthreatening manner. (3; MR; IM; MH; PS; TR)
   1 This would be ganging up on the client.
   3 This evasion and refusal to answer would have the psychologic effect of removing the nurse from the group.
   4 The nurse's behavior is not the issue; the situation should be turned back to the client's behavior.

213. **2** Accidental ligation of a ureter is a serious complication of a total abdominal hysterectomy. A decrease in urine output should be reported immediately to the surgeon. (3; MR; EV; CW; TC; WH)
   1 An apical rate of 90 falls within normal limits but should be evaluated in relation to the client's previous vital signs.
   3 A nasogastric tube is not routinely inserted.
   4 Serosanguineous vaginal drainage is to be expected.

214. **3** Because of tissue destruction, sodium ions are lost in the interstitial fluid, whereas potassium ions are liberated from the injured cells. The result is hyponatremia and hyperkalemia. (3; CJ; AN; MS; PA; IT)
   1 Blood volume decreases, and hypovolemic shock may occur.
   2 Capillary permeability is increased in burns.
   4 Fluid shifts may cause shock, but it is reversible with therapy.

215. **3** Because of fluid loss via the burned area and sodium reabsorption by the kidneys, which pulls fluid, urinary output is diminished. However, output of 30 ml per hour or less is considered a sign of shock. (3; CJ; PL; MS; PA; FE)
   1 This amount would cause overload; output is less than 30 ml per hour.
   2 This amount of fluid replacement would be inadequate, and fluid loss excessive in the newly burned client; very little fluid is left to replace losses during the first few days.
   4 This intake is excessive, as is the output; these would not be expected in the newly burned client.

216. **3** The nurse, knowing the client was combative, was negligent in not providing close supervision; a reasonable, prudent nurse would have closely observed the client to protect against self-imposed injury as well as to protect others. (2; LE; EV; MH; PS; MO)
   1 It would be unrealistic to keep a client sedated at all times.
   2 All clients should be supervised, especially those who are combative.
   4 The admitting office may have had no knowledge of the situation; therefore it was the nurse's responsibility.

217. **3** This sets appropriate limits for the client who cannot set self-limits; it rejects the behavior but accepts the client. (2; MR; IM; MH; PS; MO)
   1 This may have the effect of reinforcing the behavior rather than decreasing it.
   2 This does not show acceptance of the client, nor does it help the client control behavior.
   4 This does not deal with the problem directly. The nurse's response can confuse the client, because the client may not be aware of why the nurse is refusing to talk.

218. **3** CPR by one person is less efficient than that performed by two because of the two activities required. The 2:15 ratio is the most efficient way to provide minimally adequate tissue perfusion. (1; CJ; IM; MS; PA; CV)
    1 This ratio would be used when two people were administering CPR.
    2 Ineffective; would result in the circulation of unoxygenated blood.
    4 Ineffective; blood would not be circulated while four breaths were being administered, and thus hypoxia would result.

219. **4** An increase in total body water increases the intravascular volume and the cardiac workload; excess sodium intake contributes to fluid retention and edema. (2; MR; AN; MS; PA; CV)
    1 Limiting sodium will not reduce the edema already present; it will prevent additional fluid retention.
    2 Limiting sodium will not have a diuretic effect; it will prevent additional fluid retention.
    3 Same as answer 1.

220. **3** An interference with bile flow into the intestine will lead to increasing inability to tolerate fatty foods. The unemulsified fat remains in the intestine for prolonged periods, and the result is inhibition of stomach emptying with possible gas formation. (2; CJ; AS; MS; PA; GI)
    1 Melena is tarry stools associated with upper GI bleeding; diarrhea would be associated with increased intestinal motility.
    2 Coffee-ground emesis is usually indicative of gastric bleeding; it is not associated with cholecystitis.
    4 Gnawing pain when the stomach is empty is associated with duodenal ulcers.

221. **4** Bleeding disorders are common when bile does not flow through the intestine. Vitamin K, a fat soluble vitamin requiring bile salts for its absorption, is needed by the liver to synthesize prothrombin. (2; CJ; AS; MS; PA; GI)
    1 Prostaglandins regulate platelet aggregation and control inflammation and vascular permeability.
    2 This is untrue; platelets aggregate at the site of injury.

3 Diaphragmatic excursion itself does not put pressure on the suture line; deep breathing does result in pain.

222. **2** Exploration of the common bile duct may cause edema; a T-tube prevents the edema from obstructing the duct. (3; CJ; AN; MS; TC; GI)
    1 The cystic duct is ligated when the gallbladder is removed.
    3 The T-tube will not prevent the formation of an abscess.
    4 A T-tube can be used to inject dye for a cholangiogram, but it is not inserted for that purpose.

223. **2** A colostomy does not function for 2 to 4 days postoperatively because of the lack of peristalsis. (3; CJ; EV; MS; TC; GI)
    1 Bowel sounds will be absent until peristaltic activity returns.
    3 This would indicate an interference with circulation to the stoma; the stoma should be cherry red.
    4 This would indicate gastric bleeding, which is abnormal.

224. **4** Any other action would be an invasion of privacy. The marital status has no bearing on the needs of the client at this time. (2; MR; AS; MH; PS; TR)
    1 The client's marital status has no bearing on the course of labor.
    2 There is no indication at this time that the client requires this referral.
    3 This action would be an invasion of privacy.

225. **4** With the head and chest elevated, gravity promotes respiratory excursion; alternating side-lying positions allows for pulmonary drainage and expansion. (2; CJ; PL; PE; PA; RE)
    1 This would permit the abdominal viscera to impinge on the diaphragm, impeding lung expansion.
    2 It is difficult to maintain a 5-week-old infant in this position. In addition this position would not promote rest.
    3 This position would make it difficult for the lungs to expand, causing difficulty in breathing.

226. **1** Clients use delusions as a defense and cannot be argued out of them. The nurse's response did not demonstrate acceptance and only added to the client's anxiety and agitation. (2; CJ; EV; MH; PS; MO)
2 Maximum clinical effectiveness of antidepressants takes approximately 4 to 6 weeks; therefore, psychotropic drug therapy must be combined with psychotherapy and therapeutic milieu on an inpatient unit.
3 There is nothing to indicate that treatment had not been started toward relieving these symptoms.
4 The client should have a one-to-one relationship with staff before attempting to relate to other clients on the unit.

227. **1** The therapeutic level of lithium carbonate is very close to the toxic level. Therefore it is vital that blood levels of the drug be monitored twice a week during the acute phase and bimonthly once the client is on a maintenance dosage. (3; CJ; EV; MH; PA; DR)
2 Lithium does not affect fluid retention; monitoring daily weights is not necessary.
3 Lithium does not affect the leukocyte levels; monitoring the leukocyte count is unnecessary.
4 Psychomotor activity should be normal once the maintenance dosage is achieved; careful monitoring of psychomotor activity is not a major priority.

228. **4** This is recommended to keep weight gain (up to 24 lb) in balance and to control blood pressure. (3; MR; PL; CW; ED; HP)
1 Fats should be limited because they could cause an accumulation of unwanted adipose tissue.
2 Decreasing protein intake is not advised for clients with cardiac problems.
3 Increasing sodium intake is not advised for clients with cardiac problems.

229. **2** This provides the opportunity for paternal-infant bonding. Handling the infant may reduce some of the father's anxiety. (3; MR; PL; CW; PS; EC)
1 Although helpful, this does not meet the need for paternal-infant bonding.
3 This does not recognize the father's anxiety; also, he may not be ready to absorb this information.
4 This is a simplistic approach to the father's emotional needs and does not deal with the real situation.

230. **2** Whole milk does not meet the infant's need for vitamin C and iron. Also, it contains high amounts of protein and sodium, which may be harmful. (3; MR; PL; PE; ED; GI)
1 Whole milk contains adequate fats; the calcium content is $3^1/_2$ times that found in human milk.
3 Whole milk contains adequate thiamin; the sodium content is three times that found in human milk.
4 Whole milk contains adequate carbohydrates; the protein content is three times that found in human milk.

231. **3** The mismatched blood cells are attacked by antibodies, and the hemoglobin released from the ruptured erythrocytes plugs the kidney tubules; such kidney involvement results in backache. (3; CJ; AS; MS; PA; BI)
1 This symptom is not common to transfusion reactions.
2 Same as answer 1.
4 Same as answer 1.

232. **2** The cessation of renal function is usually evidenced by a decrease in output to less than 400 ml/24 hours. (2; CJ; AS; MS; PA; RG)
1 Although this symptom is related to the renal system, its presence does not indicate kidney damage.
3 Same as answer 1.
4 Same as answer 1.

233. **3** Hyperkalemia occurs in renal failure. Because the kidneys are damaged, the body does not excrete K+. (2; CJ; AS; MS; PA; RG)
1 Calcium excess would produce renal calculi and pathologic fractures.
2 Hyponatremia would cause headache, muscle weakness, apathy, and abdominal cramps.
4 Calcium deficiency would be manifested by tingling of the nose, ears, and fingertips, along with muscle spasms and tetany.

234. **2** The waste products of protein metabolism are the main cause of uremia. The degree of protein restriction is determined by the severity of the disease. (3; MR; IM; MS; ED; RG)
1 Fluid restriction may be necessary to prevent edema, heart failure, or hypertension; fluid does not directly influence uremia.
3 Sodium is often restricted to control fluid retention, not uremia.
4 Potassium is restricted to prevent hyperkalemia, not uremia.

235. **1** If fluid is not draining properly, the client should be positioned from side to side or with the head raised; or manual pressure should be applied to the lower abdomen to facilitate drainage by the use of external pressure and gravity. (3; CJ; IM; MS; TC; RG)

2 This deficit is not enough to require notifying the physician.

3 The client's position may be changed prn; a supine position does not facilitate drainage by the use of gravity.

4 The physician removes the cannula.

236. **2** When one's efforts toward meeting a goal are blocked or thwarted, frustration results. The child with special needs may be constantly thwarted in trying to meet developmental needs, especially in an environment where certain achievements beyond the child's ability are expected. (2; CJ; AN; MH; PS; BA)

1 This is an external factor that has little to do with the child's ability to deal with limitations.

3 This does not occur.

4 This is not a frequent occurrence.

237. **3** Medically, during the first stage of detoxification, nausea, anorexia, and hypertension are experienced. (3; CJ; AS; MH; PA; SA)

1 Psychomotor hyperactivity, not lethargy, and hypertension are experienced during this stage.

2 Hypertension, not hypotension, and agitation are experienced during this stage.

4 Hypertension, hyperactivity, and tachycardia, not bradycardia, are experienced during this stage.

238. **2** Increasing cerebral edema may predispose the client to convulsions; therefore stimuli of any kind should be minimized. (2; CJ; PL; CW; TC; HP)

1 Magnesium sulfate would be used; calcium gluconate is its antidote.

3 A cesarean delivery may not be needed; however, this is a medical decision.

4 This is a medical, not a nursing, decision; the client will likely receive intravenous magnesium sulfate to promote diuresis.

239. **3** The situation is so traumatic that the individual is unable to organize or use past coping behaviors and cannot comprehend what occurred. (2; CJ; AS; MS; PS; CS)

1 Insufficient information is available to use this diagnosis at this time.

2 Same as answer 1.

4 Same as answer 1.

240. **3** To maximize the intake of O_2 being delivered to the nares, the individual should breathe through the nose. (3; CJ; AS; MS; TC; RE)

1 Although rest would be encouraged (the client could rest in a chair), the priority is that the client receive the O_2.

2 Two liters of O_2 per minute would not be contraindicated for a client with chronic obstructive pulmonary disease (COPD); levels above 2 L should be avoided to prevent CO_2 narcosis.

4 In the adult, nasal cannulas do not come in a variety of sizes; the elastic strap is adjustable.

241. **2** The presence of secretions in the upper airway produces gurgling sounds that interfere with the free flow of air with each breath. (2; CJ; AS; MS; TC; RE)

1 Appropriate positioning would promote the drainage of mucus and saliva from the mouth.

3 Cyanosis can result from a variety of problems unrelated to the presence of secretions; suctioning should be done only when secretions are blocking the airway.

4 Suctioning is not needed in the absence of accumulated secretions.

242. **2** Leg fatigue is a common clinical manifestation caused by venous stasis and poor tissue oxygenation. (1; CJ; AS; MS; PA; CV)

1 This results from a fungus under the nail or chronic hypoxia.

3 This is indicative of thrombophlebitis.

4 Same as answer 3.

243. **2** As valves become incompetent, they allow blood to pool in the veins, which increases the hydrostatic pressure and leads to further valve destruction. (2; CJ; IM; MS; PA; CV)

1 Inflammation is a factor in thrombophlebitis, not in varicose veins.

3 Valves promote, not obstruct, the flow of blood to the heart.

4 There are no known hereditary diseases that affect only the leg muscles surrounding the veins.

244. **2** This is the manner in which the AIDS virus interferes with the individual's immunity to other infections. (2; CJ; AN; MS; PA; BI)
 1 AIDS is not an autoimmune process.
 3 This is not related to the presence of opportunistic infections or illnesses associated with AIDS; associated with the immune deficiency caused by human immunodeficiency virus (HIV) infection.
 4 Not related to opportunistic infections present with AIDS; these infections result from the immune deficiency caused by the HIV infection.

245. **1** This is a common side effect of this medication. (3; CJ; EV; MS PA; DR)
 2 Neutropenia, not leukocytosis, is associated with this drug.
 3 This is not a side effect of pentamidine.
 4 Same as answer 3.

246. **3** A wheeze indicates bronchial constriction, which could interfere with the benefits desired from aerosol pentamidine. (3; CJ; EV; MS; TC; RE)
 1 This would not be helpful in the presence of bronchoconstriction, as evidenced by the bilateral wheeze.
 2 Same as answer 1.
 4 Same as answer 1.

247. **2** By monitoring and reporting changes in the child's behavior, the physician can determine the effectiveness of the medication. (3; MR; EV; MH; PA; BA)
 1 Parents should not be encouraged to tutor children because there is usually too much emotional interaction.
 3 This child's behavior is not deliberate or easily controllable; this type of statement could lead to diminishing the child's self-esteem if control does not occur.
 4 Children need more structure and rules than adults.

248. **4** Bending increases intraocular pressure and must be avoided. (2; MR; PL; MS; TC; NM)
 1 This is not necessary.
 2 Same as answer 1.
 3 Coughing deeply increases intraocular pressure and would be contraindicated.

249. **4** Exsanguination can occur in a matter of minutes if cannulas are dislodged. (3; CJ; AN; MS; TC; RG)
 1 Although true, it is not a life-threatening situation; preventing exsanguination takes priority.
 2 Same as answer 1.
 3 Same as answer 1.

250. **2** There is a need for further teaching because blood pressure should not be taken in the affected arm. (2; MR; EV; MS; ED; RG)
 1 Indicates understanding of care; presence of bruit indicates the circulation is good and not obstructed by a thrombus.
 3 Indicates understanding of care; exsanguination can occur in a matter of minutes if the cannula is dislodged.
 4 Indicates understanding of care; these are signs of infection, which is a complication of cannulization.

251. **4** Depressed bone marrow production of formed elements of blood leads to neutropenia and increased susceptibility to infection. (2; CJ; AS; PE; PA; BI)
 1 Urine output will be within normal limits; there is no kidney involvement at this stage of the disease.
 2 There are excess, not lesser, quantities of "blasts" in the peripheral blood and bone marrow.
 3 The swallowing reflex is not affected.

252. **2** Parents' responses to their children may greatly influence decisions regarding future care. Learning about their child and the child's problem can help lessen guilt feelings. (2; CJ; PL; PE; ED; GD)
 1 This is essential for all babies.
 3 Same as answer 1.
 4 Same as answer 1.

253. **4** After a suprapubic prostatectomy there is generally leakage of urine around the suprapubic tube. This leakage creates an environment in which bacteria can flourish if the dressing is not changed frequently. (2; CJ; PL; MS; PA; RG)
 1 Uremia is caused by inadequate kidney function; it is not directly related to bladder infection.
 2 Negative pressure on the bladder may traumatize the delicate tissue; urine should flow by gravity.
 3 Clamping off the tube causes urinary stasis, which increases the risk of infection.

254. **3** Pain after a suprapubic prostatectomy may denote retention of urine as a result of blocked drainage tubes or infection, or it may be a normal response to surgery. The possibility of any complication must first be investigated. (2; CJ; EV; MS; TC; RG)
1 Analgesics can be administered after the cause of pain has been investigated.
2 Encouraging fluids without a patent drainage tube will increase pressure and discomfort; assessment should occur before implementation.
4 The need to measure vital signs is dependent upon the analgesic ordered; assessing the cause of pain takes priority.

255. **4** Keeping a record of what one eats helps limit unconscious and nervous eating by making the individual aware of intake. (2; CJ; IM; MS; ED; GI)
1 Limiting calories to 900 per day is a severe restriction and requires a physician's order.
2 Exercise causes rapid head movements, which may precipitate a Ménière's attack.
3 This is not always practical and is difficult to implement; assessment of dietary habits is the priority.

256. **3** Liquid iron preparations may stain tooth enamel, so they should be diluted and administered through a straw. (1; MR; IM; PE; PA; DR)
1 To avoid gastric irritation, iron should be given with food.
2 Constipation, rather than loose stools, often results from the administration of iron.
4 To improve absorption, iron may be given with orange juice.

257. **1** The 4-year-old can express feelings better through play than with words. (2; MR; IM; PE; PS; EH)
2 A needle is dangerous; even a play syringe would focus the child's attention on one aspect of treatment, without eliciting broader feelings.
3 This may help the nurse understand emotional problems; however, it is not as helpful as play therapy in meeting the child's emotional needs.
4 Understanding explanations requires abstract thinking; 4-year-olds think in a concrete manner and have little concept of time.

258. **3** The added cardiac workload of individuals with anemia receiving transfusions increases the risk of heart failure, leading to pulmonary edema. (3; CJ; EV; PE; PA; RE)
1 This is untrue. This problem occurs with frequent transfusions; it is not increased by anemia.
2 Same as answer 1.
4 Same as answer 1.

259. **3** This disorder interferes with the ability to perceive and respond to sensory stimuli, which causes a deficit in interpreting new sensory data, makes learning difficult, and results in learning disabilities. (2; CJ; AN; MH; PA; BA)
1 This is not necessarily true.
2 Not true; there is no mental retardation present.
4 Same as answer 1.

260. **1** Since the client is paralyzed and movement is compromised, daily inspection to determine the presence of reddened areas or lesions is necessary, (1; CJ; EV; MS; TC; IT)
2 This is helpful but does not ensure that incipient areas of breakdown will not occur; inspection is the only way to locate these.
3 This may contribute to circumscribed pressure, which can lead to skin breakdown.
4 Since sensation may be compromised, a hot water bottle should not be used.

261. **3** Until the client learns new ways of dealing with anxiety, this pattern of behavior will continue. Learning new ways to operate will break the pattern. (2; CJ; IM; MH; PS; PR)
1 This would reinforce the sick role.
2 There is a certain amount of stress in everyday family situations, and the client, not the family, must learn new coping mechanisms.
4 This would be unrealistic; the client must learn to cope with problems.

262. **3** Documentation of nursing findings during assessment is a nursing function. (2; CJ; AS; MS; PA; IT)
1 Inadequate oral hygiene has not been determined as a cause of the plaques; once daily is insufficient for anyone.
2 This is a medical intervention beyond the scope of nursing practice.
4 Candida is a frequent secondary infection in AIDS clients; it is treated when present.

263. **3** Using soap and water and ointment helps maintain skin integrity and prevent infection. (2; MR; PL; MS; ED; IT)

1 Applying an ointment to this extent is contraindicated because it would interfere with adherence of the appliance.

2 Plain water is adequate unless peroxide is specifically prescribed by the physician.

4 Vigorous rubbing may be irritating and promote conditions that contribute to infection.

264. **3** There are few physical restraints on activity postoperatively, but the client may have emotional problems resulting from the body image changes. (2; MR; PL; MS; PS; EH)

1 Swimming is not prohibited because water does not harm the stoma.

2 ADL are not resumed until 6 to 8 weeks after surgery.

4 No changes in lifestyle are necessary.

265. **3** Antidiuretic hormone (ADH) causes water retention, resulting in a decreased urine output and dilution of serum electrolytes. (3; CJ; AS; MS; PA; FE)

1 Blood volume may increase, causing hypertension and diluting the nitrogenous wastes in the blood.

2 Water retention dilutes electrolytes; client is overhydrated rather than underhydrated, so turgor is not poor.

4 ADH acts on nephron to cause water to be reabsorbed from glomerular filtrate, leading to reduced urine volume; specific gravity is elevated as a result of increased concentration.

FOCUS FOR STUDY WORKSHEET   TEST 1

Category of concern		Pathophysiology (basic science)	Pharmacology
BI	Blood and Immunity		
CV	Cardiovascular		
DR	Drug-related Responses		
EH	Emotional Needs Related to Health Problems		
EN	Endocrine		
FE	Fluid and Electrolyte		
GI	Gastrointestinal		
GD	Growth and Development		
IT	Integumentary		
NM	Neuromuscular		
RG	Reproductive and Genitourinary		
RE	Respiratory		
SK	Skeletal		
EC	Emotional Needs Related to Childbearing & Women's Health		
HC	Healthy Childbearing		
HN	High-risk Neonate		
HP	High-risk Maternal-Fetal Conditions Affecting Childbearing		
NN	Normal Neonate		
RC	Reproductive Choices		
RP	Reproductive Problems		
WH	Women's Health		
AX	Anxiety, Somatoform, and Dissociative Disorders		
CS	Crisis Situations		
DD	Dementia, Delirium, and Other Cognitive Disorders		
BA	Disorders First Evident Before Adulthood		
ED	Emotional Problems Related to Physical Health and Childbearing		
MO	Disorders of Mood		
PR	Disorders of Personality		
ES	Eating and Sleeping Disorders		
PD	Personality Development		
SD	Schizophrenic Disorders		
SA	Substance Abuse		
TR	Therapeutic Relationships		

FOCUS FOR STUDY WORKSHEET—cont'd

Nutrition	Diagnostic studies	Physical care	Emotional care

COMPREHENSIVE TEST 2: PART A

1. When being admitted for a lumpectomy the client begins to cry and states, "I found the lump several months ago but kept putting off going to the doctor because of what it could be." The nurse should reply:
   1. "You must have been very frightened."
   2. "About 80% of all lumps are found to be benign."
   3. "Cry as long as you like, you need to get it out of your system."
   4. "Ninety-five percent of all lumps are discovered by the woman herself."

2. At 4:30 PM a client who has been receiving Humulin N insulin every morning states, "I feel very nervous." The nurse observes that the client's skin is moist and cool. The most accurate interpretation of these findings would be:
   1. Polydipsia
   2. Ketoacidosis
   3. Glycogenesis
   4. Hypoglycemia

3. An obese client with diabetes mellitus is to follow a 1200 calorie ADA diet. The nurse explains that excessive weight in people with diabetes mellitus increases:
   1. Fatty acid storage
   2. Glucose oxidation
   3. Insulin requirements
   4. Cellular entry of glucose

4. A client with diabetes mellitus asks how exercise will affect insulin and dietary needs. The nurse should review how exercise:
   1. Increases the need for insulin and increases the need for carbohydrates
   2. Decreases the need for insulin and decreases the need for carbohydrates
   3. Increases the need for carbohydrates and decreases the need for insulin
   4. Decreases the need for carbohydrates but does not affect the need for insulin

5. A client with schizophrenia uses the word "worriation." The nurse should recognize its use as:
   1. Evidence of the illness while ignoring it when interacting with the client
   2. A mispronunciation, while correcting the pronunciation when interacting with the client
   3. Evidence of the illness, while clarifying the meaning with the client during the interaction
   4. A mispronunciation, while indicating to the client that the staff does not understand what it means

6. When assessing a newborn the nurse identifies a swelling on the baby's scalp. The assessment that indicates a cephalhematoma would be:
   1. Unusually wide suture line
   2. Ecchymotic area over the affected eye
   3. Swelling confined to a single skull bone
   4. Diffuse discoloration over the entire scalp

7. Lack of bile in the small intestine results in a lack of vitamin K absorption. The nurse should realize that this will be reflected in an increase in:
   1. Blood clotting
   2. Fibrin formation
   3. Prothrombin time
   4. Calcium utilization

8. A 9-year-old child is diagnosed with acute glomerulonephritis. When performing the admission history, the nurse expects to find that this child has had a recent infection caused by:
   1. *Haemophilus*
   2. *Streptococcus*
   3. *Pseudomonas*
   4. *Staphylococcus*

9. Based on the finding of hematuria, the nurse would expect the urine of a child with acute glomerulonephritis to appear:
   1. Smoky
   2. Orange
   3. Bright red
   4. Straw colored

10. Before teaching clients about nutritional needs during pregnancy, the nurse should be aware that:
    1. Carbohydrate needs are decreased during pregnancy
    2. Calorie needs increase by a maximum of 100 calories per day
    3. The need for protein increases gradually throughout pregnancy
    4. Calcium and phosphorus needs decrease gradually during pregnancy

11. At 40 weeks' gestation a client is admitted to the labor room in early labor. She asks the nurse, "What is the best position to assume during labor?" The nurse should tell her that the side-lying position:
    1. Prevents fetal hyperactivity
    2. Encourages descent of the presenting part
    3. Enhances uterine perfusion and contractions
    4. Decreases incidence of nausea and vomiting

12. A baby is admitted to the transitional nursery with a spiral scalp electrode from an internal monitor remaining in place. To remove this electrode, the nurse should:
    1. Give the electrode a quick jerk
    2. Twist the electrode clockwise until it is free
    3. Untwist the wires before pulling the electrode out
    4. Twist the electrode counterclockwise until it is free

13. An adolescent who has sustained deep partial-thickness burns of the face because of excessive exposure to the sun exclaims, "Prom night is only 4 weeks away, I'll never be healed!" The nurse's best response would be:
    1. "The eschar will be healed in 2 weeks."
    2. "Liquid makeup base can cover the area."
    3. "Recovery will take approximately 3 weeks."
    4. "The edema will remain for approximately 3 weeks."

14. The primary goal for placing a client dying of cancer in a hospice program is to:
    1. Free the client from fear related to pain
    2. Provide the newest treatments for the cancer
    3. Release the family from the burden of providing care
    4. Segregate the client with other clients who have cancer

15. The nurse can best help a client during the period immediately after a spouse's death by recommending:
    1. Crisis counseling
    2. Family counseling
    3. Marital counseling
    4. Bereavement counseling

16. To determine if a 70-year-old individual is meeting the task associated with aging, the nurse should assess that the individual has:
    1. Adapted to children leaving home
    2. Developed a personal philosophy
    3. Attained a sense of worth as a person
    4. Adjusted to life in an assisted living facility

17. A residual urine test is ordered for a client with benign prostatic hypertrophy. The nurse should instruct the client to:
    1. Collect a specimen of urine during midstream
    2. Attempt to void when a urinary catheter is in place
    3. Void after a urinary catheter is inserted and removed
    4. Empty the bladder before a urinary catheter is inserted

18. A client with gastric ulcers has an episode of vomiting blood. Because the loss of a large amount of blood can result in shock, the nurse should assess the client's blood gases for:
    1. Hypocapnea
    2. Metabolic acidosis
    3. Respiratory alkalosis
    4. Negative nitrogen balance

19. A client has a transurethral resection of the prostate. Before discharge, the nurse should plan to teach him that he should:
    1. Attempt to void every 4 hours
    2. Get OOB into a chair for several hours daily
    3. Call the physician if the urinary stream decreases
    4. Avoid vigorous exercise for at least 6 months after surgery

20. A 22-year-old with schizophrenia is admitted to the hospital. The client is poorly groomed, appears to be listening to voices, and has not spoken to anyone for several days. During the first few hospital days the nurse should plan to:
    1. Wait and see if the client approaches the staff
    2. See that the client bathes and changes clothes daily
    3. Conduct an admission assessment interview with the client
    4. Seek the client out frequently to spend short periods of time together

21. A client who has been complaining of stabbing pain in the eyes and blurring of vision is examined by an ophthalmologist, neurologist, and an internist, all of whom have found no organic cause. The client is admitted to the hospital when eye complaints increase. Nursing interventions should include:
    1. Encouraging descriptions of the eye discomfort
    2. Encouraging becoming involved with unit activities
    3. Exploring feelings about a possible impending blindness
    4. Focusing on activities while avoiding discussion of the eye discomfort

22. A client is admitted with a conversion disorder. A primary nursing intervention would be to:
    1. Talk about the physical symptoms
    2. Explore ways to verbalize feelings
    3. Focus on safe, supportive care to meet needs
    4. Explain how stress causes physical symptoms

23. A child with a congenital heart defect has a cardiac catheterization. Nursing care after this procedure should include:
    1. Encouraging early ambulation
    2. Monitoring the site for bleeding
    3. Restricting fluids until blood pressure is stabilized
    4. Comparing blood pressure in affected and unaffected extremities

24. A child with tetralogy of Fallot begins to cry frantically and experiences worsening cyanosis and dyspnea. Remembering that the child would squat if fatigued when walking or playing, the nurse should place the child in the:
    1. Orthopneic position
    2. Knee-chest position
    3. Lateral Sims' position
    4. Semi-Fowler's position

25. When assessing a client with primary open-angle glaucoma, the ocular symptom the nurse should expect the client to exhibit is:
    1. Attacks of acute pain
    2. Constant blurred vision
    3. Impairment of peripheral vision
    4. A complete loss of central vision

26. To prevent a contracture of the hip in a client with an above-the-knee amputation, the nurse should:
    1. Elevate the head of the client's bed
    2. Place pillows under the client's residual limb
    3. Encourage the client to sit in a chair as much as possible
    4. Encourage the client to lie in the prone position several times daily

27. To promote early and efficient ambulation following an above-the-knee amputation, the client should be encouraged to keep the hip:
    1. In a flexed position
    2. In functional alignment
    3. Extended and abducted
    4. Slightly raised when moving the residual limb

28. There are two factors that contribute to residual limb shrinkage: one is atrophy of the muscles, and the other is:
    1. Postoperative edema
    2. Development of skin turgor
    3. Reduction of subcutaneous fat
    4. Loss of tissue and bone during surgery

29. The nurse would know that discharge teaching for a client with glaucoma was effective when the client states, "I should:
    1. Restrict my fluid intake."
    2. Avoid bending exercises."
    3. Use mydriatics regularly."
    4. Avoid bright lights or darkness."

30. A major difference between juvenile rheumatoid arthritis and the polyarthritis of rheumatic fever is that with rheumatoid arthritis there may be:
    1. Some residual joint deformity
    2. Some permanent cardiac damage
    3. A link with the *Streptococcus* organism
    4. An exacerbation during the winter months

31. When caring for a client receiving prolonged aspirin therapy, the nurse should be alert for symptoms of:
    1. Urinary calculi
    2. Atrophy of the liver
    3. Prolonged bleeding time
    4. Premature erythrocyte destruction

32. For a 10-year-old boy with rheumatoid arthritis in a two-bed room, the best roommate would be:
    1. A 12-year-old girl with colitis
    2. A 9-year-old boy with asthma
    3. A 10-year-old girl with a fractured femur
    4. An 11-year-old boy with an appendectomy

33. Three days prior to surgery for a permanent colostomy for cancer of the colon, a client is very cooperative during all procedures, responds pleasantly when approached, and does not question staff about what is being done. From this behavior, the nurse recognizes that the client most likely:
    1. Is not verbalizing feelings about what will happen
    2. Is totally denying the illness and the need for surgery
    3. Feels reassured by frequent contacts with the nursing staff
    4. Has been fully informed by the physician about what to expect

34. Postoperative diet orders for a client following surgery for a colostomy state, "diet as tolerated." Principles that should guide food choices include:
    1. Many foods will cause all individuals with a colostomy the same discomfort
    2. More rigid dietary rules limiting food choices are needed to provide security
    3. A low-residue diet should be followed indefinitely to avoid overstimulating the intestine
    4. A return to a regular diet as soon as possible gives psychologic support and more rapid physical rehabilitation

35. During a colostomy irrigation, if a client complains of abdominal cramps, the nurse should:
    1. Clamp the tubing and allow the client to rest
    2. Reassure the client and continue the irrigation
    3. Pinch the tubing so that less fluid enters the colon
    4. Raise the irrigating can to complete the irrigation quickly

36. When a client's colostomy is located on the left side of the abdomen, the type of stool the nurse should expect would be:
    1. Liquid
    2. Moist, formed
    3. Mucus coated
    4. Pencil shaped

37. When discussing the regaining of bowel control with a client who has just had surgery for a colostomy, the nurse should emphasize the importance of:
    1. A high-protein diet
    2. An irrigation routine
    3. Managing fluid intake
    4. A soft low-residue diet

38. Since autistic children withdraw into their own world, relationships are difficult to establish. The nurse may be able to reach a child with autism by:
    1. Body contact, such as cuddling
    2. Providing a quiet, safe place for rocking
    3. Encouraging participation in group activities
    4. Imitating and participating in the child's activities

39. When assessing a child with autism, the nurse would expect the child to show:
    1. Sad, blank facial expressions
    2. Flapping of hands and rocking
    3. Lack of response to any stimulus
    4. Inappropriate smiling with flat emotions

40. When using play therapy with a child with autism, the nurse should:
    1. Play music and dance with the child
    2. Talk to the child while holding hands
    3. Provide mechanical and inanimate objects for play
    4. Provide brightly colored toys and blocks that can be held

41. Pregnancy-induced hypertension is first suspected in a pregnant woman when there is:
    1. Fluctuation of the BP
    2. Presence of albuminuria
    3. An excessive weight gain
    4. Progressive bilateral ankle edema

42. The nurse would know that dietary teaching for a client with pregnancy-induced hypertension was effective when the client says, "I should follow a diet that includes:
    1. High sodium and calories and low protein."
    2. Low sodium and calories and high protein."
    3. Normal sodium with ample calories and protein."
    4. Moderate sodium, low calories, and ample protein."

43. A client with pregnancy-induced hypertension is hospitalized and is receiving magnesium sulfate (MgSO$_4$) by IV push. Before administering each dose, the nurse should assess the client's:
    1. Temperature and pulse rate
    2. Respirations and patellar reflex
    3. Blood pressure and apical pulse
    4. Urinary output relative to fluid intake

44. With severe pregnancy-induced hypertension, changes in blood values include an elevation of the hematocrit. The nurse should understand that this results from:
    1. Vasodilation caused by an alteration in circulating fluid
    2. Agglutination of red cells caused by membrane fragility
    3. Hemoconcentration caused by a decrease in plasma volume
    4. Hemodilution of pregnancy caused by increases in blood volume

45. An 8-year-old is diagnosed as having type 1 diabetes mellitus. The nurse understands that type 1 diabetes:
    1. Does not always require insulin
    2. Involves early vascular changes
    3. Occurs more often in obese children
    4. Begins more rapidly than adult-onset diabetes

46. The physician orders 20 units of Humulin R insulin for a child with diabetes mellitus. The vial reads, 1 ml = 100 units of Humulin R insulin. If an insulin syringe is not available, the nurse should use a regular syringe and administer:
    1. 0.6 ml
    2. 0.4 ml
    3. 0.3 ml
    4. 0.2 ml

47. A 10-year-old child is diagnosed as having type 1 diabetes mellitus. As part of the teaching plan the nurse should include that insulin needs will decrease when:
    1. Puberty is reached
    2. An infection is present
    3. There is an emotional stress
    4. Active exercise is performed

48. Following surgery on the neck a client should be placed in a high-Fowler's position to:
    1. Avoid strain on the incision
    2. Promote drainage of the wound
    3. Provide stimulation for the client
    4. Reduce edema at the operative site

49. Following head and neck surgery for cancer of the tongue the client complains that the neck dressing is tight. The nurse should:
    1. Assess for signs of constriction
    2. Observe the dressing for bleeding
    3. Explain that the tight dressing is necessary
    4. Loosen the dressing to relieve the pressure

50. For clients who are terminally ill, the most important factor relative to therapeutic nurse-client relationships is the nurse's:
    1. Feelings about the situation
    2. Knowledge of the grieving process
    3. Recognition of the family's ability to cope
    4. Previous experience with terminally ill clients

51. The food combinations that can be included on a low-residue diet include:
    1. Baked fish, macaroni with cheese, strained carrots, fruit gelatin, milk
    2. Stewed chicken, baked potato with butter, strained peas, white bread, plain cake, milk
    3. Creamed soup and crackers, omelet, mashed potatoes, bran muffin, orange juice, coffee with milk
    4. Lean roast beef, buttered white rice with egg slices, white bread with butter and jelly, tea with sugar

52. A 36-year-old pregnant woman accompanied by her husband is admitted to labor and delivery, and fetal monitoring is instituted. When a fetus is being monitored, the nurse must realize that:
    1. Internal monitoring will be used in the latter part of labor
    2. The machinery can be very frightening to the laboring couple
    3. The mother may need a mild sedative every 4 hours for comfort
    4. Older primigravidas have more complications than younger women

53. A client with a history of endometriosis delivers a healthy baby. She expresses concern that the symptoms associated with endometriosis will return now that her pregnancy is over. The nurse's best response would be:
    1. "Pregnancy usually cures the endometriosis."
    2. "Endometriosis will usually cause an early menopause."
    3. "A hysterectomy will be necessary if the symptoms recur."
    4. "Breastfeeding your baby will delay the return of symptoms."

54. A client is breastfeeding her infant and complains that her breasts are swollen and painful. When teaching her about breastfeeding, the nurse should assist her in preventing engorgement in the future by telling her to:
    1. "Use a bottle for feeding when you are experiencing discomfort."
    2. "Limit nursing to 4 to 6 minutes on each breast, four times a day."
    3. "Nurse the baby frequently and for at least 10 minutes on each breast."
    4. "Feed the baby four times a day. This will prevent rapid filling of the breast."

55. When teaching a client about activities after discharge following a laryngectomy, the nurse should explain to the client that:
    1. Only humidified air should be breathed
    2. The daily intake of fluid should be limited
    3. A stomal cover should be worn over the stoma
    4. Mucus plugs can be removed with cotton-tipped swabs

56. The nurse plans interventions for a client with smoke inhalation based on a negative chest x-ray and arterial blood gases that show a Po_2 of 70 mm Hg, a Pco_2 of 45 mm Hg, and pH of 7.35 and the physician's orders. These interventions should include:
    1. Bronchial suctioning and bronchodilators
    2. Bronchodilators, coughing, and deep breathing
    3. Mechanical ventilation and bronchial suctioning
    4. Coughing and deep breathing and humidified oxygen

57. When performing tracheal suctioning for a client with a tracheostomy, the nurse should:
    1. Preoxygenate the client before suctioning
    2. Apply negative pressure as the catheter is being inserted
    3. Be sure the cuff of the tracheostomy is inflated during suctioning
    4. Instill acetylcysteine (Mucomyst) into the tracheostomy prior to suctioning to loosen secretions

58. When performing tracheostomy care, the nurse must:
    1. Place the client in the semi-Fowler's position
    2. Maintain sterile technique during the procedure
    3. Monitor the client's temperature after the procedure
    4. Use Betadine to clean the inner cannula when it is removed

59. At the end of the first trimester of pregnancy a client complains of feeling tired. The nurse recognizes that this is probably related to the normal cardiovascular changes which:
    1. Increase BP
    2. Increase hematocrit
    3. Increase blood volume
    4. Decrease cardiac output

60. During a prenatal class the nurse can help the participants understand an advantage of breast-feeding by explaining that:
    1. Breastfeeding inhibits ovulation in the mother
    2. Allergic responses are diminished in breastfed infants
    3. Breastfed infants adhere more easily to a 4-hour schedule
    4. Breast milk has a larger concentration of protein than does cow's milk

61. The nurse teaches a couple about care of their newborn who has been circumcised. The nurse would know that the teaching was effective when the father says, "We should:
    1. Observe for fussy behavior."
    2. Leave the infant undiapered."
    3. Apply petrolatum gauze to the penis."
    4. Notify the clinic if yellow exudate occurs."

62. The physician prescribes an estrogen-progestin oral contraceptive for a client. The nurse would know that teaching was effective when the client verbalizes that she should observe for the side effects of:
    1. Nausea, rash, and bleeding
    2. Lethargy, syncope, and tachycardia
    3. Hypertension, calf and breast tenderness
    4. Bradycardia, visual changes, and hypertension

63. When teaching parents about handling a child's attack of croup at home, the nurse recognizes that any action taken must be directed toward:
    1. Dilation of the bronchi
    2. Interruption of the spasm
    3. Reduction of the inflammation
    4. Depression of the cough center

64. The nurse teaches a mother that she can best help her toddler learn to control his or her own behavior by:
    1. Rewarding good behavior
    2. Setting limits and being consistent
    3. Punishing the child for misbehavior
    4. Allowing the child to learn by mistakes

65. The personality of a client with an obsessive-compulsive disorder is probably characterized by:
    1. Marked emotional maturity
    2. Elaborate delusional system
    3. Rapid, frequent mood swings
    4. Doubts, fears, and indecisiveness

66. The nurse should suspect lead-induced renal damage to the proximal tubules when a urinalysis of a $5^1/_2$-year-old demonstrates the presence of:
    1. Albumin
    2. Calcium
    3. Potassium
    4. Phosphate

67. A 3-year-old child is developmentally delayed. This conclusion is reinforced when the nurse observes that the child is unable to:
    1. Catch a ball
    2. Copy a square
    3. Balance on one foot
    4. Use a spoon effectively

68. A client calls the emergency department of the hospital after taking 24 sleeping tablets. By calling the emergency department during the very act of a suicide attempt the client has demonstrated:
    1. A need for attention
    2. A need to punish others
    3. An ambivalence about death
    4. An inability to stick to a decision

69. A client comes to the mental health clinic very depressed and with a high level of anxiety. The client expresses feelings of bitterness, hopelessness, helplessness, and despair. During the beginning phase of the relationship, the nurse would expect this client to respond to interpersonal approaches with:
    1. Anger
    2. Insight
    3. Elation and happiness
    4. Silence and withdrawal

70. During the beginning phase of a therapeutic relationship it is important that there is a clear understanding of the participant's roles because the client:
    1. Should understand what will be discussed
    2. Will then be able to develop trust in the relationship
    3. Should not have to guess about either person's role
    4. Will know that the nurse is interested and will be helpful

71. Two depressed clients are sharing a room. The health team has established a goal of increased socialization for each client. The action that would be most effective in facilitating interaction between these two client is:
    1. Taking them to a unit Bingo game together
    2. Putting a puzzle together with them in their room
    3. Exploring their reluctance to engage in conversation
    4. Suggesting that they watch television together in their room

72. Sertraline hydrochloride (Zoloft) has been ordered for a depressed client. When teaching about the drug the nurse should include the fact that:
    1. The drug can cause a hypertensive crisis
    2. The drug interferes with the reuptake of norepinephrine
    3. It may take several weeks before the effects of the drug will be evident
    4. Yogurt, bananas, and Chianti wine should be avoided when taking the drug

73. To prevent external rotation of a lower extremity, the nurse should place a pillow or sandbag:
    1. Under the client's lower affected leg
    2. By the ankle of the client's affected leg
    3. On the outside of the knee of the affected hip
    4. On the outside of the knee of the affected leg

74. A client with a history of alcoholism resumes drinking and returns to an in-house alcohol treatment program. On the client's return to the facility the nurse's best response would be:
    1. "You will die from postnecrotic cirrhosis if you continue to drink. Doesn't that bother you?"
    2. "You made some progress. Perhaps next time you can abstain for a longer period of time."
    3. "Hospitalization is useless unless you comply with the health team's recommendations."
    4. "You are an intelligent man. Certainly you must understand what you are doing to your health."

75. The most significant influence on many clients' perception of pain is their:
    1. Age and sex
    2. Overall physical status
    3. Intelligence and economic status
    4. Previous experience and cultural values

COMPREHENSIVE TEST 2: PART B

76. A client with chronic renal failure is to be treated with continuous ambulatory peritoneal dialysis (CAPD). This is done because it:
    1. Provides continuous contact of dialyzer and blood to clear toxins by ultrafiltration
    2. Exchanges and cleanses blood by correction of serum electrolytes and excretion of creatinine
    3. Decreases need for immobility of the client as it clears toxins in short intermittent periods
    4. Uses the peritoneum as a semipermeable membrane to clear toxins by osmosis and diffusion

77. The physician orders famotidine (Pepcid) 20 mg IVPB q12h. On hand is a vial labeled 10 mg/1 ml. The nurse should administer:
    1. 0.50 ml
    2. 1.0 ml
    3. 1.5 ml
    4. 2.0 ml

78. A 2-year-old child is admitted with multiple fractures and bruises and abuse is suspected. The nursing assessment that most supports this diagnosis in this child is:
    1. Bed wetting
    2. Thumb sucking
    3. Underdevelopment for age
    4. Demand for physical closeness

79. If there is a suspicion of child abuse, the nurse must:
    1. Report suspicions to the police
    2. Refer parents to a therapy group
    3. Report suspicions to the physician
    4. Elicit more information from parents

80. When caring for a $3^1/_2$-year-old child who is on bed rest, the nurse can help meet developmental needs by:
    1. Giving the child a stuffed animal
    2. Providing a coloring book and crayons
    3. Providing a set of large building blocks
    4. Taking the child to the playroom between naps

81. Because spasmodic croup may recur, the nurse's discharge teaching should include instructing the parents that if the child develops symptoms they should:
    1. Mechanically induce vomiting
    2. Call the emergency squad immediately
    3. Administer the prescribed antihistamine
    4. Take the child to the bathroom and run a hot shower

82. The mother of a 3-year-old child is concerned about how to handle temper tantrums. The nurse teaches the mother that temper tantrums:
    1. Should be ignored because they are a normal occurrence
    2. Frequently require counseling by a child guidance counselor
    3. Subside quickly if the mother holds the child during the tantrum
    4. Can be limited in frequency by providing a protective, nonstressful environment

83. For a client with an obsessive-compulsive personality disorder it is most important that the nurse:
    1. Allow the client sufficient time to carry out the ritual
    2. Promote reality by showing that the ritual serves little purpose
    3. Try to ascertain the meaning of the ritual by discussing it with the client
    4. Interrupt the ritual to demonstrate that the ritual does not control what happens

84. Recognizing that mothers whose children chronically ingest lead share certain characteristics, the nurse could best help prevent a recurrence by:
    1. Discussing with the mother ways to renovate her home to remove sources of lead
    2. Educating the mother about the dangers of lead ingestion and the type of treatment required
    3. Initiating referrals to appropriate social and public health service agencies for the total management of her problem
    4. Helping the mother recognize factors in her maternal-child interactions and in the home environment that predispose her child to pica

85. When a client has a tracheostomy tube and is on a ventilator, the tracheostomy tube must:
    1. Have an inner cannula
    2. Be changed every week
    3. Be cleansed once a day
    4. Have a low-pressure cuff

86. When scheduling segmental postural drainage treatments, the nurse should realize that the least appropriate time of day to receive this treatment is:
    1. At bedtime
    2. After a meal
    3. Before a meal
    4. On awakening

87. A client arrives in the postanesthesia care unit immediately following a segmental resection of the right lower lobe of the lung, with a chest tube drainage system in place. The nurse caring for the client should:
    1. Add 3 to 5 ml of sterile saline to the water seal chamber
    2. Raise the drainage system to bed level to check its patency
    3. Mark the time and the fluid level on the side of the drainage system
    4. Secure the chest catheter to the wound dressing with a sterile safety pin

88. A client returns to the unit fully awake following a bronchoscopy and biopsy. The nurse should:
    1. Provide ice chips to reduce swelling
    2. Advise the client to cough frequently
    3. Evaluate the presence of a gag reflex
    4. Advise the client to stay flat for 2 hours

89. The most effective way for the nurse to loosen secretions for a client with an endotracheal tube in place is by:
    1. Chest physiotherapy
    2. Increasing oral fluid intake
    3. Administering humidified oxygen
    4. Instilling a saturated solution of potassium iodide

90. In the immediate postoperative period following a right pneumonectomy it would be most beneficial for a client to be placed:
    1. In the high-Fowler's position
    2. Flat in bed with the knees flexed slightly
    3. On the right side with the head slightly elevated
    4. In the left Sims' position with the bed elevated 45°

91. A client is hospitalized with a diagnosis of possible cancer of the pancreas. On admission the client asks the nurse, "Do you think I have anything serious, like cancer?" The nurse's best reply would be:
    1. "What makes you think you have cancer?"
    2. "I don't know if you do, but let's talk about it."
    3. "Why don't you discuss this with your doctor?"
    4. "Don't worry, we won't know until all the test results are back."

92. A progressive ambulation schedule is instituted for an elderly hypertensive female client the morning after surgery. The client has been receiving antihypertensive medication and morphine sulfate for pain. When getting the client out of bed, the nurse should first have her sit on the edge of the bed with her feet dangling. This action is taken because the nurse expects the client's adaptation may be:
    1. Abdominal pain
    2. Initial hypertension
    3. Respiratory distress
    4. Postural hypotension

93. On the second day after surgery, a client complains of pain in the right calf. The nurse should first:
    1. Apply warm soaks
    2. Notify the physician
    3. Chart the symptoms
    4. Elevate the extremity above the heart

94. After experiencing a spontaneous abortion, a client states to the nurse, "We've always wanted this baby. How come this happened to us?" The nurse should be aware that the client is exhibiting the usual initial reaction to a loss, which is:
    1. Shock and denial
    2. Despair and anger
    3. Apathy and sadness
    4. Dissociation and rationalization

95. When assessing a newborn with a meningomyelocele, the nurse should suspect the possibility of hydrocephalus if the infant's:
    1. Cry sounds high pitched
    2. Apgar score was less than 5
    3. Meningomyelocele is in the lumbosacral area
    4. Head circumference is 2 to 3 cm greater than the chest circumference

96. A toddler with a repaired spina bifida demonstrates urinary incontinence and some flaccidity of the lower extremities. The teaching plan for the parents should include the fact that:
    1. An ileal bladder will be necessary once the child is of school age
    2. An indwelling Foley catheter offers the best hope for bladder management
    3. The child will probably need an intermittent straight catheterization program
    4. The child will probably wear diapers for a lifetime, since bladder training is impossible

97. Two hours after delivery, the nurse finds that a client's fundus is firm, shifted to the right, and two fingers above the umbilicus. This would indicate:
    1. A full bladder
    2. A normal process
    3. Impending bleeding
    4. Retained secundines

98. After delivery, when checking a client's vital signs, the nurse should normally find:
    1. Bradycardia with no change in respirations
    2. Tachycardia with a decrease in respirations
    3. Elevated basal temperature with a decrease in respirations
    4. Slight lowering of basal temperature with an increase in respirations

99. Nursing care of a newborn with a cephalhematoma is directed primarily toward:
    1. Supporting the parents
    2. Recording neurologic signs
    3. Protecting the infant's head
    4. Applying ice packs to the hematoma

100. The physician tells a mother that her newborn has multiple visible birth defects. The mother seems quite composed and asks to see her baby. To assess the mother's reaction the nurse should:
    1. Bring the baby to her immediately
    2. Tell her exactly what the baby looks like before bringing the baby to her
    3. Encourage her to express and explore her feelings, bring the baby to her, and stay with her during this time
    4. Show her some pictures, give her some literature, and discuss the treatment with her before bringing the baby to her

101. An older client is apprehensive about being hospitalized. The nurse realizes that one of the stresses of hospitalization is the strangeness of the environment and activity. Extension of this stress can best be limited by:
    1. Using the client's first name
    2. Visiting with the client frequently
    3. Explaining what behavior is expected
    4. Listening to what the client has to say

102. Since sodium is the major cation controlling fluid outside the cells, diet therapy in heart failure with subsequent edema is aimed at reducing the sodium intake. When teaching about the diet, the nurse should encourage the client to exclude:
    1. Fruits
    2. Grains
    3. Vegetables
    4. Processed foods

103. During the first visit to the prenatal clinic by a pregnant woman, a pelvic examination will be performed. Teaching about this examination should include telling the client:
    1. She must relax during the examination to prevent discomfort
    2. A douche prior to the examination is necessary for cleanliness
    3. A rectal examination may be included after the pelvic examination
    4. After the examination she should direct any questions to the physician

104. The fetus of a laboring woman is at +1 station. This indicates that the fetus' head is:
    1. Not yet engaged
    2. Entering the pelvic inlet
    3. Below the ischial spines
    4. Visible at the vaginal opening

105. Emergency equipment that should be at the bedside of a client after a thyroidectomy includes:
    1. A crash cart with bedboard
    2. A tracheostomy set and oxygen
    3. An airway and rebreathing mask
    4. Two ampules of sodium bicarbonate

106. When a client returns from surgery after a thyroidectomy the nurse should assess for unilateral injury of the pharyngeal nerve by:
    1. Asking the client to speak
    2. Checking the client for neck edema
    3. Observing the client for signs of tetany
    4. Palpating the client's neck for blood seepage

107. When providing discharge instructions to a client who has had a thyroidectomy, the nurse should teach the client to observe for signs of surgically induced hypothyroidism, including:
    1. Intolerance to heat
    2. Dry skin and fatigue
    3. Insomnia and excitability
    4. Emaciation and weight loss

108. A woman is admitted in labor and is diagnosed with herpes simplex virus type 2 (HSV-2) with active lesions in the perineal area. The nurse's plan of care should include:
    1. Withholding the intake of oral fluids
    2. Obtaining a permit for a paracervical block
    3. Instructing her on bottle-feeding techniques
    4. Applying moist compresses to the perineal area

109. A client has a cesarean delivery. When performing discharge teaching, the nurse recognizes that additional teaching is required when the client says:
    1. "I can take a Percocet tablet if my incision hurts."
    2. "If I don't have a bowel movement, I can take a mild laxative."
    3. "I can begin mild exercises once my abdominal discomfort has decreased."
    4. "I don't need special perineal care because I didn't have a vaginal delivery."

110. A client in a psychiatric unit and who has been acting out for several weeks approaches the nurse and says, "I'm really sorry about how I've acted. I bet everyone thinks I'm a big fool." The nurse's best initial response would be:
    1. "You're wondering how others will react to you now."
    2. "Some clients are concerned that you might lose control again."
    3. "Everyone feels foolish sometimes. You didn't deliberately act that way."
    4. "Nobody thinks you're a fool. Everyone recognized you were really struggling to keep control."

111. Three days after admission to the hospital for meningitis, a spinal tap is done to assess a child's response to therapy. The nurse correctly interprets that the child's condition is improving when the report of the spinal fluid indicates:
    1. Decreased protein
    2. Decreased glucose
    3. Increased cell count
    4. Increased specific gravity

112. When teaching a client with pulmonary tuberculosis about recovery after discharge, the nurse should plan to reinforce that the treatment measure with the highest priority is:
    1. Having sufficient rest
    2. Getting plenty of fresh air
    3. Changing lifestyle routines
    4. Consistently taking ordered medication

113. A client sustains a crushing injury to the lower left leg and a below-the-knee amputation is performed. When monitoring for the common complication of pulmonary embolus, the nurse should assess this client for:
    1. Pain in the residual limb
    2. Diminished breath sounds
    3. Absence of the popliteal pulse
    4. Blanching of the affected extremity

114. After surgery for an amputation of a lower extremity, the residual limb is kept bandaged at all times to:
    1. Limit edema of the tissues
    2. Decrease keloid formation
    3. Prevent maceration of the skin
    4. Promote psychologic adjustment

115. During a follow-up visit after a below-the-knee amputation, the nurse would have to do further teaching when the client says:
    1. "When I sit in a chair, I put my legs out straight on an ottoman."
    2. "I apply a firm, even bandage around the end of my affected leg every day."
    3. "At night I keep a pillow under my knees because it feels more comfortable."
    4. "I press the end of my affected leg against a soft surface several times during the day."

116. If a $3^1/_2$-year-old child began receiving immunizations on schedule, the nurse would expect the child to have had the following immunizations:
    1. 2 DTaPs, 2 IVPs, rubella, measles
    2. 3 DTaPs, 3 IVPs, measles, mumps
    3. 3 DTaPs, measles, mumps, rubella
    4. 4 DTaPs, 3 IVPs, measles, mumps, rubella

117. The parents of a 3-year-old tell the nurse that their child has become a "picky eater" and has not gained much weight. An appropriate response by the nurse would be:
    1. "This is not normal; your child may be sick."
    2. "This is a fast growth period, so you need to give your child vitamins."
    3. "Preschoolers do not have large appetites because this is a slow growth period."
    4. "Preschoolers enjoy gifts; provide a reward when your child eats an entire meal."

118. When a client has gluteal edema, the nurse should not use the gluteus maximus muscle for administration of intramuscular medications mainly because at edematous sites:
    1. Deposition of an injected drug causes pain
    2. Blood supply is insufficient for drug absorption
    3. Fluid leaks from the site for long periods after injection
    4. Tissue fluid dilutes the drug before it enters the circulation

119. While assisting a client with a repaired fractured hip to transfer from the bed to a wheelchair, the nurse should remember that:
    1. During a weight-bearing transfer the client's knees should be slightly bent
    2. The appropriate proximity and visual relationship of wheelchair to bed must be maintained
    3. Transfers to and from the wheelchair will be easier if the bed is higher than the wheelchair
    4. The transfer can be accomplished by pivoting while bearing weight on both upper extremities and not on the legs

120. A surgical client has a portable wound-drainage system in place. An important nursing intervention to promote drainage includes:
    1. Irrigating the drainage tube with saline
    2. Applying warm compresses to the involved site
    3. Maintaining compression of the drainage system
    4. Keeping the involved area in a dependent position

121. The nurse knows that Alzheimer's disease is characterized by:
    1. Transient ischemic attacks
    2. Remissions and exacerbations
    3. Rapid deterioration of mental functioning because of arteriosclerosis
    4. Slowly progressive deficits in intellect, which may not be noted for a long time

122. An elderly female client with Alzheimer's disease frequently switches from being pleasant and happy to being hostile and sad without apparent external cause. The nurse can best care for the client by:
    1. Trying to point out reality to the client
    2. Avoiding the client when she is angry and sad
    3. Encouraging the client to talk about her feelings
    4. Attempting to give nursing care when the client is in a pleasant mood

123. The nurse should provide a confused client with an environment that is:
    1. Familiar
    2. Variable
    3. Challenging
    4. Nonstimulating

124. Clients who have a cognitive disorder need assistance in maintaining contact with others for as long as possible. A therapy that might help a client achieve this goal is:
    1. Psychodrama
    2. Recreation therapy
    3. Remotivation therapy
    4. Occupational therapy

125. The prime objective for nursing intervention for clients with dementia, delirium, or other cognitive disorders is to stimulate:
    1. Interaction with the environment
    2. Diminished psychologic faculties
    3. Participation in educational activities
    4. Face-to-face contact with other clients

126. The physician prescribes steroid therapy for a 4-year-old who has nephrotic syndrome. The nurse understands that the goal of this treatment is to:

1. Reduce the BP
2. Cause diuresis
3. Prevent infection
4. Provide hemopoiesis

127. Of the following lunches, the most appropriate lunch for a child on a low-sodium diet would be:
    1. Macaroni and cheese, fresh pears, V-8 juice
    2. Chicken, navy beans, fresh peaches, lemonade
    3. Cheeseburger on a bun, fresh green beans, iced tea
    4. Bacon and tomato sandwich, canned chicken noodle soup, low-sodium milk

128. A $3^1/_2$-year-old boy has been ill with nephrotic syndrome. As he begins to improve, his behavior regresses. He has been toilet-trained for more than a year but has been wetting himself lately. His mother expresses concern over his behavior. The nurse's most therapeutic response to the mother would be:
    1. "He is wetting the bed to get attention. Reprimand him when he does this."
    2. "The incontinence is due to his renal disease. It will improve as he gets better."
    3. "This is a normal response to hospitalization. Ignore his regressive behavior and be supportive of him."
    4. "He is using this regressive behavior to help him cope with hospitalization; just place him in diapers and say nothing."

129. At the time of delivery a baby's blood is typed to determine the ABO group and the presence of the Rh factor. The nurse is aware that:
    1. The Rh factor is not genetically determined
    2. Not all infants of Rh-positive fathers are Rh positive
    3. The Rh factor of the fetus is determined by the father
    4. During gestation, the Rh factor of the fetus may change

130. When the nurse brings a newborn baby to the mother, the mother comments about the milia on the baby's face. The nurse should:
    1. Tell her that all babies have them and they clear up in 2 to 3 days
    2. Instruct her to avoid squeezing them or attempting to wash them off
    3. Instruct her about proper hand washing, since the milia can be infectious
    4. Explain that these are birthmarks that will disappear within a few months

131. Two hours after a child with acute laryngitis (croup) is admitted, the nurse observes an increase in the child's respiratory and cardiac rates, increased restlessness, and substernal and intercostal retractions. The nurse, acting on these observations, should immediately:
    1. Remove secretions with suction apparatus
    2. Increase the level of oxygen being delivered
    3. Strike the child on the back to dislodge mucus
    4. Inform the physician of the child's respiratory status

132. The mother of a well child receiving a screening test for TB asks the nurse what a positive reaction would mean. The nurse's best reply would be that it indicates:
    1. A depressed immune system
    2. An active tuberculosis infection
    3. Previous exposure to the organism
    4. That a tuberculosis infection is imminent

133. A client sustains a crushing chest injury in an automobile accident and a chest tube is inserted. One symptom that is considered unique to a fat embolus in a client with a traumatic chest injury is:
    1. A decreased cardiac output
    2. Petechial hemorrhages on the thorax
    3. Red chest tube drainage of 50 ml/4 hr
    4. A decreasing central venous pressure

134. To ensure accuracy when assessing a client's blood pressure, the nurse should avoid parallax error by:
    1. Elevating the head of the bed
    2. Using an appropriate size cuff
    3. Reading the manometer at eye level
    4. Placing the cuff at the level of the heart

135. A client with a myocardial infarction is admitted to the hospital and the physician orders digoxin (Lanoxin), propranolol (Inderal), furosemide (Lasix), spironolactone (Aldactone), and warfarin (Coumadin). After 1 week, the client complains of loss of appetite and nausea. The nurse should recognize that these symptoms indicate:
    1. Adverse effects of Lanoxin
    2. Therapeutic effects of Lasix
    3. Adverse effects of Aldactone
    4. Therapeutic effects of Inderal

136. A client is anxious and the physician orders alprazolam (Xanax) 5 mg po tid. Before implementing this order, the nurse should first:
    1. Assess the apical pulse
    2. Assess the blood pressure
    3. Encourage ventilation of feelings
    4. Clarify the order with the physician

137. A pregnant woman at term is admitted to the birthing center. She is 100% effaced, 3 cm dilated, and at +1 station. Based on this assessment, the nurse identifies the client's labor as:
    1. First stage
    2. Latent stage
    3. Second stage
    4. Transitional stage

138. A woman's pregnancy has been uneventful and she has gained 25 pounds. At term her hemoglobin level is 10.6 and hematocrit level is 31%. The nurse understands that this client's hematocrit level is most likely representative of:
    1. Infection
    2. Hemodilution
    3. Nutritional deficits
    4. Concealed bleeding

139. A client asks the nurse how the urine tests that can be purchased detect pregnancy. The nurse bases a response on the fact that the hormone responsible for a positive result is:
    1. Estrogen
    2. Progesterone
    3. Human chorionic gonadotropin
    4. Human chorionic somatomammotropin

140. A 28-year-old man is admitted to the psychiatric unit for the third time in one year with a diagnosis of chronic schizophrenia, paranoid type. He shows the nurse a keychain and says it protects him from the evil forces. He quickly hides it yelling, "Don't take it away from me, it's the only thing that protects me." The nurse's best response would be:
    1. "You can keep it because I know it is important to you."
    2. "You better put it away if it's valuable or someone will take it."
    3. "I must take it away from you because you may hurt yourself."
    4. "There are no evil forces here; you are safe without the chain."

141. A client with schizophrenia, paranoid type, tells the nurse, "God singled me out and gave me special powers." The nurse recognizes that this grandiose delusion is precipitated by feelings of:
    1. Compulsiveness and fear
    2. Powerlessness and anxiety
    3. Paranoia and ego disturbance
    4. Self-esteem and accomplishment

142. A client diagnosed with schizophrenia, paranoid type, is obviously angry about being readmitted to the hospital at the insistance of the family. When exploring feelings about the readmission, the client angrily turns away and shouts, "You're one of them. Leave me alone." The nurse's best response would be:
    1. "Try not to be afraid. I will not hurt you."
    2. "I am not one of them. I am here to help you."
    3. "I can see you are upset. We can talk more later."
    4. "Your family and the staff are trying to help you."

143. A client in active labor has a cervix that is dilated 3 cm. The nurse supports her by reinforcing the breathing technique of:
    1. Pant-blow breathing
    2. Slow chest breathing
    3. Rapid chest breathing
    4. Slow abdominal breathing

144. In the second stage of labor the nurse should plan to discourage a pregnant client from holding her breath more than 6 seconds while pushing with each contraction to prevent:
    1. Fetal hypoxia
    2. Perineal lacerations
    3. Carpopedal spasms
    4. Maternal hypertension

145. Two weeks after sustaining a spinal cord injury a client begins vomiting thick coffee-ground material and appears restless and apprehensive. It is most important for the nurse to:
    1. Change the client's diet to bland
    2. Prepare for insertion of a nasogastric tube
    3. Check laboratory reports for hemoglobin level
    4. Collect a stool specimen and check for occult blood

146. A client who has sustained multiple serious injuries from a motor vehicle accident is diagnosed as having a stress ulcer. When caring for this client, the nurse should immediately report:
    1. Nausea, weakness, and headache
    2. Dyspepsia, distention, and diarrhea
    3. Complaints of thirst and warm, flushed skin
    4. Tachycardia, diaphoresis, and cold extremities

147. A college athlete sustained a severance of the spinal cord while practicing on the trampoline. The physician explained to him that he is a paraplegic. Three weeks later the client says he must get out of the hospital to practice for an upcoming tournament. The nurse should realize that the client is:
    1. Exhibiting denial
    2. Verbalizing a fantasy
    3. No longer able to adapt
    4. Extremely motivated to get well

148. The most important weak or absent reflex for the nurse to report in the evaluation of a newborn is:
    1. Gag
    2. Moro
    3. Babinski
    4. Tonic neck

149. When changing a newborn female, the nurse notices a brick-red stain on the diaper. This is:
    1. A symptom of low iron excretion
    2. To be expected in female babies
    3. A normal but uncommon occurrence
    4. Due to medication given to the mother

150. Proper positioning of an infant with hydrocephalus is essential to prevent breakdown of the scalp. A suitable position would be:
    1. Supine and Trendelenburg
    2. Positioned on either side and flat
    3. Prone, with the legs elevated about 30°
    4. Prone or supine, with the head elevated about 45°

151. An infant has a noncommunicating hydrocephalus, and a ventriculoperitoneal shunt is performed. When caring for the infant postoperatively, the nurse should:
    1. Avoid touching the valve for 24 hours
    2. Position the infant flat for about 48 hours
    3. Administer sedatives and analgesics to promote rest
    4. Encourage the parents to pick their child up to prevent crying

152. Varicose veins are usually the result of:
    1. Defective valves within the veins
    2. The formation of thrombophlebitis
    3. Atherosclerotic plaques along the veins
    4. External compression of the muscles of the legs

153. A female client is going to have sclerotherapy for varicose veins. The nurse explains that prior to the procedure the physician must be certain:
1. She understands the need to lose weight
2. She is to avoid ambulation for 3 to 5 days
3. The saphenous vein has no sign of aneurysms
4. The valves at the saphenofemoral junction are competent

154. When monitoring a client in labor, the nurse notices a gush of fluid from the client's vagina. After checking the fetal heart, the nurse should:
1. Place the client on her side and obtain her BP
2. Keep the client flat in bed and elevate her legs
3. Notify the physician immediately about the gush of fluid from the vagina
4. Place the client in a modified lithotomy position and inspect the perineum

155. When a client in labor is being infused with oxytocin (Pitocin), it is the nurse's responsibility to:
1. Flush the IV tubing if the flow slows
2. Monitor fetal heart tones every 2 hours
3. Shut off the infusion in the presence of hypertonic contractions
4. Obtain a physician's order to slow the IV in the presence of hypertonic contractions

156. When the nurse first talks with a client coming to the clinic, the type of interview that is likely to be most productive is:
1. Directive
2. Exploratory
3. Problem solving
4. Information giving

157. A mother and father are in the waiting room for their first clinic appointment for their newborn. Accompanying them is their 18-month-old toddler. At the beginning of the intake interview the infant is due for a bottlefeeding and the toddler is playing on the floor. At this time the nurse's best action would be to ask the father if he would mind:
1. Giving the baby a bottle
2. Taking the toddler for a walk
3. Participating in the discussion
4. Leaving the nurse and the mother alone

158. A 15-month-old child has had no inoculations. The father says he does not believe in them. The nurse's best response to this statement would be:
1. "You feel they may be harmful?"
2. "Scientific evidence proves you wrong."
3. "How can you risk the life of your child?"
4. "Have you discussed this with your doctor?"

159. The initial immunizations for an unimmunized 14-month-old would include:
1. Measles, rubella, and mumps (MMR) combined vaccine
2. Diphtheria and tetanus toxoids and pertussis vaccine (DTaP) and trivalent poliovirus vaccine (IPV)
3. Combined tetanus and diphtheria toxoid (Td), trivalent oral poliovirus vaccine, and tuberculin test
4. Diphtheria and tetanus toxoids and pertussis vaccine (DTaP), trivalent poliovirus vaccine (IPV), and tuberculin test

160. A pathophysiologic change underlying the production of symptoms in leukemia is:
1. Excessive destruction of blood cells in liver and spleen
2. Progressive replacement of bone marrow with fibrous tissue
3. Proliferation and release of immature white blood cells into the circulating blood
4. Destruction of red blood cells and platelets by an overproduction of white blood cells

161. A client is diagnosed with cancer of the prostate and a suprapubic prostatectomy is to be performed. In answer to the client's question, the nurse explains that a suprapubic prostatectomy differs from other surgical procedures of the prostate in that:
1. An indwelling catheter is not required after surgery
2. An incision is made directly into the urinary bladder
3. A major complication, that of sexual impotence, may occur
4. The postoperative convalescent period is shorter in time

162. To prevent bleeding after a suprapubic prostatectomy, the client should be instructed to avoid straining on defecation. Therefore, the nurse should advise him to increase his intake of:
1. Milk products
2. Ripe bananas
3. Green vegetables
4. Creamed potatoes

163. After a suprapubic prostatectomy, the client should be encouraged to walk but cautioned not to sit for prolonged periods because prolonged sitting:
1. Increases the risk of bleeding
2. Potentiates the risk of infection
3. Decreases the amount of urine
4. Produces the Valsalva maneuver

164. After a suprapubic prostatectomy the client develops signs of a postoperative wound infection and is placed on an antibiotic regimen of cefazolin (Ancef) 1 g q6h IV and gentamicin 80 mg q8h IV. When administering these drugs, the nurse should:
   1. Dissolve each of the drugs in 10 ml of diluent and administer them as an IV bolus
   2. Change the IV tubing between drugs, not allowing them to come in contact with each other
   3. Dissolve each drug in a separate liter of IV fluid and administer over the prescribed interval
   4. Mix them together and administer as one dose whenever possible to maintain the time schedule

165. A neonate is admitted to the high-risk nursery with a meningomyelocele. During the first 24 hours it would be most appropriate for the nurse to:
   1. Wash the genital area with Betadine
   2. Place baby prone in a slight Trendelenburg position
   3. Perform neurologic checks above the site of the lesion
   4. Apply disposable diapers to monitor intake and output

166. An infant who has had a surgical correction of a meningomyelocele is to be discharged. To prepare the parents to care for the infant at home, the nurse should plan to:
   1. Discuss the need to limit the infant's fluid intake to formula
   2. Demonstrate restrictive positions to prevent the infant from turning
   3. Explaining the need to provide a quiet environment to limit external stimuli
   4. Teach the parents how to do passive range-of-motion exercises to the lower extremities

167. The parents of a child who has had a surgical repair of a meningomyelocele express concern about skin care and ask what they can do to avoid problems. The nurse plans to reinforce that their child:
   1. Must be kept dry and powder applied with each diaper change
   2. Needs scrupulous cleaning and more frequent diaper changes
   3. Should have vitamin A and D ointment applied after each diaper change
   4. Does not need anything more than routine cleansing and diaper changes

168. Septra is prescribed for a child with a urinary tract infection. The nurse recognizes that the father understands how to administer this drug when he states:
   1. "This drug is given with small sips of milk."
   2. "This drug should be given with 6 to 8 ounces of water."
   3. "This drug has to be given every 4 hours to maintain a blood level."
   4. "This drug must be given with orange juice to ensure acidity of urine."

169. A child is to receive an acid-ash diet. The nurse would recognize that the mother understands the dietary teaching when she states that the child's lunch can include:
   1. Fried chicken, corn, rice, milk, peaches
   2. Egg salad sandwich, cookies, plum, milk
   3. Peanut butter sandwich, cookies, prune juice
   4. Macaroni and cheese, banana, chocolate milk

170. A child with a history of a meningomyelocele will be attending nursery school. Because of the child's problems, the mother contacts the school nurse. The nurse should advise her to:
   1. Have her child wear plastic pants during school
   2. Provide an extra supply of diapers for the child's use
   3. Come in so that the child's needs can be discussed more fully
   4. Suggest that entering nursery school should be delayed for another year

171. To reduce a fracture of the hip, a client is placed in Buck's traction before surgery. Because the client keeps slipping down in bed, increased countertraction is ordered. The nurse increases countertraction by:
   1. Elevating the head of the bed
   2. Adding more weight to the traction
   3. Using a slight Trendelenburg position
   4. Tying a chest restraint around the client

172. On the second postoperative day after an open reduction and internal fixation of a fractured hip, the client is to get out of bed into a chair. The best way to accomplish this is to:
   1. Slide the client from the bed to the chair without weight bearing
   2. Have the client stand on the unaffected leg and pivot to the chair
   3. Ask the client to put weight equally on both legs and step to the chair
   4. Lift the client from the bed to the chair with the assistance of several people

173. An 85-year-old client is alert and able to participate in care. The nurse is aware that, according to Erikson, a person's adjustment to the period of senescence will depend largely on adjustment to the developmental stage of:
    1. Intimacy vs isolation
    2. Industry vs inferiority
    3. Identity vs role diffusion
    4. Generativity vs stagnation

174. An IV is started to administer edetate calcium disodium (EDTA) to a 2-year-old child with plumbism (lead poisoning). To prevent the child from pulling out the IV, the nurse should:
    1. Keep the arms restrained
    2. Tell the child not to touch the IV
    3. Cover the IV site with an overwrap
    4. Have a family member hold the child

175. The nurse should encourage the parents of a child with plumbism (lead poisoning) to:
    1. Discourage the child's pica by providing nutritious snacks
    2. Stop the child from playing in the yard, which is next to a gasoline station
    3. Assess the home environment for all lead sources and have them removed
    4. Repeat wrist and forearm x-ray films to determine when the lead line is gone

176. The nurse would expect diagnostic studies performed on a client with hyperparathyroidism to demonstrate:
    1. Demineralization of bone
    2. Consistently low serum calcium
    3. Negative Sulkowitch test of urine
    4. Decreased urinary excretion of calcium

177. A client with arthritis is to begin long-term steroid therapy. When evaluating the effectiveness of teaching about the drug, the nurse should assess the client's understanding that:
    1. Weight loss is to be expected
    2. The urine may become discolored
    3. Steroids should be taken between meals
    4. The risk of developing infections is increased

178. A pregnant woman in labor is 9 cm dilated and wants to push. The nurse should:
    1. Have her pant-blow during contractions
    2. Place her legs in stirrups to facilitate pushing
    3. Encourage her to bear down with each contraction
    4. Review the pushing techniques taught in the Lamaze class

179. An infant has been experiencing vomiting after feedings. The physical assessment reveals poor skin turgor, a sunken anterior fontanel, an olive-shaped mass in the right upper abdomen, and epigastric distention. The nurse is aware that this infant's acid-base balance is primarily upset by:
    1. Loss of fluid via the kidneys
    2. Lack of blood supply to body cells
    3. Retention of potassium in the cells
    4. Loss of chloride ions in the vomitus

180. When feeding an infant with pyloric stenosis the nurse should be aware that after a feeding it is likely that this child will:
    1. Have loud and high-pitched bowel sounds
    2. Spit up small amounts of formula when burped
    3. Suddenly expel large amounts of diarrheal stool
    4. Exhibit peristaltic waves traversing the epigastrium

181. The priority discharge criteria for a client with anxiety would have to include that the client is able to:
    1. Verbalize positive aspects about the self
    2. Follow rules and regulations of the milieu
    3. Verbalize signs of increasing anxiety and to maintain it at a manageable level
    4. Recognize that hallucinations occur at times of extreme anxiety and can be controlled

182. A 5-year-old male child in kindergarten asks to go to the bathroom about every hour. The school nurse calls the mother to get some further information about this problem and asks:
    1. "Has your child had a physical lately?"
    2. "Does your child wet the bed at night?"
    3. "Has your child had a short attention span?"
    4. "Does your child go to the bathroom often at home?"

183. A child is diagnosed as having type 1 diabetes mellitus. The school nurse sets up a plan of care that includes:
    1. Limiting fluid intake during school hours
    2. Asking the child each day what was eaten for breakfast
    3. Noting the presence of diabetes in the file but treating the child like other children
    4. Checking daily for injuries because of participation in the physical education program

184. A client with Addison's disease is receiving cortisone therapy. In the event that the client neglects to continue the cortisone therapy, an acute adrenocortical insufficiency may occur. The predominant symptom the client should be advised to report is:
    1. Dysphagia
    2. Hypertension
    3. Muscle spasms
    4. A high body temperature

185. Clients on prolonged cortisone therapy may exhibit side effects caused by its glucocorticoid and mineralocorticoid actions. The nurse should teach the client and family to observe for side effects, which include:
    1. Hypoglycemia and anuria
    2. Hypotension and fluid loss
    3. Anorexia and hyperkalemia
    4. Weight gain and moon face

186. A female client receiving cortisone therapy for adrenal insufficiency expresses concern about the fact that she is developing signs of masculinity. The nurse should tell her:
    1. That this is due to therapy
    2. It is a further sign of the illness
    3. Not to worry, because it will disappear with therapy
    4. That this is not important, so long as she is feeling better

187. A plan of care to best meet the needs of a neglected child should include:
    1. A plan to have staff members pick up and play with the child whenever they can
    2. As consistent a caregiver as possible, with stimulation that is moderate and purposeful
    3. A vigorous schedule of stimulation geared to the infant's present level of development
    4. A schedule of care that allows the infant stimulation and physical contact by several staff members

188. Conversion disorder is the term used to describe the phenomenon wherein anxiety associated with stress or conflict has been repressed and converted into specific physical manifestations. One of the characteristics of the client's reaction to the physical symptom is:
    1. Anger
    2. Anxiety
    3. Agitation
    4. Indifference

189. A client is scheduled for an occupational therapy group. While listening to instructions for the group project, the client experiences a feeling of weakness and is unable to move the right arm. After a check of pulse and respirations, the nurse's best response would be:
    1. "Exactly when did the weakness begin?"
    2. "Would you like to leave the group for a while?"
    3. "Is this similar to what you usually experience?"
    4. "What emotion were you feeling before you felt the weakness?"

190. A female client is very upset with her diagnosis of gonorrhea and asks the nurse, "What can I do to prevent getting another infection in the future?" The nurse is aware that the teaching has been understood when the client states, "My best protection is to:
    1. Douche after every intercourse."
    2. Avoid engaging in sexual behavior."
    3. Insist that my partner use a condom."
    4. Use a spermicidal cream with intercourse."

191. A client who is 39 weeks pregnant and a diabetic is admitted to the hospital to await delivery. The nurse can best answer the client's questions about why hospitalization is necessary by recalling that in pregnant women with diabetes:
    1. Complete rest prior to the work of delivery is essential
    2. Fetal development is completed and should be monitored
    3. Fetal death may occur after the thirty-sixth week of gestation
    4. Insulin needs to be administered intravenously before labor begins

192. The nurse teaches a woman with diabetes that the oral hypoglycemic pills used prior to pregnancy cannot be used during pregnancy because:
    1. They may produce deformities in the fetus
    2. The effect of exogenous insulin on the fetus is uncertain
    3. In the latter part of pregnancy, diabetes can usually be controlled by diet alone
    4. The fetal pancreas compensates for the mother's inability to secrete adequate insulin

193. When caring for the newborn infant of a mother with diabetes, the nursery nurse should be alert for a sign of hypoglycemia, which is:
    1. Poor sucking reflex
    2. Extreme restlessness
    3. Excessive birth weight
    4. Pallor of the skin and mucosa

194. The rate of fluid replacement for a client with severe burns during the immediate hypovolemic stage is considered satisfactory if the urinary output is approximately:
1. Half the intake
2. Equal to the intake
3. One-third the intake
4. One-tenth the intake

195. To promote the nutritional status of a client during the acute phase of treatment following extensive burns, when the client is permitted to ingest food and fluids, it is most important to:
1. Encourage an increased intake of sodium
2. Limit caloric intake to decrease the work of the body
3. Reduce protein intake to avoid overtaxing the kidneys
4. Encourage drinking a variety of fluids containing vitamin C

196. In the acute phase of treatment following full-thickness burns, the nurse should be aware that:
1. Death may still occur from septicemia
2. The danger of physical complications is past
3. Because of the client's need for rest, diversional therapy must be delayed
4. Mirrors should be removed to decrease the client's anxiety about appearance

197. Activities that would be most therapeutic for the hyperactive client and that the nurse should encourage include:
1. Carving figures out of wood
2. Lacing tooled leather wallets
3. Stenciling designs on copper sheeting
4. Sanding and varnishing wooden bookends

198. A male client is noisy, loud, and disruptive. The nurse informs the client that, unless he is more quiet, he will be isolated and put in restraints, if necessary. Legally:
1. The information given the client is actually a threat
2. Restraint of the client is justified for the client's own protection
3. This client's behavior is to be expected and should be ignored
4. Clients who are hyperactive and disruptive cannot be expected to understand instructions

199. During a period of hyperactivity, a client demands to be allowed to go downtown to shop. The client does not have privileges at the present time. The nurse's best response would be:

1. "You cannot leave the unit."
2. "You'll have to ask your doctor."
3. "Not right now. I don't have a staff member to go with you."
4. "I'm sorry, you can't go. Let's look through this new catalog."

200. A client is admitted with the diagnosis of possible placenta previa. Nursing care of this client includes:
1. Inspecting for hemorrhage
2. Withholding food and fluids
3. Avoiding all extraneous stimuli
4. Encouraging ambulation with supervision

201. If a vaginal examination is to be performed on a client with possible placenta previa, the nurse must be prepared for an immediate:
1. Forceps delivery
2. Induction of labor
3. Cesarean delivery
4. X-ray examination

202. A newborn weighing 2840 g (6 lbs 4 oz) should have a daily intake of:
1. 888 ml (30 oz) of fluid and 500 calories
2. 740 ml (25 oz) of fluid and 450 calories
3. 592 ml (20 oz) of fluid and 400 calories
4. 532.8 ml (18 oz) of fluid and 375 calories

203. A nurse discovers a client lying on the floor. After ascertaining that the person is unresponsive, the nurse should:
1. Call for assistance
2. Establish an airway
3. Check the carotid pulse
4. Obtain the blood pressure

204. A client's cardiac monitor shows ventricular fibrillation. The nurse from the coronary care unit should prepare for:
1. Elective cardioversion
2. Immediate defibrillation
3. An IM injection of digoxin (Lanoxin)
4. An IV line for emergency medications

205. Because the cells are deprived of oxygen during a cardiac arrest, metabolic acidosis may develop. The nurse should be prepared to administer:
1. Regular insulin
2. Calcium gluconate
3. Potassium chloride
4. Sodium bicarbonate

206. Following abdominal surgery, a client is transferred to the postanesthesia care unit with a nasogastric tube in place. When the client vomits 90 ml of bile-colored fluid, the nurse should:
    1. Administer an antiemetic
    2. Elevate the head of the bed
    3. Check the patency of the tube
    4. Encourage the client to breathe deeply

207. A cardiac catheterization is performed on an infant. After the procedure the leg used for the catheter insertion site becomes mottled. The nurse should immediately:
    1. Elevate the leg
    2. Cover the baby with a blanket
    3. Check the pulse in the extremity
    4. Notify the physician of the situation

208. The mother of a newborn asks how long she should continue to scrupulously scrub her baby's bottles. Prior to replying, the nurse should remember that during early infancy:
    1. The gastric acidity is low and unable to provide bacteriostatic protection
    2. Infants are almost completely lacking in immunity and need sterile fluids
    3. The absence of hydrochloric acid renders the stomach vulnerable to infection
    4. *Escherichia coli*, the bacterium normally found in the stomach, does not act on milk

209. When caring for the depressed client, the nurse should keep in mind that:
    1. Clients with simple depressions rarely attempt suicide
    2. Depressed clients are potentially suicidal during the entire course of their illness
    3. Opportunities to attempt suicide are practically absent on a locked psychiatric unit
    4. Once the severe depression begins to lift, the danger of suicide is no longer a problem

210. A depressed client appears preoccupied and remains seated when it is time for the clients to go to eat. The nurse's best approach would be to:
    1. Take the client by the hand and lead the client to the dining room
    2. Overlook the client not eating and leave snacks in the client's room
    3. Tell the client that now is the time to eat, since no food will be served later
    4. Ask the client whether a tray in the room would be preferable to going to the dining room

211. A client taking lithium carbonate is going home for a 3-day weekend pass. The nurse should advise the client to:
    1. Have a snack with milk before going to bed
    2. Avoid participation in controversial discussions
    3. Adjust the lithium dosage if mood changes are noted
    4. Continue to maintain a normal sodium intake while at home

212. A client with a history of heart failure admits to the nurse that a salt-restricted diet has not been followed and increased ankle edema, orthopnea, and dyspnea on exertion are now being experienced. The nurse should be alert for other signs of fluid retention such as:
    1. Dizziness on rising
    2. Rhinitis and headache
    3. A weak and thready pulse
    4. A decreased hemoglobin and hematocrit

213. During the seventh week of pregnancy a client with a history of mild rheumatic heart disease complains of some dependent edema in her ankles. The nurse advises her to:
    1. Limit her fluid intake during the day
    2. Stop using salt for the next 3 months
    3. Elevate her legs more frequently during the day
    4. Call her physician immediately for a mild diuretic

214. A male client is admitted with a lesion in the decending colon. His history reveals intermittent constipation, hemorrhoids, ulcerative colitis, and diverticulitis. The client's family questions the nurse regarding the possibility that their father has cancer. The nurse should base a response on the knowledge that this client is predisposed to cancer because of the history of:
    1. Diverticulitis and hemorrhoids
    2. Hemorrhoids and constipation
    3. Ulcerative colitis and constipation
    4. Ulcerative colitis and hemorrhoids

215. Before a client signs an operative consent for an abdominoperineal resection, the nurse should be sure the client understands that surgery will probably result in a:
    1. Permanent ileostomy in the jejunum
    2. Permanent colostomy and impotence
    3. Temporary colostomy with diminished libido
    4. Temporary colostomy in the descending colon

216. During the immediate postoperative period after an abdominoperineal resection, the nurse should assess the client for:
1. Blood in the urine
2. Return of bowel sounds
3. Drainage on the abdominal and rectal dressings
4. Functioning of the stoma and character of drainage

217. A client develops an elevated temperature after surgery. The physician prescribes ceftriaxone (Rocephin). The nurse monitors the client's intake and output to observe for side effects of the medication. This action is taken to determine the presence of:
1. Dehydration
2. Constipation
3. Acute renal failure
4. Congestive heart failure

218. A client is diagnosed as having pregnancy-induced hypertension (preeclampsia). The nurse should maintain her on bedrest in the:
1. Lithotomy position
2. Left lateral position
3. Semi-Fowler's position
4. Dorsal recumbent position

219. A client with preeclampsia is started on an infusion of magnesium sulfate. This medication acts as:
1. A diuretic
2. A sedative
3. An anticonvulsant
4. An antihypertensive

220. When caring for a client with AIDS, the nurse should:
1. Use standard precautions
2. Employ airborne precautions
3. Plan care so direct contact is limited
4. Discourage long visits from family members

221. The friend of a client dying of AIDS tells the nurse, "Life is not worth living without my partner." To help the friend deal with the impending death of his partner, the nurse should plan to:
1. Identify the friend's support system
2. Explore the friend's psychotic thoughts
3. Reinforce the friend's current self-image
4. Refer the friend to a bereavement group

222. A 40-year-old woman in her twenty-second week of pregnancy is admitted with heavy bleeding and severe abdominal cramping. The client says to the nurse, "We wanted this baby so badly." The nurse's most therapeutic response would be:
1. "It must be difficult to lose this baby that was important to you both."
2. "A D&C will give you a new start. I bet you'll become pregnant again soon."
3. "You must be disappointed, but don't feel guilty. These things sometimes happen."
4. "It's not your fault. This is nature's way of dealing with babies that may have problems."

223. A depressed client is eating very little at this time. The nursing care plan should be directed toward assisting the client with meals. Besides encouraging nourishment, this action also:
1. Proves to the client that food can be tolerated
2. Provides the client with some special attention
3. Gets the client out of the dining room with the rest of the clients
4. Shows that the staff considers the client to be a worthwhile individual

224. When obtaining a health history, the nurse should be aware that one of the subjective symptoms of primary hypertension is:
1. Mild but persistent depression
2. Transient temporary memory loss
3. Cardiac palpitation during periods of stress
4. Occipital headache, particularly in the morning

225. A male client is diagnosed with hypertension and is started on a regimen of hydrochlorothiazide. The nurse should help him to understand that he:
1. Must adjust the medication according to his blood pressure
2. May experience impotence because it is a usual side effect
3. Will probably require the medication for the remainder of his life
4. Should omit one dose if he experiences any orthostatic hypotension

226. A client with a cerebral hemorrhage is admitted to the hospital in a coma. The highest priority for the nurse when planning care for this client would be to:
1. Monitor vital signs
2. Maintain an open airway
3. Monitor pupil response and equality
4. Maintain fluid and electrolyte balance

227. When evaluating a client's status by use of the Glasgow Coma Scale after a head injury, the nurse should know that the most serious response to pressure applied to the nailbeds would be:
    1. Flexing
    2. Localizing
    3. Extending
    4. Withdrawing

228. A elderly female client has right-sided hemiplegia and expressive aphasia. The nurse explains to the client's children that she will probably be unable to:
    1. Verbally state her wishes
    2. Express herself in writing
    3. Understand written words
    4. Recognize familiar objects

229. Six days after a client has had a cerebral hemorrhage the nurse identifies that the client's arm and leg are no longer flaccid, but spastic. Spastic paralysis could predispose this client to:
    1. Spastic colon
    2. Athetoid movements
    3. Generalized seizures
    4. Contracture deformities

230. A young woman questions the nurse concerning the effectiveness of oral contraceptives. The nurse's best response is based on the recognition that the effectiveness of any contraceptive is related to:
    1. User motivation
    2. Reliability record
    3. The simplicity of use
    4. Identified risk factors

231. A neonate born at 36 weeks' gestation, weighing 2043 g, is placed under a radiant warmer. The neonate has an infusion of D10/0.2NS running through an umbilical vein catheter at a rate of 12 ml/hr. The nurse checks each of the neonate's voidings for specific gravity, knowing that:
    1. Infants under open radiant warmers are at risk for fluid volume deficit
    2. An infusion rate of 12 ml/hr is probably inadequate to meet fluid needs
    3. At this gestational age, infants are unable to produce adequate amounts of urine
    4. Renal dysfunction is the most frequent complication affecting the preterm infant

232. A preterm infant with respiratory distress syndrome (RDS) has blood drawn for an arterial blood gas analysis. The nurse knows that infants with RDS typically present:

1. A lowered HCO_3
2. An increased Po_2
3. A decreased Pco_2
4. A lowered blood pH

233. Neomycin 1 g is ordered preoperatively for a client with cancer of the colon. The client asks why this is necessary. The best response by the nurse is:
    1. "It will decrease your kidney function and lessen urine production during surgery."
    2. "It will kill the bacteria in your bowel and decrease the risk of infection after surgery."
    3. "It is used to alter the body flora, which reduces the spread of the tumor to adjacent organs."
    4. "It is used to prevent you from getting an infection, particularly a bladder infection, before surgery."

234. A client has surgery for the creation of a colostomy. Postoperatively, if the stoma is viable the nurse would expect the color to be:
    1. Gray
    2. Brick red
    3. Pale pink
    4. Dark purple

235. The nurse would know that the client needed further teaching about preventing thrombi when the client states, "I should:
    1. Massage my legs."
    2. Increase my fluid intake."
    3. Perform range-of-motion exercises."
    4. Wear elastic stockings when out of bed."

236. When calculating an Apgar score, in addition to the heart rate, the practitioner must assess the newborn's:
    1. Muscle tone
    2. Amount of mucus
    3. Degree of head lag
    4. Depth of respirations

237. A 4-year-old child who has never been separated from the parents or siblings is admitted to the hospital. The nurse should encourage the parents to:
    1. Bring a favorite toy to the hospital for the child
    2. Allow the nurse to be the child's major caregiver
    3. Visit the child as often as the hospital's rules allow
    4. Stay with the child throughout the hospitalization

238. When a child is diagnosed as being moderately retarded, it would be most helpful for the nurse to suggest that the parents:
    1. Offer simple, repetitive tasks
    2. Concentrate on teaching detailed tasks
    3. Offer challenging, competitive situations
    4. Provide complete directions at the beginning of the task to be carried out

239. A female client who has been abusing her son is undergoing treatment to control her behavior. A statement by the client that indicates the development of some insight into her behavior as a parent would be:
    1. "I promise that I won't get so angry when my son causes trouble again."
    2. "Once my son gets straightened out, I'll be better able to control my behavior."
    3. "I think the root of the problem is when my husband comes home after drinking."
    4. "If I feel angry at my son again, I'm going to go into the bedroom and punch a pillow."

240. A client in her thirty-eighth week of pregnancy is scheduled for a nonstress test and asks if the nurse thinks it is necessary. The nurse's best reply would be:
    1. "It is a fast procedure and totally harmless."
    2. "You have doubts about this test, don't you?"
    3. "Certainly; you may have problems and we want to reduce the risks."
    4. "Your physician feels it is necessary so I think you should have it done."

241. A new mother is afraid that her heart condition will prevent her from being able to care for her baby and her home when she is discharged. The most appropriate nursing intervention is to:
    1. Suggest that her husband arrange for help at home
    2. Ask her to explain more fully why she feels this way
    3. Tell her to speak to her physician about her concerns
    4. Speak to her husband alone and explain how he can assist

242. A client with a long history of alcohol abuse is admitted to the detoxification unit of an alcohol rehabilitation center. This client should be assigned to a room:
    1. Without windows and close to the nurse's station
    2. Illuminated by adequate lighting from the corridor
    3. That is well lit and away from the areas of activity
    4. With dim lights shared by a quiet, withdrawn client

243. When a client is admitted to an alcohol-detoxification unit, the nurse assigned to do the initial interview should plan to include:
    1. An explanation of the unit's routines
    2. An explanation of the client's role on the unit
    3. A description of acceptable behavior on the unit
    4. A complete list of the unit's rules and regulations

244. A female client with a diagnosis of alcohol abuse appears disheveled and disorganized. The plan that would best gain the client's involvement in personal hygienic care would include:
    1. Drawing up a schedule with her and making certain that she adheres to it
    2. Assisting her in bathing and dressing by giving her clear, simple directions
    3. Bathing and dressing her each morning until she is willing to do it for herself
    4. Giving her a schedule and requiring her to bathe and dress herself each morning

245. When a client who is receiving peritoneal dialysis complains of severe respiratory difficulty, the most immediate nursing action should be to:
    1. Notify the physician
    2. Discontinue the treatment
    3. Change the client's position
    4. Drain fluid from the peritoneal cavity

246. A male client with a fracture associated with osteomyelitis has been immobilized for 3 weeks. The nurse realizes that he may develop renal calculi as a complication because:
    1. He has more difficulty urinating in a supine position
    2. His dietary patterns have changed since admission
    3. Lack of muscle action and normal tension cause calcium withdrawal from bone
    4. Fracture healing requires more calcium and thus increases total calcium metabolism

247. A client is waiting for a renal transplant. When teaching about the transplant, the nurse tells the client that:
    1. "Your urine production will be delayed after surgery."
    2. "The symptoms of rejection include fever, hypotension, and edema."
    3. "You will require immunosuppressive drugs daily for the rest of your life."
    4. "You will be unable to follow a full program of work and recreation, including sports."

248. When caring for a young infant with Down syndrome, the nurse recognizes that the infant will have:
    1. Difficulty in hearing
    2. High incidence of circulatory problems
    3. Proneness to respiratory tract infections
    4. A developmental lag after 1 or 2 years of age

249. The indication of Down syndrome most evident to the nursery nurse during the initial newborn assessment would be:
    1. A rounded occiput
    2. Asymmetric gluteal folds
    3. A transverse palmar (simian) crease
    4. Hypertonicity of the skeletal muscles

250. A client with benign prostatic hypertrophy tells the nurse on morning rounds that he has not voided since last night. The nurse assesses the client and determines that his bladder is distended. The nurse should:
    1. Encourage use of a urinal
    2. Force fluids to induce voiding
    3. Assist him into a warm shower
    4. Apply pressure over the pubic area

251. When assessing a client with Ménière's disease, the nurse should expect the client to experience:
    1. Diarrhea
    2. Nystagmus
    3. A decrease in pulse rate
    4. An increase in temperature

252. A 3½-year-old child with severe anemia is seen by the nurse in the clinic. In addition to weakness and fatigue, the nurse should expect the child to exhibit:
    1. Cold, clammy skin
    2. Increased pulse rate
    3. Elevated blood pressure
    4. Cyanosis of the nail beds

253. The nurse should recognize that a child with an iron deficiency may become dizzy during periods of physical activity because of:
    1. An inflammation of the inner ear
    2. Insufficient cerebral oxygenation
    3. A sudden drop in blood pressure
    4. Decreased levels of serum glucose

254. When assessing a client in labor, the nurse recognizes true labor by the occurrence of:
    1. Rectal pressure
    2. Cervical dilation
    3. Uterine contractions
    4. Leakage of fluid from the vagina

255. As part of the physical assessment of a newborn, the nurse observes for the presence of an umbilical hernia. This assessment can best be accomplished when the baby is:
    1. Crying
    2. Sucking
    3. Inhaling
    4. Sleeping

256. When obtaining a health history from a client with the diagnosis of peptic ulcer disease, the client statement the nurse should consider as a possible contributory factor is:
    1. "My blood type is A."
    2. "I smoke two packs of cigarettes a day."
    3. "I have been overweight most of my life."
    4. "My blood pressure has been high lately."

257. When assessing a client with varicose veins, the nurse should expect the client to experience:
    1. A positive Homans' sign
    2. Cramping sensations in the calf muscle
    3. Continuous edema of the affected extremity
    4. Coolness and pallor of the affected extremity

258. A client is diagnosed with Addison's disease. It is most important that the nurse reinforce with the client the need for:
    1. A special low-salt diet
    2. Restriction of physical activity
    3. Hormone replacement therapy
    4. Frequent visits to the physician

259. The presence of human chorionic gonadotropin (HCG) is the reason for a positive pregnancy test. During pregnancy this hormone is produced by the:
    1. Ovary
    2. Decidua
    3. Chorionic villi
    4. Pituitary gland

260. When teaching a client about a contraction stress test, the nurse should emphasize that it is important that prior to the test the client should:
    1. Empty her bladder
    2. Take diazepam (Valium) 5 mg PO $1/2$ hour before the test
    3. Be prepared to be in the hospital for 12 hours after the test
    4. Eat nothing for 2 hours before the test and 6 hours after the test

261. A client is receiving an H_2 antagonist medication. The nurse explains that this drug is given prophylactically during the first few weeks after extensive burns to prevent:
    1. Colitis
    2. Gastritis
    3. Stress ulcer
    4. Metabolic acidosis

262. When assessing a client experiencing pain, the nurse should be alert for a sign of an involuntary reaction to pain, which is:
    1. Crying
    2. Splinting
    3. Grimacing
    4. Perspiration

263. Immediately after a prostatectomy the nurse should:
    1. Have the client stand to void
    2. Aspirate the catheter with a bulb syringe
    3. Discourage straining for a bowel movement
    4. Notify the physician if the client does not void in 12 hours

264. A client with Ménière's disease is placed on a salt-restricted diet to reduce endolymphatic fluid. When discussing the diet with the nurse, the client expresses four food preferences. After reviewing the list of foods, the nurse tells the client that it is all right to eat:
    1. Macaroni
    2. Carrot cake
    3. Baked clams
    4. Grilled cheese

265. Before a contraction stress test the nurse should explain to the client that:
    1. The FHR will be monitored for 30 minutes prior to actual testing
    2. A double-voided urine specimen will be collected prior to the test
    3. At least six contractions must be observed before the test is discontinued
    4. She will be placed in a right lateral position, which must be maintained throughout testing

COMPREHENSIVE TEST 2: PART A

ANSWERS AND RATIONALES

1. **1** This recognizes the client's feelings by using reflective technique. (2; MR; IM; CW; PS; WH)
   2 This does not recognize the client's feelings, avoids the thrust of her comments, and may cut off communication.
   3 This provides false reassurance that crying will solve her concerns.
   4 Same as answer 2.

2. **4** The sympathetic nervous system is triggered and releases epinephrine, which causes diaphoresis and nervousness. (2; CJ; AN; MS; PA; EN)
   1 Osmotic diuresis causes thirst and an increased fluid intake; related to hyperglycemia, not hypoglycemia.
   2 Warm, dry, flushed skin and lethargy are associated with ketoacidosis.
   3 Glycogenesis, the formation of glycogen in the liver, is unrelated to these adaptations.

3. **3** Obesity causes resistance to insulin at the cellular level, and more insulin is required for the transfer of glucose across the cell membrane. (3; CJ; IM; MS; ED; EN)
   1 Incorrect; the metabolism of fatty acids is altered, and fatty acids are broken down and storage is decreased.
   2 On the contrary, more insulin is required in obesity for the oxidation of glucose.
   4 Obesity causes peripheral cellular resistance to glucose entry and therefore decreases cellular entry.

4. **3** Exercise increases the uptake of glucose by active muscle cells without the need for insulin; carbohydrates are needed to supply energy for the increased metabolic rate associated with exercise. (1; CJ; PL; MS; PA; EN)
   1 The need for insulin is decreased.
   2 Although the need for insulin is decreased, the need for carbohydrates is increased with exercise.
   4 Same as answer 2.

5. **3** This is an example of a neologism, a self-coined word whose meaning is only known to the client and must be explored. (1; CJ; IM; MH; PS; SD)
   1 Although neologisms are evidence of illness, they cannot be ignored because the word usually has significance to the individual using it.
   2 It is not simply a mispronunciation; even if it were, correcting another's pronunciation or indicating meaning is not understood can cut off communication.
   4 Same as answer 2.

6. **3** A cephalhematoma is characteristically confined to a single cranial bone, since it is a collection of blood beneath the periosteum of the bone. (1; CJ; AS; CW; PA; HN)
   1 Wide suture lines usually indicate the possibility of hydrocephaly.
   2 This may be the result of a misplaced forceps; it is not characteristic of a cephalhematoma.
   4 Skin discoloration could be present for a number of reasons, such as vacuum extraction or forceps delivery.

7. **3** Vitamin K, a fat-soluble vitamin, is necessary for the formation of prothrombin (factor II); a lack of vitamin K prolongs prothrombin time. (2; CJ; AS; MS; PA; CV)
   1 Blood clotting will decrease.
   2 Fibrin formation will decrease.
   4 Calcium utilization is not influenced by vitamin K.

8. **2** Glomerulonephritis is an immune complex disease; it is a reaction that occurs as a by-product of a streptococcal infection. (1; CJ; AS; PE; PA; RG)
   1 This is associated with conjunctivitis and meningitis, not glomerulonephritis.
   3 This is associated with many diseases of humans, but not glomerulonephritis in children.
   4 This is associated with localized suppurating infections, not glomerulonephritis.

9. 1 Smoky urine indicates the presence of a large number of red blood cells. (2; CJ; AS; PE; PA; RG)

2 Orange-colored urine is usually associated with certain foods or medications.

3 This is frank bleeding associated with trauma to the urinary tract, not glomerulonephritis.

4 Straw-colored urine is normal urine that is not concentrated.

10. 3 Increased amounts of protein are needed for growth and maintenance of maternal and fetal tissues. (2; MR; AN; CW; PA; HC)

1 There is a need for an increase in all nutrients to meet the increased caloric requirement during pregnancy.

2 RDA for calories is a minimum increase of 300/day during pregnancy.

4 Calcium/phosphorus needs increase to allow for storage and to meet the rapid demand for fetal bone deposits during the last month of pregnancy.

11. 3 In the side-lying position the gravid uterus does not impede venous return; cardiac output improves, leading to better uterine perfusion, improved uterine contractions, and fetal oxygenation. (1; MR; PL; CW; PA; HC)

1 Lying on the side does not affect fetal activity.

2 Untrue; having the client walk or squat would best accomplish this.

4 This position will not decrease nausea and vomiting, which may occur in the transitional period but are not usually present in early labor.

12. 4 The spiral electrode should be turned counterclockwise in order to remove it; the electrode is attached to the fetal scalp by twisting it clockwise. (2; CJ; IM; CW; TC; HN)

1 Improper technique; this could result in a lacerating injury to the scalp.

2 The electrode is attached by turning it clockwise.

3 Unnecessary to untwist the wires; the electrode should not be pulled, since this could cause a scalp laceration.

13. 3 Honest answer; this is the expected recovery time for an uncomplicated deep partial-thickness burn. (2; CJ; IM; MS; ED; IT)

1 There is no eschar with a deep partial-thickness burn; it occurs with full-thickness burns.

2 Unnecessary; raises anxiety by implying facial lesions will still be present in 4 weeks.

4 Edema is present for approximately 48 to 72 hours.

14. 1 Hospice care attempts to break the cycle of anxiety, fear, and pain; pain medication is given on a regular basis. (2; MR; AN; MS; PS; EH)

2 Hospice care is provided after aggressive treatment has been tried and failed; it provides care during the terminal stages of an illness.

3 Family members can be very involved in the care of the client; a hospice provides a supportive environment for the client and family members.

4 The purpose is not to isolate clients with cancer, but to allow clients to die with dignity and support.

15. 4 This involves being a part of a group of people who have also sustained a loss; members provide support to each other. (1; MR; IM; MS; PS; EH)

1 Individual counseling will not provide the degree of support that a group provides; group counseling may be more prolonged than crisis intervention.

2 The information provided did not indicate other family members.

3 Marital counseling involves both a husband and a wife.

16. 3 Developing and participating in meaningful activities and satisfaction with past accomplishments increase feelings of self-worth. (2; CJ; AS; MS; ED; GD)

1 This is a task of middle adulthood.

2 This is a task of early adulthood.

4 Not a developmental task of the aging person; not all aged people live in assisted living facilities.

17. 4 The purpose of this test is to measure how much urine remains in the bladder after voiding. (2; MR; PL; MS; PA; RG)

1 This is known as a clean-catch, or midstream, urine specimen, not a residual urine test.

2 Impossible; the urinary catheter would obstruct the flow of urine.

3 The bladder would be empty of urine at this time.

18. **2** Inadequate tissue perfusion leads to anaerobic metabolism and lactic acid production, leading to metabolic acidosis. (3; CJ; AS; MS; PA; FE)

   1 This occurs with respiratory alkalosis; it would not result from loss of blood.

   3 This may occur as a result of hyperventilation in early shock but is not a result of blood loss and resultant anaerobic metabolism.

   4 Loss of other body protein, not blood, over time would lead to negative nitrogen balance.

19. **3** An untoward effect of wound healing may be a stricture, which would interfere with urinary flow. (2; MR; PL; MS; ED; RG)

   1 The client should be urged to void every two hours and after a few minutes try again to empty the bladder thoroughly.

   2 Prolonged sitting promotes venous stasis and increases the chance of hemorrhage.

   4 Too long; vigorous exercise and heavy lifting should be avoided for at least 3 weeks after discharge from the hospital to prevent hemorrhage.

20. **4** This action will help to establish trust without unduly raising anxiety. (3; CJ; PL; MH; PS; SD)

   1 A withdrawn client will not usually approach anyone.

   2 Establishing trust takes priority unless the client is extremely dirty.

   3 The client's history demonstrates a failure to speak.

21. **4** Focusing on physical complaints that have no organic cause allows the client to continue to use the complaint to avoid facing the feelings that are really the problem. (2; MR; PL; MH; TC; AX)

   1 Client's eye discomfort is a conversion reaction; focusing on physical complaints allows client to use the complaint to avoid feelings.

   2 Much too early for this; client is too introspective to become involved with unit activities at this time.

   3 Client does not have any organic problem and is not going blind.

22. **2** The major goal is to get the client to express feelings appropriately rather than through the use of physical symptoms. (2; MR; IM; MH; PS; AX)

   1 Focusing on symptoms will only increase the symptoms and encourage their use.

   3 Not a primary goal; for a while client needs to express feelings that may threaten safety.

   4 Avoidance of feelings, not stress itself, has resulted in symptoms; expression of feelings, not an intellectual understanding of cause, is required.

23. **2** Hemorrhage is a major life-threatening complication, since arterial blood is under pressure and an artery has been entered (punctured) by a catheter. (2; CJ; IM; PE; TC; CV)

   1 Child is kept in bed at least 8 hours after procedure.

   3 Fluids may be given as soon as tolerated.

   4 Pulses, not blood pressure, must be checked for quality and symmetry.

24. **2** This has the same effect as squatting, which decreases venous return from the legs; therefore the blood returning to the heart and lungs has a higher O_2 content. (2; CJ; IM; PE; PA; CV)

   1 This position does not decrease venous return from the legs; blood returning to the heart has a lower O_2 content when in this position than it does in the knee-chest position.

   3 Same as answer 1.

   4 Same as answer 1.

25. **3** With glaucoma there is a loss of peripheral vision long before the central vision is affected. The client may also complain of seeing halos around light. (2; CJ; AS; MS; PA; NM)

   1 Primary closed-angle glaucoma causes pain.

   2 Blurred vision may be due to a refractive error; peripheral vision is affected in glaucoma.

   4 This occurs when there is damage to the central retina; peripheral vision is affected in glaucoma.

26. **4** The prone position stretches the flexor muscles, thus preventing hip flexion contractures. (2; CJ; IM; MS; PA; NM)

   1 Elevating the head of the bed would cause hip flexion, which could result in a hip flexion contracture.

   2 Elevating the residual limb would cause hip flexion, which could result in a hip flexion contracture.

   3 Sitting flexes the hips, which could result in a hip flexion contracture.

27. **2** Muscles that originate at the vertebrae or pelvic girdle and insert on the femur act to abduct, adduct, flex, extend, and rotate the femur. Normal body alignment should be maintained because it facilitates the safe and efficient use of muscle groups for balance and stability. (2; MR; IM; MS; PA; NM)
   1 This position does not approximate normal body alignment; hip flexion will alter the center of gravity and promote the development of a hip flexion contracture.
   3 This position does not approximate normal body alignment; abduction of the residual limb will alter the center of gravity.
   4 This interferes with the development of a normal gait; muscles that originate at the vertebrae and pelvic girdle should be used to move the residual limb.

28. **3** Subcutaneous fat is reduced by the pressure of the initial constrictive bandage and the socket of the prosthesis. (3; CJ; AN; MS; PA; NM)
   1 Edema is limited and contributes minimally to the size of the postoperative residual limb.
   2 Restoration of skin turgor does not affect residual limb size.
   4 Tissue and bone excised remain constant; after surgery there is no additional loss.

29. **2** Exercise should not include bending and the Valsalva maneuver, which might increase intraocular pressure. (2; MR; EV; MS; ED; NM)
   1 Fluids may be taken as desired because they have no effect on intraocular pressure.
   3 Mydriatics are contraindicated in glaucoma because they dilate the pupil, which increases intraocular pressure.
   4 Lighting conditions have no effect on intraocular pressure.

30. **1** Polyarthritis of rheumatic fever is transitory and does not cause deformity. Rheumatoid arthritis is chronic and causes changes in joints. (1; CJ; AN; PE; PA; SK)
   2 Cardiac damage is often associated with rheumatic fever.
   3 The etiology of rheumatic fever is related to a previous occurrence of strep throat; rheumatoid arthritis is unrelated.
   4 Juvenile rheumatoid arthritis involves chronic inflammation of the joints; exacerbations are most often related to stress.

31. **3** Aspirin interferes with platelet aggregation, thereby lengthening bleeding time. (2; CJ; EV; MS; TC; DR)
   1 Urate excretion is enhanced by high doses of aspirin.
   2 Aspirin is readily broken down in the GI tract and liver.
   4 Aspirin inhibits platelet aggregation; it does not destroy erythrocytes.

32. **4** Ten-year-old boys prefer the company of the same sex and age group. Also, the client needs to avoid stressful situations that would tend to increase exacerbations. (2; CJ; EV; PE; PS; GD)
   1 Same-sex roommates are desirable for companionship and to maintain boy/girl separateness of this age group.
   2 Asthmatic children may have severe respiratory difficulties; this may be too stressful for the client who needs rest.
   3 Same-sex roommates are desirable for companionship and to maintain privacy needs.

33. **1** A diagnosis of cancer and a colostomy both drastically alter a person's self-image and body image. People react differently to this stress, often finding it difficult to express their concerns verbally; however, their actions may demonstrate an awareness of the situation. (2; CJ; EV; MH; PS; EP)
   2 There is not enough information to determine this.
   3 Same as answer 2.
   4 Same as answer 2.

34. **4** A diet as close as possible to normal after a colostomy is recommended because individuals will discover their own food intolerances and should eat accordingly. (2; CJ; PL; MS; ED; GI)
   1 Each person is an individual and reacts differently to foods.
   2 Rigid dietary regulations usually increase anxiety; return to normally tolerated foods provides security.
   3 A low-residue diet is not necessary; once healing occurs, a diet with adequate residue promotes peristalsis and colostomy functioning.

35. 1 Rapid instillation of fluid into the colon may cause abdominal cramps. By clamping the tubing, the nurse allows the cramps to subside so the irrigation can be continued. (2; CJ; EV; MS; TC; GI)

  2 Emotional support will not interrupt the physical adaptation of abdominal cramps; the irrigation must be temporarily interrupted.

  3 Although this may reduce the force of the fluid, it will not eliminate the flow of fluid completely; the irrigation should be temporarily interrupted.

  4 This is contraindicated; this will increase the force of flow, which will increase the abdominal cramps.

36. 2 A colostomy located on the left side of the abdomen most likely would involve the descending colon. Since most but not all of the fluid would be absorbed, the stool would be moist and formed. (3; CJ; AS; MS; PA; GI)

  1 This would be associated with a colostomy involving the ascending colon.

  3 Stools are not usually covered with mucus; they may be moist but not mucoid.

  4 This would be associated with conditions that narrow the intestinal lumen; this is not usually associated with a colostomy.

37. 2 Colostomy irrigations done daily at the same time help establish normal patterns of bowel evacuation. (2; MR; IM; MS; ED; GI)

  1 Initially after surgery, protein promotes healing; protein intake has no relationship to bowel control.

  3 Although fluid is important to prevent hard stools, it will not help the client regain bowel control; a daily regimen is the priority.

  4 A soft, low-residue diet is not necessary; it should be as close to normal as possible.

38. 4 One begins by trying to enter the world where the child's attention is currently focused; this is a way of making human contact, since the child's usual contacts are inanimate objects. (2; CJ; IM; MH; PS; BA)

  1 Autistic children generally cannot tolerate cuddling and will become rigid when anyone attempts to do so.

  2 This would have no effect on the nurse's ability to reach the child; rather it would reinforce the withdrawal.

  3 The autistic child is unable to participate in group activities.

39. 2 Isolated, unrelated activities predominate. The child's behavior reflects withdrawal or feelings of destructive rage. (2; CJ; AS; MH; PS; BA)

  1 The facial expression is blank; sadness would be a response to the external world, from which the child has withdrawn.

  3 The autistic child seems to overrespond to stimuli in the environment.

  4 The autistic child rarely if ever smiles.

40. 3 Self-isolation and disinterest in interpersonal relationships lead the autistic child to find security in nonthreatening, impersonal objects. (3; MR; IM; MH; PS; BA)

  1 This would be too threatening to an autistic child.

  2 Touching the child might prove to be too threatening.

  4 These children do not respond to bright-colored toys and blocks as other children do unless there is movement involved.

41. 3 Weight gain caused by fluid retention is the earliest objective sign of mild pregnancy-induced hypertension. (3; CJ; AS; CW; PA; HP)

  1 Continued elevations are significant; emotional upset, anxiety, and other factors may cause fluctuations or variations in blood pressure.

  2 This may occur; however, it usually becomes evident after weight gain and a progressive increase in BP.

  4 Ankle edema progresses as the signs of pregnancy-induced hypertension worsen

42. 3 The latest concept concerning pregnancy-induced hypertension is that this condition is a consequence of salt loss during pregnancy and poor protein intake. The recommendations therefore call for a diet containing normal sodium, high protein, and a sufficient number of calories. (3; MR; EV; CW; ED; HP)

  1 Low protein is contraindicated for normal fetal growth; there is no indication for increasing sodium.

  2 Lowering the intake of calories and sodium is detrimental to both fetus and mother.

  4 There is an additional requirement of 300 calories per day during pregnancy.

43. **2** The cumulative effects of magnesium sulfate include depressed respirations and an absent or weak knee-jerk reflex. (2; CJ; EV; CW; PA; DR)
    1 Temperature and pulse are not affected by administration of $MgSO_4$.
    3 The BP is monitored after administration of $MgSO_4$; the apical pulse is not relevant.
    4 Urinary output is increased after administration of $MgSO_4$.

44. **3** In severe pregnancy-induced hypertension, fluid is drawn from the plasma into the tissues and the blood becomes more concentrated. This is reflected in the elevated hematocrit level. (2; CJ; AN; CW; PA; HP)
    1 Vasodilation would not alter the ratio of cells to fluid volume.
    2 Agglutination of red blood cells does not occur.
    4 The hemodilution results in a reduced hematocrit, since there is more blood volume than there are cells.

45. **4** One of the characteristic differences between type 1 and type 2 diabetes is the rapid onset of the disease. Type 1 diabetes is often first diagnosed during acute ketoacidosis. (1; CJ; AN; PE; PA; EN)
    1 Juveniles with diabetes are insulin dependent.
    2 Vascular changes are complications associated with long-standing diabetes.
    3 Although adult-onset diabetes (type 2) often occurs in obese individuals, diabetes occurs in children of thin or normal build.

46. **4** 100 units : 1 ml = 20 units : x ml
    $$100x = 20$$
    $$x = \frac{20}{100} = \frac{1}{5} = 0.2 \text{ ml}$$
    (2; CJ; IM; PE; TC; DR)
    1 This dose is too large.
    2 Same as answer 1.
    3 Same as answer 1.

47. **4** Exercise reduces the body's need for insulin. Increased muscle activity accelerates the transport of glucose into the muscle cells, thus producing an insulin-like effect. (2; MR; PL; PE; ED; EN)
    1 With increased growth and associated dietary intake, the need for insulin increases.
    2 An infectious process, if severe enough, may require increased insulin.
    3 An emotional upset is a stress that increases the need for insulin.

48. **4** This position minimizes the discomfort associated with venous engorgement. It also promotes venous drainage by gravity, minimizing edema. (3; CJ; IM; MS; PA; RE)
    1 This position would neither increase nor decrease strain on the suture line.
    2 Drainage from the wound would not be affected.
    3 Providing stimulation would not be a priority; this position would not affect the degree of stimulation.

49. **1** If the dressing is too tight, impaired cerebral circulation may result. (2; CJ; EV; MS; PA; CV)
    2 Bleeding would not cause the client to complain of tightness.
    3 This is untrue; impaired cerebral circulation may result from a tight dressing.
    4 The dressing may be loosened or removed only if indicated by the physician.

50. **1** To be truly effective in the relationship with the client, the nurse must know and understand personal feelings about terminal illness and death. (2; MR; AN; MH; PS; CS)
    2 When dealing with terminal illness, knowledge alone is not enough to ensure an effective nurse-client relationship.
    3 Although the family is an important part of the client's support system, the client's feelings are more important to the relationship.
    4 Previous experiences could be positive or negative and would not guarantee an effective nurse-client relationship.

51. **4** This grouping of foods does not contain high-residue fruits, vegetables, or whole grains, which are irritating to the intestinal mucosa, cause bulk, and increase peristalsis. (3; CJ; PL; MS; PA; GI)
    1 This choice includes vegetables and grain, which leave increased residue.
    2 Same as answer 1.
    3 This choice includes whole-grain foods, which leave increased residue.

52. **2** Nurses can become very blasé about the equipment used in labor and forget that it may be frightening for the layperson. (2; CJ; EV; CW; PS; EC)
    1 Internal monitoring is used if adequate readouts cannot be obtained on an external monitor.
    3 Sedation is never given on a routine basis to the client in labor.
    4 This is not universally true; older primigravidas may have totally uncomplicated labors.

53. **4** Lactation delays ovarian function after delivery. It will also therefore delay the symptoms of endometriosis. (2; MR; IM; CW; PA; WH)
 1 Pregnancy temporarily suppresses ovarian function; the aberrant endometrial tissue is still present.
 2 Endometriosis may lead to sterility; it does not cause menopause.
 3 Conservative medical therapy will be used first; a hysterectomy is only a last resort.

54. **3** Frequent nursing reduces the possibility of engorgement. A 10-minute period provides for complete emptying of the breast. (1; MR; PL; CW; ED; HC)
 1 A relief bottle will prevent emptying of the breasts; this will increase pain and swelling.
 2 This does not provide for complete emptying of the breasts.
 4 This will not decrease engorgement.

55. **3** A stomal cover or scarf allows air to move in and out of the trachea but prevents particles of dirt or insects from entering the stoma. (2; MR; IM; MS; ED; RE)
 1 Not necessary; maintenance of hydration keeps normal secretions liquified and mobile so they can be expelled.
 2 Fluids should not be limited; adequate fluids help to liquify respiratory secretions.
 4 Cotton-tipped swabs should not be placed in the trachea because cotton threads may be inhaled.

56. **4** These interventions expand the alveoli, move secretions toward the mouth to be expectorated, and increase the amount of oxygen being delivered to the alveolar capillary beds. (3; MR; PL; MS; TC; RE)
 1 Bronchodilators are not indicated at this time.
 2 Same as answer 1.
 3 Mechanical ventilation is not indicated at this time.

57. **1** Administration of 100% oxygen for a few minutes prior to suctioning reduces the risk of hypoxia, the major complication of suctioning. (3; CJ; IM; MS; TC; RE)
 2 Negative pressure is applied as the catheter is withdrawn.
 3 Tracheostomy cuffs are indicated when a client is on mechanical ventilation.

 4 When ordered, this drug is usually given by inhalation, not instillation and must also be accompanied by a bronchodilator.

58. **2** The tracheostomy site is a portal of entry for microorganisms. Sterile technique must be used; the most advantageous system is a closed tracheal suctioning catheter system. (3; CJ; IM; MS; TC; RE)
 1 The high-Fowler's position promotes maximum aeration of the lungs.
 3 Body temperature is not related to the suctioning procedure.
 4 The cannula, if it is not disposable, is generally cleaned with peroxide and saline.

59. **3** The nurse should expect an increase in blood volume by as much as 40% above prepregnant levels. During pregnancy, fluid in all body compartments increases. (3; CJ; AN; CW; PA; HC)
 1 The BP remains essentially unchanged throughout pregnancy.
 2 The hematocrit decreases as a result of the hemodilution of pregnancy.
 4 An increase in cardiac output is seen as early as the end of the first trimester, because of increased blood volume.

60. **2** The antibody system is not functioning in neonates. Antibodies are transferred from the mother in breast milk. (1; MR; IM; CW; ED; HC)
 1 Lactating mothers rarely ovulate for the first 9 weeks postpartum; however, they may any time after that.
 3 Because of the higher carbohydrate content of breast milk, infants wake more easily; carbohydrate is digested more rapidly.
 4 Breast milk has 1.1 g protein/100 ml; cow's milk has 3.5 g/100 ml; whole cow's milk is unsuitable for infants.

61. **3** Petrolatum gauze helps control bleeding and prevent adherence of the diaper. (2; MR; EV; CW; ED; NN)
 1 Fussy behavior is normal for a few hours after the procedure.
 2 This is not practical with a male infant.
 4 Yellow exudate is normal; it is not part of an infectious process.

62. **3** The woman must watch closely for symptoms associated with side effects of these medications. Estrogen-progestin contraceptives have been associated with thrombophlebitis (calf pain) and breast malignancy (breast tenderness from estrogen-supported tumors), as well as cardiovascular changes (hypertension). (3; MR; EV; CW; ED; RC)
  1 Nausea and rash are not associated with using estrogen-progestin contraceptives; however, breakthrough bleeding is a major side effect.
  2 Lethargy, syncope, and tachycardia are not side effects of oral contraceptives.
  4 Bradycardia and visual changes are not side effects; hypertension is a major side effect.

63. **2** Spasm must be interrupted or hypoxia will occur. (2; CJ; AN; PE; ED; RE)
  1 The problem in croup is laryngeal spasm, not constriction of bronchi.
  3 This is not the priority; the spasm must be interrupted immediately.
  4 Same as answer 3.

64. **2** Children learn socially acceptable behavior when consistent, reasonable limits that provide guidelines are established. (2; MR; IM; PE; ED; GD)
  1 Rewards should not always be necessary for good behavior; they will become expected.
  3 Authorities vary on their attitudes about punishment; punishment should not become the major means of teaching children to control their behavior.
  4 This is not always safe or reasonable for very young children.

65. **4** These disorders are characterized by anxiety and minor distortions of reality. The anxiety results in an inability to reach a decision, because all alternatives are threatening. (2; CJ; AS; MH; PS; PR)
  1 Just the opposite is true; part of emotional maturity is the ability to relate to people, and these people have difficulties in this area.
  2 This would be indicative of severe emotional illness, not an anxiety disorder.
  3 This would be indicative of a mood disorder.

66. **1** Albumin is not normally excreted in the urine. When found, it indicates renal disease. (1; CJ; EV; PE; PA; RG)
  2 Excess calcium is normally excreted.
  3 Potassium is normally excreted by the kidneys to maintain electrolyte balance.
  4 Excess phosphate is normally excreted.

67. **4** This task should be accomplished by 2-year-old children. (2; CJ; AS; PE; ED; NM)
  1 This is a task that is expected of a 4-year-old child.
  2 Same as answer 1.
  3 Same as answer 1.

68. **3** Calling for help during a suicide attempt demonstrates the client's unconscious will to live or be stopped from dying; the contrasting feelings of wanting to die and yet wanting to live demonstrate ambivalence. (2; CJ; AN; MH; TC; CS)
  1 Seeking help is not always an attention-getting device.
  2 This is a cry for help rather than an expression of anger or an attempt to punish anyone else.
  4 The client obviously had the intention of suicide, but the wish to live was apparently stronger than the wish to die.

69. **4** Depressed clients frequently reject initial attempts to establish a relationship in the early (orientation) phase of the nurse-client interaction; silence is a form of rejection. (2; CJ; AN; MH; PS; MO)
  1 Anger usually occurs during the working phase of the relationship.
  2 Clients rarely have insight into their problems at this stage of their illness.
  3 A depressed client would not be elated.

70. **3** This understanding clarifies the settings for the relationship and establishes boundaries; allows client to focus on the relationship rather than roles. (2; MR; AN; MH; TC; TR)
  1 This may or may not be true and is not related to an understanding of roles.
  2 An understanding of roles is only one factor among many needed before the client can develop trust.
  4 Same as answer 1.

71. **2** Assisting them to work on a puzzle together provides an opportunity for interaction; this is a noncompetitive activity that requires both interaction and some degree of cooperation. (3; MR; IM; MH; TC; MO)
  1 This gets them out of their room but does not facilitate interaction.
  3 This intervention would do little to facilitate mutual interaction.
  4 Watching television does not foster social interaction.

72. 3 It may take several weeks to achieve a therapeutic level with this selective serotonin-reuptake inhibitor. (3; MR; IM; MH; ED; DR)

1 Hypertensive crises do not occur with this drug.

2 This drug inhibits serotonin uptake but has little effect on norepinephrine receptors.

4 There are no food restrictions for clients who take this drug.

73. 3 Since prevention of external rotation is a function of the hip joint, support is necessary at that point to promote functional alignment. (1; CJ; IM; MS; PA; SK)

1 This would not prevent external rotation of the hip; associated hip and knee flexion could increase pain and trauma.

2 This would not prevent external rotation of the hip.

4 Same as answer 2.

74. 2 This response helps to reinforce small gains and provides encouragement for the future. (2; MR; IM; MH; PS; SA)

1 Totally negative response that is also incorrect, since postnecrotic cirrhosis is usually the result of viral hepatitis.

3 This negative response fails to recognize the client's role in rehabilitation.

4 A judgmental statement that fails to recognize that education and intelligence frequently do not influence or modify behavior.

75. 4 Interpretation of pain sensations is highly individual and is based on past experiences, which include cultural values. (2; CJ; AN; MH; PS; PD)

1 Age and sex affect pain perception only indirectly because they generally account for past experience to some degree.

2 Overall physical condition may affect one's ability to cope with stress; but unless the nervous system were involved, it would not greatly affect perception.

3 Intelligence is a factor in understanding pain, so it can be better tolerated, but it does not affect the perception of intensity; economic status has no effect on pain perception.

ANSWERS AND RATIONALES COMPREHENSIVE TEST 2: PART B

76. 4 Diffusion moves particles from an area of greater to an area of lesser concentration; osmosis moves fluid from an area of lesser to an area of greater concentration of particles. (3; CJ; AN; MS; PA; RG)

1 The principle of ultrafiltration involves a pressure gradient, which is associated with hemodialysis, not peritoneal dialysis.

2 Peritoneal dialysis cleanses the peritoneal cavity directly and the blood indirectly.

3 Dialysate does not clear toxins in a short time; exchanges may occur four to six times daily.

77. 4 Calculate the dosage using ratio and proportion.

$$\frac{20mg}{10mg} = \frac{xml}{1ml}$$

$$10x = 20$$
$$x = 2 \div 10$$
$$x = 2ml$$

(2; CJ; IM; MS; TC; DR)

1 Inaccurate dose; this is too low.

2 Same as answer 1.

3 Same as answer 1.

78. 3 This is often seen in abused children; occurs as a result of emotional stress as well as from neglect of physical needs. (2; CJ; AS; PE; PA; ED)

1 The task of nighttime bladder training may not be completed until 4 or 5 years of age and sometimes even later; this is not pathologic.

2 This is not noteworthy because many children, not just those who are abused, continue to suck their thumb even as late as 4 years of age.

4 Abused children do not seek physical closeness because their needs for comfort have not been met in the past.

79. 1 The nurse is mandated by law to report suspected child abuse; when reported to the police, they will determine the law enforcement agency or department of social services that is responsible for the process of substantiation and proof of abuse. (2; LM; IM; PE; TC; EH)

2 This is not the prime safety action at this time.

3 The nurse must comply with the mandated state law, because all 50 states require the nurse to be a mandated reporter.

4 Assessment is an ongoing process throughout treatment; but legally the nurse is bound to report the suspected abuse.

80. **2** Hand-eye coordination activities are suitable for preschoolers. (2; CJ; IM; PE; ED; GD)
    1 This could meet a security need but would not meet a 3-year-old child's developmental needs.
    3 This is inappropriate play for a child on bed rest.
    4 The child is limited to bed rest in this situation.

81. **4** Immediate treatment for croup is mist therapy; a steamy room may alleviate the spasm. (2; MR; PL; PE; PA; RE)
    1 Vomiting may result in aspiration in an already compromised child.
    2 If mist therapy (steamy bathroom) is effective, this will not be needed.
    3 Antihistamines have no therapeutic value in croup.

82. **4** Tantrums are the result of frustration, stress, and confusion about the demands of the environment; limiting these factors reduces the occurrence of tantrums. (2; MR; IM; PE; ED; EH)
    1 They are normal for this age, but attention is required to protect the child from injury and to limit stressful situations.
    2 Professional counseling is indicated only if conservative care is ineffective or there is evidence of pathology.
    3 This is rarely effective and provides secondary gains for this behavior.

83. **1** Rituals are a means for the individual to control anxiety. If not permitted to carry out the ritual, the client will probably experience unbearable anxiety. (3; CJ; IM; MH; PS; PR)
    2 The client understands this already but is unable to stop the activity.
    3 These clients have no idea what the ritual means; only that they must continue with it.
    4 This would have the effect of increasing anxiety in the client, possibly to panic levels.

84. **1** Active sharing of responsibility will prove most helpful. It will ensure that lead sources are removed. (3; MR; IM; PE; ED; NM)
    2 This will not resolve etiologic factors or accomplish prevention.
    3 This is a good idea, but does not guarantee action; concrete action should be taken first.
    4 This omits the need to remove lead from the environment; therefore, it will not ensure prevention.

85. **4** A low-pressure cuff prevents constriction of the capillary bed, preventing tracheal necrosis. (3; CJ; PL; MS; TC; RE)
    1 The tracheostomy tube can be a single-lumen tube or have both an inner and outer cannula.
    2 A tracheostomy tube, whether it is a single-lumen tube or has both an inner and outer cannula, does not have to be changed weekly; it is usually changed every 2 to 3 weeks as necessary.
    3 The tracheostomy should be cleaned every 8 hours and whenever necessary.

86. **2** Productive coughing induced by postural drainage can cause nausea and vomiting. (2; CJ; PL; MS; PA; RE)
    1 Since coughing must be encouraged after treatment, sleep is postponed; but as breathing is facilitated, sleep may then be more restful.
    3 Approximately 1 hour before meals is a preferred time for postural drainage; the resulting cough and mucus production will be less likely to affect dietary intake.
    4 Upon awakening, mucus secretions are plentiful and tenacious; postural drainage at this time would be most beneficial.

87. **3** The fluid level and time must be marked so that the amount of drainage in the chest tube drainage system can be evaluated. (1; CJ; IM; MS; TC; RE)
    1 The amount of sterile water used to create a water seal depends on the drainage system used and is usually more than 3 to 5 ml; once the water seal is created, the nurse usually does not add water.
    2 The drainage system must be kept below chest level to promote drainage of the pleural space so that the lung can expand.
    4 The catheter is secured by skin sutures, not to the dressing itself.

88. **3** After administration of a local anesthetic during a bronchoscopy, fluids and food should be withheld until the gag reflex returns. (2; CJ; EV; MS; TC; RE)
    1 Ice chips must not be given until the gag reflex returns.
    2 Coughing should not be encouraged; it might initiate bleeding from the site of the biopsy.
    4 To allow drainage and minimize the possibility of aspiration, the client should be kept in a semi-Fowler's position.

89. 3 Because the client has an endotracheal tube in place, secretions can be loosened by the administration of humidified oxygen and by frequent turning. (2; CJ; PL; MS; PA; RE)
  1 This would be too vigorous for a client who needs an endotracheal tube.
  2 A client with an endotracheal tube in place is not permitted fluids by mouth.
  4 Potassium is never instilled into the lungs.

90. 3 To maintain normal expansion of the remaining lung after a pneumonectomy, the client should be positioned on the operative side or the back. (3; CJ; IM; MS; PA; RE)
  1 A high-Fowler's position may cause the client to slip down in the bed, diminishing thoracic excursion.
  2 Keeping the client flat will decrease lung expansion; gatching a bed may cause peripheral circulatory complications.
  4 The client should not be placed on the unaffected side; this will impede lung expansion.

91. 2 The nurse should demonstrate to the client a recognition of the verbalized concern and a willingness to listen. (3; MR; IM; MH; PS; TR)
  1 The client did not state this as the diagnosis; this response puts the client on the defensive.
  3 Avoiding the question indicates that the nurse is unwilling to listen.
  4 This could increase anxiety and would not reduce worry; furthermore, it cuts off communication and denies feelings.

92. 4 Following the administration of certain antihypertensives or narcotics, the client's neurocirculatory reflexes may have some difficulty adjusting to the force of gravity when assuming an upright position. Postural or orthostatic hypotension occurs and there is a temporarily decreased blood supply to the brain. (2; CJ; PL; MS; TC; DR)
  1 Abdominal pain will not be prevented by the intervention described.
  2 Hypertension does not occur.
  3 Respiratory distress is an adverse effect of morphine but is not prevented by the intervention described.

93. 2 Pain in the calf may be a sign of thrombophlebitis, a possible postoperative complication. If the thrombus becomes dislodged, it may lead to pulmonary embolism. Any client with this complaint should immediately be confined to bed, and the physician notified. (1; CJ; AN; MS; TC; CV)
  1 Application of heat is a dependent nursing function.
  3 Charting does not take precedence over notifying the physician of a potentially serious complication.
  4 The leg should not be elevated above heart level without a physician's order; gravity may dislodge the thrombus, creating an embolism.

94. 1 Initial disbelief and denial help protect the ego from the pain of reality in a stressful situation. (3; CJ; EV; MH; PS; CS)
  2 This may result from guilt or feelings of inadequacy because of the loss, but occurs later.
  3 Once the initial shock is over, these are the usual results as the self realizes the loss.
  4 There is no evidence of either dissociation or rationalization.

95. 3 Hydrocephalus complicates approximately 90% of lumbosacral meningomyeloceles. (2; CJ; AS; PE; PA; NM)
  1 A shrill, high-pitched cry often accompanies progressive hydrocephalus; however, it may also indicate other neurologic problems.
  2 Hydrocephalic infants may or may not have a low Apgar score.
  4 This is normal for a newborn.

96. 3 Most children with spinal cord damage resulting from spina bifida can be managed successfully with this approach. (2; MR; PL; PE; ED; NM)
  1 Most children with spinal cord damage from this defect can be managed successfully with intermittent straight catheterization.
  2 This is an inaccurate statement, and the least desirable approach because of recurrent urinary tract infections.
  4 This is a devastating and inaccurate statement to make to any young infant's parents.

97. **1** A distended bladder usually displaces the fundus upward and toward the right. (1; CJ; EV; CW; TC; HC)
2 The normal position of the fundus is at the level of the umbilicus or below, in the midline, rather than shifted to the right.
3 The fundus is firm; therefore bleeding at this time is not a problem.
4 If parts of the placenta and/or membranes were retained, bleeding would be present.

98. **1** In the postpartum period a slower-than-normal pulse rate can be anticipated as a result of a combination of factors, such as emotional relief and satisfaction, and rest after labor and delivery and decreased cardiovascular workload (2; CJ; AS; AP; CW; PA; HC)
2 Bradycardia is more likely; respirations generally are unchanged.
3 The temperature may rise slightly, but respirations usually are unchanged.
4 Same as answer 3.

99. **1** Parents need support and reassurance that their child is not permanently damaged. (3; CJ; AN; PE; PS; EH)
2 Cephalhematomas do not cause impaired neurologic functioning.
3 No special protection of the head is required; routine safety measures are adequate.
4 Cephalhematomas resolve spontaneously; no ice is applied.

100. **3** Allowing the client time to talk about her feelings and staying with her when she sees the baby for the first time provide support, acceptance, and understanding. (3; CJ; AS; MH; PS; CS)
1 This does not give the nurse a chance to assess the mother's feelings.
2 This does not give the nurse a chance to assess the mother's feelings; anomalies are difficult to describe accurately in words.
4 Showing pictures may not be helpful, and discussing treatment is premature.

101. **3** Explaining procedures and routines decreases the client's anxiety about the unknown. (1; CJ; IM; MH; PS; TR)
1 The nurse should not confuse the role of professional with that of being a friend; the client should be called by the appropriate title (Mr., Miss., Ms., Mrs., etc.) unless the client requests otherwise.

2 The nurse should not confuse the role of professional with that of being a friend; "visiting" has a social connotation.
4 Although therapeutic, this does not change the fact that the hospital environment is strange to the client.

102. **4** Processed foods generally have sodium added to enhance the taste and help preserve the food. (1; MR; PL; MS; ED; CV)
1 Most fruits have a low sodium content.
2 Although grain products contain sodium, the content is much less than in processed food.
3 Most vegetables have a low sodium content; however, carrots and celery should be avoided.

103. **3** This is usually done to palpate any masses or detect abnormalities in the rectum and is done after the vaginal examination to avoid contamination; gloves are changed between vaginal and rectal examinations. (2; MR; IM; CW; ED; HC)
1 The client may be unable to relax and will feel she is powerless if told she must do something.
2 Douching or vaginal irrigation is avoided during pregnancy unless specifically ordered by the physician.
4 The client should be encouraged to ask questions of both the physician and the nurse in order to reinforce treatment plans for health education.

104. **3** A + 1 station indicates that the fetal head is 1 cm below the ischial spines. (2; CJ; AS; CW; PA; HC)
1 This would be designated as 0 station.
2 The head is now past the points of engagement, which are the ischial spines.
4 The head must be at +3 to +5 to be visible at the vaginal opening.

105. **2** Acute respiratory obstruction can result from edema, nerve damage, or tetany. (2; CJ; PL; MS; PA; RE)
1 A cardiac arrest is not expected following surgery; heart failure could result if the hyperthyroidism were not treated.
3 This would be ineffective because the obstruction would be beyond the oropharynx.
4 Unnecessary; acidosis is not expected following thyroid surgery.

106. **1** If the pharyngeal nerve is damaged during surgery, the client will be hoarse and have difficulty speaking. (2; CJ; EV; MS; PA; EN)

    2 Edema occurs from the trauma of surgery, not pharyngeal nerve injury.

    3 This would indicate removal of the parathyroids, not pharyngeal nerve injury.

    4 This assesses for hemorrhage, not pharyngeal nerve injury.

107. **2** Dry skin is caused by decreased glandular function, and fatigue results from decreased metabolic rate. (2; MR; EV; MS; ED; EN)

    1 This is associated with hyperthyroidism because of the increased metabolic rate.

    3 Same as answer 1.

    4 Same as answer 1.

108. **1** This is part of preparation for abdominal surgery; this client has active herpes, which necessitates doing a cesarean delivery to protect the baby. (2; CJ; PL; CW; PA; HP)

    2 A paracervical block is not used in a cesarean delivery.

    3 A client with herpes may breastfeed; however, this is not an optimum time for teaching.

    4 Lesions should be kept dry.

109. **4** After a cesarean birth, the client has a vaginal discharge the same as the client who has delivered vaginally; pericare should be done to prevent ascending infection. (2; MR; EV; CW; ED; HP)

    1 Percocet or a similar analgesic is often ordered.

    2 Mild laxatives are permitted after delivery if there is no bowel movement.

    3 There is nothing to contraindicate this.

110. **1** This best clarifies the client's major concern and encourages discussion of feelings. (2; MR; IM; MH; PS; MO)

    2 The nurse cannot legitimately speak for other clients; this response can also increase the client's anxiety about the future.

    3 Poor use of empathy, which cuts off further communication, since the nurse really agrees the client acted foolishly.

    4 False reassurance; the nurse cannot legitimately speak for other staff members and clients.

111. **1** Decreased protein in spinal fluid indicates lessening of infection; meninges are becoming less inflamed. (3; CJ; EV; PE; PA; NM)

    2 Glucose levels would be normal.

    3 Cell count would be decreased.

    4 Specific gravity would be decreased.

112. **4** Tubercle bacilli are particularly resistant to treatment and can remain dormant for long periods; drugs must be taken consistently, or more drug-resistant forms recolonize and flourish. (2; CJ; PL; MS; PA; RE)

    1 Although a balance between activity and rest is desirable, compliance with chemotherapy is the the highest priority.

    2 Although fresh air is desirable and sunlight is not conducive to tubercle bacilli multiplication, compliance with chemotherapy is the highest priority.

    3 The source of infection is usually unknown, and a change in lifestyle not necessary.

113. **2** Emboli can occur with crushing injuries of the extremities; lodging of the thrombus in the pulmonary system would result in decreased breath sounds. (2; CJ; AS; MS; PA; RE)

    1 This is not related to a pulmonary embolus but to severed nerve endings in the residual limb.

    3 A thrombus lodged in the pulmonary tree would not affect the popliteal pulse.

    4 A pulmonary embolus would not interfere with arterial circulation to the distal portion of the affected extremity.

114. **1** Pressure prevents fluid shift into the interstitial compartment; this promotes shrinkage of the residual limb to facilitate use of a prosthesis. (2; CJ; AN; MS; PA; SK)

    2 Bandaging would not affect the body's formation of a scar or keloid.

    3 Maceration of skin would occur only if the bandage were saturated with fluid; not a desirable outcome.

    4 The presence of a dressing will not alter the client's adjustment to removal of a body part.

115. **3** Indicates lack of understanding of self-care; a pillow may promote a flexion contracture of the hip and knee and interfere with use of a prosthesis and ambulation. (1; MR; EV; MS; TC; SK)

    1 Appropriate; this avoids pooling of blood and edema in the extremities.

    2 Appropriate; this prevents edema and promotes residual limb shrinkage.

    4 Appropriate; this prepares the residual limb for weight bearing and use of a prosthesis.

116. **4** These are completed by 15 months of age if the child is on schedule. (3; CJ; AS; PE; PA; BI)
   1 If on schedule, 4 DTaPs and 3 IPVs, as well as mumps immunization, would be completed.
   2 If on schedule, 4 DTaPs and 3 IPVs, as well as rubella immunization, would be completed.
   3 If on schedule, the child would also have received 3 IPVs.

117. **3** This is a normal occurrence because growth slows down after the first year of life and the preschooler eats less. (2; MR; IM; PE; ED; GD)
   1 This would be alarming to the mother; decreased appetite does not necessarily indicate illness.
   2 Untrue; this is a period of slow growth.
   4 This encourages manipulative behavior on the child's part.

118. **2** Fluid in the interstitial spaces impairs circulation, leading to slowed absorption of drugs as well as predisposing to skin breakdown. (2; CJ; AN; MS; TC; IT)
   1 The pain caused by injection is influenced by the type and volume of the drug, not the site.
   3 Interstitial fluid may leak from edematous tissue, but this is not the rationale for altering sites.
   4 The dilution of the drug does not significantly affect absorption.

119. **2** The wheelchair should be angled close to the bed so the client will have to make only a simple pivot on the stronger leg. When the wheelchair is within the client's visual field, the client will be aware of the distance and direction that the body must navigate to transfer safely and avoid falling (3; CJ; IM; MS; TC; SK)
   1 If the knees are flexed, the client may be unable to support his or her weight on the unaffected leg.
   3 Moving a client back to bed in this situation would encompass moving against gravity.
   4 The large muscles of the legs rather than the arms should be used to prevent muscle strain.

120. **3** Self-contained suction devices (such as Hemovac or Jackson Pratt) for wound drainage must be compressed for the suction to work. (2; CJ; PL; MS; TC; IT)

   1 Drainage tubes are generally not irrigated by nurses.
   2 Application of heat is a dependent function and may increase inflammatory edema after surgery.
   4 A dependent position impairs venous return and increases edema.

121. **4** Alzheimer's disease is an insidious atrophy of the brain resulting in a gradually diminished intellect. (3; CJ; AS; MH; PA; DD)
   1 TIAs may precede a cerebral vascular accident; this is unrelated to Alzheimer's disease.
   2 Alzheimer's is a progressive, deteriorating disease.
   3 Alzheimer's is a slow, chronic deterioration of the brain; the role of arteriosclerosis is unclear.

122. **4** Since these clients do experience a lability of mood, it is best to attempt to establish a relationship and give care when they are feeling receptive. (3; MR; PL; MH; PS; DD)
   1 Clients with this disorder have limited contact with reality.
   2 This rejects the client when the client needs the nurse most.
   3 This may be of limited help; the client may be unable to do it.

123. **1** Sameness provides security and safety and reduces stress for the client. (3; CJ; PL; MH; PS; DD)
   2 Clients with this disorder do not do well in a constantly changing environment.
   3 A challenging environment would increase anxiety and frustration.
   4 A nonstimulating environment would promote the client's diminishing intellect.

124. **3** Clients with long-term psychiatric problems who have limited contact with reality can usually still become involved with a remotivation therapy group. The demands of this type of group are limited and self-confining. (3; CJ; AN; MH; PS; DD)
   1 This is suitable for working through emotional problems; these clients are unable to follow the dramatization of emotions.
   2 The objective of such therapy is to develop social skills; these goals are inappropriate for clients with this disorder.
   4 The objective of this therapy is to perform the activities of daily living.

125. **1** Clients are encouraged to interact with their environment by focusing their attention on some common "emotionally safe" article or activity that most clients can recognize and talk about. (2; CJ; PL; MH; PS; DD)
2 This is more appropriate for clients who have a schizophrenic disorder than for those with dementia, delirium, or other cognitive disorder.
3 The focus is on interpersonal skills and becoming competent or maintaining competence in the activities of daily living.
4 They do have face-to-face contact with other clients, but that is not the objective of the group.

126. **2** Although the exact mechanism is unknown, steroids produce diuresis in almost all children with nephrotic syndrome. (2; CJ; IM; PE; PA; DR)
1 Hypertension is not a common finding with nephrotic syndrome.
3 Steroids will not prevent infection and will in fact mask the symptoms of infection and delay treatment.
4 Steroids have no effect on the production of blood cells.

127. **2** Fresh or dried fruits and vegetables and meat are lower in sodium than canned foods and cured meats. (3; CJ; PL; PE; ED; FE)
1 Cheese and canned juices have high sodium content and should be avoided.
3 Cheese is a high-sodium food; the bun would not be allowed unless it was low-sodium.
4 Bacon, bread, and canned soup all have high sodium content and should be avoided.

128. **3** Regression frequently occurs during and after hospitalization; guilt about his regression should be avoided, but this behavior should not be encouraged. (2; MR; IM; PE; ED; EH)
1 Although punishment is a form of attention, it will not help the child overcome the problem causing the behavior.
2 Nephrotic syndrome is not associated with neurogenic control of the bladder.
4 This will shame the child; accepting the child's regressive behavior but not encouraging it is the best response.

129. **2** A heterozygous father who is Rh positive coupled with a heterozygous Rh-positive or Rh-negative mother may produce an Rh-negative infant. (3; CJ; AN; CW; PA; HN)
1 The Rh factor is a genetically determined trait; it cannot be altered by time.
3 Rh factor is a genetically determined trait; it is influenced by both parents.
4 Same as answer 1.

130. **2** These are tiny plugged sebaceous glands, and attempts to remove them will further irritate them; they will disappear by themselves. (1; MR; IM; CW; ED; NN)
1 This is not true because many infants do not have them; the mother may look for validation of this statement in other babies.
3 The white material is not pus and is not infectious.
4 These are not birthmarks; they result from maternal hormonal influences and are temporary.

131. **4** A tracheostomy may be necessary to maintain an open airway. (2; MR; IM; PE; TC; RE)
1 The symptoms are not indicative of increased secretions; suctioning can precipitate sudden laryngospasm.
2 Increased O_2 therapy would be ineffective with a severe spasm of the airway.
3 This is ineffective for laryngeal spasms.

132. **3** Indicates a past exposure or infection with the organism that is presently dormant. (3; CJ; IM; PE; ED; BI)
1 A positive response does not indicate the status of the immune system.
2 A positive response does not necessarily indicate active tuberculosis (TB) infection; PPD administered to an individual with active TB could cause a very severe reaction.
4 PPD does not predict forthcoming exposure or infection; it only indicates past exposure to the organism.

133. **2** Petechiae on the chest and shoulders indicate fat emboli after fractures. (3; CJ; AN; MS; PA; RE)
1 Not specific for fat embolus only; this may occur with emboli of any origin, such as from thrombophlebitis.
3 Not indicative of pulmonary embolus; drainage is within the amount expected and is not indicative of pulmonary hemorrhage.
4 Not related to fat embolus; it is possible that there could be an increase in central venous pressure.

134. 3 A parallax error is the apparent displacement of an observed object, in this instance the indicators on the manometer, because of the position of the observer. (1; CJ; AN; MS; TC; CV)

1 This is not associated with parallax error.

2 If this were not done, an inaccurate reading would result, but it would not be caused by a parallax error.

4 Same as answer 2.

135. 1 Toxic levels of Lanoxin stimulate the medullary chemoreceptor trigger zone, resulting in nausea and subsequent anorexia. (3; CJ; EV; MS; TC; DR)

2 The therapeutic effect of Lasix is increased urinary output with a reduction in blood pressure.

3 The therapeutic effects of Aldactone, an aldosterone antagonist, are increased urinary output and a reduction in blood pressure; adverse effects include hyperkalemia.

4 Inderal inhibits beta-adrenergic stimulation, reducing tachydysrhythmias; nausea and vomiting are side effects, not therapeutic effects.

136. 4 Therapeutic doses of alprazolam (Xanax) range from 0.75 mg to 4 mg daily; the extreme daily dose is 0.5 to 10 mg daily; the physician should be called because this dose is excessive. (3; LE; EV; MS; TC; DR)

1 Unsafe; the ordered dose is excessive and it must be questioned before administering.

2 Same as answer 1.

3 Clarifying the order is the priority; the ordered dose should not be administered before or after ventilation of feelings.

137. 1 The first stage of labor is from the onset of true labor until the cervix is fully dilated. (2; CJ; AS; CW; PA; HC)

2 There is no latent stage of labor; this is the early phase of the first stage of labor.

3 The second stage of labor is from complete dilation to birth of the baby.

4 There is no transitional stage of labor; transition is the last phase of the first stage of labor.

138. 2 The increased circulating blood volume during pregnancy is reflected in a lowered hematocrit. (2; CJ; AN; CW; PA; HC)

1 This does not lead to a lowered hematocrit.

3 The history indicates no prenatal problems, and her weight gain is adequate.

4 In the absence of other significant symptoms, concealed bleeding is highly unlikely.

139. 3 This hormone is produced by the chorionic villi of the developing embryo; it is found only in blood and urine of pregnant women. (1; MR; AN; CW; PA; HC)

1 Unrelated to pregnancy test; this is a female sex hormone produced by the ovaries and placenta.

2 Produced by the corpus luteum and placenta, this hormone prepares the endometrium for implantation and maintains pregnancy; not measurable in urine.

4 This is a placental growth hormone that does not appear in urine.

140. 1 The key chain poses no threat to the client or others; this increases his sense of security and decreases anxiety. (3; MR; IM; MH; TC; SD)

2 This statement could add to the client's anxiety and would not assist in building trust.

3 There is no evidence to support any danger from the key chain; removing it at this time will increase anxiety.

4 Client has not had time to develop trust in nurse and would have difficulty with this statement; denies and belittles client's feelings.

141. 2 These are the feelings that precipitate use of this behavior; only by being someone special with extraordinary powers can security be increased and anxiety controlled. (2; CJ; AN; MH; PS; SD)

1 Fear in itself does not precipitate grandiose delusions; compulsiveness is not a feeling but a behavior.

3 Feelings of paranoia may precipitate grandiose delusions, but ego disturbance is not a feeling.

4 If the client had these feelings, there would be little need to be someone else.

142. 3 This statement recognizes the client's feelings while providing time to sort them out. (2; MR; EV; MH; TC; SD)

1 Requires great trust on the part of the client, which may or may not be justified at this time; client feels betrayed and is angry.

2 Same as answer 1.

4 Same as answer 1.

143. **2** Contractions are less intense at this level, allowing slower chest breathing. (1; MR; IM; CW; PA; HC)
  1 Used during transition, 8 to 10 cm dilation.
  3 This is used for more intense contractions and cervical dilation of 6 to 7 cm.
  4 This is used with cervical dilation of 4 to 7 cm.

144. **1** Prolonged holding of breath at this stage decreases placental/fetal oxygenation. (2; MR; PL; CW; TC; HC)
  2 This occurs with rapid expulsion of the baby.
  3 This can occur with hyperventilation, not holding of breath.
  4 This is not caused by prolonged breath holding.

145. **2** The client should have a nasogastric tube inserted to prevent aspiration and keep the stomach decompressed. (2; CJ; IM; MS; TC; GI)
  1 Diet change requires a physician's order; clients who are vomiting may have food withheld.
  3 This information is important; however, prevention of aspiration takes priority.
  4 This would be indicated at the next bowel movement; however, maintenance of vital functions is most important.

146. **4** These signs are a result of sympathetic nervous system stimulation and could be indicative of hemorrhage from perforation and require immediate surgical intervention. (3; CJ; IM; MS; PA; GI)
  1 These complaints should be noted; however, they are not indicative of potential priority problems.
  2 These complaints should be noted, but they do not indicate an emergency situation that would threaten life.
  3 These complaints should be noted because they may indicate other health problems; however, the nurse's primary observation should be for symptoms of perforation and shock.

147. **1** Denial is a pattern of defense often demonstrated in the self-protective stage of adaptation to illness. Thoughts and feelings are so painful and provoke such anxiety that the client rejects the existence of the paraplegia. (2; CJ; AS; MH; PS; CS)
  2 From the information available, it cannot be assumed that the client is fantasizing; a fantasy is the transformation of undesirable experiences into imagined events to fulfill an unconscious wish or need.
  3 Denial is a method of psychologic adaptation.
  4 Motivation must have realistic goals in mind; the client is in denial.

148. **1** Absent or diminished gag reflex could be life threatening. The infant might aspirate mucus or formula. (2; CJ; AN; CW; TC; NN)
  2 This is important but it may be delayed because the mother may have been anesthetized; the gag reflex is of primary importance.
  3 Same as answer 2.
  4 Same as answer 2.

149. **3** The brick-red color is caused by albumin and urates that are concentrated because of dehydration, which is normal in the first 10 days. (3; CJ; AN; CW; ED; NN)
  1 Iron is eliminated via the gastrointestinal tract.
  2 This is unrelated to the sex of the infant; it is not hormonally based.
  4 No medication used in delivery would cause this discoloration.

150. **4** The infant can be positioned on the back or abdomen to allow for a routine change of head position. The head is elevated to decrease the intracranial pressure by gravity. (2; CJ; IM; PE; TC; NM)
  1 Trendelenburg positioning would be contraindicated, because it might aggravate the ICP.
  2 The head is elevated to minimize the increased pressure through gravity.
  3 The head is elevated to decrease the intracranial pressure by gravity.

151. **2** A flat position helps prevent problems associated with too rapid reduction of intracranial fluid. (3; CJ; IM; PE; TC; NM)
  1 Checking and pumping the valve provide a means of assessing and promoting function of the shunt.
  3 Sedatives and analgesics are avoided. They can mask signs of impending loss of consciousness.
  4 Initially, positioning flat is important to prevent serious complications.

152. **1** Varicose veins are dilated veins that occur as a result of incompetent valves. Varicosities may be due to numerous factors, including heredity, prolonged standing (which puts strain on the valves), and abdominal pressure on the large veins of the lower abdomen. (2; CJ; AN; MS; PA; CV)
2 Thrombophlebitis is usually a sequela of varicose veins.
3 Atherosclerotic plaques usually occur in arteries, not veins.
4 This is unrelated; this is the rationale for elastic stockings; their action limits venous pooling.

153. **4** Since the superficial vein (saphenous) will be obliterated, it is first necessary to determine whether the deep veins will be capable of supporting the return circulation. (1; MR; AS; MS; PA; CV)
1 Weight loss is desired; however, it is not a prerequisite for sclerotherapy.
2 Bed rest would promote stasis and thrombus formation and should be avoided.
3 This is insignificant; this vein is generally obliterated with sclerotherapy.

154. **4** Rupture of the membranes and the gush of fluid can carry the umbilical cord downward. Immediate placement in the lithotomy position and inspection may lead to identification of prolapse and prevention of fetal distress. (2; CJ; EV; CW; TC; HC)
1 These are routine intrapartal nursing measures.
2 The supine position may decrease blood flow and cause hypoxia in the fetus as well as hypotension in the mother.
3 The gush of fluid is due to rupture of membranes; unless it is meconium stained or followed by the cord, this is normal and needs no medical intervention.

155. **3** Hypertonic contractions of the uterus, if allowed to continue, can lead to fetal distress and uterine rupture; therefore the infusion should be discontinued so the hypertonic contractions cease. (2; LE; EV; CW; PA; DR)
1 The IV should be carefully monitored with an automatic pump to ensure a regulated and continuous flow.
2 Fetal heart tones should be monitored more frequently (q 15 min) if a fetal monitor is not used.
4 The resulting delay could lead to uterine rupture; the nurse should discontinue the infusion of oxytocin.

156. **2** The first step in the problem-solving process would be exploration so client needs could be identified. (2; CJ; AS; MH; PS; TR)
1 Without exploring client needs first, the nurse would not know what directions the client needed.
3 Without exploring client needs first, the nurse would not know the problems that needed solving.
4 Without exploring client needs first, the nurse would not know what information was needed.

157. **3** Inclusion in the interview will avoid a feeling of ostracism for the father and will foster his cooperation. (2; MR; IM; MH; PS; TR)
1 Observing one parent feed the baby does not provide the nurse an opportunity to assess family interaction.
2 Removing the father from the situation decreases his participation.
4 The father is part of the family, and his feelings will affect the mother as well.

158. **1** This allows the father to express his feelings and is nonjudgmental. (1; MR; IM; PE; PS; BI)
2 Direct contradiction often causes defensive reactions and decreases future cooperation.
3 This value-laden statement will place the father on the defensive.
4 The father, as the parent, has a right to make his own decisions; this question will place him on the defensive.

159. **4** The schedule for immunization of children not immunized in early infancy is altered and adapted from the schedule followed for infants. The tuberculin test, normally given at 1 year of age, is added to the first of the DTaP and IPV series. (3; CJ; PL; PE; ED; BI)
1 MMR is usually not given before 12 to 15 months of age. In the unimmunized child this will be given 1 month after the initial series is begun.
2 The tuberculin test, which is usually given at 1 year of age, will be added to the first series of immunizations for an unimmunized 14-month-old.
3 The adult-type tetanus and diphtheria toxoid (Td) is only given to children older than 6 years of age.

160. 3 Acute leukemia is an excessive, uncontrolled production of immature white blood cells that compete for nutrients and eventually crowd the bone marrow, preventing formation of other blood cells. (2; CJ; AN; PE; PA; BI)

1 The liver and spleen are invaded by leukemic cells.

2 Proliferating cells depress bone marrow production of the formed elements of blood.

4 RBCs and platelets are crowded out by proliferation of leukemic cells.

161. 2 With a suprapubic prostatectomy an incision is made directly into the bladder via the abdomen so that bladder abnormalities can be corrected concurrently with prostate removal; other prostatic surgery uses the transurethral route. (2; MR; AN; MS; ED; RG)

1 An indwelling catheter is used with all prostatic surgery to promote urinary drainage; the trauma of surgery causes localized edema that constricts the urethra.

3 This is not a probable complication of a suprapubic prostatectomy.

4 The transurethral approach usually has a shorter convalescent period because there is no abdominal incision.

162. 3 Green vegetables provide bulk that helps to prevent constipation by increasing intestinal peristalsis. (2; MR; IM; MS; TC; RG)

1 Milk and milk products can be constipating.

2 Bananas are constipating.

4 Creamed potatoes contain milk, which is constipating.

163. 1 Sitting raises pressure at the operative site and reduces venous return, which increases the risk of hemorrhage. (3; MR; IM; MS; TC; RG)

2 Infection is related to inadequate surgical or medical asepsis, not sitting.

3 Decreased fluid intake will decrease the amount of urinary output.

4 Holding the breath and bearing down (Valsalva maneuver) is associated with voiding and defecation, not sitting.

164. 2 These drugs are not compatible and cannot be mixed; tubing should be changed between drugs or separate secondary lines should be used for each drug. (3; CJ; IM; MS; TC; DR)

1 Unsafe; these drugs are not compatible; an intravenous bolus would be too concentrated and compromise the vein.

3 A liter of fluid is too much of a diluent; each drug should be diluted in 50 to 150 ml of fluid.

4 Unsafe; these drugs are not compatible.

165. 2 This would be the best position for preventing pressure on the sac. (2; CJ; IM; CW; TC; HN)

1 Betadine is too caustic.

3 Assessment of area below the defect is essential to determine motor, urinary, and bowel function.

4 Diapers should not be applied because they might irritate or contaminate the sac.

166. 4 The affected limbs should be exercised to promote circulation and prevent atrophy. (2; MR; PL; PE; PA; NM)

1 Fluids should be encouraged to provide adequate kidney function and prevent constipation.

2 Normal development should be encouraged; child's motion should not be restricted.

3 Child needs stimulation to develop mentally and socially.

167. 2 These children often have frequent dribbling of urine; they need frequent skin care and diaper changes to prevent skin breakdown. (2; MR; PL; PE; TC; NM)

1 This is not sufficient to replace frequent cleansing and diaper changes.

3 Insufficient; the need is for frequent diaper changes.

4 Untrue; constant dribbling of urine and seepage of feces cause skin breakdown unless areas are cleansed frequently.

168. 2 This is a sulfa drug; water must be encouraged to prevent crystallization in the kidneys. (2; MR; EV; PE; ED; DR)

1 Large amounts of water should be given to prevent crystallization in the kidneys.

3 This drug maintains the blood level for 8 to 12 hours; it is an intermediate-acting drug.

4 Orange juice causes an alkaline urine; water is the best fluid to be administered with this drug.

169. 3 All these foods are included in an acid ash diet. (3; MR; EV; PE; PA; RG)

1 Milk and peaches are not included in an acid ash diet.

2 Milk is not included in an acid ash diet.

4 Bananas and milk are not included in an acid ash diet.

170. 3 This allows the nurse to include the mother in assessing the child's specific needs and enables the nurse to observe how the mother deals with them. (3; MR; PL; PE; PA; NM)

1 Plastic pants encourage bacterial growth and increase susceptibility to urinary tract infection.

2 Extra diapers do not provide a solution to other problems that the child may have.

4. This is not necessary; a personal discussion with the mother can address the needs of the child.

171. 3 Elevating the foot of the bed uses gravity and the client's weight for countertraction. (2; CJ; IM; MS; PA; SK)

1 This would decrease countertraction.

2 This would increase traction.

4 This would have no effect on countertraction.

172. 2 Weight bearing on the unaffected leg will help maintain muscle strength; weight bearing on the affected leg is initially limited because it can disrupt the repair. (2; CJ; PL; MS; TC; SK)

1 Use of the unaffected leg should be encouraged to maintain muscle strength.

3 Contraindicated; weight on the affected leg could disrupt the repair.

4 Independence should be promoted; use of the unaffected leg maintains muscle strength.

173. 4 This stage precedes integrity vs despair; Erikson theorized that how well people adapt to a present stage depends on how well they adapted to the immediately preceding stage. (2; CJ; AN; MS; PS; GD)

1 This is the stage of young adulthood; it precedes generativity vs stagnation, not integrity vs despair.

2 This is the stage of the school-age child; it precedes identity vs role diffusion, not integrity vs despair.

3 This is the stage of adolescence; it precedes intimacy vs isolation, not integrity vs despair.

174. 3 Securing the intravenous site and putting protection around it decreases the likelihood that the line will be pulled out (2; CJ; IM; PE; TC; FE)

1 Restraints are a last resort; they only cause more anxiety and agitation as child attempts to get free.

2 Verbal instructions are not sufficient for a 2-year-old child.

4 Although family should be involved in care, the staff, not the family, is legally responsible for preventing the child from pulling out the intravenous line.

175. 3 All sources of lead must be removed from the home if the problem is to be controlled; sources include lead-painted surfaces and old plumbing that has lead solder. (1; MR; AS; PE; ED; NM)

1 Although pica must be controlled, this alone will not eliminate the environmental risks; in addition, pica is usually not related to hunger.

2 Although leaded gasoline and its fumes are present at the gas station, it is not feasible that the child was poisoned from this source.

4 Successful lead chelation is based on blood lead levels; changes in bone take longer to evaluate.

176. 1 The parathyroid gland regulates serum levels of calcium; calcium would be mobilized from bone in hyperparathyroidism and the serum calcium level increased. (3; CJ; AN; MS; PA; EN)

2 Serum calcium is elevated.

3 The test would be positive because of high urinary calcium.

4 Urinary excretion of calcium is increased, and calculi result.

177. 4 Steroid therapy decreases eosinophils, lymphocytes, and reticulocytes, resulting in depressed immunity and a greater risk for infection. (2; CJ; EV; MS; PA; DR)

1 Sodium is retained, resulting in fluid retention and weight gain.

2 Steroids have no effect on the color of urine.

3 Steroids increase production of hydrochloric acid and should be taken with food or an antacid to avoid ulcer formation.

178. **1** Pushing before cervical dilation is complete can lead to cervical trauma; pant blowing inhibits pushing. (2; MR; IM; CW; TC; HC)

2 It is too early to push; the cervix is not fully dilated.

3 Same as answer 2.

4 At this time client is completely introverted and would be unreceptive to any teaching or review techniques.

179. **4** Loss of gastric secretions, which normally contain sodium, chloride, and potassium, may result in metabolic alkalosis. (3; CJ; AN; PE; PA; FE)

1 Electrolyte deficits, rather than urinary excretion, precipitate an acid-base imbalance.

2 Electrolyte deficits, rather than inadequate blood supply, precipitate an acid-base imbalance.

3 With vomiting there is a depletion of potassium.

180. **4** Left-to-right peristalsis is noted as the stomach tries to force milk/formula into the duodenum. (3; CJ; AS; PE; PA; GI)

1 There is minimal bowel activity, since little milk/formula passes through the pyloric sphincter.

2 Projectile vomiting, not spitting up, is a classic manifestation of pyloric stenosis.

3 This is rare, since little milk/formula passes through the pyloric sphincter into the duodenum.

181. **3** This outcome would result from teaching the client to recognize situations that provoke anxiety and how to institute measures to control its development. (2; CJ; EV; MH; TC; AX)

1 Not a priority; client probably had little difficulty in this area.

2 Same as answer 1.

4 No evidence was presented to indicate client was hallucinating.

182. **4** If this behavior persists outside the schoolroom as well, the nurse can then pursue the need for a physical examination to test for possible problems such as diabetes. (2; CJ; AS; PE; PA; EN)

1 This would be done after finding out if frequent urination is also occurring at home.

2 Although enuresis is common in male children, the concern is frequent urination during the day.

3 This could be pertinent, but not most pertinent to the present problem.

183. **3** It is very important to be aware and have documentation, but it is more important that the child be treated in the same way as other children. (2; CJ; PL; PE; PA; GD)

1 This could cause physical and psychological problems; fluid should not be restricted because the child could become dehydrated.

2 This would be unnecessary and bring undue attention to the problem.

4 Overprotection or overattention could be detrimental to the child's development.

184. **4** When there are not enough circulating glucocorticoids and mineralocorticoids to sustain normal functioning of the body, the following symptoms occur: hypotension, fever, pallor, tachycardia, and cyanosis, an Addisonian crisis. (2; MR; EV; MS; ED; EN)

1 This does not occur in an Addisonian crisis.

2 Hypotension, not hypertension, is a sign of an Addisonian crisis.

3 Muscle spasms do not occur in an Addisonian crisis; the client usually progresses into a coma.

185. **4** Prolonged steroid therapy may produce Cushing's syndrome. Signs include slow wound healing, buffalo hump, hirsutism, weight gain, hypertension, acne, moon face, thin arms and legs, and behavioral disturbances. (3; MR; IM; MS; ED; EN)

1 Cortisone therapy has a glucocorticoid action, which increases blood glucose levels.

2 Hypertension and fluid retention occur.

3 Hyperkalemia occurs with Addison's disease, not Cushing's syndrome.

186. **1** Some cortisol derivatives possess 17-keto-steroid (androgenic) properties, which result in masculinization. (3; MR; IM; MS; ED; DR)
    2 Masculinization is not part of the disease; it results from the androgens present in cortisol.
    3 Saying not to worry denies the client's concerns; masculinization results from the therapy and will not go away.
    4 This response denies the client's feelings.

187. **2** A consistent caregiver enhances the formation of a trusting and mutually satisfying relationship between the child and the nurse. (2; CJ; PL; PE; PS; EH)
    1 Overstimulation should be avoided.
    3 Same as answer 1.
    4 A consistent caregiver enhances the development of trust.

188. **4** The development of the symptom is the unconscious method of reducing the anxiety. Because the symptom is meeting this need, it does not create anxiety itself but is passively accepted. (2; CJ; AN; MH; PS; PR)
    1 There is no anger; symptoms are passively accepted.
    2 There is no anxiety; the conflict is resolved by the physical symptom.
    3 There is no agitation; symptoms are passively accepted.

189. **4** This response focuses the client on the relationship between emotion and physical symptoms in a nonthreatening, accepting manner. (2; MR; AS; MH; PS; PR)
    1 The nurse knows when the weakness began so it is redundant to ask.
    2 This would provide a secondary gain; it implies sympathy and the client avoids an undesired activity.
    3 This does not help pinpoint what the person was feeling when the weakness happened.

190. **3** The nurse's best response is one that is realistic; once people become sexually active they usually remain sexually active; a condom, although not 100% effective, is the best protection against gonorrhea in a sexually active person. (2; MR; EV; CW; SI; WH)
    1 Douching has no proven protective effect against sexually transmitted disease; excessive douching can actually alter the natural environment of the vagina and may even promote an ascending infection.
    2 Although this is the best way to prevent a sexually transmitted disease, it is not the most realistic response to a sexually active person.
    4 Spermicidal cream has no protective effect against sexually transmitted diseases; spermicidals kill sperm and limit the risk of pregnancy.

191. **3** Fetal death may occur in diabetic mothers after 36 weeks of gestation; it can result from acidosis and placental dysfunction; cesarean delivery or induction may be used as necessary. (3; CJ; IM; CW; ED; HP)
    1 Exercise and ambulation are needed to promote adequate circulation and prevent thromboembolism.
    2 Fetal growth continues as long as placental functioning is still intact.
    4 This is not a routine procedure; insulin is administered according to need.

192. **1** The effects of oral hypoglycemics are not well known; such agents may be teratogenic. (2; MR; IM; CW; ED; HP)
    2 Oral hypoglycemics are not exogenous insulin.
    3 There is often a need for larger amounts of insulin in the latter part of pregnancy.
    4 The fetal pancreas does not compensate for the mother's diabetes but it does hypertrophy because of increased insulin secretion to cover increased circulating glucose.

193. **1** Feeding difficulties are due to hypoglycemic effects on the fetal CNS. (3; CJ; AS; CW; ED; HN)
    2 This may be related to hypoxia, not lowered blood sugar.
    3 Excessive birth weight is common but does not indicate hypoglycemia.
    4 This may be related to prematurity; it is generally not related to hypoglycemia.

194. **3** Since a great deal of intravascular fluid is lost during the first 48 hours through evaporation and in the exudate and edema, urinary output is not expected to equal the intake but increases from that of the first day. An output of less than 30 ml per hour is an indication of shock. (3; CJ; EV; MS; PA; FE)
    1 If half the intake is excreted, insufficient fluid is left to replace losses.
    2 This would not allow for replacement of fluid loss due to burns.
    4 This would probably indicate inadequate kidney perfusion, shock, or kidney damage.

195. **4** Vitamin C is essential for wound healing. It provides a component of intercellular ground substance that develops into collagen and is necessary to build supportive tissue. (2; CJ; IM; MS; PA; IT)
    1 To prevent excess fluid retention, which would increase the cardiovascular workload, sodium intake should be regulated.
    2 Decreasing calories could increase the work of the body; this would promote catabolism of body tissue.
    3 To help in repairing damaged tissue, protein intake should be increased.

196. **1** The skin is the first line of defense against infection. When much of it is destroyed, the individual is vulnerable to infection. (2; CJ; PL; MS; PA; IT)
    2 Complications such as infection and contractures may still occur during the acute phase and as the client is healing.
    3 Diversional therapy as tolerated may be helpful physically and emotionally.
    4 Removing mirrors can increase anxiety about body image and appearance and lead the client to conclude that the situation is even worse than it is.

197. **4** Activities that release tension and use up energy can decrease anxiety. (2; MR; PL; MH; PS; MO)
    1 This activity requires too much concentration, and the client may use the tools in a self-injurious manner in the process.
    2 This activity requires sitting still for prolonged periods and a dexterity that the client would probably find impossible at this time.
    3 This activity requires too much concentration.

198. **1** A threat is a type of assault that is an intentional tort. (3; LE; EV; MH; PS; MO)
    2 Restraints would be cruel, illegal, and unnecessary for this client.
    3 The client's behavior may be expected but should be dealt with directly; behavior should never be ignored.
    4 This generalization draws a conclusion that may not be true.

199. **4** Clients who are hyperactive are easily diverted. It is best to use this behavior rather than precipitate a confrontation. (2; MR; IM; MH; PS; MO)
    1 This response shows no consideration of how the client may feel.
    2 This response shifts responsibility to the physician; the nurse should know that a shopping trip is unrealistic at this time.
    3 This response does not deal with reality and only postpones having to deal directly with the problem.

200. **1** To prevent further maternal and fetal complications, clients must be continuously observed for blood loss by the monitoring of external bleeding and the counting and weighing of pads. (2; CJ; AS; CW; TC; HP)
    2 This would be necessary only if bleeding were continuous and profuse; a cesarean delivery might be necessary.
    3 This is unnecessary; there is no indication that the client is preeclamptic or that cerebral irritation is present.
    4 To minimize further placental separation, the client would be kept on complete bed rest.

201. **3** A vaginal examination might precipitate severe bleeding, which would be life threatening to the mother and infant and necessitate an immediate cesarean delivery. (2; CJ; PL; CW; TC; HP)
    1 This might lead to further placental separation and severe bleeding before the fetus could be delivered.
    2 The vaginal examination might precipitate severe bleeding; there would be no time for induction of labor.
    4 This would not be a priority after a vaginal examination, which can precipitate severe bleeding; an x-ray examination would not reveal placental separation, only fetal size and position.

202. **4** An infant should receive 60 calories and 88.8 ml (3 oz) of fluid per 454 g (1 lb) daily. (2; CJ; PL; CW; ED; NN)
 1 This is too much fluid and too many calories for an infant weighing 2840 g (6 lb 4 oz).
 2 Same as answer 1.
 3 Same as answer 1.

203. **1** The first step of cardiopulmonary resuscitation, after determining unresponsiveness, is calling for immediate assistance. (1; CJ; IM; MS; TC; CV)
 2 Establishing an airway, assessing for breathing and circulation, and initiating rescue breathing would be done after calling for immediate assistance.
 3 This would done after calling for immediate assistance.
 4 This is not a priority and would not be done until after breathing and circulation were established.

204. **2** When ventricular fibrillation is verified, the first intervention is defibrillation. It is the only measure that will terminate this lethal dysrhythmia. (2; CJ; EV; MS; PA; CV)
 1 Elective cardioversion delivers a shock during the R wave; since there is no R wave in ventricular fibrillation, the dysrhythmia would continue and death would result.
 3 Digitalis preparations are not used in the treatment of ventricular dysrhythmias.
 4 If not already in place, an IV line should be inserted as soon as the client is defibrillated.

205. **4** In the absence of oxygen, the body derives its energy anaerobically. This results in a buildup of lactic acid. Sodium bicarbonate, an alkaline drug, will help neutralize the acid, raising the pH. (1; CJ; PL; MS; PA; FE)
 1 Insulin is used in the treatment of diabetes mellitus; it lowers blood sugar by facilitating the transport of glucose across cell membranes.
 2 Calcium gluconate is used primarily in the treatment of hypocalcemia.
 3 Although potassium is essential for cardiac function, it will not correct acidosis.

206. **3** A nasogastric tube attached to suction removes gastric secretions and prevents vomiting. However, if it becomes clogged, secretions may accumulate, leading to distention, nausea, and vomiting. (2; CJ; EV; MS; TC; GI)
 1 An antiemetic should be administered if nausea persists after the patency of the nasogastric tube is established.
 2 To promote drainage of vomitus and prevent aspiration, the client should be initially turned on the side.
 4 Deep breathing will not prevent vomiting if the nasogastric tube is not patent.

207. **3** Some mottling is expected because of the circulatory disruption and arterial spasm. Further assessment (e.g., palpation of the pedal pulse) is done to rule out total occlusion. (1; CJ; EV; PE; PA; CV)
 1 Elevation of the leg would be contraindicated. Elevation might support bleeding from the puncture site.
 2 Mottling would be generalized if due to the external temperature; a blanket would interfere with observation.
 4 Other observations should be made before the physician is notified.

208. **1** The low gastric acidity in newborns predisposes them to GI infections. (3; CJ; AN; PE; ED; GI)
 2 This is untrue; the infant is born with passive immunity from maternal antibodies.
 3 There is hydrochloric acid in the gastric juices, but not enough to protect the infant.
 4 *Escherichia coli* is a normal intestinal bacterium; it is not found in the stomach.

209. **2** Feelings of hopelessness, helplessness, and isolation dominate the emotional state of the depressed client. The ability to attempt to act out suicide ideation frequently does not occur until psychomotor depression begins to lift. (1; CJ; AN; MH; PS; MO)
 1 This is not true; these clients frequently attempt suicide.
 3 A person intent on self-destruction will find a way on any type of unit.
 4 This is when the danger is greatest; there is more energy at this time to follow through on a plan.

210. 1 Preoccupied clients are usually not aware of external events. The client has not refused to eat but has simply not responded to external stimuli. Taking the client by the hand to the dining room simply puts the client where the food is. (3; MR; IM; MH; PS; MO)

   2 The client may be too preoccupied to eat anything; part of the intervention should be directed toward meeting client's nutritional needs.

   3 The client probably would not care and probably would not respond.

   4 This would allow a withdrawal pattern of behavior to continue.

211. 4 Lithium decreases sodium reabsorption by the renal tubules. If sodium intake is decreased, sodium depletion can occur. In addition, lithium retention is increased when sodium intake is decreased; a low-sodium intake can lead to lithium toxicity. (3; MR; IM; MH; ED; DR)

   1 This would not have any effect on the lithium therapy.

   2 If the client is well enough to go home for 3 days, participation in controversial discussions is not contraindicated.

   3 Clients should never adjust the dosage of prescribed medication without the physician's approval.

212. 4 An increase in the extracellular fluid volume can cause a relative decrease in the hemoglobin and hematocrit by dilution of the blood. (3; CJ; AS; MS; PA; FE)

   1 This occurs when the pooling of blood in the peripheral vessels causes hypotension; it rarely occurs with hypervolemia.

   2 Headache might accompany overhydration, but rhinitis would not.

   3 An increased fluid volume in the intravascular compartment (overhydration) will cause the pulse to feel full and bounding.

213. 3 The dependent edema in the ankles is normal. It results from the increased pressure of the uterus on venous return. Elevating the legs encourages venous return. (1; MR; IM; CW; ED; HC)

   1 This can be harmful; increased circulating blood volume during pregnancy must be maintained.

   2 This is contraindicated; salt is necessary to retain fluid for the increased circulating blood volume during pregnancy.

   4 Diuretics are not used during pregnancy; they may decrease the circulating blood volume.

214. 3 Chronic irritation and slower fecal transit time are both risk factors for cancer of the colon. (2; CJ; AN; MS; PA; GI)

   1 Chronic irritation associated with diverticulitis presents a risk, but hemorrhoids do not.

   2 There is no correlation with hemorrhoids, although the slower transit time with constipation is a risk factor.

   4 Although irritation is a risk factor, there is no correlation with hemorrhoids.

215. 2 A large portion of bowel and rectum are removed; during the perineal portion of the surgery, nerves involved in penile erection may be damaged. (2; LE; EV; MS; ED; GI)

   1 An ileostomy will not be performed, since the lesion is in the descending colon.

   3 A colostomy in an abdominoperineal resection is permanent, since the rectum is removed; libido will not be affected, but sexual functioning may be.

   4 The descending colon is removed; the colostomy will be permanent.

216. 3 Excessive drainage on the abdominal and/or rectal dressings may indicate hemorrhage at the incisional sites. (3; CJ; EV; MS; TC; GI)

   1 Although this could indicate trauma to the urinary tract, it is unlikely to occur; observing for incisional hemorrhage is a priority.

   2 Peristalsis will not return for several days.

   4 The colostomy will not function until peristalsis returns in approximately 3 to 5 days.

217. **4** Rocephin is nephrotoxic, and the client should be observed for decreased urinary output. (3; CJ; EV; MS; TC; DR)
    1 Rocephin does not cause dehydration.
    2 Rocephin may cause diarrhea, not constipation.
    3 Rocephin does not affect the heart.

218. **2** With pregnancy-induced hypertension (PIH), vasospasms occur, compromising blood flow to the placenta; placing the client on her side prevents the weight of the gravid uterus from obstructing venous return to the heart; thus cardiac output improves, renal flow increases, and O_2 perfusion to the uterus is enhanced. (2; CJ; IM; CW; TC; HP)
    1 Does not remove the weight of the gravid uterus from the vena cava; venous return is impaired, and cardiac output lessens with sequential decrease in renal flow, thus limiting O_2 perfusion to the placenta.
    3 Same as answer 1.
    4 Same as answer 1.

219. **3** The target tissue of $MgSO_4$ is the myoneural junction; it decreases acetylcholine, thereby depressing neuromuscular transmission, which prevents seizures. (2; CJ; AN; CW; TC; DR)
    1 Untrue; however, the client must have good kidney function (at least 30 ml/hour) in order to excrete $MgSO_4$ and prevent toxicity.
    2 It is often given along with sedation, but it has no sedative effect.
    4 It has a minimum hypotensive effect.

220. **1** The Centers for Disease Control state that standard precautions should be used for all clients; precautions that include gloves, gown, mask, and goggles should be worn when there is a risk for exposure to blood or body secretions. (1; CJ; PL; MS; TC; BI)
    2 There is no indication that airborne precautions are necessary.
    3 Unacceptable; this would isolate the client.
    4 Same as answer 3.

221. **1** Identifying the support system will decrease the person's feelings of isolation. (1; MR; PL; MS; PS; EH)
    2 Normal grieving does not involve psychotic thoughts.
    3 The concern is about loss and loneliness, not self-image.
    4 This should be done after the death of the friend, not before.

222. **1** This response acknowledges the loss and the grieving process. It also encourages ventilation through acceptance. (2; MR; IM; MH; PS; CS)
    2 This response does not recognize the loss; cuts off communication.
    3 Guilt feelings were never expressed by the client; this response may reflect the nurse's feelings.
    4 This minimizes the loss and may reflect the nurse's feelings. It also plants thoughts of a less-than-perfect fetus.

223. **4** Spending time with clients communicates to them that the staff members feel they are worthy of their attention and that someone cares. (2; MR; IM; MH; PS; MO)
    1 There is nothing to indicate that the client has a delusion regarding food.
    2 Special attention is not the purpose; the goal is to increase the client's self-esteem, self-concept, and self-worth.
    3 The goal is eventually to have the client relate to the other clients, not to get away from them.

224. **4** This is caused by increased vascular tension and damage to the vessels when hypertension is prolonged. (2; CJ; AS; MS; PA; CV)
    1 A nonspecific response; this is not physiologically related to increased arterial blood pressure.
    2 This occurs with transient ischemic attacks, which may be a later consequence of hypertension.
    3 This is a common physiologic effect of increased adrenaline released from the adrenal medulla during stress.

225. **3** If medication is necessary to control primary hypertension, it is usually a lifetime requirement. (1; MR; PL; MS; PA; CV)
   1 The client should not adjust dosage without the physician's direction.
   2 May occur with some antihypertensive medications but not hydrochlorothiazide.
   4 The drug should not be stopped; orthostatic hypotension can be controlled by a slow change of body position.

226. **2** A patent airway is the priority since the airway may become occluded in the unconscious client. (1; CJ; PL; MS; TC; RE)
   1 This is not the highest priority, although it is an important nursing function.
   3 Same as answer 1.
   4 Same as answer 1.

227. **3** The inability to withdraw from a painful stimulus indicates the greatest neurologic impairment in relation to the other options; it receives a rate of 2; the greater the injury the less purposeful the movement. (3; CJ; AN; MS; PA; NM)
   1 This movement indicates a response to pain that is more purposeful than extension; it receives a rate of 3.
   2 This movement indicates a response to pain that is more purposeful than extension; it receives a rate of 5.
   4 This movement indicates a response to pain that is more purposeful than extension; it receives a rate of 4.

228. **1** This is a characteristic of expressive aphasia from damage to Broca's area in the dominant hemisphere. (2; MR; IM; MS; PA; NM)
   2 This is known as agraphia; it is not a description of aphasia.
   3 This is known as alexia or dyslexia; it is not a description of aphasia.
   4 This is known as agnosia; it is not a description of aphasia.

229. **4** Spasticity causes muscles to flex and results in fixed flexion or contractures. (2; CJ; AN; MS; PA; NM)
   1 The immobility, not the spasticity, would lead to constipation rather than spastic colon.

   2 Although athetosis can be associated with CVA, it is not caused by spasticity.
   3 Although seizures can be associated with CVA, they are not caused by muscular spasticity.

230. **1** Conception will not be prevented unless the user is motivated to use the method properly and consistently. (1; CJ; AS; CW; ED; RC)
   2 This is not relevant if the method is not used properly and consistently by the woman.
   3 No matter how simple, the method must be used consistently.
   4 Risk factors have little influence on the effectiveness of the contraceptive method.

231. **1** Open radiant warmers cause excess fluid loss without electrolyte loss. (3; CJ; EV; CW; PA; HN)
   2 This infusion rate is appropriate for this size infant based on a rate of 150 ml/kg/day.
   3 An infant at 36 weeks is able to produce sufficient quantities of urine but is unable to concentrate urine effectively.
   4 Seldom true; respiratory distress syndrome is the most frequent complication.

232. **4** Hypoxia from inadequate O_2/CO_2 exchange leads to anaerobic metabolism with accumulation of acid byproducts. (3; CJ; AS; CW; PA; HN)
   1 Acidosis, not alkalosis, is present; carbonic acid will be elevated.
   2 Po_2 is decreased because of inadequate lung surface area available for diffusion of gases.
   3 Pco_2 increases because of inadequate lung surface area available for diffusion of gases.

233. **2** This is a factual answer; Neomycin provides preoperative intestinal antisepsis. (1; CJ; IM; MS; TC; GI)
   1 The desired effect of this drug is unrelated to kidney function.
   3 It will not prevent metastasis of tumor to other areas.
   4 This is not the purpose of administering this medication.

234. **2** This describes the stoma that has adequate vascular perfusion. (2; CJ; AS; MS; PA; GI)
   1 Indicates inadequate perfusion of the stoma.
   3 Same as answer 1.
   4 Same as answer 1.

235. 1 This would be unsafe if a thrombus were developing because it could dislodge, causing a fatal embolus. (2; CJ; EV; MS; ED; CV)

2 Fluids decrease blood viscosity, reducing the risk of thrombus formation.

3 This prevents venous stasis and promotes muscle tone; it propels venous blood toward the heart, facilitated by venous one-way valves.

4 These physically compress the veins, which prevents venous stasis, lowering the risk of thrombus formation.

236. 1 The five areas that are assessed when calculating the Apgar score are heart rate, respiratory effort, muscle tone, reflex irritability, and color. (2; CJ; AS; CW; PA; NN)

2 This is not a function tested with an Apgar score.

3. Same as answer 2.

4. The rate, not the depth, is assessed in an Apgar score.

237. 3 The 4-year-old child has developed trust but still needs frequent support from the parents. (1; MR; IM; PE; PS; EH)

1. The parents may bring a toy, but their presence to provide support and reinforce trust is more important.

2. The parents should participate in their child's care as much as possible, so there will be no interference with the trust relationship and to provide support.

4. This is appropriate for an infant who is just developing trust in the parents; hospitalization at 4 years of age should not interfere with this important aspect of personality development.

238. 1 For a child who is moderately retarded, simple repetitive tasks provide all the challenge needed. (2; MR; IM; MH; PS; BA)

2. This would be asking too much of a moderately retarded child.

3. Same as answer 2.

4. Moderately retarded children will not be able to follow many instructions given at a single time.

239. 4 This response demonstrates some insight; the client assumes the responsibility for her behavior and devises a preliminary plan of action. (2; MR; EV; MH; PS; TR)

1. This response does not show insight; it places blame on the son and promises behavior that is probably beyond her ability.

2. This response does not show insight but instead places responsibility for her abuse on the son's behavior.

3. Same as answer 2.

240. 2 This reply encourages the client to discuss fears and anxieties. (1; MR; IM; MH; PS; ED)

1. This cuts off communication and does not allow the client to express fears and anxiety.

3. This does not encourage the client to discuss the situation further. The mention of risk may frighten the client.

4. Opinions or value judgments should not be expressed by the nurse. The nurse should deal only with the client's feelings.

241. 2 Information seeking is the first step in problem solving. (2; MR; IM; MH; PS; ED)

1. This is presumptuous and expensive; the nurse should not make decisions for the client.

3 This shifts the responsibility to the physician.

4 This assumes that the husband will solve the problem; it violates the confidence between nurse and client.

242. 3 A well-lit and quiet room helps reduce the fears and illusional experiences of the client during alcoholic withdrawal. (3; CJ; PL; MH; PS; SA)

1 The nurses' station is usually a busy place; a room nearby is not the ideal location for the alcoholic client experiencing delirium. Noises can be frightening and may stimulate hallucinations or illusions.

2 Bright lights from the corridor can cast shadows on the walls and ceiling of a darkened room, increasing stimulation and illusions of frightening objects.

4 Dim lights in the room increase stimulation, producing illusions and hallucinations; strangers may increase the client's fear, restlessness, and confusion.

243. 1 This would provide some security because the client would know what to expect at different periods during the day. (2; CJ; PL; MH; PS; SA)

2 This would be inappropriate and would probably increase the client's anxiety. There is no one prototype of a client's role.

3 This would be inappropriate and would increase the client's anxiety and serve little purpose. Necessary limits should be individually set, not set by regulation.

4 This would be inappropriate and would be somewhat overwhelming. Many of the regulations would not even apply to the client.

244. 2 This action provides the disorganized client with the necessary structure to encourage participation and support self-image. (2; CJ; PL; MH; PS; SA)

1 This would increase the client's anxiety and foster withdrawal. It would also decrease the client's level of functioning.

3 This would increase dependency and add to the client's self-doubt.

4 Same as answer 1.

245. 4 When respiratory distress occurs, possibly from pressure of the dialysate on the diaphragm, fluid should be removed and the client's vital signs and status observed. (3; MR; EV; MS; TC; RG)

1 The physician should be notified after immediate action is taken.

2 Treatment is discontinued only if ordered.

3 This may be indicated after the solution is drained and the diaphragmatic pressure decreased.

246. 3 All clients who are confined to bed for any considerable period risk losing calcium from bones. This is precipitated in the urine and causes calculi. (2; CJ; AN; MS; PA; RG)

1 Although this may occur from inability to assume a normal anatomic position and the emotional impact of using a urinal, it usually does not predispose a client to the development of renal calculi unless fluid intake is low and/or stasis occurs.

2. There is no indication that the client's diet has changed.

4 The presence of a healing fracture does not increase total calcium metabolism; however, there will be increased deposition of bone at the fracture site.

247. 3 Immunosuppressive agents are administered to reduce the immune system's tendency to reject the transplanted organ. (2; MR; IM; MS; ED; RG)

1 Urine production occurs almost immediately.

2 Although fever and edema would occur, hypotension would not; an increased BP would usually be due to fluid retention.

4 This is untrue; recreation and exercise are encouraged. Only contact sports should be avoided.

248. 3 Infants with Down syndrome have decreased muscle tone, which compromises respiratory expansion as well as the adequate drainage of mucus. These factors contribute to increased susceptibility to upper respiratory tract infections. (2; CJ; AS; PE; PA; RE)

1 Impaired hearing is not an expected problem in Down syndrome.

2 Cardiac, not circulatory, problems are common in children with Down syndrome.

4 Slowed development is usually apparent before this time.

249. 3 A simian crease is a common clinical manifestation. It is readily observable when present. (1; CJ; AS; PE; ED; NM)

1 Many children who do not have Down syndrome also have rounded occiputs.

2 This is not a characteristic of children with Down syndrome, but of children with congenital hip dislocation.

4 Children with Down syndrome usually manifest hypotonicity of skeletal muscles.

250. 3 Warm water will often relax the urinary sphincter, enabling a client to void. (2; CJ; IM; MS; PA; RG)

1 The client has already indicated an inability to void.

2 Since the bladder is already distended, increased fluid intake will only increase pressure and may result in hydronephrosis.

4 Pressure over a distended bladder induces pain, which causes muscular contraction of the urinary sphincters.

251. **2** Jerky lateral eye movement (nystagmus), particularly toward the involved ear, occurs. (2; CJ; AS; MS; PA; NM)
    1 This is not usually associated with Ménière's disease.
    3 Same as answer 1.
    4 Same as answer 1.

252. **2** Inadequate oxygenation increases demands on the heart. This leads to tachycardia as the body tries to compensate. (2; CJ; AS; PE; PA; BI)
    1 Anemia is usually caused by iron deficiency rather than by blood loss that could cause cold, clammy skin.
    3 This is not generally an adaptation associated with decreased hemoglobin.
    4 This results from excess carboxyhemoglobin; pallor is more common with anemia.

253. **2** Decreased oxygen-carrying capacity of the blood may lead to hypoxia during exercise, when oxygen demand is greater. (2; CJ; AN; PE; PA; BI)
    1 Although this may be a cause of dizziness, it is not directly related to anemia.
    3 Same as answer 1.
    4 Same as answer 1.

254. **2** False labor does not produce cervical dilation; true labor does. (2; CJ; AS; CW; ED; HC)
    1 Rectal pressure may be associated with other situations, such as hemorrhoids, diarrhea, or constipation.
    3 Irregular contractions (Braxton Hicks) may occur and are not true labor.
    4 Urine may appear to leak from the vaginal orifice during false or true labor.

255. **1** Increased intraabdominal pressure associated with crying, coughing, or straining will cause protrusion of the hernia. (1; CJ; AS; CW; ED; NN)
    2 This does not increase intraabdominal pressure.
    3 The lowering of the diaphragm may increase intraabdominal pressure slightly but not enough to cause protrusion of the hernia.
    4 Same as answer 2.

256. **2** Smoking increases the acidity of gastrointestinal secretions, which damages the mucosal barrier. (1; CJ; AS; MS; PA; GI)
    1 While blood type O is more frequently associated with duodenal ulcer, type A has no significance.
    3 This is unrelated to peptic ulcer disease.
    4 This is not directly related to peptic ulcer disease.

257. **2** Because of the dilation in the veins and concomitant decrease in arterial flow, the client may experience heaviness or muscle cramps in the legs. Edema, if present, can be relieved by elevating the legs. (2; CJ; AS; MS; PA; CV)
    1 Homans' sign is present in deep vein thrombosis.
    3 Edema may be decreased when the extremity is elevated.
    4 These signs may indicate early arterial occlusion.

258. **3** Clients with Addison's disease must take glucocorticoids regularly to enable them to adapt physiologically to stress and prevent an Addisonian crisis, a medical emergency similar to shock. (2; MR; PL; MS; ED; EN)
    1 Sodium should be taken as desired because hyponatremia frequently occurs from diminished mineralocorticoid secretion.
    2 Activity is permitted as tolerated.
    4 Frequent visits are not indicated after control is established.

259. **3** Human chorionic gonadotropin (HCG) is only found in pregnancy; it is produced by the chorionic villi of the developing placenta. (1; CJ; AS; CW; PA; HC)
    1 HCG is produced by chorionic villi; the ovary is generally quiescent as pregnancy progresses.
    2 HCG is produced by chorionic villi; decidua is the name for the endometrium during pregnancy.
    4 HCG is produced by chorionic villi.

260. **1** The CST will take 1 to 2 hours, during which time the client is confined to bed. Movement on and off a bedpan should be avoided. (2; MR; IM; CW; ED; HP)
    2 Valium could interfere with the results of the CST, since the fetus would be sedated.
    3 The client may go home 1 hour after the test.
    4 No food restrictions are indicated for this test.

261. **3** An ulcer of the upper GI tract is related to the excessive secretion of stress-related hormones, which increases hydrochloric acid production. H$_2$ antagonists decrease acid secretion. (2; MR; IM; MS; ED; DR)
　1 This is not a complication of burns.
　2 Same as answer 1.
　4 This is not a complication of burns unless hypermetabolism or renal failure exists; it is not treated with H$_2$ antagonists.

262. **4** Perspiration is an involuntary physiologic response. It is mediated by the autonomic nervous system under a variety of circumstances, such as rising ambient temperature, high humidity, stress, and pain. (1; CJ; AS, MS; PA; NM)
　1 This is a voluntary emotional response.
　2 This is a voluntary action that may limit tension on the abdomen, reducing pain.
　3 This is a result of voluntary contraction of the facial muscles, a common response to pain.

263. **3** Straining applies pressure to the operative site. (3; CJ; IM; MS; TC; RG)
　1 A retention catheter is routinely put in place.
　2 To prevent trauma, negative pressure should not be exerted on the bladder.
　4 Same as answer 1.

264. **1** Prepared without salt, this food has the least sodium. (1; MR; PL; MS; ED; NM)
　2 This food choice has a high sodium content, which promotes fluid retention and increases endolymphatic fluid in the cochlea.
　3 Same as answer 2.
　4 Same as answer 2.

265. **1** This is done to measure baseline FHR variability and to observe any FHR alteration without oxytocin-induced stress. (2; MR; IM; CW; ED; HP)
　2 There is no indication for this; the test is concerned only with observing the FHR.
　3 This is incorrect; the test involves monitoring the fetal heart during three uterine contractions within a 10-minute period.
　4 The semi-Fowler's position with a left-sided tilt is the position of choice.

FOCUS FOR STUDY WORKSHEET   TEST 2

Category of concern		Pathophysiology (basic science)	Pharmacology
BI	Blood and Immunity		
CV	Cardiovascular		
DR	Drug-related Responses		
EH	Emotional Needs Related to Health Problems		
EN	Endocrine		
FE	Fluid and Electrolyte		
GI	Gastrointestinal		
GD	Growth and Development		
IT	Integumentary		
NM	Neuromuscular		
RG	Reproductive and Genitourinary		
RE	Respiratory		
SK	Skeletal		
EC	Emotional Needs Related to Childbearing & Women's Health		
HC	Healthy Childbearing		
HN	High-risk Neonate		
HP	High-risk Maternal-Fetal Conditions Affecting Childbearing		
NN	Normal Neonate		
RC	Reproductive Choices		
RP	Reproductive Problems		
WH	Women's Health		
AX	Anxiety, Somatoform, and Dissociative Disorders		
CS	Crisis Situations		
DD	Dementia, Delirium, and Other Cognitive Disorders		
BA	Disorders First Evident Before Adulthood		
ED	Emotional Problems Related to Physical Health and Childbearing		
MO	Disorders of Mood		
PR	Disorders of Personality		
ES	Eating and Sleeping Disorders		
PD	Personality Development		
SD	Schizophrenic Disorders		
SA	Substance Abuse		
TR	Therapeutic Relationships		

FOCUS FOR STUDY WORKSHEET—cont'd

Nutrition	Diagnostic studies	Physical care	Emotional care

Index

Fluid intake
  in benign prostatic hypertrophy, 624
  of newborn, 194
  postoperative, 472
Fluid loss
  in burn injury, 343
  in pediatric diarrhea, 334
Fluid shift in burn, 564
Fluids in intravenous fluid therapy, 465
Fluke, 521
Focal infection, 452
Folate deficiency, 498
Folic acid, 484
Folklore of health care agency, 11
Follicle-stimulating hormone, 176-177, 546
Follicular phase of menstrual cycle, 176
Fontanel, 194
Food cravings during pregnancy, 180
Foot
  clubfoot and, 328-329
  of newborn, 195
Foramen ovale, 179
Forced expiratory volume in 1 second, 502
Forceps birth, 210
Forebrain, 570
Foreign object aspiration, 342, 348-349
Formal commitment, 40
Formal operational stage of development, 45
Formula, infant, 198, 311
Four-point alternate crutch gait, 587
Fracture
  as birth injury, 218
  extremity, 603-605
  hip, 605
  jaw, 526
  in multiple myeloma, 601
  skull, 588
  toddler and, 342, 347-348
Fresh frozen plasma, 486
Freud psychodynamic theory, 43-44
Frontal lobe, 571
  tumor of, 590
Frostbite, 476
Frotteurism, 96
FSH. See Follicle-stimulating hormone.
Fugue, dissociative, 95
Full liquid diet, 472
Full-thickness burn, 343, 563
Functional encopresis, 69-70
Fundal height in estimating date of birth, 182
Fungal infection, 453
  antifungals for, 455-456
  respiratory, 503
  in ringworm, 372
Furniture polish poisoning, 346
Furosemide, 483
Fusiform aneurysm, 496

G

Gabapentin, 580
Gag reflex, 196
Gait
  developmental dysplasia of hip and, 329
  of toddler, 340
Galactosemia, 331
Gallbladder, 519
Gallstones, 530-531
Gamete, 177
Gamma ray therapy, 474
Gangrene, 626
Gas exchange, 502
Gas gangrene, 626
Gasoline poisoning, 346
Gastrectomy, 529
Gastric juice, 518
Gastroenteritis, 631-632
Gastroesophageal reflux disease, 527
Gastrointestinal series, 524
Gastrointestinal system, 517-544
  acute pancreatitis and, 532-533
  age-related characteristics of, 306-307
  appendicitis and, 537-538

Gastrointestinal system—cont'd
  celiac disease and, 354
  changes during pregnancy, 180
  changes during puerperium, 189
  chemical principles of, 520
  cholelithiasis and cholecystitis and, 530-531
  colorectal cancer and, 541-542
  colostomy irrigation and care, 523
  Crohn's disease and, 538-539
  diverticular disease and, 540-541
  endoscopy of, 523
  enemas and, 524
  esophageal cancer and, 527-528
  functions of, 517-518
  gastroesophageal reflux disease and, 527
  gastrointestinal series and, 524
  hemorrhoids and, 543-544
  hepatic cirrhosis and, 535-537
  hepatitis and, 534-535
  hernias and, 544
  hiatal hernia and, 528
  Hirschsprung's disease and, 320-321
  in hypertrophic pyloric stenosis, 320
  intestinal obstruction and, 540
  intussusception and, 331-332
  jaw fracture and, 526
  liver cancer and, 537
  malformations of, 316-318
  microorganisms in, 520-521
  of newborn, 193
  oral cancer and, 526-527
  pancreatic cancer and, 533-534
  paracentesis and, 525-526
  parenteral replacement therapy and, 525
  peptic ulcer disease and, 528-530
  peritonitis and, 543
  pharmacology of, 521-523
  physical principles of, 519
  psychologic factors and, 52
  stomach cancer and, 530
  structures of, 518-519
  tube feeding and, 524-525
  ulcerative colitis and, 539-540
Gastrostomy, 524, 528
Gate-control theory of pain, 449
Gavage, 524-525
Gender identity disorder, 97-98
Gene, 177-178
General adaptation syndrome, 13
General anesthetics, 467-468
Generalized anxiety disorder, 92
Generalized seizure, 593
Generativity versus stagnation, 44
Genetic counseling, 357
Genetics
  of mental illness, 41
  of panic disorder, 42
Genital stage of psychodynamic development, 44
Genitalia of newborn, 195
Genitourinary system, 613-626
  acute renal failure and, 619-620
  adenocarcinoma of kidney and, 622
  benign prostatic hypertrophy and, 624-625
  bladder tumor and, 623-624
  chronic renal failure and, 620-621
  continuous bladder irrigation and, 617
  displaced urethral openings and, 328
  exstrophy of bladder and, 327-328
  functions of, 613
  glomerulonephritis and, 622-623
  male reproductive system and, 615-616
  microorganisms of, 616
  pharmacology of, 616-617
  prostate cancer and, 625
  psychologic factors and, 52
  structures of, 613-615, 614f
  testicular cancer and, 625-626
  urinary catheterization and, 617
  urinary tract infection and, 617-618
  urolithiasis and nephrolithiasis and, 618-619

GERD. See Gastroesophageal reflux disease.
Gestational age, 194
Gestational diabetes, 212-213, 555
Gestational hypertension, 199-201
Giardia lamblia, 521
Glands
  autonomic functions of, 574
  integumentary, 560
  of male reproductive system, 615
Glargine, 546
Glasgow Coma Scale, 586
Glaucoma, 610-611
Glial cell, 41
Glioblastoma, 590
Glioma, 590
Global aphasia, 591
Globulin, 520
Glomerular filtration, 306
Glomerular filtration rate, 615
Glomerulonephritis, 622-623
Glomerulus, 613, 614f
Glossopharyngeal nerve, 572t, 585
Glucagon, 545
Glucocorticoids, 548
  for preterm labor, 207
Gluconeogenesis, 518
Glucose
  age-related characteristics of, 306
  blood, 477
  diabetes mellitus and, 555
  metabolism of, 517
  muscle contraction and, 578
  screening during pregnancy, 183
  storage as fat, 518
Gluten-sensitive enteropathy, 354
Glycogenesis, 517, 518
Glycogenolysis, 517, 518
Goals, leadership and, 17
Goblet cell, 518
Gold therapy, 474
Gonadal dysgenesis, 315
Gonadotropin-releasing hormone, 225
Gonads, 225-226, 615
Gonorrhea, 632-633
Good Samaritan Laws, 17
Goodell's sign, 180
Gouty arthritis, 599
Gram-negative microorganisms, 453
Gram-positive microorganisms, 453
Grand mal seizure, 593
Grandiose delusional disorder, 82-83
Granulocyte, 477
Grasp reflex, 196
Graves' disease, 551-552
Gray matter, 570, 573f
Greenstick fracture, 347, 603
Griseofulvin, 456
Group, 8-11
Group A streptococci, 370
Group membership, 10
Growth and development, 446-449
  of adolescent, 374-375
  of infant, 309-311
  of middle-aged adult, 446-447
  of middle-older adult and older-older adult, 448-449
  of preschooler, 359-360
  principles of, 306-307
  of school-age child, 366-367
  of toddler, 340-341
  of young adult, 446
  of young-older adult, 447-448
Growth hormone overproduction, 548
Growth spurt, 374
Guillain-Barré syndrome, 598
Gums, 180
Guthrie blood test, 330
Gynecoid pelvis, 184
Gynecomastia, 194, 322